Clinical Urogynaecology

Edited by

Stuart L Stanton FRCS FRCOG
Professor of Reconstructive Pelvic Surgery and Urogynaecology and Consultant Gynaecologist, St George's Hospital, London, UK

Ash K Monga BMedSci MRCOG
Consultant Gynaecologist, Subspecialist in Urogynaecology, The Princess Anne Hospital, Southampton University Hospitals Trust, Southampton, UK

Foreword by

David Warrell FRCOG
Retired Urogynaecologist formerly of St Mary's Hospital, Manchester, UK

SECOND EDITION

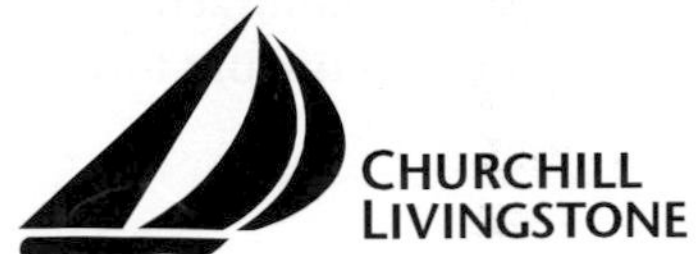

London • Edinburgh • New York • Philadelphia • St Louis • Sydney • Toronto 2000

Dedicated to Julia, Claire, Talia, Jo, Tamara and Noah
SLS

Dedicated to my mother and father and to Suzanne
AKM

Churchill Livingstone
An imprint of Harcourt Publishers Limited

First published 2000

ISBN 0443 039496

Cataloguing in Publication Data:
Catalogue records for this book are available from the British Library and the US Library of Congress.

Note
Medical knowledge is constantly changing. As new information becomes available, changes in treatment, procedures, equipment and the use of drugs become necessary. The editors, authors, contributors and the publishers have, as far as possible, taken care to ensure that the information given in this text is accurate and up to date. However, readers are strongly advised to confirm that the information, especially with regard to drug usage, complies with the latest legislation and standards of practice.

Typeset by J&L Composition Ltd, Filey, North Yorkshire

Printed in Spain

For Harcourt Publishers Limited:

Commissioning Editor: Miranda Bromage
Project Development Manager: Lucy Hamilton
Design Direction: Ian Dick, Deborah Gyan

The Publisher's Policy is to use **paper manufactured from sustainable forests**

Contents

Contents

Contributors

Paul Abrams MD FRCS
Professor of Urology, Bristol Urological Institute, Southmead Hospital, Bristol, UK

Kate Anders RGN
Clinical Nurse Specialist, Urogynaecology Unit, King's College Hospital, London, UK

Phillip A Barksdale MD
Urogynaecologist, The Louisiana Incontinence and Pelvic Reconstruction Center, Womans Hospital, Baton Rouge, Louisiana, USA

Christian G Barnick MRCOG
Lecturer and Senior Registrar, Department of Obstetrics and Gynaecology, St Bartholomew's and The Royal London School of Medicine and Dentistry, The Royal London Hospital, London, UK

Thomas B Bolton BSc PhD (Lond) BVetMed MA (Oxon) MRCVS FAcadSci
Professor and Head, Department of Pharmacology and Clinical Pharmacology, St George's Hospital Medical School, University of London, London, UK

Karen Brown MBBS MRCOG
Consultant Gynaecologist, Royal Victoria Infirmary, Newcastle upon Tyne, UK

Nicolas P Bryan FRCS
Specialist Registrar, St James's University Hospital, Leeds, UK

Richard C Bump MD
Professor and Chief, Division of Gynecologic Specialties, Duke University Medical Center, Durham, North Carolina, USA

Linda D Cardozo MB ChB MD FRCOG
Professor of Urogynaecology, Department of Obstetrics and Gynaecology, King's College Hospital, London, UK

Charlotte Chaliha MB BChir
Specialist Registrar, Department of Obstetrics and Gynaecology, Kingston Hospital, Kingston upon Thames, UK

Christopher R Chapple BSc MD FRCS (Urol)
Consultant Urological Surgeon, Royal Hallamshire Hospital, Sheffield, UK

Kate E Creed PhD DSc
Associate Professor of Physiology, Division of Veterinary and Biomedical Science, Murdoch University, Perth, Australia

Sarah M Creighton MD MRCOG
Consultant Obstetrician and Gynaecologist, University College London Hospitals, London, UK

Geoffrey W Cundiff MD
Associate Professor, Director of Division of Gynecologic Specialties, Johns Hopkins Medicine, Baltimore, Maryland, USA

Alfred Cutner MD MRCOG
Consultant Gynaecologist, The University College London Hospitals, London, UK

Prokar Dasgupta MSc (Urol) FRCS
Specialist Registrar in Urology, Department of Urology, Colchester General Hospital, Colchester, UK

John M Davison MSc MD MRCOG
Professor of Obstetric Medicine and Consultant Obstetrician and Gynaecologist, University of Newcastle upon Tyne, Royal Victoria Infirmary, Newcastle upon Tyne, UK

John O L DeLancey MD
Norman F Miller Professor of Gynecology; Professor, Department of Obstetrics and Gynecology, University of Michigan Medical School, Ann Arbor, Michigan, USA

Joy Dixon MRCOG
Obstetrician and Gynaecologist, Oxford Clinic, Christchurch, New Zealand

Sheila L B Duncan MD FRCOG
Reader and Consultant in Obstetrics and Gynaecology (Retired), University of Sheffield, Jessop Hospital for Women, Sheffield, UK

John M Fitzpatrick MCh FRCSI FRCS
Consultant Urologist and Professor of Surgery, Department of Surgery/Urology, Mater Misericordiae Hospital and University College, Dublin, Ireland

Clare J Fowler MSc FRCP
Reader in Clinical Neurology, Institute of Neurology, University College, London, UK
Consultant in Uro-Neurology, The National Hospital for Neurology and Neurosurgery, University College London Hospitals Trust, London, UK

David Gordon MD
Director, Urogynecology Unit, Lis Maternity Hospital, Tel Aviv Medical Center, Tel Aviv, Israel

Emma Gorton MRCOG
Senior Registrar, Obstetrics and Gynaecology Department, The Royal Surrey County Hospital, Guildford, UK

Derek J Griffiths BA PhD
Medical Scientist, Griffiths Urodynamics and Pro-Continence Consulting, Edmonton, Alberta, Canada

Bernard Haylen MD FRCOG FRANZCOG CU
Urogynaecologist, St Vincent's Clinic, Sydney, Australia

Michael M Henry MB FRCS
Consultant Surgeon, Chelsea and Westminster Hospital, London, UK
Consultant Surgeon, Royal Marsden Hospital, London, UK

Paul Hilton MB BS MD FRCOG
Consultant Gynaecologist, Subspecialist in Urogynaecology, Royal Victoria Infirmary, Newcastle upon Tyne, UK
Senior Lecturer in Urogynaecology, University of Newcastle upon Tyne, UK

John Hindmarsh MD FRCS FEBU
Consultant Urologist, South Cleveland Hospital, Middlesbrough, UK

David M Holmes BSc MD FRCOG
Consultant Obstetrician and Gynaecologist, Cheltenham General Hospital, Cheltenham, UK

W Glenn Hurt MD
Professor, Department of Obstetrics and Gynecology, Medical College of Virginia, Virginia Commonwealth University, Richmond, Virginia, USA

Gerald J Jarvis MA (Oxon) FRCS FRCOG
Consultant Urogynaecologist, Department of Urogynaecology, St James's University Hospital, Leeds, UK

Con J Kelleher MD MRCOG
Consultant Obstetrician and Gynaecologist, St Thomas's Hospital, London, UK

John Kelly FRCS FRCOG
Consultant Obstetrician and Gynaecologist, The Birmingham Women's Hospital, Birmingham, UK

Richard Kerr-Wilson FRCS FRCOG
Consultant Obstetrician and Gynaecologist, Cheltenham General Hospital, Cheltenham, UK

Bjørn Klevmark MD PhD
Professor Emeritus of Urology, Department of Urology, Rikshospitalet, University of Oslo, Norway

Robert J Krane MD
Chairman, Department of Urology, Massachusetts General Hospital, Harvard Medical School, Boston, Massachusetts, USA

Sigurd Kulseng-Hanssen MD PhD
Head, Department of Gynaecology and Obstetrics , Bærum Hospital, Bærum, Norway

Jo Laycock PhD FRSP
Chartered Physiotherapist, The Culgaith Clinic, Culgaith, Penrith, UK

Andrew J Macaulay MD MSc MRCPsych
Consultant Psychiatrist, The Cardinal Clinic, Windsor, UK
Consultant Psychiatrist, Wexham Park Hospital, Slough, UK

James Malone-Lee MD FRCP
Professor of Medicine, Department of Medicine, Whittington Campus, Royal Free and University College Medical School, London, UK

Hansjörg Melchior MD
Professor and Director, Department of Urology, Klinikum Kassel, Germany

Ash K Monga BMedSci MRCOG
Consultant Gynaecologist, Subspecialist in Urogynaecology, The Princess Anne Hospital, Southampton University Hospitals Trust, Southampton, UK

John F B Morrison MB ChB BSC PhD FRCSEd FI Biol
Chairman, Departments of Physiology and Pharmacology, Faculty of Medicine and Health Sciences, United Arab Emirates University, UAE

Tony Mundy MS FRCS FRCP
Professor and Director of Urology, Institute of Urology and Nephrology, Middlesex Hospital, London, UK

Peggy A Norton MD
Professor and Chief, Division of Urogynecology and Pelvic Reconstructive Surgery, Department of Obstetrics and Gynecology, University of Utah School of Medicine, Salt Lake City, Utah, USA

Christine Norton MA RGN
Nurse Specialist (Continence), St Mark's Hospital, Northwick Park and St Mark's NHS Trust, Harrow, UK

Alison B Peattie MB ChB MRCOG
Consultant Obstetrician and Gynaecologist, Countess of Chester Hospital, Chester, UK

Charlotta Persson-Jünemann MD
Head of Pediatric Urology, Department of Urology, Klinikum Kassel, Kassel, Germany

Eckhard Petri MD PhD
Professor and Chair, Department of Gynaecology and Obstetrics, Klinikum Schwerin, Schwerin, Germany

Stanislav Plevnik DSc Dipl Eng
Honorary Research Fellow, Department of Obstetrics and Gynaecology, St George's Hospital Medical School, University of London, London UK
Development Scientist, Ljubljana, Slovenia

Stephen C Radley FRCS(Ed) MRCOG
Senior Registrar, Department of Obstetrics and Gynaecology, Central Sheffield University Hospital Trust, Sheffield, UK

Sanjay Razdan MD
Lecturer in Urology, Department of Urology, University of Michigan Medical Center, Ann Arbor, Michigan, USA

Fran Reader FRCOG MFFP BASRT Accred
Consultant in Family Planning and Reproductive Health Care, The Ipswich Hospital NHS Trust, Ipswich, UK

P Julian R Shah FRCS
Senior Lecturer and Honorary Consultant Urologist, Academic Unit, Institute of Urology, Institute of Urology and Nephrology, University College, London, UK
Consultant Urologist to The Spinal Cord Injuries Unit, Royal National Orthopaedic Hospital, Stanmore, UK

Mike B Siroky MD
Director of Neuro-Urology, Department of Urology, Boston University School of Medicine, Boston, Massachusetts, USA

Anthony R B Smith MD FRCOG
Consultant Urogynaecologist, St Mary's Hospital, Manchester, UK

Stuart L Stanton FRCS FRCOG
Professor of Reconstructive Pelvic Surgery and Urogynaecology and Consultant Gynaecologist, St George's Hospital, London, UK

Abdul H Sultan MD MRCOG
Consultant Obstetrician and Gynaecologist, Mayday University Hospital, Croydon, UK

Thelma M Thomas MRCP MRCGP
The Surgery, Eastmead Avenue, Greenford, Middlesex, UK

John A Thornhill MCh FRCSI
Consultant Urologist, The Adelaide and Meath Hospital, Dublin, Ireland

Michael J Torrens MBBS BSc MPhil ChM FRCS
Chairman of Neurosurgery, Hygeia Hospital, Athens, Greece
Honorary Consultant Neurosurgeon, Frenchay Hospital, Bristol, UK

Sandra R Valaitis MD FACOG
Assistant Professor of Obstetrics and Gynecology, Director of Urogynecology, The University of Chicago Hospital, Chicago, Illinois, USA

Suzie N Venn MS FRCS (Urol)
Senior Registrar, Institute of Urology, Middlesex Hospital, London, UK

Eboo Versi MD
Chief, Division of Urogynaecology, Brigham Women's Hospital, Boston, Massachusetts, USA

David B Vodušek MD DSc
Professor of Neurology and Medical Director, Division of Neurology, University Medical Center, Ljubljana, Slovenia

L Lewis Wall MD DPhil
Director, Division of Gynecology, Urogynecology and Reconstructive Pelvic Surgery, Cedars-Sinai Medical Center, Los Angeles, California, USA

Kate Wang RN
Urogynaecology Nurse Manager, Urogynaecology Unit, St George's Hospital, London, UK

Alan J Wein MD
Professor and Chair, Division of Urology, University of Pennsylvania Health System, Philadelphia, USA

Christopher R J Woodhouse MB FRCS FEBU
Reader in Adolescent Urology, Institute of Urology, University College, London, UK
Consultant Urologist, The Royal Marsden Hospital, London, UK

Peter H L Worth FRCS
Consultant Urologist, University College London Hospitals, London, UK
Honorary Senior Lecturer, Institute of Urology, University College, London, UK

Foreword

It gives me a great deal of pleasure to write the foreword to a book whose contents reflect the considerable advances made during my professional life in the care of women suffering from urinary incontinence and genital tract prolapse. It has long been recognised that these problems were usually the consequences of pregnancy and childbirth and it was customary for the obstetrician/gynaecologist to manage them. Faecal incontinence and defaecation difficulties were ill understood and neglected by gynaecologist and surgeon alike. The aetiology of urinary incontinence was speculative and the arguments as to the supports of the genital tract swayed back and forth between the importance of pelvic floor muscle versus parametrial ligaments. Diagnosis of the cause of urinary incontinence was clinical and the choice of treatment empiric, often with a poor outcome. Prolapse was treated by vaginal surgery with reasonable results.

During the last four decades, there has been considerable progress in the understanding and management of disorders of the bladder and lower bowel function and the relation of these to prolapse of the genital tract. Knowledge is continually being acquired about the underlying pathologies. Diagnosis is precise and is the basis for rational treatment. Therapy is evaluated and the possibility of identifying women whose health is particularly at risk from childbirth damage is starting to emerge.

It is interesting to speculate how these advances have come about. I believe a major factor has been that individuals from many different disciplines have contributed their specialist knowledge and have been prepared to work together on these problems. Throughout my working life, I have always been impressed and often humbled by the enthusiasm and dedication that they have brought to the care of women whose life has been blighted by incontinence. This book is a major work documenting the current state of knowledge in the areas of medicine now termed urogynaecology and it is noteworthy that the authors come from no less than seventeen different disciplines. It is always difficult for a multi-author textbook to achieve a consistent theme and the editors are to be congratulated on producing one which has successfully accomplished this and which will be of great value to both the newcomer and the experienced practitioner.

David W Warrell MD FRCOG
Retired Urogynaecologist, formerly of St Mary's Hospital, Manchester, UK

Preface

This book's predecessor was published 15 years ago. Urogynaecology is now an accepted specialty, both within obstetrics and gynaecology and within other disciplines of medicine. There are now at least 33 recognised urogynaecology fellowship centres worldwide. The Royal College of Obstetricians and Gynaecologists recognises five units for subspecialty training in the United Kingdom, of which St George's was the first. International organisations, such as the International Continence Society and the International Urogynecological Association, and national societies, such as the American Urogynecologic Society, flourish in many countries of the world, with annual meetings and journals to support urogynaecology.

The historical concept of three separate anatomical divisions of the pelvic floor – urological, gynaecological and colorectal – is rejected in favour of the philosophy that the pelvic floor is one functional unit, best managed by close collaboration between the three specialties. Such collaboration serves the interests of patients and researchers alike. The eventual goal for the Third Millennium is training in all benign pelvic floor disorders with a fellowship programme of urology, gynaecology and colorectal surgery, culminating in the subspecialty of pelvic floor reconstruction.

The range of subjects has expanded since the first edition and 11 chapters have been added. There are over 20 new international contributors. These changes reflect global practice and the increased emphasis on evidence-based medicine, the importance of audit, conservative management before surgery, the role of laparoscopy and adequate training in urogynaecology. The increased reliance on evidence-based medicine will lead to a more scientific basis for treatment. A chapter on clinical neurophysiology highlights the importance of neuropathic conditions in urogynaecology and a new chapter on the alimentary tract emphasises the close relationship of the pelvic floor to colorectal disorders.

We should like to thank our colleagues, from both within and outside St George's Hospital, London, and Princess Anne Hospital, Southampton, who have referred patients to us, and particularly to thank for their support, advice and collaboration Chris Woodhouse of the Institute of Urology, Devinder Kumar, Doug Maxwell and Peter Millard of St George's Hospital, and to the Audio-Visual Department of St George's Hospital Medical School. Our research fellows have long been a source of stimulus, new ideas and argument – all of which are respected and acknowledged. Wendy Nash has been a tireless and long-suffering personal assistant who, together with Diana Davy, has played a vital role in the preparation of this book. Our special thanks are due to Miranda Bromage and Lucy Hamilton of Harcourt Publishers who have seen us through changes in publishing houses and patiently cajoled us into meeting all our deadlines. Our final thanks go to our authors whose patience and friendship we have strained in chapter re-writes and deadline demands. We are very grateful for these and hope this book will justify their efforts.

Stuart L Stanton
Ash K Monga

October 1999

Basic science

SECTION

1

Anatomy

JOHN O L DELANCEY

GENERAL EMBRYOLOGY

Development of the kidneys and ureters

The urinary tract develops from two separate primordia. The bladder and urethra arise from the primitive cloaca, and the kidneys and ureters from the metanephros. During the embryonic period from 3 to 7 weeks each kidney develops from a ridge which forms on the dorsal body wall lateral to the midline. These raised areas are composed of intermediate mesoderm, and are called the nephrogenic ridges. A wave of development within the nephrogenic ridge passes from its cranial to its caudal end. First a series of tubules and a duct form in the uppermost portion, called the pronephros, which soon undergoes regression. Next, just caudal to the pronephros, the mesonephric (Müllerian) tubules and duct form as the second phase of development (Fig. 1.1). Subsequently, the most caudal of the three portions of the nephrogenic ridge forms the metanephros, which is destined to become the adult kidney, and collecting system (Fig. 1.2). It arises from two primordia: a metanephric blastema which will form the kidney, and the ureteric bud which becomes the calyces, renal pelvis and ureter. Although the metanephros originally arises from the mesonephros, it eventually develops a separate origin from the urogenital sinus (Fig. 1.3) which foreshadows the separate entries of the ureter and ejaculatory duct into the lower urinary tract in the mature individual. The kidney, which arises in the pelvis, ascends during subsequent development to take its position in the thoracolumbar region. Failure of this process results in the not uncommon pelvic kidney.

Development of the bladder and urethra

During early development, beginning at about 15 days following fertilization, the embryo is formed by

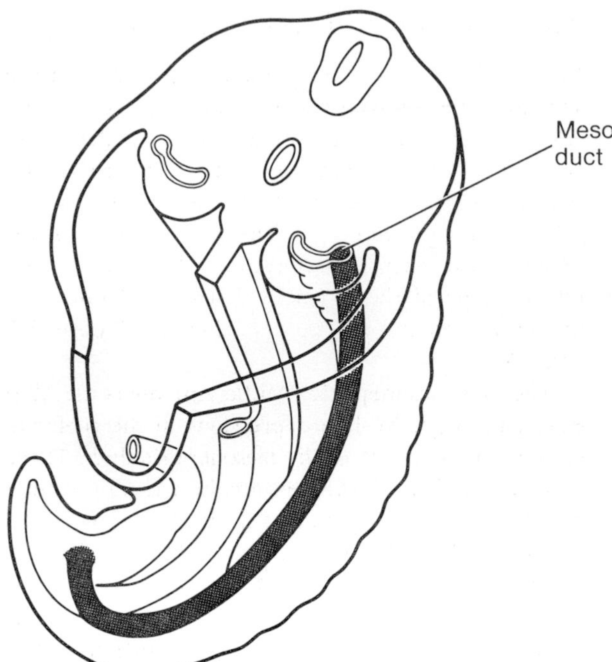

Fig. 1.1 Embryo 28 days (5 mm crown–rump length) after fertilization. Mesonephric duct has reached cloaca and cranially lies within urogenital ridge. Positions of some tubules associated with mesonephric duct are indicated. From Gosling et al (1982), with permission.

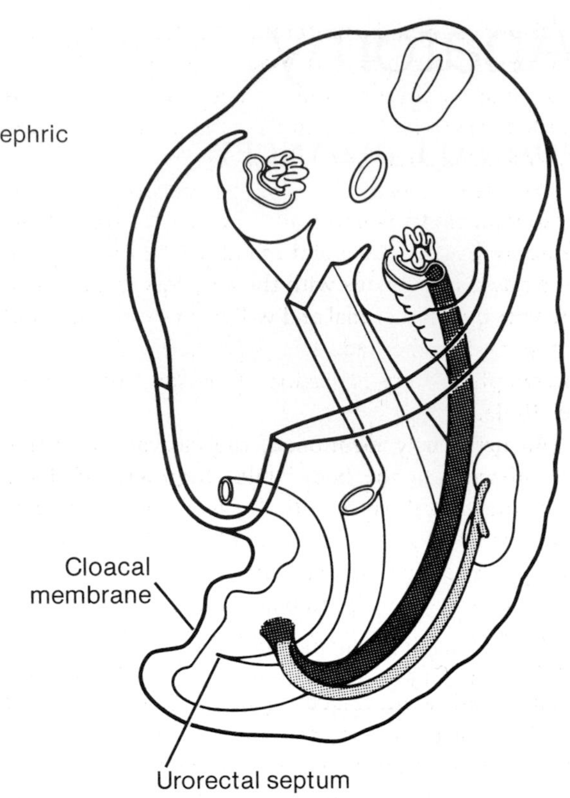

Fig. 1.2 Embryo approximately 32 days (8 mm crown–rump length) after fertilization. Definitive ureter and mesonephric duct share a common opening into partially divided cloaca. Cloacal membrane and urorectal septum are indicated. Note that ureter has induced formation of kidney from metanephrogenic blastema. From Gosling et al (1982), with permission.

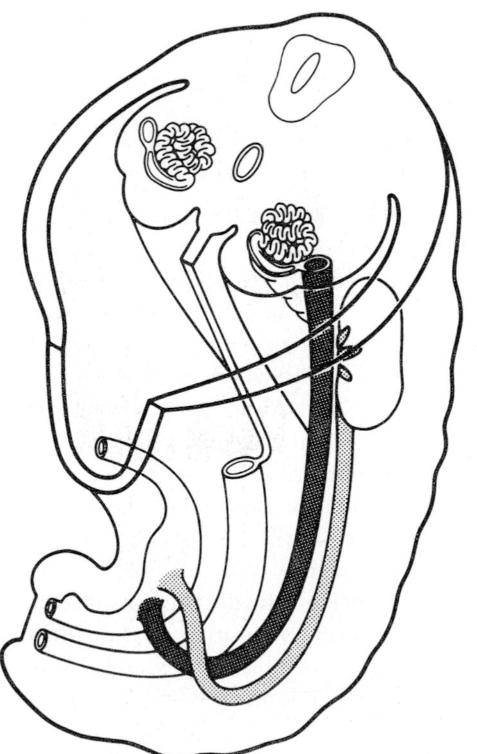

Fig. 1.3 By the 37th day (14 mm crown–rump length) cloaca has been divided into ventral urogenital and dorsal alimentary parts. In addition, kidney has continued to ascend and undergo medial rotation. From Gosling et al (1982), with permission.

three layers: endoderm, mesoderm, and ectoderm. A gap in this three-layered arrangement occurs in the caudal end of the embryo where the endoderm and ectoderm fuse without an intervening mesoderm. This region forms the cloacal membrane, which lies just caudal to the body stalk (Fig. 1.2). A reservoir develops above the cloacal membrane formed by the junction of the hindgut, and the allantois. The ventral allantois is a tubular-shaped endodermal outgrowth of the yolk sac, which it begins to form between 17 and 19 days after fertilization and lies in the body stalk. At its caudal end it is fused with the hindgut.

The wedge of tissue which lies at the junction of the allantois and the hindgut is called the urorectal septum. It grows caudally between the allantois and hindgut, until it reaches the cloacal membrane, thereby dividing the cloaca into an anterior urogenital sinus and posterior anorectum (Fig. 1.2). This also divides the cloacal membrane into the urogenital membrane and anal membrane. The urorectal septum will become the perineal body in the adult.

At about this time, the mesodermal borders of the cloacal membrane thicken. Lateral to the cloaca these thickenings form the urethral folds, and at the cranial end of the membrane, the genital tubercle. Further growth of the urethral folds and genital tubercle leads to the formation of the penis and urethra in the male, and the labia and clitoris in the female.

As the cloaca is being partitioned, the mesonephric ducts enter into the ventral wall of the cloaca (Fig. 1.3). This point of entry into the urogenital sinus is continuous with the allantois and is called the vesicourethral canal and will form the urethra and bladder in the adult. The sinus below the mesonephric ducts is destined to become the vaginal vestibule.

As previously mentioned, the cloacal membrane lies adjacent to the body stalk. Ingrowth of tissue from the lateral aspects of the body wall separates these structures and is responsible for the lower portion of the abdominal wall. Failure of this aspect of development gives rise to bladder exstrophy.

There are four different embryological primordia within the urogenital sinus which develop into the female urethra and bladder (Dröes 1974). These are: the detrusor muscle, trigonal muscle, urethral smooth muscle, and urethral striated muscle primordia (Fig. 1.4). Although the urethra and bladder form a single continuous mass on gross inspection, microscopically and functionally, there are important differences in the musculature from one region to another. These differences are explained by their different embryologic derivations. In both the male and female, there is a fifth prostatic primordium, but in the female adult this fails to provide any significant structure and therefore will not be discussed here.

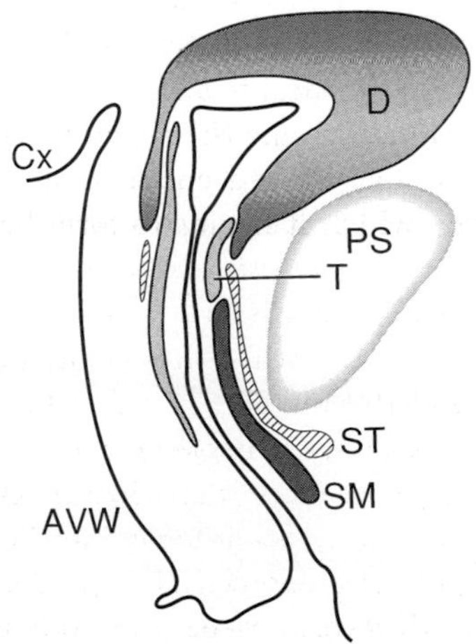

Fig. 1.4 Schematic drawing of the vesicourethral primordia in a 20 cm fetus. AVW, anterior vaginal wall; CX, cervix; D, detrusor primordium; PS, pubic symphysis; SM, smooth muscle primordium; ST, striated primordium; T, trigonal primordium. With permission, W B Saunders Co.

Gonadal and genital tract development

During the fifth week, genital ridges make their appearance as thickenings of coelomic epithelium just lateral to the mesonephros and together these two areas form the urogenital ridge. Here, the reproductive tracts take origin, with the mesonephric ducts gaining ascendancy in the male, and paramesonephric ducts developing in the female. The relationships of these systems, and development of the female internal genitalia are shown in Figures 1.5 and 1.6.

The paramesonephric (Müllerian) ducts develop from paired groove-like depressions in the coelomic epithelium, adjacent to the mesonephric duct. These paramesonephric ducts develop in a cranial caudal direction, and fuse in the midline in the region where the uterus is destined to develop. The fused lower uterovaginal primordia indent the wall of the urogenital sinus as the Müllerian tubercle. This, in turn, induces the formation of the distal portion of the vagina, so that its proximal portion is derived from the mesoderm of the uterovaginal primordium, and the distal portion from the endoderm of the urogenital sinus.

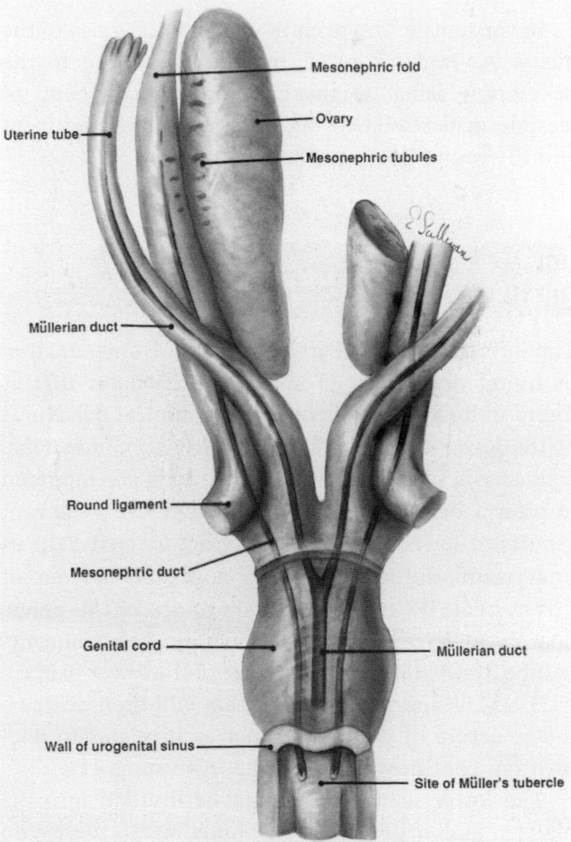

Fig. 1.5 Early relationships of the Müllerian and Wolffian systems early in development.

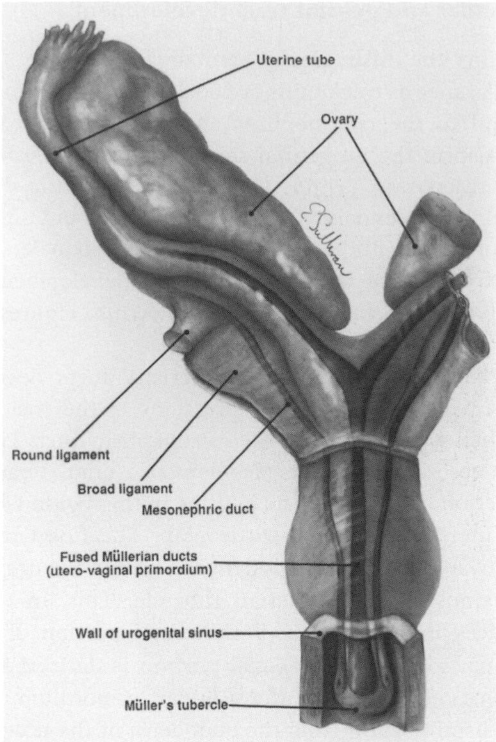

Fig. 1.6 Same relationships as Figure 1.5, later in gestation.

In the female, the primitive gonad gives rise to the ovary. As it develops, it remains connected to the developing labia by the gubernaculum, a band of mesoderm destined to become the ovarian ligament and the round ligament.

FUNCTIONAL ANATOMY OF THE LOWER URINARY TRACT

The intimate relation between structure and function in living organisms is one of the common themes found in biology. The anatomy and clinical behaviour of the lower urinary tract exemplify this immutable connection. The following descriptions are intended to offer a brief overview of some clinically relevant aspects of lower urinary tract structure that help us understand the normal and abnormal behaviour of this system. Because of the importance of the pelvic floor to lower urinary tract function, my comments will be divided into the structure of the lower urinary tract organs and a separate section will then describe the structure of the pelvic floor as it relates to micturition, continence and pelvic organ support.

The lower urinary tract can be divided into the bladder and urethra. At the junction of these two continuous, yet discrete structures, lies the vesical neck. This hybrid structure represents that part of the lower urinary tract where the urethral lumen traverses the bladder wall before becoming surrounded by the urethra. It contains portions of the bladder muscle, and also elements which continue into the urethra. It is considered separately because of its functional differentiation from the bladder and the urethra. The spatial relationships of this region are illustrated in Figure 1.7 and displayed in Table 1.1.

Bladder

The bladder is made up of the detrusor muscle, covered by an adventitia, with serosa over its dome, and lined by a submucosa and transitional epithelium. The muscular layers of the detrusor are not discrete but, in general, the outer and inner layers of the detrusor musculature tend to be longitudinal, with an intervening circular-oblique layer.

Two prominent bands on the dorsal aspect of the bladder form one of the prominent landmarks of detrusor musculature (Gil Vernet 1968). They are derived from the outer longitudinal layer and pass beside the urethra to form a loop, the detrusor loop, on its anterior aspect. On the anterior aspect of this loop, some detrusor fibres leave the region of the vesical neck and attach to the pubic bones and pelvic walls. These are called the pubovesical muscles and will be discussed below.

Trigone

Within the bladder there is a visible triangular area known as the vesical trigone whose apices are formed by the ureteral orifices and the internal urinary meatus. The base of the triangle, the interureteric ridge, forms a useful landmark in identifying the ureteric orifices. This triangular elevation is caused by the

Table 1.1 Topography of urethral and paraurethral structures[ab]

Approximate location[c]	Region of the urethra	Paraurethral structures
0–20	Intramural urethra	Urethral lumen traverses the bladder wall
20–60	Midurethra	Sphincter urethrae muscle Pubovesical muscle Vaginolevator attachment
60–80	Perineal membrane	Compressor urethrae muscle Urethrovaginal sphincter muscle
80–100	Distal urethra	Bulbocavernosus muscle

[a]Smooth muscle of the urethra was not considered.
[b]From DeLancey (1986), with permission from the American College of Obstetricians and Gynecologists.
[c]Expressed as a percentage of total urethral length.

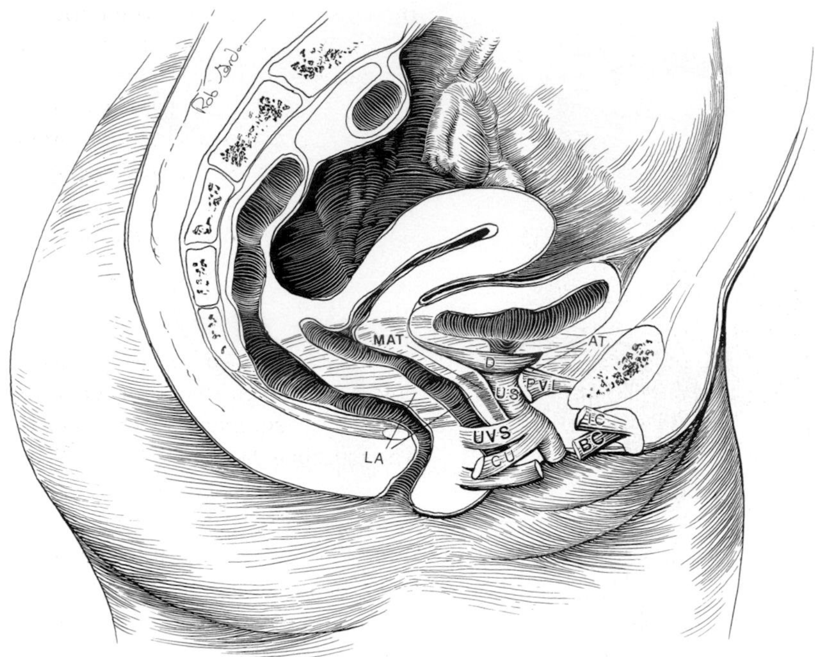

Fig. 1.7 The lower urinary tract, including the striated urogenital sphincter muscle. From DeLancey (1986), with permission.

presence of a specialized group of smooth muscle fibres which lie within the detrusor and arise from a separate embryological primordium, as previously noted. They are continuous above, with the ureteral smooth muscle (Woodburne 1965), and below they continue down the urethra. In addition to their visible triangular elevation, these muscle fibres form a ring inside the detrusor loop at the level of the internal urinary meatus (Huisman 1983) (Fig. 1.8). Some fibres continue down the dorsal surface of the urethra and lie between the ends of the U-shaped striated sphincter muscles of the urethra. These smooth muscle fibres of the trigone are clearly separable from those of the detrusor by the smaller size of their fascicles and the greater content of surrounding connective tissue. The mucosa over the trigone frequently undergoes squamous metaplasia and therefore differs from that in the rest of the bladder. The circumferential distribution of the trigonal ring fibres at the vesical neck might contribute to closure of the vesical neck's lumen at this area, but its role has yet to be fully elucidated.

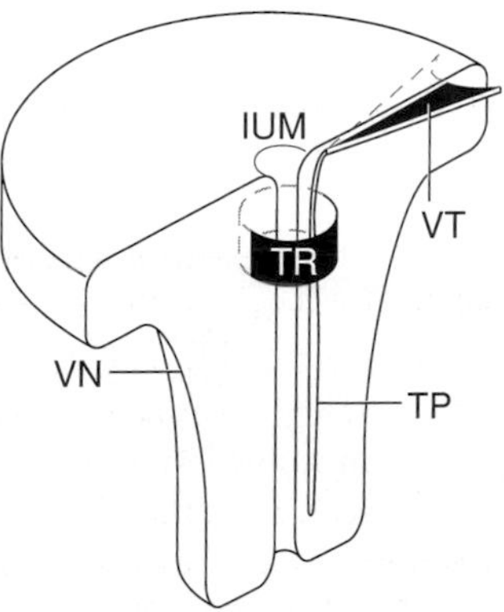

Fig. 1.8 Schematic diagram of the trigonal musculature within the bladder base and urethra (cut in sagittal section). IUM, internal urinary meatus; TP, trigonal plate; TR, trigonal ring; VN, vesical neck; VT, vesical trigone. With permission, W B Saunders Co.

Urethra

The urethra holds urine in the bladder and is therefore an important structure that helps determine urinary continence. It is a complex tubular viscus extending below the bladder. In its upper third it is clearly separable from the adjacent vagina, but its lower portion is fused with the wall of the latter structure. Embedded within its substance are a number of elements that are important to lower urinary tract dysfunction. Their locations are summarized in Table 1.1 (DeLancey 1986).

Striated urogenital sphincter

The outer layer of the urethra is formed by the muscle of the striated urogenital sphincter (Figs 1.9 and 1.10) which is found from about 20 to 80% of total urethral length (measured as a percentage of the distance from the internal meatus to the external

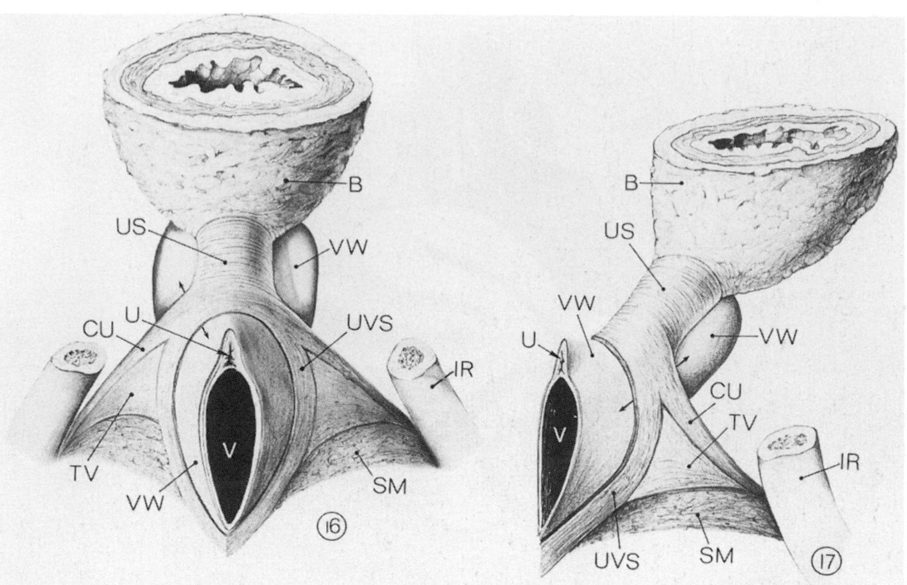

Fig. 1.9 Striated urogenital sphincter muscle seen from below after removal of the perineal membrane and pubic bones Including US, urethral sphincter; UVS, urethrovaginal sphincter; CU, compressor urethrae. Bladder (B), ischiopubic ramus (IR), transverse vaginae (TV) muscle, smooth muscle (SM), urethra (U), and vagina (V), vaginal wall (VW). From Oelrich (1983), with permission.

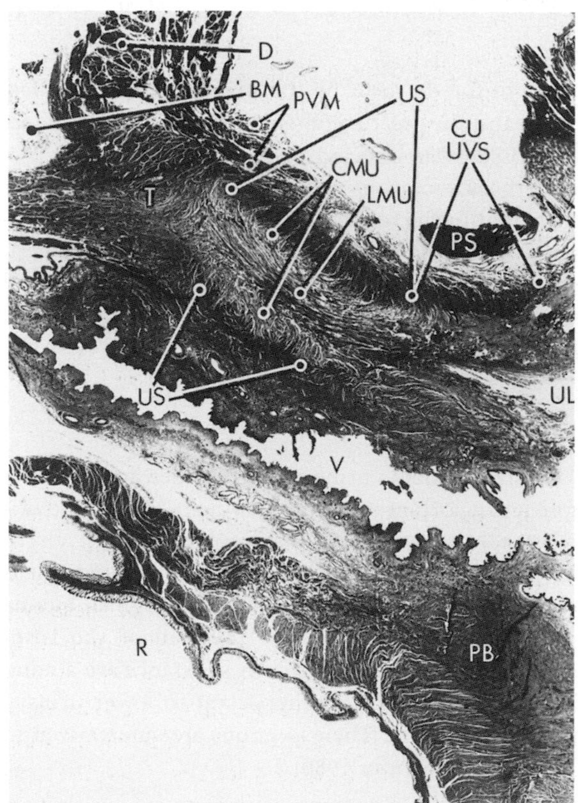

Fig. 1.10 Sagittal section from a 29-year-old cadaver. Cut just lateral to the midline and not quite parallel to it. The section contains tissue nearer the midline in the distal urethra where the lumen can be seen then at the vesical neck. BM, bladder mucosa; CMU, circular smooth muscle of the urethra; CU, compressor urethrae; D, detrusor muscle; LMU, longitudinal smooth muscles of the urethra; PB, perineal body; PS, pubic symphysis; PVM, pubovesical muscle; R, rectum; T, trigonal ring; UL, urethral lumen; US, urethral sphincter; UVS, urethrovaginal sphincter; V, vagina. From DeLancey (1986), with permission.

meatus). In its upper two thirds, the sphincter fibres lie in a primarily circular orientation, while distally, they leave the confines of the urethra and either encircle the vaginal wall as the urethrovaginal sphincter, or extend along the inferior pubic ramus above the perineal membrane (the urogenital diaphragm) as the compressor urethrae. This muscle is composed largely of slow-twitch muscle fibres (Gosling et al 1981) which are well suited to maintaining the constant tone this muscle exhibits, as well as allowing voluntary increases in urethral constriction during times when increased closure pressure is needed. In the distal urethra, this striated muscle compresses the urethra from above, and proximally, it constricts the lumen. Studies of skeletal muscle blockade suggest that this muscle is responsible for approximately one third of resting urethral closure pressure (Rud et al 1980).

Urethral smooth muscle

The smooth muscle of the urethra is contiguous with that of the trigone and detrusor, but can be separated from these other muscles on embryological, topographical and morphological grounds (Huisman 1983, Dröes 1974). It has an inner longitudinal layer, and a thin outer circular layer, with the former being by far the more prominent of the two (Fig. 1.11). They lie inside the striated urogenital sphincter muscle, and are present throughout the upper four fifths of the urethra. The configuration of the circular muscle suggests a role in constricting the lumen, and the

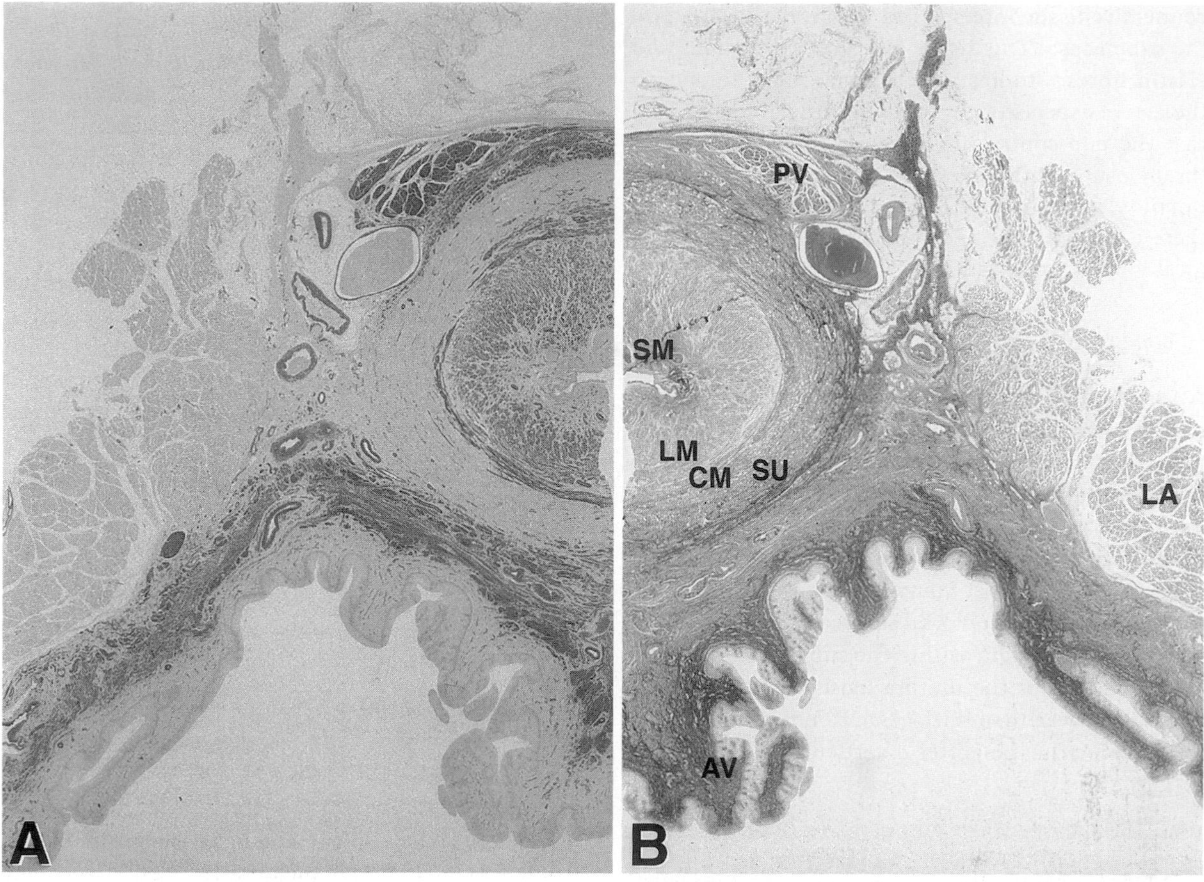

Fig. 1.11 Axial mid-urethral actin immunoperoxidase histologic section for smooth muscle (**A**) and mirrored Mallory Trichrome histologic section (**B**) from the same specimen. A few small blood clots are identified in the submucosa (SM). The longitudinal (LM) and circular (CM) smooth muscle of the urethra, the pubovesical muscle (PV), and the smooth muscle layer of the anterior vaginal wall (AV) are easily identified on the actin-stained immunoperoxidase preparation whereas the striated urogenital sphincter muscle (SU) does not stain with actin. From Strohbehn et al (1996), with permission.

longitudinal muscle may help shorten and funnel the urethra during voiding.

Submucosal vasculature

Lying within the urethra is a surprisingly well developed vascular plexus which is more prominent than one would expect for the ordinary demands of so small an organ (Berkow 1953). These vessels have been studied in serial reconstruction by Huisman (1983) who has demonstrated the presence of several specialized types of arteriovenous anastomoses. They are formed in such a way that the flow of blood into large venules can be controlled to inflate or deflate them. This would assist in forming a water-tight closure of the mucosal surfaces, and offer the possibility of rapid increases in their filling from the pressure on the abdominal vessels which supply them. Occlusion of the arterial inflow to these venous reservoirs has been shown to influence urethral closure pressure (Rud et al 1980). In addition, these appear to be hormonally sensitive (Huisman 1983), and may help to explain some individuals' response to oestrogen supplementation.

Mucosa

The mucosal lining of the urethra is continuous above with the transitional epithelium of the bladder, and with the non-keratinizing squamous epithelium of the vestibule below. Its lining consists of these two types of epithelium, with the point of transition lying at different places, varying from the lower third of the urethra, to a level above the internal urinary meatus. This mucosa shares a common derivation from the urogenital sinus with the lower vagina and vestibule. Like these other areas, its mucosa is hormonally sensitive, and undergoes significant change depending on its state of stimulation.

Connective tissue

In addition to the contractile and vascular tissue of the urethra, there is a considerable quantity of connective tissue interspersed within the muscle, and the submucosa. This tissue has both collagenous and elastin fibres. Studies which have sought to abolish the active aspects of urethral closure have suggested that the non-contractile elements contribute to urethral closure (Huisman 1983). It is difficult, however, to study these tissues' function specifically, because there is no specific way to pharmacologically or surgically block their action.

Glands

A series of glands are found in the submucosa primarily along the dorsal (vaginal) surface of the urethra (Huffman 1948). They are most concentrated in the lower and middle thirds, and vary in number. The location of urethral diverticula, which are derived from cystic dilation of these glands, follows this distribution, being most common distally, and usually originating along the dorsal surface of the urethra. In addition, their origin within the submucosa indicates that the fascia of the urethra must be stretched and attenuated over their surface, and indicates the need for its approximation after diverticular excision.

Vesical neck

The term 'vesical neck' is a regional and functional one, as previously discussed, and does not refer to a single anatomical entity. It denotes that area at the base of the bladder, where the urethral lumen passes through the thickened musculature of the bladder base. Therefore, it is sometimes considered as part of the bladder musculature, but also contains the urethral lumen studied during urethral pressure profilometry. It is a region where the detrusor musculature, including the detrusor loop, surrounds the trigonal ring and the urethral meatus.

The vesical neck has come to be considered separately from the bladder and urethra because it has unique functional characteristics. Specifically, sympathetic denervation or damage of this area results in its remaining open at rest (McGuire 1986), and when this happens in association with stress incontinence, simple urethral suspension is often ineffective in curing this problem (McGuire 1981).

Innervation

The innervation of the bladder and urethra are the subject of Chapter 2 and will not be covered here.

Functional terms

There are a number of terms which have arisen to describe functional units within the vesicourethral unit based upon radiographic observations of the activities of these viscera. The term extrinsic continence mechanism, or external sphincteric mechanism, usually refers to that group of structures which respond when an individual is instructed to stop their urine stream. The two phenomena observed during this effort are a constriction of the urethral lumen by the striated urogenital sphincter, and an elevation of the vesical neck caused by contraction of the levator ani muscles, as will be described below. The intrinsic continence mechanism, then, consists of the structures which lie within the vesical neck, and which are not specifically activated by contraction of the voluntary muscles. It is this system which fails in patients whose vesical neck can be seen to be open at rest.

PELVIC FLOOR

The position and mobility of the bladder and urethra are recognized as important to urinary continence (Hodgkinson 1953). Because these two organs are limp and formless when removed from the body they must depend upon attachments to the pelvic floor for their shape and position. Fluoroscopic examination has shown that the upper portion of the urethra and vesical neck are normally mobile structures while the distal urethra remains fixed in position (Muellner 1951; Westby et al 1982). These aspects of support and fixation are determined by the pelvic floor muscles and fasciae, and a knowledge of these relationships is important to our understanding of lower urinary tract function.

The pelvic floor consists of several components lying between the pelvic peritoneum and the vulvar skin. These are (from above downward): the peritoneum, viscera and endopelvic fascia, levator ani muscles, perineal membrane and external genital muscles. The eventual support for all of these structures comes from their connection to the bony pelvis and its attached muscles. The viscera are often thought of as being supported by the pelvic floor, but are actually a part of it. Through such structures as the cardinal and uterosacral ligaments, and the pubocervical fascia, the viscera play an important role in forming the pelvic floor.

Endopelvic fascia

The viscero–fascial layer

The top layer of the pelvic floor is provided by the endopelvic fascia that attaches the pelvic organs to the pelvic walls, thereby suspending the pelvic organs (Ricci & Thom 1954; Uhlenhuth & Nolley 1957; DeLancey 1992). Because this layer is a combination of the pelvic viscera and the endopelvic fascia, it will be referred to as the viscero–fascial layer. It is common to speak of the fasciae and ligaments alone, separate from the pelvic organs as if they had a discrete identity, yet unless these fibrous structures have something to attach to (the pelvic organs), they cannot hold anything up.

On each side of the pelvis the endopelvic fascia attaches the uterus and vagina to the pelvic wall (Figs 1.12–14). This fascia forms a continuous sheet-like mesentery extending from the uterine artery at its cephalic margin to the point at which the vagina fuses with the levator ani muscles below. The part which attaches to the uterus is called the parametrium and that which attaches to the vagina, the paracolpium.

The parametria are made up of what we clinically refer to as the cardinal and uterosacral ligaments (Range & Woodburne 1964; Campbell 1950). These are two different parts of a single mass of tissue. The uterosacral ligaments are the visible and palpable medial margin of the cardinal–uterosacral ligament complex. Opposite the external cervical os the sheet of tissue that attaches the genital tract to the pelvic wall arbitrarily changes name from the parametrium to the paracolpium. Although we name these tissues 'ligaments' and 'fasciae' they are not the same type of tissue seen in the 'fascia' of the rectus abdominus muscle or the ligaments of the knee, both of which are made of dense regular connective tissue. These supportive tissues contain prominent blood vessels; nerves and fibrous connective tissue can be thought of as mesenteries that supply the genital tract bilaterally. Their composition reflects their combined function as neurovascular conduits as well as supportive structures.

The structural effect of this arrangement is most evident when the uterine cervix is pulled downward with a tenaculum, as is done during a D and C, or pushed downward during a laparotomy. After a certain amount of descent within the elastic range of the fascia, the parametria become tight and arrest further cervical descent. Similarly, downward descent of the vaginal apex after hysterectomy is resisted by the paracolpia. The fact that these ligaments do not limit the downward movement of the uterus in normal healthy women is attested to by the observation that

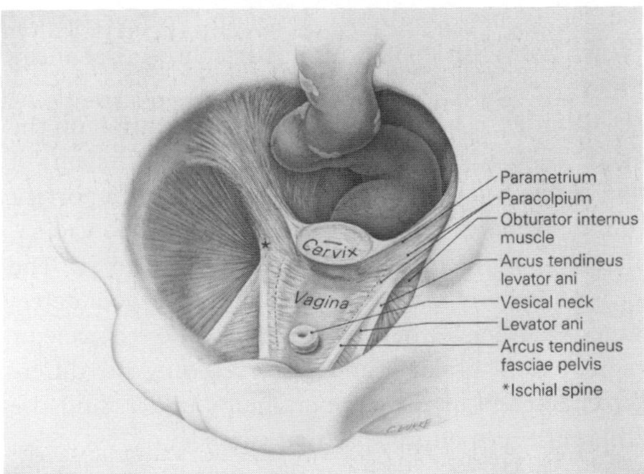

Fig. 1.12 Supportive tissues of the cervix and upper vagina. Bladder has been removed above the vesical neck. From Delancey (1992), with permission.

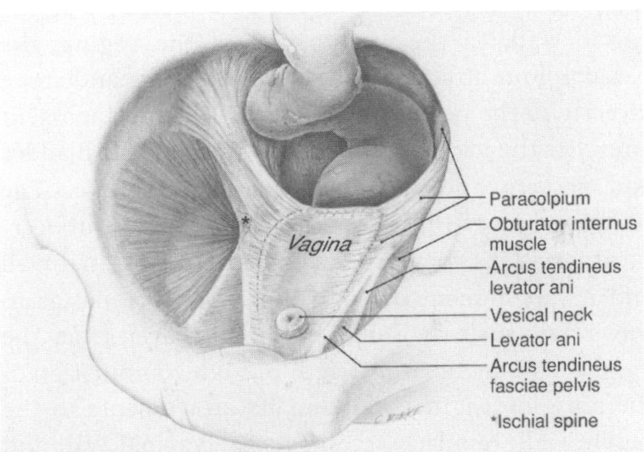

Fig. 1.13 Vagina and supportive structures drawn from dissection of 56-year-old cadaver after hysterectomy. The paracolpium extends along the lateral wall of the vagina. From DeLancey (1992), with permission.

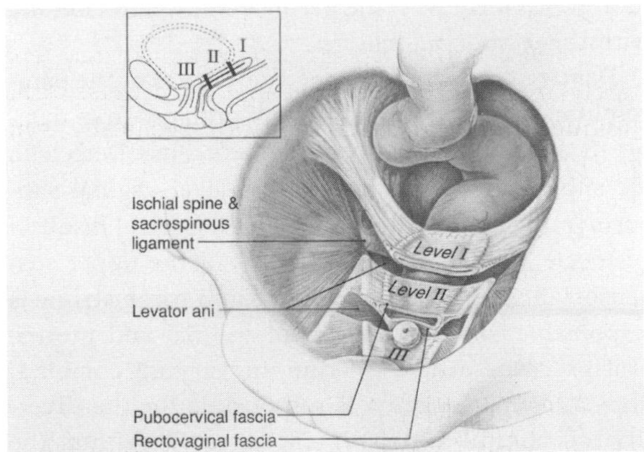

Fig. 1.14 Level I (suspension) and Level II (attachment). In Level I the paracolpium suspends the vagina from the lateral pelvic walls. Fibres of Level I extend both vertically and also posteriorly towards sacrum. In Level II vagina is attached to arcus tendineus fasciae pelvis and superior fascia of levator ani. From DeLancey (1992), with permission.

the cervix may be drawn down to the level of the hymen with little difficulty (Bartscht & DeLancey 1988).

Although it is traditional to focus attention on the ligaments that suspend the uterus, the attachments of the vagina to the pelvic walls are equally important and are responsible for normal support of the vagina, bladder and rectum, even after hysterectomy. The location where these supports are damaged determines whether a woman has a cystocele, rectocele or vaginal vault prolapse and understanding the different characters of this support helps understand the different types of prolapse that can occur.

The upper two thirds of the vagina is suspended and attached to the pelvic walls by the paracolpium after hysterectomy (DeLancey 1992). This paracolpium has two portions (Fig. 1.14). The upper portion (Level I) consists of a relatively long sheet of tissue that suspends the vagina by attaching it to the pelvic wall. In the mid-portion of the vagina, the paracolpium attaches the vagina laterally and more directly to the pelvic walls (Level II). This attachment stretches the vagina transversely between the bladder and rectum and has functional significance. The structural layer that supports the bladder ('pubocervical fascia') is composed of the anterior vaginal wall and its attachment through the endopelvic fascia to the pelvic wall. It is not a separate layer from the vagina, as sometimes inferred, but is a combination of the anterior vaginal wall and its attachments to the pelvic wall. Similarly, the posterior vaginal wall and endopelvic fascia (rectovaginal fascia) form the restraining layer that prevents the rectum from protruding forward blocking formation of a rectocele. In the distal vagina (Level III) the vaginal wall is directly attached to surrounding structures without any intervening paracolpium. Anteriorly, it fuses with the urethra, posteriorly with the perineal body, and laterally with the levator ani muscles.

Damage to the upper suspensory fibres of the paracolpium causes a different type of prolapse from damage to the mid-level supports of the vagina. Defects in the support provided by the mid-level vaginal supports (pubocervical and rectovaginal fasciae) result in cystocele and rectocele, while loss of the upper suspensory fibres of the paracolpium and parametrium is responsible for development of vaginal and uterine prolapse. These defects occur in varying combinations and this variation is responsible for the diversity of clinical problems encountered within the overall spectrum of pelvic organ prolapse.

Pelvic diaphragm

Any connective tissue within the body may be stretched by subjecting it to constant force. Skin expanders used in plastic surgery stretch the usually dense and resistant dermis to extraordinary degrees and flexibility exercises practised by dancers and athletes elongate leg ligaments with as little as 10 minutes of stretching a day. Both of these observations underscore the malleable nature of connective tissue when subjected to force over time. If the ligaments and fasciae within the pelvis were subjected to the continuous stress imposed on the pelvic floor by the great weight of abdominal pressure, they would stretch. This stretching does not occur because the pelvic floor muscles close the pelvic floor and carry the weight of the abdominal and pelvic organs, preventing constant strain on the ligaments.

Below the viscero–fascial layer is the levator ani group of muscles (Dickinson 1889) (Fig. 1.15). They have a connective tissue covering both superior and inferior surfaces called the superior and inferior fasciae of the levator ani. When these muscles and their fasciae are considered together, the combined structure is called the pelvic diaphragm. The levator ani consists of two portions: the pubovisceral muscle and the iliococcygeus muscle (Lawson 1974). The pubovisceral muscle is a thick U-shaped muscle whose ends arise from the pubic bones on either side of the midline and passes behind the rectum forming a sling-like arrangement. This portion includes both the pubococcygeus and puborectalis portions of the levator ani. Laterally, the iliococcygeus arises from a fibrous band on the pelvic wall (arcus tendineus levator ani) and forms a relatively horizontal sheet that spans the opening within the pelvis and forms a shelf on which the organs may rest.

The pubovisceral muscle has several components. The pubococcygeus muscle is the most cephalic portion of the levator and passes from the pubic bones to insert on the inner surface of the coccyx and comprises only a small portion of the overall levator complex. Clinicians have often referred to the entire pubovisceral muscle under the term pubococcygeus. The pubococcygeus portion of the levator ani muscles actually connects two relatively immovable structures (pubis and coccyx) and, therefore, could not be expected to contribute substantially to supporting the pelvic organs. The puborectalis portion of the pubovisceral muscle passes beside the vagina; the lateral vaginal walls are attached to it. The muscle then continues dorsally where some fibres insert into the rectum between the internal and external sphincter, while others pass behind the ano-rectal junction. The vagina attaches to the medial portion of the pubovis-

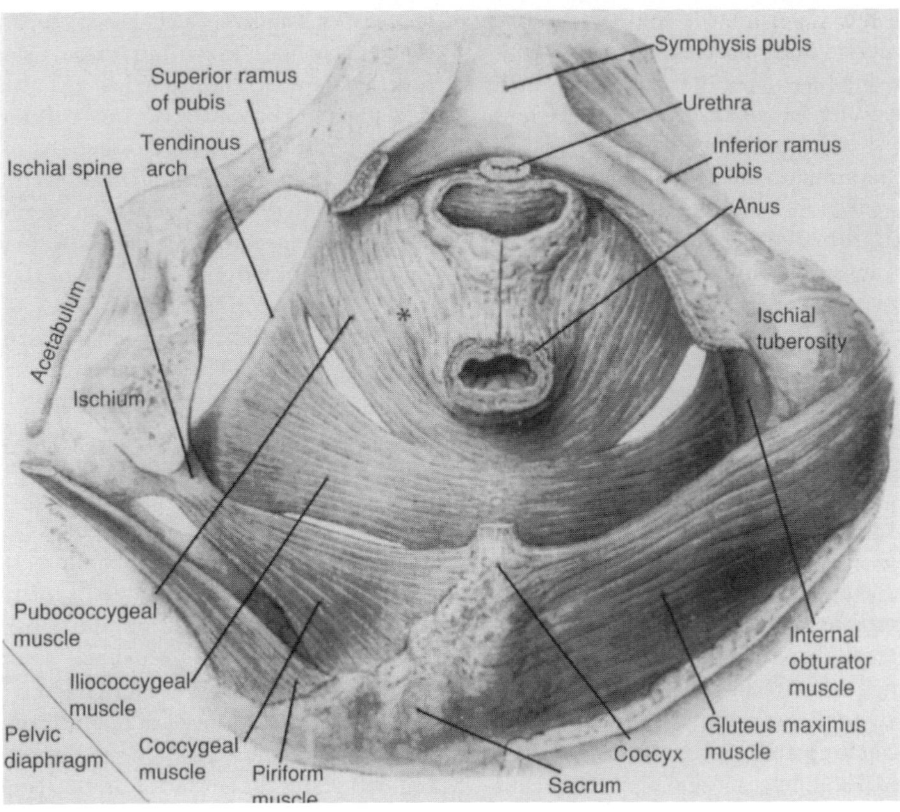

Fig. 1.15 Levator ani muscles seen from below. That portion of the pubococcygeus which inserts into the rectum and forms a 'U' behind it is called the puborectalis. From DeLancey (1997), with permission.

ceral muscle and the fibres between the vagina and pubic bone are referred to as the pubovaginalis muscle. These muscle fibres are responsible for elevating the urethra during pelvic muscle contraction, but muscle fibres of the levator have no direct connection to the urethra itself.

The opening within the levator ani muscle, through which the urethra and vagina pass (and through which prolapse occurs), is called the urogenital hiatus of the levator ani. The rectum also passes through this opening, but because the levator ani muscles attach directly to the anus and external anal sphincter, it is not included in the name of the hiatus. The hiatus, therefore, is bounded ventrally (anteriorly) by the pubic bones, laterally by the levator ani muscles and dorsally (posteriorly) by the perineal body and external anal sphincter. The normal baseline activity of the levator ani muscle keeps the urogenital hiatus closed. It squeezes the vagina, urethra and rectum closed by compressing them against the pubic bone and lifts the floor and organs in a cephalic direction.

The levator ani muscles constantly contract (Parks et al 1962). This continuous contraction is similar to the continuous activity of the external anal sphincter muscle and closes the lumen of the vagina in a similar way to that in which the anal sphincter closes the anus. This constant action eliminates any opening within the pelvic floor through which prolapse could occur and forms a relatively horizontal shelf on which the pelvic organs are supported (Berglas & Rubin 1953; Nichols et al 1970).

The interaction between the pelvic floor muscles and the supportive ligaments is critical to pelvic organ support. As long as the levator ani muscles function properly, the pelvic floor is closed and the ligaments and fascia are under no tension. The fasciae simply act to stabilize the organs in their position above the levator ani muscles. When the pelvic floor muscles relax or are damaged, the pelvic floor opens and the vagina lies between the high abdominal pressure and low atmospheric pressure. In this situation it must be held in place by the ligaments. Although the ligaments can sustain these loads for short periods of time, if the pelvic floor muscles do not close the pelvic floor, the connective tissue must carry this load for long periods of time and will eventually fail to hold the vagina in place.

This support of the uterus has been likened to a ship in its berth floating on the water attached by ropes on either side to a dock (Paramore 1918). The ship is analogous to the uterus, the ropes to the ligaments, and the water to the supportive layer formed by the pelvic floor muscles. The ropes function to hold the ship (uterus) in the centre of its berth as it rests on the water (pelvic floor muscles). If, however, the water level were to fall far enough that the ropes would be required to hold the ship without the support of the water, the ropes would all break. The analogous situation in the pelvic floor involves the pelvic floor muscles supporting the uterus and vagina that are stabilized in position by the ligaments and fasciae. Once the pelvic floor musculature becomes damaged and no longer holds the organs in place, the connective tissue fails because of its significant overload.

Perineal membrane and external genital muscles

In the anterior portion of the pelvis, below the pelvic diaphragm, is a dense triangular-shaped membrane containing a central opening called the perineal membrane (the urogenital diaphragm). It lies at the level of the hymenal ring, and attaches the urethra, vagina, and perineal body to the ischiopubic rami. Just above the perineal membrane are the compressor urethrae and urethrovaginal sphincter muscles, previously discussed as part of the striated urogenital sphincter muscle.

The term perineal membrane replaces the old term urogenital diaphragm, reflecting more accurate anatomical information (Oelrich 1983). Previous concepts of the urogenital diaphragm show two fascial layers, with a transversely oriented muscle in between (the deep transverse perineal muscle). Observations based on serial histology and gross dissection, however, reveal a single connective tissue membrane, with muscle lying immediately above. The correct anatomy explains the observation that pressures during a cough are greatest in the distal urethra (Hilton & Stanton 1983; Constantinou 1985), where the compressor urethra and urethrovaginal sphincter can compress the lumen closed in anticipation of a cough (DeLancey 1988).

Position and mobility of the urethra

When the importance of urethral position to determining urinary continence was recognized, anatomical observations revealed an attachment of the tissues around the urethra to the pubic bones. These connections were referred to as the pubourethral ligaments (Zacharin 1968), and found to be continuous with the connective tissue of the urogenital diaphragm (Milley & Nichols 1971). Further studies (Richardson et al 1981; DeLancey 1988, 1994) have expanded on these observations and revealed several separate structural elements contained within these tissues that have functional importance to urinary continence.

As mentioned earlier in this chapter, the support of the urethra is dynamic rather than static. Fluoroscopic and topographic observations (Muellner 1951; Westby et al 1982) suggest that urethral position is determined by both attachments to bone and also to the levator ani muscles. The role of the urethral supportive tissue's connection to the levator ani is probably more important than previously thought for the following reasons. The resting position of the proximal urethra is high within the pelvis, some 3 cm above the inferior aspect of the pubic bones (Noll & Hutch 1969) (Fig.1.16) and above the insertion of the 'posterior pubourethral ligaments' which attach near the lower margin of the pubic bones (Zacharin 1968). Maintenance of this position would best be explained by the constant muscular activity of the levator ani (Parks et al 1962). In addition, the upper two thirds of the urethra is mobile (Muellner 1951; Jeffcoate & Roberts 1952; Westby et al 1982) and under voluntary control. At the onset of micturition, relaxation of the levator ani muscles allows the urethra to descend, and obliterates the posterior urethrovesical angle (Fig. 1.16). Resumption of the normal tonic contraction of the muscle at the end of micturition returns the vesical neck to its normal position.

Some of the control of the proximal vesical neck's position and mobility, therefore, must come from activity of the levator ani muscles and connections of the periurethral tissues to the fibrous elements of the pelvic wall ('ligaments and fasciae'). From these

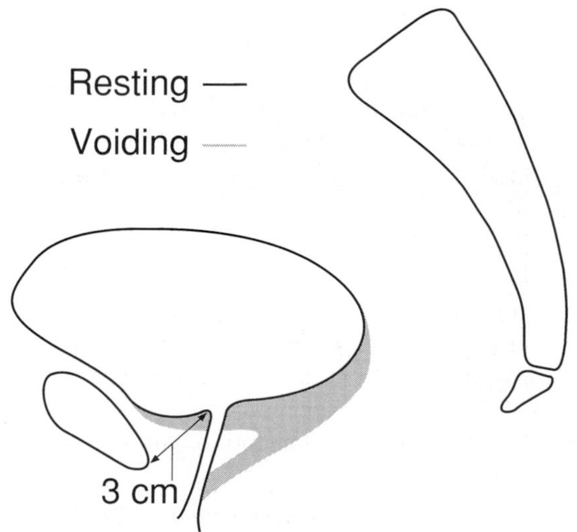

Fig. 1.16 Topography and mobility of the normal proximal urethra and vesical neck based upon resting and voiding in nulliparae. From Delancey (1988), with permission.

observations, the support of the urethra would seem to involve both voluntary muscle and inert elements. This is in fact what examination of this region reveals (DeLancey 1988, 1994). Recent observations demonstrating that patients with stress incontinence have neurological damage to the pelvic floor support the importance of the levator ani to urinary continence (Smith et al 1989). In addition, functional testing reveals that continence during increases in abdominal pressure decrease when the pelvic muscles are paralysed (Bump 1991). There does not appear to be a one-to-one relationship between denervation and stress incontinence, and so the relative role of the muscular and fascial tissues in urethral support remains to be clarified.

The anterior vaginal wall and urethra arise from the urogenital sinus, and are intimately connected. The support of the urethra depends not on attachments of the urethra itself to adjacent structures, but upon the connection of the vagina and periurethral tissues to the muscles and fascia of the pelvic wall. Surgeons are most familiar with seeing this anatomy through the space of Retzius and this view is also helpful in understanding urethral support (Fig. 1.17). On either side of the pelvis, the arcus tendineus fascial pelvis is found as a band of connective tissue attached at one end to the lower sixth of the pubic bone, 1 cm from the midline, and at the other end to the ischial spine. In its anterior portion this band lies on the inner surface of the levator ani muscle which arises some 3 cm above the arcus tendineus fasciae pelvis. Posteriorly, the levator ani arises from a second arcus, the arcus tendineus fasciae levatoris ani, which fuses with the arcus tendineus fasciae pelvis near the spine.

The layer of tissue that provides urethral support has two lateral attachments: a fascial attachment and a muscular attachment (Figs 1.18 and 1.19). The fascial attachment of the urethral supports connects the periurethral tissues and anterior vaginal wall to the arcus tendineus fasciae pelvis and have been called the paravaginal fascial attachments by Richardson (Richardson et al 1981). The muscular attachment connects these same periurethral tissues to the medial border of the levator ani muscle. (This connection was referred to as the vaginolevator attachment in the author's previous work (DeLancey 1986). These attachments allow the normal resting tone of the levator ani muscle to maintain the position of the vesical neck, supported by the fascial attachments (Fig. 1.20). When the muscle relaxes at the onset of micturition, it allows the vesical neck to rotate downwards to the limit of the elasticity of the fascial attachments, and then contraction at the end of micturition allows it to resume its normal position.

Also within this region are the pubovesical muscles. These are extensions of the detrusor muscle (Gil Vernet 1968; Woodburne 1968; DeLancey 1989). They lie within some connective tissue, and when both muscular and fibrous elements are considered together, they are called the pubovesical ligaments in much the same way that the smooth muscle of the ligamentum teres is referred to as the round ligament

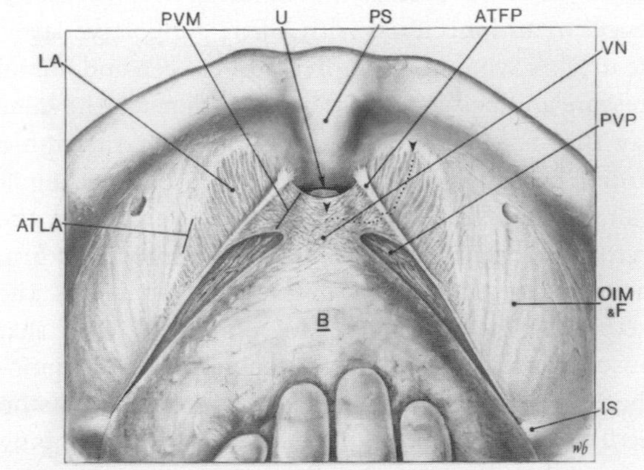

Fig. 1.17 Space of Retzius (drawn from cadaver dissection). Pubovesical muscle (PVM) can be seen going from vesical neck (VN) to arcus tendineus fasciae pelvis (ATFP) and running over the paraurethral vascular plexus (PVP). ATLA, arcus tendineus levator ani; B, bladder; IS, ischial spine; LA, levator ani muscles; OIM & F, obturator internus muscle and fascia; PS, pubic symphysis; U, urethra. Dotted lines indicated plane of section of Figure 16. From DeLancey (1989), with permission.

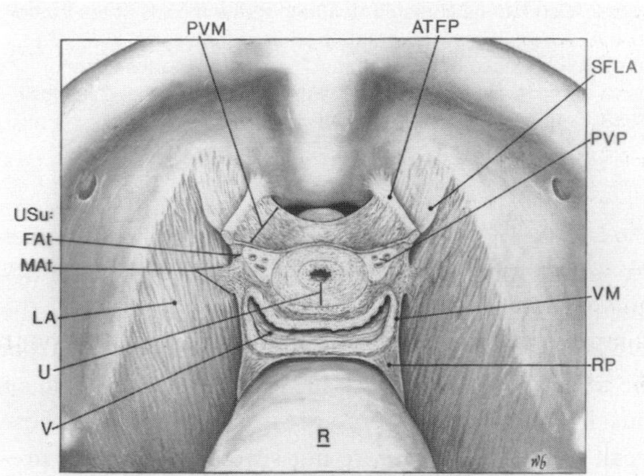

Fig. 1.18 Relationship of the supportive tissues of the urethra (USu) to the pubovesical muscles (PVM). Cross-section of the urethra (U), vagina (V), arcus tendineus fasciae pelvis (ATFP), and superior fascia of levator ani (SFLA) just below the vesical neck (drawn from cadaver dissection). Pubovesical muscles (PVM) lie anterior to urethra and anterior and superior to paraurethral vascular plexus (PVP). The urethral supports (USu) ('the pubo-urethral ligaments') attach the vagina and vaginal surface of the urethra to the levator ani muscles (MAt, muscular attachment) and to the superior fascia of the levator ani (FAt, fascial attachment). Additional abbreviations: LA, levator ani muscles; R, rectum; RP, rectal pillar; VM, vaginal wall muscularis. From DeLancey (1989), with permission

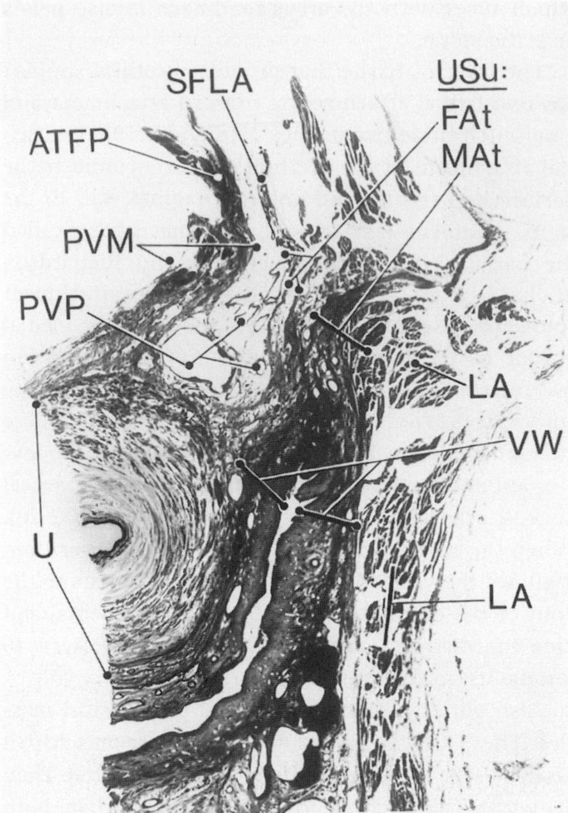

Fig. 1.19 Cross-section of the urethra (U), vaginal wall (Vw), and levator ani muscles (LA) from the right half of the pelvis taken just below the vesical neck. The pubovesical muscles (PVM) can be seen anterior to the urethra and the periurethral vascular plexus (PVP) and attach to the arcus tendineus fasciae pelvis (ATFP). Urethral supports (USu) run underneath (dorsal to) the urethra and vessels. Some of its fibres (MAt) attach to the muscle of the levator ani (LA), while others (FAt) are derived from the vaginal wall (VW) and vaginal surface of the urethra (U) and attach to the superior fascia of the levator ani (SFLA). Magnification × 5. From DeLancey (1989), with permission.

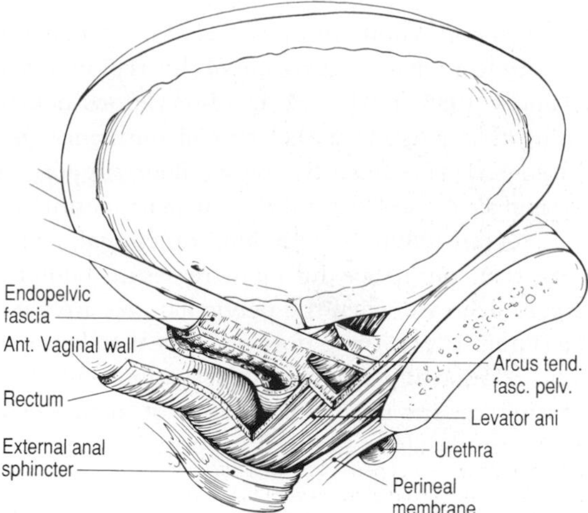

Fig. 1.20 Lateral view of the pelvic floor structures related to urethral support seen from the side in the standing position, cut just lateral to the midline. Note that windows have been cut in the levator ani muscles, vagina, and endopelvic fascia so that the urethra and anterior vaginal walls can be seen. From DeLancey (1994), with permission.

(Figs 1.10, 1.11, 1.17 and 1.18). Although sometimes the terms pubovesical ligament and pubourethral ligament have been considered to be synonymous, the pubovesical ligaments are different structures from the urethral supportive tissues. Fibres of the detrusor muscle are able to undergo great elongation and these weak tissues are therefore not suited to maintain urethral position under stress. In addition, they run in front of the urethra rather than underneath it, where one would expect supportive tissues to be found. It is not surprising, therefore, that these detrusor fibres are no different in stress incontinent patients than those without this condition (Wilson et al 1983). The actual supportive tissues of the urethra, as described above, are separated from the pubovesical ligament by a prominent vascular plexus, and are easily separated from them. Rather than supporting the urethra, the pubovesical muscles may be responsible for assisting in vesical neck opening at the onset of micturition by contracting to pull the anterior part forward, as some have suggested (Power 1954).

This mechanism influences incontinence, not by determining how high or how low the urethra is, but how it is supported. In examining anatomic specimens, simulated increases in abdominal pressure reveal that the urethra lies in a position where it can be compressed against the supporting hammock by rises in abdominal pressure (Fig. 1.20). In this model, it is the stability of this supporting layer rather than the height of the urethra that determines stress continence. In an individual with a firm supportive layer, the urethra would be compressed between abdominal pressure and pelvic fascia (Fig. 1.21) in much the same way that you can stop the flow of water through a garden hose by stepping on it and compressing it against concrete. If, however, the layer under the urethra becomes unstable and does not provide a firm backstop for abdominal pressure to compress the urethra against concrete, the opposing force that causes closure is lost and the occlusive action diminished. This latter situation is similar to trying to stop the flow of water through a garden hose by stepping on it while it lies on soft soil.

The structural and functional aspects of the body must always be in agreement. As new functional observations are made of the lower urinary tract, it will be necessary to re-examine our anatomical concepts, and doubtless some of the structural arrangements described in this chapter will be corrected,

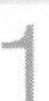

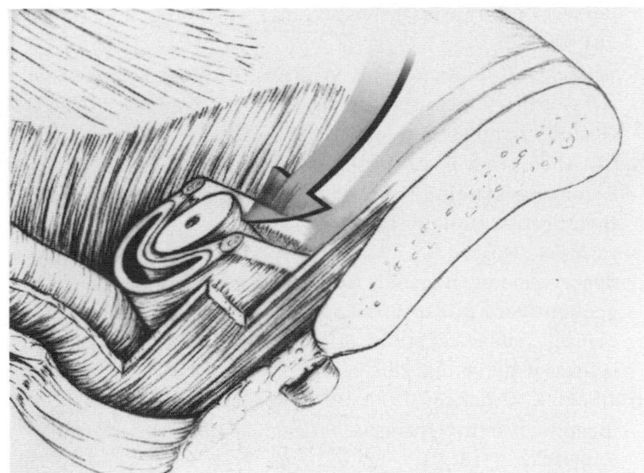

Fig. 1.21 Lateral view of pelvic floor with the urethra, vagina and fascial tissues transected at the level of the vesical neck drawn from three-dimensional reconstruction indicating compression of the urethra by downward force (arrow) against the supportive tissues indicating the influence of abdominal pressure on the urethra (arrow). From DeLancey (1994), with permission.

expanded upon, and improved. This will continue to enhance our ability to understand the variety of patients with lower urinary tract dysfunction, and improve our ability to restore normal urinary control.

ACKNOWLEDGMENT

Figures 1.7, 1.10 and 1.16 are reprinted with permission from the American College of Obstetricians and Gynecologists.

REFERENCES

Anson B 1950 Atlas of Human Anatomy. WB Saunders, Philadelphia

Bartscht K D, DeLancey J O L 1988 A technique to study cervical descent. Obstetrics and Gynecology 72: 940–943

Berglas B, Rubin I C 1953 Study of the supportive structures of the uterus by levator myography. Surgery, Gynecology and Obstetrics 97: 677–692

Berkow S G 1953 The corpus spongiosum of the urethra: its possible role in urinary control and stress incontinence in women. American Journal of Obstetrics and Gynecology 65: 346–351

Bump R C, Huang K C, McClish D K et al 1991 Effect of narcotic anesthesia and skeletal muscle paralysis on passive dynamic urethral function in continent and stress incontinent women. Neurourology and Urodynamics 10: 523–532

Campbell R M 1950 The anatomy and histology of the sacrouterine ligaments. American Journal of Obstetrics and Gynecology 59: 1–12

Constantinou C E 1985 Resting and stress urethral pressures as a clinical guide to the mechanism of continence in the female patient. Urologic Clinics of North America 12: 247–258

DeLancey J O L 1986 Correlative study of paraurethral anatomy. Obstetrics and Gynecology 68: 91–97

DeLancey J O L 1988 Structural aspects of the extrinsic continence mechanism. Obstetrics and Gynecology 72: 296–301

DeLancey J O L 1989 Pubovesical ligament: A separate structure from the urethral supports (pubo-urethral ligaments). Neurourology and Urodynamics 8: 53–62

DeLancey J O L 1992 Anatomic aspects of vaginal eversion after hysterectomy. American Journal of Obstetrics and Gynecology 166: 1717–1728

DeLancey J O L 1994 Structural support of the urethra as it relates to stress urinary incontinence: the hammock hypothesis. American Journal of Obstetrics and Gynecology 170: 1713–1720

DeLancey J O L 1997 Surgical anatomy of the female pelvis. In: Rock J A, Thompson J D (eds) TeLinde's Operative Gynecology, 8th edn. Lippincott Raven, Philadelphia

Dickinson, R L 1889 Studies of the levator ani muscle. American Journal of Diseases of Women 22: 897–917

Dröes, J T H P M 1974 Observations on the musculature of the urinary bladder and urethra in the human foetus. British Journal of Urology 46: 179–185

Gil Vernet S 1968 Morphology and function of the vesico-prostato-urethral musculature. Edizioni Canova Treviso, Italy

Gosling J A, Dixon J S, Critchley H O D, Thompson S A 1981 A comparative study of the human external sphincter and periurethral levator ani muscles. British Journal of Urology 53: 35–41

Gosling J A, Dixon J, Humpherson J R 1982 Functional anatomy of the urinary tract. Gower Medical Publishing, London.

Hilton P, Stanton S L 1983 Urethral pressure measurement by microtransducer: The results in symptom-free women and in those with genuine stress incontinence. British Journal of Obstetrics and Gynaecology 90: 919–933

Hodgkinson CP 1953 Relationships of the female urethra in urinary incontinence. American Journal of Obstetrics and Gynecology 65: 560–573

Huffman J 1948 Detailed anatomy of the paraurethral ducts in the adult human female. American Journal of Obstetrics and Gynecology 55: 86–101

Huisman A B 1983 Aspects on the anatomy of the female urethra with special relation to urinary continence. Contributions in Gynecology and Obstetrics 10: 1–31

Jeffcoate T N A, Roberts H 1952 Observations on stress incontinence of urine. American Journal of Obstetrics and Gynecology 64: 721–738

Lawson J O N 1974 Pelvic anatomy I: pelvic floor muscles sphincters. Annals of the Royal College of Surgeons of England 54: 244–252

Lawson J O N 1974 Pelvic anatomy II: anal canal and associated sphincters. Annals of the Royal College of Surgeons of England 54: 288–300

McGuire E J 1981 Urodynamic findings in patients after failure of stress incontinence operations. Program of Clinical Biology Research 78: 351–360

McGuire, E J 1986 The innervation and function of the lower urinary tract. Journal of Neurosurgery 65: 278–285

Milley P S, Nichols D H 1971 Relationship between the pubo-urethral ligaments and the urogenital diaphragm in the human female. Anatomy Record 170: 81–83

Muellner S R 1951 Physiology of micturition. Journal of Urology 65: 805–810

Nichols D H, Milley P S, Randall C L 1970 Significance of restoration of normal vaginal depth and axis. Obstetrics and Gynecology 36: 251–256

Noll L E, Hutch J A 1969 The SCIPP line – An aid in interpreting the voiding lateral cystourethrogram. Obstetrics and Gynecology 33: 680–689

Oelrich T M 1983 The striated urogenital sphincter muscle in the female. Anatomy Record 205: 223–232

Paramore R H 1918 The uterus as a floating organ. In: Paramore R H The statics of the female pelvic viscera. H K Lewis, London, ch 2, pp 12–15

Parks A G, Porter N H, Melzak J 1962 Experimental study of the reflex mechanism controlling muscles of the pelvic floor. Diseases of the Colon and Rectum 5: 407–414

Power R M H 1954 An anatomical contribution to the problem of continence and incontinence in the female. American Journal of Obstetrics and Gynecology 67: 302–314

Range R L, Woodburne R T 1964 The gross and microscopic anatomy of the transverse cervical ligaments. American Journal of Obstetrics and Gynecology 90: 460–467

Ricci J V, Thom C H 1954 The myth of a surgically useful fascia in vaginal plastic reconstructions. Quarterly Review of Surgical Obstetrics and Gynecology 2: 261–263

Richardson A C, Edmonds P B, Williams N L 1981 Treatment of stress urinary incontinence due to paravaginal fascial defect. Obstetrics and Gynecology 57: 357–362

Rud T, Anderson K E, Asmussen M, Hunting A, Ulmsten U 1980 Factors maintaining the intraurethral pressure in women. Investigative Urology 17: 343–347

Smith A R B, Hosker G L, Warrell D W 1989 The role of partial denervation of the pelvic floor in the aetiology of genitourinary prolapse and stress incontinence of urine: a neurophysiological study. British Journal of Obstetrics and Gynaecology 96: 24–28

Strohbehn K, DeLancey J O L 1996 The anatomy of stress incontinence. In: Operative Techniques in Gynecologic Surgery. 2: 5–16

Uhlenhuth E, Nolley G W 1957 Vaginal fascia a myth? Obstetrics and Gynecology 10: 349–358

Westby M., Asmussen M, Ulmsten U 1982 Location of maximum intraurethral pressure related to urogenital diaphragm in the female subject as studied by simultaneous urethrocystometry and voiding urethrocystography. American Journal of Obstetrics and Gynecology 144: 408–412

Wilson P D, Dixon J S, Brown A D G, Gosling J A 1983 Posterior pubo-urethral ligaments in normal and genuine stress incontinent women. Journal of Urology 130: 802–805

Woodburne R T 1968 Anatomy of the bladder and bladder outlet. Journal of Urology 100: 474–487

Woodburne R T 1965 The ureter ureterovesical junction and vesical trigone. Anatomy Record 151: 243–249

Zacharin R F 1968 The anatomic supports of the female urethra. Obstetrics and Gynecology 21: 754–759

Neurophysiology

JOHN F B MORRISON AND MICHAEL J TORRENS

INTRODUCTION

Most forms of incontinence are due to a disturbance of neuromuscular function. Following many years of structurally based theories of the genesis of incontinence, this may seem an extreme view. However, it is becoming more and more realistic (see Bock & Whelan 1990). An understanding of physiology is paramount in this field, and an overview of the subject which attempts to bring together clinical and experimental aspects on the anatomy, physiology and pharmacology of the lower urinary tract in man and animals is also helpful (Torrens & Morrison 1987). The physiology of the lower urinary tract shows species differences, as might be expected, and mechanisms elucidated in some species may operate to a variable extent in others. Thus some of Barrington's oft-quoted reflexes (Barrington 1914, 1921, 1925, 1931) are known not to operate in man, and some experimentalists have doubts as to whether they all exist even in the cat. Experimental models on animals can be used to elucidate mechanisms underlying observations that are common to man and animals, but relatively few attempts have been made to exploit the potential value of these models. This chapter is designed, however, not as a critical view of these models, but as a simple guide to the significance of the nervous system in incontinence.

MICTURITION CYCLE

Bladder filling and voiding may be represented as a pressure–volume loop (Fig. 2.1). It can be divided into various components as described in the legend to the figure. In addition, the urethra goes through a related, reciprocal cycle of activity, remaining closed during bladder filling and opening during voiding. The most important physiological properties of the lower urinary tract are to contract and relax at the

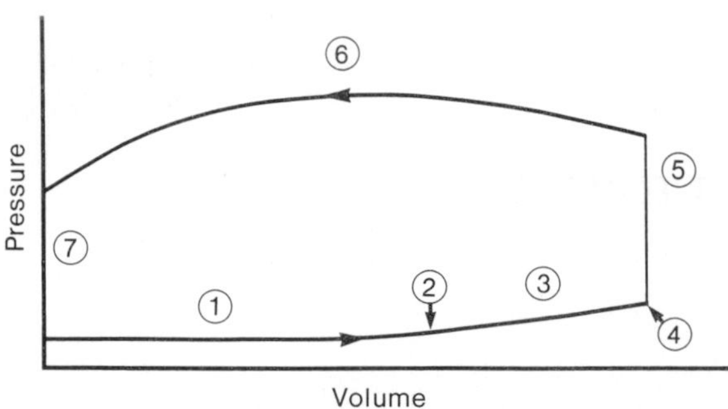

Fig. 2.1 Micturition cycle represented as pressure–volume loop. Various phases, indicated by numbers, are: 1. Accommodation – partly because of intrinsic properties of bladder wall and partly because of unconscious nerve-mediated inhibition. 2. First conscious sensation – mediated by tension receptors, since no rise in detrusor pressure is necessary. 3. Postponement – cortical function, lost in certain cerebral lesions. 4. Initiation of voiding coordinated by pontine micturition centres. 5. Isometric, detrusor contraction – phase before flow starts, usually short in female. 6. Sustained detrusor contraction – phase in which detrusor pressure remains relatively constant throughout voiding. 7. Relaxation phase – majority of which occurs after voiding has ended. In some cases detrusor pressure may rise as bladder neck closes (isometric 'aftercontraction').

right times. Abnormal function is best described in terms of the observed overactivity or underactivity of the appropriate parts of the system. Certain passive or mechanical factors may be relevant, but they are relatively less important.

Filling phase

The normal bladder fills without much significant rise in intravesical pressure. It has been suggested that during the collecting phase the bladder behaves as if it were a hollow sphere of passive viscoelastic material (Griffiths 1980). This is an admittedly mechanical analogy. The process of accommodation (Fig. 2.1) to increasing volume may be related in part to the physical properties of the bladder wall, but it is also influenced by the intrinsic tone of the smooth muscle and by the extent of nerve-mediated inhibition. The pressure–volume relationship during filling is usually observed by a cystometrogram, and is dependent on the rate of filling (Klevmark 1977, 1980). Under these circumstances the relationship is best described in terms of compliance. Compliance is defined as the change in pressure for a given change in volume and as a measurement is not subject to terminological confusion. The normal bladder is highly compliant over the usual volume range, and low compliance is abnormal.

Compliance is a measure of the elastic properties of all the components of the bladder wall, including elastic tissue and smooth muscle. Tone refers to the contribution made to compliance by muscle, as distinct from elastic tissue, and cannot be assessed without inducing a paralysis or complete relaxation of the detrusor muscle. The tone of the bladder is generally regarded as being myogenic, being uninfluenced by anesthesia or ganglionic blockade (Ruch 1979); it is possible that the myogenic activity may be reduced by sympathetic impulses, and there is some evidence that, at least in the cat, muscular tone may be reduced by sympathetic activity, causing the bladder to become more compliant (Edvardsen 1967; Gjone 1966).

The tone of the smooth muscle therefore contributes to compliance, but is not equivalent to it. Tone, or tonus, is a concept that is best avoided in clinical practice, at least until methods are available to discriminate between the elastic and muscle contributions to compliance. Terms such as hypertonic and hypotonic should also not be used.

The urethra remains closed during the filling phase, the intraurethral pressure being greater than the intravesical pressure. Often, although not always, the electromyographic activity of the pelvic floor muscles increases as the bladder fills. It is assumed that the striated muscle of the urethral sphincter behaves similarly.

Voiding phase

The filling and voiding phases should always be considered together when classifying function. Towards the end of the filling phase the sensation of bladder fullness is consciously appreciated. This sensation leads to the voluntary postponement of micturition, and some time later an appropriate place and position for voiding is chosen, which is a function of the cerebral hemispheres. A normal person should be able to initiate a void regardless of the volume in the bladder. The sequence of events is said to be a relaxation of the pelvic floor with descent of the bladder base and reduction of intraurethral pressure, followed by contraction of the bladder. In fact, the events are probably initiated at the same time, the bladder taking longer to respond. The bladder neck opens as the intravesical pressure exceeds the intraurethral pressure. Further than this, the control of bladder neck function in the female has not been fully identified.

The voiding contraction should be sustained until the bladder is empty. The intravesical pressure during voiding, which should be more or less constant, depends on the rate at which the urine can be discharged. In females with a high urine flow rate, the pressure may be low. In some cases it may hardly change from the resting level, but this does not mean that the bladder is acontractile, as will be discussed later. The compliance of the urethra can be defined in a similar way to that of the bladder, as a function of the intraurethral pressure and urethral diameter. It is not a parameter that can be measured easily, but it is a useful concept. Urethral compliance during voiding depends on normal relaxation of the urethral sphincter muscle and on normal urethral distensibility. Decreased compliance may produce urethral obstruction, rare in the female. Increased compliance, producing a 'baggy' urethra, may be relatively common. The pathological significance of this latter condition has not been fully appreciated.

CENTRAL NERVOUS SYSTEM INFLUENCES

The most important co-ordination centres for micturition are situated in the brainstem, especially the dorsolateral pontine tegmentum. Various adjacent areas may have slightly differing functions, but the net effect is that the pontine tegmentum contains the origin of the final common path for co-ordinated bladder and sphincter activity (Fig. 2.2). The effects of neurological lesions are explained in the legend. The organization of the central nervous system in relation to micturition has been reviewed by Nathan (1976), Fletcher & Bradley (1978), Torrens & Morrison (1987) and Morrison (1997, 1999).

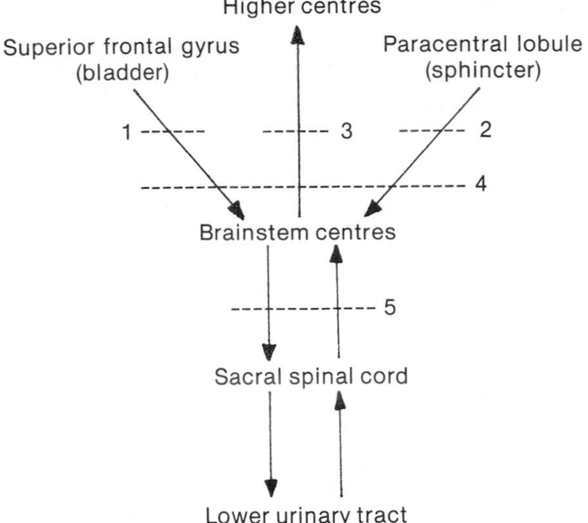

Fig. 2.2 Simplified scheme of interaction of various levels of nervous system in micturition. Location of certain possible nervous lesions are denoted by numbers and explained in the following. 1. Lesions isolating superior frontal gyrus prevent voluntary postponement of voiding. If sensation is intact, this produces urge incontinence. If lesion is large and destroys more of frontal lobe, there will be loss of social concern about incontinence. 2. Lesions isolating paracentral lobule, often with hemiparesis, will cause spasticity of urethral sphincter and retention. This will be painless if sensation is also abolished. 3. Pathways of sensation are not known accurately. In theory, isolated lesion of sensation above brainstem would lead to unconscious incontinence. Defective conduction of sensory information would explain enuresis. 4. Lesions above brainstem centres lead to involuntary voiding that is coordinated with sphincter relaxation. 5. Lesions below brainstem centres but above sacral spinal cord lead, after period of bladder paralysis, to involuntary 'reflex' voiding that is not coordinated with sphincter relaxation (detrusor/sphincter dyssynergia).

Normal sensation

Humans experience a number of sensations that arise from the lower urinary tract. Sensations arising from the urethra are usually felt more acutely than those arising from the bladder, and this is probably due to the relative density of innervation of these two regions. The distal urethra gives rise to sensations of touch, temperature and pain, and receives a somatic innervation akin to the skin. The proximal urethra also responds to touch and temperature and can give rise to pain, but in addition there are a number of sensations specifically related to the lower urinary tract, of which the sensation of imminent micturition probably arises from this site. There are no muscle spindles in the periurethral muscle, but some do exist in the pelvic floor of man.

Sensations relating to the level of normal distension and to overdistension of the bladder arise from sensory endings in the bladder itself, and these sensations include proprioceptive sensations such as the first sensation of distension during cystometry and the desire to micturate, and the more noxious sensations of urgency or of overt pain. Sensations arising from the bladder are usually located deep to the skin and either in the suprapubic area or in the perineum, but may also extend into the thighs. Afferent nerve fibres from the bladder and proximal urethra pass through the hypogastric and pelvic nerves to enter the upper lumbar and mid-sacral cord in man, where they make contact with ascending neurones that initiate sensation and with the autonomic cell columns that influence reflex behaviour. Apart from a few Pacinian corpuscles that detect transmitted vibration, the main sensory endings have no defined structure and are the terminations of unmyelinated and small myelinated fibres. The unmyelinated endings occur particularly in the submucosa, and some actually penetrate the epithelium of the bladder. The endings located in muscle are believed to monitor the tension in the bladder or the vesical ligaments and are responsible for the sensations associated with distension. During cystometry in cats, these afferents begin to discharge when the bladder is about 30% full, i.e. at a point in the pressure–volume curve that corresponds to the first sensation during cystometry in humans. These afferents respond to high pressures as well as low ones, and it seems likely that they mediate the noxious sensation associated with overdistension as well as the innocuous proprioceptive sensations (Jänig & Morrison 1986).

Abnormal sensation: afferent hypersensitivity in inflammatory states

Recently there have been a series of studies in rats (see Morrison 1999) that indicate the presence of unmyelinated afferents in the mucosa that are sensitive to changes in the composition of urine, and to inflammatory mediators. Many of these afferents are sensitive to distension, and can increase their sensitivity to mechanical stimulation following the luminal application of potassium, high osmolality and low pH solutions, and also respond to capsaicin and a number of endogenous mediators, such as Neurokinin A (derived for nerve endings), or ATP (released for the urothelium – see Ferguson et al 1997). In addition, Nerve Growth Factor, released by smooth muscle in the hypertrophied bladder, can also increase afferent sensitivity, which may account for reports of hyperexcitability of bladder reflexes in this state (Dmitreva & McMahon 1996). The effect of hypersensitive afferents is that the reflex behaviour of the bladder increases, and there is a lower threshold of sensation, both characteristic of inflammatory states. The interesting result of these experiments is that there are a series of mediators present in the urothelium, submucosal nerves and the smooth muscle, all of which can increase the responsiveness of the afferent population that signals bladder volume.

There is good evidence in man and animals that the lateral columns of the white matter subserve the sensations of bladder filling and desire to micturate and of pain, while the dorsal columns subserve innocuous sensations arising from the urethra and pelvic floor muscles. The lateral column pathway appears to originate mainly from the deeper layers of the dorsal horn which receive primary afferents from viscera, and from areas of the ventral horn (McMahon & Morrison, 1982a, b). Bladder sensations are sometimes referred to somatic areas (skin or muscle), particularly in the suprapubic and perineal regions. The explanation of referred sensations from viscera was provided by Ruch in 1946 in his 'Convergence-Projection Theory' (Ruch 1979); this suggested that sensations elicited by impulses in visceral nerves were felt in the somatic areas innervated by spinal segments which received the visceral inputs. Ruch believed that ascending spinal neurones received inputs from viscera and from somatic areas, and that impulses in such pathways were interpreted by the brain as coming primarily from the somatic area. In the case of the bladder, there is ample evidence that impulses in some ascending spinal pathways may arise from the urinary tract as well as from skin or muscle innervated from the same segments. Somatovisceral convergence of this type may therefore explain referred sensations from the bladder; where this phenomenon occurs in neurones which project locally in the cord, this mix of sensory inputs may be responsible for automatic micturition, such as is seen in paraplegic patients or animals (McMahon & Morrison 1982b; Sasaki et al 1994). In normal subjects the somatic inputs may be inhibited, probably by descending pathways from the brain that can reduce the amounts of transmitter released by primary afferents. A fuller account of the sensory systems that transmit impulses from the viscera can be found in *The Physiology of the Lower Urinary Tract* by Torrens & Morrison (1987).

Sensation is difficult to assess objectively in the clinic. The first sensation during cystometry is a useful guide, and the volume at which it occurs depends to some extent on the state of contraction or relaxation of the bladder smooth muscle. The integrity of sensory pathways can be checked by monitoring responses evoked from the bladder or urethra (Rockswold & Bradley 1977). An attempt has been made to quantify the urethral electrical threshold by Powell & Feneley (1980). The normal threshold was 4–8 mA for their bipolar stimulating catheter. Abnormal threshold correlated well with pathological states. The bulbocavernosus reflex latency has also been used to test reflex pathways elicitable from afferents in the pudendal nerve. The variations in technique and interpretation of this test are discussed by Fowler & Fowler (1987).

Brain centres

Analysis of the effects of ablation, stimulation and tumour growth in humans, reinforced by stimulation studies in animals, has revealed areas in the brain with an influence on micturition. The cortical control of the lower autonomous centres has developed in proportion to the social significance of micturition in animals and humans. The cortical areas involved in humans are the superior frontal gyrus and the adjacent anterior cingulate gyrus. Lesions in these areas reduce or abolish both the conscious and unconscious inhibition of the micturition reflex. The bladder tends to empty at a low functional capacity. Sometimes the patient is aware of the sensation of urgency, and sometimes micturition may be entirely unconscious. The lesions may not, however, abolish the social distress caused by incontinence. These areas, which have now been localized by functional magnetic resonance imaging, are supplied by the anterior cerebral and pericallosal arteries, spasm or occlusion of which produces incontinence. Similar symptoms occur in more generalized cerebral disorders such as atrophy and hydrocephalus.

Localized lesions rather more posteriorly, in the paracentral lobule, may produce retention rather than incontinence because of a combination of impaired sensation and spasticity of the pelvic floor. Many areas of the subcortical brain have been described as influencing micturition (Torrens 1995). The highest autonomous centres probably exist in the septal and preoptic areas (Nathan 1976) and project to the reticular formation of the brainstem, especially the pons, where a succession of researchers have recognized a region which appears essential for normal reflex and voluntary control of the bladder (Barrington 1921, 1925; de Groat 1975; Fletcher & Bradley 1978; Holstege 1992; Torrens & Morrison 1987). Other areas may also influence this pathway (Fig. 2.3). Although it is tempting to localize brain function topographically into specific areas, this is manifestly not the way the brain works. Rather, there is a continuous interaction of inhibitory and facilitatory activity that finally summates to produce discharge of the appropriate motor neurones.

Descending tracts

The descending influences from the reticular formation of the brainstem pass caudally in the reticulospinal tracts. Their location in humans is not entirely clear. The fibres may be laterally close to the insertion of the dentate ligaments (Hitchcock et al 1974) or more medially between the lateral corticospinal tract and the intermediolateral grey matter of the spinal cord (Nathan 1976; McMahon & Morrison 1982c). Kuru (1965) suggests that the fibres causing detrusor contraction and detrusor relaxation are separated into the lateral and ventral reticulospinal tracts respectively, and in a similar way fibres activating and inhibiting the urethral sphincter mechanism may travel separately in the ventral and medial reticulospinal tracts. The excitatory pathways can be traced to the rostral pons, and the inhibitory pathways to the midline raphe nuclei and the nucleus gigantocellularis reticularis in the medulla (McMahon & Spillane 1982; Morrison & Spillane 1986; Lumb & Morrison 1986).

Sacral micturition centre

It is generally considered that the motor neurones supplying both the bladder and the sphincter mechanism are located in the grey matter of the sacral spinal cord. Certainly, stimulation of this area can evoke a bladder contraction. Unlike the centres in the brain, this area cannot coordinate parasympathetic, sympathetic, and somatic activity. When it is disconnected from the brain, there is a tendency for bladder and sphincter contraction to occur together. This uncoordinated contraction is described as dyssynergia. The initial effect of spinal transaction is detrusor paralysis or areflexia. After a variable time, reflex detrusor contraction develops. This delay emphasizes the importance of supraspinal control of the sacral neurones.

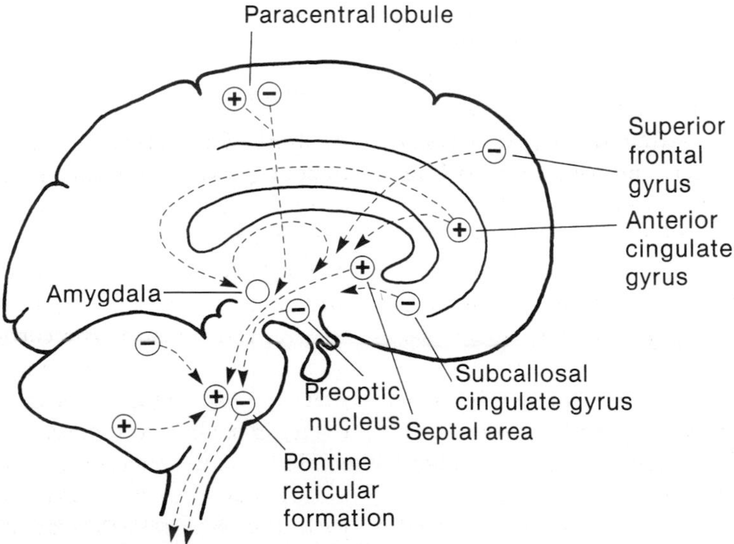

Fig. 2.3 Simplified representation of cerebral areas involved in micturition. Multiplicity of interactions makes it easy to appreciate why subject should be left to the research physiologist. +, facilitation; –, inhibition. From Torrens & Feneley (1982), with permission.

Transection presumably causes many synaptic sites of these neurones to be vacated, and the cells cannot discharge again until the sites have been reoccupied.

The parasympathetic preganglionic cell bodies innervating the bladder are found at the lateral edge of the anterior horn of the spinal cord. The cell bodies of the somatic efferent neurones to the urethral sphincter mechanism are situated anteromedially in a group in the anterior horn of the spinal cord. These cells seem to be relatively unaffected in, for example, motor neurone disease. They also seem to continue to function soon after spinal cord injury. The cells innervating the sphincter are located about one cord segment higher than those that supply the bladder.

PERIPHERAL INNERVATION

The possible organization of the peripheral nervous system in relation to the lower urinary tract is summarized in Fig. 2.4 and explained in the legend. It is likely that this interpretation will require modification as knowledge advances.

Innervation of detrusor

The parasympathetic fibres in the anterior sacral roots (S2 to S4) are the principal motor supply to the detrusor. Shishito (1961) has demonstrated a few efferent fibres in the posterior roots. These preganglionic parasympathetic nerves run out through the sacral and pelvic plexuses to the autonomic ganglia lying both outside and inside the wall of the bladder. Here, the majority of the final interaction between the sympathetic and parasympathetic systems occurs. The human detrusor muscle is richly supplied with presumed cholinergic nerve fibres, the density of the innervation being such that the majority of muscle cells are individually supplied with nerves (Gosling 1979). The density of this innervation may well be related to the fact that the detrusor is under direct nervous control, in many ways more like striated muscle than like the smooth muscle of the intestine. Because the ganglia from which these nerves arise are located close to the bladder, it is technically almost impossible to denervate the organ. The section of preganglionic nerve fibres will only 'decentralize' the detrusor. Unlike certain experimental animals, the human detrusor does not contain many noradrenergic nerves. Those that do exist are mainly around the bladder base. If the sympathetic nervous system does have a significant effect on the detrusor, this effect must take place at the ganglia, where a profuse sympathetic innervation has been observed.

Because sympathectomy caused no demonstrable difference in bladder function, the sympathetic nervous system was dismissed by some earlier researchers as being responsible only for vasomotor activity. Learmonth (1931) showed that stimulation of

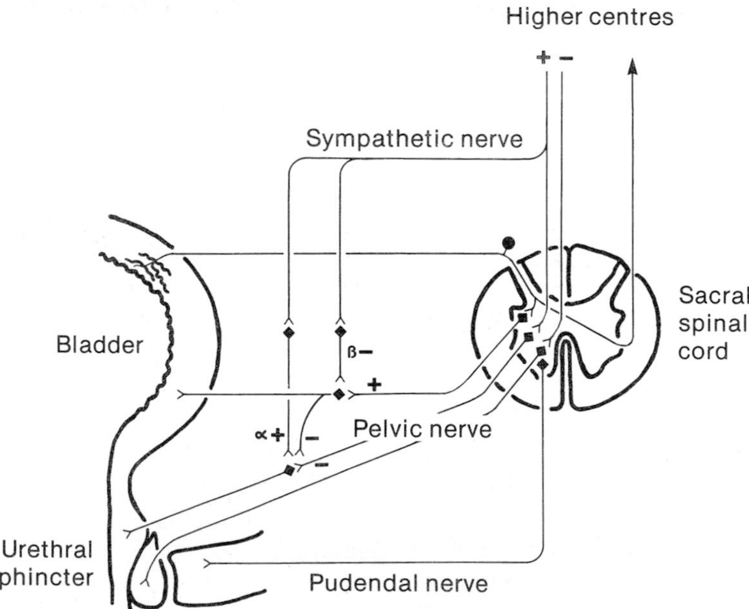

Fig. 2.4 Summary of possible organization for peripheral nervous supply to lower urinary tract. Preganglionic parasympathetic fibres and postganglionic sympathetic fibres both synapse with ganglion cells close to, and within, bladder wall. Arrangement in relation to urethra may be morphologically similar but functionally different. Somatic nerve supply to intramural urethral striated muscle runs with pelvic nerve (and is vulnerable during pelvic surgery).

the presacral nerve was followed by contraction of the region of the bladder neck and trigone. He also allowed himself to be injected with epinephrine (adrenaline), which he noted caused a prolonged bladder relaxation. Sundin & Dahlstrom (1973) developed a technique for measuring bladder relaxation and showed that sympathetic (hypogastric nerve) stimulation produced an initial contraction that was followed by a prolonged relaxation of the bladder. The initial contraction could be reduced to one third by the administration of α-adrenergic blocking drugs, and the subsequent bladder relaxation was entirely abolished by β-adrenergic blocking drugs. In theory, therefore, there may be peripheral sympathetic inhibition of the bladder, which assists urine storage by accommodation. However, it is indisputably true that extensive lumbar sympathectomy in the human does not interfere with continence or obviously affect the ability to store urine, although retrograde ejaculation is well documented. It therefore appears that central inhibition is more important for accommodation than are the activities of the sympathetic nervous system.

Stimulation of parasympathetic fibres in the sacral nerves produces sustained detrusor contraction. The threshold for this response is higher than that required for an effect on the striated urethral sphincter (Fig. 2.5), perhaps because the nerve fibres involved are of a smaller calibre. Conversely, section or ablation of sacral nerves will temporarily abolish activity of the detrusor. Activity tends to return, and the rate and extent of recovery are greater the more proximal the denervation and the less extensive the damage. It is also more likely for normal function to return if part of the nerve supply has been completely damaged (for example, single level sacral nerve ablation) than when all of the nerve supply has been partly damaged (for example, central prolapsed disc).

The physiological response to nerve damage depends on whether motor or sensory fibres are involved. If sensory fibres only are ablated, there is impairment of detrusor contractility, but the bladder pressure remains low. If motor fibres alone or motor and sensory fibres together are involved, the effect is a decrease in detrusor contractility but an increase in the bladder pressure with time. An explanation for this increased bladder pressure, and consequently decreased compliance, has been suggested by Norlen et al (1976). In the cat, preganglionic parasympathetic denervation leads to a reinnervation of the pelvic postganglionic neurones by cholinergic preganglionic sympathetic efferents. This results in the conversion of the normal relaxation response to hypogastric stimulation into a contractile one thus the bladder contracts instead of relaxing when the sympathetic nerves are stimulated (de Groat & Kawatani, 1989). Although no profuse vesical adrenergic innervation exists in humans, it is possible that a similar effect could occur at the peripheral ganglia.

Innervation of urethra

Noradrenergic sympathetic nerve fibres have been identified in relation to the male preprostatic urethra

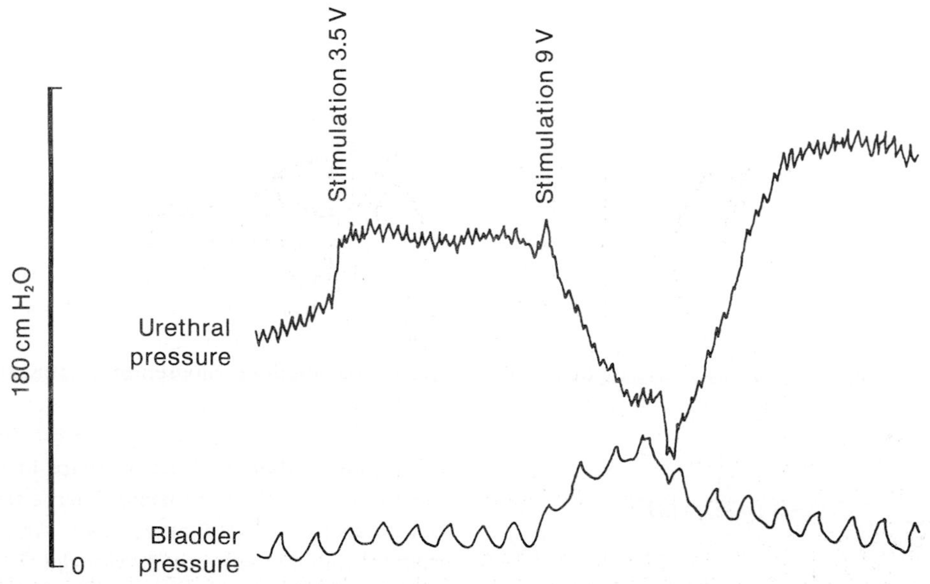

Fig. 2.5 Urethral and bladder pressure responses to sacral nerve stimulation in female. Urethral response has two components, contraction at low voltage and relaxation at higher voltage. From Torrens (1978), with permission.

but are not common in the female urethra at all. In contrast, the dominant innervation of the longitudinal urethral smooth muscle in the female is cholinergic. Despite this discrepancy the majority of the measurable resting urethral pressure in both sexes can be abolished by the use of α-sympathetic blocking drugs. This has led to the conclusion that the functional innervation of the urethral smooth muscle is adrenergic, despite the fact that in the mid-urethra there is no significant adrenergic innervation demonstrable morphologically.

All this serves to emphasize how far apart the morphological and physiological studies are at present. It may be that there are α-adrenergic receptors on the urethral smooth muscle but no nerves to produce the transmitter. On the other hand, α-adrenergic effects may occur at the level of the pelvic ganglia. It is also likely that α-adrenergic blocking drugs have effects on neuromuscular transmission that are not conventionally recognized. Phenoxybenzamine (Dibenyline) in particular is not a 'clean' drug.

There are two groups of striated muscle fibres in relation to the urethra that Gosling (1979) calls intramural and periurethral. The intramural striated muscle is supplied by myelinated fibres from S2 to S4 that run with the pelvic nerve. This explains why it is not affected by pudendal block or pudendal neurectomy. The periurethral striated muscle is part of the pelvic floor and is supplied by the pudendal nerve, also S2 to S4. The reflex control of the periurethral skeletal muscle of the rat has been examined recently by Fedirchuk et al (1991, 1994) and Morrison et al (1995).

The effect of stimulation on the urethra depends on the voltage applied (Fig. 2.5). Experiments in humans (Torrens 1978) have shown that the response to a low voltage is one of sphincter contraction. As the voltage is increased and another population of fibres perhaps stimulated, the urethra relaxes. This is a peripherally integrated and specific effect, since it occurs on stimulation of the distal end of a cut nerve and does not require any contemporaneous bladder contraction. Transection of the sacral nerves, including parasympathetic and somatic fibres, reduces the voluntary contractility of the urethral sphincter but does not reduce the resting pressure unless the denervation is very extensive. It is further evidence for the importance of a sympathetic nervous effect.

NEUROTRANSMITTERS AND HORMONES

It was shown in the previous section that some confusion exists when the functions of nerves and receptors are compared. The understanding of this aspect of physiology is very much in evolution. Some of the reasons why progress is slow in this field are given in the following list:

1 Individual nerves may produce more than one neurotransmitter.
2 Neurotransmitters may act on more than one type of receptor, producing different actions.
3 Neurotransmitters may act in different ways at the same receptor site according to their concentration.
4 Neurotransmitters may interact with one another.
5 There are considerable species differences in both neurotransmitters and receptors.

An example of fundamental controversy is the question of the principal neurotransmitters to the detrusor muscle. The postganglionic parasympathetic fibres are presumed to be cholinergic in that they are associated with identifiable acetylcholinesterase. However, if the transmitter is acetylcholine, it should be blocked by atropine. Although some species are atropine sensitive, perhaps the majority are not. This has led to the suggestion that another substance may be the principal neurotransmitter, or alternatively the receptors on bladder muscle may have more nicotinic than muscarinic characteristics, or perhaps some receptors are not accessible to freely circulating atropine. Suggestions for alternative transmitters include 5-hydroxytryptamine, purine nucleotides such as adenosine triphosphate (ATP), prostaglandins and peptides.

Neuropeptides such as Substance P (SP) and vasoactive intestinal polypeptide (VIP) are found in the bladder but their precise role is unclear. SP and VIP are amongst the neuropeptides that have been identified in bladder efferents, and VIP is present in some peripheral cell bodies in the paracervical and pelvic ganglia, and in axonal terminals around pelvic ganglion cells (Torrens & Morrison 1987). Indomethacin (a prostaglandin synthetase inhibitor) inhibits the atropine-resistant contraction to nerve contraction and the responses to SP, and the conclusion has been made that SP may be the non-adrenergic non-cholinergic (NANC) transmitter in the guinea-pig bladder. Sjogren et al (1982) however did not support the view that SP was an excitatory transmitter in the rabbit, guinea-pig or rat. In the human, SP has an excitatory effect on strips of bladder muscle, but the effects of transmural nerve stimulation are not antagonized by SP-antagonists. An SP antagonist that inhibited contractions induced by a submaximum dose of SP had no effect on the response to electrical field stimulation. The possibility that SP might act as a local modulator of neurotransmission however cannot be excluded, and this role has been attributed to VIP in the guinea-pig bladder (Johns 1979). VIP appears to have either no action or some relaxatory effect on the smooth muscle of the bladder, depending partly on the species (Johns 1979; MacKenzie & Burnstock 1984; Levin, Jacoby & Wein 1981). According to MacKenzie & Burnstock (1984), it is unlikely that VIP is a NANC transmitter in the bladder; this view is based on comparisons of the effects of erogenous VIP and the effects of intramural nerve stimulation in the rabbit. Of these putative NANC transmitters, the most likely candidate for excitatory transmission in the bladder would appear to be ATP (Burnstock 1986). Burnstock had suggested in 1972 that the NANC transmitter in the pelvic supply to the bladder was ATP, despite evidence that the nerve-mediated response was not reduced after development of tachyphylaxis to ATP. Using quinacrine fluorescence histochemistry, Burnstock and colleagues (1978) demonstrated what they believed to be purinergic nerves in guinea-pig bladder; electrical stimulation of these nerves released ATP from the bladder, and this release was blocked by tetrodotoxin (which blocks the nerve impulse by antagonizing the voltage-dependent Na channel), but not by neurotoxins that destroy adrenergic neurones. Support for the purinergic transmission hypothesis came from a study by Downie & Dean (1977). The contractile effect of ATP on the bladders of animals and humans was demonstrated by Levin, Jacoby & Wein (1981); in this study large concentrations (0.1–1 mmol/litre) ATP were required. NANC transmission in the bladder can be inhibited by drugs that block Ca++ entry into cells. There is less evidence concerning the other contenders for NANC transmission (Torrens & Morrison 1987).

Oestrogen can influence the smooth muscle of the urethra by modifying spontaneous activity and the responses to α-adrenoceptor stimulation (Callahan & Creed 1985). In a number of species, the urethra shows spontaneous contractile activity, which is reduced following the administration of oestrogens, possibly due to uncoupling of electrical activity between smooth muscle cells rather than a decreased activity of individual cells. Phenylephrine (an α-adrenoceptor agonist) contracted the urethra, and oestrogens increased the sensitivity in some but not all species. It is not clear whether the effect of oestrogen on continence in elderly women is due to trophic actions on epithelia or to the smooth muscle effects referred to above.

DETRUSOR CONTRACTILITY

The detrusor muscle is a functional syncytium and also has an intramural nerve plexus. There are thus two ways in which the stimulus to contract can be propagated throughout the bladder wall. In some species a pacemaker centre exists from which depolarization can spread. In humans there is no evidence for the existence of such a pacemaker. Observations of the response to direct electrical stimulation and the existence of the high density of innervation described earlier suggest that contraction is likely to be initiated at much the same time throughout the organ.

Differential contraction of the various areas of the bladder, especially around the base, has sometimes been postulated to explain the opening of the bladder neck. Such a phenomenon could be due to selective neuropharmacological effects. There may be no need to look for a morphological explanation. However, very little evidence has yet been collected, and this whole area remains obscure.

Bladder contraction depends both on an intact nerve supply and on the characteristics of the muscle. In a clinical context the bladder may be normal, overactive or underactive. The typical manifestation of detrusor overactivity is the appearance of frequent, involuntary, but otherwise characteristic bladder contractions. These are associated typically with either a disturbance of nervous control or with an obstructed outflow tract. Conversely, detrusor underactivity is characterized by delayed, poorly sustained, or absent contraction, associated with neural depletion or muscle damage. The excitability of the micturition reflex was recently examined in a conference in Oslo (see Morrison 1995)

The contractility of detrusor muscle is judged usually from the pressure it can generate during voiding. However, this pressure depends not only on the integrity of nerve and muscle but also on the potential flow rate of urine. The higher the flow, the lower the pressure. Only if flow is zero is the pressure directly proportional to the strength of muscle contraction, which is then isometric. Griffiths (1980) has classified detrusor contractions as strong or weak (on the basis of the isometric detrusor contraction pressure) and as fast or slow (on the basis of the speed of shortening of muscle, extrapolated from a flow-related coefficient).

In clinical practice the more useful concept is that of the isometric detrusor contraction pressure (P iso). This can be measured by sudden occlusion of the urethra during micturition. Not all females may be able to contract the urethral sphincter voluntarily to achieve this. Mechanical occlusion may be necessary. The detrusor pressure should rise when flow stops. If no such rise occurs, it may mean that a bladder has relatively impaired contractility, and retention will be more likely after any operation that raises urethral resistance.

REFERENCES

Barrington F J F 1914 The nervous mechanism of micturition. Quarterly Journal of Experimental Physiology 8: 33–71

Barrington F J F 1921 The relation of the hind brain to micturition. Brain 44: 23–53

Barrington F J F 1925 The effect of lesions of the hind and mid-brain on micturition in the cat. Quarterly Journal of Experimental Physiology 15: 181–202

Barrington F J F 1931 The component reflexes of micturition in the cat. Brain 54: 177–188

Bock G, Whelan J (eds) 1990 Neurobiology of Incontinence. Ciba Foundation Symposium, John Wiley & Sons, Chichester

Burnstock G 1986 The changing face of autonomic neurotransmission. Acta Physiologica Scandinavica 126: 67–91

Burnstock G, Cocks T, Crowe R, Kasakov L 1978 Purinergic innervation of the guinea-pig urinary bladder. British Journal of Pharmacology 63: 125–138

Callahan S M, Creed K E 1985 The effects of oestrogens on spontaneous activity and responses to phenylephrine of the mammalian urethra. Journal of Physiology 358: 35–46

de Groat W C 1975 Nervous control of the urinary bladder of the cat. Brain Research 87: 201–211

de Groat W C, M Kawatani 1989 Reorganisation of sympathetic preganglionic connections in cat bladder ganglia following parasympathetic denervation. Journal of Physiology 409: 431–449

Dmitreva N, McMahon, S B 1996 Sensitisation of visceral afferents by nerve growth factor in the adult rat. Pain 66: 87–97

Downie J W, Dean D M 1977 The contribution of cholinergic postganglionic neurotransmission to contractions of the rabbit detrusor. Journal of Pharmacology and Experimental Therapeutics 203: 417–425

Edvarsen P 1967 Nervous control of urinary bladder in cats. Acta Neurologica Scandinavica 43: 543–563

Fedirchuk B, Shefchyk S J 1991 Effects of electrical stimulation of the thoracic spinal cord on bladder and external urethral sphincter activity in the decerebrate cat. Experimental Brain Research 84: 635–642

Fedirchuk B, Downie J W and Shefchyk S J 1994 Reduction of perineal evoked excitatory postsynaptic potentials in cat lumbar and sacral motoneurons during micturition. Journal of Neuroscience 14: 6153–6159

Ferguson D R, Kennedy I, Burton T J 1997 ATP is released from rabbit urinary bladder epithelial cells – a possible sensory mechanism. Journal of Physiology 505: 503–511

Fletcher T F, Bradley W E 1978 Neuroanatomy of the bladder/urethra. Journal of Urology 119: 153–160

Fowler C J, Fowler C 1987 Clinical neurophysiology. In: Torrens M J, Morrison JFB (eds) The Physiology of the Lower Urinary Tract. Springer-Verlag, London, pp 309–332

Gjone R 1966 Peripheral autonomic influence on the motility of the urinary bladder in the cat. Acta Physiologica Scandinavica 66: 72–80

Gosling J A 1979 The structure of the bladder and urethra in relation of function. In: Turner-Warwick R, Whiteside C G (eds) Symposium on Clinical Urodynamics, Urology Clinics of North America 6: 31–38

Griffiths D J 1980 Urodynamics. Hilger, Bristol.

Hitchcock E, Newsome D, Salama M 1974 The somatotopic representation of the micturition pathways in the cervical cord of man. British Journal of Surgery 61: 395–401

Holstege G 1992 Neuronal organisation of micturition. Neurourology and Urodynamics 11: 273–277

Jänig W, Morrison J F B 1986 Functional properties of spinal visceral afferents supplying abdominal and pelvic organs, with special emphasis on visceral nociception. In: Cervero F, Morrison J F B (eds) Progress in Brain Research. Vol. 67: Visceral Sensation. Elsevier, Amsterdam, pp 87–114

Johns A 1979 The effect of vasoactive intestinal polypeptides on the urinary bladder and taenia coli of the guinea-pig. Canadian Journal of Physiology and Pharmacology 57: 106–108

Klevmark B 1977 Motility of the urinary bladder in cats during filling at physiological rates. II. Effects of extrinsic bladder denervation on intraluminal tension and intravesical pressure patterns. Acta Physiologica Scandinavica 101: 176–184

Klevmark B 1980 Motility of the urinary bladder in cats during filling at physiological rates. III. Spontaneous rhythmic bladder contractions in the conscious and anaesthetised animal. Influence of distension and innervation. Scandinavian Journal of Urology and Nephrology 14: 219–224

Kuru M 1965 Nervous control of micturition. Physiology Reviews 45: 425–494

Levin R M, Jacoby R, Wein A J 1981 Effect of adenosine triphosphate on contractility and adenosine triphosphatase activity of the rabbit urinary bladder. Molecular Pharmacology 19: 525–528

Learmonth J R 1931 A contribution to the neurophysiology of the urinary bladder in man. Brain 54: 147–176

Lumb B M and Morrison J F B 1986 Electrophysiological evidence for an excitatory projection from ventromedial forebrain structures on to raphe- and reticulo-spinal neurones in the rat. Brain Research 380: 162–166

MacKenzie I. Burnstock G 1984 Neuropeptide action on the guinea-pig bladder: a comparison with the effects of field stimulation and ATP. European Journal of Pharmacology 105: 85–94

McMahon S B, Morrison, J F B 1982a Spinal neurones with long projections activated from the abdominal viscera. Journal of Physiology 322: 1–20

McMahon S B, Morrison J F B 1982b Two groups of spinal interneurones that respond to stimulation of the abdominal viscera. Journal of Physiology 322: 21–34

McMahon S B, Morrison J F B 1982c Factors that determine the excitability of parasympathetic reflexes to the bladder. Journal of Physiology 322: 35–44

McMahon S B, Spillane K 1982 Brainstem influences on the parasympathetic supply to the urinary bladder of the cat. Brain Research 234: 237–249

Morrison J F B 1995 The excitability of the micturition reflex. Scandinavian Journal of Urology and Nephrology Suppl. 175: 21–26

Morrison J F B 1997 Central nervous control of the bladder. pp 129–150. In: Jordan D (ed) Vol Central Nervous Control of Autonomic Function In: Burnstock G (series ed) The Autonomic Nervous System. Overseas Publishers Association, Amsterdam BV, and Harwood Academic Publishers.

Morrison J F B 1999 The activation of bladder wall afferent nerves. Experimental Physiology 84: 131–6

Morrison J F B, Sato A, Sato Y, Yamanishi T 1995 The influence of afferent inputs from skin and viscera on the activity of the bladder and the skeletal muscle surrounding the urethra in the rat. Neuroscience Research 23: 195–205

Morrison J F B, Spillane K 1986 Neuropharmacological studies on descending inhibitory controls over the micturition reflex. Journal of the Autonomic Nervous System Suppl. 1: 393–397

Nathan P W 1976 The central nervous connections of the bladder. In: Williams D I, Chisholm G (eds) The Scientific Foundations of Urology. Heinemann Medical Books, London.

Norlen L, Dahlstrom A, Sundin T, Svedmyr N 1976 The adrenergic innervation and adrenergic receptor activity of the feline urinary bladder and urethra in the normal state and after hypogastric and/or parasympathetic denervation. Scandinavian Journal of Urology and Nephrology 10: 177–184

Powell P H, Feneley R C L 1980 The role of urethral sensation in clinical urology. British Journal of Urology 52: 539–541

Rockswold G L, Bradley W E 1977 The use of evoked electromyographic responses in diagnosing lesions of the cauda equina. Journal of Urology 118: 629–631

Ruch T C 1979 The pathophysiology of pain. In: Ruch T C, Patton H D (eds) Physiology and Biophysics. 20th edn. Saunders, Philadelphia, pp 272–324

Sasaki M, Morrison J F B, Sato Y, Sato A 1994 Effect of mechanical stimulation of the skin on the external urethral sphincter muscles in anaesthetised cats. Japanese Journal of Physiology 44: 575–590

Shishito S 1961 Experimental studies on the innervation of the urinary bladder. Urologia Internationalis 12: 254–269

Sjogren C, Andersson K E, Husted S, Mattiasson A, Moller-Madsen B 1982 Atropine-resistance of the transmurally stimulated, isolated human bladder. Journal of Urology 128: 1368–1371

Sundin T, Dahlstrom A 1973 The sympathetic innervation of the urinary bladder and urethra in the normal state and after parasympathetic denervation at the spinal root level. Scandinavian Journal of Urology and Nephrology 7: 131–149

Torrens M J 1978 Urethral sphincteric responses to stimulation of the sacral nerves in the human female. Urologia Internationalis 33: 22–26

Torrens M J 1995 Suprapontine influences on the micturition reflex. Scandinavian Journal of Urology and Nephrology 29: supp. 175: 11–13

Torrens M J, Feneley F C L 1982 In: Illis L S, Sedgwick E M, Glanville H J (eds) Rehabilitation of the Neurological Patient. Blackwell Scientific Publications, Oxford

Torrens M J, Morrison J F B, 1987 The Physiology of the Lower Urinary Tract. Springer-Verlag, London, p 355

SECTION 1
CHAPTER
3

Mechanism of continence

PAUL HILTON

INTRODUCTION

Urinary incontinence may be defined as 'a condition in which involuntary loss of urine is a social or hygienic problem, and is objectively demonstrable' (Abrams et al 1990). Continence, then, is the ability to retain urine within the bladder between voluntary acts of micturition. From these definitions it is self-evident that continence is dependent on 'the powers of urethral resistance exceeding the forces of urinary expulsion'. This concept was first expressed by Barnes (1940), and first proven by Enhorning (1961), who showed that continence was maintained when the maximum urethral pressure exceeded the bladder pressure or when the urethral closure pressure was positive. Normal micturition may be said to result from the controlled reversal of this equilibrium, and incontinence from its uncontrolled reversal. The important aspects of the control of continence, therefore, are firstly those factors which maintain low intravesical pressure and, secondly, those which ensure that the urethral pressure remains high – or at least higher than intravesical pressure – at all times during the filling and storage phases of the micturition cycle.

PHYSIOLOGY OF THE LOWER URINARY TRACT

Behaviour of the bladder

The intravesical pressure is dependent upon a number of factors (see Fig. 1) including the following:

- The hydrostatic pressure at the bladder neck
- The transmission of intra-abdominal pressure
- The tension in the bladder wall itself.

The hydrostatic pressure at the bladder neck

Liquid in the bladder, when in hydrostatic equilibrium, has a vertical gravitational pressure gradient, and the measured pressure must therefore be referred to a standard level. For clinical practice the intravesical pressure is defined as the pressure in the bladder

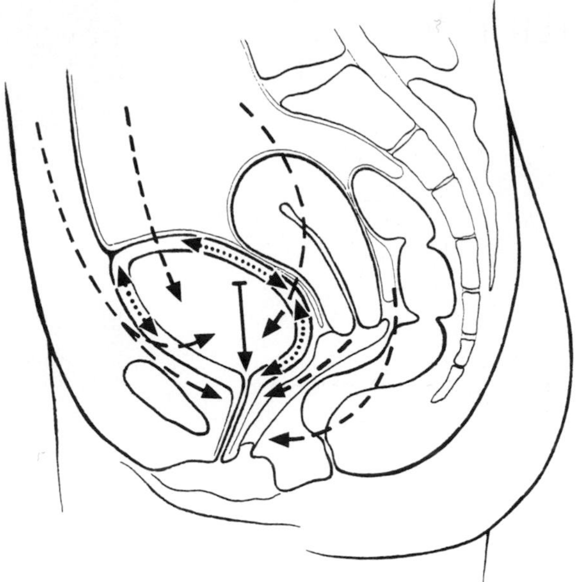

Fig. 3.1 Factors determining the intravesical pressure, and which are therefore of relevance to the maintenance of urethral closure pressure. Solid line shows hydrostatic pressure at the bladder neck; broken line shows transmission of intra-abdominal pressure; dotted line shows passive and active tension in the bladder wall.

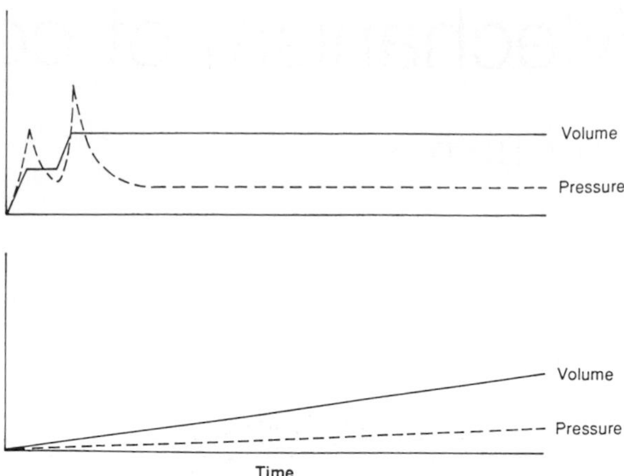

Fig. 3.2 The behaviour of the bladder in terms of pressure and volume changes with time during rapid stepwise filling (above) and slow continuous (physiological) filling (below).

with respect to atmospheric pressure measured at the level of the upper border of the symphysis pubis. In terms of the maintenance of continence, the critical pressure is that acting at the bladder neck, tending to work against the closure forces of the urethra. This has a hydrostatic element dependent on the head of fluid above it; this, of course, increases with increasing bladder volume, though rarely amounts to more than 10 cm H_2O.

The transmission of intra-abdominal pressure

The bladder is normally an intra-abdominal organ, and is therefore subject to pressures transmitted from adjacent viscera and elsewhere within the abdominal cavity. This is not of great importance in the resting situation since pressures transmitted to the bladder are low and generally are transmitted equally to bladder neck and proximal urethra. This effect may, however, be critical in the maintenance of continence in the face of stress (see below).

The tension in the bladder wall itself

This is in part a passive phenomenon related to the distensibility or viscoelastic properties of the bladder wall itself, and in part an active phenomenon due to the contractility of the detrusor muscle and its neurological control.

Viscoelasticity of the bladder During rapid stepwise filling of the bladder the detrusor pressure rises rapidly and afterwards decays exponentially with time (see Fig. 3.2A); this time dependence is similar to that expected of a passive viscoelastic solid. However, under the near static conditions of physiological filling, the detrusor's behaviour is more accurately described as elastic. That is to say, the detrusor pressure rises little as the bladder volume increases from zero to functional capacity (see Fig. 3.2B).

Contractility of the bladder and its neural control The neurological control of detrusor contractility is dependent upon a sacral spinal reflex under control of several higher centres (see Ch. 2). This basic reflex arc is best considered as a loop (see Fig. 3.3) extending from sensory receptors within the bladder wall, through the pelvic plexus and via visceral afferent fibres travelling with the pelvic splanchnic nerves; it enters the spinal cord in the S2 to S4 level, via internuncial neurones within the cord synapsing with cell bodies in the intermediolateral grey area of the same sacral levels, and thence via parasympathetic fibres in the pelvic splanchnic nerves through the pelvic plexus to the smooth muscle cells of the detrusor. The stretch receptors or proprioceptors within the bladder wall are in effect connected in series with muscle cells and are therefore stimulated by both passive stretch and by active contraction of the detrusor. Once a critical level of stretch is achieved, impulses pass in the afferent limb of the reflex arc, and the resultant efferent discharge leads to a detrusor contraction.

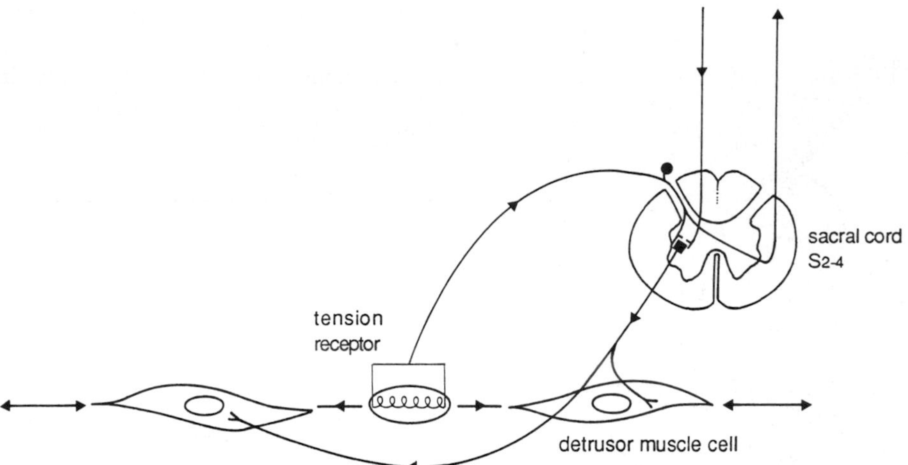

Fig. 3.3 The basic visceral reflex arc concerned in detrusor contractility.

The higher control over the basic visceral reflex arc is mediated through descending pathways from the pontine reticular formation. Although both excitatory and inhibitory centres have been located in this region, their net effect is primarily an inhibitory one, and their normal influence is therefore to prevent contraction of the detrusor, and thus to encourage the maintenance of a low intravesical pressure during the filling phase of the micturition cycle.

Urethral closure mechanisms

In order to maintain continence, it is vital not only that the intravesical pressure should remain low during the storage phase of the micturition cycle, but also that the urethral lumen should seal completely. Zinner et al (1976) described three components of urethral function necessary to achieve this hermetic property:

- Urethral inner wall softness
- Inner urethral compression
- Outer wall tension

Urethral inner wall softness

Whilst the closure of any elastic tube can be obtained if sufficient compression is applied to it, the efficiency of closure is dramatically increased if its lining possesses the property of plasticity, or the ability to mould into a watertight seal.

There has been much debate over the morphological components which contribute to the functional characteristics of softness, compression and tension in the urethra. Several authors have commented on the vascularity of the urethra and pointed out that the submucosal vascular plexi far exceed the requirements of a blood supply for the organ. Some have suggested a significant vascular contribution to urethral closure (Huisman 1983; Rud et al 1980) although others have found no specific features to suggest an important occlusive role for the urethral vascular supply (Gosling et al 1983). Nevertheless, whatever the contribution of the urethral blood supply to the measured intraluminal pressure, it is likely to be of significance as regards the plasticity of the urothelium and submucosa.

Inner urethral compression and outer wall tension

The structures leading to inner wall compression by virtue of their contribution to outer wall tension can be quantified in terms of the urethral pressure profile (see Fig. 3.4). These structures may include the intramural elastic fibres, the intrinsic smooth and striated muscle and the extrinsic or periurethral striated muscle. Tanagho and colleagues, extrapolating from urethral pressure studies in dogs, suggested that approximately 50% of the resting urethral pressure was due to striated muscle components (Tanagho et al 1969a; Tanagho et al 1969b). From urethral pressure studies undertaken at various stages during radical pelvic surgery Rud and colleagues showed that approximately one third of the resting urethral pressure is due to striated muscle effects, one third to smooth muscle effects, and one third to its vascular supply (Rud et al 1980).

Whatever the relative importance of the above factors to active wall tension, it should be remembered that these same structures also contribute a passive or elastic tension, together with the supporting elements of collagen and elastin.

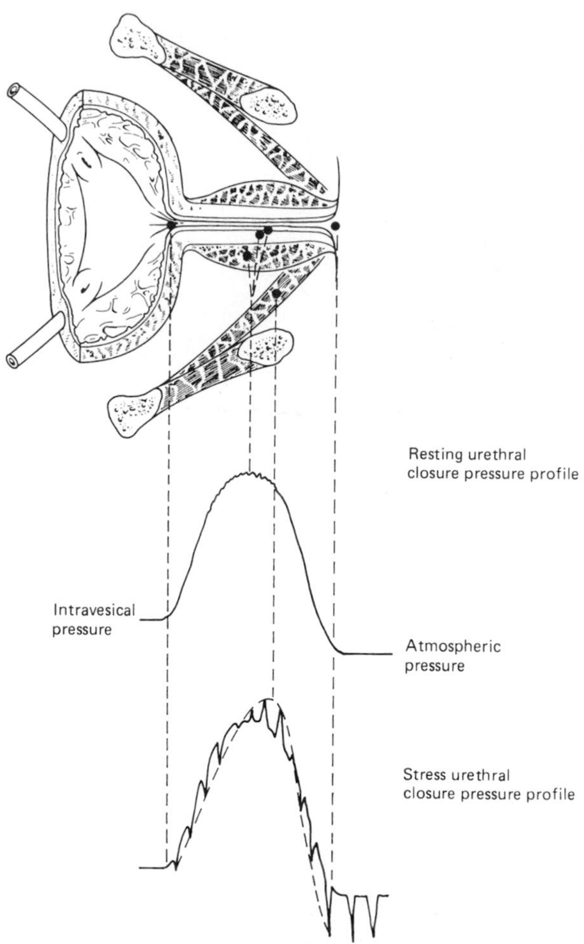

Fig. 3.4 (top) Schematic drawing of the female bladder and urethra in coronal section. Below are shown urethral closure pressure profiles at rest (middle) and on stress (bottom) to demonstrate the morphological and functional correlation. From Hilton (1990), with permission.

The usual level of continence in the female is not, as one might expect, in the mid-urethra at the level of maximum resting pressure, but at the bladder neck. This region in the female has no sphincteric circular smooth muscle and is virtually devoid of striated muscle; it would therefore seem that the passive elastic tension is the most important factor leading to closure at the bladder neck and proximal urethra (see Fig. 3.4 – top/middle). It is recognized, however, that 20–50% of women have incompetence at the bladder neck level (Hilton & Stanton 1983; Versi et al 1986; Versi 1991), and depend on distal mechanisms for continence (Versi et al 1990).

In the mid-urethra the most prominent structural feature is the intrinsic striated muscle or rhabdosphincter. Electron microscopic and histochemical evidence suggests that this may be responsible for the bulk of active urethral tone at rest (Gosling & Dixon 1979). Electromyographic studies (Anderson 1984), histochemical evidence (Gosling et al 1981) and urethral pressure measurements (Hilton & Stanton 1983) all suggest that the periurethral striated muscles have their maximum effect at a level slightly distal to that of the resting urethral pressure profile (see Fig. 3.4 middle/bottom) and do not contribute greatly to the maintenance of continence at rest. It is likely, however, that these distally located extrinsic striated muscles, both the pubococcygeus, and the compressor urethrae (DeLancey 1990) play a significant role in the maintenance of urethral closure in the face of increased intra-abdominal pressure.

THE NORMAL MICTURITION CYCLE

The main function of the bladder is to convert the continuous excretory process of the kidneys into a more convenient, intermittent process of evacuation. In order to achieve this, the bladder must serve firstly as an efficient low pressure reservoir with a competent sphincter, and alternately as a contractile pump with a low resistance outflow tract. From the background information contained in Chapters 1 and 2, and earlier sections of this chapter, it is now possible to discuss the mechanisms whereby urine is retained within the bladder during the filling and storage phases and evacuated during the voiding phase of the normal micturition cycle (see Fig. 3.5).

Filling and storage phase

The bladder normally fills with urine by a series of peristaltic contractions at a rate of between 0.5 and 5 ml/min; under these conditions the bladder pressure increases only minimally. Even during the course of cystometry at rapid filling rates, in normal individuals the pressure rises by no more than 15 cm H_2O from empty to cystometric capacity.

Urethral closure, meanwhile, is maintained by the combined passive and active effects of its smooth and striated muscle components, its elastic content, and its blood supply. The hermetic efficiency is accentuated by the softness of its mucosa.

During the early stages of bladder filling, proprioceptive afferent impulses from stretch receptors within the bladder wall pass via the pelvic nerves to sacral dorsal roots S_2–S_4. These impulses ascend in the cord via the lateral spinothalamic tracts and a detrusor motor response is subconsciously inhibited by descending impulses from the subcortical micturition centres (see Fig. 3.5a).

As the bladder volume increases, further afferent impulses ascend to the cerebral cortex, and the sen-

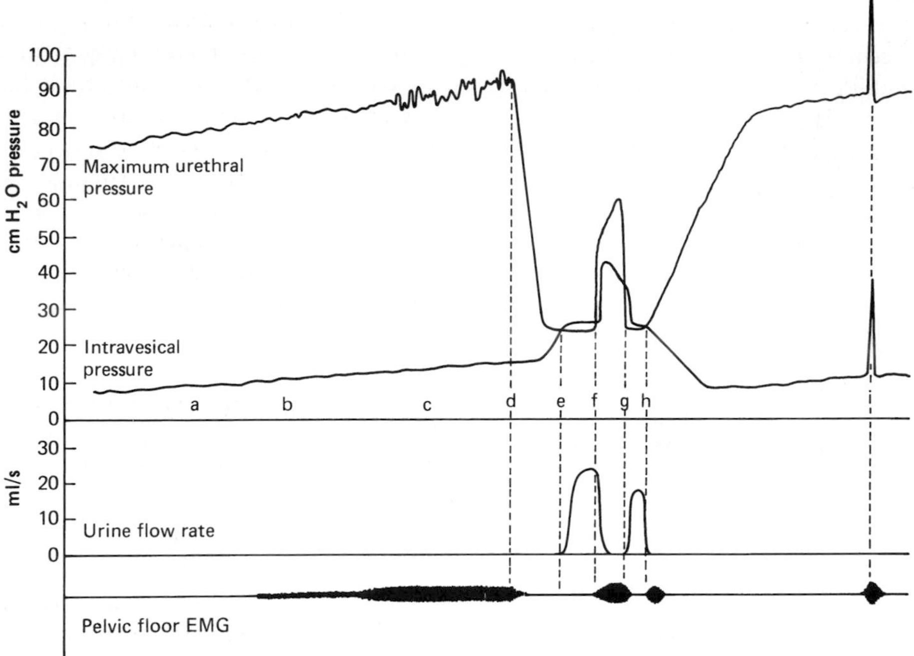

Fig. 3.5 The normal micturition cycle showing changes in urethral and intravesical pressure, urine flow rate and pelvic floor electromyogram (EMG). (a) Phase of subconscious inhibition; (b) phase of conscious (suppressible) inhibition; (c) phase of reinforced (unsuppressible) inhibition; (d) initiation or transition; (e) voiding; (f) interruption of micturition by pelvic floor contraction; (g) resumption of micturition; (h) end of void; (i) increase in intra-abdominal pressure due to a cough. From Hilton (1986), with permission.

sation of bladder filling, associated with the desire to micturate, is first consciously appreciated usually at between 200 and 300 ml or half the functional bladder capacity. The inhibition of detrusor contraction is now cortically mediated, although the desire to void may be further suppressed to subconscious levels again, given sufficient distracting afferent stimuli. Whilst descending impulses inhibit preganglionic parasympathetic cell bodies in the sacral cord, there may also be excitatory effects on the sympathetic neurones in the thoracolumbar region. This will cause increased efferent discharge to the β-adrenoreceptors within the bladder (and/or further inhibition within the pelvic plexus of parasympathetic fibres to the bladder), leading to its relaxation, and to α-adrenoreceptors in the proximal urethra (and/or further excitation within the pelvic plexus of post-ganglionic parasympathetic fibres to the urethra), leading to a slight increase in urethral pressure (see Fig. 3.5b).

With further filling, impulses within the visceral afferent fibres accompanying the sympathetic efferents to thoracolumbar roots T_{10}–L_2 ascend to the cerebral cortex, and a further desire to void is appreciated; reinforced conscious inhibition of micturition then occurs whilst a suitable site and posture for micturition are sought. During this time, in addition to the cortical suppression of detrusor activity, there may also be a voluntary pelvic floor contraction in an attempt to maintain urethral closure; this may be evidenced by a further increase in urethral closure pressure and by marked fluctuations in urethral pressure (Asmussen & Ulmsten 1976) as the sensation of urgency becomes increasingly severe (see Fig. 3.5c).

Initiation phase

When a suitable time, site and posture for micturition are selected, the process of voiding commences. This may be considered in two phases – the initiation or transition from the non-voiding state and micturition itself. Several theories have been propounded to explain the transition phase, although the process is perhaps best viewed as combining features of several of these (Bradley et al 1974; Denny-Brown & Robertson 1933; Hutch 1965; Lapides 1958; Tanagho & Miller 1970).

Relaxation of the pelvic floor may be shown to occur early in the process, both radiologically and electromyographically; it is likely that simultaneous relaxation of the intrinsic striated muscle also occurs, since a marked fall in intraurethral pressure is seen before the intravesical pressure rises, during both voluntary and provoked voiding (Karlson 1953) and the same has been shown in response to sacral nerve stimulation (Torrens 1976) (see Fig. 3.5d).

A few seconds later the descending inhibitory influences from the cerebral cortex acting on the sacral micturition centre are suppressed, allowing a rapid discharge of efferent parasympathetic impulses via the pelvic nerves to cause contraction of the detrusor, and probably also to pull open the bladder neck and shorten the urethra. Simultaneous inhibition of the efferent sympathetic discharges via the thoracolumbar outflow to the pelvic plexus probably also occurs, encouraging detrusor contraction and urethral relaxation. Depending on the relationship between the force of detrusor contraction and the residual urethral resistance, the intravesical pressure may rise to a variable extent (usually less than 60 cm H_2O). When the falling urethral and increasing intravesical pressures equate, urine flow will commence (see Fig. 3.5e).

Voiding phase

The application of physical laws to explain the mechanism of continence is often considered inappropriate and misleading. In considering the bladder during micturition, however, the law of Laplace may be useful. It states that the pressure (P) in a vessel varies directly with the mural tension (T), and inversely with the radius (R). Since the bladder at the initiation of micturition takes on a nearly spherical shape, and has walls which are thin in comparison to its radius, its behaviour may be usefully expressed by the basic formula of the law as applied to a sphere:

$$P = 2T/R$$

As the mural tension rises in the absence of voiding, the intravesical pressure also rises. When a critical opening pressure is achieved, urine will start to flow and the bladder radius will fall. The pressure, however, usually remains constant during voiding, and the mural tension therefore must fall. Once initiated, therefore, the process of micturition requires little to sustain it. Whilst active tension is required throughout, the effectiveness of detrusor contraction increases as the muscle fibres shorten and therefore decreasing forces are required as micturition proceeds (Zinner et al 1976).

If micturition is voluntarily interrupted midstream, this is usually achieved by a contraction of the periurethral striated muscle of the pelvic floor. In association with this contraction the urethral pressure rises rapidly to exceed the intravesical pressure and therefore urine flow stops. The detrusor, being a smooth muscle, is much slower to relax, and therefore goes on contracting against the closed sphincter. That is to say, an isometric contraction occurs, and again applying the law of Laplace, the intravesical pressure rises (see Fig. 3.5f). If micturition is resumed by relaxation of the pelvic floor, both urethral and intravesical pressures will return to their previous voiding state (see Fig. 3.5g).

At the end of micturition the intravesical pressure gradually falls as urinary flow diminishes (see Fig. 3.5h). The pelvic floor and intrinsic striated muscle are contracted and flow is interrupted in mid-urethra; the few drops of urine left in the proximal urethra are milked back into the bladder by the intrinsic mechanisms discussed above which contribute to the hermetic closure of the urethra and bladder neck competence. Simultaneously, the subconscious inhibition of the sacral micturition centre is reapplied as the filling phase of the cycle recommences.

Mechanism of stress continence

The above discussion of the normal micturition cycle relates to the events occurring in a patient essentially at rest, and assumes that intravesical pressure is unaffected by extravesical influences. Acute intra-abdominal pressure rises due to coughing, or more sustained pressure variations due to straining or movement, would easily exceed the normal resting maximum urethral closure pressure and result in incontinence unless additional influences were brought to bear on the mechanism of continence.

The factors which maintain the positive urethral pressure at rest (i.e. which ensure that the urethral pressure exceeds the bladder pressure) have been considered above. This positive closure pressure is also maintained in symptom-free women in the face of intra-abdominal pressure rises (see Fig. 3.5i) by at least two mechanisms.

Firstly there is a passive or direct mechanical transmission of the intra-abdominal increase to the proximal urethra. This effect is dependent upon the normal spatial relationships between the bladder and urethra, and on their fixation in a retropubic position by the posterior pubourethral ligaments, and the muscular and fascial attachments of the anterior vaginal wall (DeLancey 1990). The extent of this transmission of intra-abdominal pressure to the urethra may be quantified by means of urethral pressure profiles recorded during stress (see Fig. 3.6) (Henriksson et al 1977a; Henriksson et al 1977b; Hilton & Stanton 1983; Hilton 1983). The pressure transmission ratio is defined as the increment in urethral pressure as a percentage of the simultaneously recorded increment in intra-abdominal pressure. This parameter may be recorded at several points along the urethra, and a pressure transmission profile can be constructed which details the transmission of intra-abdominal pressure rises from bladder neck to external urethral meatus (Hilton 1990; Hilton & Stanton 1983). Using this technique, it has been shown that in normal women transmission of intra-abdominal pressure rises is effective throughout the proximal three quarters of the urethral length, i.e. throughout that portion of the urethra lying above the urogenital diaphragm (see Fig. 3.6) (Hilton 1983).

Secondly, there may be an active or neuromuscular effect on transmission which may be important in stress continence. It may also be shown by simultaneous bladder and urethral pressure measurements that in a region around the third quarter of the functional urethral length, pressure transmission ratios often exceed 100% (see Fig. 3.6). It has been suggested that the high transmission ratios may reflect a reflex contraction of the pelvic floor in response to stress, augmenting urethral closure. The finding of fast-twitch muscle fibres within the pubococcygeus muscle which might be recruited under such circumstances is obviously compatible with this suggestion (Gosling et al 1981; Gosling & Dixon 1979; Koelbl et al 1989). Certainly, the observed pressure changes do fit closely with the current concepts of the anatomy of the region, and an active neuromuscular element in the maintenance of normal stress continence is accepted by many authors. Rud, however, has demonstrated that this accentuated pressure transmission is maintained following curarization, thus throwing doubt on its being a striated muscle effect (Rud 1981). Alternatively, this may be an entirely passive effect, perhaps due to kinking of the urethra as the intra-abdominal pressure rises, as a result of the relative mobility of its proximal part, and fixation of its lower part, below the level of the so-called 'knee of the urethra' (Westby et al 1982) where it enters the perineal membrane (DeLancey 1986).

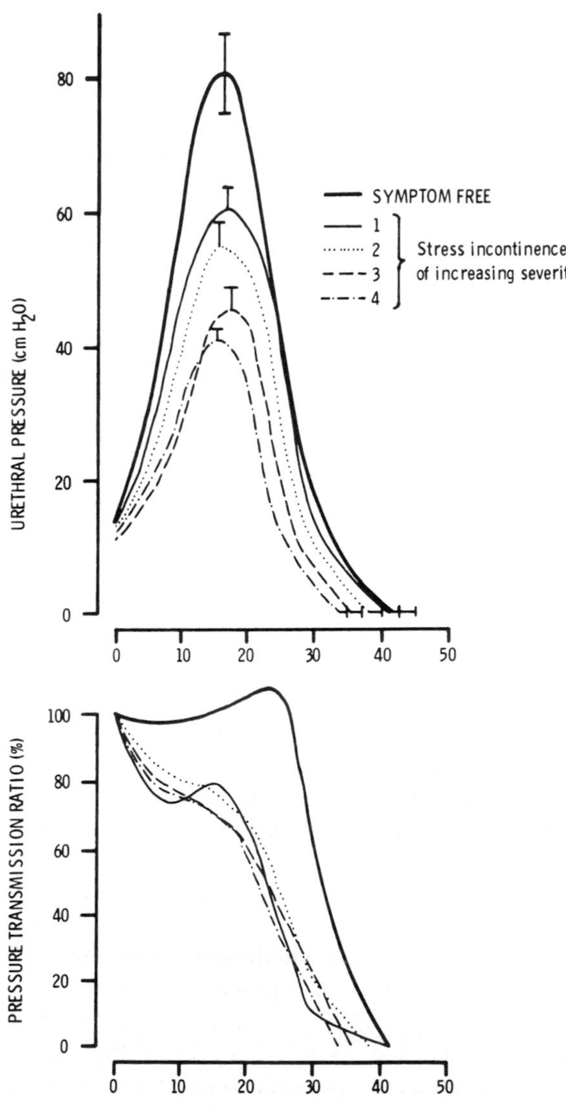

Fig. 3.6 (top) Average resting urethral pressure profiles and (bottom) pressure transmission profiles in a group of symptom-free women and four groups with stress incontinence of varying severity. From Hilton & Stanton (1983), with permission.

PATHOPHYSIOLOGY OF URINARY INCONTINENCE

General considerations

The pathophysiology of several causes of incontinence is considered in greater detail in this volume in chapters relating to individual conditions. Here, general comments are made in so far as the pathophysiology relates to abnormalities of the micturition cycle as described above.

Assuming an intact lower urinary tract, urine flow occurs only when the intravesical pressure exceeds the maximum urethral pressure, or when the maximum urethral closure pressure becomes zero or negative. In general terms this may occur as a result of:

1 A fall in urethral pressure associated with an increase in intravesical pressure. This is seen in normal voiding or in many cases of detrusor instability, primarily those of idiopathic or psychosomatic origin, or those resulting from neurological lesions above the level of the pontine micturition centre. (See Chapter 20.)
2 An increase in intravesical pressure associated with an increase in urethral pressure, the latter being insufficient to maintain a positive closure pressure. This is seen in detrusor instability with associated detrusor sphincter dyssynergia,

resulting from neurological lesions above the sacral but below the pontine micturition centre. (See Chapters 21 and 39.)

3 An abnormally steep rise in detrusor pressure during bladder filling. This situation is considered by some workers to be analogous to detrusor instability, but is perhaps better considered as impaired bladder compliance. This may be seen in chronic inflammatory conditions such as tuberculosis or interstitial cystitis and also following pelvic irradiation. A similar situation also accounts for the incontinence often seen in chronic urinary retention, where the bladder pressure rises acutely at the end of filling. (See Chapters 21 and 22.)

4 A loss of urethral pressure alone, without any coincident change in intravesical pressure, as in urethral instability. (See Chapters 2, 19 and 39.)

5 Where on stress the intravesical pressure rises to a greater extent than the intraurethral pressure as in stress incontinence. This effect may arise from inherent weakness of the urethra itself (intrinsic sphincter incompetence), or more commonly from impairment of urethral support (genuine stress incontinence). (See Chapter 19.) There is increasing evidence that this defect may result, in part at least, from a degree of denervation of the pelvic floor, as a normal part of ageing and as a consequence of childbirth (Anderson 1984; Deindl et al 1993; Deindl et al 1994; Smith et al 1989a; Smith et al 1989b; Snooks et al 1985). Alterations in the biochemistry or mechanical properties of pelvic connective tissues are also known to occur progressively with increasing age; the endocrine effects of pregnancy may also accelerate this process (Sayer et al 1990; Landon et al 1989; Versi et al 1988).

REFERENCES

Abrams P, Blaivas J, Stanton S, Andersen J 1990 The standardisation of terminology of lower urinary tract function. British Journal of Obstetrics and Gynaecology 97: suppl. 6

Anderson R 1984 A neurogenic element to urinary genuine stress incontinence. British Journal of Obstetrics and Gynaecology 91: 41–46

Asmussen M, Ulmsten U 1976 Simultaneous urethrocystometry by a new technique. Scandinavian Journal of Urology and Nephrology 10: 7–11

Barnes A 1940 The method for evaluating the stress of urinary incontinence. American Journal of Obstetrics and Gynecology 40: 381–390

Bradley W, Timm T, Scott F 1974 Innervation of the detrusor muscle and urethra. Urological Clinics of North America 1: 3–27

Deindl F, Vodusek D, Hesse U, Schussler B 1993 Activity patterns of pubococcygeal muscles in nulliparous continent women. British Journal of Urology 72: 46–51

Deindl F, Vodusek D, Hesse U, Schussler B 1994 Pelvic floor activity patterns: comparison of nulliparous continent and parous urinary stress incontinent women. A kinesiological EMG study. British Journal of Urology 73: 413–417

DeLancey J 1986 Correlative study of paraurethral anatomy. Obstetrics and Gynecology 68: 91–97

DeLancey J 1990 Anatomy of the urethral sphincters and supports. In: Drife J O, Hilton P, Stanton S L (eds) Micturition. Springer-Verlag, London, pp. 3–16

Denny-Brown D, Robertson, E 1933 On the physiology of micturition. Brain 56: 149–190

Enhorning G 1961 Simultaneous recording of the intravesical and intraurethral pressure. Acta Chirurgica Scandinavica suppl. 276: 1–68

Gosling J, Dixon J 1979 Light and electron microscopic observations on the human external urethral sphincter. Journal of Anatomy 129: 216

Gosling J, Dixon J, Critchley H, Thompson S 1981 A comparative study of human external sphincter and periurethral levator ani muscle. British Journal of Urology 53: 35–41

Gosling J, Dixon J, Humpherson J 1983 Functional Anatomy of the Urinary Tract. Churchill Livingstone, Edinburgh pp. 51–52

Henriksson L, Ulmsten U, Andersson K 1977a The effects of changes in posture on the urethral closure pressure in healthy women. Scandinavian Journal of Urology and Nephrology 11: 201–206

Henriksson L, Ulmsten U, Andersson K 1977b The effects of changes in posture on the urethral closure pressure in stress incontinent women. Scandinavian Journal of Urology and Nephrolgy 11: 207–210

Hilton P 1983 Urethral pressure measurement on stress: a comparison of profiles on coughing and straining. Neurourology and Urodynamics 2: 55–62

Hilton P 1986 The mechanism of continence. In: Stanton S L, Tanagho E A (eds) Surgery for Female Incontinence. Springer-Verlag, Berlin pp. 1–21

Hilton P 1990 Urethral pressure profilometry in the female. In: George N, O'Reilly P, Weiss A (eds) Diagnostic Techniques in Urology. W B Saunders, Pennsylvania pp. 309–335

Hilton P, Stanton S 1983 Urethral pressure by microtransducer: the results in symptom-free women and in those with genuine stress incontinence. British Journal of Obstetrics and Gynaecology 90: 919–933

Huisman A 1983 Aspects of the anatomy of the female urethra with special relation to urinary continence. In: Ulmsten U (ed.) Contributions to Gynaecology and Obstetrics: Female stress incontinence, Vol. 10. Karger, Basel pp. 1–31

Hutch J 1965 A new theory of the anatomy of the internal urethral sphincter and physiology of micturition. Investigative Urology 3: 36–58

Karlson S 1953 Experimental studies on the functioning of the female urinary bladder and urethra. Acta Obstetrica et Gynaecologica Scandinavica 32: 285–307

Koelbl H, Strassegger H, Riss P, Gruber H 1989 Morphologic and functional aspects of pelvic floor muscles in patients with pelvic relaxation and genuine stress incontinence. Obstetrics and Gynecology 74: 789–795

Landon C, Smith A, Crofts C, Trowbridge E 1989 Biomechanical properties of connective tissue in women with stress incontinence of urine. Neurourology and Urodynamics 8: 369–370

Lapides J 1958 Structure and function of the internal vesical sphincter. Journal of Urology 80: 341–353

Rud T 1981 The striated pelvic floor muscles and their importance in maintaining urinary continence. In: Zinner N, Sterling A (eds) Female Incontinence. Liss, New York, pp. 105–112

Rud T, Andersson K-E, Asmussen M, Hunting A, Ulmsten U 1980 Factors maintaining the intraurethral pressure in women. Investigative Urology 17: 343–347

Sayer T, Hosker G, Dixon J, Warrell D 1990 Stress incontinence – a dual etiology. International Urogynecology Journal 1: 178–179

Smith A, Hosker G, Warrell D 1989a The role of partial denervation of the pelvic floor in the aetiology of genitourinary prolapse and stress incontinence of urine. A neurophysiological study. British Journal of Obstetrics and Gynaecology 96: 24–28

Smith A, Hosker G, Warrell D 1989b The role of pudendal nerve damage in the aetiology of genuine stress incontinence in women. British Journal of Obstetrics and Gynaecology 96: 29–32

Snooks S, Badenoch D, Tiptaft R, Swash M 1985 Perineal nerve damage in genuine stress urinary incontinence. British Journal of Urology 57: 422–426

Tanagho E, Miller E 1970 Initiation of voiding. British Journal of Urology 42: 175–183

Tanagho E, Myers F, Smith D 1969a Urethral resistance, its components and implication, I – smooth muscle components. Investigative Urology 7: 136–149

Tanagho E, Myers F, Smith D 1969b Urethral resistance, its components and implication. I – striated muscle components. Investigative Urology 7: 195–205

Torrens M 1976 Urethral sphincter response to stimulation of the sacral nerves in the human female. Urology International 33: 22–26

Versi E 1991 The significance of an open bladder neck in women. British Journal of Urology 68: 42–43

Versi E, Cardozo L, Brincat M, Cooper D, Montgomery J, Studd J 1988 Correlation between urethral physiology and skin collagen in postmenopausal women. British Journal of Obstetrics and Gynaecology 95: 147–152

Versi E, Cardozo L, Studd J 1986 The urinary sphincter in the maintenance of female continence. British Medical Journal 292: 166–167

Versi E, Cardozo L, Studd J 1990 Distal urethral compensatory mechanisms in women with an incompetent bladder neck who remain continent. Neurourology and Urodynamics 9: 579–590

Westby M, Asmussen M, Ulmsten U 1982 Location of maximum intraurethral pressure related to urogenital diaphragm in the female subject as studied by simultaneous urethrocystometry and voiding urethrocystography. American Journal of Obstetrics and Gynecology 144: 408–412

Zinner N, Ritter R, Sterling A 1976 The mechanism of micturition. In: Williams D I, Chisholm G D (eds) Scientific Foundations of Urology. Heinemann, London, pp. 39–51

SECTION 1
CHAPTER

4

Theory of pharmacology

THOMAS B BOLTON AND KATE E CREED

INTRODUCTION

The transport of urine from its site of formation in the kidney to its eventual voiding is largely controlled by the activity of smooth muscle cells located in the walls of the urinary tract. Waves of contraction pass down the ureters from the pelvices of the kidney to expel the urine into the bladder. Here it is accommodated by an increase in volume which occurs with little increase in intravesical pressure. At some socially convenient time contraction of the detrusor muscle (associated with relaxation of the urethra) causes urine to pass along the urethra to the exterior. The activity of the smooth muscle during storage of urine in the bladder, and during micturition, is controlled by autonomic nerves acting upon it and their effects are modified by hormonal influences.

SMOOTH MUSCLE PROPERTIES

Passive and active electrical properties

The smooth muscle cells of the lower urinary tract are small, spindle-shaped cells which are arranged into bundles. The gross arrangement is described in Chapter 1. Like smooth muscles in the gastrointestinal tract they have inherent myogenic activity and small spontaneous contractions occur. Excitation spreads through the tissue owing to low resistance electrical pathways between muscle cells. In all species studied, including guinea-pig, rabbit, dog, wallaby, monkey and human, spike-like action potentials can be recorded with micro-electrodes from strips of detrusor muscle. They occur at intervals of 6–30 per min, superimposed on a resting membrane potential of −30 to −42 mV and normally have an overshoot of up to 20 mV. The action potentials arise abruptly from the resting potential but the recovery phase shows species variation. In the guinea-pig the membrane potential returns immediately to the resting level (Creed 1971a) but in the rabbit the spike is followed by an after hyperpolarization which may have a second depolarization superimposed (Creed et al 1983) which is similar to human cells. The pattern of activity in the bladder base or trigone and urethra of rabbits is similar to that of the detrusor muscle (Callahan & Creed, 1985). In pig urethral muscle cells, outward potassium currents were detected, but no appreciable calcium inward current (Brading et al 1996). In the guinea-pig urethra, the mean resting membrane potential (–42 mV) is slightly greater than for detrusor cells (–36 mV) and bursts of 20 to 30 spikes which last 7 to 10 s occur at intervals of up to 6 min (Callahan & Creed 1981). These bursts may be superimposed on a progressive depolarization or plateau which develops so that the discharge is not unlike that occurring in the ureter. In this muscle an initial spike may be followed by one or more smaller spikes carried on a plateau which lasts about a second before repolarization occurs (Kuriyama et al 1967).

As in other smooth muscle cells, the upstroke of the action potential is not affected by tetrodotoxin but is reduced by Mn^{2+}, low extracellular Ca^{2+}, or Ca antagonists such as nifedipine and verapamil. The spike is therefore due to Ca^{2+} entry across the membrane (Creed 1971b). This has been confirmed on individual smooth muscle cells of the bladder with the patch clamp technique (Klöckner & Isenberg 1985b). Calcium channels in guinea-pig urinary bladder have a conductance of 5–8 pS in physiological calcium concentrations; calcium current is activated by depolarization but within 50 ms substantially inactivates (Nakayama & Brading 1993b; Klöckner 1996). A prolonged open state of the calcium channel can be evoked by polarization to positive potentials (Nakayama & Brading 1993a). Repolarization is due to K^+ outward current, part of which may be activated by calcium which enters during the upstrokes of the spikes and which may also be released within the cell (Klöckner & Isenberg 1985a). Potassium channels sensitive to ATP within the cell and modulated by muscarinic receptor activation are also present (Bonev & Nelson 1993). The ureter has a well-developed sodium–calcium exchange process (Aickin et al 1984) and this may be of significance in the plateau phase of the action potential which is sodium sensitive (Shuba 1981). The plateau in guinea-pig ureter has been ascribed to slowly inactivating inward Ca^{2+}-current, Na^+-dependent late inward current, and a weakly developed delayed rectifier K-current; repetitive spiking on the plateau has been ascribed to rapid reactivations of inward calcium current which are followed by repolarizations due to Ca^{2+}-activated K-current (Imaizumi et al 1989).

The smooth muscle cells of all parts are not electrically independent but form an electrical syncytium. This allows the propagation of spikes for at least limited distances in the bladder and along the whole of the length of the ureter. The spread of spikes and contraction in the detrusor (at a rate of 3–6 cm/s in the guinea-pig) produces a small phasic contraction of the region involved. The region is presumably rather limited in normal bladders (Bramich & Brading 1996) so that significant rises in intravesical pressure do not occur; in the hyperactive bladder more extensive spread may occur with larger rises in intravesical pressure, the urge to void, and incontinence.

The electrical syncytium arises because the interiors of adjacent smooth muscle cells are linked by regions (possibly nexuses) of low electrical resistance. These allow current to pass between adjacent smooth muscle cells and give rise to the cable properties of strips of detrusor smooth muscle (Creed 1971a; Creed et al 1983). Weak hyperpolarizing currents applied at one end of a muscle strip can be recorded by an intracellular electrode several millimetres away. The length constant (the distance for decay to 37% of the evoked potential) for detrusor muscle of guinea-pig is 1.7 mm and of rabbit is 2.15 mm and lies within the range found for other smooth muscles (Creed 1979b).

Contraction is triggered by the action potential and the resting tone of the muscle reflects the frequency of spontaneous action potentials. Unlike the gastrointestinal tract, the cells of the detrusor muscle seem to be relatively insensitive to stretch but the frequency of action potentials can be modified by drugs, neurotransmitters, and hormones which may either increase or decrease the frequency of action potential discharge and so alter tone or contractile activity.

Contraction and relaxation

Contraction of smooth muscle cells is controlled by the level of free ionized calcium concentration in the cells which affects the tension developed by the contractile proteins of smooth muscle. However, other second messengers and mechanisms as yet unknown may well modify this primary control. In urinary smooth muscle, the spike or action potential seems to be the main determinant of tension. The entry of calcium during the upstroke of the spike has three important effects on tension. Firstly, the calcium entering the cell raises $[Ca^{2+}]_i$. Secondly, it is very likely that calcium entry triggers further calcium release within the cell (calcium-induced calcium release, Ganitkevich & Isenberg 1992) i.e. there is an amplification process which allows $[Ca^{2+}]_i$ to rise more than would be expected simply from the amount of calcium entering during the upstroke of the action potential. Conclusive evidence for such a process is lacking but the strong calcium buffering properties of the interior of the cell probably make such a process essential. Finally the entering calcium, or a portion of it, may be sequestered in store from whence it can be released by a subsequent action potential. This loading of the calcium store may be important for longer-term changes in tension since it involves charging a reservoir from which calcium is potentially able to be released at a later stage.

Tension in response to an action potential is phasic, i.e. it increases and soon declines. In general, initial tension generated by a constant excitatory influence applied for several minutes to detrusor smooth muscle is not well sustained, i.e. the tonic tension mechanisms of the detrusor muscle are not well-developed although a small amount of tonic tension can be maintained (Brading 1987).

It is clear from the above that contraction of urinary smooth muscle is largely brought about by the entry of calcium into the cell through voltage-dependent calcium channels responsible for the upstroke of the spike, possibly aided by release of calcium from stores within the cell. These two processes are modulated by excitatory influences which include neurotransmitter released from nerves, local and circulating hormones, and drugs. Most excitatory neurotransmitters and hormones increase the frequency of spike discharge (and so increase tension) by depolarizing the cells. This is generally brought about by an increase in the permeability of the cell membrane to ions; sodium, potassium, and calcium are almost certainly involved; increases in chloride permeability and decreases in potassium permeability are also possible. ATP applied to single bladder cells opens channels in the membrane which are permeable to Ca^{2+}, Na^{+} and K^{+}ions. The resulting inward current is responsible for the depolarization normally observed (Schneider et al 1991). The links between receptor activation and channel opening, which causes increase in permeability, depolarization and spiking, have been little investigated in bladder but are probably similar to those in other smooth muscles. Some receptors for stimulant substances may be an integral part of the ion channel they open: others may be linked to channel opening by second messengers or G-proteins. The mechanisms involved are probably of several types and include modulation of voltage-dependent calcium channel function either directly by receptor activation (Yoshino et al 1996), or indirectly via complex effects on other voltage-dependent membrane conductances (see Shuba 1981). Release of calcium from stores may also follow receptor activation (Mostwin 1985). In this case the second messenger, D-myoinositol 1,4,5 trisphosphate, may be involved (Iacovou et al 1990; Creed et al 1991); it is formed by the action of a triphosphoinositide phosphodiesterase, phospholipase C, on an integral membrane phospholipid, phosphatidylinositol 4,5 bisphosphate. The release of calcium from stores by activation of muscarinic receptors reduces calcium-activated potassium current which normally contributes to repolarization of the membrane (Yoshino et al 1996).

Activation of receptors for acetylcholine (muscarinic receptors), adenosine triphosphate (ATP), substance P, prostaglandins, histamine and serotonin (5HT) all cause contraction. Several of these stimulants have been shown to accelerate spike discharge and depolarize detrusor smooth muscle (Creed 1971b; Callahan & Creed 1986; Yoshino et al 1996). Both acetylcholine and ATP elevate intracellular Ca concentrations (Oike et al 1998; Wu et al 1995). In the urethra, activation of α-adrenoreceptors by noradrenaline has similar effects but in detrusor an inhibitory effect via β-adrenoreceptors predominates. Prostaglandins at concentrations that are too low to produce contraction or changes in membrane potential enhance responses of the bladder of guinea-pigs to acetylcholine or to nerve stimulation, possibly by facilitating Ca movements. Caffeine, which releases Ca^{2+} from intracellular stores in smooth muscles of the gut, can produce a hyperactive bladder with urge incontinence, presumably by facilitating calcium release within the cell.

The mechanisms involved in relaxation of smooth muscle by various agents, including non-adrenergic non-cholinergic (NANC) inhibitory transmitter(s) are not well established. β-receptor activation, by accelerating calcium storage or extrusion from the cell, may reduce tension, although some inhibitory effect seems to be via a reduction in action potential frequency (Creed 1971b). Sodium nitroprusside and nitroso-containing compounds increase cyclic guanosine monophosphate (cGMP) levels in other smooth muscle and accelerate calcium pumping from the cell; atrial natriuretic peptide also increases cGMP levels but evidence for such actions in urinary muscle is lacking.

Recently there has been considerable interest in a class of drugs, 'K^{+}-channel openers', of which cromakalim can be regarded as the best known example. They inhibit action potential discharge and so cause existing tension to fall; the tension increment to excitatory influences impinging on the muscle is also attenuated. The effect in the bladder is to reduce contractile activity (Malmgren et al 1990; Creed & Malmgren

1993) and to increase membrane permeability to K^+ which causes hyperpolarization (Foster et al 1989). Interest in cromakalim and other potassium-channel openers stems from their possible usefulness in the treatment of bladder instability.

INNERVATION OF THE MUSCLES OF THE LOWER URINARY TRACT

Retention and elimination of urine is controlled by fibres in the hypogastric (sympathetic) and pelvic (parasympathetic) nerves to smooth muscle (Langley & Anderson 1895) and the pudendal (somatic) nerve to urethral striated muscle. The hypogastric nerves extend from the ventral mesenteric ganglia which in turn receive fibres from the sympathetic chains at lumbar roots 2–5. The parasympathetic nerves leave the spinal cord, mostly in sacral roots 1, 2 and 3, and partially combine to form the pelvic nerves which lie beside the urogenital branch of the internal pudendal arteries on each side of the rectum. The hypogastric and pelvic nerves come together to form the pelvic plexus, a loose network of nerve fibres and ganglion cells on the lateral aspects of the bladder base. From there nerve fibres supply the ureters, bladder and urethra as well as the rectum and genital organs. The pelvic plexus extends as the vesical plexus onto the surface of the bladder, and ganglion cells, probably cholinergic, have been reported within the walls of several species including human (Dixon et al 1983). The pudendal nerves also exit from the spinal cord in sacral roots 1–4. They then pass caudoventrally on the medial side of the superficial gluteal muscle and emerge at the distal end of the urethra in females and at the crura of the penis in males. Several small branches run along the ventral surface of the striated muscle of the membranous urethra from its caudal end and enter the muscle at intervals.

The pelvic plexus was believed to be a simple parasympathetic relay but, from work on the effects of nerve stimulation in animals, it became clear that modification of inputs and interaction between pelvic and hypogastric nerves occurs there (de Groat & Saum 1976). This is supported by anatomical studies, which have revealed many adrenergic endings on the ganglion cells (Hamberger & Norberg 1965), and by intracellular recording from ganglion cells in the pelvic plexus of guinea-pigs and rabbits, which has revealed a number of different patterns of response to stimulation of the nerves (McLachlan 1977). Some cells are selectively excited by either hypogastric or pelvic nerve inputs and in other cells stimulation of the hypogastric nerve depresses excitatory post-synaptic potentials (epsp) evoked by pelvic nerve stimulation. A similar inhibition can be produced by administration of noradrenaline (Akasu et al 1988). In the cat vesical plexus both excitatory (nicotinic) and inhibitory (muscarinic) cholinergic psp have been recorded in response to focal stimulation (Gallagher et al 1982). Considerable facilitation of the epsp produced in response to repetitive pelvic nerve stimulation is seen with high but not low frequencies suggesting that the ganglia act as 'high pass filters' (de Groat & Booth 1980).

Such results suggest that, at least in these species, parasympathetic cholinergic pathways provide the major excitatory input to the ganglia via nicotinic receptors. These can be modified by inhibitory adrenergic inputs acting mainly on α-adrenoreceptors. Immunohistochemical examination of ganglia has revealed that they contain several peptides, especially dynorphin, VIP and NPY (Morris & Gibbins 1987). These sometimes occur within the same cell but it is not known if they co-exist with noradrenaline or acetylcholine (Keast 1992). A complete understanding of the system must await more information on the patterns of innervation, time courses of responses and the nature of the transmitters within the plexus.

Parasympathetic nervous system and bladder contraction

Stimulation of the pelvic nerves produces contraction of the detrusor muscle, resulting in an increase in intravesical pressure. In most animal species studied, the response is only partially blocked by the muscarinic cholinergic antagonist, atropine, suggesting that all the nerves are not cholinergic. The bladders of humans and monkeys contain a lower proportion of atropine resistant fibres (Cowan & Daniel 1983) and the pelvic nerve to healthy human bladders is probably exclusively cholinergic (Sibley 1984). There is no evidence from electrical or mechanical recording for inhibitory innervation to the detrusor muscle.

Records taken with the double sucrose gap have confirmed that excitatory responses of the bladder occur in two stages (Creed et al 1983; Callahan & Creed 1986). Stimulation of nerves in detrusor strips from guinea-pig and rabbit reveal an initial excitatory junction potential (ejp) with a superimposed spike followed by a late depolarization. All the responses are abolished by tetrodotoxin, which blocks nerve, but not smooth muscle, action potentials and only the late depolarization is blocked by atropine or enhanced by neostigmine. Acetylcholine, which increases the rate of spontaneous action potentials with little change in membrane potential, produces a sustained increase in tone. Non-adrenergic non-cholinergic (NANC) innervation is responsible for the large ejp and initial contraction. In tissues from human and monkey bladders, the initial ejp is relatively much smaller and the contraction tends to be slower.

Over the years there have been many attempts to identify the NANC transmitter of the bladder. Most of the evidence now points to ATP released by purinergic nerves and acting on P_{2x} receptors (Burnstock et al 1972). ATP produces a rapid contraction, marked depolarization and increase in action potential frequency. The ATP analogue, α-β methylene ATP, which desensitizes P_{2x} receptors, abolished the nerve-evoked ejp recorded from rabbit, guinea-pig and pig with the double sucrose gap (Fujii 1988; Creed et al 1991). This has recently been confirmed with micro-electrode recording (Bramich & Brading 1996). Suramin, a drug used against trypanosomes, has been reported to block, selectively, purinergic receptors including those on guinea-pig bladder (Hoyle et al 1990). However, the drug does not have an inhibitory effect on all species and tends to increase spontaneous activity (Creed et al 1994).

In other tissues innervated by the autonomic nervous system, including the myenteric plexus and the smooth muscle of the small intestine, there is evidence that peptides may act as neurotransmitters. In the lower urinary tract, nerves containing peptides including substance P, calcitonin gene-related peptide and neuropeptide Y have been identified (Gibbins et al 1987). Substance P contracts the detrusor muscle in all species studied and accelerates spontaneous action potentials recorded from the smooth muscle cells; vasoactive intestinal peptide produces relaxation and decreased action potential frequency in some species only; other peptides such as somatostatin, neurotensin and leu-enkephalin produce small, inconsistent responses (Sjögren et al 1982; Sjögren et al 1985; Callahan & Creed 1986). Responses to peptides are slow and it is unlikely that they are excitatory neurotransmitters but some may act as modulators of transmitter release or action as reported for the intestine. Conclusive evidence must await the development of specific inhibitors to these peptides.

Sympathetic nervous system and urine retention

The role of the sympathetic nervous system in micturition has been debated for many years. However, there is some evidence that it facilitates storage of urine by constricting the proximal urethra and inhibiting the tone of the detrusor muscle (Elliott 1907; Satchell & Vaughan 1988). The hypogastric nerves which end on the ganglion cells or on the smooth muscle are considered to be predominantly adrenergic, though in some species cholinergic and other nerve types have been identified (Taira 1972). Recent electrophysiological studies have confirmed that the proximal urethra of the rabbit receives excitatory innervation involving the three neurotransmitters, adenosine triphosphate (ATP), acetylcholine and noradrenaline (Creed et al 1997).

Pharmacological experiments indicate that the action of the adrenergic transmitter, noradrenaline, on the lower urinary tract can be separated into contraction through α-adrenoreceptors and inhibition through β-receptors. The predominance of α-receptors in the bladder base and urethra and β-receptors on the detrusor muscle would support the suggestion that sympathetic activity promotes urine retention. However, there are few adrenergic nerves to the smooth muscle cells of the bladder of several species, including human (Dixon et al 1983) and close arterial injection of noradrenaline or stimulation of hypogastric nerves has little effect on vesicular pressure. Although noradrenaline reduces the frequency of spontaneous action potentials recorded with micro-electrodes from detrusor muscle of guinea-pig, this only occurs with high concentrations (5×10^{-5} M) (Creed 1971b). On the other hand, the proximal urethra receives a dense adrenergic innervation and stimulation of the hypogastric nerves produces an increase in the urethral pressure which is abolished by the α-adrenergic antagonist, phentolamine (Creed 1979a). Close arterial injection of noradrenaline or the more specific α-adrenergic agonist, phenylephrine, also produces a large increase in urethral pressure in many species and increases the dynamic functional length of the urethra in normal and incontinent women (Schreiter et al 1976). Phenylephrine or noradrenaline triggers action potentials in the guinea-pig and rabbit urethra (Callahan & Creed 1981; Creed et al 1997).

In addition to excitatory fibres, the proximal urethra, unlike the bladder, receives inhibitory innervation. This is often only observed when the smooth muscle tone is raised either spontaneously or by drugs. A rapid transient relaxation can be recorded in many species in response to stimulation of nerves in the wall (Dokita et al 1991; Hashimoto et al 1993). This is blocked by nitric oxide synthetase inhibitors, such as L-NAME, suggesting that it results from the action of nitric oxide, or a substance which easily gives rise to it. A more prolonged relaxation may also occur which is due to the β-action of noradrenaline. It is unknown if the nitrergic nerves are activated by hypogastric or pelvic nerve inputs, and the role of these nerves in micturition has not been determined.

Oestrogens are used in the treatment of urinary incontinence in postmenopausal patients and in spayed bitches (Salmon et al 1941; Osborne et al 1972). They have been shown to act by increasing closure of the urethra by preventing or reversing atrophy of the mucous membrane but there is now evidence that they also modify the spontaneous activity of the smooth muscle cells and increase their sensitivity to chemical agents including α- adrenergic agonists. In the rat ureter there is facilitation by oestrogen treatment of responses to adrenaline (Raz et al 1972) and in anaesthetized dogs oestrogens produce a marked increase in sensitivity of the urethra to phenylephrine (Creed 1983). A similar shift is seen in contractile responses of isolated urethral strips of dogs and wallabies though no significant change occurs in guinea-pig and rabbit strips (Callahan & Creed 1985). In women the increase in dynamic functional length of the urethra produced by phenylephrine was enhanced after 10 days' treatment with oestradiol (Schreiter et al 1976).

The premenstrual phase in women may be accompanied by incontinence. This also occurs in pregnancy when the progesterone level is elevated. Progesterone treatment has no significant effect on contraction of the urethra of dogs or rabbits to phenylephrine (Hodgson et al 1978; Creed 1983). However, in the rat ureter (Raz et al 1972) and in the uterus of several species, progesterone facilitates β-adrenergic responses and may act in this way in the urethra.

The membranous urethra and external sphincter

The distal two thirds of the urethra (the membranous urethra) contains an inner layer of smooth muscle, running predominantly longitudinally, and an outer sheath of circularly orientated striated muscle (Huisman 1983). Reports in the literature concerning a 'urogenital diaphragm' external to the urethra originally described by Henle (1873) are not supported anatomically (Oelrich 1980; Kaye et al 1997) and the striated muscle sheath is now believed to act as the external urethral sphincter under voluntary control (Thind 1995). The role of the smooth muscle in continence is unclear but it may act to bunch up the soft urethral lining so that the lumen is closed.

The longitudinal smooth muscle receives innervation in the pelvic nerve which sends out branches proximal to the pelvic plexus. These pass through the striated muscle to the inner layers. There appear to be no branches from the genital nerve bundles which run caudally from the pelvic plexus on the outer surface of the urethra. A rich cholinergic network and less dense adrenergic network has been demonstrated among the smooth muscle cells (Gosling et al 1977; Klück 1980). The predominant response to nerve stimulation is contraction via muscarinic cholinergic receptors (Creed, unpublished). A small adrenergic contraction may also be present and some nitrergic relaxation can be seen when the tone is raised.

Stimulation of the intramural nerves in the striated muscle of dog or guinea-pig produces rapid action potentials and contractions characteristic of striated muscles (Creed et al 1998). These are completely blocked by curare which acts on nicotinic cholinergic receptors. It has been suggested that the striated muscle receives innervation in both pelvic and pudendal nerves (Elbadawi & Schenk 1974). However, pelvic nerve stimulation only produces slow urethral contractions which are not affected by curare whereas all responses to pudendal nerve stimulation are abolished by curare (Creed et al 1998).

REFERENCES

Aickin C C, Brading A F, Burdyga T V 1984 Evidence for sodium – calcium exchange in the guinea-pig ureter. Journal of Physiology 347: 411–430

Akasu T, Tsurusaki M, Nishimura T, Tokimasu T 1988 Norepinephrine inhibits calcium action potential through α_2-adrenoceptors in rabbit vesical parasympathetic neurons. Neuroscience Research 6: 186–190

Bonev A D, Nelson M T 1993 Muscarinic inhibition of ATP-sensitive K+ channels by protein kinase C in urinary bladder smooth muscle. American Journal of Physiology 265: C1723–C1728

Brading A F 1987 Physiology of bladder smooth muscle. In: Torrens M, Morrison J (eds) Physiology of the Lower Urinary Tract. Springer-Verlag, Berlin, pp 161–191

Brading A F, Teramoto N, Nakayama S et al 1996 The relationship between the electrophysiological properties of lower urinary tract smooth muscles and their function in vivo. In: Bolton T B, Tomita T (eds) Smooth Muscle Excitation. Academic Press, London, chap. 33 pp 403–415

Bramich N J, Brading A F 1996 Electrical properties of smooth muscle in the guinea pig urinary bladder. Journal of Physiology 492: 185–198

Burnstock G, Dumsday B, Smythe A 1972 Atropine resistant excitation of the urinary bladder: the possibility of transmission via nerves releasing a purine nucleotide. British Journal of Pharmacology 44: 451–461

Callahan S M, Creed K E 1981 Electrical and mechanical activity of the isolated lower urinary tract of the guinea-pig. British Journal of Pharmacology 74: 353–358

Callahan S M, Creed K E 1985 The effects of oestrogens on spontaneous activity and responses to phenylephrine of the mammalian urethra. Journal of Physiology 358: 35–46

Callahan S M, Creed K E 1986 Non-cholinergic neurotransmission and the effects of peptides on the urinary bladder of guinea pigs and rabbits. Journal of Physiology 374: 103–115

Cowan W D, Daniel E E 1983 Human female bladder and its cholinergic contractile function. Canadian Journal of Physiology and Pharmacology 61: 1236–1246

Creed K E 1971a Membrane properties of the smooth muscle membrane of the guinea pig urinary bladder. Pflügers Archives 326: 115–126

Creed K E 1971b Effects of ions and drugs on the smooth muscle cell membrane of the guinea pig urinary bladder. Pflügers Archives 326: 127–141

Creed K E 1979a The role of the hypogastric nerve in bladder and urethral activity of the dog. British Journal of Pharmacology 65: 367–375

Creed K E 1979b Functional diversity of smooth muscle. British Medical Bulletin 35: 243–247

Creed K E 1983 Effect of hormones on urethral sensitivity to phenylephrine in normal and incontinent dogs. Research in Veterinary Science 34: 177–181

Creed K E, Ishikawa S, Ito Y 1983 Electrical and mechanical activity recorded from rabbit urinary bladder in response to nerve stimulation. Journal of Physiology 338: 149–164

Creed K E, Ito Y, Katsuyama H 1991 Neurotransmission in the urinary bladder of rabbits and guinea pigs. American Journal of Physiology 261: C271–C277

Creed K E, Malmgren A 1993 The effect of cromakalim on the electrical properties of and [86Rb+] efflux from normal and hypertrophied rat bladder. Clinical & Experimental Pharmacology and Physiology 20, 215–221

Creed K E, Callahan S M, Ito Y 1994 Excitatory transmission in the mammalian bladder and the effects of suramin. British Journal of Urology 74: 736–743

Creed K E, Oike M, Ito Y 1997 The electrical properties and responses to nerve stimulation of the proximal urethra of the male rabbit. British Journal of Urology 79: 543–553

Creed K E, Van der Werf B A, Kaye K W 1998 Innervation of the striated muscle of the membranous urethra of the male dog. Journal of Urology 159: 1712–1716

de Groat W C, Booth A M 1980 Inhibition and facilitation in parasympathetic ganglia of the urinary bladder. Federation Proceedings 39: 2990–2996

de Groat W C, Saum W R 1976 Synaptic transmission in parasympathetic ganglia in the urinary bladder of the cat. Journal of Physiology 256: 137–158

Dixon J S, Gilpin S-A, Gilpin C J, Gosling J A 1983 Intramural ganglia of the human urinary bladder. British Journal of Urology 55: 195–198

Dokita S, Morgan W R, Wheeler M A, Yoshida M, Latifpour J, Weiss R M 1991 N^G-nitro-L-arginine inhibits non-adrenergic, non-cholinergic relaxation in rabbit urethral smooth muscle. Life Sciences 48: 2429–2436

Elbadawi A, Schenk E A 1974 A new theory of the innervation of bladder musculature. Part 4. Innervation of the vesicourethral junction and external urethral sphincter. Journal of Urology 111: 613–615

Elliott T R 1907 The innervation of the bladder and urethra. Journal of Physiology 35: 367–445

Foster C D, Speakman M J, Fujii K, Brading A F 1989 The effects of cromakalim on the detrusor muscle of human and pig urinary bladder. British Journal of Urology 63: 284–294

Fujii K 1988 Evidence for adenosine triphosphate as an excitatory transmitter in guinea-pig, rabbit and pig urinary bladder. Journal of Physiology 404: 39–52

Gallagher J P, Griffith W H, Shinnick-Gallagher P 1982 Cholinergic transmission in cat parasympathetic ganglia. Journal of Physiology 332: 473–486

Ganitkevich V Ya, Isenberg G 1992 Contribution of Ca^{2+}-induced Ca^{2+} release to the $[Ca^{2+}]_i$ transient in myocytes from guinea-pig urinary bladder. Journal of Physiology 458: 119–137

Gibbins I L, Furness J B, Costa M 1987 Pathway specific patterns of the co-existence of substance P, calcitonin gene related peptide, cholecystokinin and dynorphin in neurons of the dorsal root ganglia of the guinea pig. Cell and Tissue Research 248: 417–437

Gosling J A, Dixon J S, Lendon R G 1977 The autonomic innervation of the human male and female bladder neck and proximal urethra. Journal of Urology 118: 302–305

Hamberger B, Norberg K-A 1965 Studies on some systems of adrenergic synaptic terminals in the abdominal ganglia of the cat. Acta Physiologica Scandinavica 65: 235–242

Hashimoto S, Kigoshi S, Muramatsu I 1993 Nitric oxide-dependent neurogenic relaxation in isolated dog urethra. European Journal of Pharmacology 231: 209–214

Henle J 1873 Handbuch der systematischen Anatomie des Menchen. Braunschweig: F. Vieweg and sons

Hodgson B J, Dumas S, Bolling D R, Heesch C M 1978 Effect of oestrogen on sensitivity of rabbit bladder and urethra to phenylephrine. Investigative Urology 16: 67–69

Hoyle C H V, Knight G E, Burnstock G 1990 Suramin antagonizes responses to P2-purinoceptor agonists and purinergic nerve stimulation in the guinea pig urinary bladder and taenia coli. British Journal of Pharmacology 99: 617–621

Huisman A B 1983 Aspects of the anatomy of the female urethra with special relation to urinary continence. Contributions to Gynecology and Obstetrics 10: 1–3

Iacovou J W, Hill S J, Birmingham A T 1990 Agonist-induced contraction and accumulation of inositol phosphates in the guinea-pig detrusor: evidence that muscarinic and purinergic receptors raise intracellular calcium by different mechanisms. Journal of Urology 144: 775–779

Imaizumi Y, Muraki K, Watanabe M 1989 Ionic currents in single smooth muscle cells from the ureter of the guinea-pig. Journal of Physiology 411: 131–159

Kaye K W, Milne N, Creed K E, Van der Werf B A 1997 The 'urogenital diaphragm', external urethral sphincter and radical prostatectomy. Austalian and New Zealand Journal of Surgery 67: 40–44

Keast J R 1992 Connectivity and neurochemistry of pelvic ganglia. Proceedings of the Australian Neurosciences Society 3: 43–44

Klöckner U 1996 Voltage-dependent L-type calcium channels in smooth muscle cells. In: Bolton T B, Tomita T (eds) Smooth Muscle Excitation. Academic Press, London, chap. 1 pp 1–12

Klöckner U, Isenberg G 1985a Action potentials and net membrane currents of isolated smooth muscle cells (urinary bladder of the guinea pig). Pflügers Archives 405: 329–339

Klöckner U, Isenberg G 1985b Calcium currents of cesium loaded isolated smooth muscle cells (urinary bladder of the guinea-pig). Pflügers Archives 405: 340–348

Klück P 1980 The autonomic innervation of the human urinary bladder, bladder neck and urethra: a histochemical study. Anatomical Record 198: 439–447

Kuriyama H, Osa T, Toida N 1967 Membrane properties of the smooth muscle of guinea-pig ureter. Journal of Physiology 191: 225–238

Langley J N, Anderson H K 1895 The innervation of the pelvic and adjoining viscera. Part II: The bladder. Journal of Physiology 19: 71–84

McLachlan E M 1977 Interaction between sympathetic and parasympathetic pathways in the pelvic plexus of the guinea pig. Proceedings of the Australian Physiological and Pharmacological Society 8: 15P

Malmgren A, Andersson K-E, Andersson P O, Fovaeus M, Sjögren C 1990 Effects of cromakalim (BRL 34915) and pinacidil on normal and hypertrophied rat detrusor in vitro. Journal of Urology 143: 828–834

Morris J L, Gibbins I L 1987 Neuronal colocalization of peptides, catecholamines and catecholamine synthesizing enzymes in guinea pig paracervical ganglia. Journal of Neuroscience 7: 3117–3130

Mostwin J L 1985 Receptor operated intracellular calcium stores in the smooth muscle of the guinea pig bladder. Journal of Urology 133: 900–905

Nakayama S, Brading A F 1993a Evidence for multiple open states of the Ca^{2+} channels in smooth muscle cells isolated from the guinea-pig detrusor. Journal of Physiology 471: 87–105

Nakayama S, Brading A F 1993b Inactivation of the voltage-dependent Ca^{2+} channel current in smooth muscle cells isolated from the guinea-pig detrusor. Journal of Physiology 471: 107–127

Oelrich T M 1980 The urethral sphincter muscle in the male. American Journal of Anatomy 158: 229–246

Oike M, Creed K E, Onoue H, Tanaka H, Ito Y 1998 Increase in calcium in smooth muscle cells of the rabbit bladder induced by acetylcholine and ATP. Journal of the Autonomic Nervous System 69: 141–147

Osborne C A, Low D G, Finco D R 1972 Canine and feline urology. Saunders, Philadelphia

Raz S, Zeigler M, Caine M 1972 Hormonal influence on the adrenergic receptors of the ureter. British Journal of Urology 44: 405–410

Salmon U J, Walter R I, Geist S H 1941 The use of oestrogens in the treatment of dysuria and incontinence in post-menopausal women. American Journal of Obstetrics and Gynecology 42: 845–851

Satchell P, Vaughan C 1988 Hypogastric nerve activity to the feline bladder during slow filling. Journal of the Autonomic Nervous System 25: 41–47

Schneider P, Hopp H H, Isenberg G 1991 Ca^{2+} influx through ATP-gated channels increments $[Ca^{2+}]_i$ and inactivates I_{Ca} in myocytes from guinea-pig urinary bladder. Journal of Physiology 440: 479–496

Schreiter F, Fuchs P, Stockamp K 1976 Estrogenic sensitivity of α-receptors in the urethral musculature. Urologica Internationalis 31: 13–19

Shuba M F 1981 Smooth muscle of the ureter: the nature of excitation and the mechanisms of action of catecholamines and histamine. In: Bülbring E, Brading A F, Jones A W, Tomita T (eds) Smooth Muscle, an assessment of current knowledge. Arnold, London, pp 377–384

Sibley G N A 1984 A comparison of spontaneous and nerve-mediated activity in bladder muscle from man, pig, and rabbit. Journal of Physiology 354: 431–443

Sjögren C, Andersson K-E, Husted S 1982 Contractile effects of some polypeptides on the isolated urinary bladder of guinea pig, rabbit and rat. Acta Pharmacologica et Toxicologica 50: 175–184

Sjögren C, Andersson K-E, Mattiasson A 1985 Effects of vasoactive intestinal polypeptide on isolated urethral and urinary bladder smooth muscle from rabbit and man. Journal of Urology 133: 136–140

Taira N 1972 The autonomic pharmacology of the bladder. Annual Review of Pharmacology 12: 197–208

Thind P 1995 The significance of smooth and striated muscles in sphincter function of the urethra in healthy women. Neurourology Urodynamics 14: 585–618

Wu C, Wallis W R J, Fry C H 1995 Purinergic activation induces a transient rise of intracellular Ca^{2+} in isolated human detrusor myocytes. Journal of Physiology 489: 136p.

Yoshino M, Tsutai K, Yabu H 1996 Muscarinic action on smooth muscle membrane of guinea pig urinary bladder. In: Bolton TB, Tomita T (eds) Smooth Muscle Excitation. Academic Press, London, chap. 18 pp 215–225

Epidemiology of micturition disorders

SANDRA R VALAITIS AND THELMA M THOMAS

INTRODUCTION

To estimate the prevalence of micturition disorders, it is necessary to clearly define the specific disorder of interest, and to be able to include all cases in the total population at risk. However, most information about micturition disorders has so far been based on studies of patients presenting to hospital clinics. Some other studies have selected specific groups of the population to study, such as elderly nursing home patients (Ouslander et al 1982), nursing students (Wolin 1969), or a highly motivated group of volunteers suffering from incontinence (Wyman et al 1987). This results in an incomplete picture of the morbidity of these disorders due to incomplete reporting of all cases in the community, and is further complicated by the fact that some patients with urinary complaints do not seek medical advice. For instance, Norton et al (1988) found that 25% of patients referred to a urogynaecology clinic for evaluation had waited more than five years to seek professional help. Thomas et al (1980) found that only one third of women complaining of moderate to severe incontinence were receiving assistance from medical or social services. Roberts et al (1998) found that men were twice as likely to seek treatment as women for urinary incontinence symptoms. Nonetheless, only 29% of men and 13% of women with incontinence had actually sought treatment for such complaints. However, a study by Brocklehurst (1993) found more optimistic observations that 52% of patients suffering from incontinence sought immediate treatment from their local practitioners, and an additional 31% sought advice later. Although this study is encouraging, there are still large numbers of patients who wait to seek treatment for their micturition difficulties, believing that their symptoms may be a normal part of ageing or feeling too embarrassed to talk about the problem.

Prevalence (the proportion of a defined population with the symptom or disorder in question) is the most commonly used measure for chronic conditions. Incidence rates (or the number of new cases over a given period of time) may be more appropriate than prevalence for short-lived symptoms such as frequency and dysuria due to cystitis or 'urethral syndrome'. However, if these attacks are considered part of an ongoing process with intermittent bacteriuria (Smith 1981) then prevalence may, once again, be the more appropriate measure, though difficult to establish without a persisting marker of the condition.

Estimates of prevalence have little meaning unless a clear definition of the symptom or disease in question is stated. Without this it is impossible either to interpret individual studies or to make comparisons between studies. The definition may be derived arbitrarily before embarking on a study. This is a valid method provided the definition is clearly specified and rigidly adhered to throughout the study. However, the definitions of various urinary complaints differ greatly between studies. For instance, in one study incontinence was defined as any episode of leaking, or wet or damp pants in the past (Brocklehurst 1993), and in another study it was defined as at least one episode of leaking per week (Wyman et al 1987).

An alternative approach is to use a population survey to arrive at a definition. This definition, based on the formal data collected, can then be used in further studies. An example of this method of establishing a definition is the study by Osborne (1976), who asked a group of 600 working women aged 35–60 years to complete questionnaires about bladder habits. Likewise, Wolin (1969) asked over 4000 American nursing students to complete a questionnaire about their bladder habits.

The agreed definition must, for epidemiological purposes, be one which can be easily applied on a large scale. Therefore, it needs to be simple and unambiguous, and should not depend on the results of hospital-based or invasive diagnostic techniques. Although such additional measures may be used later to validate results, attempts to include them in surveys will seriously limit response rates and provide biased results based only on largely self-selected groups of the population.

For many reasons few studies of micturition disorders have been able to give reproducible estimates of the prevalence of urinary complaints in the general population; however in this chapter, we will try to present the data that does exist to this regard and stress the degree of magnitude of these problems in all age groups.

PREVALENCE OF MICTURITION DISORDERS

Urinary symptoms other than incontinence

Relatively little information about micturition disorders can be gained from routine statistics. Table 5.1 shows the findings of the National Morbidity Survey Report (RCGP 1981–82) general practice consultation rates per 100 for women. McGrother et al (1987) carried out a major study of the health and social status of 1097 elderly persons aged 75 years and over living at home in Melton Mowbray, Leicestershire. The prevalence of urinary symptoms is shown in Table 5.2.

An American study (Diokno et al 1986) included those aged 60 years or over, and reported much higher levels of urinary symptoms. It is likely this is a reflection of different definitions, though true differences cannot be totally ruled out.

Urinary symptoms are particularly common in patients with generalized neurological disease, especially multiple sclerosis (see Table 5.3). In order to investigate aspects of management, a study was carried out to determine the prevalence of symptoms attributable to neuropathic bladder in an outer London population (Thomas et al 1988). Of the 305 patients interviewed with chronic neurological disease, 97 (83%) of the 117 men and 161 (86%) of the 188 women had urinary symptoms in the preceding six months. Details of some studies are summarized in Table 5.4.

Dysuria

Acute attacks of dysuria are common in women of childbearing age. Walker et al (1981) carried out a postal survey of 7700 women aged 20–54 years in four London general practices. Of the 4100 who replied, 52% had complained of symptoms of acute dysuria at some time in their lives, 20% had in the previous

Table 5.1 General practice consultation rates.

Symptoms	Prevalence per 100 women (all ages)
Cystitis/urinary infection	62.5
Incontinence of urine	6.0
Dysuria	7.4
Frequency	7.2
Haematuria	1.8

From RCGP (1981–82), with permission.

Table 5.2 Prevalence of urinary symptoms in sample aged 75 and over (n=1097).

	Male %	Female %
Urgency	3.3	6.2
Diurnal frequency	5.0	4.3
Nocturia	3.9	3.3
Painful micturition	1.9	1.8
Post-micturition dribble	2.5	–

From McGrother et al (1987), with permission.

year, and 10% had more than one episode in the last 12 months. In a study of women of childbearing age, Rees (1978) showed that 35.6% had symptoms definitely suggestive of cystitis and a further 23% had possible attacks.

Frequency

More studies have described the prevalence of micturition disorders in postmenopausal and/or elderly patients. Milne et al (1972) found that 235 of a random sample of 200 women aged between 62 and 90 years living in a defined area of Edinburgh had increased frequency. Nocturia was reported by 58% of the women, 10% getting up more than twice. In a general practice based study of 375 women aged 65 years and over, Brocklehurst et al (1972) reported that 61% had nocturia.

Voiding difficulties

In patients without neurological conditions, there have been few studies assessing the incidence of voiding difficulties. Sommer et al (1990) sent questionnaires to 600 women aged 20–70 years, and found that few of them reported obstructive symptoms such as

Table 5.3 Prevalence of urinary symptoms in patients with neurological disease.

Symptom	Multiple Sclerosis (N = 142*) No. (%)	Other Neurological Conditions (N = 53*) No. (%)	Total (N = 195*) No. (%)
Frequency	25 (17.6)	8 (15.1)	33 (16.9)
Nocturia	49 (34.5)	19 (18.9)	59 (30.3)
Urgency	56 (39.4)	22 (41.5)	78 (40.0)
Dysuria	13 (9.2)	6 (11.3)	19 (9.7)
Haematuria	13 (9.2)	6 (11.3)	19 (9.7)
Incontinence	76 (53.5)	39 (56.6)	106 (54.4)
Poor stream	44 (31.0)	6 (11.3)	50 (25.6)
Incomplete emptying	41 (28.9)	16 (30.2)	57 (29.2)
Dribbling	53 (37.3)	18 (34.0)	71 (36.4)
Straining	79 (55.6)	26 (49.1)	105 (53.8)

*14 patients with multiple sclerosis and 19 with other diagnoses had indwelling catheters. 12 patients with multiple sclerosis and 21 with other diagnoses were using other appliances. Full details are not available for six patients. From Thomas et al (1988), with permission.

Table 5.4 A summary of selected studies of the prevalence of urinary incontinence in subjects living at home.

Authors	Study group	Method	Prevalence
Brocklehurst (1993)	4007 adults 30 years and over	Postal questionnaire	6.6% men 14% women
Diokno et al (1986)	1955 Americans aged 60 or over	Structured interview	19% males 38% females
Iosif & Bekassy (1984)	902 Swedish 61-year-old women	Postal questionnaire	29.2% incontinent 12% stress 8% urge 10% mixed
Jolleys (1988)	977 women aged 25 and over	Postal questionnaire	41% overall 6% always needing protection against leakage
Kok et al (1992)	719 Dutch women aged 60 or over	Postal questionnaire	23% incontinent 14% incontinent daily
McGrother et al (1987)	1097 elderly aged 75 and over	Structured interview	5% males 7% females
Milsom et al (1993)	10 000 randomly selected Swedish women from 7 birth cohorts	Postal questionnaire	24.6% 1900 cohort 13.9% 1920 cohort 12.1% 1940 cohort
O'Brien et al (1991)	7300 randomly selected adults 35 years and older	Postal questionnaire	4.4% men 16.4% women
Thomas et al (1980)	7767 Women aged 15 years or over	Postal questionnaire	10% incontinent twice or more per month

hesitancy, intermittent or poor stream. Brocklehurst et al (1972) found that 13% of the women in their study reported scalding and 3% had difficulty passing urine. Another study by Moore et al (1991) asked 528 women attending a general gynaecology clinic to complete an anonymous questionnaire and found that 85% of them usually crouched over a public toilet. They took these findings further and performed urodynamic studies in a crouching and sitting position and found a 21% reduction in average urine flow rate and a 149% increase in residual urine volume in the crouching position. Stanton et al (1983) reviewed the urinary symptoms of 600 consecutive women attending a urodynamic clinic and found that symptoms of voiding difficulty were unreliable. Voiding difficulties were actually proven in only 87 women of 195 who complained of such problems. However, there is little data available on the urinary habits of women without voiding difficulties.

Urinary incontinence

The prevalence of urinary incontinence in women has been shown to vary widely from 2–57% (Brocklehurst et al 1972; Crist et al 1972) in subjects living at home, and 0.2–91% (Knox 1979; McLaren et al 1981) in institutionalized patients. Some of the more recent studies determining the prevalence of urinary incontinence are outlined in Tables 5.5 and 5.6. The wide range of the numbers is likely to be a reflection of the different methods and definitions used in these studies. Clearly, however, urinary incontinence of some degree is common. One or more episodes of stress incontinence, defined as urine loss with coughing, laughing, sneezing, or excitement seems to be a fairly general experience even for young women. However, the suggestion that 16% of 421 American nursing students were incontinent daily (Wolin 1969) has not been replicated in other studies. Incontinence is commonest in certain patient groups and is associated with disabilities such as reduced mobility, cerebrovascular disease or neurological disease (Table 5.5).

The Royal College of Physicians of London (1995) separated urinary incontinence into two categories, regular and total incontinence, to further assess prevalence rates. Regular incontinence was described as a condition of slight dampness, whereas total incontinence also included more severe forms requiring special protection or curtailing lifestyle. In their review they found that the prevalence of both categories increased with age and was more common in women than men. Also, they found a trend of increasing rates of incontinence in institutionalized inhabitants when compared to a population living at home (Table 5.6).

Milsom et al (1993) studied 10 000 randomly selected women from seven different birth cohorts between 1900 and 1940 who resided in Goteborg, Sweden, and found a statistically significant linear increase in incontinence with age. However, unlike Thomas et al's study (1980), no distinction was made between the various types of incontinence (e.g. stress or urge incontinence). The duration of oral contraceptive use or menopausal status did not affect the prevalence of incontinence. The delivery of at least one child and a history of hysterectomy did have a positive effect on the prevalence of incontinence.

Table 5.5 A summary of selected studies of the prevalence of urinary incontinence in subjects living in institutions and other groups.

Authors	Study group	Prevalence
Campbell et al (1985)	559 subjects 65 years or over	11.6% overall 21.7% in those over 80 years
Hellstrom et al (1990)	974 85-year-old men and women	37% overall
Masterson et al (1980)	404 male and female residents of 11 Scottish old people's homes	17% severe 19% occasional
McLaren et al (1981)	121 female psychogeriatric patients	91% incontinent at least once in three weeks
Ouslander et al (1982)	954 nursing home patients	50% incontinent (73% of these were female)
Sier et al (1987)	363 patients aged 65 or over admitted to medical and surgical services of a university hospital	35% incontinent (44% female 48% over 75)
Thomas et al (1980)	Population of two London boroughs (including institutionalized)	0.2% in women 15–64 years 2.5% in women over 65 years
Thomas et al (1981)	Geriatric patients General wards	29% 10%
Thomas et al (1988)	Patients with neurological disorders	54% with multiple sclerosis 57% with other disorders

Table 5.6 Percentage of the population who have urinary incontinence. Based on an average of data.

	Age (years)	% incontinent
Women living at home	15–44	5–7
	45–64	8–15
	65 and over	10–20
Men living at home	15–64	3
	65 and over	7–10
Both sexes together living in institutions		
Residential homes		25
Nursing homes		40
Hospital (elderly and elderly mentally infirm)		50–70

From RCP (1995), with permission.

Thom (1998) reviewed English literature reporting the prevalence of incontinence in adults. Twenty-one studies were selected to compare the prevalence of incontinence based on frequency, age and gender. He found that incontinence was 1.3~2 times greater in older women than in older men. Overall, reported rates were higher if in-person interviews were used for data collection. This reflects that patients are more likely to admit incontinence when specifically asked about these embarassing symptoms.

There are no international comparisons of indices of urinary incontinence based on clearly defined and comparable criteria. Anecdotal accounts suggest that urinary incontinence may not be a common problem among people who squat to void and need to be able to direct their stream accurately (Shepherd 1980). Varying approaches to toilet training in childhood may have an impact on the prevalence of urinary incontinence in later life. One study from Pakistan found that women using a commode type of toilet had a greater rate of urinary incontinence (28.5%) than those using a squatting posture (12.3%) (Shershah & Ansari 1989). Some authors have concluded that Chinese women may have fewer problems with urinary incontinence than white women (Zacharin 1977). Brieger et al (1996) in a telephone survey of women in Hong Kong determined that the prevalence of incontinence in Chinese women was similar to the prevalence of incontinence reported in white women by other investigators (Thomas et al 1980; Jolleys 1988). In this Hong Kong study there was a response rate of only 25%, which introduces a selection bias; however, they found an overall prevalence of stress incontinence of 22% and urge incontinence or urgency in 15%. The authors concluded that despite the low response rate, the notion that urinary incontinence is rare in the Hong Kong Chinese population should be reconsidered.

Age

The study by the MRC Epidemiology and Medical Care Unit on the prevalence of urinary incontinence was based on the definition of 'regular' urinary incontinence as 'involuntary excretion or leakage in inappropriate places or at inappropriate times twice or more a month, regardless of the quantity of urine lost' (Thomas et al 1980). Figure 5.1 shows the prevalence of urinary incontinence by 10-year age groups in women 15 years and over, and the proportion of each age group reporting the symptoms of urge and stress incontinence. Prevalence in women changed little between the ages of 3 and 64 years but fell in those aged 65–74 and rose in those aged 75 and over. The lowest prevalence, in the 65–74-year-old group, was consistent in all the practices surveyed and seems to be accounted for by the less frequent occurrence of stress incontinence in the older age groups. This was previously noted by Brocklehurst et al (1972). The prevalence of urge incontinence alone was similar between the ages of 15 and 54 years but increased after this age. Stress incontinence alone, without

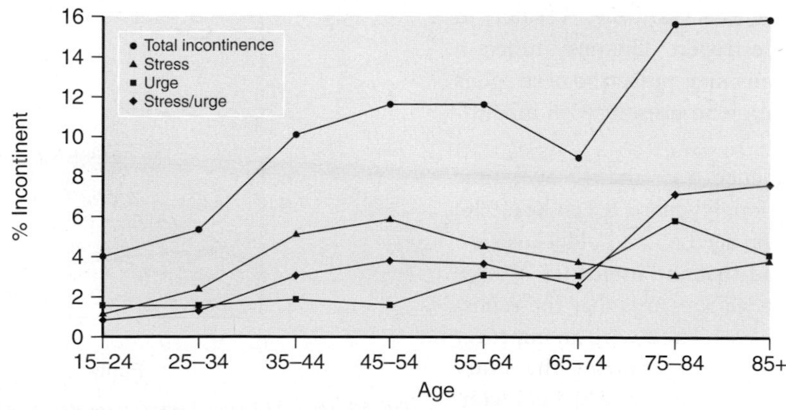

Fig. 5.1 The prevalence of stress, urge and stress/urge incontinence in women by age.

symptoms suggestive of bladder instability, was reported by only 85 of the women aged 15–64 years with regular urinary incontinence and was even less common above this age.

In comparing rates of incontinence in the general community, Brocklehurst (1993) found from a postal questionnaire that 14% of 2124 women polled suffered at some point from incontinence symptoms. Similarly, Thomas et al (1980) found that 8.5% of women aged 15–64 years, and 11.6% of women aged 65 and over suffer from incontinence. Diokno et al (1986) studied the prevalence of incontinence in non-institutionalized elderly aged 60 years or over, and found that 37.7% of women suffered from incontinence, many of them suffering from mixed (stress and urge) incontinence. Campbell et al (1985) found similar results but included institutionalized patients in their study, and demonstrated that with increasing age, greater numbers of women suffered from incontinence related to confusion, but the most frequent symptom was stress in those aged 65–79, and urge in those aged 80 or over.

Due to the increasing prevalence of urinary incontinence in elderly women it would be beneficial to be able to identify risk factors associated with the development of this condition. Brown et al (1996) looked at the prevalence of urinary incontinence in 7949 community-dwelling women whose mean age was 76.9 years. They found a 41% prevalence of urinary incontinence (loss of urine at least once a month) with 14% reporting daily leakage. Forty-two percent of women with incontinence considered it a problem. The risk factors they identified as most significantly associated with this prevalence included age (odds ratio (OR) 1.3), prior hysterectomy (OR 1.4), a higher body mass index (OR 1.6), a history of stroke (OR 1.9), diabetes (OR 1.7), chronic obstructive pulmonary disease (OR 1.4), or chronic illness (OR 1.6). Faster gait speed was associated with a decreased rate of incontinence (OR 0.8). Interestingly enough, the prevalence of daily incontinence was twice greater in women who used oral oestrogen. This may reflect a selection bias as physicians may prescribe oestrogens more frequently to women who present with incontinence symptoms.

The rates of incontinence may change over time within a specific population. Nygaard & Lemke (1996) studied a cohort of women aged 65 and older over a 6 year time span and found that the incidence of urge incontinence increased with age, and that the remission of urge incontinence correlated with an improvement in activities of daily living. During the study period, the remission rates for urge and stress incontinence were 22% and 25%, respectively, reflecting the dynamic state of the prevalence of incontinence complaints in a given population.

Parity

The results by parity in those aged 15 years or more from Thomas et al's study (1980) are shown in Figure 5.2. Even in this large survey, the numbers within subcategories of urinary incontinence in different parity groups are sometimes small, and some caution is therefore necessary in interpreting the results. Urge incontinence may be a little commoner in the parous than nulliparous, but within the parous there is no obvious increase in the prevalence of urge incontinence with increasing parity. The rise in the prevalence of incontinence with parity is due to a rise in the prevalence of stress (and stress/urge) incontinence. The effects of parity on the prevalence of urinary incontinence are independent of the effects of age.

A similar study was carried out 10 years later by Jolleys (1988) in a general practice in Leicestershire. A postal questionnaire was sent to 937 women over 25 years old and was completed by 833 (89%). Questions were asked about urinary leakage and how often it occurred, and also about other factors such as obstetric history. The overall prevalence was 41% with 6% of women reporting that they always needed to wear protection against leakage. The overall prevalence of 41% is comparable with the results of the MRC postal survey (Thomas et al 1980) where an overall preva-

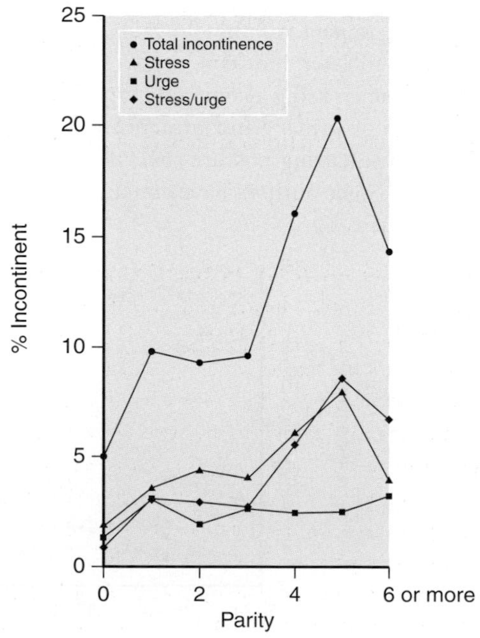

Fig. 5.2 The prevalence of stress, urge and stress/urge incontinence in women by parity.

lence of 28% was reported but the definition used would have excluded the most minor degrees of incontinence included in Jolleys' study.

Jolleys found an increasing prevalence of incontinence with increasing parity. Urinary incontinence was common even in the nulliparous, involving 17%. She found that contrary to expectation, a higher proportion of women who had carried out daily postnatal exercises reported leakage than those who had not. The explanation for this was that these patients might have been more keen to do the exercises if they had difficulties with incontinence before delivery, however prenatal incontinence rates were not documented.

Wilson et al (1996) reviewed data from 1505 completed questionnaires sent to women who were 3 months postpartum. The questionnaires inquired about prevalence, type and frequency of urinary incontinence, and other urinary symptomatology, both at the time of completing the questionnaire and previously as related to the preceding pregnancy and delivery. At 3 months postpartum, 34% reported urinary incontinence. Nineteen per cent of primiparous patients reported a history of incontinence before their pregnancy. Women who performed pelvic floor exercises (PFE) had higher rates of incontinence (36.9% doing PFE compared to 28.5% of women who were not). The four most important variables associated with urinary incontinence were pregnancy body mass index, parity (odds ratio increased after four deliveries), daily PFE during pregnancy, and mode of delivery. There was an increased rate of incontinence in women who had spontaneous or forceps vaginal deliveries compared to those who received caesarean section. This last factor may explain why many women are now requesting caesarean delivery to preserve their pelvic floor function (Sultan & Stanton 1996).

Nocturnal enuresis

Epidemiological studies of bedwetting and associated symptoms in children have provided useful information about the natural history of enuresis (DeJonge 1973; Forsythe & Redmond 1974; Miller et al 1974; Essen & Peckham 1976), but relatively little is known about the natural history of urinary incontinence in younger and middle aged adults. Moore et al (1991) reviewed the urodynamic records of 1000 consecutive men and women and found that 63% of the men with urodynamically proven detrusor instability had a history of primary enuresis, as opposed to only 38% of the women. Urinary incontinence has been reported to be transient in up to a third of incontinent elderly patients (Willington 1969; Milne et al 1970; Yarnell & StLeger 1979). This was not confirmed by the findings of the MRC Epidemiology and Medical Care Unit Study, where only one in nine of those aged 65 and over were dry at follow-up interview after one year. This difference may be due to the different definitions used in the studies.

FAECAL INCONTINENCE

Although this chapter deals with the prevalence of micturition disorders, the association of urinary incontinence with faecal incontinence, especially in the elderly, cannot be ignored. In a study by Ouslander et al (1982) of elderly nursing home patients, 64% of those with urinary incontinence had concomitant faecal incontinence. Similarly, in an American study of elderly patients admitted to a medical or surgical service in an acute care hospital in Los Angeles, Sier et al (1987) found that 59% of the patients with urinary incontinence were incontinent of stool. They admitted that this high frequency of faecal symptoms may be related to the pathophysiological mechanisms producing urinary incontinence or to the administration of laxatives in these patients. In a study of community dwelling subjects in New Zealand, 65 years old and over (Campbell et al 1985), faecal incontinence was estimated to occur in 3.1% of the population studied. More recently, Kok et al (1992) found 4.2% of 60–84-year-olds and 16.9% of those 85 years old and over suffered from faecal incontinence in a population of community-residing women in the Netherlands. Similarly the Royal College of Physicians found prevalence rates of 0.4–15% in home-dwellers, with increasing rates directly related to age and institutionalization (RCP 1995). The increasing prevalence of this symptom in the elderly complicates their care and provides further embarrassment to those who suffer from this condition.

SEVERITY AND SERVICE IMPLICATIONS

Knowledge of the prevalence and severity of micturition symptoms, especially incontinence, establishes a baseline for the planning and assessment of services. However, assessments of prevalence vary between studies due to differences in definitions, population selection, and hesitancy to report symptoms. Although many women might not consider themselves to have problems warranting medical intervention, a few would certainly welcome more active management than they are receiving. About 90% of the incontinent women had been so for longer than a year. Less than 20% had any investigation other than examination of a mid-stream urine specimen. For those in receipt of services, there was, nevertheless, evidence of considerable room for improvement (Thomas et al 1981), which is a finding reported from other areas (Slack 1981).

Ideally, the effectiveness of management methods, whether by nursing, medical or surgical means, should be assessed by randomized controlled trials using clearly defined outcome measures. The advantages of using an objective urodynamic outcome measure must be weighed against those of a subjective clinical assessment. Whatever measure is used it should be made 'blindly' (i.e., without knowledge of the method of treatment). Subjective assessments of surgical success should, therefore, be made by someone other than the surgeon who carried out the procedure.

Investigations such as urodynamic measurements should only be carried out routinely when there is a clear understanding of their value in improving diagnosis and management (Cardozo & Stanton 1980; Jarvis et al 1980). Hilton & Stanton (1981) have suggested that invasive investigations of urinary incontinence could be avoided in a proportion of incontinent elderly women (60% in their series) if an algorithmic method of assessment were used. The use of randomized controlled trials in assessing the indication of urodynamics has not been sufficiently exploited.

Even so, it is difficult to predict whether an objective assessment of an acceptable cure will accurately estimate the patient's satisfaction with the treatment. Wan et al (1993) pointed out, in their article assessing stress leak point pressure as a diagnostic tool for assessment of incontinence in children, that researchers and patients should not necessarily trust arbitrary scales that rate the degree of incontinence. Moderate wetness in one patient, may be considered severe for another. Similarly, two pads soaked daily may be no better than four damp pads. The physician must not forget the patient's needs and ability to cope with the problem.

Quality of life issues are of utmost importance in assessing the patient's ability to deal with her symptoms of disordered micturition. Urinary incontinence, for example, can be a cause of great discomfort, loss of self-esteem, and withdrawal from social activities. Grimby et al (1993) used the Nottingham Health Profile to assess the effect of urinary incontinence on quality of life and found that women with urinary incontinence had higher scores in the domains of emotional and sleep disturbances, and social isolation than age-matched controls. In a study by Macaulay et al (1987) patients with sensory urgency were found to be more anxious than those with genuine stress urinary incontinence (GSI). Patients with detrusor instability had significantly higher scores in the hysteria scale than those with sensory urgency or GSI. Wyman et al (1987) found that women with incontinence had greatest difficulties with self-perception and daily activities, especially circumstances involving unfamiliar places, long distance travel, physical recreation, and vacation. One fifth of these patients felt they smelt and one ninth experienced a compromise in sexual relations. Aside from the emotional and social aspects of dealing with urinary incontinence, there is also an economic burden to these patients in terms of laundering soiled clothing, frequent changing of pads, and using other continence aids.

Finally, the role of the physician in eliciting the symptoms of various micturition disorders from patients and in proceeding to diagnose and treat the cause of the disorder should be reiterated. Brocklehurst (1993) analyzed a Market and Opinion Research (MORI) poll commissioned by the British Association for Continence Care, and found only 22% of the patients who sought medical advice for their incontinence from general practitioners were actually examined by the physician. The majority of GPs (54%) took a urine sample, 42% referred the patients to a specialist, and 36% prescribed tablets. In a related study by Jolleys & Wilson (1993) only 30% of 1284 general practitioners polled in the United Kingdom felt very confident in diagnosing and managing incontinence and 80% of them felt their training in continence promotion was inadequate. This likely explains O'Brien et al's (1991) findings that, of the patients who actually approached their general practitioner with complaints of incontinence, only 20% were evaluated in the previous year, and 30% had never had any form of assessment of the problem. Briggs & Williams (1992) expanded further on this and found that, of 101 general practitioners polled, 42 had never used a continence advisor for their elderly patients over 65 years of age. The question is whether there is a lack of such referral services available for a growing population of patients in need.

Due to the increasing numbers of elderly people in society and their increased life expectancy (especially in women, who more frequently suffer from incontinence) it is anticipated that the demands for services capable of dealing with continence awareness and managing micturition disorders will greatly increase. Therefore, as caregivers, physicians must be prepared to handle these problems on a larger scale. Also, many estimates on health care costs have found that incontinence and related disorders are expensive to society in general. It is believed that urinary incontinence accounts for approximately 2% of health care costs in the United States (Hu 1990) and Sweden (Ekelund et al 1993). More recently, Hu et al (1994) reported a 60% increase in this cost, estimating that 1.2 billion dollars are spent annually in the community and 5.2 billion, in nursing homes. Therefore, in these times of cost containment, we must look for more effective and comprehensive methods of dealing with these economically and socially challenging problems.

REFERENCES

Brieger G M, Yip S K, Hin L Y, Chung T K H 1996 The prevalence of urinary dysfunction in Hong Kong Chinese women. Obstetrics and Gynecology 88: 1041–1044

Briggs M, Williams E S 1992 Urinary incontinence. British Medical Journal 304: 255

Brocklehurst J C 1993 Urinary incontinence in the community – analysis of a MORI poll. British Medical Journal 306: 832–834

Brocklehurst J C, Fry J, Griffiths L L, Kalton G 1972 Urinary infection and symptoms of dysuria in women aged 45–64 years: their relevance to similar findings in the elderly. Age and Ageing 1: 41–47

Brown J S, Seeley D G, Fong J, Black D M, Ensrud K E, Grady D, for the Study of Osteoporotic Fractures Research Group 1996 Urinary incontinence in older women: who is at risk? Obstetrics and Gynecology 87: 715–721

Campbell A J, Reinken J, McCosh L 1985 Incontinence in the elderly: prevalence and prognosis. Age and Ageing 14: 65–70

Cardozo L D, Stanton S L 1980 Genuine stress incontinence and detrusor instability – a review of 200 patients. British Journal of Obstetrics and Gynaecology 87: 893–896

Crist T, Shingleton H M, Koch G G 1972 Stress incontinence and the nulliparous patient. Obstetrics and Gynecology 40: 13–17

DeJonge G A 1973 Epidemiology of enuresis. In: Clinics in Developmental Medicine. William Heinemann Medical Books, London

Diokno A C, Brock B M, Brown M B, Herjog A R 1986 Prevalence of urinary incontinence and other urological symptoms in the noninstitutionalised elderly. Journal of Urology 136: 1022–1025

Ekelund P, Grimby A, Milsom I 1993 Urinary incontinence. Social and financial costs high. British Medical Journal 306: 1344

Essen J, Peckham C 1976 Nocturnal enuresis in childhood. Developmental Medicine and Child Neurology 16: 577–589

Forsythe WI, Redmond A 1974 Enuresis and spontaneous cure rate study. Archives of Disease in Childhood 49: 259–263

Grimby A, Milsom I, Molander U, Wiklund I, Ekelund P 1993 The influence of urinary incontinence on the quality of life of elderly women. Age and Ageing 22: 82–89

Hellstrom L, Ekelund P, Milsom I, Mellstrom D 1990 The prevalence of urinary incontinence and use of incontinence aids in 85-year-old men and women. Age and Ageing 19: 383–389

Hilton P, Stanton S L 1981 Algorithmic method for assessing urinary incontinence in elderly women. British Medical Journal 282: 940–942

Hu T 1990 Impact of urinary incontinence on health care costs. Journal of the American Geriatric Society 38: 292–295

Hu T, Gabelko K, Weis KA, Fogarty TE, Diokno AC, McCormick KA 1994 Clinical guidelines and cost implications – the case of urinary incontinence. Geriatric Nephrology and Urology 4: 85–91

Iosif C S, Bekassy Z 1984 Prevalence of genito-urinary symptoms in the late menopause. Acta Obstetrica et Gynecologica Scandinavica 63: 257–260

Jarvis G J, Hall S, Stamp S, Millar D R, Johnson A 1980 An assessment of urodynamic examination in incontinent women. British Journal of Obstetrics and Gynaecology 87: 893–896

Jolleys J V 1988 Reported prevalence of urinary incontinence in women in a general practice. British Medical Journal 296: 1300–1302

Jolleys J V, Wilson J V 1993 G P's lack confidence. British Medical Journal 306: 1344

Knox J D E 1979 Ambulant incontinent patients in general practice. Nursing Times 75: 1133–1135

Kok A L M, Voorhorst F J, Burger C W, VanHouten P, Kenemans P, Janssens J 1992 Urinary and faecal incontinence in community-residing elderly women. Age and Ageing 21: 211–215

Macaulay A J, Stern R S, Holmes D M, Stanton S L 1987 Micturition and the mind: psychological factors in the aetiology and treatment of urinary symptoms in women. British Medical Journal 294: 540–543

McLaren S M, McPherson F M, Sinclair F, Ballinger B R 1981 Prevalence and severity of incontinence among hospitalized female psychogeriatric patients. Health Bulletin (Edinburgh) 38: 62–64

McGrother C W, Castledon C M, Duffin J, Clarke M 1987 A profile of disordered micturition in the elderly at home. Age and Ageing 16: 105–110

Masterson G, Holloway E M, Timbury G C 1980 The prevalence of incontinence in local authority homes for the elderly. Health Bulletin (Edinburgh) 38: 62–64

Miller F J W, Court S D M, Knox E G, Brandon S 1974 The School Years in Newcastle on Tyne. Oxford University Press, London

Milne J S, Hope K, Williamson J 1970 Variability in replies to a questionnaire on symptoms of physical illness. Journal of Chronic Diseases 2: 805–810

Milne J S, Williamson J, Maule M M, Wallace E T 1972 Urinary symptoms in older people. Modern Geriatrics 2: 198–212

Milsom I, Ekelund P, Molander U, Arvidsson L, Areskoug B 1993 The influence of age, parity, oral contraception, hysterectomy and menopause on the prevalence of urinary incontinence in women. Journal of Urology 149: 1459–1462

Moore K H, Richmond D H, Parys B T 1991 Sex distribution of idiopathic detrusor instability in relation to childhood bedwetting. British Journal of Urology 68: 479–482

Moore K H, Richmond D H, Sutherst J R, Imrie A H, Hutton J L 1991 Crouching over the toilet seat: prevalence among British gynaecological outpatients and its effect upon micturition. British Journal of Obstetrics and Gynaecology 98: 569–572

Norton P A, MacDonald L D, Segwick P M, Stanton S L 1988 Distress and delay associated with urinary incontinence, frequency and urgency in women. British Medical Journal 297: 1187–1189

O'Brien J, Austin M, Sethi P, O'Boyle P 1991 Urinary

incontinence: prevalence, need for treatment, and effectiveness of intervention by nurse. British Medical Journal 303: 1308–1312
Osborne J L 1976 Post-menopausal changes in micturition habits and in urine flow and urethral pressure studies in: The Management of the Menopause and Post-menopausal Years. MTP, Lancaster, 285–289
Ouslander J G, Kane R L, Abrass I B 1982 Urinary incontinence in elderly nursing home patients. Journal of the American Medical Association 248: 1194–1198
RCGP Office of Population Censuses and Surveys 1981–82. DHSS morbidity statistics from general practice third national study, studies on medical and population subjects, No. 36.
R C P 1995 Report. Incontinence, causes, management and provision of services. The Royal College of Physicians of London, May 1995.
Rees D L P 1978 Urinary tract infection. In: Clinics in Obstetrics and Gynaecology. W B Saunders, London 5: 169–192
Roberts R O, Jacobsen S J, Rhodes T et al 1998 Urinary incontinence in a community-based cohort: prevalence and health care-seeking. Journal of the American Geriatrics Society 46: 467–72
Shepherd A 1980. In: Incontinence and its Management. Croom Helm, London, 156–159
Shershah S, Ansari R L 1989 The frequency of urinary incontinence in Pakistani women. Journal of the Pakistan Medical Association 39: 16–17
Sier H, Ouslander J, Orzeck S 1987 Urinary incontinence among geriatric patients in an acute-care hospital. Journal of the American Medical Association 257: 1767–1771
Slack P 1981 Incontinence – a forward look. Nursing Times, (suppl) 77
Smith P 1981 The urethral syndrome. In: Clinics in Obstetrics and Gynaecology. W B Saunders, London 8: 161–172
Sommer P, Bauer T, Nielsen K K et al 1990 Voiding patterns and prevalence of incontinence in women. A questionnaire survey. British Journal of Urology 66: 12–15
Stanton S L, Ozsoy C, Hilton P 1983 Voiding difficulties in the female: prevalence, clinical and urodynamic review. Obstetrics and Gynecology 61: 144–147
Sultan A H, Stanton S L 1996 Preserving the pelvic floor and perineum during childbirth – elective caesarean section? British Journal of Obstetrics and Gynaecology 103: 731–734
Thom D 1998 Variation in estimates of urinary incontinence prevalence in the community: effects of differences in definition, population characteristics, and study type. Journal of the American Geriatrics Society 46: 473–80
Thomas T M, Gibson M, George M, Parikshak N, Meade T W 1988 The prevalence of urinary symptoms in patients with chronic neurological disease. Community Medicine 10: 124–29
Thomas T M, Karran O D, Meade T W 1981 Management of urinary incontinence in patients with multiple sclerosis. Journal of the Royal College of General Practitioners 31: 286–298
Thomas T M, Plymat K R, Blannin J, Meade T W 1980 Prevalence of urinary incontinence. British Medical Journal 281: 1243–1245
Walker M, Heady J A, Shaper A G 1981 Prevalence of urinary tract infection symptoms in women. Journal of Epidemiology and Community Health 35: 152
Wan J, McGuire E J, Bloom D A, Ritchey M L 1993 Stress leak point pressure: a diagnostic tool for incontinent children. Journal of Urology 150: 700–702
Willington F L 1969 Problems of urinary incontinence in the aged. Gerontology 11: 330–350
Wilson P D, Herbison R M, Herbison G P 1996 Obstetric practice and the prevalence of urinary incontinence three months after delivery. British Journal of Obstetrics and Gynaecology 103: 154–161
Wolin L H 1969 Stress incontinence in young healthy nulliparous female subjects. Journal of Urology 101: 545–549
Wyman J F, Harkins S W, Choi S C, Taylor J R, Fantl J A 1987 Psychosocial impact of urinary incontinence in women. Obstetrics and Gynecology 70: 378–381
Yarnell J W G, StLeger A L 1979 The prevalence, severity, and factors associated with urinary incontinence in a random sample of the elderly. Age and Ageing 8: 81–85
Zacharin R F 1977 'A Chinese anatomy' – the pelvic supporting tissues of the Chinese and Occidental female compared and contrasted. Australian and New Zealand Journal of Obstetrics and Gynaecology 17: 1–11

SECTION

2

Investigation

Physical aspects of urodynamic investigations

DEREK J GRIFFITHS

INTRAVESICAL PRESSURE

Effect of gravity

The intravesical pressure, unlike some of the other 'pressures' measured in urodynamics, is a true *fluid* pressure. Because of gravity, it is different at different levels within the bladder. In practice the actual effect of gravity depends on whether the bladder pressure is measured with a catheter-tip transducer in the bladder or with an external transducer in communication with the bladder via a water-filled catheter (see below and Griffiths 1980, 1996).

External pressure transducer

With an external transducer the reading does not depend significantly on the level of the catheter opening within the bladder. It does however depend on the height of the external transducer with respect to the bladder. To standardize the reading the transducer should be positioned so that, when it is opened to the atmosphere to establish the zero reading, the water meniscus is at the level of the upper edge of the symphysis pubis (International Continence Society 1979, 1988). This requirement can be a nuisance if the patient moves or is moved during the procedure. The main advantage of an external transducer is that the zero reading and the calibration can be checked without removing the catheter. The weakest link is the water-filled tube connecting it to the bladder. Knocking the tube, for example, causes artefacts in the pressure reading. If the catheter kinks, or the opening of the lumen into the bladder becomes blocked, then the measurement may be poor (Fig. 6.1A) or even fail entirely (Fig. 6.1E). This tends to occur when the bladder is nearly empty – at the beginning of a filling cystometry, or at the end of a voiding study.

Catheter-tip pressure transducer

In contrast, a catheter-tip transducer must be zeroed when it is exposed to atmospheric pressure, before it is introduced into the bladder. It is important *never* to 'push the zero button' after the catheter is in the bladder, since this would make it impossible to establish the correct values of intravesical and detrusor pressure. The reading of this type of transducer does depend on the level of the catheter tip within the bladder, and should in principle be corrected by adding on the vertical distance above the upper border of the symphysis pubis. However, the error due to omission of this correction is unlikely to exceed 10 cm H_2O, which is no greater than other errors (see below). The main practical advantage of catheter-tip transducers is that they are unaffected by knocks, and the

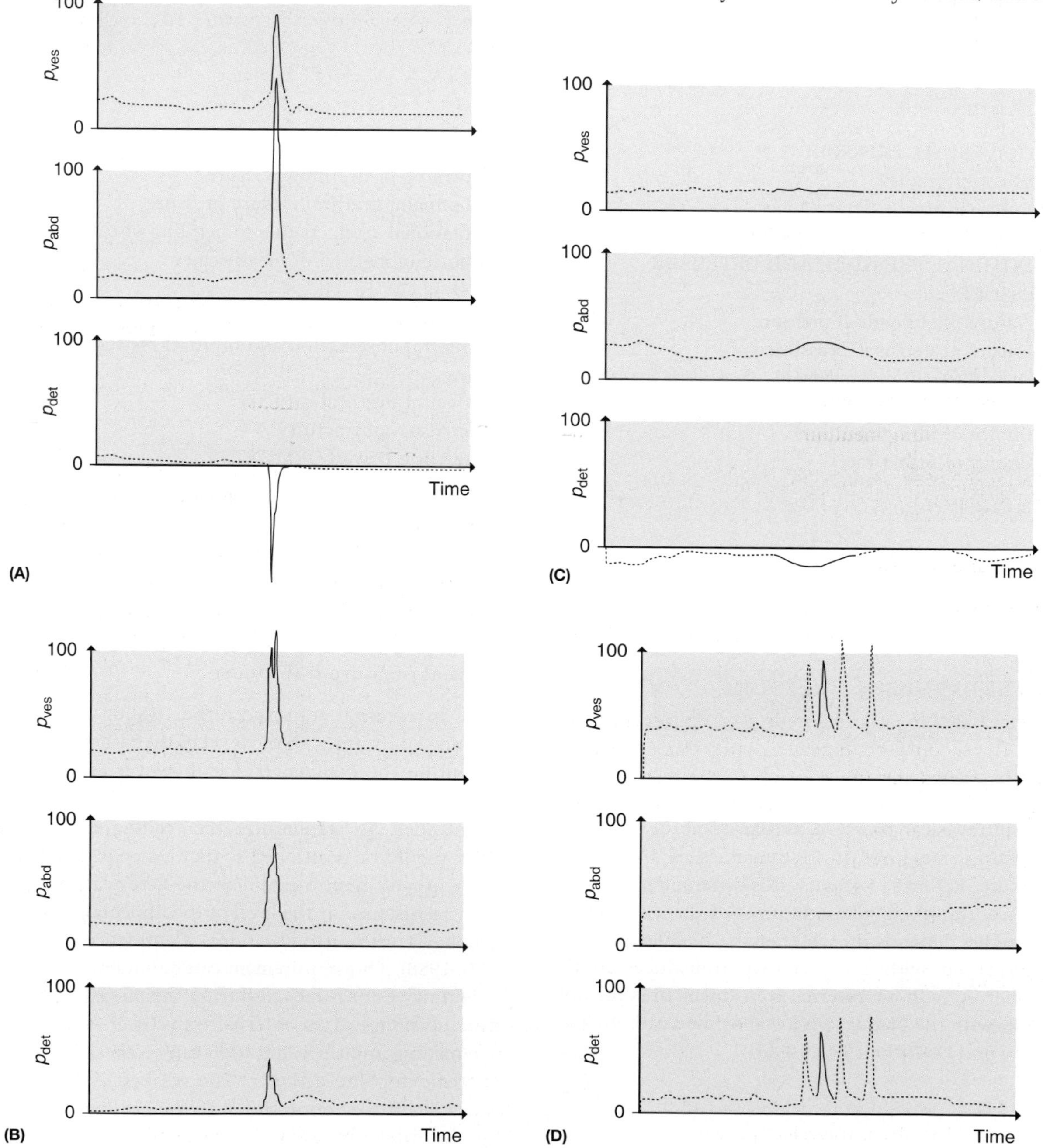

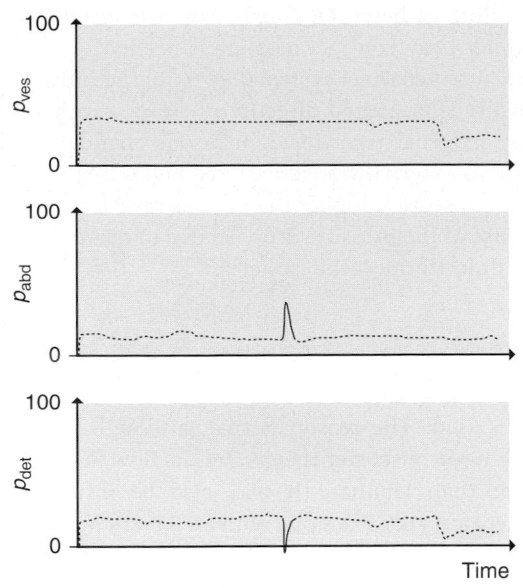

Fig. 6.1 Examples of artefacts in pressure (Modur 1993). **(A)** Abdominal pressure change (cough) unequally transmitted to bladder (p_{ves}): and rectum (p_{abd}): underregistration in p_{ves} channel. **(B)** Abdominal pressure change (cough) unequally transmitted to bladder and rectum: underregistration in p_{abd} channel. **(C)** Phasic contractions of rectum. **(D)** Rectal catheter not functioning (coughs not registered). **(E)** Bladder catheter not functioning (cough not registered).

main disadvantage is that the zero and calibration cannot easily be checked.

ABDOMINAL PRESSURE AND DETRUSOR PRESSURE

Nature of abdominal pressure

The abdominal pressure is the contribution to the intravesical pressure that is not due to the bladder wall itself, i.e. it is the net effect of forces exerted on the bladder by its abdominal surroundings. Obviously the abdominal pressure is not a true fluid pressure. It can only be estimated, and this is usually done by measuring the pressure in the rectum. This procedure is very liable to artefacts because, (a) the rectum is not normally fluid-filled, so that no true fluid pressure exists inside it, and (b) even if a true fluid pressure were to be measured, it would not be exactly the same as the desired abdominal pressure.

Nature of detrusor pressure

The detrusor pressure is formed by subtracting the abdominal pressure from the intravesical pressure (International Continence Society 1979, 1988). It is intended to represent the contribution of forces in the bladder wall to the intravesical pressure and to help distinguish detrusor contractions from abdominal pressure variations.

In principle the zero point of the detrusor pressure is correct only if the transducers for the intravesical and rectal pressures are at the same level and are correctly zeroed (see above and Griffiths 1996). This is easy to arrange with external transducers but more difficult with catheter-tip transducers.

Difficulties in measurement

Among the difficulties that may arise when measuring the abdominal pressure are the following:

1 No general abdominal pressure may exist; the external pressure exerted on the rectum may differ from that exerted on the bladder.
2 The rectal pressure may be greater than the abdominal pressure because the rectum has its own tone or is contracting. Regular rectal contractions are easily recognized because they are not present in the intravesical pressure and appear as a mirror image in the detrusor pressure (Fig. 6.1C). A steady rectal tone results in an unusually low or even negative detrusor pressure.
3 In order for the catheter to measure a real (fluid) pressure in the rectum, its opening must be immersed in water or a similar liquid. To prevent dispersion of the water and blockage of the catheter opening, the end of the catheter may be enclosed in a loosely fitting, non-inflated balloon, or else extra water should be flushed through the catheter whenever necessary. The working of the catheter should be frequently checked by observing whether variations in abdominal pressure (due, for example, to respiration or coughing) are subtracted out completely in the detrusor pressure (Fig. 6.1B, 6.1D). Display of all three pressure traces (intravesical, abdominal and detrusor) is important to check catheter functioning and to identify artefacts.

FILLING CYSTOMETRY

Description

In filling cystometry (see Ch. 9) the intravesical pressure is recorded while the bladder is filled with either liquid or gas. It is good practice to record the abdominal and detrusor pressures as well. The end result is a graph showing the three pressures as functions of time. If the bladder is filled at a steady rate, then the same graph also represents the pressures as functions of bladder volume (see Fig. 6.3, below). Obviously, any urine remaining in the bladder before filling is started must be allowed for; if filling is very slow, natural urine production may have to be considered too.

Bladder compliance

The inverse slope of the graph of detrusor pressure vs. volume represents a volume increase divided by the corresponding rise in detrusor pressure. It is called the compliance of the bladder. Since the slope of the graph changes as the bladder is filled, interpretation of the numerical value of the compliance is complicated. However, normal bladders show hardly any measurable detrusor pressure rise during filling to capacity at a medium rate (i.e. they have a high compliance), while a detrusor pressure rise much greater than 10 cm H_2O suggests an abnormally low compliance. A rise to above 40 cm H_2O, without leakage through the urethra, is seen in some types of neuropathy and is associated with upper tract damage. In these cases the low compliance is probably active in origin (due to increased detrusor muscle tone), but in other cases it may be due to structural changes in the bladder wall, resulting in reduced passive elasticity.

Choice of filling medium

One- and two-channel systems

The choice of filling medium – gas or liquid – is bound up with the choice of system and the size of the filling catheter. Of course, for videourodynamics a liquid X-ray contrast medium is needed.

In a two-channel system (Fig. 6.2B) the intravesical pressure is measured directly by either a catheter-tip or an external transducer. In a one-channel system (with an external transducer, see Fig. 6.2A) the measured pressure is higher than the intravesical pressure because of the pressure drop needed to drive the infusion fluid through the catheter.

Effect of turbulence and viscosity

The pressure drop can be quite high whether water or gas is used. The reason is that, although gas has a much lower viscosity than water, its flow is turbulent rather than laminar. (It may also be infused at a higher rate.) For example, with an 8 French gauge filling catheter of typical length and wall thickness, and at a steady filling rate of 100 ml/min, the recorded pressure might be roughly 20 cm H_2O higher than the intravesical pressure. With X-ray contrast medium the pressure drop may be considerably higher because of the higher viscosity; a solution with as low a viscosity as possible should be used.

Because this pressure difference is quite large and depends on the infusion rate, the recorded pressure varies unpredictably unless the infusion rate is kept strictly constant. With water this problem is usually avoided altogether by using a two-channel system. With gas a one-channel system is often used for simplicity; in that case the pressure drop can be reduced by using a larger filling catheter.

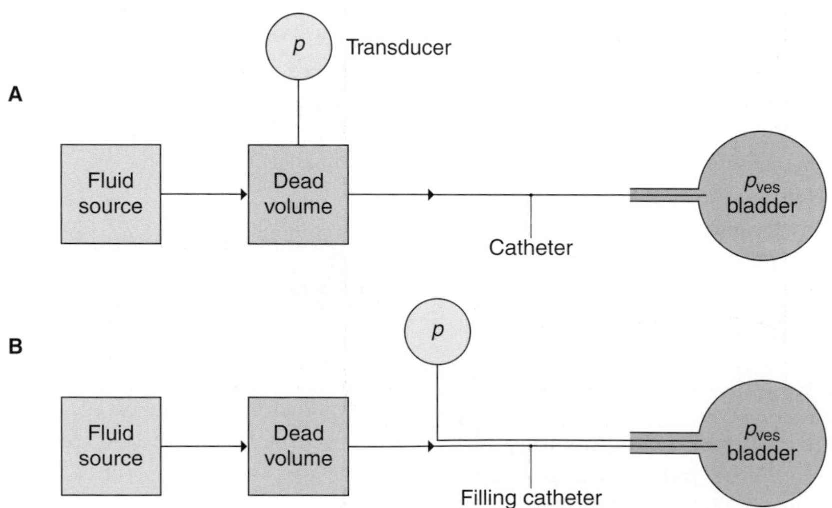

Fig. 6.2 Schematic diagrams of measuring systems for filling cystometry. **(A)** One-channel system. **(B)** Two-channel system; in a two-channel system the pressure transducer may be either external or catheter-mounted.

Effect of gas compressibility

If the intravesical pressure changes, as during a detrusor contraction, the difference in compressibility between gas and water may become important. With water, the volume in the bladder remains essentially the same, whatever the change in intravesical pressure. With gas however the volume falls by about 10% for every 100 cm H_2O rise in pressure. Thus, if 500 ml of gas is introduced into the bladder and a contraction to 100 cm H_2O then develops, the bladder volume decreases to 450 ml. The volume in the bladder is thus not exactly equal to the volume of gas introduced, and the detrusor contraction is not strictly isovolumetric.

Smoothing of rapid pressure changes in gas cystometry

With a one-channel system, the compressibility of gas coupled with the dead space on the bladder side of the pump and in the connecting tubing (Fig. 6.2A), is potentially capable of causing a more serious artefact. The pressure is actually measured in the dead space. When the bladder contracts, some of the gas in it is forced backwards through the catheter into the dead space, until the pressure there becomes equal to the intravesical pressure. When the bladder relaxes, gas flows back through the catheter into the bladder. Because of the resistance of the catheter, these gas flows and the corresponding changes in the measured pressure take time to accomplish, so that fast changes in intravesical pressure cannot be followed; i.e. a smoothed-out version of the intravesical pressure changes is recorded. If the smoothing time constant is longer than 0.1 s it is difficult to record coughs and abdominal straining accurately.

With the 8 French gauge catheter considered above, the smoothing time constant becomes longer than 0.1 s if the dead-space volume exceeds 10 ml. With a 10 French gauge catheter the dead space could be twice as large for the same time constant. With care, therefore, smoothing problems can usually be avoided in practice.

Advantages and disadvantages of gas cystometry

Other disadvantages of gas as a cystometry medium are undetected leakage, which can make the recorded bladder volume even more unreliable (Gleason & Reilly 1979), and the fact that gas cannot be used for a subsequent voiding study. One advantage of gas is the easy simultaneous registration of an intraurethral EMG signal. Nevertheless, gas cystometry as normally practised should be considered only as a quick and convenient screening examination; water cystometry with a two-channel system is technically superior.

Choice of filling rate

Viscoelastic behaviour of bladder

Quite apart from the potential artefacts just discussed, the behaviour of the bladder itself depends on the rate of filling. The faster the filling rate, the higher the detrusor pressures that are developed. If

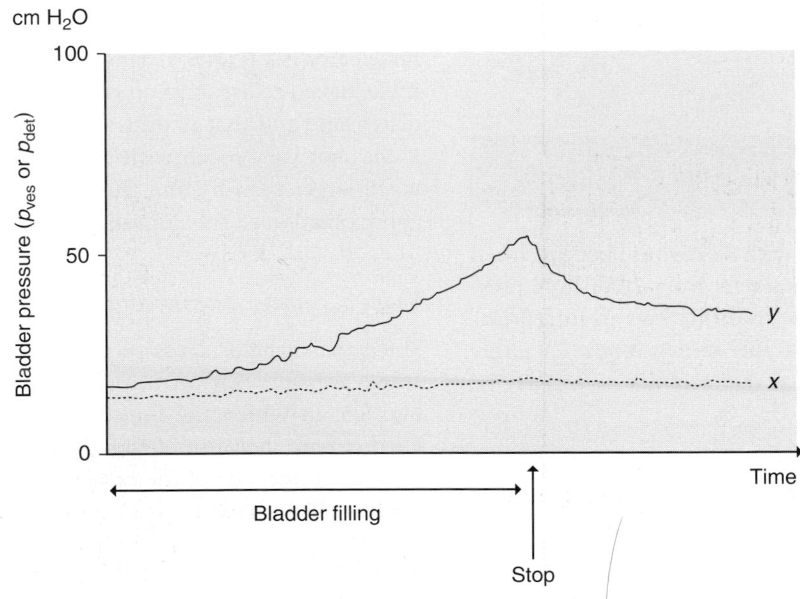

Fig. 6.3 Bladder pressure as measured during filling cystometry. x, small pressure rise, little pressure relaxation when filling is stopped; y, large pressure rise (low-compliance bladder), significant pressure relaxation after filling stops.

fast filling is interrupted, the detrusor pressure gradually 'relaxes' back towards a lower value that corresponds more closely to what would have been measured at the same volume during very slow filling (see Ch. 9, Cystometry and Videocystourethrography). With a 'medium' rate of filling (10–100 ml/min, International Continence Society 1979, 1988), two situations typically arise (Fig. 6.3).

1. ***Normal compliance*** The pressure rise during filling is small (e.g. < 5 cm H_2O) (apart from obvious detrusor contractions); i.e. the bladder has a normal, high compliance. In this case the potential fall in pressure that can occur during relaxation is obviously limited to less than 5 cm H_2O, and in practice is usually even smaller. The measured pressures are thus quite similar to those that would have been measured at a much slower filling rate.

2. ***Low compliance*** The pressure rises more steeply during filling (e.g. by > 20 cm H_2O); i.e. the bladder has a low compliance. In this case there is potentially more room for relaxation, and in my own experience it can nearly always be observed. One can look at this in two ways: (a) the filling rate is too fast, so that unphysiologically high pressures are being generated, or (b) the low compliance is abnormal and a sign of a pathological condition. The fact that low compliance may be associated with upper tract damage supports the second view. Clearly it would be useful to be able to distinguish a passive (viscoelastic) from an active (hypertonic) cause of the low compliance, but this is usually impossible because the actual relaxation appears to be very similar in both cases. If phasic detrusor contractions can also be detected, then an active cause is likely.

URETHRAL PRESSURE

The pressure measured with a catheter inside a closed urethra is different in character from a true fluid pressure, and this gives rise to difficulties in interpretation. The mere use of the term *urethral pressure* implies some assumptions that may not necessarily be valid.

Meaning of urethral pressure

Definition

Imagine an open urethra, filled with a fluid, and concentrate attention on one point along its length (Fig.

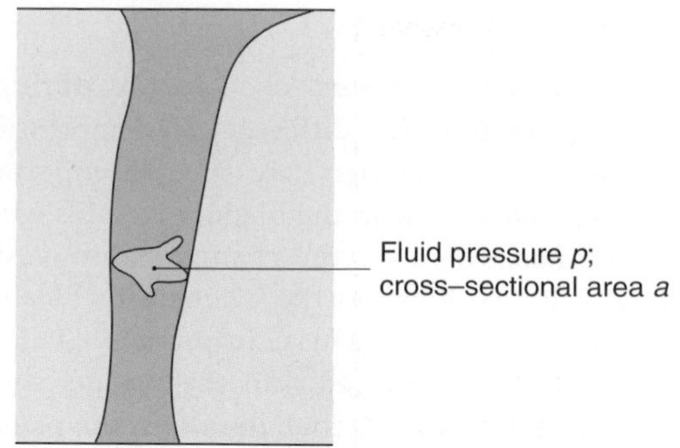

Fig. 6.4 Fluid-filled urethra with non-circular lumen. When fluid pressure is *p*, lumen cross-sectional area is a at the point shown.

6.4). If the pressure of the fluid rises, the urethra is forced further open and vice versa; thus there is a relation between the fluid pressure and the lumen area (Fig. 6.5). If the fluid pressure is reduced, the lumen eventually closes (at the point in question) when the pressure is p_o. If the pressure in the fluid nearby were gradually raised from a low value, the lumen would begin to open when it reached p_o. Thus p_o is the lowest pressure at which leakage can occur past the given point, and it is therefore the urethral pressure that we are interested in when assessing incontinence (see Ch. 13). Notice that p_o is a true fluid pressure and so cannot vary if, for example, the catheter used to measure it is rotated within the urethra.

Measurement with a catheter

In practice p_o cannot be directly measured. Instead, a catheter of finite cross-sectional area, *a*, is inserted in the urethra, and measures the pressure, *p*, when the lumen area is *a* (Fig. 6.5). Obviously, $p > p_o$. However, if we make the assumption that the urethra is highly distensible and that it seals well when it closes, then *p* does not vary much with *a* (Fig. 6.6); thus *p* is not much larger than p_o, and the measurement is a good approximation to the desired urethral pressure.

Shape of catheter cross-section

Since the catheter cross-section is round, the measured pressure may in principle differ from that in Fig. 6.5, in which the lumen has its natural shape. Furthermore, because of this distortion a transducer located on one side of the catheter may give different readings if the catheter is rotated within the urethra, even though the desired urethral pressure p_o does not itself depend on orientation. Provided that the assumption of high distensibility is valid, however, these effects should be small. The rotational varia-

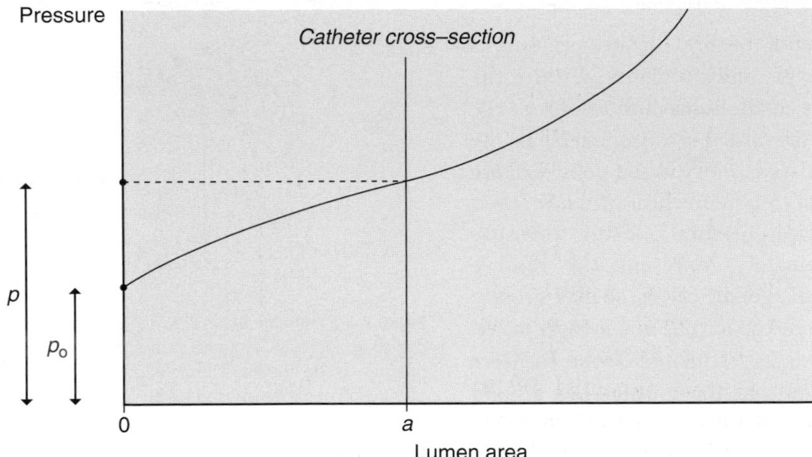

Fig. 6.5 Possible relation between fluid pressure and lumen area at point shown in Fig 6.4. p_o: fluid pressure needed to open lumen at this point; p: pressure that would be measured by catheter of cross-sectional area a, ignoring any difference between natural form of urethral cross-section (Fig. 6.4) and that of catheter. Here p is significantly greater than p_o, showing that this urethra is not particularly highly distensible.

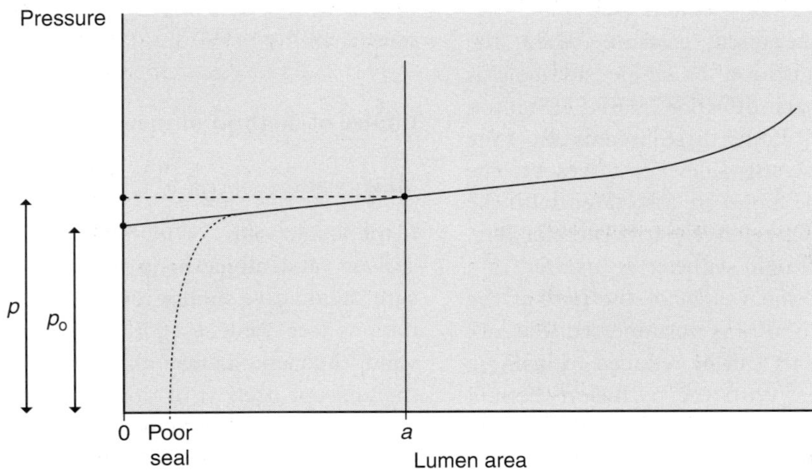

Fig. 6.6 Possible relation between fluid pressure and lumen area for highly distensible urethra. Full curve: urethra seals well and p is approximately equal to p_o. Broken curve: if seal is poor, lumen may remain open at zero (atmospheric) pressure, so that p_o does not even exist at ordinary pressures.

tions sometimes observed probably result from a different type of distortion, as discussed below.

Urethral sealing

If the urethra is not highly distensible, any catheter will significantly overestimate the urethral pressure p_o. If the urethra does not seal properly, p_o may not even exist within the normal range of pressures, and leakage can then always occur past the point in question, whatever the pressure reading given by a urethral catheter (Fig. 6.6). In this case the concept of urethral pressure has little meaning and there is no point in trying to measure it. How well the urethra seals is partly determined by the softness of its inner wall, as discussed by Zinner et al (1980).

Maximum urethral closure pressure

Definition and properties

The urethral pressure p_o varies from point to point along the urethra, so forming the urethral pressure profile. Only if the fluid pressure in the bladder exceeds the maximum value of p_o can leakage via the urethra take place. The difference between this maximum urethral pressure and the intravesical pressure is known as the maximum urethral closure pressure. As long as the maximum urethral closure pressure is greater than zero, leakage cannot occur. The actual value of the maximum closure pressure (above zero) is a measure of the reserve capacity of the urethra to resist leakage.

Validity of measurements with catheter

In practice, the maximum urethral closure pressure is estimated from catheter measurements within the urethra and is subject to the same limitations as the measurement of the urethral pressure itself. If the assumptions of high distensibility and a good seal are valid at the point of maximum urethral pressure, then the estimated maximum urethral closure pressure does indeed approximately represent the reserve capacity to prevent leakage; otherwise it may grossly overestimate the reserve capacity. Thus a high maximum closure pressure, as estimated from catheter measurements, suggests that the urethra has a good capacity to resist leakage but cannot by itself guarantee it.

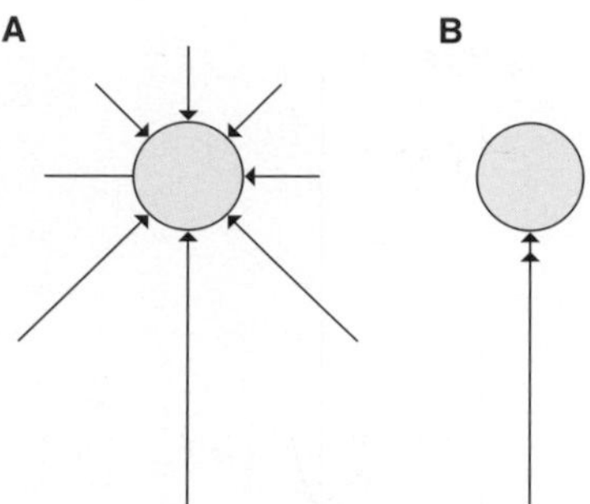

Fig. 6.7 If a catheter with a side-mounted transducer or a single perfusion side-hole is rotated in the urethra, it may register a higher pressure in one orientation than in others. **(A)** Schematic diagram of distribution of forces exerted by by urethral wall on catheter in this situation. **(B)** Resultant of these forces, i.e. net sideways force exerted by urethral wall on catheter at the point in question. ('Sideways' here means perpendicular to the axis of the catheter and the urethra.)

Rotational artefacts due to bending of catheter

The rotational effects sometimes observed with the catheter-tip and perfusion methods (see Table 6.1) involve a higher measured pressure when the catheter-mounted transducer or single side-hole is oriented in one particular direction (Hilton & Stanton 1981a, see also Ch. 13). Under these circumstances the urethra is exerting strong sideways forces on the catheter (Fig. 6.7). The forces are associated with the attempted bending of a relatively stiff catheter (Fig. 6.8), and arise if a straight catheter is inserted in a curved urethra, or if the weight of the part of the catheter outside the urethra is unsupported (Plevnik et al 1985). This artefact can be reduced by using a very flexible catheter. With the perfusion method rotational effects are much reduced if multiple side-holes are used but it remains difficult to know what pressure is being measured. The problem can be eliminated entirely by using an end-hole instead of a side-hole (Griffiths 1985).

Choice of method of measurement

Validity of the concept of urethral pressure

If the assumptions of high distensibility and a good seal are valid, all methods of measuring urethral pressure should give similar results within their own limitations (see Table 6.1). If the assumptions are not valid, the methods may all give different results, but the concept itself is of doubtful validity. Obviously then it is difficult to choose a 'best' method, although

Table 6.1 Methods of measuring urethral pressure.

Advantages	Disadvantages
1. Membrane/balloon catheter	
(a) measures real fluid pressure	(a) large size: (i) large cross-section exaggerates difference between measured p and p_o (ii) length smooths out pressure profile
(b) no rotational effects	(b) sensitive to knocks if water-filled
(c) fast response to pressure changes	(c) sensitive to temperature changes if air-filled
2. Catheter-tip transducer	
(a) small size	(a) does not measure real fluid pressure, so subject to artefacts: (i) recessed transducer reads too low (Hilton & Stanton 1981b) (ii) shows rotational effects (Hilton & Stanton 1981a; see discussion in text)
(b) fast response	(b) older types rather fragile
(c) not sensitive to knocks	(c) older types tended to drift
3. Perfusion (Brown-Wickham) method	
(a) fairly small measuring site	(a) slow response to rising pressure can cause distortion (Fig. 6.9)
(b) direct measure of real leakage pressure	(b) sensitive to knocks
(c) simple and robust	(c) rotational effects, depending on catheter stiffness and number of side-holes
(d) dependence on perfusion rate	(d reading depends on perfusion rate allows distensibility check

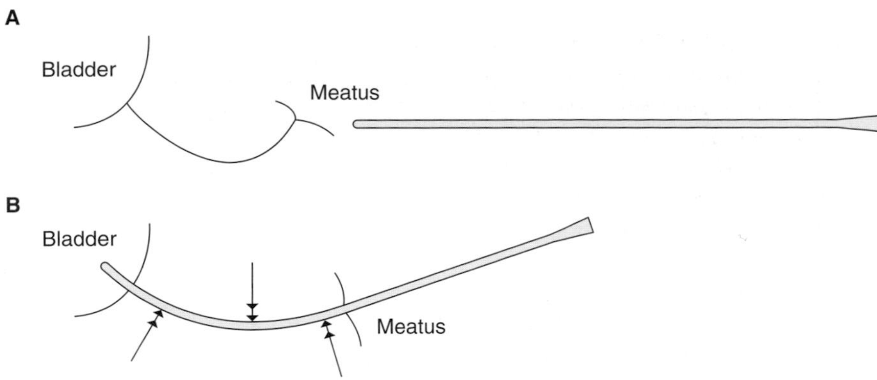

Fig. 6.8 (**A**) Curved urethra and straight catheter. (**B**) When the catheter is inserted into the urethra, both assume a common intermediate curvature. Arrows show schematically the distribution of net sideways forces that the urethra must exert on the catheter to bend it to this curvature.

the perfusion method stands out as being closest to an ideal measurement of the leakage pressure (see below).

Checks of the validity of the concept

An indirect indication of whether a given urethra seals well can be gained by measuring the urethral softness (Plevnik et al 1981). In practice, however, a direct measurement of the capacity to resist leakage, preferably with no catheter in the urethra, is better in cases where the assumptions of high distensibility and a good seal are questionable. A suitable method is the leak point pressure discussed below. Failing this, the perfusion method (see Table 6.1) provides the most direct estimate of the leakage pressure. Variation of the perfusion rate allows the distensibility of the urethra to be estimated (Griffiths 1985): if the reading is essentially independent of perfusion rate then the urethra is highly distensible. If perfusion is carried out through an end-hole rather than a side-hole, then in the proximal urethra the perfusion fluid escapes to the bladder through an uncatheterized part of the urethra, so that the pressures measured refer to the urethra without a catheter present. In fact, if perfusion is stopped entirely the recorded pressure falls until it reaches p_o. Thus in the proximal urethra the true urethral pressure at a point near the catheter tip can be directly recorded, provided that it remains steady for long enough to be measured. From a fundamental point of view therefore the perfusion method is almost ideal; in practice it has disadvantages, the most serious of which is the slow response to rising pressure (Fig. 6.9) (see Abrams et al 1978), which may make it unsuitable for measurements during stress (e.g. coughing) unless special precautions are taken.

Practical limitations of static urethral pressure measurements

Quite apart from these fundamental physical considerations, it is obvious that, under the conditions in which leakage is likely, functional changes in the urethral pressure (e.g. relaxation or tightening of the urethral and periurethral muscles, or 'transmission' of abdominal pressure changes to the urethra) are likely to occur. Static urethral pressure measurements give little or no information about these changes. Measurements during stress induced by coughing or straining give more information in principle but demand a measuring system with a high speed of response to pressure changes and also a reliable means of securing the measuring catheter inside a mobile urethra.

Valsalva leak point pressure

Measurement of the leak point pressure during a sustained Valsalva manoeuvre offers a very direct way of assessing the ability of the urethra to prevent leakage under stress. The intravesical pressure is measured during a series of sustained Valsalva manoeuvres of successively greater intensity. The leak point pressure is the intravesical pressure at which leakage is first observed. (In some centres the abdominal pressure is measured instead of the intravesical pressure.)

Normally the walls of the proximal urethra are *coapted* at rest (i.e. the urethral pressure is greater than zero) and are subject to abdominal pressure changes. In this case the proximal urethra cannot be opened by abdominal straining, because the urethral pressure rises in parallel with the intravesical pressure, no matter how high it becomes. Therefore, if leakage is observed at a finite Valsalva leak point pressure, then either the proximal urethra is not closed at rest or abdominal pressure changes are not fully

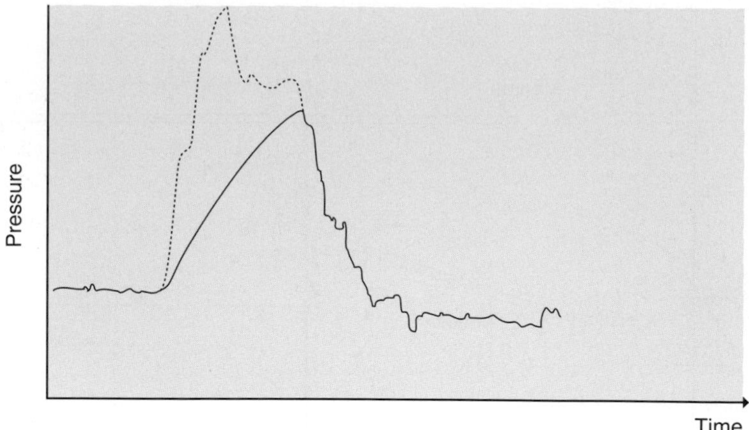

Fig. 6.9 Distortion of urethral pressure profile which can occur with a poorly designed perfusion system. Broken curve: true course of pressure profile. Solid curve: measured profile, showing typical 'sawtooth' distortion.

transmitted to the proximal urethra. Failure of pressure transmission may be associated with urethral mobility under straining, although this is is not necessarily so.

URINE FLOW RATE

Definition and properties

The rate of flow of urine (or other liquid) is the volume voided per second (see Ch. 11). This is not quite as straightforward as it sounds, since the volume leaving the bladder per second may differ from the volume per second flowing in the external stream some 30 cm beyond the urethral meatus, and may differ still more from what is recorded by a flowmeter intercepting the stream. Obviously there is a delay before changes in the rate of flow out of the bladder are recorded by the flowmeter. To some extent it can be allowed for. However, a weak link in most flowmeters is the collecting funnel, which adds a further, variable delay that depends on the direction and angle of the stream. This can cause extra dips and peaks in the flow curve (Scott 1973; Rollema 1981). Consequently, isolated peaks in an otherwise smooth flow curve should be regarded as possible artefacts (Grino et al 1993).

Methods of measurement

Once the fluid has been collected, the flow rate can be measured in many different ways, each with its own peculiarities. The methods are of two main types.

Type 1: Direct measurement of flow rate The flow rate itself is measured and the voided volume calculated by integrating it with respect to time (Table 6.2). Type 1 methods can respond very rapidly to flow rate variations. However, to take full advantage of their speed the collecting funnel must be carefully designed or even abolished altogether (Ask et al 1985). Their main disadvantage is that, if a dribbling flow rates is too small to be registered, the voided or leaked volume will be underestimated.

Type 2: Measurement of voided volume The voided volume is measured and the flow rate calculated by differentiation with respect to time (Table 6.2). Type 2 methods tend to be slower in response, but time constants of about 0.2–0.3 s are attainable and this is probably short enough, given the limitations of most collecting funnels. Knocking the collecting vessel often produces a flow artefact.

PRESSURE-FLOW STUDIES OF MICTURITION

Aim

These are simultaneous, combined measurements of pressure and flow rate during voluntary or involuntary voiding. Usually the aim is to investigate the relation between the bladder pressure (intravesical or detrusor) and the corresponding flow rate. The basics of pressure-flow studies are discussed in Griffiths (1995).

Flow delay

The main complication is that the measured flow rate is delayed with respect to the bladder pressure that

Table 6.2 Methods of measuring urine flow rate.

Advantages	Disadvantages
Type 1 (Measurement of flow rate)	
1. Rotating disk (Dantec; Ask et al 1985)	
(a) direct measurement of the flow rate itself	(a) reading depends on density of liquid (water, X-ray contrast)
(b) quickness of response to changes, subject to limitations of funnel, if any	(b) may miss dribbling flows and underestimate voided volume
(c) insensitivity to mechanical disturbances such as knocks	(c) motor unit should be kept dry (older models)
	(d) difficult to clean
2. Air displacement method	
(a) measures flow rate (not volume)	(a) seems complicated and slow but has been improved
(b) not sensitive to knocks	
3. Electromagnetic	
(a) measures flow rate (not volume)	(a) zero tends to drift
(b) insensitive to knocks	(b) needs priming with water
4. Mechanical balance (Wiest, older models)	
(a) measures flow rate	(a) reading depends on liquid density
(b) small, waterproof transducer can be placed in normal toilet bowl	(b) not very accurate
	(c) needs priming, levelling and careful zero check
Type 2 (Measurement of voided volume)	
1. Weight of collected fluid (many different models use this principle)	
(a) simple	(a) reading depends on liquid density
(b) fast response	(b) sensitive to knocks
2. Pressure at bottom of collecting vessel	
(a) cheap and robust	(a) reading depends on liquid density
	(b) sensitive to knocks
	(c) slower response to changes
3. Electrical capacitance of immersed dipstick	
(a) cheap and robust	(a) sensitive to knocks
(b) relatively insensitive to properties of voided liquid	(b) slower response because of need to damp level disturbances
	(c) with insufficient damping, level oscillation artefacts
	(d) may need priming
	(e) apparently less accurate

Lists of advantages and disadvantages are not complete but based on personal observation and experience.

produces it. The delay should in principle be allowed for when analysing pressure-flow relations, especially if there are rapid variations of flow rate and bladder pressure. In principle the flow delay may be variable; it may depend for example on the flow rate. In practice satisfactory results are usually obtained by assuming a constant delay time of 0.5–1 s, depending on the equipment used (Schäfer 1983b).

Urethral obstruction and urethral resistance to flow

Urethral obstruction

Urethral obstruction may be due either to urethral overactivity or to faulty mechanics (International Continence Society 1988). In young patients extreme urethral or external meatal stenosis can occasionally cause mechanical obstruction (Griffiths & Scholtmeijer 1982), and a urethral catheter exaggerates the degree of obstruction. In adult patients, mechanical urethral obstruction is rare; if encountered it may be iatrogenic in origin. A poor urine flow is usually caused by a weak detrusor contraction and/or incomplete urethral relaxation (urethral overactivity). Such functional abnormalities may be either neurogenic or psychogenic in nature. Characteristically they are rather variable, resulting in complicated, changing patterns of pressure and flow.

Urethral resistance

If mechanical obstruction is suspected it may be important to have an objective measure of the elevated urethral resistance to flow. Unfortunately, the term urethral resistance tends to suggest (in analogy to the flow of electricity) something that is caused by energy losses due to viscosity and turbulent flow, and on this basis various different 'resistance factors' have been proposed, which purport to give a numerical value for the resistance. In fact, fluid flow through the urethra is not analogous to the flow of electricity, and the main part of the urethral 'resistance' is not usually due to viscous or turbulent energy losses (see discussion by Schäfer 1985). In particular, a finite pressure is needed to open up the urethra and so to allow any flow at all (Fig. 6.10). (This pressure is sometimes called the minimum urethral opening pressure, but a term that better describes what is actually measured is the minimum voiding detrusor pressure, $p_{det.min.void}$; International Continence Society 1997). Because the situation is quite different from the electrical analogy, the older resistance factors have little theoretical basis or clinical relevance.

Graphical and numerical expression of urethral resistance

Since urethral resistance means the relation between bladder pressure and urine flow rate for a given urethra, irrespective of its physical origin, a graphical method of expressing it is to be preferred (International Continence Society 1988) (see Fig. 6.10). If, however, a numerical value for the resistance is required (e.g. for statistical analysis), then there are several possibilities, including some newer resistance factors which are more soundly based than the older factors because they take $p_{det.min.void}$ into account.

Methods

1. ***Detrusor pressure at maximum flow*** For a normal, highly distensible urethra the detrusor pressure itself is quite a good measure of the urethral resistance. Often the maximum flow rate occurs when urethral overactivity is minimal, so that the detrusor pressure at maximum flow represents mainly the mechanical contribution to the urethral resistance. Certainly, if the detrusor pressure at maximum flow is low (< 20 cm H_2O), then mechanical obstruction can probably be ruled out, while if it is elevated (> 40 cm H_2O) then mechanical obstruction is possible but not proved.

An abnormally low detrusor pressure at maximum flow (< 10 cm H_2O) corresponds to a low urethral resistance, which may sometimes be clinically significant. However, even a normal value is already quite low (20–30 cm H_2O), so that a low value may be an artefact caused by small errors in the intravesical or abdominal pressure.

2. ***Obstruction nomogram*** It is helpful to judge the detrusor pressure at maximum flow in conjunction with the maximum flow rate itself, and this can be done graphically (Fig. 6.10). The nomogram shown was developed for assessing prostatic obstruction in men (Abrams & Griffiths 1979) and is not very suitable for women, who fall in nearly every case in either the unobstructed or the equivocal regions. A similar but revised nomogram is suggested by the International Continence Society as a provisional standard (International Continence Society 1997).

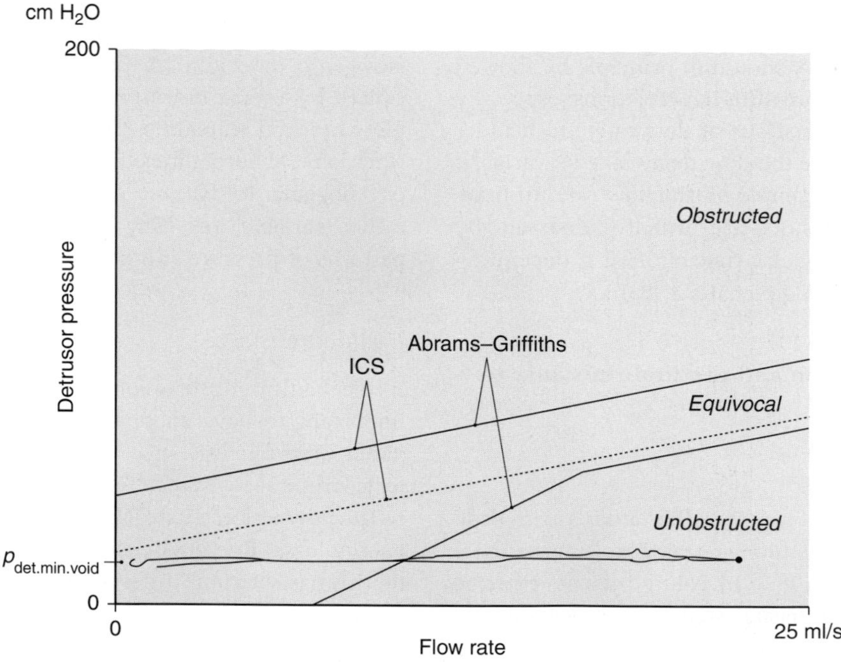

Fig. 6.10 Pressure/flow plot showing the minimum voiding detrusor pressure $p_{det.min.void}$, the Abrams–Griffiths obstruction nomogram and the ICS provisional nomogram for definition of urethral obstruction. The position of the maximum flow point (filled circle) shows that this micturition is classified as unobstructed by either nomogram.

A similar nomogram developed for male patients by Schäfer (the linear PURR, 1990) provides more grades of obstruction. Only a few of the lower grades are useful for women.

3. ***Maximum voiding detrusor pressure*** Because of the way that the bladder responds to urethral changes, the highest detrusor pressure is often attained not when the flow is maximum but when the urethra is least relaxed, that is, most nearly shut off. This maximum voiding detrusor pressure is then close to the isovolumetric detrusor pressure and gives more information about bladder function than about urethral resistance (see below).

4. ***Group-specific urethral resistance factor*** For patients of a given type, the voiding pressure–flow relationships tend to resemble one another, and in this case it may be possible to draw a series of average pressure–flow relationships that represent in an empirical way different degrees of urethral resistance in the group. Figure 6.11 shows such curves for a large group of adults, both obstructed and non-obstructed. All points on any one curve correspond, on average, to the same value of the urethral resistance. The detrusor pressure at the zero-flow point has been chosen to represent this resistance (URA) numerically. The curves for URA are based on measurements in both men and women, the pressure–flow curves for women tending to fall in the lower part of the figure. Because URA gives a very fine grading of urethral resistance, it is able in principle to detect differences between urethral resistance in different women, which are too small for the obstruction nomogram and the linear PURR to detect. However, for gynaecological studies it would be better to construct new curves based on measurements in a large group of adult women only.

URA can be calculated by computer but, since it is based on the maximum flow rate and the detrusor pressure at maximum flow, it can also be read off from the curves in Fig. 6.11.

Effect of urethral catheter

Even in young girls an 8 French gauge urethral catheter usually has very little mechanical effect on the urethral resistance (Griffiths & Scholtmeijer 1982). In a minority, with distal urethra or meatus calibrating at about 20 French gauge or less, it can cause significant obstruction. In true obstructive stenosis (calibre less than 16 French gauge) it exaggerates the degree of anatomical obstruction. For most patients, especially adults, this mechanical artefact is less important than the psychological one: the presence of a urethral catheter is just one of the circumstances surrounding a urodynamic examination that affect micturition by inhibiting both complete urethral relaxation and full development of the detrusor contraction.

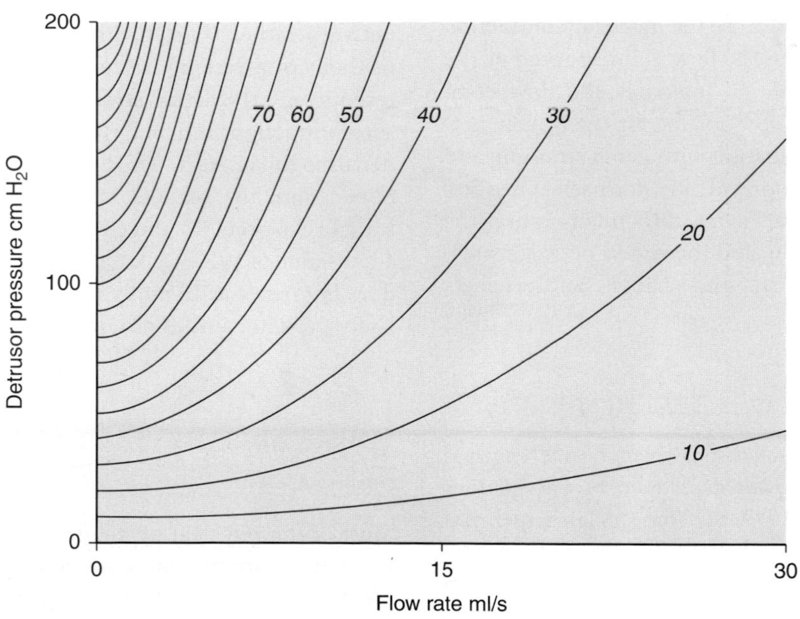

Fig. 6.11 Nomogram for estimating group-specific resistance factor URA from maximum flow rate (horizontal axis) and corresponding detrusor pressure (vertical axis). Each curve corresponds to a constant value of URA. The lower curves are labelled with this value in cm H_2O. For the upper curves URA continues to increase in steps of 10 cm H_2O.

Detrusor contractility

Aspects of contractility

Detrusor contractility has two different aspects: (a) the strength of the detrusor contraction; and (b) how well the contraction is sustained. An elevated postvoid residual urine is nearly always due to premature fading of the detrusor contraction, before the bladder is empty (Abrams & Griffiths 1979). Therefore residual urine reflects how well the contraction is sustained. The contraction strength is related to the flow rate developed. For example, a weak contraction will usually produce only a low urine flow rate, even if there is no urethral obstruction. (Of course, a low flow rate may alternatively be the result of urethral obstruction with a normal detrusor contraction strength.)

Strength of the detrusor contraction: isovolumetric detrusor pressure

If voiding is suddenly interrupted by sphincter action, the detrusor pressure often rises rapidly to a higher value. This behaviour reflects a fundamental myogenic property of the contracting detrusor – a trade-off between the pressure generated and the flow delivered. The detrusor pressure attained on stopping, the isovolumetric detrusor pressure, is in principle a more reliable measure of the strength of the detrusor contraction than the pressure during voiding, which depends also on the flow rate and therefore on the urethral resistance (Griffiths 1980, 1991). In practice, however, such a 'stop test' may be difficult to interpret because the detrusor contraction may be inhibited when the flow is interrupted or the patient may be unable to interrupt the flow completely, leading to too low a value for the isovolumetric pressure. In a micturition with much straining and little obvious development of detrusor pressure, interpretation is even more difficult because the interruption in the flow and the rise in detrusor pressure are masked by irregular changes and artefacts caused by straining.

Mechanical power and Watts factor (WF)

Another approach to detrusor contraction strength is via the mechanical power developed by the bladder (Abrams & Griffiths 1979; Schäfer 1983a), which has the advantage that it can be followed throughout micturition and does not require any special manoeuvres by the patient. Although the mechanical power alone (flow rate × detrusor pressure) is not in fact satisfactory, analysis of the myogenic behaviour of the bladder shows that a certain combination of detrusor pressure, flow rate and bladder volume (the Watts factor, WF) approximately represents the strength of the detrusor contraction (Griffiths et al 1986; Griffiths 1991). WF has units of $\mu W/mm^2$ (power developed per unit of bladder surface area). It includes a contribution representing the internal muscular processes as well as the purely mechanical power. Numerically (and conveniently) it is approximately equal to 1/10 of the isovolumetric pressure that would be measured (in cm H_2O) in a stop test.

WF can be calculated by computer. Since it varies throughout the course of micturition, the maximum value, or the value at maximum flow, can be used to characterize the strength of the detrusor contraction in that micturition. A value of WF much below 2 $\mu W/mm^2$ implies that the detrusor is hardly contracting at all. A value of, for example, 16 $\mu W/mm^2$ corresponds to a very strong contraction. Because of the way WF is constructed, a micturition in which the detrusor pressure is low but the flow is good may well correspond to an adequate detrusor contraction. Suppose, for example, that the detrusor pressure is 20 cm H_2O and the flow rate is 21 ml/s when the bladder volume is 300 ml. Under these conditions the calculated value of WF is 6 $\mu W/mm^2$. This certainly represents a reasonably good detrusor contraction: the corresponding isovolumetric detrusor pressure would be 60 cm H_2O.

WF, like other urodynamic variables, must not be calculated blindly. For example, if abdominal straining results in artefactual peaks in the recorded detrusor pressure, the value of WF should be examined in between rather than during these peaks. Like other methods of assessing detrusor contractility, WF represents only the actual strength of the current detrusor contraction and not the potential ability of the detrusor to contract. Thus a strong contraction, sustained until the bladder is empty, implies that contractility aspects (a) and (b) are both good. However, a low value of WF, or a large volume of residual urine, does not necessarily imply that the bladder could not contract better under other circumstances.

DESIRABLE DEVELOPMENTS

Most of the physical principles that are important in lower-tract urodynamics are understood, at least in theory. In actual practice some problems remain:

1 Because the physical principles are moderately complicated and are not completely understood

by all practising urodynamicists, measurements are quite commonly interpreted incorrectly.
2 Critical examination of measurements often reveals artefacts caused by poor technique or poor choice of methods. Even in experienced hands a complete urodynamic examination without artefacts is rare.

The solution to these problems is better education of urodynamicists in the underlying physical principles, the choice and use of equipment, and the recognition and elimination of artefacts. Further, the current wave of computerization of equipment may offer the opportunity to develop 'intelligent' machines that will recognize common errors and artefacts and prompt the operator to correct them before it is too late (Modur 1993).

ACKNOWLEDGMENT

The revision of this chapter was supported by a grant from the Alberta Heritage Foundation for Medical Research. I am grateful to Dr Pradeep Modur for allowing me to reproduce the examples shown in Fig. 6.1.

REFERENCES

Abrams P H, Griffiths D J 1979 The assessment of prostatic obstruction from urodynamic measurements and from residual urine. British Journal of Urology 51: 129–134

Abrams P H, Martin S, Griffiths D J 1978 The measurement and interpretation of urethral pressures obtained by the method of Brown and Wickham. British Journal of Urology 50: 33–38

Ask P, Engberg A, Oberg P A, Spangberg A 1985 A short-time-delay urinary flowmeter. Neurourology and Urodynamics 4: 247–256

Gleason D, Reilly R 1979 Gas cystometry. In: Clinical urodynamics. Urological Clinics North America 6: 143–148

Griffiths D J 1980 Urodynamics: The mechanics and hydrodynamics of the lower urinary tract. Adam Hilger, Bristol

Griffiths D J 1985 The pressure within a collapsible tube, with special reference to urethral pressure. Physics in Medicine and Biology 30: 951–963

Griffiths D J 1991 Assessment of detrusor contraction strength or contractility. Neurourology and Urodynamics 10: 1–18

Griffiths D J 1995 Basics of pressure-flow studies. World Journal of Urology 13: 30–33

Griffiths D J 1996 Pressure-flow studies of micturition. Urologic Clinics of North America 23: 279–297

Griffiths D J, Scholtmeijer R J 1982 Precise urodynamic assessment of meatal and distal urethral stenosis in girls. Neurourology and Urodynamics 1: 89–95

Griffiths D J, Constantinou C E, Van Mastrigt R 1986 Urinary bladder function and its control in healthy females. American Journal of Physiology 251: R225–R230

Grino P B, Bruskewitz R, Blaivas J G, Siroky M B, Andersen J T, Cook T, Stower E 1993 Maximum urinary flow rate by uroflowmetry: automatic or visual interpretation? Journal of Urology 149: 339–341

Hilton P, Stanton S L 1981a Urethral pressure measurement by microtransducer. II. An analysis of rotational variation. (Proceedings of eleventh annual meeting of International Continence Society, Lund, Sweden) pp 70–71

Hilton P, Stanton S L 1981b Urethral pressure measurement by microtransducer. IV. The effect of transducer design on the urethral profile. (Proceedings of eleventh annual meeting of International Continence Society, Lund, Sweden) pp 120–121

International Continence Society 1979 First, second and third reports on the standardisation of terminology of lower urinary tract function. Journal of Urology 121: 551–554

International Continence Society 1988 Standardisation of terminology of lower urinary tract function. Neurourology and Urodynamics 7: 403–427

International Continence Society 1997 Standardisation of terminology of lower urinary tract function: Pressure-flow studies of voiding, urethral resistance, and urethral obstruction. Neurourology and Urodynamics 16: 1–18

Modur P N 1993 Pattern recognition in urodynamics: an application to cystometry. MSc thesis, University of Alberta, Canada, pp 122–130

Plevnik S, Vrtacnik P, Rakovec S, Janez J 1981 Urethral softness distribution in the female urethra. (Proceedings of eleventh annual meeting of International Continence Society, Lund, Sweden) pp 84–86

Plevnik S, Janez J, Vrtacnik P, Brown M 1985 Directional differences in urethral pressure recordings: contributions from the stiffness and weight of the recording catheter. Neurourology and Urodynamics 4: 117–128

Rollema H J 1981 Uroflowmetry in males. Doctoral thesis, State University of Groningen, Netherlands, pp 40–42

Schäfer W 1983a Detrusor as the energy source of micturition. In: Hinman F Jr (ed) Benign Prostatic Hypertrophy. Springer-Verlag, New York, pp 450–469

Schäfer W 1983b The contribution of the bladder outlet to the relation between pressure and flow rate during micturition. In: Hinman F Jr (ed) Benign Prostatic Hypertrophy. Springer-Verlag, New York, pp 470–496

Schäfer W 1985 Urethral resistance? Urodynamic concepts of physiological bladder outlet function during voiding. Neurourology and Urodynamics 4: 161–201

Schäfer W 1990 Principles and clinical application of advanced urodynamic analysis of voiding function. Urologic Clinics of North America 17: 553–566

Scott F B 1973 Correlation of flow rate profile with diseases of the urethra in man. In: Lutzeyer W and Melchior H (eds) Urodynamics. Springer-Verlag, New York

Zinner N, Sterling A M, Ritter R C 1980 Role of inner urethral softness in urinary continence. Urology 16: 115–117

History and examination

STUART L STANTON

INTRODUCTION

Early description of disease relied much on the ability of the clinician to accurately record the history and clinical examination; confirmatory investigations were rudimentary, most information being provided by histological specimens either removed at operation or at post mortem. Complex and sophisticated investigations have gradually evolved, but we still rely on the history and examination to provide the framework for diagnosis.

HISTORY

Most history taking uses the patient's own words and is written in prose. More use is made now of a structured questionnaire entered directly onto a computer. This method has the following advantages:

1. Questioning is consistent without omission of data. This is important before an operation as the patient's recall of symptoms afterwards is frequently incomplete.
2. Recording is consistent within the department by different doctors.
3. It allows an efficient and rapid method of dealing with a large patient throughput.

A variety of questionnaires have been developed. There is significant evidence to show that the bladder is an unreliable witness and that at best history and examination indicate the nature and severity of the problem but will not necessarily give an accurate diagnosis (Bates et al 1973). Jarvis et al (1980) showed that clinical diagnosis was accurate in only 65% of cases. Cardozo & Stanton (1980) found that stress and urge incontinence were complaints in 55% of patients with urethral sphincter incompetence and in 35% of patients with detrusor instability. Farrar et al (1975) showed that symptom analysis, or the use of symptom complexes, was more accurate, reaching 96% accuracy in the diagnosis of some conditions. In a very selective group, Videla & Wall (1998) found that USI was confirmed in 97% of women fulfilling very strict criteria for the diagnosis of stress incontinence. However, where patients present to primary health care teams, symptoms of stress and urge incontinence are sufficiently predictable to enable the general practitioner to commence conservative treatment without the need for urodynamic studies (Largo-Jansen et al 1991). The severity of symptoms and their impact on the patient are impossible to assess with objective studies, and well validated questionnaires are essential to determine the quality of life. In developing a scale for measuring the impact of incontinence on a woman's daily life, an Incontinence Impact Questionnaire and a Urogenital Distress Inventory have been developed by the Continence Program For Women Research Group (Shumaker et al 1994). Both questionnaires include symptoms of prolapse and incontinence, so a range of pelvic problems are covered. They have been widely used in monitoring treatment.

Black et al (1996) developed a questionnaire to provide a measurement of stress incontinence for use in surgical studies, but this was less helpful for patients with mixed symptoms. Two further quality of life questionnaires need mentioning: The Bristol Female Urinary Tract Symptoms questionnaire covers all symptoms but has 33 items and is tediously long (Jackson et al 1996). A questionnaire developed by Kings College Hospital has been well validated for quality of life, but is less effective for severity of symptoms (Kelleher et al 1997).

Our first questionnaire was developed in 1978 (Cardozo et al 1978) and then modified by Krieger (personal communication, 1982) and by others since. The history includes urological, neurological, gynaecological, bowel, medical, psychiatric, drug and past history questions and is graded for frequency of occurrence of symptoms and their severity but does not include quality of life.

Urological

Incontinence (Table 7.1)

The most common presenting symptom at a urogynaecology clinic is incontinence, which needs careful evaluation. Stress incontinence is a symptom and sign and not a diagnosis. It must be distinguished from urgency leading to urge incontinence. Incontinence has to be defined: is it intermittent or continuous, precipitated by effort, present at rest, on seeing running water or putting the key in the door, on intercourse or orgasm, as the patient stands up, or at night? The severity of incontinence is measured by the number of changes of incontinence pads.

Postmicturition dribble This occurs after micturition as the patient stands up and may be due to urethral diverticulum or alteration of vaginal anatomy following resection of the rectum.

Continuous incontinence This occurs with an ectopic urethra, epispadias, urinary fistula or retention with overflow. Frontal lobe lesions may produce a lack of social awareness and lead to incontinence at an inappropriate time and place.

Urgency

This is the sudden desire to void, which, if uncontrolled or unfulfilled, may result in urge incontinence. Urgency on its own is a commonplace symptom. Bungay et al (1980) found that 20% of women between 30 and 64 years of age had urgency. The common causes are indicated in Table 7.2.

Frequency

This is defined as more than seven times during the day and nocturnal frequency is arousal from sleep twice or more at night. Urgency and frequency are often linked, and it is tempting to think that there

Table 7.1 Conditions causing incontinence.

Condition	Symptom
USI (GSI)	Stress incontinence
Detrusor instability	Stress incontinence, urgency, and urge incontinence, frequency and nocturia, enuresis, urgency on inserting the key in the door, seeing running water, drinking coffee or on orgasm
Urethral diverticulum	Postmicturition dribble
Fistula	Continuously wet
Urinary retention	Frequency, stress incontinence and continuously wet
Voiding difficulty	Poor or intermittent stream, hesitancy, incomplete emptying, straining to void

Table 7.2 Causes of urgency, urge incontinence and frequency.

Urgency/urge incontinence & frequency	Additional causes of frequency
Urinary tract infection	Increased fluid intake
Upper motor neurone lesion	Impaired renal function
Irritative mucosal lesion	Reduced bladder capacity
Urethral syndrome	Pelvic mass
Detrusor instability	Chronic residual urine
Habit	Diabetes insipidus
	Diabetes mellitus
	Increased age
	Diuretic therapy
	Hypothyroidism
	Hypercalcaemia
	Hypokalaemia

may be a vicious circle of frequency leading to urgency leading to more frequency. We have shown that the operative cure of one is associated with the cure of the other (Stanton et al 1976). The common causes of frequency are indicated in Table 7.2.

The incidence can be charted by a patient using a urinary diary or frequency/volume chart (Fig. 7.1) that records input and output volumes with a note of episodes of urgency and leakage.

Voiding difficulty

Most women are completely unaware of their voiding ability and potential; they have little concept of stream velocity or cast distance. They are aware of

DAY: THURSDAY . 22. 4.

TIME	INTAKE (ml)	OUTPUT (ml)	LEAKAGE ACTIVITY	Amount	Urge	Wet Bed
01.10		120cc			Yes	
02.50		120cc			Yes	
05.10		120cc			Yes	
07.35		90cc			Yes	
08.35	240cc	60cc			Yes	
09.25		60cc			Yes	
10.30			Sneezed	Soaked Underwear		
10.55	240cc					
11.30		90cc			Yes	
12.50		90cc			Yes	
1.00	240cc					
2.15	240cc	90cc			Yes	
3.15	240cc		Coughed	Few drops		
4.45		90cc			Yes	
6.10			Coughing	Soaked Underwear		
6.35		60cc			Yes	
7.00			Getting out of bath	Emptied bladder		
7.30	240cc					
9.00		120cc			Yes	
9.10	240cc					
10.00		210cc			Yes	
10.30		180cc			Yes	
11.05		60cc				
TOTAL	1680cc	1560cc				

Fig. 7.1 Urinary diary showing daily input and output, timing and amount of leakage and whether or not associated with urgency. What activity has precipitated this can be recorded.

hesitancy, difficulty in voiding, poor stream, having to stand to void, and incomplete emptying, but these symptoms may be uncommon. The prevalence of symptoms of confirmed voiding disorders in new attenders at a urogynaecology clinic is 12%. A further 2% had asymptomatic voiding difficulty (Stanton et al 1982). No single symptom seemed to accord more accurately with the clinical situation, but 'poor stream' was the most common. Hesitancy is an uncommon symptom, but its postpartum prevalence in a group of healthy women without previous urological abnormality is 8–10% (Stanton et al 1980). Acute retention, which is the most serious symptom, needs to be defined and is 'an inability to empty the bladder which may be painful or painless, requiring catheterization for relief.' The volume removed should be noted and should be at least 50% of the functional bladder capacity. Hilton & Laor (1989) found that a poor urinary flow or intermittent stream are more reliable than the other symptoms and correlated better with urodynamic parameters.

Neurological

The occurrence of bladder disturbances due to neurological disease makes it imperative that a neurological history and examination are completed. Questions should be directed towards general neurological disease, and particularly motor and sensory abnormalities affecting sacral roots S2, 3 and 4. The common neurological diseases are multiple sclerosis, peripheral neuropathy associated with diabetes mellitus, cerebrovascular accidents, Parkinsonism and autonomic dysreflexia (with symptoms of sweating, palpitations and headaches). The patient should be questioned about blurred or double vision, back pain, disturbance of balance, alteration in bowel control, lower limb sensation and motor power.

Gynaecological

Because of the close embryological, anatomical and physiological relationships between the urological and genital tracts, lesions of either may affect both.

The urothelium is oestrogen-sensitive and dependent. This means that urological symptoms will vary with the menstrual cycle and bladder function has been found to change correspondingly (Shimonowitz et al 1997). The symptomatic and cytological changes associated with postmenopausal oestrogen deficiency are well known.

The association of genital prolapse with stress incontinence is established. About 40% of patients with urethral sphincter incompetence will have significant anterior vaginal descent (Cardozo & Stanton 1980).

The relationship between urological symptoms and gynaecological surgery is important. Occasional repair of uncomplicated prolapse may cause postoperative urethral sphincter incompetence, believed to result from operative interference and postoperative scarring of the urethral sphincter mechanism. In a pre- and postoperative study of anterior colporrhaphy and vaginal hysterectomy for prolapse, with or without stress incontinence, we could find no evidence of increase in symptoms of postoperative urgency and frequency (Stanton et al 1982). Thakar et al (1998), in preliminary findings on a study on the effects of hysterectomy on bladder and bowel, found a significant reduction in symptoms of nocturia and stress incontinence after hysterectomy. There was no difference in bowel function. Colposuspension may cause dyspareunia, groin pain and symptoms and signs of enterocele and rectocele. Frequency and urgency are usually decreased following colposuspension, but they may arise de novo, with or without detrusor instability.

Cyclical variation of detrusor instability with urge incontinence and frequency coinciding with menstruation has been reported by Wall & Warrell (1989). These symptoms responded satisfactorily to mefenamic acid given before and during menstruation.

Ovarian and uterine enlargement may cause frequency and sometimes urinary retention when impaction occurs. Endometriosis involving the bladder can lead to frequency, urgency and cyclical haematuria. Frequency and urgency may also be associated with pelvic inflammatory disease.

Bowel symptoms include: frequency of bowel emptying, constipation, incomplete bowel emptying requiring vaginal or anal digitation or splinting, and a feeling of prolapse. Incontinence may vary from soiling, lack of flatal control or frank incontinence.

Medical

Any condition increasing abdominal pressure – for example, constipation or chronic cough – may induce stress incontinence due to urethral sphincter incompetence by altering the pressure gradient between bladder and proximal urethra. Cardiac and renal failure will produce frequency, and diabetes mellitus and inspidus should be considered when polydipsia and polyuria or frequency appear.

Psychiatric history taking is discussed in detail in Chapter 35. For elderly patients who may have dementia, a dementia score to determine the awareness and degree of understanding and cooperation is helpful in their assessment (Table 7.3). The patient's appearance and behaviour at the interview, mood state, form and content of 'talk', and intelligence and orientation are important observations. Various self-administered psychiatric questionnaires are available for patient assessment, e.g. the Wakefield Self-Assessment of Depression Inventory (WDI) to detect depression; Middlesex Hospital Questionnaire (MHQ) to detect neuroticism; and the Minnesota Multiphasic Personality Inventory (MMPI) to detect personality change. Referral to a psychiatrist is advisable where psychiatric disease is suspected.

Drug

The current drug regimen is important. Drugs taken for gynaecological symptoms or other conditions may affect the lower urinary tract. In the case of diuretics, it is important to confirm that the patient is taking the drug at the correct time, as sometimes nocturia can be caused by late administration of a diuretic.

Non-steroidal anti-inflammatory drugs and cyclophosphamide can cause cystitis-like symptoms. Alpha-adrenergic blockers may aggravate stress incontinence, and tricyclic antidepressants, in a sensitive patient, can lead to voiding difficulties.

Past

The obstetrical history should include parity, method of delivery, and weight of the largest infant. The length of labour may be incorrectly recalled by the patient and may not be helpful.

All past major surgery, particularly pelvic and back surgery, should be recorded. Urinary tract infection and its treatment should be enquired about, and whether or not positive bacterial culture was obtained before treatment.

Table 7.3 Dementia score.

1.	Age
2.	Time (nearest hour)
3.	Address for recall at end
4.	Year
5.	Name of this hospital
6.	Recognize two people
7.	D.O.B. (day & month sufficient)
8.	Year of start of World War I
9.	Name of present monarch
10.	Count back from 20–1
10a.	Recall address

EXAMINATION

It is important, at the outset, to place the patient at ease by reassuring her that no embarrassment should be felt if she is incontinent during the course of the examination. The attitude and demeanour of the patient and any obvious personality or mental disorder should be noted. The height and weight of the patient are recorded and a simple 'score' made of her mobility (for example, walks unaided, requires a walking stick, or is restricted to a wheelchair).

Neurological

A simplified neurological examination should be performed on all patients. The pupils are tested for pupillary reflex and nystagmus; the lower limbs are tested for tone, power, reflex and sensation, paying attention particularly to sacral root dermatomes S2–S4 (Fig. 7.2); the back is examined for lesions such as spina bifida (overt or occult Fig. 7.3), and spondylosis. A rectal examination is carried out to assess anal sphincter tone.

Special neurological tests to confirm an intact sacral reflex include stroking the skin lateral to the anus to elicit contraction of the external anal sphincter and tapping and squeezing the clitoris, which will produce a contraction of the ischio- and bulbocavernosus muscles.

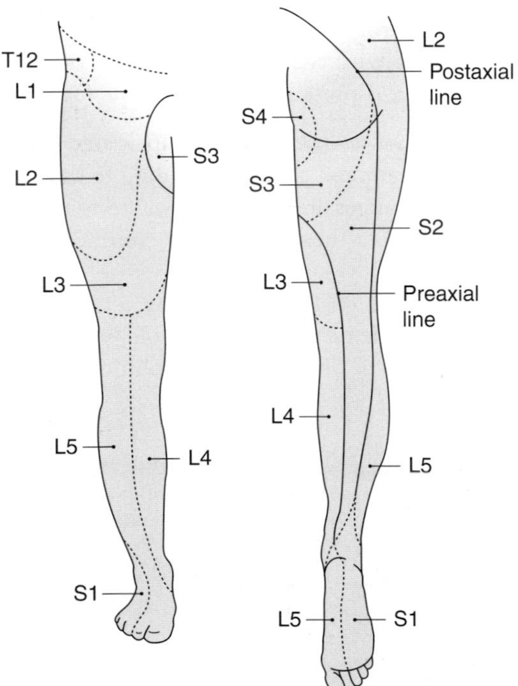

Fig. 7.2 Cutaneous distribution of lumbar and sacral nerve roots.

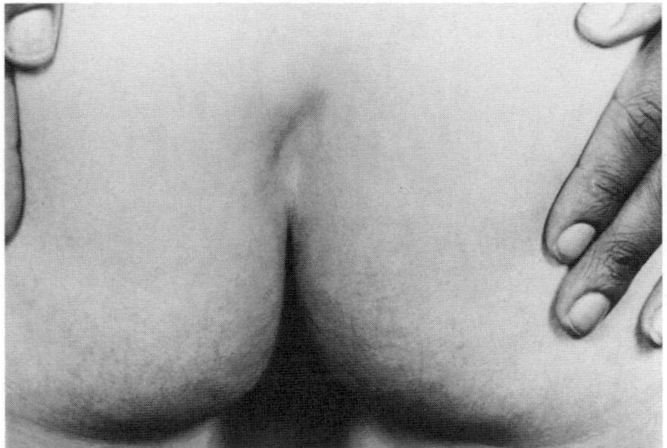

Fig. 7.3A Sacral hollow found overlying spina bifida occulta of S2 to S4.

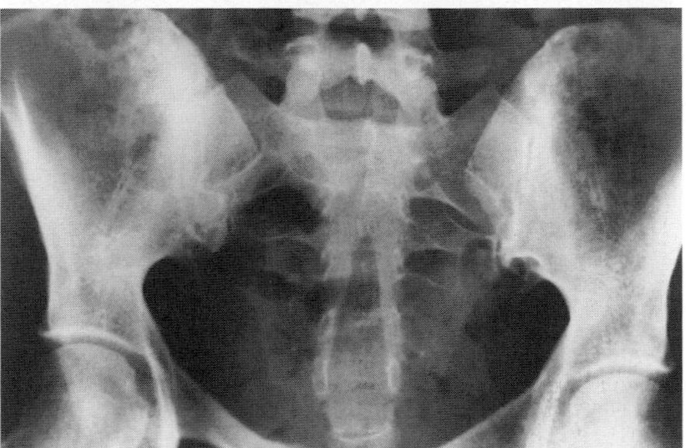

Fig. 7.3B Radiograph showing spina bifida occulta of S2 to S4.

Referral to a neurologist is advised if the neurological history and examination are abnormal or when upper or lower motor neurone lesions are detected on cystometry.

Gynaecological

As part of the abdominal examination, renal enlargement and a palpable bladder should be detected. Vulval excoriation will give some indication of the severity of incontinence. A bimanual examination will allow ballottement of the bladder by the vaginal finger and a crude estimate may be made of the residual urine. Congenital abnormalities such as epispadias (Fig. 7.4) will be evident but an ectopic ureter may be more difficult to detect. The presence of stress incontinence may be detected in the supine or erect position and is more noticeable when the patient has a comfortably full bladder. Undue 'wetness' within or around the vagina needs differentiation between a healthy vaginal discharge (which is clear or opalescent and asymptomatic) and pathological vaginal discharge (which is creamy or yellow and may be offensive, and is associated with symptoms of vaginal discomfort and the presence of vaginitis) and an ectopic ureter or fistula.

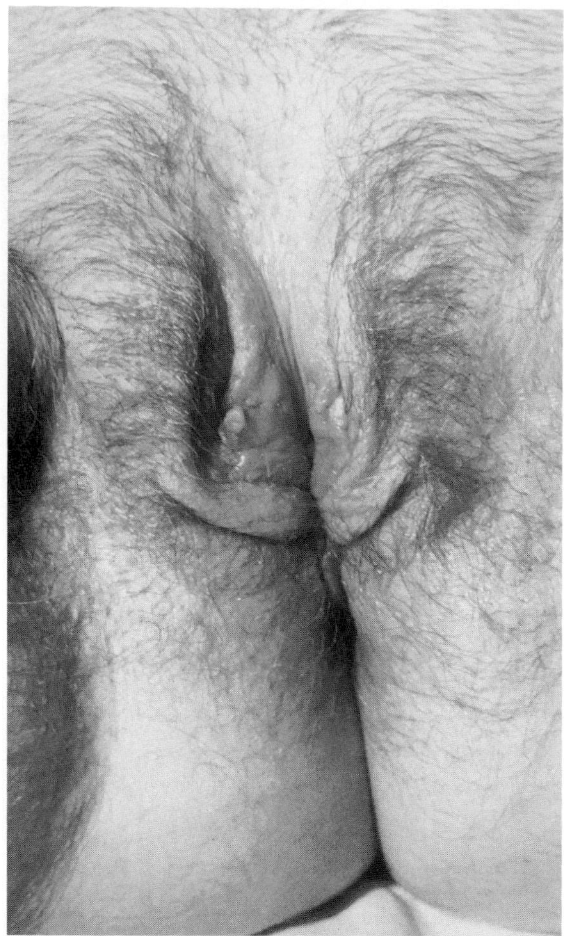

Fig. 7.4 Epispadias showing separation of clitoris and local absence of pubic hair indicating the underlying defect.

Any atrophic genital change is noted and the capacity and mobility of the vagina is determined by attempting to elevate the lateral fornix towards the lateral pelvic side wall and the ipsilateral ileopectineal ligament. This may be compromised by past pelvic surgery and may limit the choice of subsequent bladder neck surgery.

The urethra is examined for tenderness, discharge and fixity. An adjacent anterior vaginal wall mass may be either a urethral diverticulum or a paraurethral or vaginal cyst. A bimanual examination will confirm the presence of abnormal pelvic organs or masses and detect any bladder enlargement.

Genital prolapse, comprising descent of the anterior or posterior vaginal wall and uterus or vault, may be detected on coughing and straining with the use of a Sims or similar speculum in the supine and erect position. Some clinical grading of prolapse is important. Anterior vaginal prolapse is divided into cystocele and cystourethrocele – a urethrocele on its own is very rare. Vault descent often cannot be differentiated from enterocele, and sometimes the distinction is only academic because the true nature of the prolapse may only be revealed at surgery. Descent may be Grade 1 – within the vagina; Grade 2 – to the introitus; Grade 3 – beyond the introitus.

To provide a more scientific assessment of prolapse the ICS Standardization Committee produced a site-specific system for prescribing, quantifying and staging pelvic floor descent (Fig. 7.5A,B,C) (Bump et al 1996). It has been validated and takes about 3 to 4 minutes. Stages have been described in accordance with the staging of pelvic organ prolapse as follows:

- 0 No prolapse and all points are 3 cm above the hymen.
- I All points are more than 1 cm above the hymen.
- II Maximal prolapse point protrudes to or beyond 1 cm above the hymen but not more than 1 cm below.
- III Maximal prolapse point protrudes beyond 1 cm below hymen but less than 2 cm less than the total vaginal length.
- IV Maximal prolapse point protrudes the length of the vagina with complete inversion of the vagina and cervix if present.

The pelvic floor muscle is carefully palpated to determine its strength and gauged according to the Oxford Scale which ranges from 0 where there is no movement, to 5 where there is a strong contraction (Laycock 1994).

The examination is concluded by a rectal examination to exclude rectal or anal pathology, to quantify a rectocele and to determine anal sphincter integrity and tone.

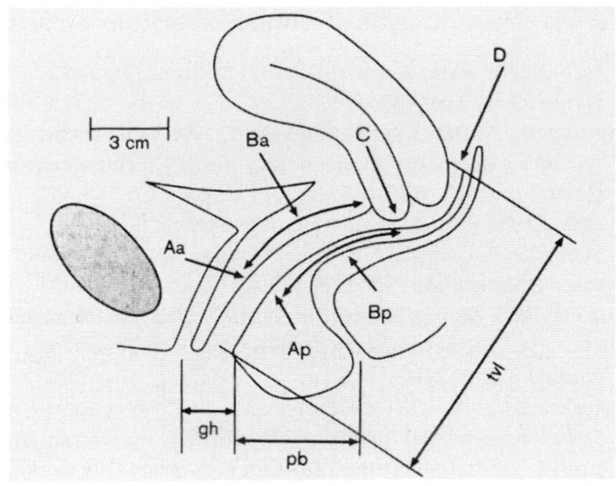

(A)

(B)

anterior wall **Aa**	anterior wall **Ba**	cervix or cuff **C**
genital hiatus **gh**	perineal body **pb**	total vaginal length **tvl**
posterior wall **Ap**	posterior wall **Bp**	posterior fornix **D**

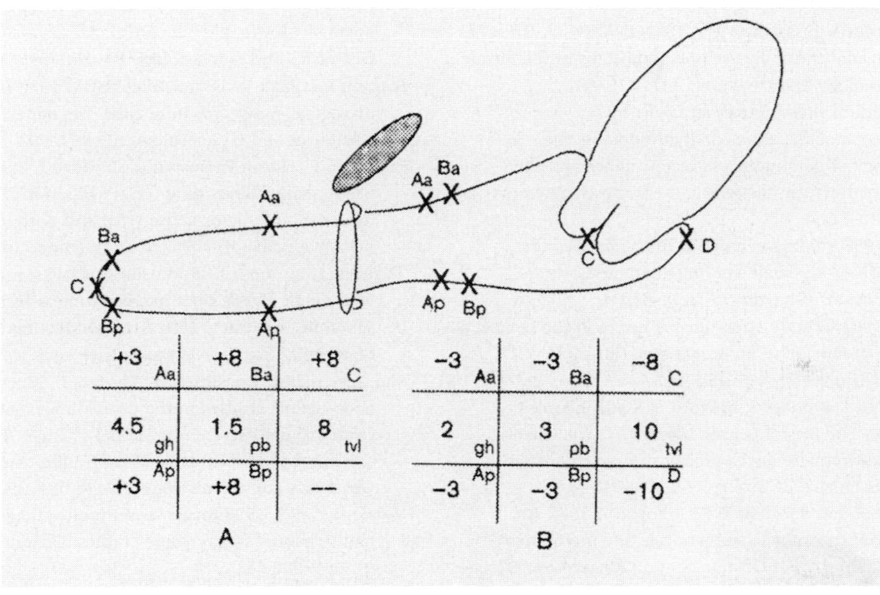

(C)

Fig. 7.5 ICS prolapse classification. **A** Nine points of measurement used for the pelvic organ prolapse quantification: two on the anterior vaginal wall (Aa, Ba), one on the most distal part of the cervix (C), the posterior vaginal fornix (D), two points on the posterior vaginal wall (Bp, Ap), the genital hiatus (gh), the perineal body (pb), and the total vaginal length (tvl). **B** A 3 × 3 grid for recording quantitative description of pelvic organ support. Negative numbers are used for points cranial to the hymen and positive numbers for points caudal or distal to the hymen. **C** Grid and line diagram: A – demonstrating Stage IV eversion of the post-hysterectomy vagina. The most distal point of the anterior wall (Ba), vaginal cuff scar (C) and the most distal point of the posterior wall (Bp) are all in the same position (+8). Points Aa and Ap are maximally distal (+3). Vaginal length is 8 cm, genital hiatus 4.5 cm and the perineal body is 1.5 cm. B – Normal support (Stage 0 prolapse) without hysterectomy. Points Aa, Ba, Ap and Bp are all –3 as there is no descent of the anterior and posterior vaginal walls. The lowest point of the cervix (C) is 8 cm (–8) proximal to the hymen and the posterior fornix is 2 cm above this (–10) Vaginal length is 10 cm, genital hiatus is 2 cm and the perineal body 3 cm. From Bump et al (1996), with permission.

REFERENCES

Bates C P, Loose H, Stanton S L 1973 Objective study of incontinence after repair operations. Surgery, Gynecology and Obstetrics 136: 17–22

Black N, Griffiths J, Pope C 1996 Development of a symptom severity index and a symptom impact index for stress incontinence in women. Neurourology and Urodynamics 15: 630–640

Bump C, Mattiasson A, Bo K et al 1996 The standardisation of terminology of female pelvic organ prolapse and pelvic floor dysfunction. American Journal of Obstetrics and Gynecology 175: 10–17

Bungay G T, Vessey M P, McPherson C K 1980 Study of symptoms in middle life with special reference to the menopause. British Medical Journal 281: 181–183

Cardozo L, Stanton S L 1980 Genuine stress incontinence and detrusor instability: a review of 200 patients. British Journal of Obstetrics and Gynaecology 87: 184–190

Cardozo L, Stanton S L, Bennett A E 1978 Design of a urodynamic questionnaire. British Journal of Urology 50: 269–274

Farrar D J, Whiteside C G Osborne J L, Turner-Warwick R T 1975 A urodynamic analysis of micturition symptoms in the female. Surgery, Gynecology and Obstetrics 141: 875–881

Hilton P 1981 Urethral pressure measurement by microtransducers: observations on methodology, the pathophysiology of genuine stress incontinence and the effects of its treatment in the female. M D thesis. University of Newcastle-upon-Tyne

Hilton P, Laor D 1989 Voiding symptoms in the female: the correlation with urodynamic voiding characteristics. Neurourology and Urodynamics 8: 308–310

Hodgkinson C P 1963 Urinary stress incontinence in the female: a programme of preoperative investigations. Clinics in Obstetrics and Gynaecology 6: 154–177

Jackson S, Donovan I, Brookes S, Eckford S, Swithinbank L, Abrams P 1996 The Bristol Female Lower Urinary Tract Symptoms questionnaire development and psychometric testing. British Journal of Urology 77: 805–812

Jarvis G J, Hall S, Stamp S, Millar D R, Johnson A 1980 An assessment of urodynamic examination in the incontinent woman. British Journal of Obstetrics and Gynaecology 87: 893–896

Kelleher C J, Cardozo L D, Khullar V, Salvatore S 1997 A new questionnaire to assess the quality of life of urinary incontinent women. British Journal of Obstetrics and Gynaecology 104: 1374–1379

Largo-Jansen A, Debruyne F, Van Weel C 1991 Value of the patient's case history in diagnosing urinary incontinence in general practice. British Journal of Urology 67: 569–572

Laycock J 1994 Clinical evaluation of the pelvic floor. In: Schussler B, Laycock J, Norton P, Stanton S L (eds) Pelvic Floor Re-education. Springer-Verlag, London, p. 42–48

Shimonovitz S, Monga A, Stanton S L 1997 Does the menstrual cycle influence cystometry? International Urogynecology Journal 8: 213–216

Shumaker S A, Wyman J F, Uebersax J S, McClish D, Fantl J A 1994 Health-related quality of life measures for women with urinary incontinence: the Incontinence Impact Questionnaire and the Urogenital Distress Inventory. Continence Program in Women (CPW) Research Group. Quality of Life Research 3: 291–306

Stanton S L, Williams J E, Ritchie D 1976 The colposuspension operation for urinary incontinence. British Journal of Obstetrics and Gynaecology 83: 890–895

Stanton S L, Kerr-Wilson R, Harris V G 1980 Incidence of urological symptoms in normal pregnancy. British Journal of Obstetrics and Gynaecology 87: 897–900

Stanton S L, Hilton P, Norton C, Cardozo L et al 1982 Clinical and urodynamic effects of anterior colporrhaphy and vaginal hysterectomy for prolapse with and without incontinence. British Journal of Obstetrics and Gynaecology 89: 459–463

Thakar R, Stanton S L, Robinson G, Clarkson P, Shah K, Manyonda I 1998 Does hysterectomy affect bladder and bowel function? Abstract, 28th Annual Meeting of International Continence Society, Jerusalem

Van Geelen J M, Doesburg W, Thomas C, Martin C 1981 Urodynamic studies in the normal menstrual cycle: the relationships between hormonal changes during the menstrual cycle and the urethral pressure profile. American Journal of Obstetrics and Gynecology 141(4): 384–392

Videla P, Wall L 1998 Stress incontinence diagnosed without multi-channel urodynamic studies. Obstetrics and Gynecology 91: 965–968

Wall L, Warrell D W 1989 Detrusor instability association with menstruation. Case report. British Journal of Obstetrics and Gynaecology 96: 737–738

General urological investigations

CHRISTOPHER R J WOODHOUSE

INTRODUCTION

Urology and gynaecology are closely related specialties. The gap that now exists will not be closed by this chapter, but by a knowledge of the barest outline of 'urological' investigation one specialist may get a little insight into the workings of a near neighbour.

URINE INVESTIGATIONS

Dipsticks

The examination of urine has a pedigree as old as medicine. There can be no investigation that is as cost-effective as the 'stick' test of urine. The most widely used general stick test costs only a few pence and its slowest component takes 45 s to react. Eight parameters are tested in a qualitative and, in seven, a semi-quantitative way. There can be no justification for failing to stick test the urine of all new patients.

The components of the stick test are:

- pH
- Blood
- Ketones
- Bilirubin
- Glucose
- Urobilinogen
- Protein
- Nitrites.

There is not space to review the significance of positive results from these tests. All are important in their different ways and will indicate a particular line of further investigation.

Urine culture and the mid-stream urine (MSU)

Urine is normally sterile. On stick testing, the presence of nitrites is highly suggestive of infection (but the finding of protein, contrary to popular superstition, is not). Bacteria reduce urinary nitrates to nitrites. The bacteria and urine must be in contact for long enough for this reaction to occur; in effect this means 'incubation' in the bladder for 1 to 2 hours and so the test may never become positive in patients with the gross frequency of bacterial cystitis. It is of most value with the first specimen passed in the morning.

A stick test for urinary leucocyte esterase is also available (Cytur). A positive result correlates with 10 or more leucocytes per millilitre. A positive result in both tests indicates a significant urinary infection but is still not a substitute for urine culture.

Urine for culture must be collected and stored without contamination. The system for collecting a mid-stream urine (MSU) is well-known and therefore often neglected. The labia must be held apart while the perineum is cleaned with sterile water or soft soap (not disinfectant which may contaminate the specimen). Occasionally the patient may have so copious a vaginal discharge that a swab or tampon may have to be inserted to keep the periurethral area clear. The middle part of the urinary stream is collected in a sterile bottle.

The specimen must be sent to the laboratory for microscopy and culture within 2 hours. If delay is unavoidable, because, for example, the patient is collecting the specimen at home, it may be kept in the ordinary fridge at 4°C for up to 2 days.

In the laboratory, microscopy allows the estimation of the number of bacteria, red and white blood cells. Bacteria can usually be seen on high power light microscopy when more than 30 000 organisms per ml are present; thus virtually all cases of urinary infection should have visible bacteria. Occasional blood cells are a normal component of urine because there is a constant daily loss of blood into the urinary tract. More than 5 white blood cells per ml constitutes significant pyuria.

On culture, a pure growth of bacteria is indicative of infection of the urine. The number of bacteria and the number of white cells should only be considered in association with the clinical circumstances. It is assumed that each colony found on culture has arisen from a single organism. Traditionally, a count of 10^5 organisms per ml is taken as the level for infection. This may well be relevant in a patient with no symptoms but not in one with gross frequency and dysuria: if a patient has appropriate symptoms and a pure culture of less than 10^5 organisms, she may still be suffering from bacterial cystitis (see Chapter 29).

Other findings on microscopy

Microscopy of a urine specimen less than 4 hours old can provide a wealth of diagnostic information. In urological practice, the commonest finding is of asymptomatic haematuria. The finding of red blood cells on microscopy must always be taken as seriously as if the blood were visible to the patient.

In patients over 50 years old with microscopic haematuria, the incidence of significant findings is between 10% and 20%, most of which are malignancies.

In those under 50 years the incidence is 2 to 10%, usually due to stones, specific infections (eg: bilharzia, TB), and various forms of nephritis, while cancer is a rare finding.

The gynaecologist will often be faced with this problem and should consider referral of all such patients to a urologist without delay. There are several myths about microscopic and gross haematuria that must be laid to rest if serious mistakes are to be avoided.

1 Even a single episode must be investigated as cancers frequently bleed only once and then remain quiescent for many months.
2 Haematuria must never be blamed on infection unless there is a positive urine culture. Even with a positive culture, painless haematuria may well have another cause, the bacteruria being coincidental.
3 Dipstick haematuria requires investigation even if the microscopy is negative. The red cells may well have undergone lysis by the time the urine reaches the laboratory.
4 Microscopic proteinuria and haematuria together are far more likely to be caused by glomerulonephritis than by urinary infection.
5 The normal urinary tract does not bleed, even in the presence of full anticoagulation. Therefore haematuria should not be blamed on anticoagulants, aspirin or blood dyscrasias unless appropriate investigations of the urinary tract have proved to be negative.

Cytology (Figs 8.1 and 8.2)

Neoplasms of the urinary tract (particularly those of transitional cell origin) shed surface cells into the urine. The cells may be collected from the urine after microfiltration and identified by Papanicolaou stain-

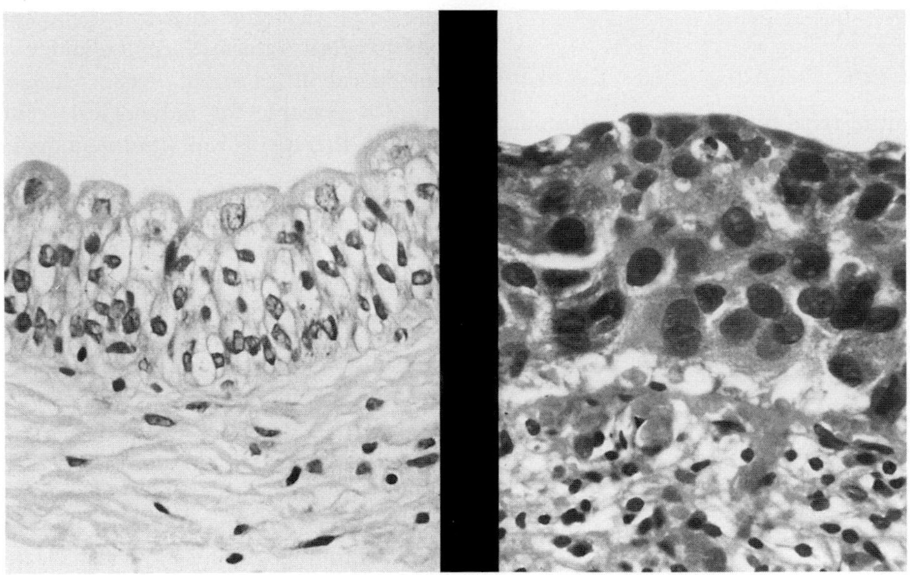

Fig. 8.1 Haemotoxylin- and eosin-stained sections of normal urothelium (left) and carcinoma *in situ* (right).

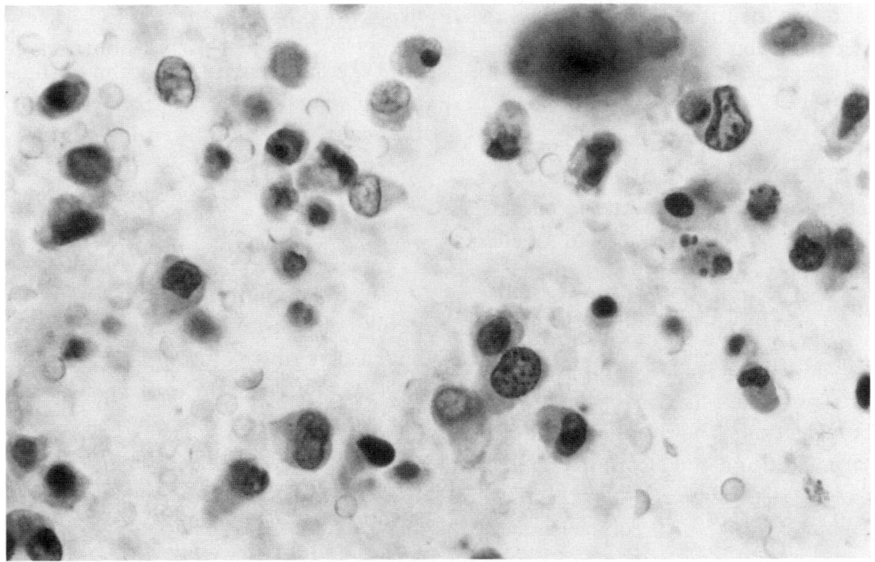

Fig. 8.2 Malignant transitional cells similar to those in Fig. 8.1 (right) from microfiltered and Papanicolaou-stained urine.

ing. Cells may be found in any urine, but the second full specimen passed in the morning usually has the highest concentration. The test is a useful screen for transitional cell carcinoma of the urothelium. It should always be ordered for patients with painless haematuria or unexplained painful frequency. Carcinomas that are well differentiated may shed cells that are too similar to normal transitional cells to be identifiable. Very deeply invasive cancers may have too small a surface area to shed enough cells to identify. As so often, a positive investigation is significant while a negative one does not rule out cancer.

Bladder tumour antigens

Bladder carcinomas also shed antigens of varying specificity into the urine. Testing the urine with appropriate agglutinating antibodies can detect the presence of cancers with a specificity and sensitivity similar to that achieved by cytology. A commercial kit (Bard BTA test) that can be used in the clinic is now available and is cheaper than cytology.

BLOOD INVESTIGATIONS

The measurement of renal function is important, at a crude level, in all patients undergoing major surgery. In a few urological patients and in patients receiving chemotherapy, a precise measurement of renal function is essential.

The simplest screen of renal function is estimation of the plasma electrolytes urea and creatinine. It is reasonable to accept that a patient with normal values in these parameters has good enough kidneys for major surgery. The urea and creatinine do not rise until about two thirds of the renal function has been lost.

When an accurate measure of renal function is needed it is usual to measure the glomerular filtration rate (GFR). Its direct measurement is not possible in clinical practice and so it is measured indirectly by the clearance of a substance which is freely filtered and not handled at all by the tubules. For many years, creatinine clearance has been used. For this it is necessary to measure the concentration in plasma and in a 24 h urine collection.

Creatinine clearance measurement is rather cumbersome and a 24 h urine collection is open to error. When the facilities are available it is better to measure the clearance of ethylene ditetra acetic acid labelled with Cr^{51} (Cr^{51}EDTA). This compound fulfils the criteria for measurement of GFR. It is injected intravenously and, after the first 10 min, its clearance from the blood stream has a linear relationship with the GFR. Blood samples are taken at two or three fixed intervals after the injection. The activity counts of the whole blood are made and the clearance rate calculated. The method is more accurate than creatinine clearance and, of course, quicker. Errors arise if the injection extravasates or if the patient is oedematous and the isotope can accumulate outside the circulating blood.

RADIOLOGICAL INVESTIGATIONS

In the last 10 years the technology of 'imaging' has undergone a revolution. The intravenous urogram (IVU) has been moved from its pre-eminent position in urology to being one of many equals. Increased sophistication has made it even more important to decide the question that is to be answered and to select the investigation accordingly.

Imaging investigations may be roughly divided into those that give anatomical and those that give physiological information. Radiology gives mainly anatomical information. Recent developments have made it possible for radiological techniques to be used for therapy as well (interventional radiology).

The intravenous urogram

Preparation

Most radiology departments have given up routine preparation before an IVU. Some give a laxative on the night before, especially if the patient is known to be constipated; most recommend 4 h of starvation. Dehydration is seldom used and is dangerous in patients with renal failure, diabetes or multiple myeloma. High doses of modern contrast media combined with tomography allow visualization of the urinary tract through the overlying bowel shadows.

The plain film

All IVUs start with a plain film of the kidneys, ureters and bladder. Aside from the non-urological lesions, the main value is to identify stones which would be obscured by the contrast.

Physiology of contrast media

Intravenous contrast medium has two main components: a radio-opaque part which is based on iodine and a carrying solution which is usually based on sodium. There is little to choose between the commercially available media.

With normal renal function at least 300 mg/kg of iodine are needed and double in renal failure. This is a volume of 70–100 ml. Currently used solutions are isotonic and cause fewer side-effects than the older hyperosmolar contrasts. Even this osmolar load is dangerous in the sick infant and as it gives little useful information in this group the IVU has rightly disappeared from neonatal practice.

In a few patients the injection is complicated by a 'reaction' which may be severe or even fatal. It is of unknown aetiology but is at least partly related to the concentration of dissociated iodine ions. It is not a true allergy as it may occur with first exposure and may not be repeated on subsequent exposures. It begins within a few minutes of injection and consists of vasodilatation, urticaria and bronchospasm. The blood pressure may drop and cardiac arrest occasionally follows. Treatment should be started at once with intravenous hydrocortisone and antihistamine. Intubation and ventilation may be necessary. If the reaction is mild, subsequent IVUs should be covered with prophylactic hydrocortisone and antihistamine. If the reaction is severe the investigation should not be repeated.

In isotonic solutions the concentration of dissociated iodine ions is very low. The isotonicity means that the unpleasant sensations of contrast injection are minimal. The bound iodine makes reactions and other side-effects uncommon. These media are safer but, inevitably, more expensive. They should always be used in children, the elderly and in patients with diabetes, renal failure or cardiac disease. In most departments they are used as a routine for all patients.

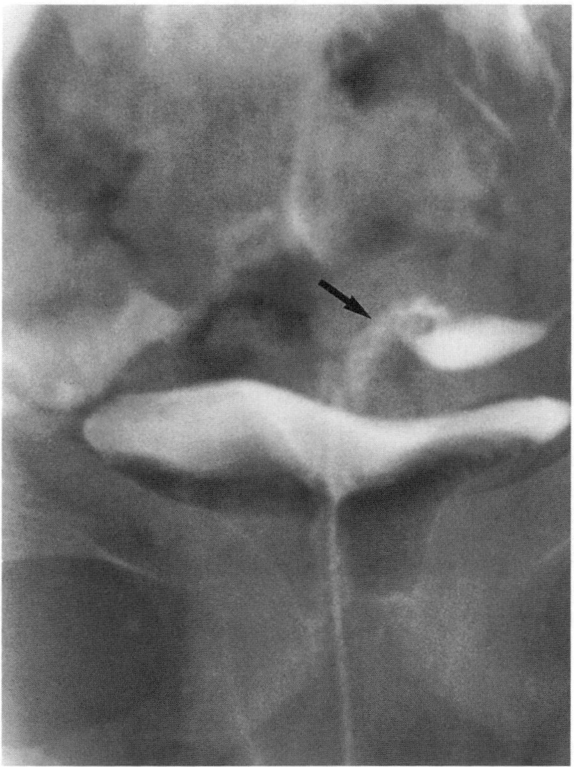

Fig. 8.3 Retrograde ureterogram of the left ureter showing a ureterovaginal fistula.

The urogram

The urogram provides excellent anatomical but little physiological information. The first phase, the nephrogram, is seen as the contrast is being filtered and passing down the tubules. The whole renal outline should be seen. A delayed nephrogram indicates diminished blood supply; a prolonged one indicates renal obstruction or acute tubular necrosis.

In the second phase, the contrast, providing it has been concentrated adequately by the nephrons, fills the calyces, renal pelvis and ureter. Their overall size and shape are seen.

It is a serious error to try to derive physiological information from this phase of the examination. Although the concentration of contrast depends on renal function, there are so many other factors involved that apparently poor concentration cannot be attributed to low GFR. Likewise, it must be absolutely understood that dilatation of the collecting system is not synonymous with obstruction.

The third phase occurs when the bladder fills. The patient should begin the IVU with an empty bladder. If this is done, the contrast will fill the bladder and give a good view of its outline. However if there is residual urine, the contrast will sink to the bottom of the bladder and the outline will be false. Furthermore, unless many oblique films are taken, it cannot be certain that the whole periphery is seen. The fact that more than 30% of IVUs on patients with invasive bladder cancer show no abnormality is an indication of the limited value of the bladder films.

The patient should be allowed to fill the bladder as much as possible before being sent to void in private.

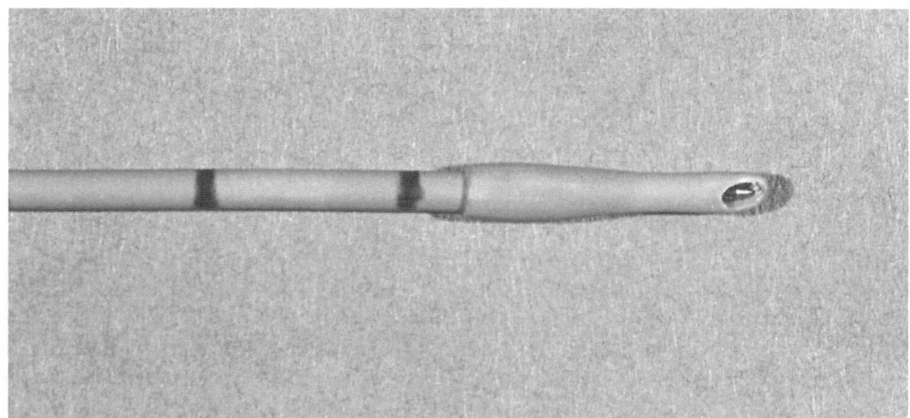

Fig. 8.4 Bulb-ended (Chevassu) ureteric catheter for retrograde ureterograms.

The film taken after micturition is often the best for showing small filling defects such as neoplasms. The residual contrast is open to much misinterpretation. If the bladder empties completely it shows that there is no residue; if emptying is incomplete it may only mean that in the embarrassing circumstances of the examination the patient did not manage to empty the bladder completely.

When patients have hydroureter it is useful to note whether the upper tracts empty after micturition. Obstructed ureters will not, while those whose emptying is prevented by high bladder pressure usually do. In any case, the urine in the dilated upper tracts acts as a residue and, regardless of other factors, will predispose to infection.

Micturating cystourethrogram (MCU)

This examination is of most value when combined with a cystometrogram (Ch. 9). In women its principal use is in the detection of vesico–ureteric reflux and, very occasionally, urethral diverticula (Ch. 10).

Ureterograms

As the technique of IVU has improved, the requirement for ureterogram has diminished. If a ureter draining a functioning kidney is poorly visualized on IVU, the IVU should be repeated, if necessary with a higher dose of contrast, with preparation of the bowel and abdominal compression. Should this fail, the ureter can be filled by a retrograde catheter at cystoscopy or antegradely after a percutaneous puncture of the renal pelvis.

Retrograde ureterogram is useful to identify fistulae and lower ureteric carcinomas (Fig. 8.3). It should be avoided in the obstructed ureter as there is a risk of causing upper tract infection. The only exception to this general advice is when the obstruction is thought to be an untreatable cancer and the clinician does not want to introduce a nephrostomy. Its role lessens all the time and the ureteroscope is taking over as it allows visualization, biopsy and endoscopic surgery.

If the examination is to be done, it should not be spoilt by poor circumstances. The ureteric orifice should be catheterized with a bulb-ended catheter (Fig. 8.4). The injection of contrast should be watched on the image intensifier and, when lesions are seen, static films should be taken for subsequent review. A high-quality image intensifier, with a memory and print capacity, is essential. Modern, mobile machines now fulfil these criteria and it is most convenient to do such imaging in theatre or in a dedicated radiological procedures room.

Antegrade puncture of the renal pelvis is done under local anaesthetic in X-ray. A large obstructed pelvis is quite easy to hit without any special aids. A smaller target requires X-ray or ultrasonic guidance. Once the needle is in position, contrast is injected. When injecting contrast either up or down a ureter, very high pressures can be generated and the pelvis ruptured: the examiner should remember not to push too hard on the syringe. If the system is obstructed the residual urine should be aspirated before injection.

Antegrade ureterogram gives much better visualization of the upper urinary tract. If the system is obstructed, the needle is replaced by a small catheter to provide continuous drainage. Percutaneous nephrostomy has now become the investigation and emergency treatment of choice for the obstructed kidney, especially when infection is present. In cases of doubtful obstruction, antegrade can be combined with a pressure measurement during perfusion (see below).

Computed tomography (CT scan)

In urology, CT is used for the definition of cancers and their metastases. In the pelvis, CT has not yet replaced the examination under anaesthetic for the definition of operability. In the retroperitoneum, however, no other investigation can give comparable information. Three-dimensional reconstruction programmes for spiral CT scanners have reduced the radiation exposure and immeasurably improved the imaging of this area.

The only conflict is in the assessment of pelvic lymph nodes. CT scanning is unreliable for the identification of nodes that are less than 1 cm in diameter. So far, magnetic resonance imaging (MRI) seems to be no better. (For a fuller discussion of CT and MRI, see Chapter 10.)

ULTRASOUND

Ultrasound has been widely used in obstetrics and gynaecology for many years. For medical imaging, frequencies of 1–10 megahertz (MHz) are used. Sound waves are reflected at every tissue interface but the amount of reflection depends on the difference in their mechanical properties. The intensity of reflection is proportional to the square of the difference of their acoustic impedances. Thus the interface between two soft tissues is poor, while that between soft tissue and fluid is good. Waves of this frequency do not penetrate bone or stones so the image beyond these structures is blank, the so-called acoustic shadow. In the pelvis, ultrasonography is done through a full bladder so that the urine provides an interface with the soft tissue; it is of limited use in patients who have no bladder or are unable to keep it full.

External beam ultrasound will identify the majority of bladder carcinomas, providing the bladder is full and the whole wall is scanned. However, it is not consistent enough to exclude definitely the presence of a carcinoma. It cannot, therefore, replace the cystoscopy in patients with haematuria or on follow-up for bladder carcinoma. As a screen for patients with non-specific symptoms it is useful; for example, in men with benign prostatic hypertrophy it has proved more useful than an IVU. It is very much better than radiography and safer than catheterization for the measurement of post-void residual urine (Ch. 14).

In the upper urinary tract it can distinguish between solid renal lesions, which are always significant, and cystic ones, which are almost never significant, with 98% confidence (Fig. 8.5). In renal carcinoma, ultrasound can identify renal vein and vena caval invasion. Dilatation and sites of obstruction, especially stones, are easily seen. Needles can be placed accurately with ultrasound guidance for aspiration and biopsy.

Because it is safe and painless, it is particularly useful to monitor the progress of a disease. It is often necessary to use other modalities to establish a diagnosis, for example renal obstruction. Thereafter serial ultrasounds can be used to watch the changes with treatment.

It must always be remembered that ultrasound is a clinical investigation. In some countries, particularly Germany, ultrasound is performed by the clinician. It is almost impossible, in urological practice, to look at the hard copy to confirm or refute the ultrasonographer's opinion. The clinician, therefore, must trust the ultrasonographer sufficiently to act on his or her opinion. The investigation is useless when done by an unknown stranger with no knowledge of the specialty in general or the patient in particular.

ISOTOPE SCANS AND RENOGRAPHY

Many compounds whose renal handling has been defined can be labelled with radioactive isotopes. After injection, their passage through the urinary tract can be followed by renography or scintigraphy on gamma camera. These investigations give physiological and some anatomical information.

Renography

The plotting of radioactivity counts will provide a graph of the isotopes' passage. Poor renal uptake (as

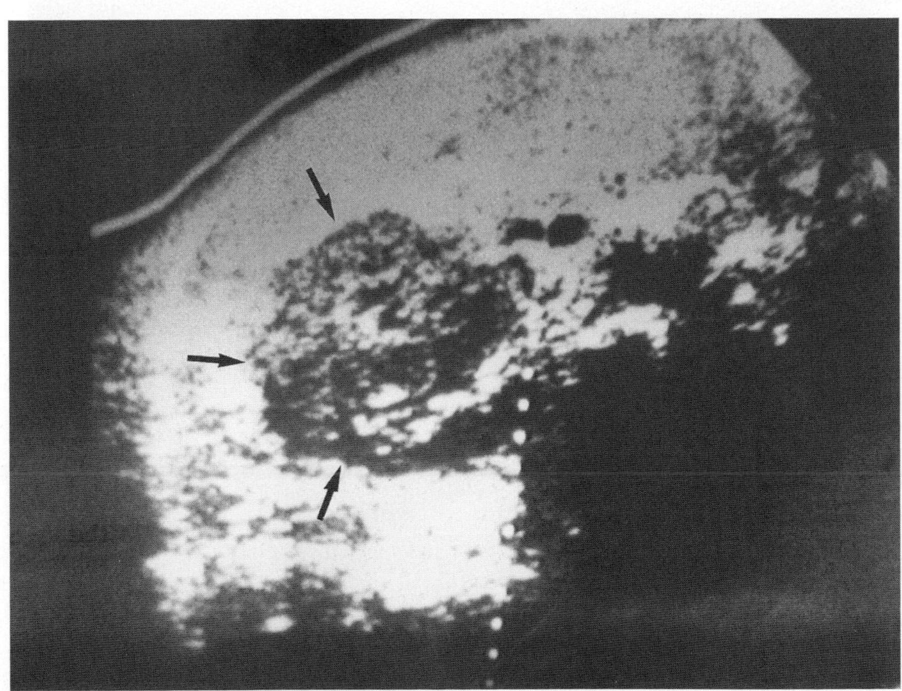

Fig. 8.5 Ultrasound scan of a kidney with an echogenic mass at the upper pole (left) typical of adenocarcinoma.

in vascular disease) and delayed clearance (as in obstruction) are seen. ^{131}I-Hippuran was the first compound in general use. It has now been replaced by ^{99m}Tc-DTPA and MAG 3 (see below) which also give excellent gamma camera pictures. MAG 3 produces better images and a more accurate differential function, but is more expensive.

Scintigraphy

Two types of compound are commonly used for scintigraphy and the information they provide is totally different.

DTPA and MAG 3

^{99m}Technetium-diethylene-triamine-penta-acetic acid (DTPA) and mercapto-acetyl-triglycine (MAG 3) are wholly filtered by the glomeruli and are ignored by the tubules. Therefore, once they have been taken up, their clearance depends on the drainage system of the kidney. Serial gamma camera pictures, combined with scintigraphy counts, can identify points of obstruction within small areas of the kidney, at the pelviureteric junction or in the ureter. In doubtful cases, the picture can be clarified by increasing the urine flow with frusemide (Fig. 8.6).

The initial uptake of DTPA and MAG 3 depends on

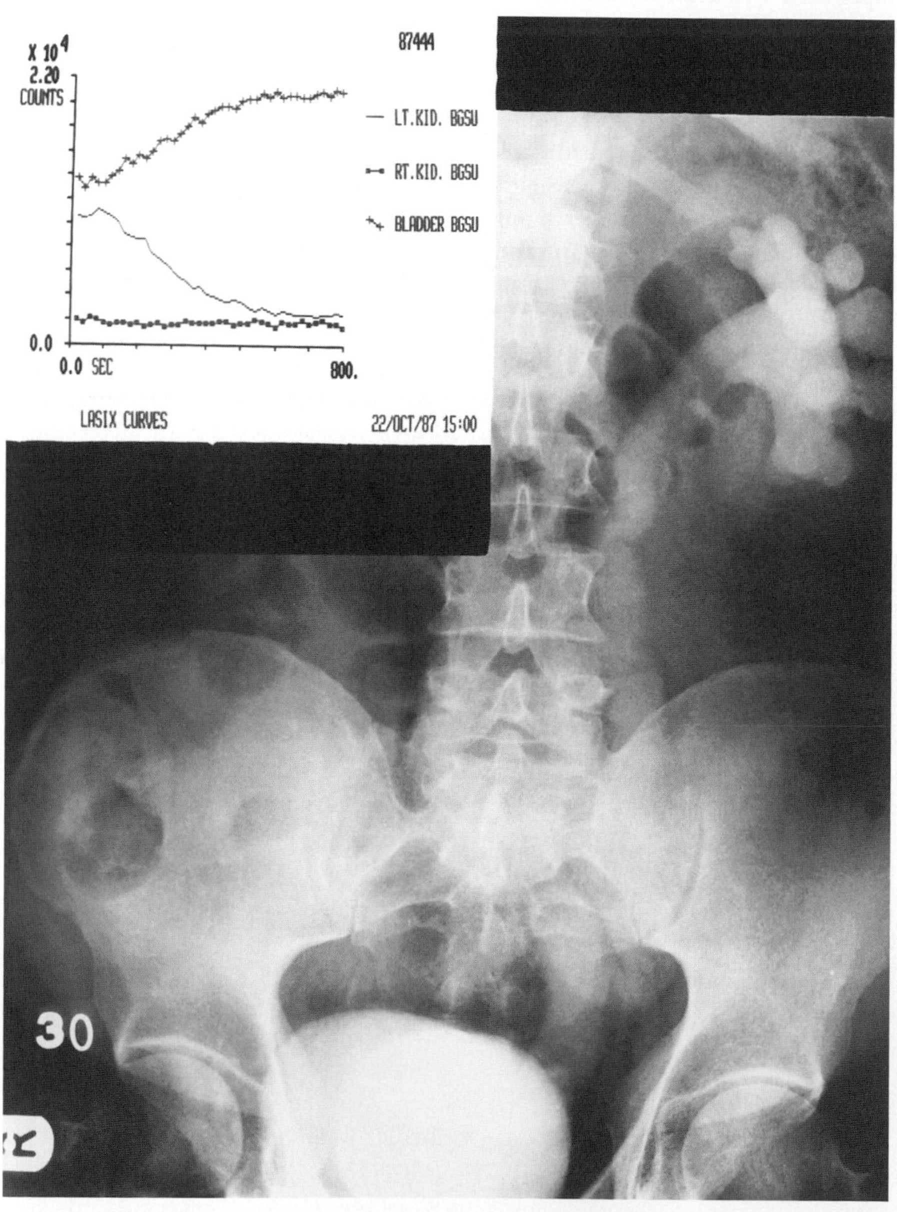

Fig. 8.6 IVU of a patient with left hydronephrosis and hydroureter. The DTPA renogram, superimposed, shows that there is good clearance of the isotope after frusemide, indicating that the left system is not obstructed.

the glomerular filtration rate. Therefore the relative contribution of each kidney to the overall function can be calculated. However, it must be remembered that the function is measured under the prevailing conditions and does not predict what will happen to function after treatment. On the assumption that treatment will not make the function worse, the test can sometimes be used to identify kidneys that still have useful function and therefore should not be sacrificed. The IVU cannot be used for this purpose.

DMSA

^{99m}Technetium-dimer-capto-succinate (DMSA) is excreted slowly through the tubules and is almost independent of the transport system. Immediate uptake depends on renal function and so much the same information is given as in the early pictures of the DTPA or MAG 3. Later pictures identify functioning tissue: it is therefore used to see renal scars and to distinguish tumours from pseudo-tumours (Fig. 8.7).

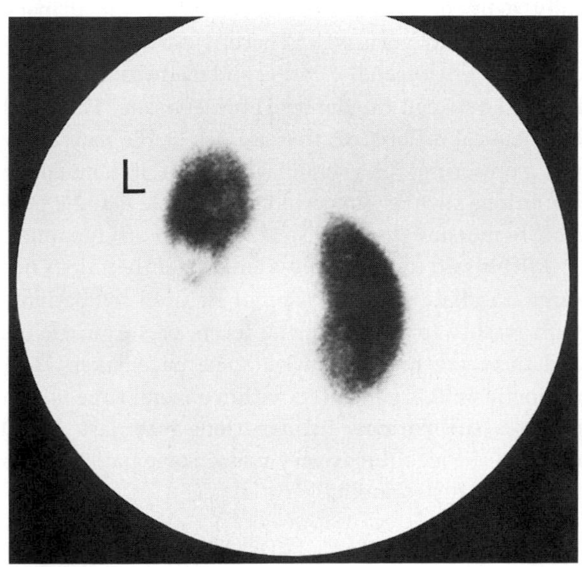

Fig. 8.7 DMSA isotope scan of a patient with unilateral reflux nephropathy. One kidney is small and scarred.

Bone scan

^{99m}Technetium-labelled methylene diphosphonate is taken up by osteoblastic activity in bones. Positive areas of uptake are, therefore, seen in areas of inflammation, infection, degeneration and metastasis. It is not specific but remains the best and earliest method of identifying bone metastases. In carcinoma of the prostate, it will be positive up to 6 months before bone lesions can be seen on X-ray.

ANTEGRADE PRESSURE STUDIES (WHITAKER TEST)

It has already been said that a dilatated urinary tract is not necessarily obstructed (as in Fig. 8.6, for example). Diagnosis of obstruction takes up much urological effort and is made more difficult by the absence of a clear mathematical definition. Even where a diagnostic system is recognized, there is a large 'grey area' of equivocal obstruction.

If there is a 'gold standard' for obstruction it is the antegrade pressure/flow study devised by Whitaker. The apparatus is shown diagrammatically in Figure 8.8. The measurement made is the pressure difference between the renal pelvis and the bladder when the former is perfused at a constant rate of 10 ml/min. The test is done with the bladder full and empty, as

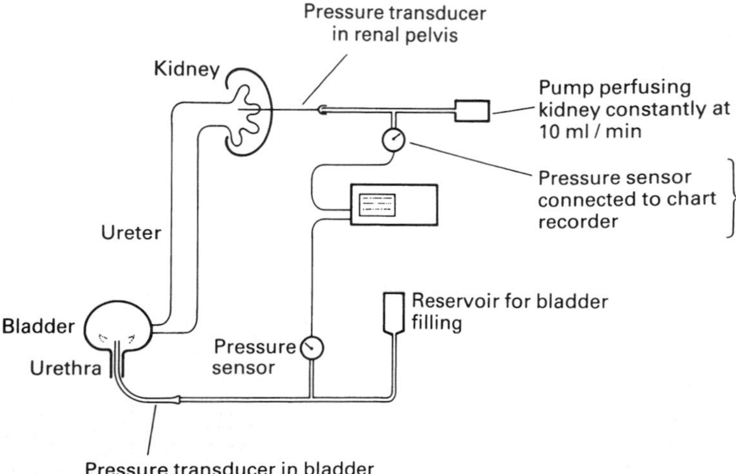

Fig. 8.8 Diagram of the apparatus for a Whitaker pressure/flow study. (From Thompson F D, Woodhouse C R J 1987 *Disorders of the Kidney and Urinary Tract*. Edward Arnold, London, with permission.)

some obstructions are only apparent when it is full. A pressure differential of less than 15 cm water means unobstructed, up to 22 cm is equivocal and above that means obstructed.

This test has the serious disadvantage that it requires a percutaneous nephrostomy and a urethral catheter. In units where it is performed frequently, it is accurate and reproducible. There are a small number of false positives and negatives. Many of the cases that show equivocal obstruction on other tests give the same result with the Whitaker test, which may lead to the conclusion that the kidney is partly obstructed for part of the time.

In practice, most clinicians will begin the investigation of a dilatated system with an isotope study using frusemide. If the function of the kidney is good, the dilatation not of long standing and the test result in accordance with the clinical findings, no further confirmation is necessary. If these criteria are not fulfilled, especially with a poorly functioning kidney and a chronically dilatated system, a Whitaker test is indicated. In a few patients with very difficult problems it is reasonable to monitor the differential function over a year: a kidney that maintains its function is unlikely to have significant obstruction.

MAGNETIC RESONANCE IMAGING (MRI)

The MRI imaging machine measures the response of hydrogen nuclei to varying magnetic fields and radio frequencies. The magnetic resonance is altered by the biochemical environment of the atoms and by their position in the magnetic field.

These physical properties are converted into visual and biochemical information of clinical relevance by computer software similar to that developed for CT scanning.

MRI produces finer anatomical detail than the CT scanner. Furthermore, as the direction of the magnetic field is infinitely variable, the body can be scanned in any axis. Small magnetic coils are now available to allow examination of the pelvic organs through the rectum (endorectal coils). Contrast media are occasionally used.

The role of this medium in urology, especially in a hospital that already has a CT scanner, has yet to be fully defined. The anatomical detail of the urinary tract is shown very well. There is particularly good distinction between the cortex and medulla of the kidney and between tumour and normal tissue. The small biochemical differences that are detectable may allow the monitoring, or even diagnosis, of inflammatory conditions such as glomerulonephritis. It may be possible to measure flow and so be useful in urodynamics.

MRI is said to be harmless and certainly it does not carry a radiation risk. It cannot be used for patients with freshly implanted metal joints or surgical clips and there are problems with some pacemakers. The magnetic field is generated within a metal tube which encloses the patient. Examinations may last 30–60 min and the machine is very noisy. Some patients suffer from claustrophobia.

FURTHER READING

Amis E S, Newhouse J H (eds) 1991 Essentials of Uroradiology. Little, Brown, Boston

Mundy A R, Stephenson T P, Wein A J (eds) 1994 Urodynamics – principles, practice and application, 2nd edn. Churchill Livingstone, Edinburgh

Newall R G (ed) 1990 Clinical Urinalysis. Ames Division, Miles Ltd, Stoke Poges

Retik A B (ed) 1990 Paediatric urinary tract obstruction. Urologic Clinics of North America vol 17.2

Theologides A D, Jameson R M, Scott A 1971 The reliability of urinary cytology. British Journal of Urology 43: 598–602

Whitaker R H 1973 Methods of assessing obstruction in dilated ureters. British Journal of Urology 45: 15–21

Cystometry and videocystourethrography

PEGGY A NORTON

INTRODUCTION

Urodynamic testing is often necessary to diagnose correctly the type of urinary incontinence and to identify the most appropriate treatment options. Cystometry is the central test in urodynamics, by which bladder storage and emptying functions can be studied. The term 'cystometry' literally means 'to measure the bladder', including the pressures originating within and outside the bladder; and the paper tracing produced is a cystometrogram (CMG). There are simple cystometric techniques which are widely available, and performing these tests is within the scope of many physicians who provide primary care to women. Combined with a good history and physical examination, simple cystometry can provide a presumptive diagnosis and the formulation of an initial treatment scheme, especially if the treatments are conservative in nature. Complex cystometry requires special training and equipment, and is performed by persons with a special expertise in incontinence usually in a tertiary care setting. Understanding complex cystometry will help the physician understand when such testing is indicated, and will improve his or her technique in simple cystometry.

Before describing the technique of cystometry, it is important to consider these points:

- Cystometry should augment but not replace the clinical assessment of the incontinent woman. The test cannot evaluate some important social or quality of life issues, and cannot replace the physician–patient interaction in deciding symptom priority and treatment options. Cystometry cannot be read like an electrocardiogram: the study must be conducted by clinicians familiar with the history and physical findings, so that testing can be individualized according to the patient's symptoms.
- Cystometry is conducted in artificial, laboratory settings which may not reflect the 'real life' settings in which our patients experience urinary incontinence. Therefore, failure to demonstrate incontinence as described by the patient does not imply that the patient is unreliable in her history.

Rather, we have failed to reproduce the circumstances which provoke incontinence in her real life.

- Tests should be performed if they will influence or alter the diagnosis, if risk factors need assessment, and if management might be altered by information from testing. If the history and examination point to a simple (presumptive) diagnosis and treatment scheme, then cystometry may not be necessary. A healthy woman with occasional stress incontinence might enquire about initial non-surgical options. As long as inexpensive, low risk options can be offered which improve her condition, cystometric testing will not alter the management of such an individual.
- The aim of urodynamic testing is to gain information about bladder function. In truth, we measure the physical properties of the bladder (capacity, pressure, volume, and compliance) and make inferences about function. The measurement may adversely affect function, such as the woman who voids in an abnormal pattern only because she is being observed in a testing situation. We must always consider whether the measurement of physical bladder properties corresponds to function or dysfunction in our patients.

CYSTOMETRY

This urodynamic test has many variations depending on the purpose of the evaluation. In the *storage* function of the urinary bladder, increasing bladder volume should be accepted without a significant increase in bladder pressure. Although a normal bladder may initiate small detrusor contractions during normal filling, these are easily suppressed by the individual and are often asymptomatic. Bladder dysfunction may be seen during the storage phase when detrusor contractions cannot be inhibited, resulting in the sensation of urgency, urge incontinence, or pain. Loss of urine in the absence of detrusor contractions may occur with increased intra-abdominal pressure (stress incontinence).

In the *emptying* function of the urinary bladder, voluntary contraction of the detrusor muscle is coordinated with relaxation of the urethral sphincter, allowing efficient micturition at a time and place of the woman's own choosing. Disorders of emptying in women are less common than in men, but may be seen after anti-incontinence surgery.

Indications for cystometry

Cystometry is usually performed in conjunction with other urodynamic testing, and it is the major diagnostic test to distinguish detrusor instability from genuine stress incontinence. Indications for simple cystometry include the evaluation of women with clear-cut symptoms of urge or stress incontinence, especially those who are interested in conservative management and who have not had previous treatment failures. Simple cystometry can provide information on bladder sensation, bladder capacity, may differentiate urge from stress incontinence, and may indicate that further testing is needed. Consideration of surgical intervention is an important indication for cystometry. In some clinicians' hands, simple cystometry confirming stress incontinence after a careful history and examination may be sufficient to offer anti-incontinence surgery to the female patient. However, it is remarkable how many women undergo surgery for symptoms that are clearly urge incontinence. It may be that some of the benefit of complex urodynamic testing is to consult with someone trained to carefully differentiate types and severity of continence, and to weigh potential risks and benefits of treatments available.

Complex cystometry should be the first-line evaluation in women with mixed or unclear symptoms, failed therapies including previous anti-incontinence procedures, known or suspected neurological disorders, history of radical pelvic surgery or pelvic irradiation, significant voiding complaints, and women with significant pelvic organ prolapse. Some authors have suggested studying women who are at special risk for diagnostic or therapeutic errors (Bump et al 1993), such as elderly women or black women (because of a higher prevalence of urge incontinence). Cystometry may evaluate risk factors such as potential voiding dysfunction after anti-incontinence surgery, impaired voiding which may be adversely affected by anticholinergic medications, and high detrusor pressures which may lead to upper tract damage. Cystometry is not very helpful in the evaluation of interstitial cystitis, recurrent cystitis, urinary fistula, or urethral diverticulum.

Measurement of bladder pressure

The pressure in the bladder results from forces within the bladder and outside the bladder. Simple cystometry measures the bladder pressure (vesical pressure, or P_{ves}) in centimetres of water, that pressure which would move a column of water so many centimetres above the pubic symphysis. In subtracted cystometry, an additional measurement is made of intra-abdominal pressure (P_{abd}), usually measured as vaginal or rectal pressure (Fig. 9.1). Subtracting abdominal pressure from bladder pressure therefore calculates the pressure in the bladder which originates from the bladder itself (detrusor pressure or P_{det}); thus, P_{ves} minus P_{abd} = P_{det}. This calculation can result artifactual errors; for example, abdominal pressure may be recorded in the absence of intravesical pressure, leading to a *negative* detrusor pressure. Also, fluctuations in rectal recording can produce a negative abdominal pressure in the absence of intravesical pressure, thus the urodynamic machine calculates a detrusor pressure which is an artefact. These errors may be avoided by recording both P_{ves} and P_{abd}.

In women, abdominal pressure may be measured in the rectum or in the vagina. Many women find the vaginal catheter more comfortable, but errors can occur from catheter movement in women with significant prolapse. Rectal catheters may become blocked by faeces, and rectal contractions may be interpreted incorrectly as detrusor contractions by an inexperienced urodynamicist.

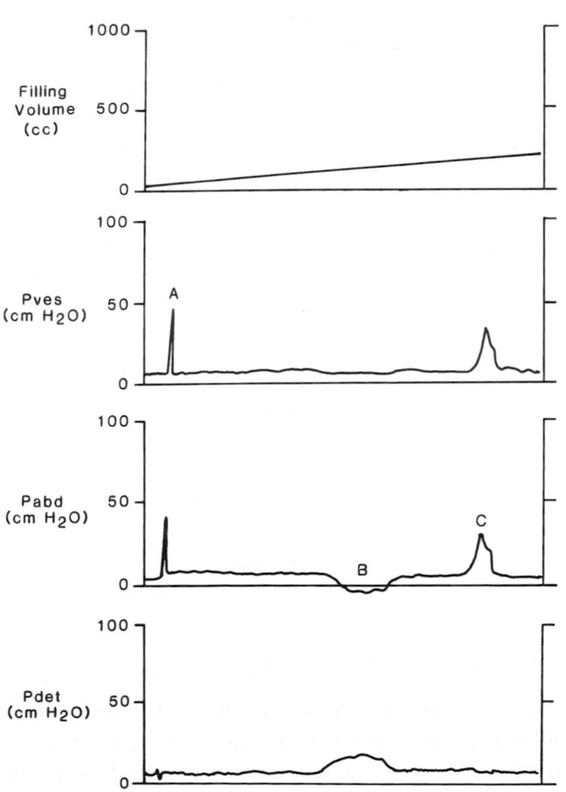

Fig. 9.1 Subtracted cystometry. A cough is reflected in the vesical and abdominal channels (**A**); an artifactual rise in detrusor pressure (**B**); and Valsalva manoeuvre (**C**).

Technical points

There are many variations on the technique of cystometry. The urodynamicist must carefully describe the conditions of testing and reporting these result according to the recommendations of the International Continence Society (Abrams et al 1988):

- Access: urethral or suprapubic
- Filling medium: water, saline, radiological contrast agents, or carbon dioxide gas
- Fluid temperature: cold, room temperature, or body temperature
- Position of patient: supine, sitting, or standing
- Filling speed: slow (10 ml/min), medium (10–100 ml/min), or fast (> 100 ml/min). Calibrated pumps greatly assist in control of filling speed
- Transducer: pressure is converted to electronic signals via a pressure transducer; external fluid column zeroed to the symphysis; or microtip transducers mounted in the catheter tip
- Number and source of signals: pressure from bladder, abdomen, urethra; flow, EMG, filling volume; calculated detrusor pressure
- Catheters: number, size. Multilumen catheters may deliver filling volumes and measure bladder and urethral pressures via separate ports.

The routine cystometrogram in women consists of room temperature water instilled via urethral *microtip transducer* catheters or a separate filling catheter at 80–100 ml/min in the sitting or standing position. Additionally, provocative manoeuvres are used to determine whether detrusor contractions can be suppressed. These are often aimed at reproducing conditions which provoke symptoms in the individual, and may include Valsalva, coughing, heel bouncing, standing up, rapid fill or cooler temperatures, listening to running water or washing hands. Neurologically compromised individuals undergo testing in conditions which optimize bladder function: warm water is instilled at a physiological rate of 10 ml/min, and filling is begun without emptying the postvoid residual, which can be calculated later.

Detrusor activity

What is a clinically significant detrusor contraction? In the past, an arbitrary value of 15 cm H_2O was suggested. Normal women may experience detrusor contractions at various times in the day, these are rapidly suppressed and do not produce symptoms or incontinence (Heslington & Hilton 1996.) During filling cystometry, a detrusor contraction in the range of 15 cm H_2O which is immediately suppressed and which does

not reproduce symptoms may be normal. Conversely, some women with severe incontinence may leak urine during testing with only small increases in their detrusor pressures, but reproducing symptoms. Contractions due to uninhibitable detrusor activity are phasic; high pressures (over 40–60 cm H_2O) may be related to upper tract damage over time (McGuire et al 1981). A multichannel cystometrogram demonstrating urge incontinence is shown in Fig. 9.2.

Bladder compliance

In the normal bladder, initial bladder pressures are low and rise only slightly with the initiation of filling. The normal bladder wall is able to accept increasing bladder volumes without substantial increases in bladder pressures, a process called adaptation. *Compliance* describes the relationship of change in volume to change in pressure, or Δ volume/Δ pressure. With further filling, the elastic and viscoelastic properties reach their maximal stretch and further increases in volume result in increases in pressure. Women with abnormal bladder compliance have a progressive tonic increase in detrusor pressure with filling which does not subside with cessation of filling (Fig. 9.3). If filling is too rapid, a normal bladder may transiently be unable to accommodate to increasing volume – cessation of filling in these individuals should result in falling detrusor pressure at this same bladder volume.

Normal subtracted cystometry – filling

Instructions for performing subtracted cystometry are outlined in Table 9.1 and in Fig. 9.4. Approximate normal results are listed in Table 9.2.

Abnormal subtracted cystometry – filling

Conditions associated with *urine loss* which can be determined on filling cystometry include detrusor overactivity (detrusor instability or detrusor hyperreflexia), and stress urinary incontinence. Conditions associated with *abnormal sensation* include sensory urgency (symptoms of urgency without uninhibitable detrusor activity on provocation) and low compliance (change in volume/change in pressure greater than 100 ml/cm H_2O). (See Chs 20, 27 and 28.)

Abdominal leak point pressure

McGuire and associates (1993) have suggested a simple concept to evaluate the type and severity of stress incontinence. In the absence of detrusor activity, the amount of intravesical pressure which overcomes the urethral continence mechanism is termed the abdominal leak point pressure. In 1923, Bonney observed that minimal pressure was required to overcome the continence mechanism in women with severe stress incontinence compared to women with less severe symptoms. Urethral pressure profilometry has not

Table 9.1 Technique for filling cystometry in women (multichannel).

1. After voiding with a comfortably full bladder, place the patient in supine lithotomy position or a birthing chair; clean the urethral orifice, and insert a catheter to measure the *postvoid residual*. This may be done using the filling catheter; if using narrow microtip transducer catheters, a separate catheter should be used.
2. Insert the intravesical pressure catheter, and the separate filling catheter if used. Insert the intra-abdominal pressure catheter into the vagina or rectum. Secure both catheters to the thigh with tape. The catheters should have previously been sterilized and zeroed to atmospheric pressure.
3. Place the patient into the desired position for filling and ask her to cough. Adjust the transducers or catheters to obtain identical deflections in the bladder and abdominal channels, with minimal movement in the detrusor channel. Reduce pelvic organ prolapse if significant. *Record initial bladder and abdominal pressures.*
4. Begin filling, usually 80 ml/min. The patient should remain quiet without movement, and should report symptoms and cooperate in provocative tests. *Record the volume at first desire to void.*
5. Perform first set of provocative manoeuvres. Check to see that subtraction continues to be optimal. *Record any urgency, pain, or incontinence.* Keep track of filling volume, because special tests such as leak point pressure are to be performed at set volumes.
6. Continue filling. *Record strong desire to void, and maximum desire to void.* Filling should be stopped when the patient can hold no more fluid and can no longer delay micturition. If capacity is reached at low volumes, the patient should be encouraged to accept more filling volume, especially if her functional bladder capacity on frequency/volume charts is higher.
7. At cystometric capacity, repeat provocative tests. Record the detrusor pressure after pressures equilibrate to obtain bladder compliance (change in volume/change in pressure.) *Record any abnormal sensation, urgency, or incontinence. Record the provocation, patient reaction to event, detrusor pressure at the point of leakage, and the bladder leak point pressure.*

Table 9.2 Normal cystometric values in women.

- Residual urine less than 50 ml; less than 100 ml in older women
- First desire to void at least 150 ml, usually 200 ml
- Strong desire to void at 300–400 ml
- Maximum desire to void 400–600 ml
- No pain, urgency, or incontinence
- No uninhibitable detrusor contractions, despite provocation
- Bladder compliance 20–100 ml/cm H_2O
- Spontaneous voiding due to a voluntary detrusor contraction less than 50 cm H_2O which is sustained throughout voiding
- Maximum flow rate greater than 15 ml/s > 150 ml fluid voided

Modified from Wall et al (1993)

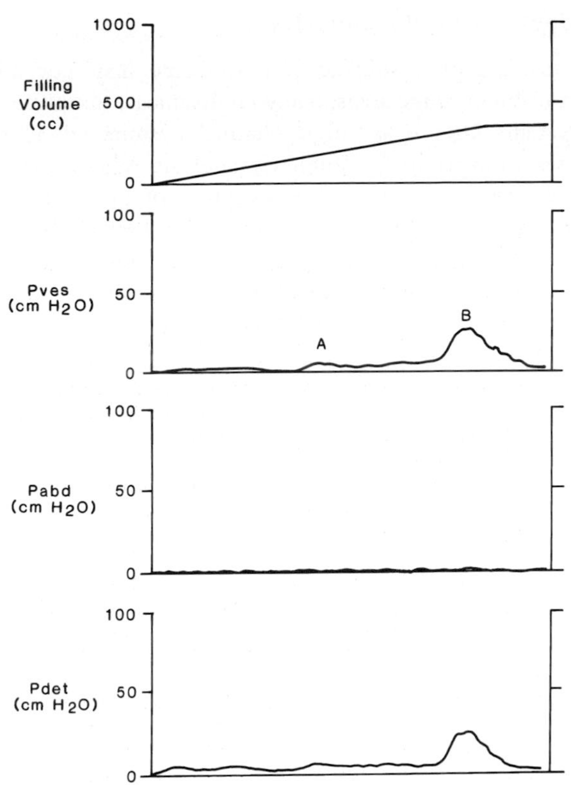

Fig. 9.2 Subtracted cystometry demonstrating detrusor instability. At FDV, a small contraction is seen (**A**); at 300 ml, the patient has an uninhibitable contraction (**B**) and leakage of urine.

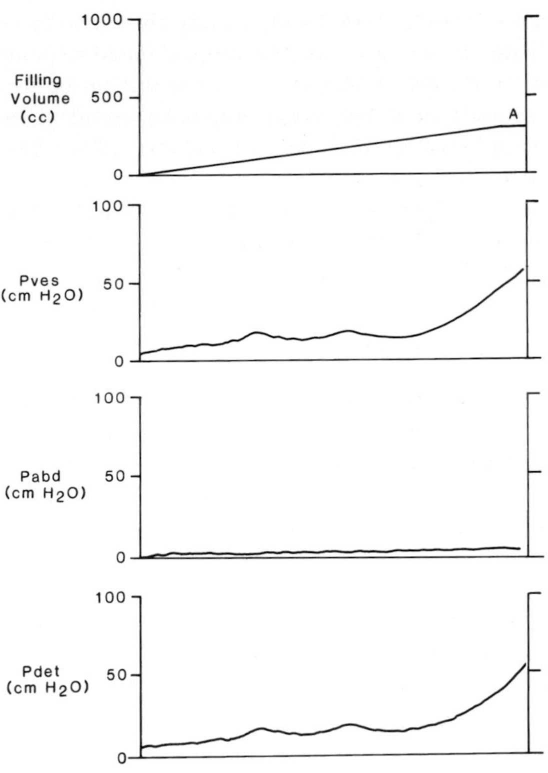

Fig. 9.3 Subtracted cystometry demonstrating poor compliance even when filling is halted (**A**).

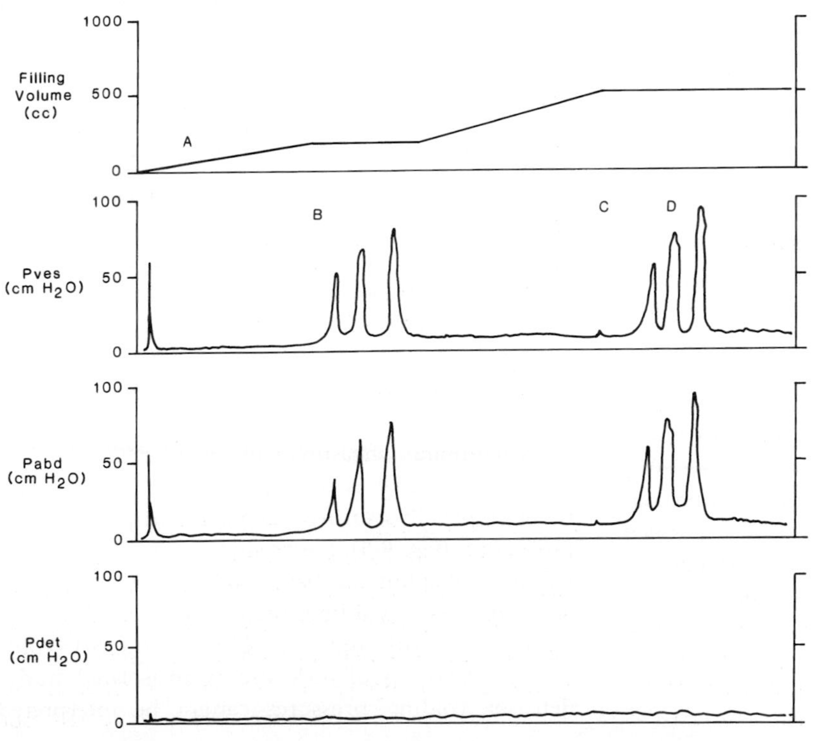

Fig. 9.4 Normal subtracted cystometry. At FDV (150 ml), the patient is asked to perform provocative manoeuvres (**A**). At 200 ml, filling is halted (**B**) and the patient does not leak with Valsalva efforts (**C**). At MDV (500 ml), provocative and Valsalva manoeuvres are repeated (**D**).

been very helpful in distinguishing these two types of patients, nor at predicting surgical outcome (Summitt et al 1994). Leak point pressure was introduced as a urodynamic test which might be useful in the evaluation of stress incontinence, but has not been fully evaluated to date.

Bump et al (1995) found that the Valsalva leak point pressure was reproducible as long as the catheter size was held constant. Heritz & Blaivas (1995) also described good inter-observer reproducibility, as did Song et al (1995). In McGuire's original description of Valsalva leak point pressure, 76% of women with intrinsic sphincter deficiency had a VLPP less than 60 cm H_2O, and all had a value less than 90 cm H_2O (McGuire et al 1993). The correlation between a low VLPP and a low maximum urethral closure pressure (MUCP) is poor in most studies. Finally, the greatest usefulness of such a test would allow the surgeon to select women who would not benefit from a standard retropubic urethropexy and who should be treated with injectables or slings. Although the correlation between the diagnosis of intrinsic sphincter deficiency and a low VLPP is good, there are few outcome studies as yet to identify a VLPP value which predicts surgical outcome. In the absence of anterior wall prolapse, few would argue that values greater than 100 cm H_2O represent hypermobile type stress incontinence.

At a standardized volume (200 ml in many reports), the patient is asked to Valsalva with progressively greater effort (see Fig. 9.4). The lowest effort which produces incontinence is termed the abdominal leak point pressure. If no incontinence is produced, she is asked to cough with increasing force (cough leak point pressure). The actual values will depend on the experience of each urodynamic laboratory, but low leak point pressures (less than 60 cm H_2O) are associated with intrinsic sphincter deficiency, high leak point pressures (greater than 90) with hypermobile-type SUI, and intermediate values (60–90 cm H_2O) sometimes are indicative of combined hypermobile and intrinsic sphincter deficiency. However useful, abdominal leak point pressure should only be viewed as an adjunct to history and careful examination of the woman with stress urinary incontinence.

Abdominal leak point pressure should not be confused with 'detrusor leak point pressure', which refers to high detrusor pressures in neurologically abnormal patients. Detrusor leak point pressure has been correlated with upper tract damage in these individuals (McGuire et al 1981).

Single channel cystometry

Since complex subtracted cystometry may not be available in some areas, many clinicians use simplified systems known as single channel cystometry. This uses an inexpensive single channel intravesical pressure apparatus, with the advantage of providing a tracing record of the study but the disadvantage of only measuring bladder pressure. This simple system is not appropriate for studying complex patients, and precludes many provocative manoeuvres and voiding studies.

Several researchers have reported reasonable correlations between the simple system and the gold standard of multichannel subtracted cystometry. Sand et al (1991) showed that two simple tests approached a single multichannel test for the diagnosis of detrusor instability. Scotti and Myers (1993) reported a positive predictive value of 87% for single channel cystometry compared to 84% for multichannel studies for the diagnosis of genuine stress incontinence in women. It is important to note that the individuals reporting favourable results with simple testing are trained urogynaecologists, and may overestimate the success which the primary care physician may obtain. On the other hand, no fancy laboratory can replace the care provided by the concerned physician who is familiar with the patient and her treatment goals.

Voiding cystometry

The bladder's role in micturition is one of providing the energy for intravesical pressure and of coordinating with the urethra to facilitate flow. When pressure is exerted on urine in the bladder, the energy of intravesical pressure is converted to the energy of flow of urine out of the urethra. Approximately one third of women referred for urodynamics void with detrusor pressure, one third utilize strain or Valsalva, and one third void via urethral relaxation alone, the intravesical pressure being almost negligible in these individuals. If flow is suddenly stopped, a pressure rise is seen in the bladder that theoretically represents the maximum pressure that can be generated by the bladder.

Synchronous measurement of bladder pressure and uroflowmetry is used to evaluate voiding dysfunction, usually seen in women after anti-incontinence procedures (Fig. 9.5). Electromyography of the external urethral sphincter may be added to these studies to further assess voiding; these studies are discussed elsewhere in this text (see Chs 15 and 24). Voiding cystometry is of little use as an isolated study: detrusor voiding pressures cannot be interpreted without measurements of flow resulting from detrusor contraction. Furthermore, it can be difficult for women to void in a testing situation, and an environment conducive to voiding would include smaller calibre catheters, the opportunity to sit on a commode, and as much privacy as is practical.

Special tests during voiding cystometry include:

- Assessment of possible obstruction. Although nomograms exist to describe the relationship between detrusor voiding pressure and urinary flow rate in men (Abrams-Griffiths), there is no comparable nomogram for women. Obstruction may be said to exist in a woman with a maximum detrusor voiding pressure (P_{det} max) greater than 60 cm H_2O with no flow, or 80 cm H_2O with low flow rates (less than 15 ml/s) (Fig. 9.6).
- Assessment of inadequate voiding with straining (bladder pressure for voiding arising from abdominal pressure, not detrusor pressure), involuntary urethral sphincter contraction during detrusor voiding (detrusor–sphincter dyssynergia), or atonic bladder. Impaired contractility is often seen in conjunction with detrusor hyperreflexia in the elderly, and is one argument for performing complex urodynamics when evaluating elderly women with urinary incontinence (Resnick & Yalla 1987).
- Assessment of potential voiding dysfunction after surgery: studies have suggested P_{det} max less than 20 cm H_2O. In the *isometric detrusor test*, the patient is asked to suddenly interrupt the flow of urine, and an increase in detrusor pressure suggests that the individual may be able to generate a similar increase against the relative obstruction of surgery (Norton & Stanton 1988).

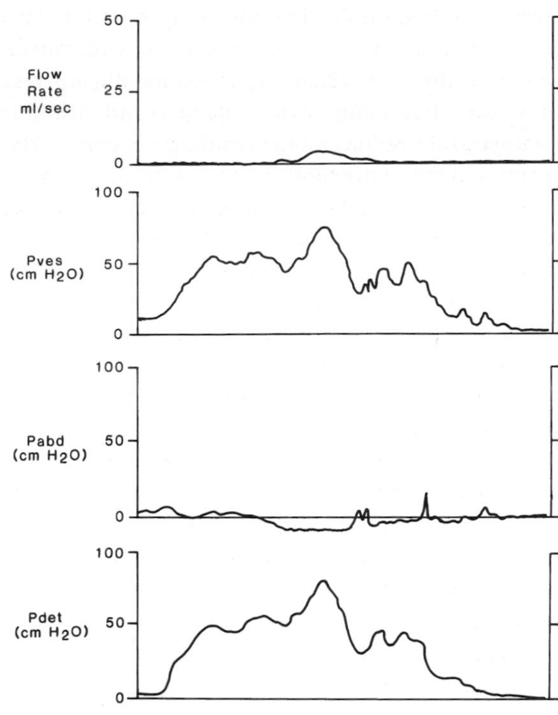

Fig. 9.6 Voiding study demonstrating obstruction. This patient's post-operative voiding difficulties include high detrusor voiding pressures and low flow rates.

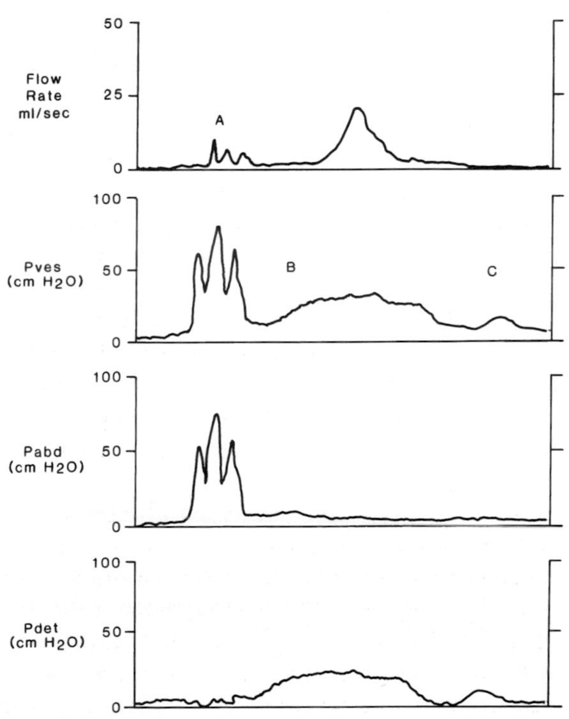

Fig. 9.5 Voiding study. Initially the patient strains to void (**A**) but then initiates a detrusor contraction (**B**) which produces a smooth curve of flow. A small after contraction may be seen (**C**).

VIDEOCYSTOURETHROGRAPHY

This technique combines the pressure dynamics of the cystometrogram with the visual dynamics of the voiding cystogram. Cystometry is performed with radio-opaque contrast as the filling medium, measuring pressures with direct observation of bladder filling and empyting. Both the radiological image and the pressure tracing can be recorded simultaneously on videotape, or videocystourethrography or 'VCU' (not to be confused with 'VCUG' or voiding cysturethrogram). VCU allows the clinician to directly observe the effects of bladder events: the position and conformation of the bladder neck in relation to the pubic symphysis, bladder neck closure during rest and stress, diverticuli of the bladder and urethra, vesicoureteral reflux, and voiding events. The dynamics of flow interruptions and urethral milkback can be seen, as well as coordination of intravesical pressure with urethral opening. In short, VCU is a wonderful tool for understanding bladder filling and emptying. It is much more costly, technical, time-consuming, space-demanding, and available only in some tertiary referral centres.

Although VCU is critical in the evaluation of men with neurologic bladder dysfunction, its role is less important in the evaluation of women with primary bladder dysfunction (Stanton et al 1988). VCU in women may have some advantage over subtracted cystometry in cases of suspected vesicoureteral reflux, although VCUG may supplement the cystometry. Women with complex neurological disorders or severe voiding dysfunction may also benefit from VCU because the effects of high detrusor pressure are seen on the ureters and ureterovesical junction. The logistics of VCU may include more personnel and equipment than ordinary subtracted cystometry and such an audience makes normal voiding difficult for most women in these circumstances. Modification of the fluoscopy system to allow voiding on a commode is most likely to obtain voiding results in female patients.

INDICATIONS FOR VCU

Clearly VCU is a useful clinical tool, but its use is controversial. Some busy urodynamic units use the technique exclusively; others, not at all. VCU has often been held as the 'gold standard' by many urodynamicists, but its advantage over subtracted cystometry has not been demonstrated in clinical trials. However, there are specific situations in which VCU is of great advantage over routine subtracted cystometry. If bladder outlet obstruction is diagnosed on subtracted pressure-flow studies (high detrusor voiding pressure, no/low flow), VCU can identify the site of obstruction. VCU remains an important research tool, but probably is not necessary for the vast majority of women presenting with incontinence.

REFERENCES

Abrams P, Blaivas J, Stanton S, Andersen J R 1988 The standardisation of terminology of lower urinary tract function. Scandinavian Journal of Urology and Nephrology Supplement 114: 5–18

Bump R C 1993 Racial comparisons and contrasts in urinary incontinence and pelvic organ prolapse. Obstetrics and Gynecology 81: 421–425

Bump R, Elser D, Theofrastus J, McClish D 1995 Valsalva leak point pressures in women with genuine stress incontinence: reproducibility, effect of catheter caliber, and correlations with other measures of urethral resistance. American Journal of Obstetrics and Gynecology 173: 551–557

Heritz D, Blaivas J 1995 Reliability and specificity of the leak point pressure. Journal of Urology 153: 492

Heslington K, Hilton P 1996 Ambulatory monitoring and conventional cystometry in asymptomatic female volunteers. British Journal of Obstetrics and Gynaecology 103: 434–441

McGuire E, Woodside J, Borden T, Weiss R 1981 The prognostic value of urodynamic testing in myelodysplastic patients. Journal of Urology 126: 205–209

McGuire E, Fitzpatrick C, Wan J et al 1993 Clinical assessment of urethral sphincter function. Journal of Urology 150: 1452–1454

Norton P, Stanton S 1988 Isometric detrusor test as a predictor of postoperative voiding difficulties. Neurourology and Urodynamics 7: 287–88

Resnick N, Yalla S 1987 Detrusor hyperactivity with impaired contractile function: an unrecognized but common cause of incontinence in elderly patients. Journal of the American Medical Association 257: 3076–3080

Sand P, Brubaker L, Novak T 1991 Simple standing incremental cystometry as a screening method for detrusor instability. Obstetrics and Gynecology 77: 453–457

Scotti R, Myers D 1993 A comparison of the cough stress test and single-channel cystometry with multichannel urodynamic evaluation in genuine stress incontinence. Obstetrics and Gynecology 81: 430–433

Song J, Rozanski T, Belville W 1995 Stress leak point pressure: a simple and reproducible method utilizing a fiberoptic microtransducer. Urology 46: 81–84

Stanton S, Krieger M, Ziv E 1988 Videocystourethrography: its role in the assessment of incontinence in the female. Neurourology and Urodynamics 7: 172–173

Summitt R, Sipes D, Bent A, Ostergard D 1994 Evaluation of pressure transmission ratios in women with genuine stress incontinence and low urethral pressure: a comparative study. Obstetrics and Gynecology 83: 984–988

Wall L, Norton P, DeLancey J 1993 Practical urodynamics In: Wall L, Norton P, DeLancey J Practical Urogynecology. Williams and Wilkins, Baltimore, MD, p 99

SECTION 2
CHAPTER

10

Radiology and MRI

ASH K MONGA AND STUART L STANTON

Imaging investigations play a crucial role in identifying the normal and abnormal anatomy of the pelvic floor and help in the assessment of urinary incontinence, prolapse and faecal incontinence. They also allow the indirect assessment of function of the urinary tract and pelvic floor. There are three main modalities employed: radiology, ultrasound and magnetic resonance. In this chapter we will discuss the use of radiology and MRI; ultrasound is discussed in Ch. 14. Some of the available imaging techniques are research tools, but may have clinical implications in the future.

RADIOLOGY

Plain films

Plain radiographs of the abdomen and pelvis may be taken to investigate a visible abnormality or as part of an intravenous urogram. The following conditions may cause incontinence or are related to its treatment.

Epispadias and bladder exstrophy are congenital anomalies with a characteristic separation of pubic bones observed on a plain film (Fig. 10.1). Traumatic symphysial separation usually occurs after road traffic accidents. Avulsion of the pelvic ring is often associated with injury to other pelvic soft tissue structures. Less marked symphysial separation may also persist after symphysiotomy during vaginal delivery.

Urinary retention may be found during investigation of a lower abdominal mass and has to be distinguished from ascites or an ovarian cyst. The 'fluid level' shown here is due to a urinary tract infection by gas producing organisms.

Osteitis pubis is a well recognized complication of the Marshall–Marchetti–Krantz procedure. The increasing use of bone anchors for suspension and sling type procedures may also increase the risk of this complication. Figure 10.2 demonstrates osteomyelitis in both pubic rami which required curettage.

The artificial urinary sphincter (Fig. 10.3) is shown in activated mode; although contrast is present in the pump and reservoir it is absent from the cuff. This woman presented with recurrent incontinence despite her sphincter and had a malfunctioning cuff.

Radio-opaque bladder calculi can also be identified (Fig. 10.4).

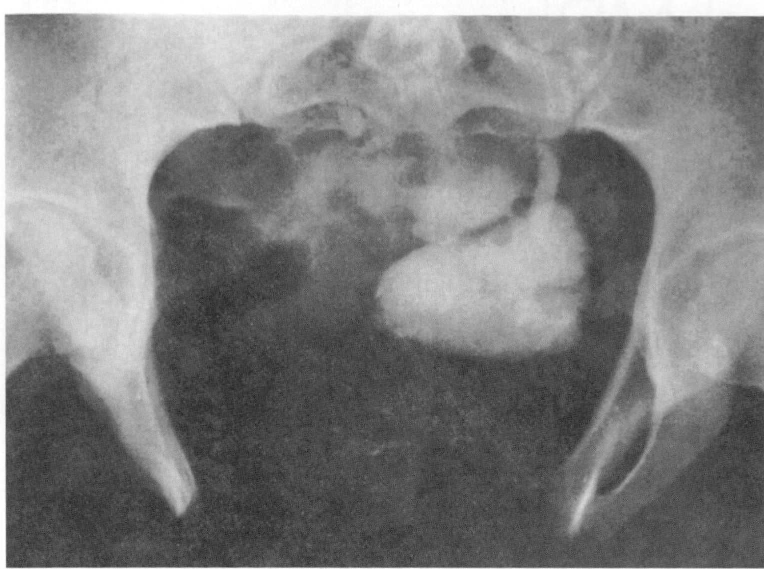

Fig. 10.1A Pelvis in bladder exstrophy showing widely separated pubic bones resulting from outward rotation of pubis and innominate bones. There is contrast in the reconstructed bladder.

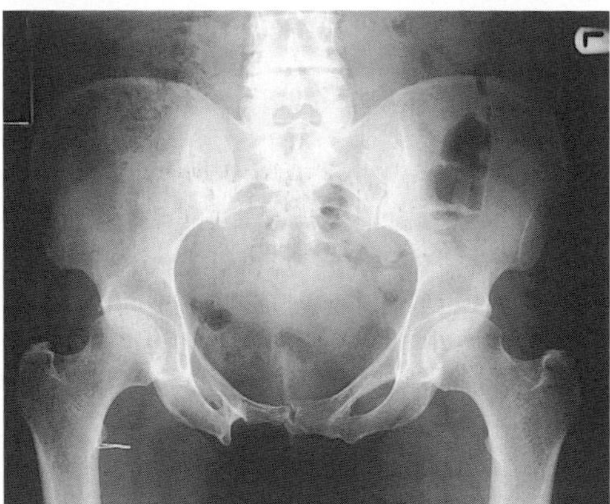

Fig. 10.1B Radiograph showing pubic diastasis

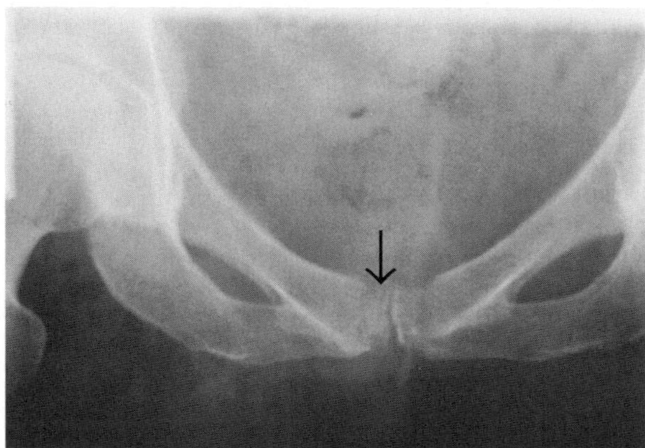

Fig. 10.2 Osteomyelitis of pubis resulting from osteitis pubis following Marshall-Marchetti-Krantz procedure. Arrow shows area of osteomyelitis

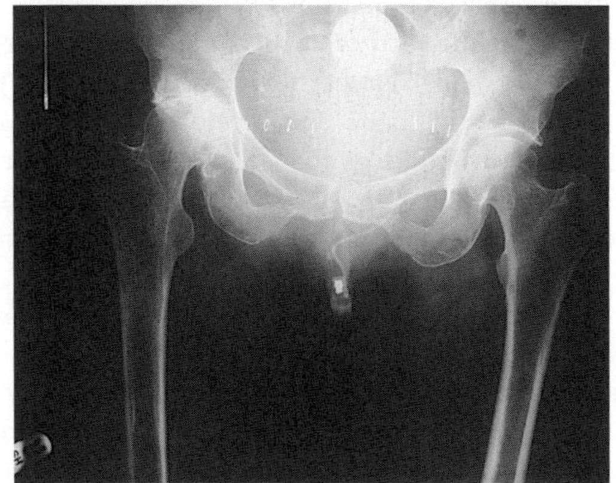

Fig. 10.3 Activated artificial urinary sphincter (AMS 800) showing reservoir, cuff and pump filled with contrast.

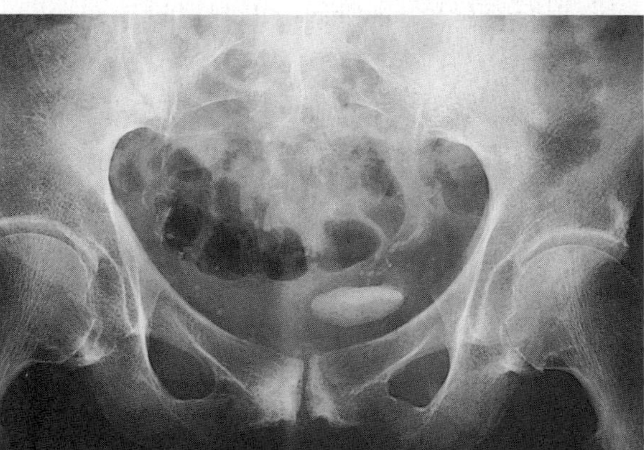

Fig. 10.4 Plain film showing radio-opaque bladder calculi.

Vertebral column radiographs

Vertebral column radiographs include plain lateral and anteroposterior plain films, myelograms and spinal angiograms. With respect to the urinary tract, Table 10.1 outlines the conditions that may be investigated.

Sacral agenesis (Fig. 10.5) will produce urinary symptoms only if three or more sacral segments are absent. Spina bifida occulta which is found in up to 50% of the population without any clinical significance, will produce symptoms and signs if the cord is tethered by an abnormally thick filum terminale. If the cord is bifurcated by a spur or bone or cartilage growing from the back of the vertebral body, as in diastomatomyelia, symptoms and signs of neuropathic bladder will present as the child grows: upward movement of the conus medullaris produces traction on nerve roots from the bony spur or tethered filum.

Trauma to the spinal cord, intra- or extramedullary tumours and extradural abscess will cause disturbance of micturition, the precise form dependent on the level and extent of the lesion. Lumbar spinal stenosis which is a combination of degeneration of the intervertebral disc and osteoarthritic change producing osteophytes along the posterior margins of the vertebral bodies leads to compression of the spinal cord and nerve roots (principally L4, L5 and S1. Neurogenic claudication affecting the legs and urinary retention are common symptoms; radiological changes include narrowing of the lumbar canal, shortening of the pedicles, and anteroposterior flattening of the exit foramina of the nerve roots. Myelography will show narrowing and multiple waistlike anterolateral and posterolateral indentations on the thecal sac.

Prolapsed intervertebral disc is most common at the L4–5 and L5–S1 levels. Compression of the corresponding lateral nerve roots may occur. Central compression may cause a cauda equina syndrome (Fig.

Table 10.1 Disorders involving the spinal cord that cause disturbance of micturition.

- I. Congenital
  - A. Sacral agenesis
  - B. Spina bifida occulta
  - C. Diastomatomyelia
  - D. Myelomeningocele
- II. Trauma
- III. Tumour
  - A. Intramedullary
  - B. Extramedullary
- IV. Inflammatory
  - A. Extradural abscess
  - B. Spinal arachnoiditis
- V. Spinal lumbar canal (stenosis)
- VI. Prolapsed intervertebral disc
- VII. Spondylolisthesis

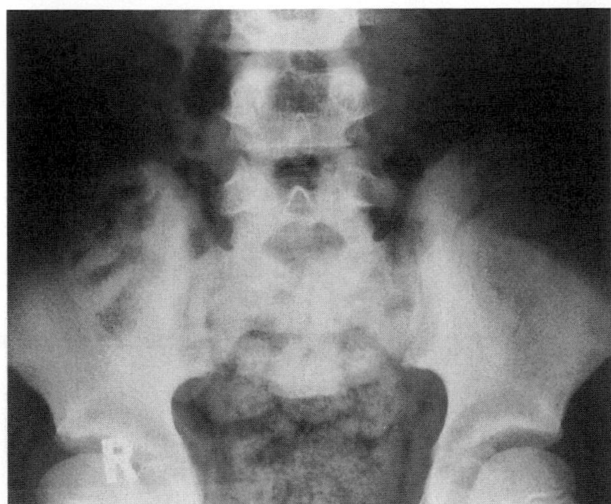

Fig. 10.5 Sacral agenesis.

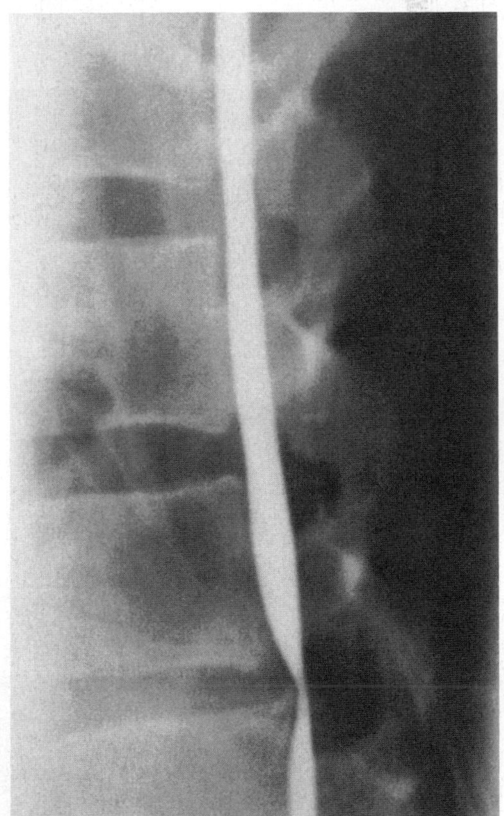

Fig. 10.6 Prolapsed intervertebral disc with compression of spinal cord.

10.6). Spondylolisthesis (Fig. 10.7) commonly of L5 slipping on S1 will mainly cause frequency.

Intravenous urography (IVU)

IVU will delineate the kidneys, ureters and bladder. Congenital and acquired anatomical abnormalities are elucidated. In addition ureteric reflux can be visualized. Urogynaecological indications for IVU include:

1. Haematuria
2. Abnormal urine cytology
3. Suspected urinary tract calculus
4. Continuous incontinence
5. Suspected ureteric obstruction or ureterovaginal fistula
6. Neuropathic bladder
7. Recurrent urinary tract infection
8. Prior to cancer surgery
9. Persistent 'vaginal discharge'.

The following conditions may be identified using intravenous urography. An ectopic ureter is bilateral in 5–25% of cases and is more common in women than men. The ectopic opening may be detected by careful vaginal examination or cystourethroscopy. Incontinence will only occur if the ectopic opening is distal to the bladder neck or into the vagina.

Hydronephrosis and hydroureter may be sequelae to outflow obstruction and vesicoureteric reflux. They are an index of renal function. Figure 10.8 demonstrates obstruction of the right ureter following inadvertent ligation at hysterectomy.

Ureterovaginal and vesicourethral fistulae can also be demonstrated using this technique.

Bladder imaging

Radiological investigation of bladder function in women has undergone many changes since cystography was first used at the beginning of the century. Early cystography consisted of anteroposterior views using a manual cassette changer. Fluoroscopy was used in the 1920s allowing oblique and lateral views but the radiation dose was unacceptably high. Chain cystography was introduced in the 1930s and lateral views were used extensively in the 1950s. The development of image intensification allowed a longer period of screening with much lower radiation exposure and a record of the dynamic act of micturition could be stored.

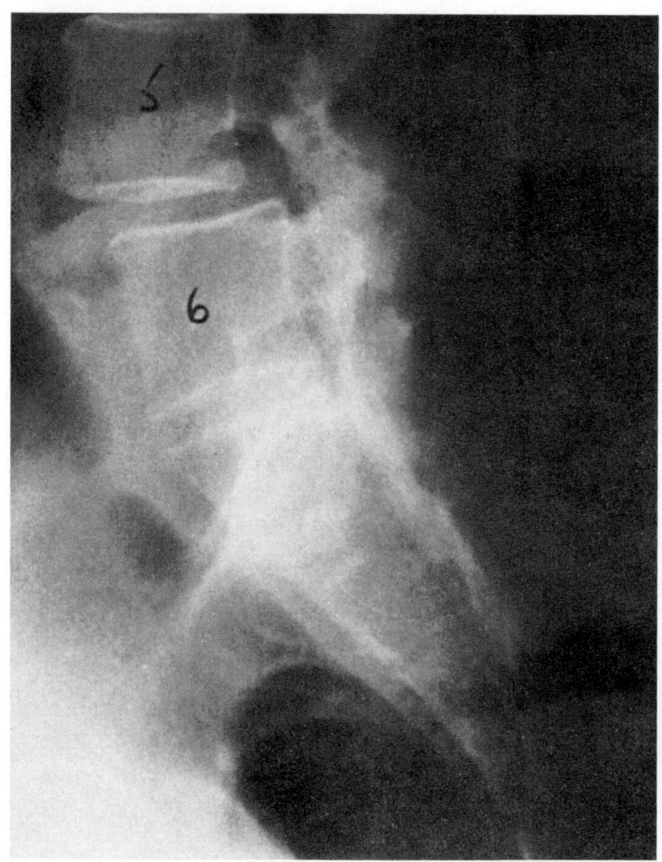

Fig. 10.7 Spondylolisthesis with slipping forward of L5 on L6.

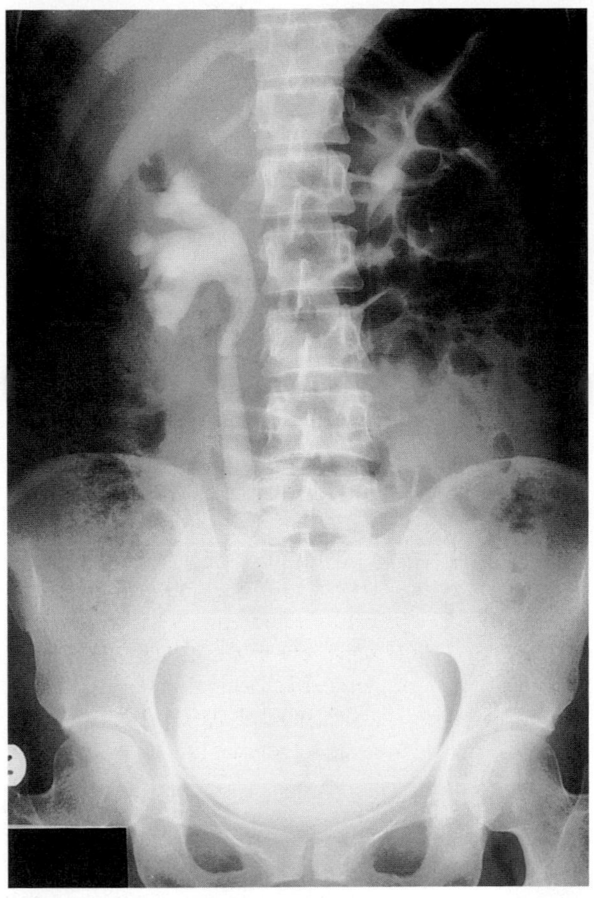

Fig. 10.8 Intravenous urogram showing obstruction of the right ureter.

The static cystogram lateral views led to the theories on the posterior urethrovesical angle which remained unchallenged for 20 years (Jeffcoate & Roberts 1952). However, a change in emphasis away from morphological towards physiological measurements and the pioneering work by Enhorning (1961) with urethral and bladder pressure measurements led to the development of a combination of cineradiographic screening of the bladder during micturition, with simultaneous measurement of urethral and bladder pressures (Enhorning et al 1964). Bates et al (1970) refined the use of videocystourethrography. The techniques for bladder imaging may be classified as shown in Table 10.2.

Table 10.2 Classification of bladder imaging techniques.

I. Static radiograph
   A. Erect
      1. Oblique
      2. Lateral
      3. Anteroposterior
   B. Sitting
II. Micturition cystography
III. Videcystourethrography

Static radiography

This is usually carried out as part of a more dynamic investigation and is rarely used in isolation. The lateral erect position will demonstrate the relationship of the bladder, bladder neck and urethra to the symphysis. An oblique erect non-straining radiograph is shown in Fig. 10.9; the bladder neck is open and contrast is in the proximal urethra. Without simultaneous bladder and abdominal pressure recordings, it is difficult to differentiate between (1) an uninhibited detrusor contraction, (2) leakage of contrast in response to coughing caused by urethral sphincter incompetence, (3) voluntary voiding and (4) a bladder neck held open by fibrosis and incomplete milkback. The role of the posterior urethrovesical angle is disputed. To outline the urethra and determine its anatomical relationship to the bladder and symphysis, a metallic bead chain may be introduced into the urethra and bladder and radiographs taken at rest and strain. This technique has largely been superseded by non-invasive ultrasound.

Micturition cystography

Micturition cystography consists of radiological screening of the bladder in the sitting or standing positions. Continuous imaging is preferable as micturition is a dynamic process. Micturition cystography may be used to demonstrate vesicoureteric reflux (Fig. 10.10), vesicovaginal fistula (Fig. 10.11), bladder diverticulum (Fig 10.12) and urethral diverticulum (Fig. 10.13). Without simultaneous pressure measurement it is difficult to diagnose the cause of incontinence. Marked descent of the bladder with residual urine associated with third degree uterine descent and descent of the anterior vaginal wall is illustrated in Fig. 10.14.

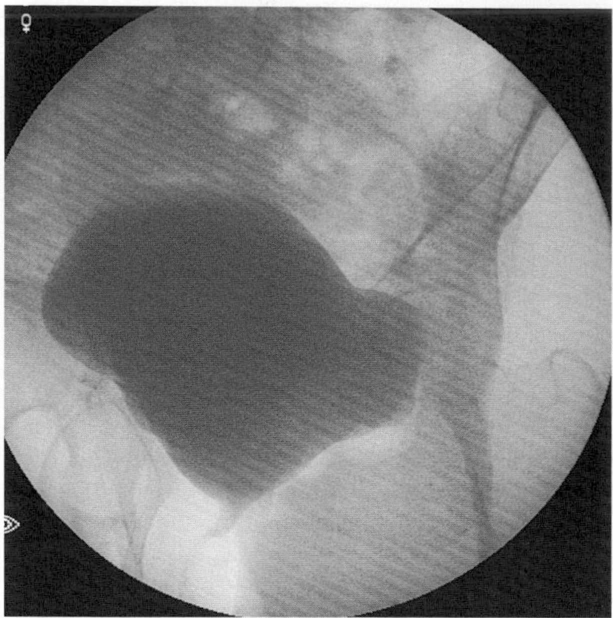

Fig. 10.9 Oblique erect non-straining radiograph showing open bladder neck and contrast in the proximal urethra.

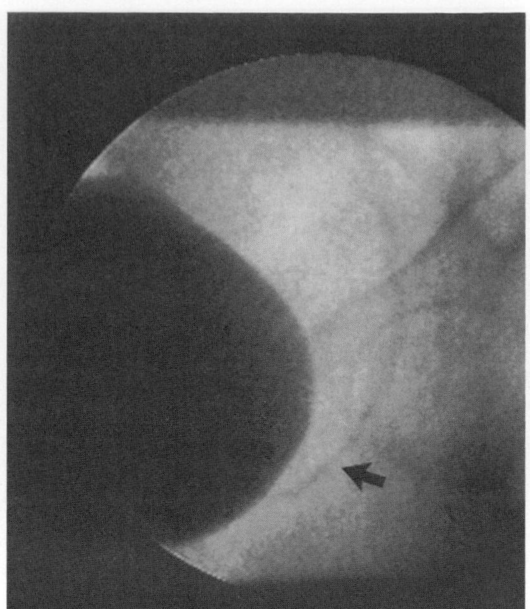

Fig. 10.10 Micturition cystogram showing left vesicoureteric reflux.

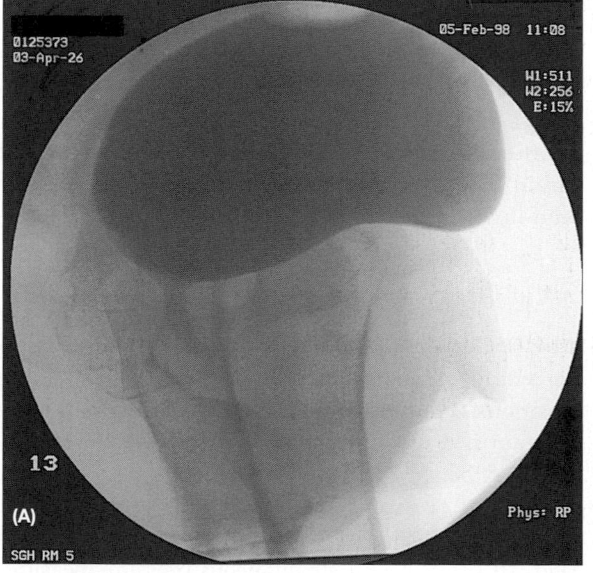

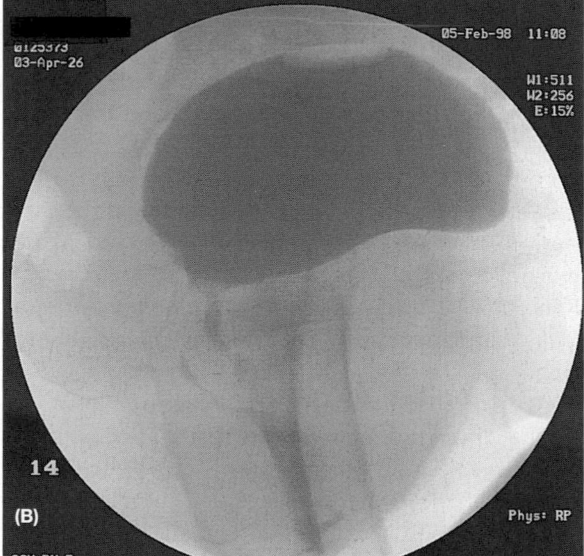

Fig. 10.11 Micturition cystogram showing (**A**) vesicovaginal fistula and (**B**) contrast pooling in the upper vagina.

(A)
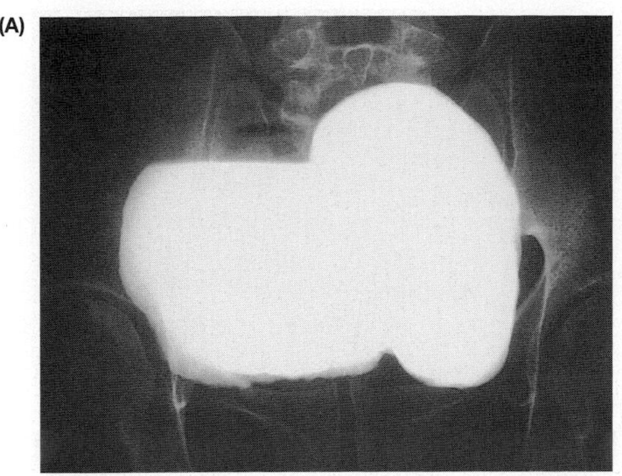
(B)
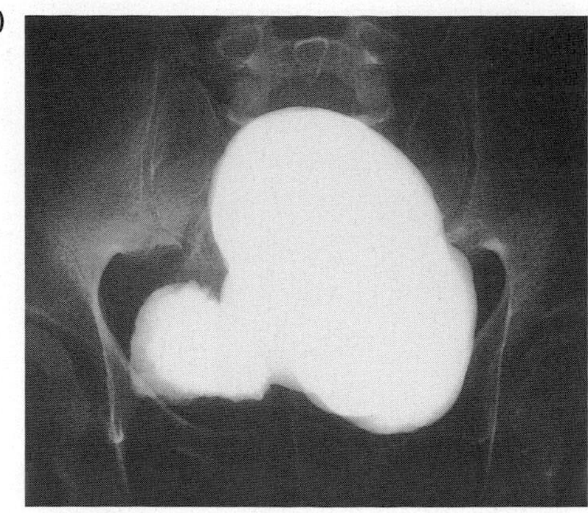

Fig. 10.12 Micturition cystogram showing (**A**) bladder and diverticulum filled with contrast and (**B**) diverticulum after completion of voiding.

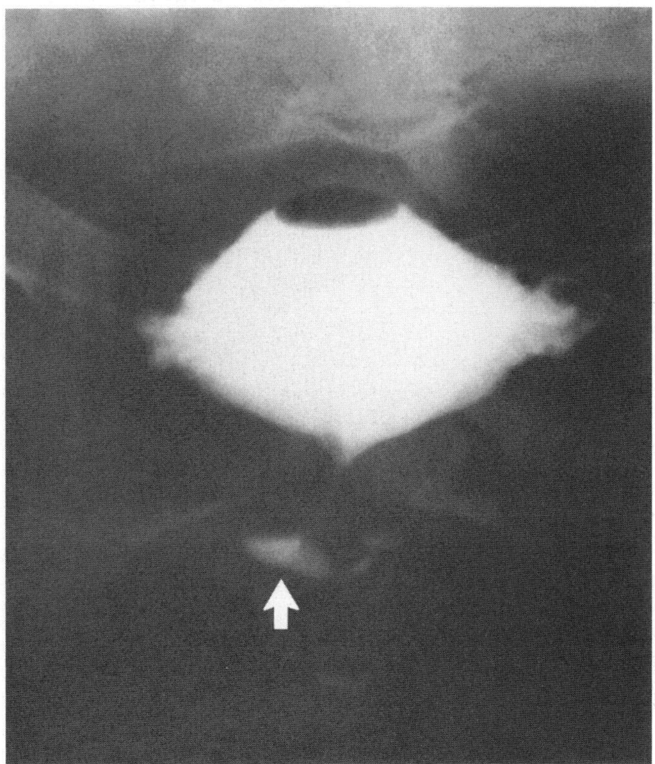

Fig. 10.13 Micturition cystogram showing urethral diverticulum.

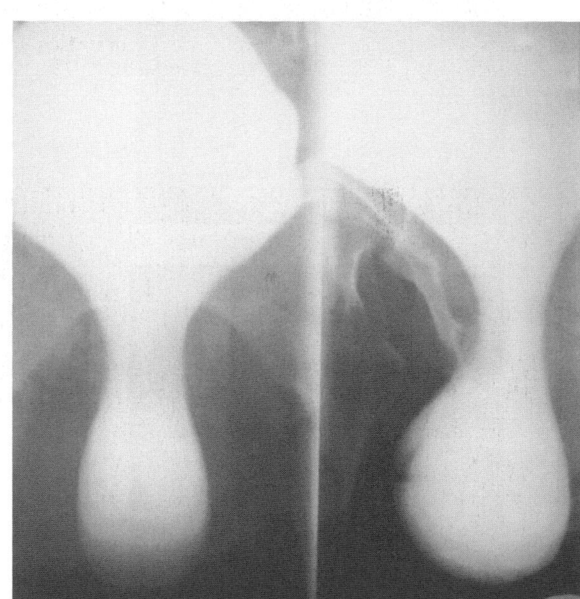

Fig. 10.14 Micturition cystogram showing marked cystocele. Left, anteroposterior view. Right, lateral view.

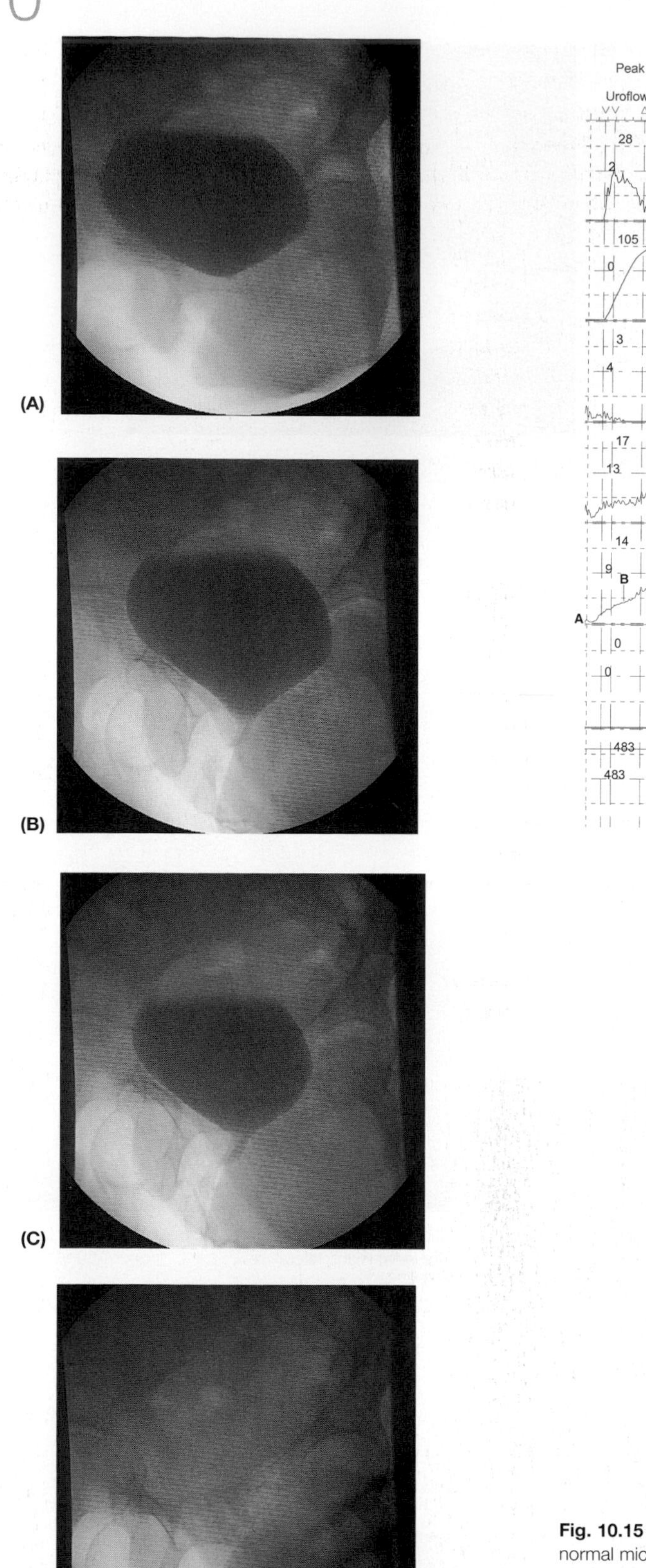

Fig. 10.15 Series of still frames from videocystourethrogram showing normal micturition. (**A**) Bladder full of contrast prior to voiding. (**B**) Bladder neck opening and contrast visible in proximal urethra. Detrusor pressure beginning to rise. (**C**) Contrast outlining the whole urethra with continued detrusor pressure rise. (**D**) End of micturition with detrusor pressure falling to zero.

Videocystourethrography

The technique is the synchronous radiological screening of the bladder and measurement of bladder and abdominal pressure during bladder filling and voiding. If a radio-opaque filling medium is used during cystometry (see Ch. 9 for a methodological description), then the lower urinary tract can be visualized by X-ray screening with an image intensifier. There are only a few situations in which VCU provides more information than cystometry. In the erect position the patient is asked to cough; bladder base descent and leakage of contrast medium per urethram can be evaluated. During voiding bladder morphology can be assessed; vesicoureteric reflux, trabeculation and diverticula should be noted. Indications include:

1 Previous failed continence surgery
2 Voiding disorder
3 Neuropathic bladder
4 Recurrent urinary tract infection
5 Suspected vesicovaginal fistula.

A series of still frames from a normal videocystourethrogram is shown in Fig. 10.15. The importance of videocystourethrography is illustrated in the following cases of incontinence. Figure 10.16 demonstrates incontinence caused by urethral sphincter incompetence; the bladder neck is open, and leakage is seen with a cough sequence in progress. There is no evidence of uninhibited detrusor contraction. Uninhibited detrusor activity is demonstrated in Fig. 10.17. Voiding difficulties may be identified by a trace showing delayed first sensation, a large bladder capacity, and a minimal detrusor pressure rise. External urethral sphincter spasm or distal urethral stenosis may be present (Fig. 10.18). Figure 10.19 shows how apparently normal voiding may occur without a detrusor contraction, owing to a rise in abdominal pressure and relaxation of the pelvic floor. A urethral diverticulum is demonstrated.

Colporecto-cystourethrography

This technique was first described in 1962 (Bethoux and Bory) and has been reintroduced for pelvic floor evaluation. Radio-opaque media are instilled into bladder, vagina and rectum simultaneously and images obtained during rest and straining. This is believed to allow an indirect assessment of pelvic floor movement and deficiency. The technique has, as yet, no clinical application and is associated with a high radiation dose. Although many investigators are treating asymptomatic prolapse uncovered by this technique normal findings in controlled trials are unavailable. Other investigators also visualize the small bowel simultaneously to perform 'four-contrastography' (Altringer et al 1995). Figure 10.20 shows small bowel descent within a vaginal vault prolapse.

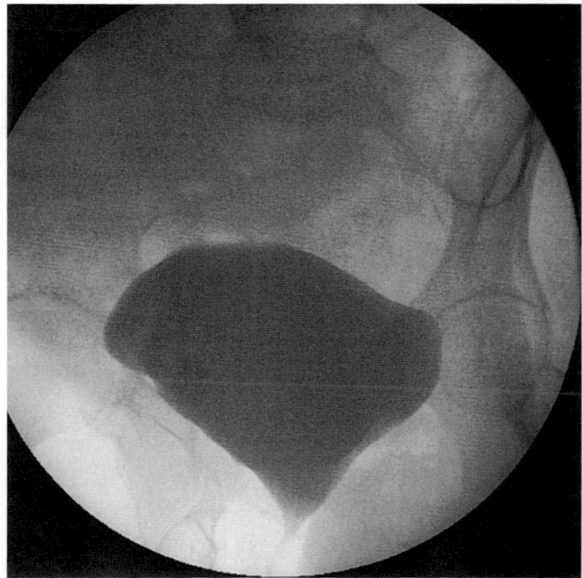

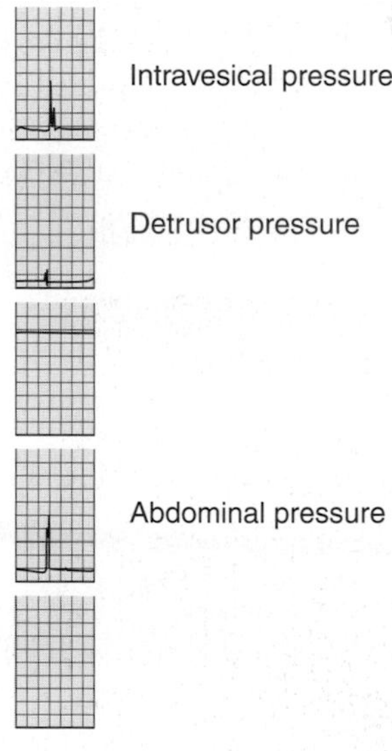

Fig. 10.16 Videocystourethrogram showing genuine stress incontinence with contrast within the urethra with abdominal pressure rise.

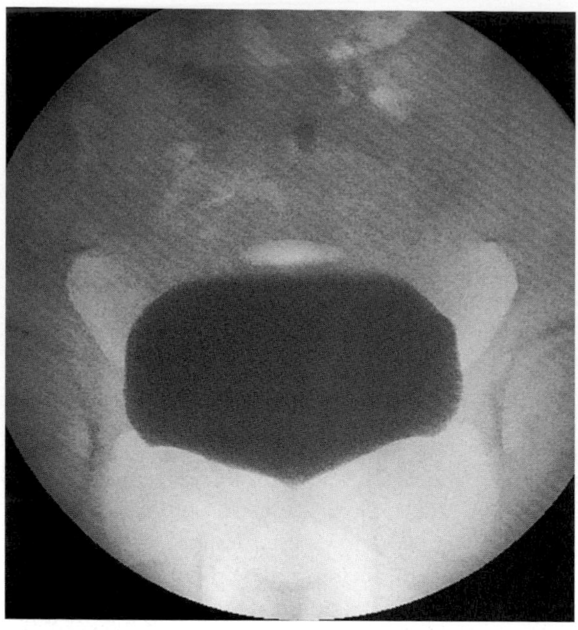

Fig. 10.17 Videocystourethrogram showing uninhibited bladder contractions during bladder filling.

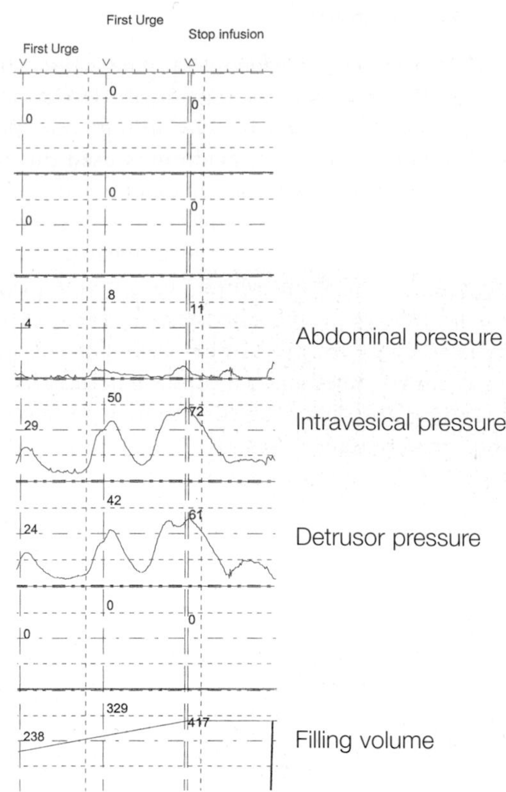

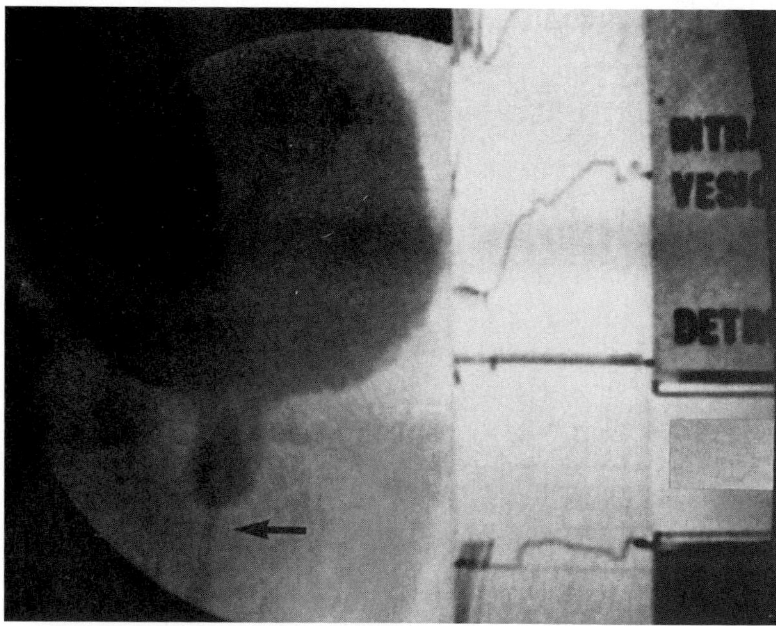

Fig. 10.18 Videocystourethrogram image during voiding with detrusor pressure exceeding 70 cm H_2O and a flow rate of 8 ml/s. There is a narrowing of the distal urethra as a result of distal urethral stenosis.

Evacuation proctography

Defaecation following barium paste instillation into the rectum allows dynamic assessment of evacuation. Rectocele can be identified and quantified (Fig. 10.21). If there is a large bowel motility insufficiency then conventional rectocele repair will not succeed in aiding emptying. This is an important investigation in patients with the symptom of incomplete emptying and a clinical rectocele. Unfortunately the amount of barium trapped at the end of defaecation does not correlate with the symptom of incomplete emptying (these techniques are discussed further in Ch. 38).

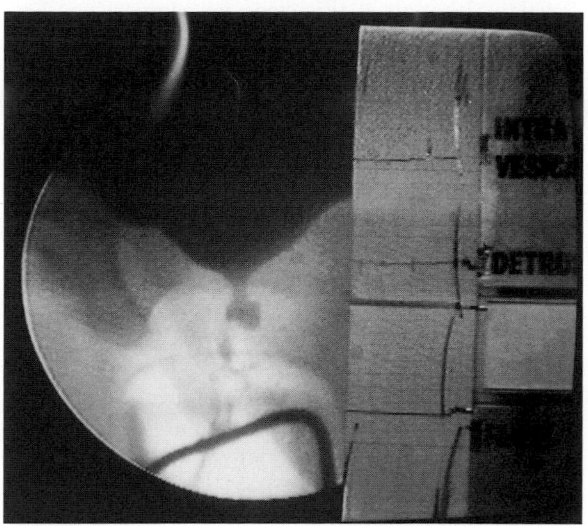

Fig. 10.19 Videocystourethrogram image showing normal voiding resulting from increase in abdominal pressure with pelvic floor relaxation but without rise in detrusor pressure. Urethral diverticulum is present.

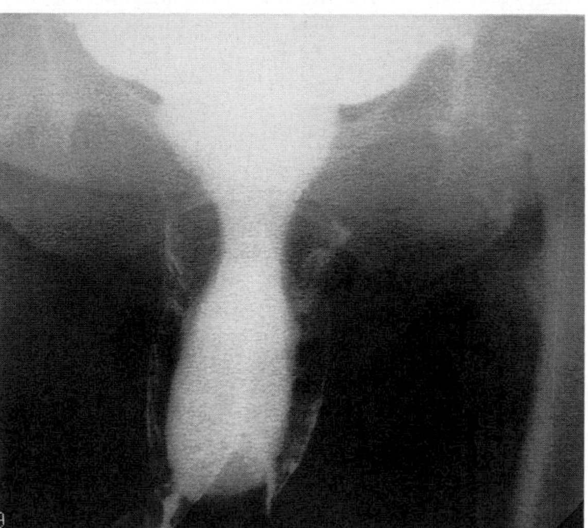

Fig. 10.20 Colporecto-cystourethrogram image showing small bowel descent within a vaginal vault prolapse.

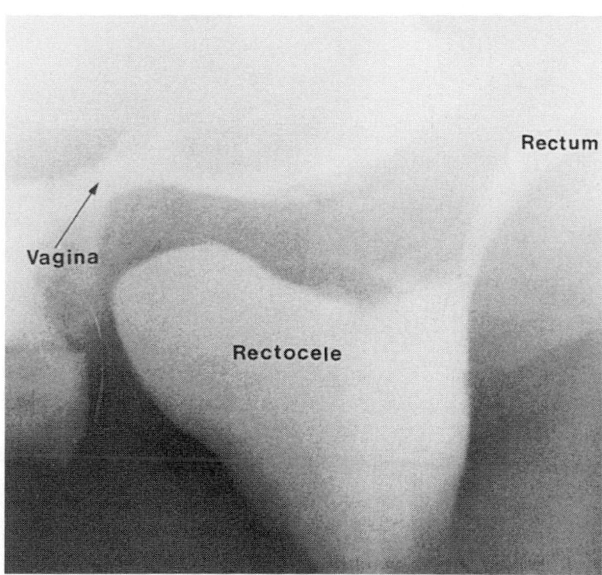

Fig. 10.21 Barium defaecogram showing rectocele.

MAGNETIC RESONANCE IMAGING (MRI)

MRI is a non-invasive and non-ionizing technique that produces images of excellent contrast. The fine detail achieved is superior to ultrasound. Despite the development of dynamic fast scan images, the collated images are still not real-time as slices are taken several seconds apart and the patient must remain very still. However MRI provides excellent visualization of anatomy.

Klutke et al (1990) compared MRI of women with stress urinary incontinence with those from continent controls and demonstrated that the urethropelvic ligaments in the former group were directed obliquely and more horizontal in the controls. Women with genuine stress incontinence had more anterior wall prolapse and a 'U' rather than a 'H' shaped vagina. Strohbehn et al (1996) have harvested the urethra and surrounding structures from 13 female cadavers (age 21–81 years) and fixed them in buffered formalin. High resolution T1 and T2 images were obtained and Mallory trichrome stained histological sections were prepared in planes corresponding to the MRI sections. Histology and anatomy were compared using side by side correlation of projected images and by superimposing projected images. T2 images of the cadaveric urethra revealed distinct layers. From the centre to the periphery a series of concentric rings were visible: an inner bright ring, the mucosa; a dark ring, the submucosa; an outer bright ring, the smooth muscle of the urethra in a loose connective tissue matrix and a peripheral dark ring; the striated urogenital sphincter (Fig. 10.22). Using a vaginal endocoil the authors obtained similar pictures in a living female. Although at this stage no comparisons have been made between continent and incontinent women, this type of imaging may shed some light on anatomical changes in incontinence.

Attempts have been made to quantify prolapse in the anterior, middle and posterior compartments and also pelvic floor movement from rest to maximum Valsalva. The measurements have used a line from the inferior border of the symphysis pubis to the last coccygeal joint as a reference (Yang et al 1991). Monga et al (1994) used these measurements before and after sacrocolpopexy (Fig. 10.23). They were unable to predict postoperative genuine stress incontinence but were able to predict women who would develop postoperative rectocele. To date all the uses are research based and clinical application for this expensive technique requires evaluation. However, pelvic floor MRI can demonstrate muscle asymmetry, muscle defects and volume estimation.

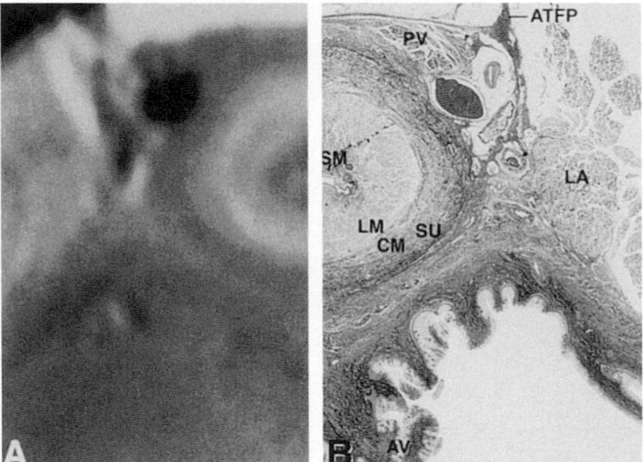

Fig. 10.22 MRI and comparative histology of the striated urethral sphincter.

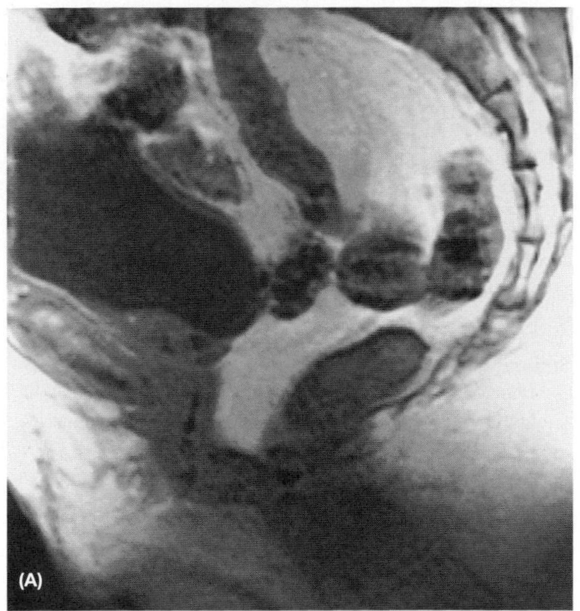

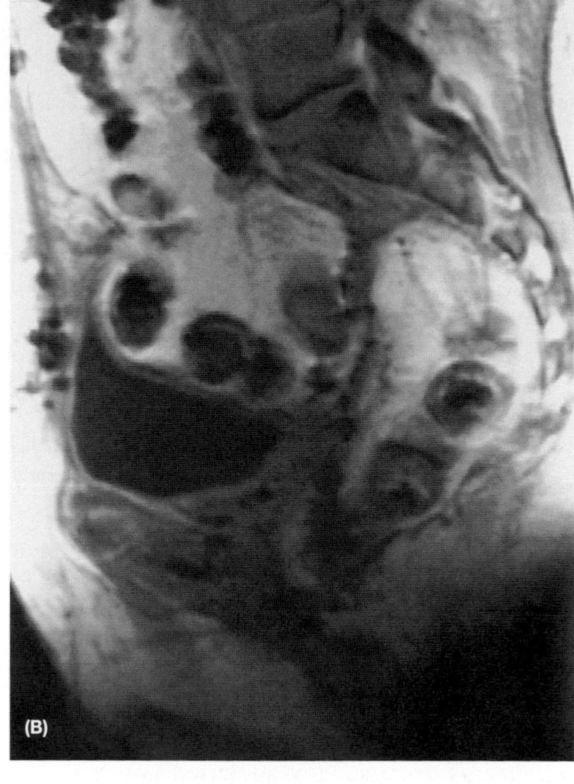

Fig. 10.23 MRI images of a female pelvis. (**A**) Demonstrating vault prolapse and (**B**) after sacrocolpopexy with mesh attachment between the vaginal vault and sacrum.

REFERENCES

Altringer W E, Saclarides T J, Dominguez J M 1995 Four contrast defecography; pelvic floor-oscopy Diseases of the Colon and Rectum 38: 695–698

Bates C P, Whiteside C G, Turner-Warwick R 1970 Synchronous cine/flow/cystourethrography with special reference to stress and urge incontinence. British Journal of Urology 42: 714–723

Bethoux A, Bory S 1962 Les mecanismes statiques visceraux pelviens chez la femme: a la lumiere de l'exploration fonctionelle du dispositif en position debout. Annales de Chirurgie 16: 887–916

Debus-Thiede G 1994 Magnetic resonance imaging of the pelvic floor. In: Schussler B, Laycock J, Norton P, Stanton S (eds) Pelvic floor re-education, Springer-Verlag, London pp 78–82

Enhorning G 1961 Simultaneous recording of intravesical and intraurethral pressures. Acta Chirurgica Scandinavica (suppl) 27: 61–68

Enhorning G, Miller A E, Hinman F 1964 Urethral closure studies with cineroentgenography and simultaneous bladder-urethral pressure recording. Surgery, Gynecology and Obstetrics 118: 507–516

Jeffcoate N, Roberts H 1952 Stress incontinence. British Journal of Obstetrics and Gynaecology 59: 685–720

Klutke C, Golomb J, Barbaric Z, Raz S 1990 The anatomy of stress incontinence: magnetic resonance imaging of the female bladder neck and urethra. Journal of Urology 563–566

Monga A K, Heron C W, Stanton S L 1994 How does sacrocolpopexy affect bladder function and pelvic floor anatomy? A combined urodynamic and MRI approach. Neurourology and Urodynamics 13: 378–380

Strohbehn K, Quint L E, Prince M R, Wojno K J, Delancey J O L 1996 Magnetic resonance imaging anatomy of the female urethra: a direct histologic comparison. Obstetrics and Gynecology 88: 750–756

Yang A, Mostwin J L, Rosenshein N B, Zerhouni E A 1991 Pelvic floor descent in women: dynamic evaluation with fast magnetic resonance imaging and cinematic display. Radiology 179: 25–33

Uroflowmetry

BERNARD HAYLEN AND PAUL ABRAMS

HISTORICAL INTRODUCTION

The importance of the measurement of urine flow rates was realized half a century ago (Ballenger et al 1932). Drake (1948) made the first accurate measurements of urine flow. He used a spring balance; a pen that wrote on a kymograph was attached to one end, and a receptacle for the voided volume was attached to the other end. By rotating the kymograph drawn at a known speed, Drake obtained a trace of voided urine volume against time. He calculated the maximum urine flow rate by a measurement of the steepest part of the volume–time curve. It is evident from his description that the apparatus was relatively crude and difficult to use. Furthermore, urine flow rates had to be calculated from volume–time data. Kaufman (1957) produced a refined modification of Drake's flowmeter which still made no direct recording of flow rate.

The advent of electronics in medical instrumentation allowed the mass production of accurate and reliable recording devices. Von Garrelts (1956) designed the first of the electronic urine flowmeters, comprising a tall urine-collecting cylinder with a pressure transducer in the base. The pressure transducer measured the pressure exerted by an increasing column of urine as the patient voided, producing a direct recording of urine flow rate by electronic differentiation with time.

DEFINITIONS OF URINE FLOW RATE MEASUREMENTS

Urine flow rates are measured in millilitres per second (ml/s). Figure 11.1 denotes the different urine flow rate measurements as suggested by the Standardization Committee of the International Continence Society (1977).

METHODS OF URINE FLOW RATE MEASUREMENT

There have been many methods used for urine flow measurement, from measuring the time to void a given volume through audiometric and radio-isotopic methods to include high-speed cinematography.
In addition, flowmeters have been produced that use the principles of air displacement, resistance to gas flow, electromagnetism, photoelectricity, capacitance and a rotating disc. Flowmeters employing the principles of weight transduction, a rotating disc, and a capacitance transducer are the best known and the most completely tested and validated of the flowmeters available.

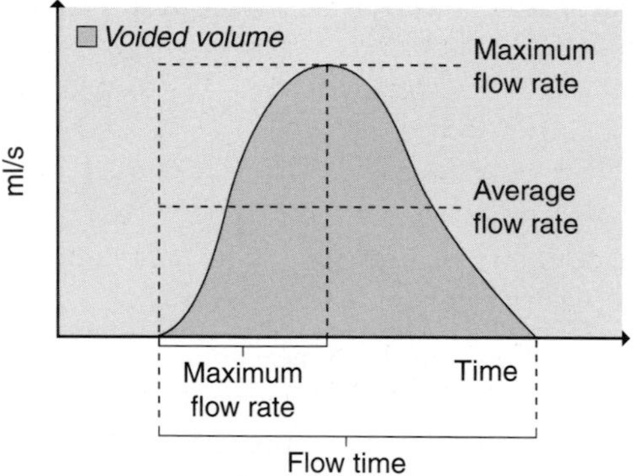

Fig. 11.1 Diagrammatic urine flow curve with measured parameters. Flow rate: the volume of fluid (ml) expelled from the bladder per second. Maximum flow rate: the maximum measured value of the flow rate. Flow time: the time over which measurable flow occurs. Flow time is easily measured if flow is continuous, unless there is a lengthy terminal dribble that may be noted but not included in the flow time. If urine flow is intermittent, the time intervals between flow episodes are not included. Volume voided: the total volume of fluid expelled via the urethra. This can be calculated from the area beneath the flow time curve. Average flow rate: the volume voided divided by the flow time. From International Continence Society (1977), with permission.

The weight transducer type of flowmeter (Fig. 11.2A) weighs the voided urine and by differentiation with time produces an 'on-line' recording of urine flow rate:

$$FR = dV/dT$$

where dV is the change in volume of urine over change in time, dT.

The rotating disc flowmeter (Fig. 11.2B) depends on a servometer maintaining the rotation of the disc at a constant speed. Urine hits the disc, and the extra power required to maintain the speed is electronically converted into a measurement of flow rate.

The capacitance flowmeter is the simplest of the three flowmeters. It consists of a funnel channelling urine into a collecting vessel. The transducer is a dipstick made of plastic and coated with metal, which dips into the vessel containing the voided urine (Fig. 11.2C).

All three types of flowmeter perform accurately and efficiently. For clinical purposes, the measured and indicated flow rate should be accurate to within +/–5% over the clinically significant flow rate range (Rowan et al 1987). The capacitance flowmeter is the least expensive to buy and has the advantage of having no moving parts, which means mechanical breakdowns are eliminated. Rotating disc flowmeters have the advantage of not requiring priming with fluid. Automatic start and stop facilities in most modern flowmeters assist by minimizing patient and staff involvement during the uroflowmetry.

CLINICAL MEASUREMENT OF URINE FLOW RATES

Women are used to voiding in circumstances of almost complete privacy. It is essential in the clinical situation that every effort is made to make the patient feel comfortable and relaxed. If these requirements are ignored, a higher proportion of patients will fail to void in a representative way. Ideally, all free uroflowmetry studies should be performed in a completely private uroflowmetry room/toilet, lockable from the inside, and out of hearing range of other staff and patients. When video studies are combined with pressure-flow recordings in a radiology department, up to 30% of women may fail to void (Arnold et al 1974).

The patient should be encouraged to attend for uroflowmetry with their bladder comfortably full. It is desirable that the measured urine flow rates should be for a voided volume within the patient's normal range. This range can be determined if, in the week

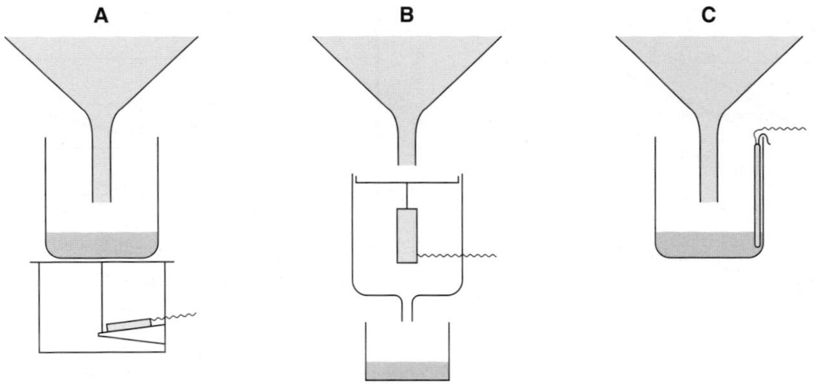

Fig. 11.2 Urine flowmeters. (**A**) Weight transducer. (**B**) Rotating disc. (**C**) Capacitance (dipstick).

before the flow study, the patient completes a frequency–volume chart (urinary diary). There are nomograms which provide normal reference ranges for urinary flow rates over a wide range of voided volumes. There is no need for multiple uroflowmetry in most women. Abnormal or unusual flow curves and urinary flow rates, however, merit repeating the study.

NORMAL URINE FLOW RATES IN WOMEN

The maximum and average urinary flow rates are the two most important parameters and are numerical representations of the flow curve. The clinical usefulness of flow rates has been attenuated by the lack of absolute values defining normal limits (Marshall et al 1983). As urinary flow rates are known to have a strong dependence on voided volume (Drake 1948; Drach et al 1979), these normal limits need to be over a wide range of voided volumes, ideally in the form of nomograms.

Previous studies on normal values for urinary flow rates in women include those of Peter & Drake (1958), Scott & McIhlaney (1961), Backman (1965), Susset et al (1973), and Walter et al (1979), Drach et al (1979), Bottacini & Gleason (1980), Fantl et al (1982) and Rollema et al (1985). Data and/or statistical analysis in these studies has not allowed effective nomogram construction. Difficulties have included small patient numbers (Susset et al, Walter et al, Bottacini & Gleason, Fantl et al, Rollema et al); the use of outmoded or less well-evaluated equipment (Peter & Drake, Drach et al) and the incompleteness of data at lower voided volumes (Backman, Drach et al) due in part to the inaccuracy of some equipment at lower voided volumes (Drach et al).

The maximum urine flow rate has been most studied. Recommended lower limits of normality range between 12 and 20 ml per second. Most commonly, a minimum rate of 15 ml per second is quoted for the same parameter if at least 150 ml (or sometimes 200 ml) has been voided. The practice of artificially imposing minimum limits for the voided volume is difficult to justify (Ryall & Marshall 1982a) and very often impractical. Women with certain states of lower urinary tract dysfunction – those in whom the urine flow rate might be most important – may not be able to hold 200 ml. Because of the strong dependency of urine flow rates on voided volume, a normal urine flow rate at 200 ml may not also be normal at 400 ml.

In a study by Haylen et al (1989a), 249 healthy and asymptomatic female volunteers (16 to 63 years), underwent uroflowmetry studies. Each woman voided once in a completely private environment over a calibrated rotating disc-type uroflowmeter; 46 voided on a second occasion. The maximum and average flow rates of the first voids were compared with the respective voided volumes. By using statistical transformations of both voided volumes and urine flow rates, relationships between the two variables were obtained. This allowed the construction of nomograms, which, for ease of interpretation, have been displayed in centile form.

Fig. 11.3A, B shows the Liverpool nomograms for the maximum and the average flow rate in women.

CLINICAL FACTORS INFLUENCING NORMAL URINE FLOW RATES

Voided volume

The use of nomograms overcomes the danger of referencing urine flow rates to any one voided volume. A maximum flow rate of 15 ml/s might fall just within the 5th centile curve at 200 ml voided volume,

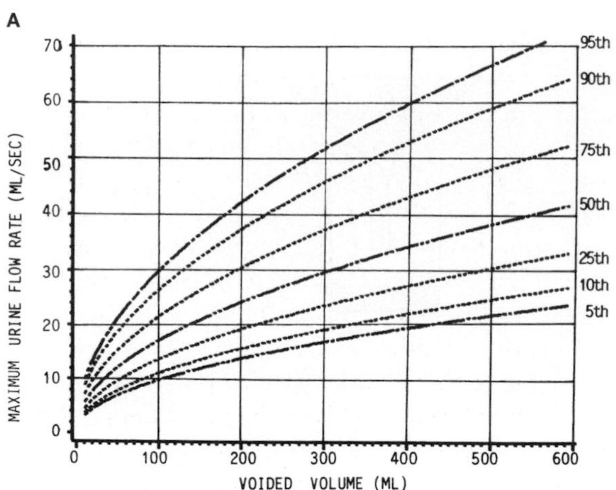

Fig. 11.3 (A) The Liverpool maximum urine flow rate nomogram for women.

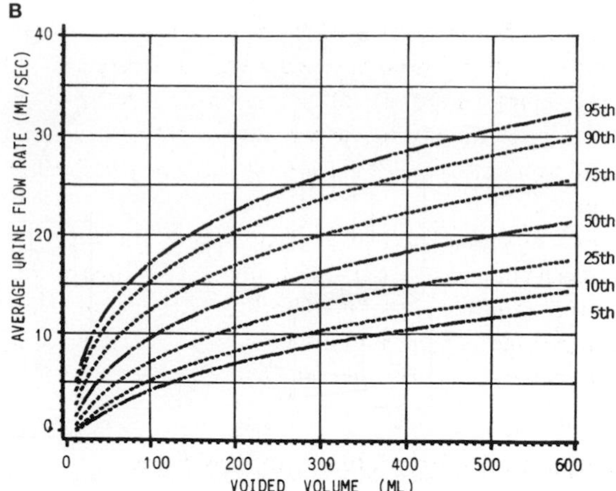

Fig. 11.3 (B) The Liverpool average urine flow rate nomogram for women. From Haylen et al (1989a), with permission.

though well below the same curve at 400 ml. The median voided volume of 171 ml in the above series highlights the need for normal reference ranges to include data at lower voided volumes.

Both the maximum and average urine flow rates had a strong and equal dependence on voided volume. The clinical use of either flow rate is equally valid. However, the centile lines onto which the maximum and average urine flow rates respectively fall for the same voided volume (centile rankings) are not interchangeable in an individual instance, due to wide variations in urine flow patterns. The closer the urine flow pattern comes to the 'ideal' flow time curve (seen in Figure 11.1), the more chance there will be that the centile rankings for the maximum and average urine flow rates are the same.

Age and parity

Haylen et al (1989a) found no significant age dependence of urinary flow rates in normal women. This agreed with the findings of Drach et al (1979) and Fantl et al (1982). There is, however, deterioration in urine flow with age in women with lower urinary tract dysfunction (Torrens 1987; Haylen et al 1995). The studies of Drach et al, Fantl et al and Haylen et al (1989a) all found that there was no significant effect of parity on flow rates in normal women, though a small deleterious effect has been noted in symptomatic women (Haylen et al 1999).

Repeated voiding

There was a remarkable consistency in the centile rankings of the paired first and second voids in the study of Haylen et al (1989a). This consistency is further witnessed in the multiple voids from a single 25-year-old normal female volunteer (Fig. 11.4). Fantl et al (1982) found no significant differences between the first and up to the sixth void in the 60 women they tested.

Clinically, in the majority of normal women, the centile rankings of successive voids will not differ widely. It is uncertain, at present, whether this is also true for women with lower urinary tract dysfunction.

Presence of a urethral catheter

The above nomograms refer to free flowmetry voids; they are not applicable where a pressure or other catheter is present in the urethra. By necessity, potentially unfavourable environmental and psychological factors are introduced when catheterization uroflowmetry is performed. Ryall & Marshall (1982b) suggested that physical obstruction was caused by the pressure catneter, with a reduction in maximum

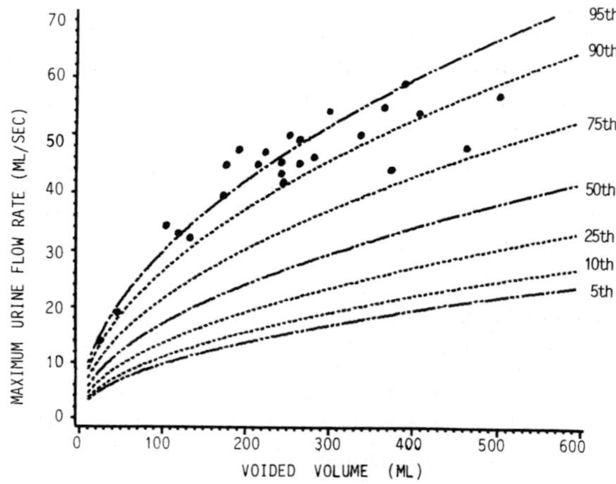

Fig. 11.4 The maximum flow rates from a large number of voids by a single 25-year-old female volunteer superimposed on the respective Liverpool nomogram. From Haylen et al (1989a), with permission.

urinary flow rate caused by the fine (diameter = 2 mm) urethral catheter used in their study of 147 symptomatic men was of the order of several ml/s. Though small, this reduction was enough to change the diagnostic categorization of one third of their subjects.

Recent studies (Cerqui A, Haylen B T and Law M G, personal communication, 1999) showed an unexpected favourable effect of a 7FG Urethral catheter of urine flow, particularly in patients with prolapse, if voiding cystometry was performed close to bladder capacity.

Comparison with male urine flow rates

In the Liverpool nomogram studies (Haylen et al 1989a), women were found to have higher urine flow rates than men at any comparative age and voided volume. This is demonstrated in Table 11.1 for the maximum urine flow rates for women and the two age groupings of men at different voided volumes.

Backman (1965) using Von Garrelts' (1957) male data and Drach et al (1979) had previously suggested that female urine flow rates were higher than male. The difference in urethral length (20 cm vs. 4 cm) between men and women according to Backman (1965) quoting Bernoulli's law relating to turbulent flow along a tube, would account for urinary flow in women being 0.38 times faster than men. As seen in Table 11.1, the maximum urine flow rates in women were on average 0.19 times higher than those of young men and 0.39 times higher than older men. The urethral length factor can then account for all the intersex differences in urine flow rates.

OTHER FACTORS INFLUENCING URINE FLOW RATES

Urine flow depends on the relationship between the bladder and urethra during voiding. The situation during voiding is the antithesis of the situation required for continence. Continence depends on intraurethral pressure being higher than intravesical pressure. For voiding to occur, intravesical pressure must exceed intraurethral pressure.

Table 11.1 Comparison of the 50th centiles for the maximum urine flow rates in women and the two age groupings of men at different voided volumes.

	100	300	500
Women	17.1	29.7	38.5
Men under 50	13.5	24.9	34.7
Men over 50	11.1	21.6	30.7

Enhorning (1961), and later Asmussen & Ulmsten (1976), showed clearly that before there was any rise in intravesical pressure, a fall in intraurethral pressure occurred. This suggests that the urethra actively relaxes during voiding rather than being passively 'blown open' by the detrusor contraction. Soon after the urethra has relaxed and pelvic floor descent has occurred, the detrusor contracts. The detrusor normally contrives to contract until the bladder is empty, producing a continuous flow curve. Many women void by urethral relaxation alone with minimal or no detrusor involvement. This method of voiding is common in women with stress incontinence.

Changes in intra-abdominal pressure also influence urine flow. Some women appear to void entirely by increasing intra-abdominal pressure, that is, by contraction of the diaphragm and anterior abdominal wall muscles.

It follows from this discussion that the urine flow may differ from normal as a result of abnormalities of the urethra or the detrusor.

Urethral factors

Anatomical factors

The narrowest part of the urethra, as shown by video studies of voiding, is usually the mid-zone. However, the urethra may become narrowed; the most common site is towards the external meatus associated with an oestrogen deficiency in the postmenopausal woman. Intrinsic bladder neck obstruction in the female is extremely rare (Turner-Warwick et al 1973). Deviation from a normally straight female urethra is most common in anterior vaginal wall prolapse and higher degrees of uterine and vaginal vault prolapse. The effect of prolapse on urine flow rates is demonstrated in Table 11.2.

Vaginal repair of the prolapse has not been shown to produce a significant alteration in postoperative flow rates, irrespective of whether or not stress incontinence was present preoperatively (Stanton et al 1982). Correction of anterior vaginal wall prolapse by a colposuspension does lead to deterioration in urinary flow rates (Stanton et al 1978).

Pathological factors

Unusual congenital conditions such as urethral duplication, urethral diverticula or urethral cysts may obstruct voiding. Infective lesions as in urethritis or infected paraurethral cysts may lead to voiding difficulties. Post-traumatic strictures and urethral neoplasms will have a similar effect. An intravaginal

Table 11.2 Effect of prolapse in symptomatic women on the median centiles for the maximum (MUFR) and average (AUFR) urine flow rates.

	Cystocele		Uterine		Rectocele		Enterocele	
	MUFR	AUFR	MUFR	AUFR	MUFR	AUFR	MUFR	AUFR
Grade 0	42	30	49	37	43	32	35	30
Grade 1	35	32	32	32	24	16	11	10
Grade 2/3	20	11	17	11	32	27	17	12

From Haylen et al (1999), with permission.

abnormality, such as a foreign body or tumour, might also obstruct micturition.

Functional factors

Abnormal urethral behaviour during voiding may lead to alteration in the urine flow rate recording. In the neurologically abnormal patient, failure of striated muscle relaxation during detrusor contraction is known as detrusor sphincter dyssynergia. In the nervous and anxious but neurologically normal patient, flow may be affected by failure to relax the pelvic floor.

Detrusor factors

Contractility

Poor detrusor contractility may be responsible for a slow flow rate. Such patients may present with urinary tract infections or urinary retention. These patients have normal urethral function as judged by pressure profilometry or radiology. Their reduced flow rates are secondary to a weak and poorly sustained detrusor contraction.

Innervation

Normal detrusor behaviour depends on normal innervation. Bladder contractions are preserved if the sacral reflex arc is intact, even when the upper motor neurones are damaged. However, if the sacral reflex arc is damaged, bladder contractions are generally absent. The only form of contractile activity possible when the lower motor neurone is damaged is locally mediated – the 'autonomous' bladder. The urine flow rates produced by the abnormally innervated bladder are usually reduced and interrupted.

Pathological factors

Although little specific literature on the subject exists, it is evident that gross disease of the detrusor will result in abnormal urine flow rates. The fibrosis resulting from irradiation, tuberculosis, cystitis, or interstitial cystitis is likely to impair detrusor contractility.

URINE FLOW RATES IN UROGYNAECOLOGY PATIENTS

Peter & Drake (1958) observed lower urine flow rates in 12 women with incontinence and prolapse than those in normal women. Bottacini & Gleason (1980) found a higher incidence of low flow rates in stress incontinent women than in normal women. The only large studies have been those of Haylen et al (1990, 1999) involving 168 and 250 women respectively, looking at the effect of urodynamic diagnosis.

Symptomatic versus asymptomatic women

Urine flow rates are significantly slower in women with symptoms of lower urinary tract dysfunction (see Table 11.3) than in normal women.

Effect of prolapse

Table 11.2 shows the progressive decline in urine flow rates with increasing grades of prolapse with the most significant decline in the presence of uterine prolapse closely followed by cystocele and enterocele. There is a much smaller effect in the presence of a rectocele.

Patients often report quicker urine flow in the early morning (after the prolapse has receded overnight with rest) and appearing slowest at the end of the day when the prolapse is most prominent.

Table 11.3 Urine flow rates overall in symptomatic women

	Symptomatic 1990	Symptomatic 1999	Asymptomatic
Mean centile maximum urine flow rate (MUFR)	31	32	50
Mean centile average urine flow rate (AUFR)	26	26	50

From Haylen et al (1990; 1999), with permission.

Table 11.4 Effect of prior hysterectomy on urine flow rate centiles.

	Number	MUFR	AUFR
No hysterectomy	124	50	31
Vaginal hysterectomy	71	23	18
Abdominal hysterectomy	25	23	20

From Haylen et al (1999), with permission.

Effect of prior hysterectomy

There is a significant decline in urine flow rates in symptomatic women with a prior hysterectomy, as seen in Table 11.4. The effect appeared the same with both vaginal and abdominal hysterectomy. Parys et al (1989) showed voiding difficulties to be a major diagnosis in symptomatic women following hysterectomy, probably due to nerve injury.

Effect of age

There is a significant deterioration of urine flow rates in symptomatic women with age. As seen in Figure 11.5, in women with neither prior hysterectomy nor prolapse (top line), the age deterioration occurs after the menopause, with distal atrophic urethral changes a possible factor. There are further progressive declines for women with either a prior hysterectomy or prolapse (centre line) and the greatest decline in women with a prior hysterectomy and higher grade prolapse. It does suggest that a large part of the decline in urine flow rates with age in symptomatic women may be due to the increased frequency of hysterectomy and prolapse in older women.

Effect of urodynamic diagnosis

All diagnostic groups are seen in Table 11.5 to have median urine flow centiles lower than 50, the median for asymptomatic women. In terms of the specific diagnostic ability of urine flow rates, the main discriminatory ability occurs with the diagnosis of voiding difficulties.

When the 5th and 10th centiles of the Liverpool nomograms were examined, it appeared that the 10th centile for the maximum urine flow rate provides the best ability to discriminate between those at higher risk of voiding difficulties (centiles 10 and under) and those women unlikely to have voiding difficulties (centiles over 10) with a sensitivity of 81% and a specificity of 92%. Normally, the final diagnosis of voiding difficulties would require the complementary information provided by a residual urine measurement and voiding cystometry.

In the largest female diagnostic group, genuine stress incontinence, over 20% will have urine flow rates under the 10th centile putting them at higher risk of voiding difficulties (Haylen et al 1990)

URINARY FLOW PATTERNS

Urine flow curves are complementary to flow rates in the assessment of voiding. Because flow curves cannot be numerically represented (except by flow rates), they are less useful for clinical comparisons than flow rates. Several patterns of flow curves can however be recognized.

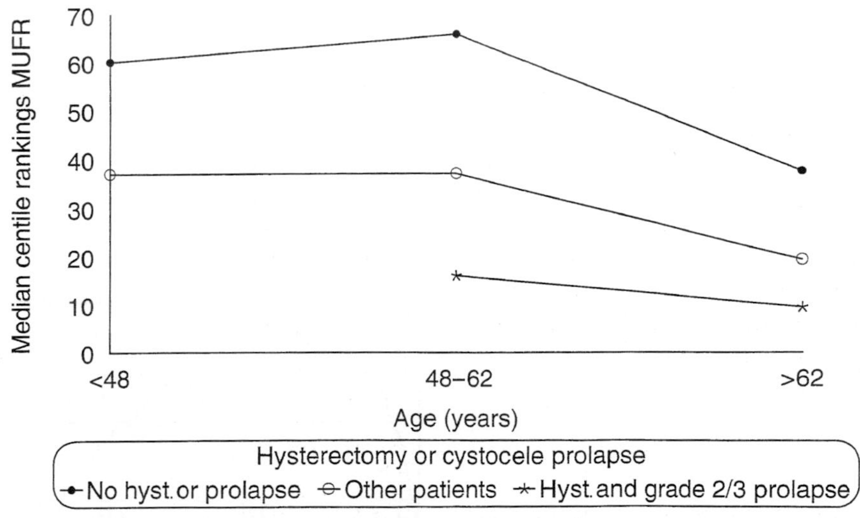

Fig. 11.5 Median centile rankings maximum urine flow rates (MUFR) according to age, depending on the presence or absence of prior hysterectomy and/or prolapse. From Haylen et al (1999), with permission.

Table 11.5 Median centiles for the MUFR and AUFR depending on final urodynamic diagnosis.

	Number	Median centile MUFR	Median centile AUFR
Genuine stress incontinence (GSI)	107	48	40
Detrusor instability (DI)	14	38	32
Voiding difficulties (VOID)	7	1	6
GSI plus DI	39	34	32
GSI plus VOID	22	3	2
DI plus VOID	14	3	2
GSI plus DI plus VOID	10	4	7
Normal	7	70	52

From Haylen et al (1999), with permission.

Normal

The **normal** flow trace (Fig. 11.6A, B) shows a symmetrical peak with maximum flow rate generally achieved within 5 seconds of the beginning of voiding. The maximum flow rate is generally 1.5–2 times the average flow rate.

A **low normal (suboptimal)** flow trace (Fig. 11.7A) shows no symmetrical peak. Maximum flow rate, somewhere between the 10th and 25th centiles, occurs early, then the flow trails off. An **abdominal strain pattern** (Fig. 11.7B) shows the influence of intermittent strain during the void.

Abnormal – continuous flow

Urine flow curves reflected in flow rates below the 5th centile may generally be regarded as abnormal; abnormality can be suspected in those curves with flow rates between the 5th and 10th centiles.

A **reduced** flow rate may be due either to a **urethral obstruction** or to a **poor detrusor contraction** (Fig. 11.8). It is necessary to perform full pressure flow studies to demonstrate the cause of a reduced urine flow rate.

A **reduced and fluctuating** flow pattern (Fig. 11.9) is usually associated with an incompletely sustained detrusor contraction, as may be seen in patients with multiple sclerosis. As well as being incompletely sustained, the maximum detrusor pressure is usually below normal; hence the reduced flow.

Abnormal – interrupted flow

Voluntary sphincter contraction

In the anxious and nervous patient the distal urethral sphincteric mechanism may close. Urine flow may decrease or stop (Fig. 11.10). Characteristically, the rate of change of flow rate is rapid, indicating sphincter closure. As was seen in Figure 11.9, when flow rate changes are due to changes in the detrusor activity, the rate of change is slow.

Detrusor sphincter dyssynergia

Detrusor sphincter dyssynergia is an involuntary phenomenon in which the expected coordination of the detrusor contraction and urethral relaxation is lost. Despite an effective detrusor contraction, the urethral mechanism remains closed for longer periods of time (up to several minutes). Detrusor sphincter

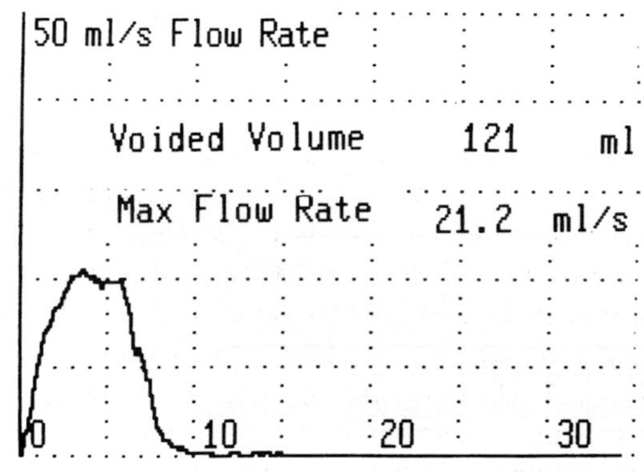

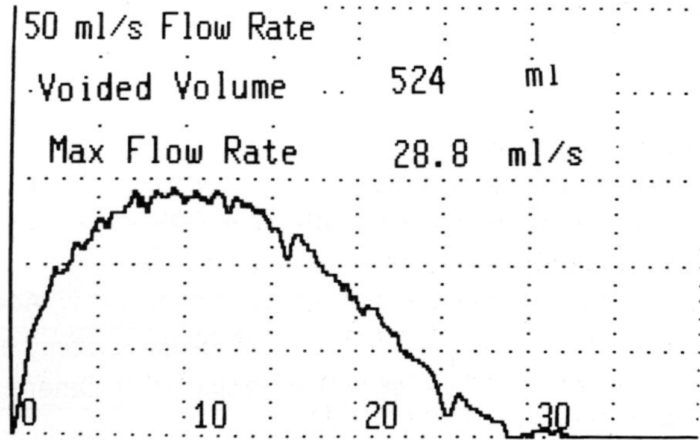

Fig. 11.6 Normal flow curves for voided volumes of **(A)** 121 ml and **(B)** 524 ml. From Haylen et al (1989a) with permission.

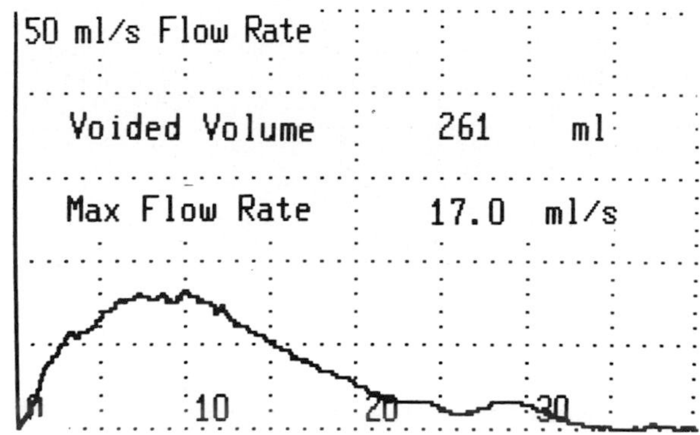

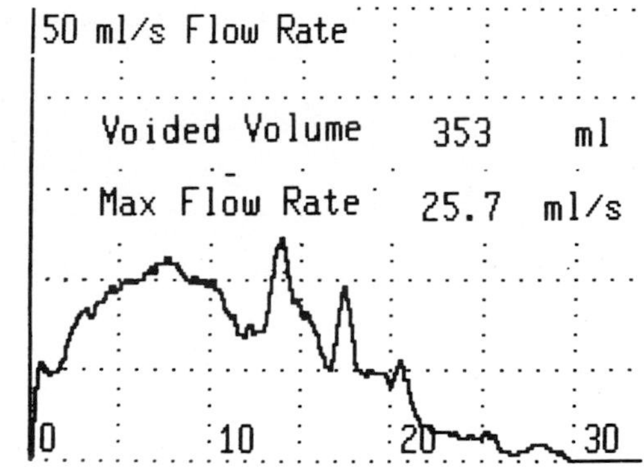

Fig. 11.7 (**A**) Low normal (suboptimal) flow curve (voided volume 261 ml). (**B**) Abdominal strain pattern (voided volume 353 ml). From Haylen et al (1989a), with permission.

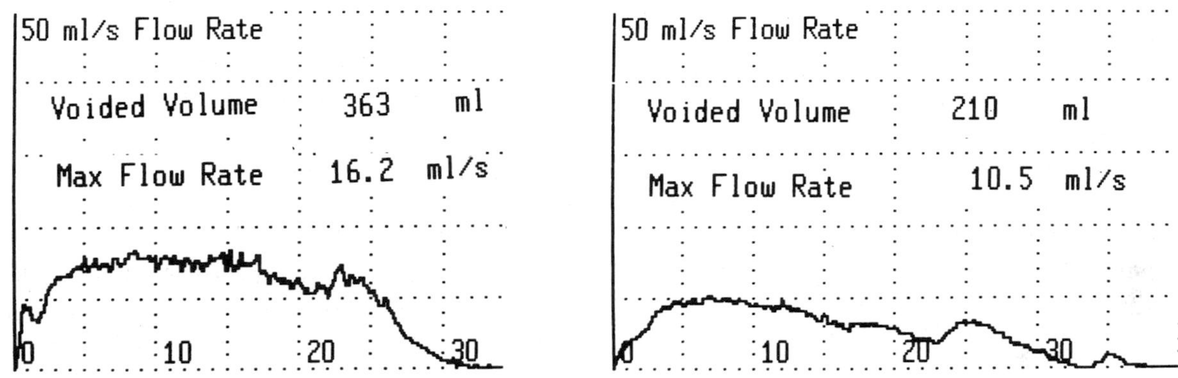

Fig. 11.8 Reduced urine flow trace caused by: (**A**) detrusor underactivity (maximum detrusor pressure 20 cm H_2O) and (**B**) outflow obstruction (meatal stenosis, maximum detrusor pressure 54 cm H_2O). From Haylen et al (1989a) with permission.

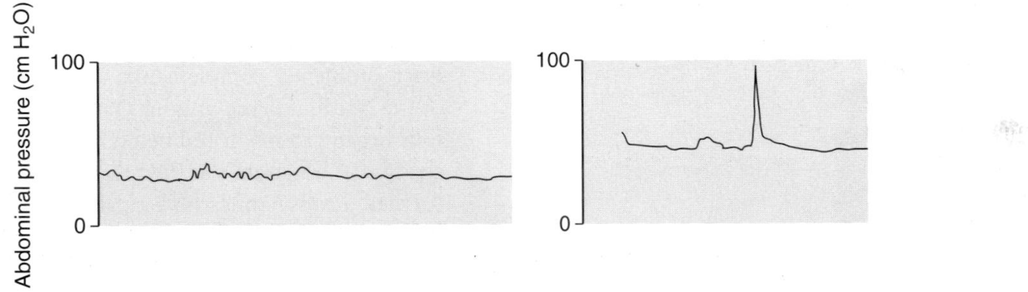

Fig. 11.9 Reduced and fluctuating urine flow trace caused by incompletely sustained detrusor contraction (as seen on intravesical pressure trace) in patient with spina bifida.

dyssynergia may result in a large residual urine together with upper tract dilatation and renal failure and is often associated with repeated infection. Detrusor sphincter dyssynergia only occurs in neurologically abnormal patients, most classically in higher spinal cord trauma. The flow rate produced by detrusor sphincter dyssynergia is usually reduced and always interrupted (Fig. 11.11).

The flow patterns that have been described in the last two sections are secondary to pathophysiological problems. The patient may modify her flow tract by straining, using abdominal wall and diaphragmatic muscles. Before a flow rate measurement, the patient should be asked whether or not she strains to void. If she does usually strain, she should be asked whether she can void without straining. If she has to strain to void, it is likely that detrusor activity is reduced or absent. If the patient claims not to void by straining, she should be asked to void in a relaxed manner and without straining. Straining produces changes in

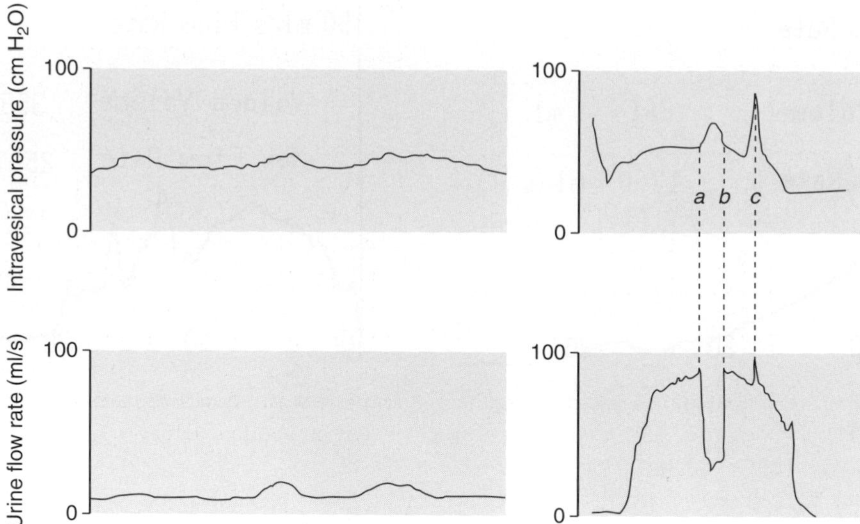

Fig. 11.10 Interrupted urine flow trace caused by voluntary sphincter contraction in anxious patient. At point *a* sphincter closes with increase in intravesical pressure and decrease in flow rate. Converse occurs at point *b*. At point *c* patient raises her intraabdominal pressure, and as sphincter is open, flow rate increases.

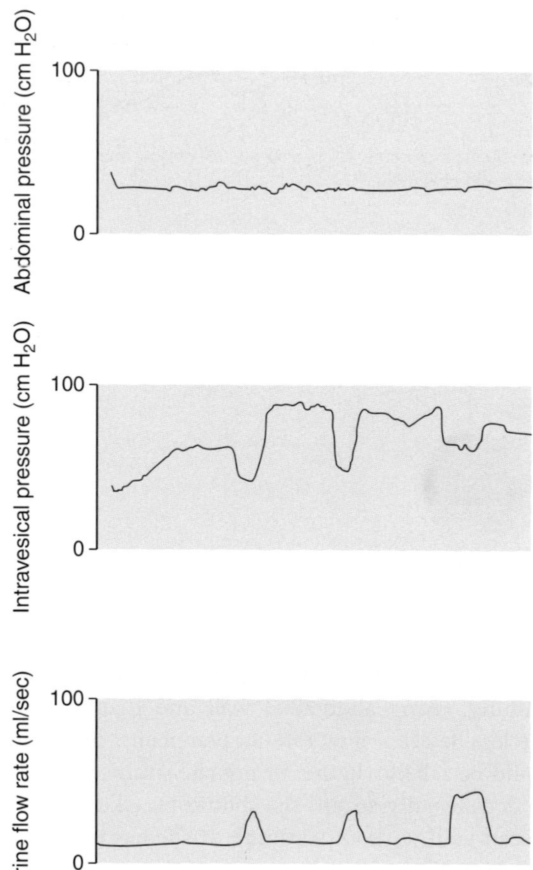

Fig. 11.11 Tracing of spinal cord-injured patient with detrusor sphincter dyssynergia. Urine flow trace is interrupted and flow only occurs when sphincter relaxes at which time intravesical pressure falls.

flow rate of moderate speed and usually the flow remains continuous (Figure 11.12). However, straining may be used by any patient with any coexisting lower urinary tract problem.

INDICATIONS FOR UROFLOWMETRY

Urine flow studies are an important screening test for voiding difficulties in all patients with lower urinary tract problems, complementary to the measurement of the residual urine volume. These problems fall into four broad groups, listed below. However, the demonstration of an abnormal flow trace is an indication for further urodynamic investigation, that is, inflow cystometry and pressure-flow studies, with or without simultaneous videocystourethrography.

Symptoms suggestive of outflow obstruction

Thirty percent of apparently normal women will describe at least one of the following symptoms of voiding difficulties (hesitancy, poor stream, need to strain to void, sense of incomplete emptying or the need to immediately revoid). This compares with urodynamic patients, 70% of whom will admit to at least one and 53% to at least two of the same symptoms (Haylen et al 1989b). Apparently normal women, who yet admit to incontinence, will also have a 30% incidence of at least one other symptom of voiding difficulties.

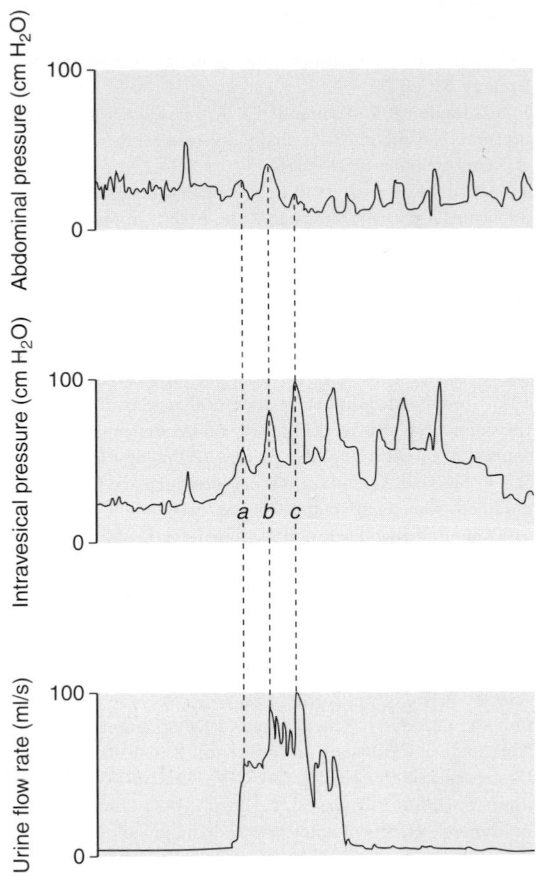

Fig. 11.12 Irregular urine flow trace of patient with normal lower urinary tract who is straining while voiding. At points *a*, *b* and *c*, patient strains with consequent increase in abdominal pressure and intravesical pressure and on each occasion urine flow rate rises.

Symptoms suggestive of bladder overactivity

Flow studies are preliminary to cystometry that is necessary to define the urodynamic abnormality responsible for the symptom complex of frequency, nocturia, urgency and urge incontinence. Anticholinergic medications will exacerbate any tendency towards urinary retention in patients with the combined diagnoses of detrusor instability and voiding difficulties.

Genuine stress incontinence

Flow studies are an important preoperative investigation in women awaiting surgery for genuine stress incontinence. Assuming genuine stress incontinence has been urodynamically proven, a normal flow rate reassures the surgeon that long-term voiding difficulties are unlikely to follow the operation to cure the stress incontinence. Since effective surgery usually results in an increase in urethral resistance in women with poor preoperative flow rates, incomplete emptying or even persistent failure to void may follow surgery (Stanton et al 1978). Therefore urine flow studies, with or without pressure-flow studies, are to be recommended before surgery.

Neuropathic lower urinary tract dysfunction

Voiding problems in patients with neuropathic lower urinary tract dysfunction consist of three main types. Patients may experience incontinence as a result of bladder instability. The main problem may be the failure to empty the bladder because of a poorly sustained detrusor contraction. Detrusor sphincter dyssynergia may prevent an effective detrusor contraction from emptying the bladder, with the consequent possible complications of recurrent infections and renal failure. Urine flow studies may suggest the origin of the problems experienced by this group of patients, although video-pressure-flow studies are desirable in almost every case.

REFERENCES

Arnold E, Brown A, Webster J 1974 Videocysturethrography with synchronous detrusor pressure and flow rate recordings. Annals of the Royal College of Surgeons 55: 90–98

Asmussen M, Ulmsten U 1976 Simultaneous urethrocystometry with a new technique. Scandinavian Journal of Urology and Nephrology 10: 7–11

Backman K-A 1965 Urinary flow during micturition in normal women. Journal of Urology 137: 497–499

Ballenger E G, Elder O F, McDonald H P 1932 Voiding distance decrease as an important early symptom of prostatic obstruction. Southern Medical Journal 25: 863

Bottacini M R, Gleason D J 1980 Urodynamic norms in women: normals versus stress incontinents. Journal of Urology 124: 659–661

Drach G W, Ignatoff J, Layton T 1979 Peak urine flow rate: observations in female subjects and comparison to male subjects. Journal of Urology 122: 215–219

Drake W M 1948 The uroflowmeter: an aid to the study of the lower urinary tract. Journal of Urology 59: 650–658

Enhorning G 1961 Simultaneous recording of intravesical and intraurethral pressure. Acta Chirurgica Scandinavica (Suppl.) 276: 1–68

Fantl J A, Smith P J, Schneider V, Hurt W F, Dunn L J 1982 Fluid weight uroflowmetry in women. American Journal of Obstetrics and Gynecology 145: 1017–1024

Haylen B T, Ashby D, Sutherst J R, Frazer M I, West C 1989a Maximum and average urine flow rates in normal male and female populations – the Liverpool nomograms. British Journal of Urology 64: 30–38

Haylen B T, Sutherst J R, Frazer M I 1989b Is the investigation of most urinary incontinence really necessary. British Journal of Urology 64: 147–149

Haylen B T, Parys B T, Anyaegbunam W I, Ashby Deborah, West C R 1990 Urine flow rates in male and female urodynamic patients compared with the Liverpool nomograms. British Journal of Urology 65: 483–487

Haylen B T, Law M G, Frazer M I 1995 Urine flow rates in urogynaecology patients. Neurourology and Urodynamics 14: 417–419

Haylen B T, Law M G, Frazer M I, Schulz S 1999 Urine flow rates and residual urine volumes in urogynaecology patients. International Urogynaecology Journal 10: 2 (in press)

International Continence Society 1977 Second report on the standardization of terminology of lower urinary tract function. British Journal of Urology 49: 207–210

Kaufman J 1957 A new recording uroflowmeter: a simple automatic device for measuring voiding velocity. Journal of Urology 78: 97–102

Marshall V R, Ryall R I, Austin M L, Sinclair G R 1983 The use of urinary flow rates obtained from voided volumes less than 150 ml in the assessment of voiding ability. British Journal of Urology 55: 28–33

Parys B T, Haylen B T, Woolfenden K A, Parsons K F 1989 Vesico-urethral dysfunction after simple hysterectomy. Neurourology and Urodynamics 8: 315–316

Peter W P, Drake W M Jr 1958 Uroflowmetric observations in gynecologic patients. Journal of the American Medical Association 166: 721–724

Rollema H J, Griffiths D J, Jones U 1985 Computer-aided uroflowmetry. Normal values in healthy women and applications in gynaecological patients. Proceedings of the International Continence Society London, pp 210–211

Rowan D, James E D, Kramer A E J L, Sterling A M, Suhel P F 1987 Urodynamic equipment: technical aspects. International Continence Society Working Party on Urodynamic Equipment. Journal of Medical Engineering and Technology 11: 57–64

Ryall R L, Marshall V R 1982a Normal peak urinary flow rate obtained from small voided volumes can provide a reliable assessment of bladder function. Journal of Urology 127: 484–487

Ryall R L, Marshall V R 1982b The effect of a urethral catheter on the measurement of maximum urinary flow rate. Journal of Urology. 128: 429–432

Scott R, McIhlaney J G 1961 Voiding rate in normal adults. Journal of Urology 128: 429–432

Stanton S L, Cardozo L, Chaudhury N 1978 Spontaneous voiding after surgery for urinary incontinence. British Journal of Obstetrics and Gynaecology 83: 149–152

Stanton S L, Hilton P, Norton C, Cardozo L 1982 Clinical and urodynamic effects of anterior colporrhaphy and vaginal hysterectomy for prolapse, with and without incontinence. British Journal of Obstetrics and Gynaecology 89: 459–463

Susset J G, Picker P, Kretz M, Jorest R 1973 Clinical evaluation of uroflowmeters and analysis of normal curves. Journal of Urology 109: 874–878

Torrens M J 1987 Urodynamics. In: Torrens M J, Morrison J F B (eds) The physiology of the lower urinary tract. Springer-Verlag, London, Chap. 9, pp 277–307

Turner-Warwick R et al 1973 A urodynamic view of the clinical problems associated with bladder neck dysfunction and its treatment by endoscopic incision and trans-trigonal posterior prostatectomy. British Journal of Urology 45: 44–59

Von Garrelts B (1956) Analysis of micturition: a new method of recording the voiding of the bladder. Acta Chirurgica Scandinavica 112: 326

Von Garrelts, B (1957) Micturition in the normal male. Acta Chirurgica Scandinavica 114: 197–210

Walter S Olesen K P, Nordberg J, Hald T 1979 Bladder function in urologically normal middle aged females. Scandinavian Journal of Urology and Nephrology 13: 249–258

Urethral function tests

DAVID M HOLMES AND ALISON B PEATTIE

INTRODUCTION

> Many techniques have been introduced, none are specific, and few are standardised.
>
> *Hodgkinson 1990*

Hodgkinson's brief statement brings into perspective the highly sophisticated technology we routinely use to test urethrovesical function. As with many of the tests we use in clinical medicine these have been accepted on the basis of their past or theoretical relevance rather than on a strict audit of their clinical value. Abnormalities are often defined without reference to a true normal range, thus making interpretation of the results arbitrary. The investigation of urinary incontinence is an area where attempts have been made to standardize investigations, but it is important for us to realize that no perfect test of urethral function has yet been devised.

History and clinical examination are used in urogynaecology to make a provisional diagnosis of the cause of lower urinary tract symptoms. Investigations establish a urodynamic diagnosis and if the two diagnoses concur this is then used as the basis for treatment.

The International Continence Society has defined detrusor instability and genuine stress incontinence (Abrams et al 1988) using twin-channel subtracted cystometry. Cystometry is thus the only diagnostic test for these conditions that, by definition, cannot be diagnosed clinically. Even experienced clinicians are only able to correctly predict the cystometric diagnosis in 65% of women using the history and clinical findings alone (Jarvis et al 1980).

The techniques described in this chapter are investigations of, rather than diagnostic tests of, urethral function. It is important to interpret their results in the light of the history, examination and possible clinical diagnoses.

Urethral function

The urethra acts not only to transmit stored urine from the bladder, but also to maintain continence. The concept that continence can only be maintained by the hydrostatic pressure in the urethra exceeding that within the bladder is not new (Barnes 1940), but does oversimplify what is a complicated physical model. Measuring intravesical pressure is a relatively easy procedure; whereas attempts to measure hydrostatic pressure within the sealed lumen of the continent urethra have been bedevilled by a failure to recognize the impossibility of doing so. Hydrostatic pressure can only be measured in an unsealed urethra, where the lumen is patent and contains fluid at the point of measurement. If the lumen is patent the urethral closure forces have been overcome and the measurement does not truly reflect the continent situation.

Two active and two passive components have been suggested to maintain continence (Enhorning 1976).

1 Active

- Active compression from the surrounding musculature
- Pressure transmission from the abdomen to the uretha

2 Passive

- The tone of the musculature of the urethral wall
- Stasis in the submucous cavernous vasculature of the urethra.

The magnitude of the compressive forces required to seal a lumen are related to the viscoelastic properties of the material surrounding it. The more elastic the material the easier it is to seal. It is recognized clinically that a rigid, scarred urethra will not seal easily (Hodgkinson 1965). A technique to quantify urethral elastance has been developed (Colstrup et al 1983) and elaborated (Lose 1991) to try and distinguish between normal and pathological urethral function. The results indicate that there are indeed differences, and that pathological subgroups exist, confirming the multifactorial nature of the pathophysiology of genuine stress incontinence.

If the inner walls of the urethra are coated with a thin layer of plastic material then the seal is maintained under lower compressive forces (Zinner et al 1976) than if the seal was dry. This plastic material may represent mucous from the paraurethral glands, or the presence of thin walled, submucous blood vessels which approximate to this function. The nature of this variable has not been fully investigated despite the development of the necessary technology (Plevnik & Vrtacnik 1980, 1981a; Plevnik et al 1981).

Urethral pressure measurement

Leakage will only occur if bladder pressure exceeds the maximum urethral pressure. This occurs if there is a relative drop in urethral pressure, a relative rise in bladder pressure or a combination of the two.

Several techniques have been used to estimate 'the idealized concepts which represent the ability of the urethra to prevent leakage' (Abrams et al 1988). These different techniques do not always give consistent results and so in reporting any investigation it is important to specify the exact method used.

TECHNIQUES OF PRESSURE MEASUREMENT

Retrograde sphincterometry

The earliest method of estimating the maximum urethral closure forces was retrograde sphincterometry (Bonney 1923). A catheter attached to a manometer tube was inserted into the distal urethra and the reservoir slowly elevated until the hydrostatic pressure overcame the urethral closure forces and allowed fluid to pass into the bladder. Although the technique has been modified to use carbon dioxide as the medium and remains in clinical use (Robertson 1974), most authorities now feel that the method is inaccurate (Tanagho 1979). Any rise in intravesical pressure or reflex rhabdosphincter activity will inevitably confuse the results due to the unphysiological nature of the investigation.

Fluid perfusion systems

Fluid perfusion systems (Toews 1967; Brown & Wickham 1969) are the commonest techniques used to estimate the pressure in the urethra. They have the benefit of being easy to use but the results vary with the technique and so it is important to report this in detail. The commonest equipment consists of an 8F catheter with two side-holes diametrically opposite each other 5 cm from the tip (Fig. 12.1) connected through a manometer tube to a pressure transducer. The catheter lumen is perfused with saline from a syringe pump or intravenous giving set whilst being

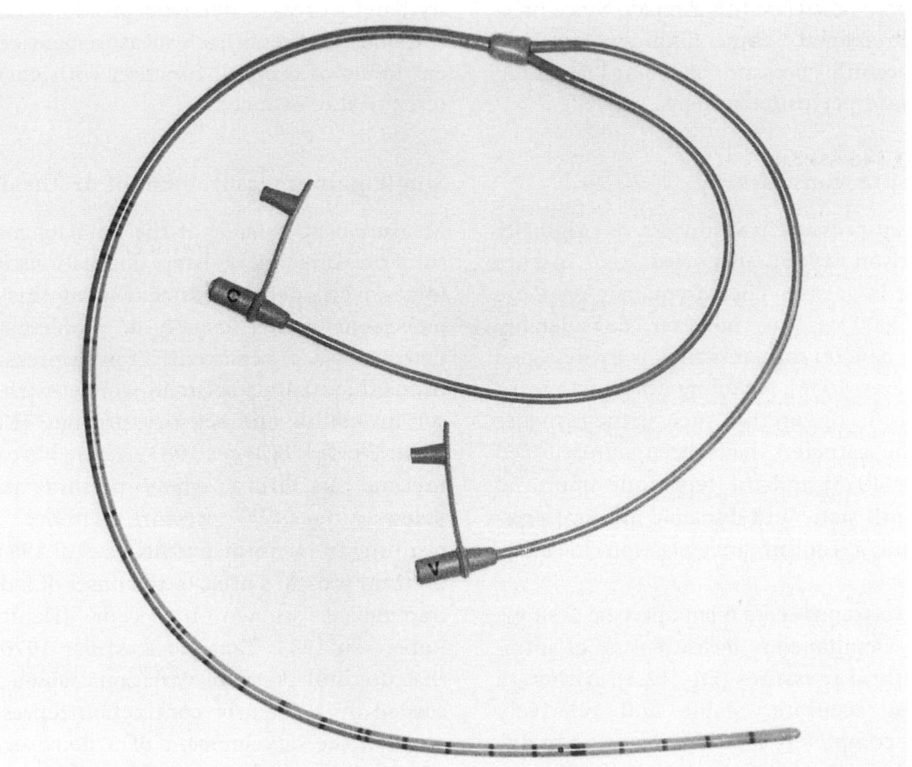

Fig. 12.1 Fluid perfusion catheter with two side-holes 5 cm from tip.

withdrawn from the bladder along the urethra at a steady rate of 5–15 cm/min (Fig. 12.2).

The frequency response of the system is low, and so cannot accurately register fast events such as coughing or reflex urethral contraction. The frequency response is determined by the rate of perfusion, a faster flow improving the response. In practice, a perfusion rate of between 1 and 5 ml/min is adequate for a catheter withdrawal rate of 5 cm/min. If the withdrawal rate is too fast, or the perfusion rate too slow, the static profile will have an asymmetric appearance with a steep slope on the proximal profile and a shallow slope on the distal profile. The closure forces in the urethra may be estimated at any point by measuring the pressure required to lift the urethral mucosa away from the side-holes of the catheter and maintain a fixed perfusion rate. Measurement of urethral pressure by such a method is indirect since the lumen has been made artificially patent and does not represent the continent situation. Even a thin, flexible catheter will inevitably distort the urethra with distortion of the results. Measurement of urethral pressure using a single side-hole gives a variable profile dependent on the catheter orientation. Undoubtedly catheter stiffness (Hertogs & Stanton 1983; Plevnik et al 1985a) contributes to this and the two side-hole catheter repre-

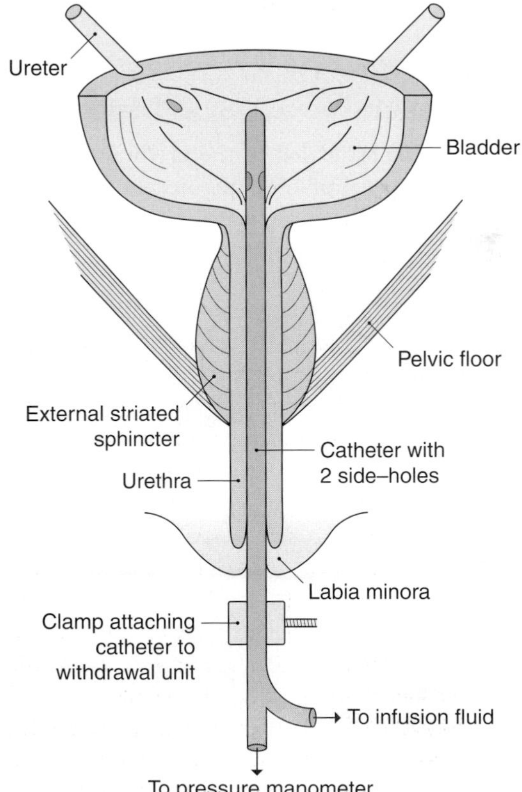

Fig. 12.2 Scheme for performing urethral pressure profile.

sents an attempt to eliminate this artefact. Since pressure is non-directional, these findings question whether intraurethral pressure is being measured accurately by fluid perfusion systems.

Microtip pressure transducers

Catheter-mounted pressure transducers, as originally described (Karlson 1953), distorted the urethra because of their large size. Their frequency response of more than 2000 Hz was, however, considerably higher than the balloon catheters they were designed to replace (Simons 1936), enabling them to record transient activity in the urethra such as the response to a cough. The catheters have been miniaturized (Millar & Baker 1973) and the technique improved (Hilton 1981) until static and dynamic urethral pressure profiles are a routine investigation in many centres.

Mounting two transducers 5 cm apart on a single catheter allows simultaneous measurement of intravesical and urethral pressures (Fig. 12.3). Although the catheter is accurate, stable and relatively robust, it is not completely flexible, resulting in different profiles from the same urethra depending on the transducer face orientation (Hilton & Stanton 1981).

APPLICATIONS OF PRESSURE MEASUREMENT

Pressure may be estimated in the urethra at a single point, as a resting profile of the urethra throughout its length or as a dynamic profile to investigate its response to stress. Each measurement reveals different facets of urethral function with varying degrees of clinical relevance.

Single point measurement of urethral pressure

Measurement is made at the point of maximum urethral pressure and registers fluctuations in the closure forces over a period of time. During this test catheter movement is not usually a problem but can be detected by a persistently lower pressure. Spontaneous fluctuations occur in women with both detrusor instability and sensory urgency (Ulmsten et al 1982; Plevnik & Janez 1983). These have been termed urethral instability, where urethral pressure falls below intravesical pressure without provocation, resulting in incontinence (Bates et al 1981). A drop in urethral pressure prior to the onset of a detrusor contraction is known to occur (Denny-Brown & Robertson 1933; Tanagho & Millar 1970). It may be that urethral pressure variations which are not succeeded by a detrusor contraction represent an early stage in the development of a detrusor contraction which is aborted before the detrusor pressure rises.

Continuous monitoring of urethral pressure has been used to investigate both women with genuine stress incontinence and those with detrusor instability (Sorensen 1991). In women with genuine stress incontinence both the mean maximum closure pressure and the mean urethral pressure were reduced from values previously obtained from healthy volunteers (Sorensen et al 1986). The urethral pressure variations were reduced in women with genuine stress

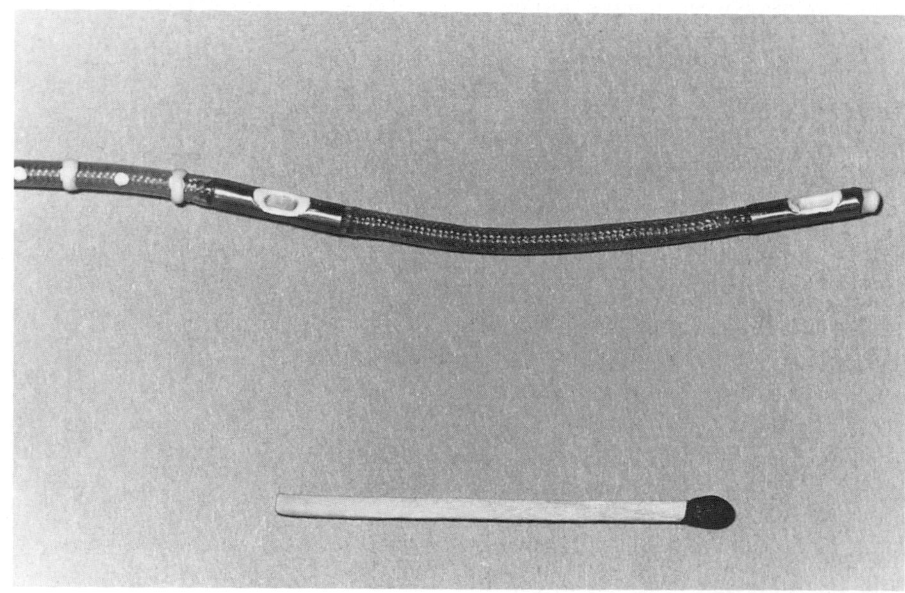

Fig. 12.3 Microtip pressure transducer catheter with match stick to give scale.

incontinence, probably reflecting the lower baseline pressure in these patients. In women with detrusor instability the pressures were all, surprisingly, within the normal range. The urethral pressure variations were, however, different with rhythmic, large drops in pressure. Although of interest, this information cannot form the basis of a test to distinguish between detrusor instability and genuine stress incontinence because of the large overlap between groups.

Ambulatory monitoring of urethral pressure may reveal further unrecognized phenomena which may be of clinical relevance though the problems of catheter stabilization at the precise point in the urethra have to be overcome.

Static urethral pressure profile

A static urethral pressure profile is produced by withdrawing the pressure measuring device through the urethra at a fixed speed (e.g. 5 cm/min). This is normally carried out with the patient in the dorsal position with a fixed volume of fluid in the bladder. The profile landmarks have been standardized by the International Continence Society (Fig. 12.4) but no conditions have been defined using this or any other profile of urethral function. The maximum urethral closure pressure is believed to be a reasonable predictor of the final cystometric diagnosis of genuine stress incontinence (Abrams et al 1978), though other authors dispute this (Versi 1990). A low maximum urethral closure pressure (MUCP) is more common throughout the length of the urethra with genuine stress incontinence, but there is no fixed level below which the diagnosis can be made. Figure 12.5 demonstrates that there is considerable overlap in the MUCP values between symptom-free women and those with the symptoms of stress incontinence (Hilton & Stanton 1983).

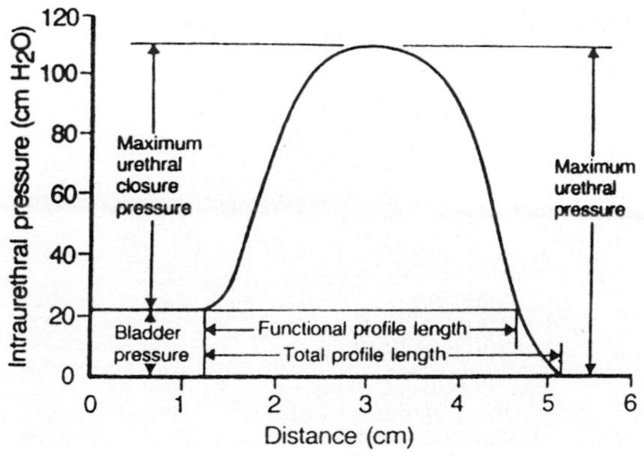

Fig. 12.4 The urethral pressure profile showing ICS recommended nomenclature.

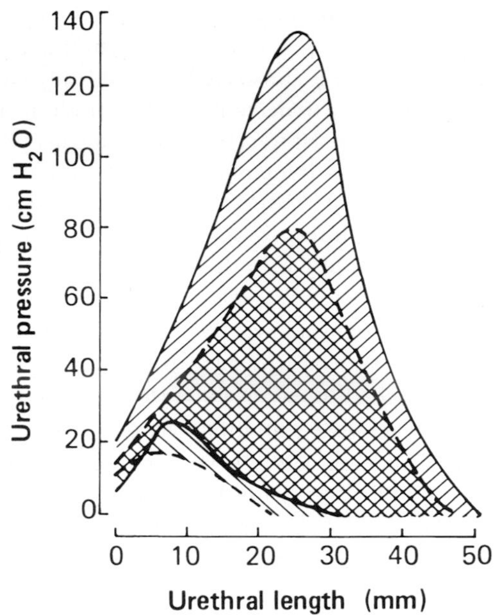

Fig. 12.5 Urethral pressure versus urethral length in normal (hatch) and stress incontinent (cross-hatch) patients.

Despite this overlap several authors have shown that a maximum urethral closure pressure of less than 20 cm H_2O found preoperatively correlates well with a poor outcome postoperatively (McGuire 1981; Sand et al 1987). This value cannot be used as a discriminatory test to decide who should be operated on, but might be used as a guide as to the type of procedure required (Blaivas & Olsson 1988; Bowen et al 1989; Koonings et al 1990). The general suggestion has been that those with a low maximum urethral closure pressure would benefit from a suburethral sling procedure (Horbach et al 1988), but confirmation of this by a controlled clinical trial has yet to be published.

Dynamic urethral pressure profile

The dynamic urethral pressure profile seems to be the most attractive method for determining the presence of urethral sphincter incompetence. The technique is the same as the static profile, except that during catheter withdrawal the woman challenges the urethral closure forces by coughing. Pressure is measured simultaneously in the urethra and bladder; the difference between the two pressures (or urethral closure pressure) at any point representing the residual safety margin for continence. As long as this value remains positive at any point in the profile then continence should, theoretically, be maintained. The technique requires the use of a twin sensor microtip pressure measuring catheter which is inserted into the bladder and slowly withdrawn whilst the woman lies supine with a fixed volume of fluid in the bladder. She is asked to cough every 3–4 s as the catheter is withdrawn at a speed of 5 cm/min. The intravesical pressure is subtracted electronically from the urethral pressure to demonstrate the urethral closure pressure profile. Hilton (1981) recommends placing the transducer at the point of maximum urethral pressure for a period of 20–30 s and then requesting the woman to cough serially about six times. In some, the repeated stress to which this manoeuvre submits the urethral sphincter causes it to relax, revealing a previously unrecognized negative closure pressure.

Urethral pressure measurement is a useful research tool giving much information about the nature of genuine stress incontinence and the method of action of physiotherapy and continence procedures. The results at present show that it provides neither a sensitive nor specific test for the presence or absence of genuine stress incontinence (Hilton & Stanton 1983; Tapp et al 1985; Shepherd et al 1985; Hanzal et al 1991; Rai & Versi 1991), and may be omitted from the routine investigation of female urinary incontinence (Blaivas et al 1982; Abrams et al 1988).

Pressure fluid bridge

Proximal urethral incompetence, either passive (in genuine stress incontinence) or active (in detrusor instability) is a prerequisite for involuntary urinary leakage but urine then has to pass the point of maximum urethral pressure to appear at the external urethral meatus. The pressure fluid bridge was the first method to objectively verify proximal urethral incompetence and distal urethral electric conductance (see later) the first for more distal incompetence.

It has been demonstrated that transmission of cough impulses to the proximal urethra occurs independent of intraluminal transmission through the fluid column created during proximal urethral incompetence (Shelley & Warrell 1965). Any method which uses pressure measurement to detect proximal urethral incompetence must be capable of distinguishing between these. The frequency response characteristics of a fluid perfusion system to extra luminal pressure transmission are much slower than intraluminal transmission, which is limited predominantly by the frequency response of the pressure transducer itself.

The equipment uses a 12 F, double lumen catheter (Brown & Sutherst 1978; Fig. 12.6). Each lumen is connected by fluid-filled, rigid polythene tubing to a pressure transducer. The other end of the inner lumen opens into the bladder, thus allowing intravesical pressure to be measured directly. Bladder volume is standardized at 150 ml. The outer lumen opens 6 cm proximally and can be used with a fluid perfusion system to estimate urethral pressure. If the catheter is inserted so that both lumina open intravesically then, on coughing, both pressure transducers will register intravesical pressure. As the catheter is slowly withdrawn, the proximal side-hole enters the proximal urethra and starts to register urethral pressure. This point acts as a landmark so that at any time the distance between the proximal opening and the bladder is known. If the proximal side-hole is placed within the urethra and the woman coughs, then two possible situations can arise.

1 If the urethra is competent down to the position of the side-hole then the pressure measured at the side-hole will be that transmitted extraluminally to maintain urethral competence. Fluid perfusion systems have low frequency response characteristics which means that they take a long time to register any changes in pressure. The slower the rate of perfusion, the slower the response time. If the perfusion system is switched off at the time of the cough then extraluminal cough pressure transmission is hardly recorded at all (Fig. 12.7).

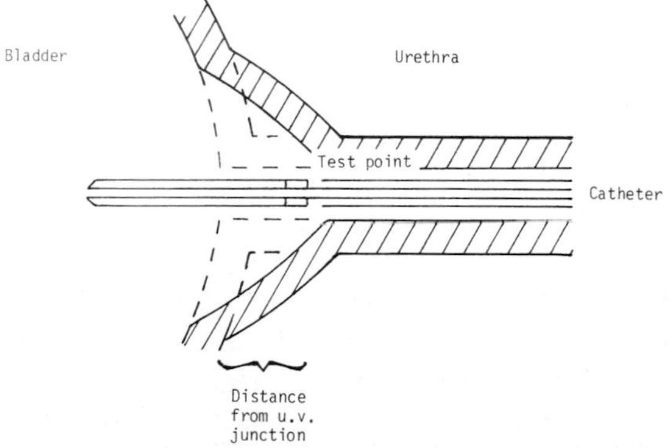

Fig. 12.6 Diagram of fluid bridge test.

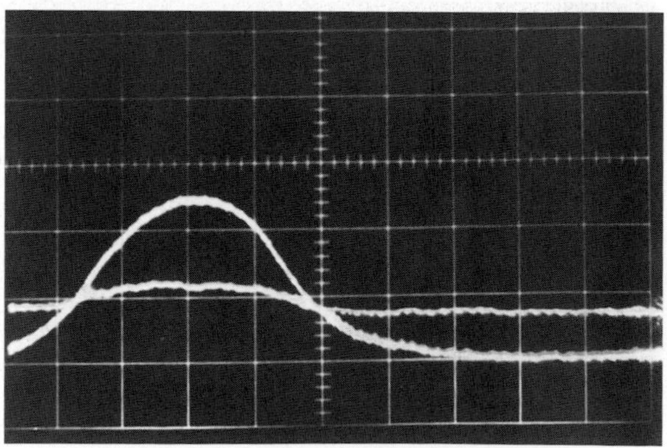

Fig. 12.7 Tracing from continent patient showing two separate traces from bladder and urethra.

2 If the urethra is incompetent to the point of measurement, then as the urethra opens a fluid column or 'fluid bridge' is established between the bladder and the pressure transducer. In this situation, the pressure measured by both transducers is intravesical, and the traces will be superimposable (Fig. 12.8). The investigation may be repeated at 0.5 cm intervals down the urethra and the extent of incompetence of the proximal urethra gauged (Murray et al 1983).

The diagnosis of urethral sphincter incompetence as arrived at by cystometry and urethral closure profile has been compared with that found by the pressure fluid bridge investigation (Sutherst & Brown 1980). A highly significant correlation was found between the absence of urinary symptoms and a negative fluid bridge investigation. Eleven out of 29 symptomatic women whose cystometric diagnosis was not genuine stress incontinence had an incompetent bladder neck during a pressure fluid bridge test giving a significant false positive rate. The mean ages of the asymptomatic control group and the study group represented pre- and post-menopausal age ranges respectively. Up to 50% of postmenopausal women seem to maintain continence despite an incompetent bladder neck as diagnosed by videocystourethrography and dynamic urethral pressure profilometry (Versi et al 1986b) and so the difference between the fluid bridge test results in symptomatic and asymptomatic women may be artefactual.

The technique has been used to assess proximal urethral competence before and after continence surgery, and this may give some information about the different methods of action of vaginal and suprapubic surgery (Murray et al 1981).

The diagnostic accuracy has been increased by performing the investigation in the erect position.

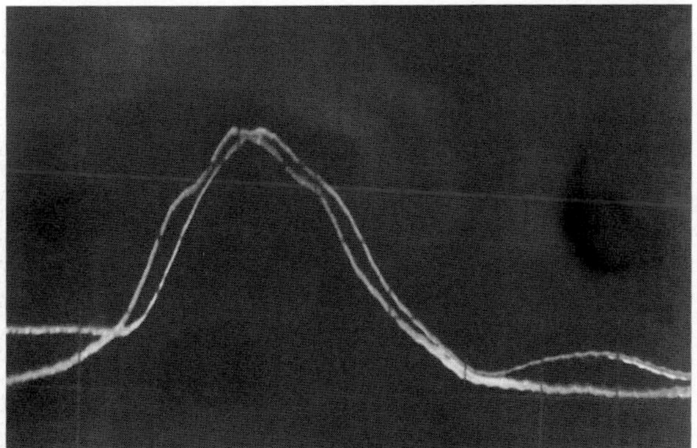

Fig. 12.8 Tracing with cough incompetence at the bladder neck and superimposition of the two traces. From Mayne & Hilton (1988), with permission.

There still remains, however, a proportion (4/27) of asymptomatic continent women with a positive fluid bridge test result at 0.5 cm from the bladder neck (Sutherst & Brown 1981). This discrepancy may be accounted for by the difference in mean age between the groups, shortening of the urethra around the catheter (Hertogs & Stanton 1983) or catheter movement relative to the whole urethra.

ELECTRIC CONDUCTANCE MEASUREMENTS

Early studies

Impedance measurements are reported to have been used by Atzler as early as 1935 in an attempt to measure cardiac stroke volume (Geddes et al 1962). The principles have been adapted to measure a number of different urological variables including ureteric flow (Harris et al 1971) bladder emptying (Denniston & Baker 1975) bladder volume (Abbey & Close 1983) and residual urine volume (Doyle & Hill 1975).

When a high frequency voltage is applied across two electrodes, the current that flows is directly related to the impedance of the material separating the electrodes. If the material is of low impedance the current will be high and vice versa. If an object of low impedance is placed within the electric field created when material of high impedance separates the electrodes then the current will fall by an amount related to the geometry and impedance of the object. When measuring urethral electric impedance, it is important to avoid exciting tissues within the electric field (Plevnik et al 1985b).

The measurement of conductivity in the proximal urethra was originally described to detect incompetence of the bladder neck mechanism using a rigid catheter onto which were mounted two ring electrodes (Plevnik & Vrtacnic 1981b). A constant, 200 millivolt (mV) peak to peak voltage was applied at 1 kHz across the electrodes, and the device placed in the urethral lumen. Any increase in the measured current passing between the electrodes in response to coughing represented a decrease in the impedance of the material within the field. Since the impedance of urine is less than that of the urethral tissue the inference is that these increases in current represented the passage of urine down to the level of the electrodes due to incompetence of the bladder neck. The current used was close to that which would stimulate the surrounding tissues, and so the electrodes were modified and its use in 50 patients reported using 100 mV at 25 kHz (Plevnik et al 1983a). No correlation with the final urodynamic diagnosis was reported. The electrodes were then mounted on a flexible catheter, and a small pilot study of this new device was reported (Hertogs & Stanton 1983). These authors felt that, because of the shortening effect seen around the catheter during videocystourethrography, there would be significant false positives and no larger series was undertaken.

A three-channel 'electric fluid bridge' has been described to track fluid down the urethra by simultaneous measurement of impedance at three different sites in the urethra (Plevnik et al 1983b). This method allows the velocity of a bolus of urine travelling down the urethra to be calculated, but is hampered by the rigidity of the catheter and the lack of any fixed reference point in the urethra. No clinical application was suggested for this device but it is the first method which could demonstrate leakage of urine throughout the urethra.

Bladder neck electric conductance (BNEC) test

Patients frequently complain of significant urgency and urge incontinence but have cystometrically normal bladders. Indeed up to 70% of people with stable bladders complain of the symptom of urgency

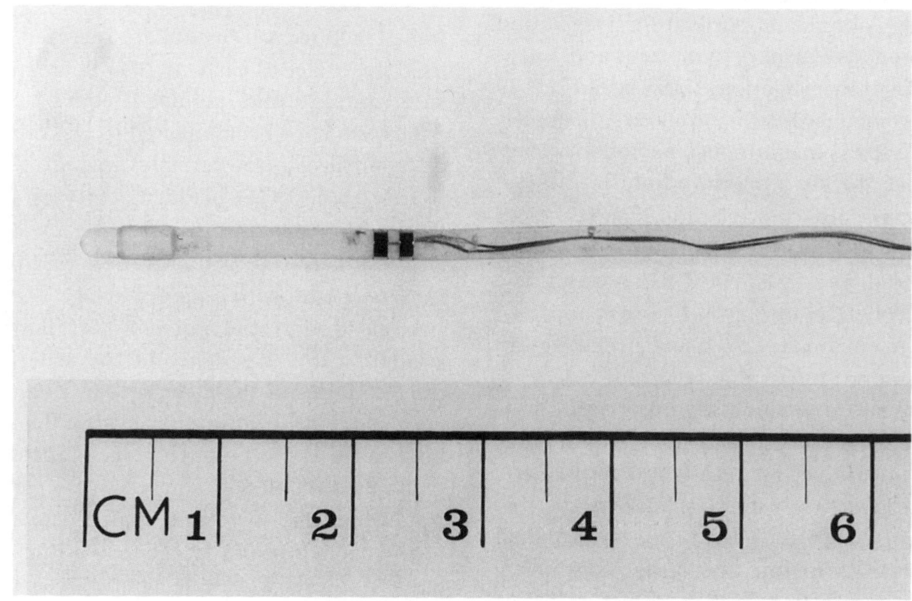

Fig. 12.9 Urethral electric conductance catheter showing ring electrodes.

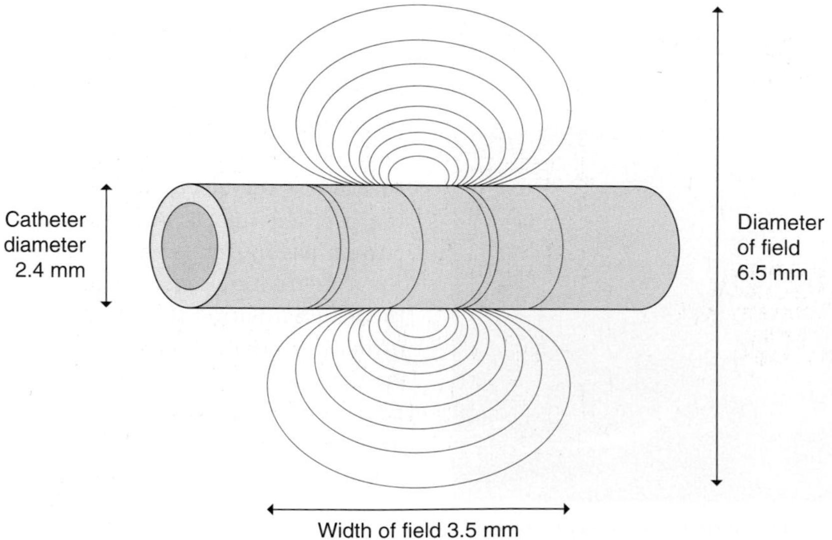

Fig. 12.10 Field of measurement of the conductivity catheter.

(Abrams 1983) and 55% complain of urge incontinence (Cantor & Bates 1980), whilst in a group of 75 women who complained of the symptom of urgency, 36 had objectively stable bladders (Jarvis et al 1980). Conventional cystometry is a specific test for detrusor instability. Since detrusor instability cannot be reliably distinguished symptomatically from 'sensory urgency', cystometry is an insensitive test for the abnormality associated with the symptoms of urgency and urge incontinence.

The use of conductivity measurements to investigate symptoms of urgency and urge incontinence has been described (Plevnik et al 1985b). A constant, 20 mV (peak to peak), 50 kHz signal is generated across two ring electrodes mounted on a flexible 7F catheter (Fig. 12.9). This generates an elliptical electric field with the electrodes immersed in saline, which extends longitudinally 0.5 mm beyond the ring electrodes, and has a maximum radial diameter of 6.5 mm (Fig. 12.10).

When the bladder contains 250 ml 0.9% saline at room temperature, if the electrodes are inserted transurethrally into the bladder a relatively high conductivity is registered. The conductivity of the urothelium is lower than that of saline and so, if the electrodes are withdrawn at a fixed speed, the current falls as the bladder neck and proximal urethra impinge on the electric field. The resultant profile is known as the urethral electric conductance profile (UECP) (Fig. 12.11). The only similarly derived profile of urethral function is the static urethral pressure profile, which has been simultaneously measured by the method of Brown and Wickham and superimposed in Figure 12.12. It can be seen that the first steep slope of the UECP represents an area previously inaccessible to investigation. Radiological studies have shown that this area is the bladder neck (Holmes 1987).

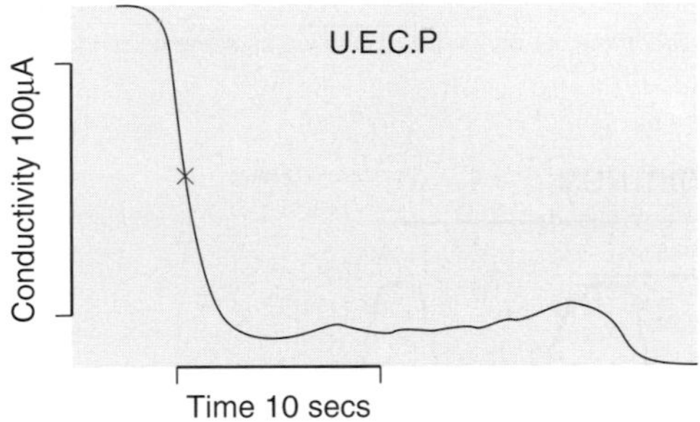

Fig. 12.11 The Urethral Electric Conductance Profile.

If the electrodes are sited at the bladder neck, then variations in conductivity may be recorded. Increases in conductivity represent opening of the bladder neck (since more saline enters the electric field), whilst decreases represent its closure. Figure 12.13 shows the simultaneous measurement of rectal and intravesical pressures with the bladder neck conductivity. The patient was asked to indicate those times when she experienced an increase in the subjective sensation of urgency (Fig. 12.13). During involuntary detrusor contractions the patient experienced urgency each time accompanied by an increase in conductivity. Urgency also occured in the absence of contractions. There is, however, a rise in conductivity each time that urgency is experienced.

This finding can be used to assess the severity of the symptom of urgency (Holmes et al 1985a). Bladder neck activity was monitored over a period of 3 min with the patient resting in the supine position with a fixed volume of 250 ml of 0.9% saline in the bladder.

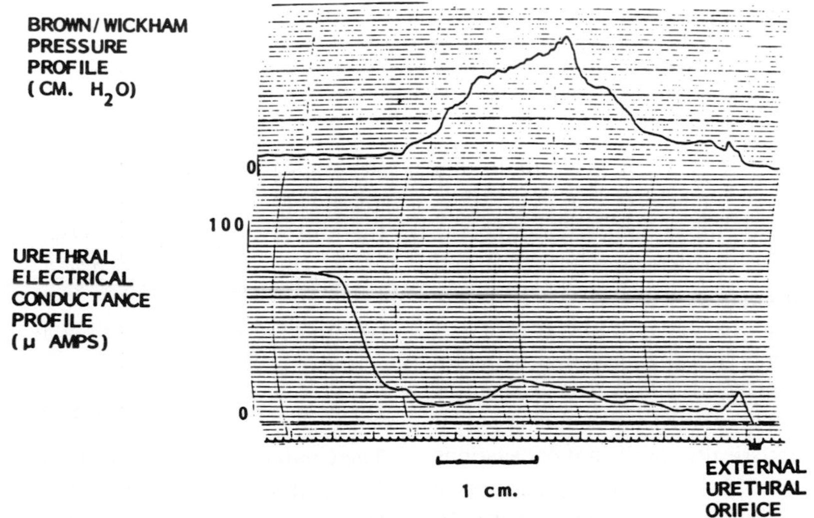

Fig. 12.12 Static urethral pressure profile simultaneously measured by Brown and Wickham method and superimposed.

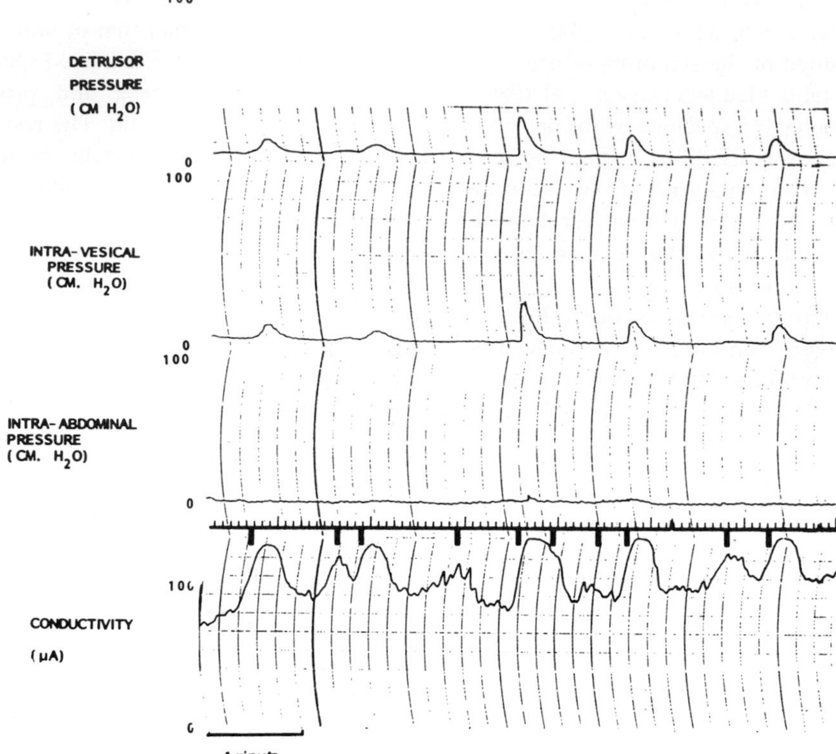

Fig. 12.13 Simultaneous measurement of rectal and intravesical pressures with the bladder neck conductivity. Solid marks along scale indicate an increase in the subjective sensation of urgency.

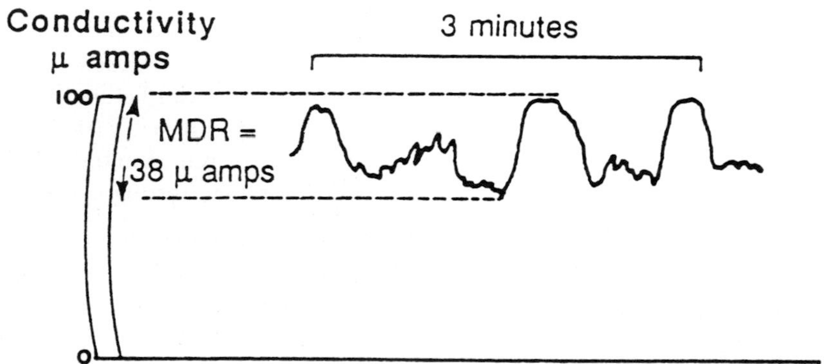

Fig. 12.14 Maximum deflection at rest (MDR).

The change in conductivity from peak to trough (maximum deflection at rest MDR) is noted (Fig. 12.14). Conventional fast fill cystometry, noting the volume at which the first desire to void (FDV) (ml) and maximum detrusor pressure rise (MPR) (cm H_2O) were recorded. The correlations between the severity of the symptom of urgency and the measured variables of FDV, MPR and MDR are illustrated in Figures 12.15, 12.16, 12.17. The results are summarized in Table 12.1. Highly statistically significant correlations with the symptoms of urgency and urge incontinence are found with the BNEC test results. The correlation with the symptom of urgency found with the BNEC test is significantly better than either cystometric variable ($p < 0.05$) (Holmes et al 1989a). This means that this test may be used not only to grade the severity of the symptoms of urgency and urge incontinence, but also to monitor its response to treatment (Peattie et al 1988a; Holmes et al 1989b).

Distal urethral electric conductivity (DUEC) test

The conductivity electrodes may also be stabilized at 1.5 cm from the external urethral meatus where they can detect urine leaking down the urethra during an exercise pad test (Fig. 12.18) (Holmes et al 1985b).

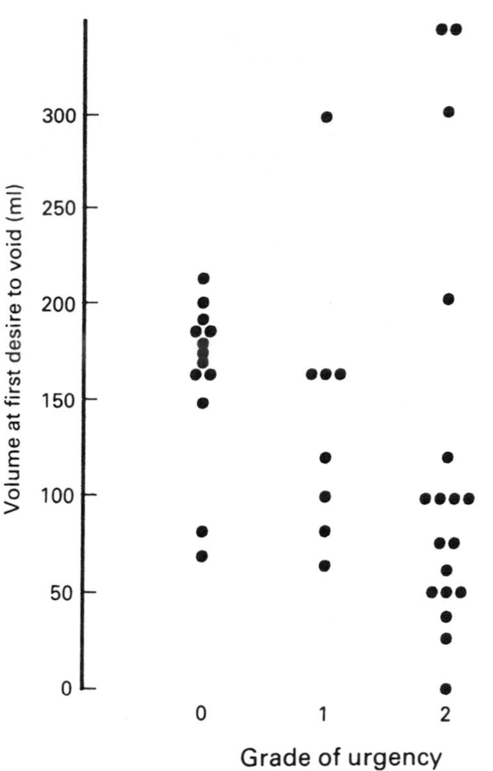

Fig. 12.15 Symptom of urgency plotted against first desire to void (FDV).

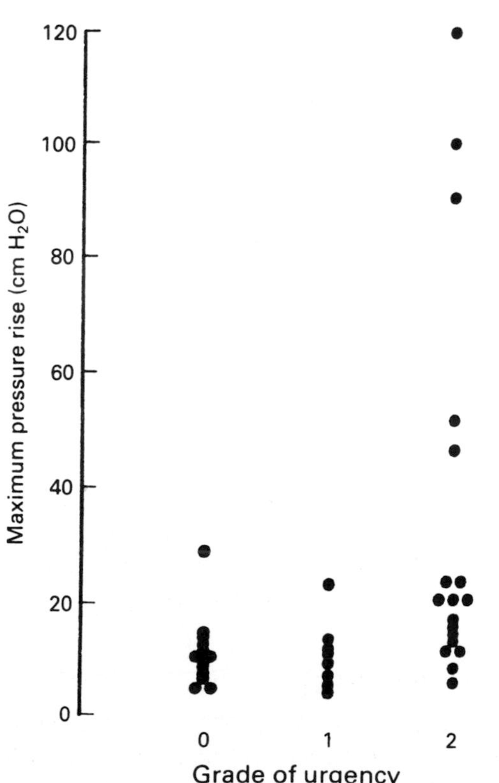

Fig. 12.16 Symptom of urgency plotted against maximum pressure rise (MPR).

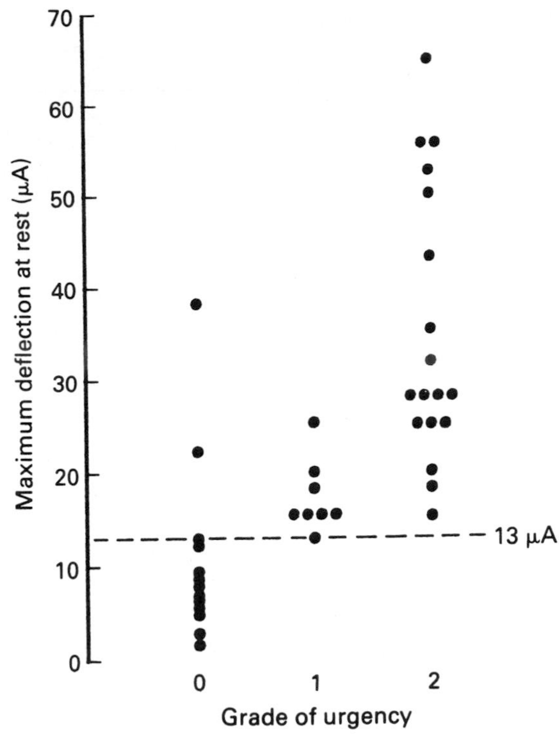

Fig. 12.17 Symptom of urgency plotted against maximum deflection at rest (MDR).

With the UEC probe in the distal urethra a positive result means urine has passed the point of maximum urethral closure pressure and the patient is, by definition, incontinent. This test is carried out with a comfortably full bladder and a sanitary towel over the perineum to absorb any leakage. The 1-hour pad test (Bates et al 1983) correlates accurately with a positive DUEC test. The latter has been modified to be carried out at a fixed bladder volume of 250 ml 0.9% saline and found to be a sensitive method of detecting urinary leakage (Mayne & Hilton 1987).

In a study to assess the possibility of using DUEC testing as a screening test 104 patients had DUEC traces in conjunction with their subtracted cystometry (Peattie et al 1988b) (Fig. 12.19). Patients complaining of incontinence were significantly more likely to have a positive DUEC test than abnormal cystometry ($p < 0.001$). DUEC testing was in agreement with cystometry in 71% cases, in 21% an additional diagnosis was made, leaving only 8% of patients where a diagnosis made at cystometry was not detected by DUEC testing. DUEC testing is more sensitive than pad detection of urinary leakage as seen by the greater pick-up rate with DUEC as compared to cystometry. The agreement of diagnosis in 71% of cases between DUEC and cystometric diagnosis and the Cohen's kappa values of 0.85–0.91 imply that the

Table 12.1 Correlation between symptom severity and urodynamic measurements.

	Subjective severity of					
	Urgency		Urge incontinence		Stress incontinence	
	τ_B	P	τ_B	P	τ_B	P
Volume at first desire to void	–0.35	<0.01	–0.19	>0.05	0.27	<0.05
Maximum pressure rise at cystometry	0.36	<0.01	0.28	<0.01	–0.07	>0.05
Maximum deflection of conductivity trace at rest	0.68	<0.0001	0.49	<0.005	–0.14	>0.05

n = 39

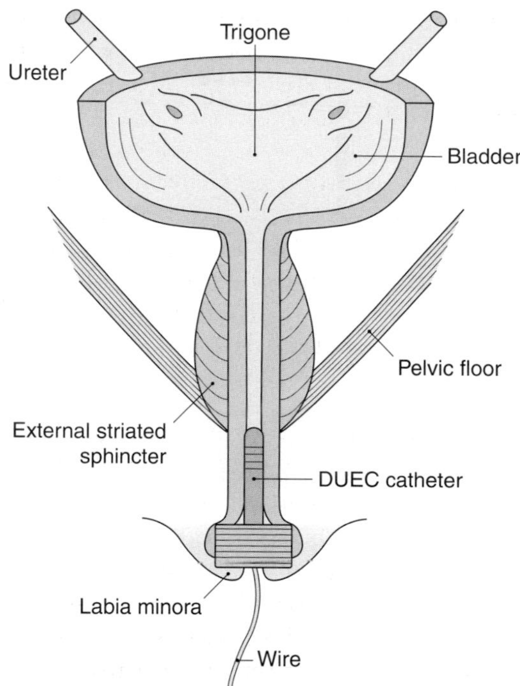

Fig. 12.18 DUEC catheter in situ.

DUEC test is a diagnostic test and could be applied in the absence of cystometry to screen an incontinent population (Peattie et al 1988b).

Intraoperative use of conductivity test

A novel use of the UEC catheter has been devised to assess the suture tension required to achieve continence during incontinence surgery (Janez et al 1985). The technique involves placing the electrodes at the proximal urethra once the elevating sutures are in position. Intra-abdominal pressure is raised until a pressure of 100 cm H_2O is registered. If the electrodes remain dry then the test is negative and the suture tension is correct. If the test is positive then the sutures require further tightening. The technique has

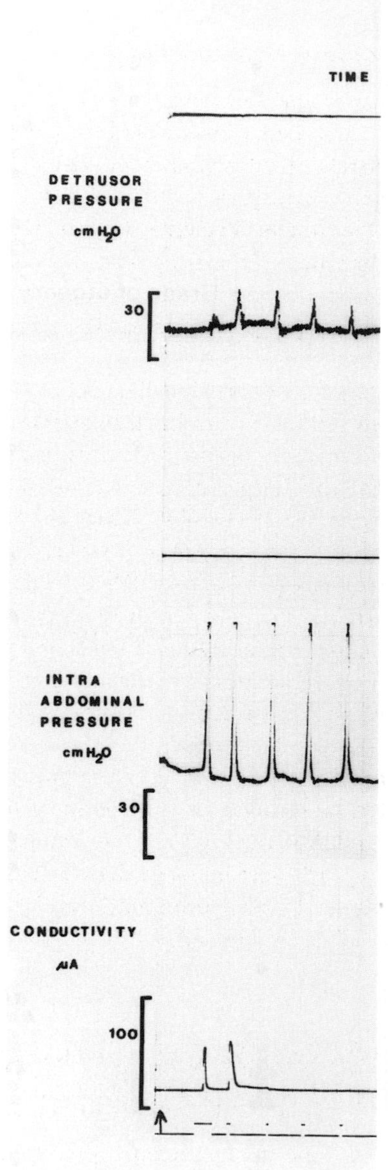

Fig. 12.19 Conductivity trace (bottom) showing positive DUEC test with leakage of urine associated with cough.

been tested on 21 patients undergoing surgical correction of their genuine stress incontinence under epidural anaesthesia, 16 during fascial sling procedures and 5 during anterior colporrhaphy. All had a positive test result initially, and 17 had a negative test after the surgery. Four had a positive test after the surgery and all of these were clinically incontinent at 6 month follow-up. Only two women had a negative test initially and were subsequently incontinent. The test seems to have a good predictive value in assessing whether the particular surgical procedure is going to be unsuccessful at the time of the surgery thus allowing an alternative procedure to be adopted at the time.

Urethral softness measurement

The compliance of the mucosal lining of the urethra is recognized to be important in the maintenance of its seal (see above). Experimental models have confirmed this, but little evidence as to its importance *in vivo* is available. Plevnik & Vrtacnik (1980) have developed a probe which utilizes the principles of conductivity measurement to measure the deformability of the urethral lining to give a variable called urethral softness. The device consists of a 10 F perspex catheter into which is cut a small chamber. The chamber has two sets of electrodes incorporated into its walls and thus can measure the conductivity of the chamber contents. Negative pressure can be applied to the chamber via a central channel which can also be used to estimate urethral pressure using the method of Brown & Wickham (1969). The probe is used as a urethral pressure sensor to locate the chamber at the point of measurement: the saline perfusion is switched off and a negative pressure applied to the chamber whilst measuring the conductivity of the contents. The depth to which the mucosa is sucked into the chamber by a given negative pressure is linearly related to changes in the conductivity of the chamber contents thus giving an estimate of its deformability. The methodology has been standardized (Plevnik et al 1981) but clinical evaulation of the results has not been pursued.

VALSALVA LEAK POINT PRESSURES

The Valsalva leak point pressure (VLPP) was first described as a method of assessing the probability of upper urinary tract damage in myelodysplasia (McGuire et al 1981).

The technique was transferred to adult continence use as an objective method of assessing the severity of urinary incontinence, but is now used to identify 'intrinsic sphincter deficiency' and measure 'urethral resistance'. Neither of these terms have been clearly defined.

The VLPPs are measured by a variety of methods. The basic principle is to observe the external urethral meatus whilst measuring the pressure generated by a Valsalva manoeuvre. The difference between resting pressure and the pressure which generates leakage is the VLPP (Fig. 12.20).

Pressure may be measured intravesically (by catheterization), intravaginally or rectally. The patient may be standing, sitting, lying down or tilted to an angle of 45°. The volume of the fluid in the bladder may be fixed or variable, (e.g. maximum cystometric capacity). The diameter of the catheter inserted into the bladder is not defined. All of these factors will affect the measurement of the VLPP (Bump et al 1995). The test has been shown to be reproducible, but until its technique is standardized (Swift & Utrie 1996) and its value objectively measured in clinical trials, its use to decide or assess clinical outcome should be discouraged.

CONCLUSIONS

Tests of urethral function do not reproduce the clinical situation, and so, as yet, have little to offer in the clinical assessment of patients with urinary incontinence. Their role has been as research tools to investigate the mechanism of continence or the actions of procedures to restore continence.

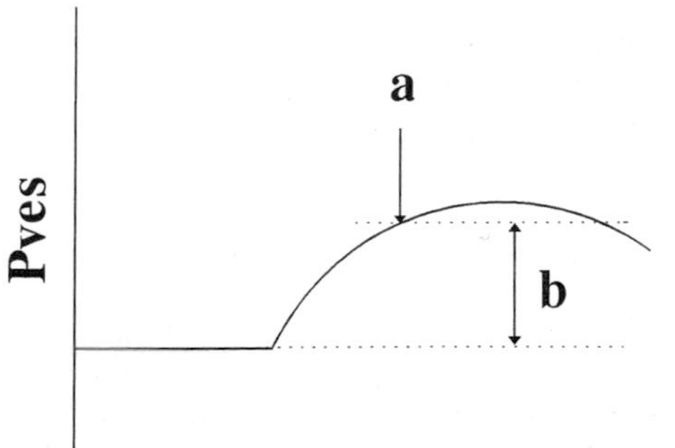

Fig. 12.20 Measurement of Valsalva leak point pressure: periurethral area is swabbed dry, after which patient is asked to bear down progressively while holding her breath. Precise instant that fluid is observed at external urethral meatus is recorded on vesical pressure with remote event marker (arrow at a). Rise in vesical pressure (p_{ves}) over baseline (b) is measured at instant leakage begins and represents the Valsalva leak point pressure. Data from Bump et al (1995), with permission.

REFERENCES

Abbey J C, Close L 1983 Electrical impedance measurement of urinary bladder fullness. Journal of Microwave Power 18 (3): 305–309

Abrams P H 1983 The clinical contribution of urodynamics. In: Abrams P H, Fenaley R C L, Torrens M (eds) Urodynamics. Springer-Verlag, Berlin, p 142

Abrams P H, Martin S, Griffiths D J 1978 The measurement and interpretation of urethral pressure profiles obtained by the method of Brown and Wickham. British Journal of Urology 50: 33–38

Abrams P H, Blaivas J G, Stanton S L, Andersen J 1988 The standardisation of lower urinary tract function. Scandinavian Journal of Urology and Nephrology (Suppl) 114: 5–19

Barnes A C 1940 The method of evaluating the stress of urinary incontinence. American Journal of Obstetrics and Gynaecology 40: 381–390

Bates C P, Bradley W E, Glen E S et al 1981 Fourth report on the standardisation terminology of lower urinary tract function. Terminology related to neuromuscular dysfunction of the lower urinary tract. British Journal of Urology 53: 333–335

Bates C P, Bradley W E, Glen E S et al 1983 Fifth report on the standardisation of terminology of lower urinary tract function. Quantification of urine loss. International Continence Society Committee for Standardisation of Terminology, Bristol

Blaivas J G, Awad S A, Bissada N et al 1982 Urodynamic procedures: recommendations of the urodynamic society. 1. Procedures that should be available for routine urologic practice. Neurourology and Urodynamics 1: 51–55

Blaivas J, Olsson C A 1988 Stress incontinence: Classification and surgical approach. Journal of Urology 139: 727–731

Bonney V 1923 On diurnal incontinence of urine in women. Journal of Obstetrics and Gynaecology of the British Empire 30: 358–365

Bowen L W, Sand P K, Ostergard D R 1989 Unsuccessful Burch retropubic urethropexy: A case controlled urodynamic study. American Journal of Obstetrics and Gynaecology 160: 452–458

Brown M, Sutherst J R 1978 Detection of fluid entry into the proximal urethra during coughing. Proceedings of 8th Meeting International Continence Society, Manchester, pp 147–150

Brown M, Wickham J E A 1969 The urethral pressure profile. British Journal of Urology 41: 211–217

Bump R C, Elster D M, Theofrastous J P, McClish D K and the Continence Program for Women Group 1995. Valsalva leak point pressure in women with genuine stress incontinence: reproducibility, effect of catheter caliber, and correlations with other measures of urethral resistance. American Journal of Obstetrics and Gynaecology 173: 551–557

Cantor T J, Bates C P 1980 A comparative study of symptoms and objective urodynamic findings in 214 incontinent women. British Journal of Obstetrics and Gynaecology 87: 889–892

Colstrup H, Mortensen S O, Kristensen J K 1983 A probe for measurement of related values of cross-sectional area and pressure in the resting female urethra. Urolological Research 11: 139–141

Denniston J C, Baker L E 1975 Measurement of urinary bladder emptying using electrical impedance. Medical and Biological Engineering 13: 305–306

Denny-Brown D, Robertson E C 1933 On the physiology of micturition. Brain 56: 149–190

Doyle P T, Hill D W 1975 The measurement of residual urine volume by electrical impedance in man. Medical and Biological Engineering 13: 307–308

Enhorning G 1976 A concept of urinary continence. Urologia Internationalis 31: 3–5

Geddes L A, Hoff H E, Hickman D M, Moore A G 1962 The impedance pneumograph. Aerospace Medicine 33: 28–33

Hanzal E, Berger E, Koelbl H 1991 Reliability of the urethral closure pressure profile during stress in the diagnosis of genuine stress incontinence. British Journal of Urology 68: 369–371

Harris J H, Therkelson E E, Zinner N R 1971 Electrical measurement of ureteral flow. In: Boyarsky S, Gottschalk C W, Tanagho E A, Zimskind P D (eds) Urodynamics. Academic Press, New York, pp 465–472

Hertogs K, Stanton S L 1983 Urethral function tests: limits to certainty. Proceedings of 13th Meeting International Continence Society, Aachen, pp 155–157

Hilton P 1981 Urethral pressure measurement by microtip transducer: observations on the methodology, the pathophysiology of genuine stress incontinence and the effects of its treatment in the female. MD Thesis, University of Newcastle-upon-Tyne

Hilton P, Stanton S L 1981 Urethral pressure measurement by microtransducer: An analysis of variance and an analysis of rotational variation. Proceedings of 11th Meeting International Continence Society, Lund, pp 69–71

Hilton P, Stanton S L 1983 Urethral pressure measurement by microtransducer: the results in symptom-free women and in those with genuine stress incontinence. British Journal of Obstetrics and Gynaecology 90: 919–933

Hodgkinson C P 1965 Stress urinary incontinence in the female. Surgery, Gynecology and Obstetrics 120: 595–613

Hodgkinson C P 1990 The renaissance of female urethrovesical function. International Urogynecology Journal 1(2): 104–108

Holmes D M 1987 Clinical and research applications of conductivity measurements in the female lower urinary tract. MD Thesis, University of Wales

Holmes D M, Plevnik S Stanton S L 1985a Bladder Neck Electric Conductance (BNEC) test in the investigation and treatment of sensory urgency and detrusor instability. Proceedings of 15th Meeting International Continence Society, London, pp 96–97

Holmes D M, Plevnik S, Stanton S L 1985b Distal Urethrel Conductance (DUEC) test for the identification of urinary leakage. Proceedings of 15th Meeting International Continence Society, London 94–95

Holmes D M, Plevnik S, Stanton S L 1989a Bladder Neck Electrical Conductivity (BNEC) test in female urinary urgency and urge continence. British Journal of Obstetrics and Gynaecology, 96: 816–820

Holmes D M, Plevnik S, Stanton S L 1989b Bladder Neck Electrical Conductivity (BNEC) test in the treatment of detrusor instability with biofeedback. British Journal of Obstetrics and Gynaecology 96: 821–826

Horbach N S, Blanco J S, Ostergard D R, Bent A E, Cornella J L 1988 A suburethral sling procedure with polytetrafluoroethylene for the treatment of genuine stress incontinence in patients with low urethral closure pressure. Obstetrics and Gynecology 71, 648–752

Janez J, Plevnik S, Vrtacnik P 1985 Prognostic value of Urethral Electric Conductance (UEC) during the surgery for stress incontinence. Proceedings of 15th Meeting International Continence Society, London, pp 93–94

Jarvis G J, Hall S, Stamp S, Millar D R, Johnson A 1980 An assessment of urodynamic examination in incontinent women. British Journal of Obstetrics and Gynaecology 87: 893–896

Karlson S 1953 Experimental studies on the functioning of the female urinary bladder and urethra. Acta Obstetricia et Gynecologia Scandinavia 32: 285–307

Koonings P P, Bergman A, Ballard C A 1990 Low urethral pressure and stress urinary incontinece in women: risk factor for failed retropublic surgical procedure. Urology 36: 245–248

Lose G 1991 Urethral pressure and power generation during coughing and voluntary contraction of the pelvic floor in females with genuine stress incontinence. British Journal of Urology 67, 580–585

McGuire E J 1981 Urodynamics findings in patients after failure of stress incontinent operations. Progress in Clinical and Biological Research. 78: 351–360

McGuire E J, Woodside J R, Borden T A, Weiss R M 1981 Prognostic value of urodynamic testing in myelodysplastic patients. Journal of Urology 126: 205–209

Mayne C J, Hilton P 1987 A comparison of Distal Urethral Electrical Conductance (DUEC) with weighed pads during a standardised exercise test. Neurourology and Urodynamics 6(3): 167–168

Mayne C J, Hilton P 1988 The distal urethral conductance test: standardisation of method and clinical reliability. Neurourology and Urodynamics 7: 55–60

Millar H D, Baker L E 1973 Stable ultraminiature catheter tip pressure transducer. Medical and Biological Engineering 11: 86–89

Murray A, Sutherst J R, Brown M 1981 Clinical application of the fluid bridge test: objective assessment of bladder neck closure before and after incontinence surgery. Proceedings of 11th Meeting International Continence Society, Lund, pp 58–60

Murray A, Sutherst J, Brown M 1983 The fluid bridge test: a refinement for measuring the severity of sphincter weakness in genuine stress incontinence. Proceedings of 13th Meeting International Continence Society, Aachen, pp 164–166

Peattie A B, Plevnik S, Stanton S L 1988a The use of Bladder Neck Electrical Conductance (BNEC) in the investigation and management of sensory urge incontinence in the female. The Journal of the Royal Society of Medicine 81: 442–444

Peattie A B, Plevnik S, Stanton S L 1988b Distal Urethral Conductance (DUEC) test: a screening test for female urinary incontinence? Neurourology and Urodynamics 7 (3): 173–174

Plevnik S, Vrtacnik P 1980 How to measure inner wall softness. Proceedings of 10th Meeting International Continence Society, Manchester 44–48

Plevnik S, Vrtacnik P 1981a How to measure inner wall softness. Progress in Clinical and Biological Research (New York) 78: 253–258

Plevnik S, Vrtacnik P 1981b Electric fluid bridge test. Proceedings of International Continence Society, Lund 56–57

Plevnik S, Janez J 1983 Urethral pressure variations. Urology 21: 207–209

Plevnik S, Vrtacnik P, Rakovec S, Janez J 1981 Urethral softness distribution in the female urethra. Proceedings of 11th Meeting International Continence Society, Lund, pp 84–86

Plevnik S, Vrtacnik P, Janez J 1983a Detection of fluid entry into the urethra by electric impedance measurement: electric fluid bridge test. Clinical Physics and Physiological Measurement (York) 4: 309–313

Plevnik S, Brown M, Sutherst J R, Vrtacnik P 1983b Tracking of fluid in urethra by simultaneous electric impedance measurement at three sites. Urology International 38: 29–32

Plevnik S, Janez J, Vrtacnik P, Brown M 1985a Directional differences in urethral pressure recordings; contributions from the stiffness and weight of the recording catheters. Neurourology and Urodynamics 4: 117–128

Plevnik S, Holmes D M, Janez J, Mundy A R, Vrtacnik P 1985b Urethral elecric conductance (UEC) – A new parameter for the evaluation of urethral and bladder function; methodology of the assessment of its clinical potential. Proceedings of 15th Meeting International Continence Society, London, pp 90–91

Rai RS, Versi E 1991 Urethral pressure profilometry. International Urogynecology Journal 2: 222–227

Robertson J R 1974 Gas cystometrogram with urethral pressure profile. Obstetrics and Gynaecology 44: 72–76

Sand P K, Bowen L W, Panganiban R, Ostergard D R 1987 The low pressure urethra as a factor in failed retropubic urethropexy. Obstetrics and Gynecology 69: 399–402

Shelley T, Warrel D W 1965 Measurement of intra-vesical and intra-urethral pressure in normal women and in women suffering from incontinence of urine. Journal of Obstetrics and Gynaecology of the British Commonwealth 72: 926–929

Shepherd A M, Lewis P A, Howell S C, Abrams P H 1985 Video screening and stress urethral profiles – unnecessary investigations in the diagnosis of genuine stress incontinence. Proceedings of 15th Meeting International Continence Society, London, pp 261–262

Simons I 1936 Studies on bladder function: The sphincterometer. Journal of Urology 35: 96–102

Sorensen S 1991 Urethral pressure and pressure variations in stress incontinent women and women with unstable detrusor. Neurourology and Urodynamics 10: 483–492

Sorensen S, Kirkeby H J, Stodkilde-Jorgensen H, Djurhuus J C 1986 Continuous recording of urethral activity in healthy female volunteers. Neurourology and Urodynamics 5: 5–16

Sutherst J R, Brown M C 1980 Detection of urethral incompetence in women using the fluid-bridge test. British Journal of Urology 52: 138–142

Sutherst J R, Brown M 1981 Detection of urethral incompetence. Erect studies using the fluid-bridge test. British Journal of Urology 53: 360–363

Swift S E, Utrie J W 1996 The need for standardisation of the Valsalva leak point pressure. International Urogynaecology Journal 7: 227–230

Tanagho E A 1979 Membrane and microtransducer catheters: their effectiveness for profilometry of the lower urinary tract. Urological Clinics of North America 6 (1): 110–119

Tanagho E A, Millar E R 1970 The initiation of voiding. British Journal of Urology 42: 175–183

Tapp A, Versi E, Cardozo L 1985 Is urethral pressure profilometry useful in the diagnosis of genuine stress incontinence? Proceedings of 15th Meeting International Continence Society, London, pp 263–264

Toews H A, 1967 Intraurethral and intravesical pressures in normal and stress-incontinent women. Obstetrics and Gynaecology 29: 613–624

Ulmsten U, Henricksson L, Josef S 1982 The unstable female urethra. American Journal of Obstetrics and Gynecology 144: 93–97

Versi E 1990 Discriminant analysis of urethral pressure profilometry data for the diagnosis of genuine stress incontinence. British Journal of Obstetrics and Gynaecology 97: 251–259

Versi E, Cardozo L D, Studd J W W, Brimcat M, O'Dowd T M, Cooper D J 1986a Evaluation of urethral pressure profilometry for the diagnosis of genuine stress incontinence. World Journal of Urology 4: 6–9

Versi E, Cardozo L D, Studd J W W et al 1986b Internal urinary sphincter in maintenance of female continence. British Medical Journal 292: 166–167

Zinner N R, Ritter R C, Sterling A M 1976 The mechanism of micturition. In: Williams D I, Chisholm G D (eds) Scientific Foundations of Urology. Heinemann, London pp 39–54

Cystourethroscopy

PETER H L WORTH

Cystourethroscopy is essentially an examination to establish if disease is present in the bladder or urethra. It is not the investigation to decide whether a bladder neck is obstructed or incompetent: this can only be satisfactorily established by urodynamic testing. It may however be of help in deciding how to operate on a patient with incontinence.

PREPARATION

Rigid or flexible cystoscopy can usually be performed without any anaesthetic. Flexible cystoscopy has the advantage that it can be used with the patient lying supine rather than in the lithotomy position, and on account of its mobility the anterior wall of the bladder can be more easily inspected. It does take time to master the technique (Fowler et al 1984). Small biopsies and diathermy can be undertaken. In a controlled trial 89% of patients preferred a flexi cystoscopy to a rigid cystoscopy (Flannigan et al 1988).

It is bad practice to carry out cystoscopy under general anaesthetic as an isolated procedure without being prepared to proceed to biopsy or diathermy, and a gynaecologist should be trained at least to be able to biopsy the bladder.

With a standard cystoscope, examination of the urethra proves difficult because the opening is not at the end of the instrument. An alternative instrument that is rigid and can be used without a general anaesthetic is the integrated cystoscope (Miller et al 1987). It is smaller than most cystoscopes and even at 17.5 Charriere (outside circumference in mm), it has an instrument channel that can take a 7 gauge catheter (Fig. 13.1).

Modern endoscopic equipment is very sophisticated. The Hopkins solid rod system to which a high quality TV camera can be attached, the solid state diathermy machines and the flexible light sources make endoscopic surgery much easier.

What instrument a gynaecologist chooses to use, will depend very much on his practice. Out-patient diagnostic cystoscopy is probably not of major interest, but bladder inspection as part of an assessment of malignant disease in the pelvis or prior to incontinent surgery, will more commonly be done under general anaesthetic and for this a rigid instrument is to be

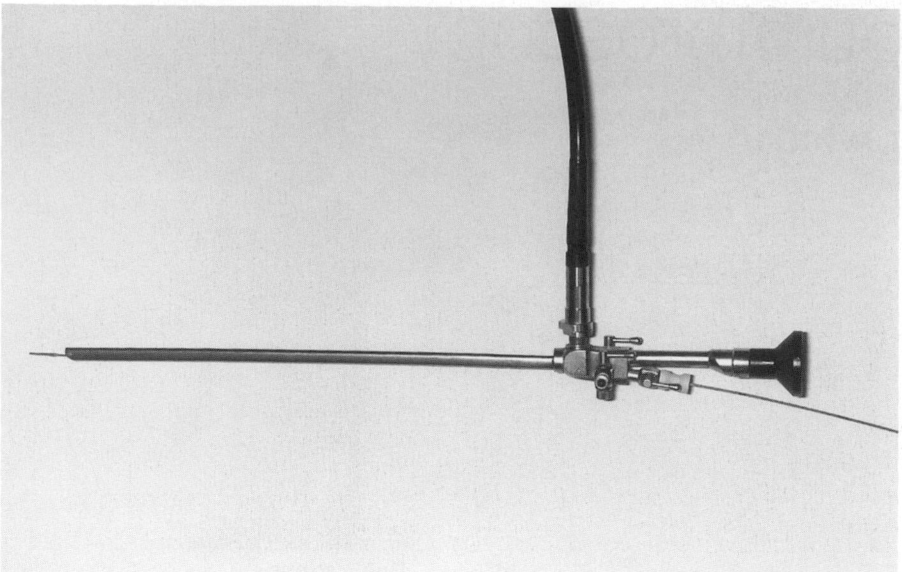

Fig. 13.1 Miller cystoscope with ureteric catheter.

preferred. It is important to have a good basic set consisting of a cystoscope, and a biopsy forcep. In addition some means of dilating the urethra is needed. An Otis urethrotome is ideal but other types of dilator, such as the Canny Ryall, Wyndham Powell or Hegar's dilators will do (Figs 13.2, 13.3). In gynaecological practice there is no need to use anything but water for bladder irrigation.

TECHNIQUE

Before the cystoscope is passed, the external urethral meatus should be inspected to exclude any local pathological condition such as a urethral caruncle or urethral mucosal prolapse. The urethra is a difficult area to examine in women and it is probably best inspected on withdrawal rather than on entry.

The instrument having been passed, the residual urine can be measured. It is not necessarily a very accurate assessment because there is no guarantee that the individual has made an effort to empty the bladder. If the bladder is full of clot, useful information cannot be gained until the clot has been washed out.

While using the 70° telescope, the first thing is to orientate oneself, identify the trigone and the interureteric bar (not always easy in women), and find the ureteric orifice. Then look for the air bubble which is always to be found in the dome of the bladder and is a useful reference point. Examine the lateral walls of the bladder in turn and look very carefully between the air bubble and the bladder neck. Try not to over distend the bladder, and be careful when emptying the bladder because in certain conditions it may cause the bladder to bleed and make re-examination very difficult. It is important to note how much fluid has gone into the bladder from the filling bag so that the capacity can be roughly assessed. Accurate measuring by emptying the bladder into a jug is not usually necessary, unless it is thought the capacity is abnormally low.

At this stage the bladder neck and upper urethra should be examined using a 30° or 0° telescope. The appearance of the bladder neck does not correlate with function and it is dangerous to draw conclusions from the endoscopic appearance. The degree of laxity may signify incompetence. The opening of a urethral diverticulum is often difficult to identify unless one knows from radiological studies where it is to be found.

GENERAL POINTS

Trabeculation

Trabeculation (Fig. 13.4) is readily recognized but interpretation of what it means is very difficult. In women it is not usually associated with obstruction and does not signify a high pressure system. When trabeculation becomes marked, sacculation may form between the trabeculae and eventually a diverticulum may be formed. When a diverticulum is present,

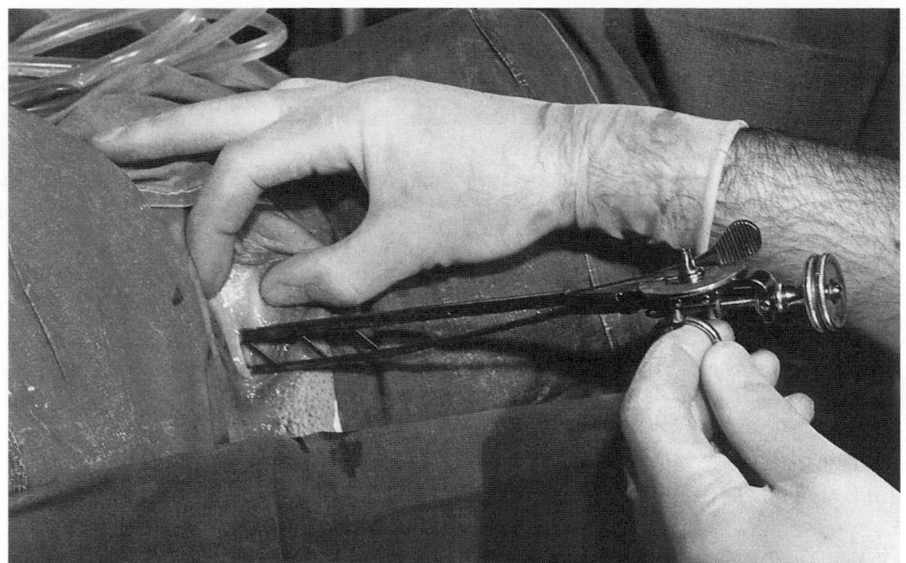

Fig. 13.2 Otis urethrotome. Shown open calibrating the urethra.

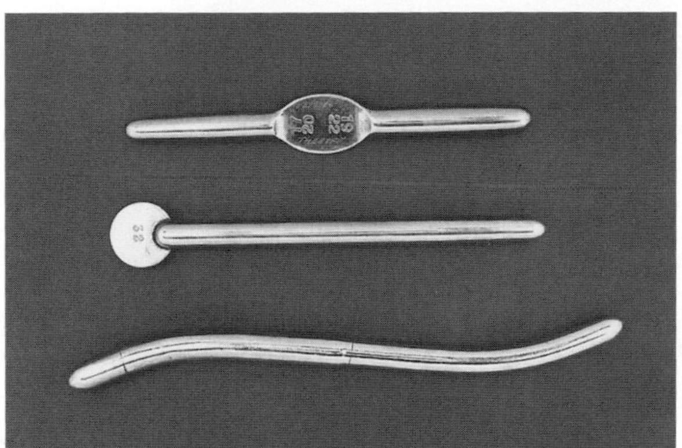

Fig. 13.3 Canny-Ryall dilator, Wyndham-Powell dilator, Hegar's dilator (From top to bottom).

attempts should be made to look inside it (not always easy), because it may be harbouring disease, e.g. a carcinoma. It is also important to locate the opening of the diverticulum in relation to the ureteric orifices.

Cystitis

Cystoscopy should be avoided in the presence of active cystitis because it is potentially dangerous and may cause bacteraemia or septicaemia. If cystoscopy is undertaken quite soon after acute cystitis has been treated the mucosa is reddened and tends to bleed on decompression.

In recurrent bouts of cystitis or urethrotrigonitis the bladder may be normal, but there may be marked squamous change on the trigone. Whether this should be treated by diathermy resection, urethral dilatation, sphincterotomy or by no action at all is debatable.

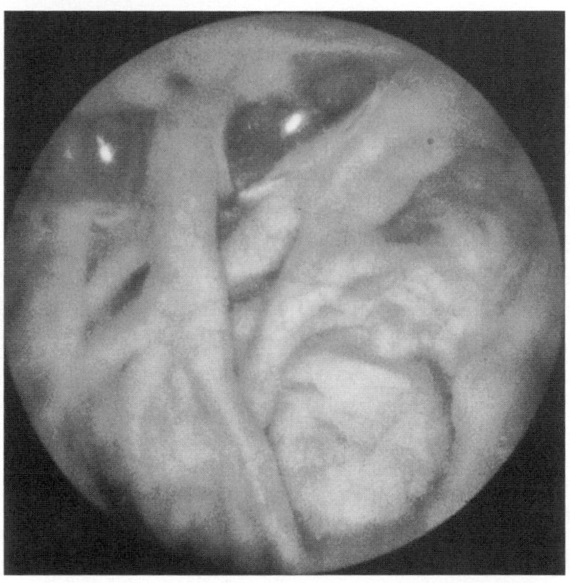

Fig. 13.4 Cystoscopic view of trabeculation.

Chronic cystitis is a collection of conditions not usually associated with bacterial infection but producing recurrent bouts of frequency and a great deal of suprapubic pain. In tuberculosis discrete red areas may be visible in the bladder, and the ureteric orifices may be rigid and open. In interstitial cystitis, linear splits which bleed on decompression, may be visible in the dome of the bladder. More often there is generalized vascularity in the dome and very often the capacity is reduced. Despite deep anaesthesia the patient may develop inspiratory stridor, or a marked tachycardia on account of the severity of the pain, which is produced as the bladder fills.

Histological diagnosis is always important and a

biopsy should be obtained of an appropriate lesion and adjacent mucosa. Care should be taken with biopsies on the posterior wall of the bladder which is quite thin and unprotected. A full thickness biopsy may enter the peritoneal cavity, and will be associated with extravasation of fluid. Biopsies of the trigone are best obtained by using a resectoscope loop.

Recurrent pyelonephritis with reflux

When ureteric reflux has been demonstrated in the prepubertal child by micturating cystourethrography, it is important to assess the position of the ureteric orifices. Often the trigone is abnormally wide, with the ureteric orifices laterally placed. In addition, the configuration of the orifice may give some guide to the possibility of the reflux ceasing – a big open ureteric orifice laterally placed is unlikely to become competent whereas a normally appearing orifice in the correct place may become competent as the child grows.

Duplications

Completely duplicated ureters usually open quite close together in the bladder, either side by side or on the ureteric ridge a short distance apart: the ureter draining through the lower orifice comes from the upper calyx of the kidney. An ectopic ureteric orifice may be near the bladder neck, but may also be found in the urethra, vagina or perineum. It may be very difficult to detect even if the patient has been given a dye, because the amount of urine being produced by that part of the kidney may be very small.

Ureterocele

A ureterocele is caused by a bag of mucosa at the lower end of the ureter and may be associated with obstruction. A ureterocele may be single and orthotopic or part of a duplex system and either orthotopic or ectopic. It has a very characteristic appearance and may be flattened when the pressure in the bladder rises, and may even prolapse back up the ureter. In a young child a ureterocele may occasionally be so big that it is seen as a mass at the urethral orifice having prolapsed out of the bladder.

Fistulae (see also Ch. 23)

Large vesicovaginal fistulae are no problem in diagnosis, but when they are small diagnosis may be difficult. Out-patient methylene blue testing may already have established that a vesicovaginal rather than a ureterovaginal fistula is present. This test involves placing three swabs in the vagina, and then filling the bladder through a catheter (better placed before the swabs are inserted), with water and methylene blue. Do not use Bonneys blue which is acidic and causes severe bladder damage. Pressure should be applied to the bladder with a catheter clamped. This may cause some leakage into the superficial swab; but if the middle swab is clean and the dye is present on the deepest swab, a vesicovaginal fistula must be present. If the swab is damp but not discoloured, a ureterovaginal fistual is present. Sometimes it is easier to find a fistula by filling the bladder, then, with speculum in the vagina, water may be seen to be spurting through the fistula. A small probe or ureteric catheter can be passed through the hole and the opening in the bladder can then be recognized. It is important to note the relationship of the fistula to the ureteric orifices and trigone.

A vesicocolic fistula can be difficult to detect. It is rarely a hole, but more often a red patch with oedematous mucosa situated high up on the left lateral wall of the bladder away from the ureteric orifice. It is unlikely to occur in a woman who has not had a hysterectomy.

Absent kidney

If a hemitrigone is seen at cystoscopy, then it is likely that the kidney is absent. This can be confirmed by ultrasound.

Ascending ureterography

Retrograde pyelography is now rarely done. Instead if the ureter is blocked ascending ureterography is carried out. This involves using a Chevassu catheter which has a conical end which is placed in the ureteric orifice and contrast injected while screening. This should accurately define the site and cause of ureteric obstruction. Be careful not to inject too much contrast (2–3 ml will fill the ureter) and only use dilute contrast because otherwise chemical irritation may make the obstruction worse and cause severe loin pain.

Bladder cancer

The majority of bladder cancers are discrete papillary tumours with an orange colour, more often than not found on the base of the bladder or above and lateral to the ureteric orifices (Fig. 13.5). Biopsy resection with a resectoscope loop effectively cures the lesion. It is important to be certain that the lesion is single

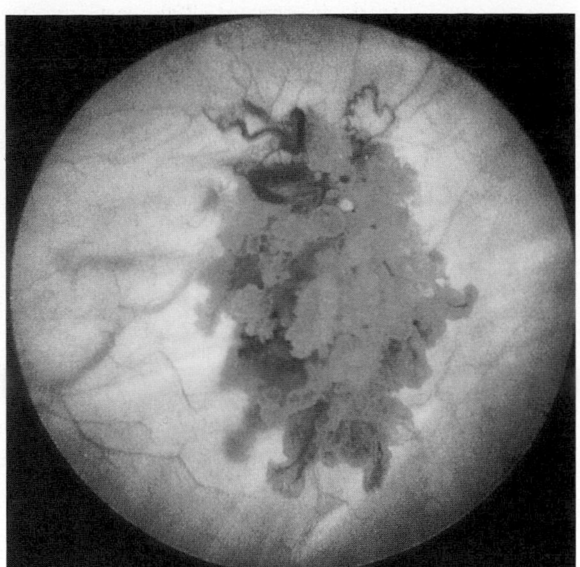

Fig. 13.5 Cystoscopic view of bladder cancer. Note the papillary nature often suggesting low grade and stage.

rather than multiple and it is necessary to inspect the mucosa around the tumour base very carefully. If it is abnormal it should be biopsied.

Solid tumours may be extensive and should have generous biopsies taken, preferably with a resectoscope loop. Tumour in the bladder may be the result of cervical cancer, and may occasionally be related to rectal cancer. They look different, they tend to be relatively flat and have an irregular surface and the mucosa may be essentially intact.

The important examination at the time of cystoscopy in the case of bladder cancer, is the bimanual examination to assess the staging of the tumour. Additional information will be gained by CT scanning. Having accurately staged and graded the tumour, a decision on management can be made.

REFERENCES

Flannigan G M, Gelister J S K, Noble J G, Milroy E J G 1988 Rigid versus flexible cystoscopy. A controlled trial of patient tolerance. British Journal of Urology 62: 537–540

Fowler C G, Badenoch D F, Thakar D R 1984 Practical experience with flexible cystoscopy in outpatients. British Journal of Urology 56: 618–621

Miller R A, Coptcoat M J, Parry J, Dawkins G, Wickham J E A 1987 The integrated cystoscope. An alternative to conventional and fibreoptic cystoscopy. British Journal of Urology 60: 128–131

Ultrasound

SARAH M CREIGHTON AND DAVID GORDON

INTRODUCTION

Ultrasound has been used for many years by obstetricians and gynaecologists, however it is only comparatively recently that it has been applied to the evaluation of the lower urinary tract in women. It has the advantages of being a non-invasive technique and without any risk of ionizing radiation. Its increasing use is in part due to its easy availability in all general gynaecological departments. Either static or dynamic images can be obtained and, particularly with the latter, prolonged observation can be made without risk to patient or examiner.

Holmes (1971) demonstrated the ease and accuracy of evaluating the static urinary bladder with transabdominal ultrasound and measured residual urine, bladder wall mobility, distortion of the bladder wall by adjacent pelvic tumours and detection and evaluation of bladder tumours. Further work continued into the assessment of incontinent female patients (White et al 1980). Other techniques were developed including the use of the perineal probe (Kohorn et al 1986), the rectal probe (Nishizawa et al 1982; Brown et al 1985) and the vaginal probe (Quinn et al 1988).

ROUTE

Ultrasound in the incontinent female has been performed using transabdominal, perineal, rectal and vaginal ultrasound probes. Perineal and abdominal probes are usually linear array. Vaginal and rectal probes may be either linear array or sector scanners. Linear array transducers used for this purpose have the disadvantages of needing a larger housing unit for the crystals and having relatively lower operating frequencies. Mechanical sector scanners require a smaller housing unit and are more acceptable to the patient. They theoretically cause less anatomical distortion and as they operate at a higher frequency, the image resolution is improved.

Abdominal

The first descriptions of bladder ultrasound used the transabdominal route (Holmes 1971; White et al 1980). The transducer is placed on the abdomen and aimed caudally below the symphysis. This technique is the most comfortable for the patient although it is often not easy to perform, particularly in obese patients. The urethrovesical junction is often hidden behind the symphysis and cannot be seen. Transabdominal scanning does not use a fixed reference when assessing bladder neck descent so any movement of the patient or transducer will introduce artefact into the measurements. Despite these difficulties, transabdominal ultrasound has been used to select patients suitable for surgical correction of genuine stress incontinence (Bhatia et al 1987). Vaginal, rectal and perineal probes were designed to overcome the technical difficulties associated with transabdominal scanning.

Rectal

The transrectal probe was initially developed to study the prostate gland (Watanabe et al 1974) and subsequently used to study the bladder and urethra (Brown et al 1983; Richmond & Sutherst 1989a). Its most recent application has been in the study of anal sphincter damage in postpartum women and the prediction of faecal incontinence. Using rectal ultrasound, a good view of the bladder and urethra is obtained and localization of the bladder neck is not difficult. However it is possible that insertion of the transducer alters the alignment of the bladder neck; Bergman et al (1988) used the Q-tip test while inserting the rectal probe and found no restriction of the urethrovesical mobility with a rectal probe a vaginal probe did restrict movement. Richmond & Sutherst (1989b) also used the rectal probe to assess the bladder neck during urodynamic studies and found no alteration in any of the parameters although this does not exclude small changes in bladder neck position. The probe itself may move during cough or Valsalva manoeuvre thus creating artefact. Another considerable disadvantage of the rectal probe is unacceptability for the patient. The probe may cause discomfort and certainly causes embarrassment.

Vaginal

The vaginal probe is more acceptable to the patient and also gives a good view of the bladder base, bladder neck, urethrovesical junction and the inferior border of the pubic symphysis (Quinn et al 1988). In some cases the precise position of the urethra cannot be identified without placing a urethral catheter. It is however probable that the probe interferes with position and function of the bladder neck and urethra and results obtained may not be representative of the true clinical picture. Wise et al (1992) performed urethral pressure profilometry with and without a vaginal probe *in situ*, and found a significant increase in maximum urethral pressure and functional urethral length both at rest and during stress in the presence of the probe. They also performed lateral bead chain urethrocystography with and without a vaginal probe in place and found that it also restricted bladder neck movement on Valsalva manoeuvre. In those women where a Foley catheter in the urethra is necessary to see the bladder neck clearly, it is likely that this will also interfere with movement on straining. Beco et al (1994) confirmed the distortion of the posterior urethrovesical angle in both transvaginal and abdominal ultrasound.

Koelbl et al (1989, 1990) have described 'introital sonography' in order to minimize some of the interference. They place the vaginal probe adjacent to the vulva just under the external urethral meatus. They claim to obtain a clear picture with this method although it is likely that there are difficulties scanning obese patients. It is often necessary to push the probe some way into the vagina to obtain a clear image and the problems of interference with function have been discussed above.

To assess bladder neck mobility the probe needs to move with the patient on Valsalva manoeuvre in order to maintain the same position in relation to the bladder neck. This is difficult with the vaginal probe as the view is easily lost and artefacts of movement created. The vaginal probe cannot be used on patients with a large cystocele, rectocele or vault prolapse as these push the probe out of the vagina on straining.

Perineal

The perineal probe (Kohorn et al 1986; Gordon et al 1989) is the least expensive and most readily available technique. A good view of the bladder and urethra is obtained and the symphysis pubis can be used as a reference point for movement (Fig. 14.1). The method is acceptable to the patient and easy to perform and is feasible even in the obese patient. There is no possibility of interfering with bladder neck position and it can be used on patients with prolapse.

The main disadvantage of perineal ultrasonography is that to visualize the urethrovesical junction, a Foley catheter may need to be inserted. This may interfere with bladder neck movement and care must be taken to ensure that the catheter is free to move and not held under tension. An extra catheterization is not necessary if the scan is performed along the routine cystometry as a catheter is already *in situ* (Gordon et al 1989). Attempts to overcome the need for catherization have been made and Schaer et al (1995) filled the bladder with contrast media (Echovist) before scanning at rest and on Valsalva manoeuvre. They found that bladder and urethral anatomy was more clearly seen and urinary leakage easier to detect. They also reported easier visualization of bladder neck funnelling although as with videocystourethrography the clinical usefulness of this may be limited.

Intraurethral

This new method uses minature transducers (20 MHz on a 6 or 9 F catheter) to visualize the urethra, external urethral sphincter and paraurethral tissues. Kirschner-Hermanns et al (1994) used this method to study continent women and women with stress incontinence. They measured sphincter size in terms of area and circumference and compared sphincter size to continence. This technique is currently only a research tool but has interesting clinical possibilities and may lead to reassessment of the role of the external urethral sphincter.

INDICATIONS FOR ULTRASOUND

Ultrasound is currently used to determine residual urine, particularly in women with voiding difficulties. It is also indicated in the investigation of the anatomy of the urethra, bladder neck and adjacent

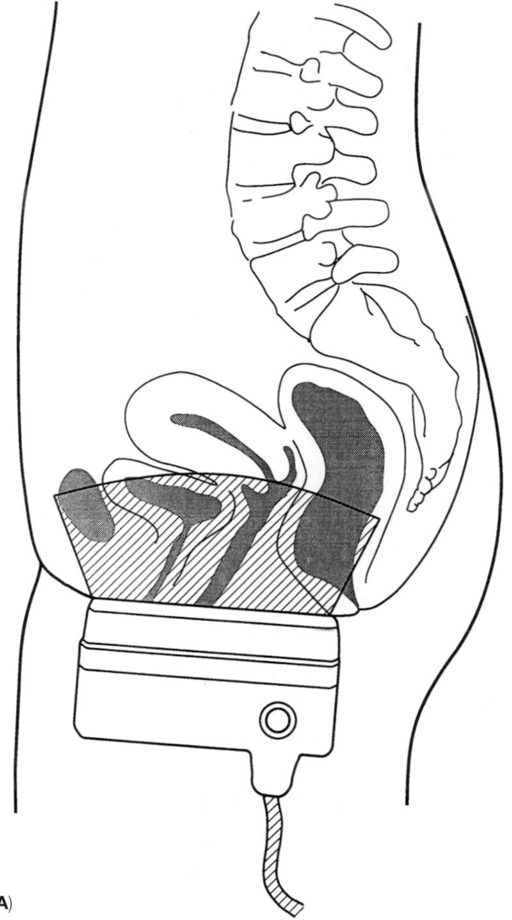
(A)

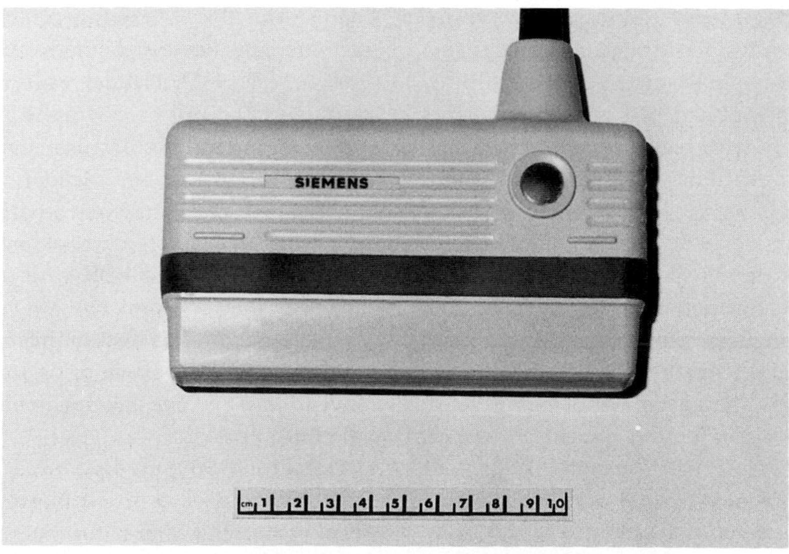

(B)

Fig. 14.1 (**A**) Diagrammatic representation of the area scanned by the perineal probe. (**B**) 3.5 MHz linear array probe suitable for perineal scanning (Siemens).

structures. More recently ultrasound has been applied to the assessment of the incontinence patient for diagnosis, selection of the correct surgical procedure and prediction of operative outcome.

Investigation of voiding difficulties

The estimation of postmicturition residual urine was described by Holmes (1967) and is the simplest use of ultrasound. It obviates the need for urethral catheterization with its risk of infection. It is indicated in the investigation of patients with voiding difficulties either idiopathic or postoperative and also occasionally following postoperative catheter removal.

The bladder is scanned in two planes and three diameters are measured. As the bladder only approaches a spherical shape when full, a correction factor has to be applied. Several different formulae have been devised with varying degrees of accuracy. Pederson et al (1975) correlated the result directly to the product of bladder height × width × depth and obtained an error rate of 24%. Poston et al (1983) multiplied the three diameters obtained by a correction factor of 0.7 and obtained a 21% error on comparison with volume voided. Probably the most commonly used formula is to multiply the product of three diameters (height × width × depth) by a figure of 0.625 (Hakenberg et al 1983). This has an error rate of 21% which is acceptable. This formula is not appropriate in women in the puerperium as the involuting uterus affects bladder shape (Benness et al 1989) and in these patients a correction factor of 0.7 gives the most accurate results.

Most of the studies evaluating ultrasound in residual urine scanning were performed using static B-mode scanners although today the majority of scans are performed using real-time ultrasound. Some of the methods with the B-mode scanner require multiple parallel scans (Beacock et al 1985) which cannot be reproduced accurately with real-time scanners. Kiely et al (1987) evaluated real-time ultrasound and found a wide range of error (+52% to −29%) and even using a different correction factor of 0.65 to give a smaller error still found a wide range. They concluded real-time ultrasound was unsuitable for any clinical purpose requiring repeated assessment of residual urine.

Most residual urine estimation is performed transabdominally. This has the advantage of being comfortable and non-invasive for the patient. However for bladder volumes of less than 150 ml it is not a reliable method. More recently, rectal and intravaginal probes have been used to give a more accurate measurement (Haylen et al 1989) although the procedure may be less acceptable for the patient.

Bladder and urethral anatomy

Urethral cysts and diverticula can be examined using ultrasound (Ganabathi et al 1994). The disadvantage of the method is that unless the opening of the diverticulum is seen, the two cannot be differentiated. It has also been found possible to visualize the external rhabdosphincter when using transabdominal ultrasound and a full bladder (De Gonzalez et al 1988) although the clinical application of this is uncertain.

Investigation of incontinence

Ultrasound has been used to demonstrate genuine stress incontinence and the presence of detrusor contractions. There have also been attempts to define bladder neck position and movement in women with stress incontinence in the assessment before and after surgical treatment.

Diagnosis

Vaginal ultrasound has been used to diagnose stress incontinence and detrusor instability in an attempt to replace routine cystometry and obviate catheterization. Quinn et al (1988) identified bladder neck opening in patients with stress incontinence although bladder neck opening has also been shown to occur in 21% of asymptomatic nulliparous women (Chapple et al 1989). The ultrasound equipment used to demonstrate this needs to have a high frame rate to image dynamic events such as bladder neck opening and such equipment is not usually part of a routine gynaecological scanning department. Detrusor instability is also associated with bladder neck opening and detrusor pressure should also be measured to distinguish this from stress incontinence. Detrusor contractions may be seen on ultrasound in some cases (Bhatia et al 1987). Bladder wall thickness measured by transvaginal ultrasonography has been proposed as a screening test for detrusor instability. Khullar et al (1996) found that the bladder wall thickness was significantly greater in women with detrusor instability, presumably due to detrusor muscle hypertrophy. The results compared well with ambulatory urodynamics as long as women with outflow obstruction were excluded. This technique was proposed as a screening test in women prior to surgery, avoiding conventional cystometry, but is not yet used in general clinical practice.

Creighton (1989) used perineal ultrasound to compare bladder neck position of women with genuine stress incontinence to continent controls. Although these results showed a tendency for the continent patients to have higher and more posteriorly positioned bladder necks than those with stress incontinence, there was a large overlap between the groups. There was no difference in bladder neck mobility. Given that we know that the aetiology of stress incontinence is multifactorial, these results are expected and it is unlikely that we could predict continence based on bladder neck position alone. Some studies have presented the rather simplistic view that bladder neck hypermobility is the cause of stress incontinence and that women cured by incontinence surgery have immobile bladder necks (Johnson et al 1992). Unfortunately patients who remain incontinent after surgery may still have fixed bladder necks on ultrasonographic examination. More recent studies using transvaginal ultrasonography have identified a difference in bladder neck mobility between continent and incontinent women but also admit that the overlap is large and clinical relevance limited (Hol et al 1995).

Beco et al (1987) has used vaginal ultrasound to study women during micturition and claim to have identified a 'prepubic muscle' which can be seen to contract before voiding in normal women and contracts to reduce urethral pressure in women with urethral instability. These findings have not been reported in any other series and have yet to be confirmed. The practical difficulties of asking the patient to void with the vaginal probe *in situ* may be a drawback to this and the presence of the probe may cause an unphysiological response.

Khullar et al (1996) have used three-dimensional ultrasound to measure urethral sphincter volume in women with genuine stress incontinence (GSI) and continent controls. Women with GSI had significantly smaller urethral sphincter volume but unfortunately the overlap with control was too great.

Assessment for surgery

Ultrasound has been used to study women before and after bladder neck surgery in an attempt to discover the reasons for failure of surgery and to make the choice of procedure more objective. Both bladder neck position and excursion have been studied.

In the past, lateral chain cystography was used to outline the urethra and bladder neck and display downward and backward movement during coughing and straining (Hodgkinson 1953). This method has been used in the assessment of surgical failure, based on the premise that if the bladder neck has not been moved upwards and backwards compared with the preoperative position that operation has been a technical failure (Stamey 1983). However radiographic evaluation of the posterior urethral angle has proved neither reliable nor consistent in clinical practice. Wall et al (1994) examined lateral chain X-rays on 98 women undergoing one of four different bladder repairs and confirmed that no useful information was obtained regarding the dynamics of incontinence or its surgical cure. The technique also has the disadvantage of radiation exposure. Measurements cannot be made directly and must be taken from an X-ray film at a later time.

Ultrasound avoids some of the risks and drawbacks of lateral chain cystography and it was hoped that it might be a more useful tool for investigating incontinence and its surgical success or failure. Ultrasound has been shown to correlate well with videocystourethrography (VCU) (Bergman et al 1988). Gordon et al (1989) compared perineal ultrasound with lateral chain cystography. They compared ultrasound views at rest and on strain with those obtained on the same patients at lateral chain X-ray and found a good correlation. They used a balloon catheter to visualize the bladder neck accurately and concluded that the good correlation showed that the catheter did not interfere with movement of the bladder base, bladder neck or urethra. Whether or not the bead chain interferes with bladder neck function has not been investigated.

Most recent studies of ultrasound in the incontinent women are purely comparisons of the technique to conventional radiological techniques (White et al 1980; Bergman et al 1988). There are few studies using the ultrasound either to identify the features of the continent patient or to assess surgical cure. Quinn et al (1989) used the vaginal probe to assess 40 women with stress incontinence before and after colposuspension. The postoperative position of the bladder neck in relation to the pubic symphysis was measured and it was found that there was no clear distinction of position for dry patients as compared with those persisting with stress incontinence.

Richmond & Sutherst (1989b) however studied 25 continent and 59 incontinent women and found greater bladder neck mobility in incontinent women when compared with continent parous women. There were also significant differences in the outcome of surgery in patients with mobile as compared with non-mobile bladder necks. They now use ultrasound to determine their choice of operative procedure (Richmond & Sutherst 1989c), performing a Burch colposuspension on those patients with a fixed bladder neck and a sling procedure on those women with bladder neck descent and rotation. This is contrary to current practice which recommends that colposuspension is the procedure of choice in women where further bladder neck elevation is possible (Stanton 1986).

Creighton (1994) also used perineal ultrasound to look at women undergoing either the Raz bladder neck suspension or a colposuspension to determine whether there were ultrasound measurements which predicted surgical success or failure (Figs 14.2, 14.3). In those women who were not cured by colposuspension there was no difference in bladder neck elevation

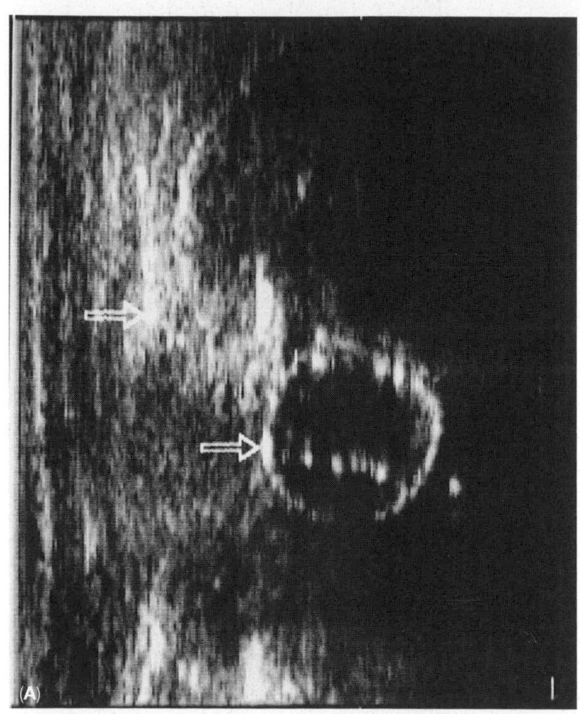

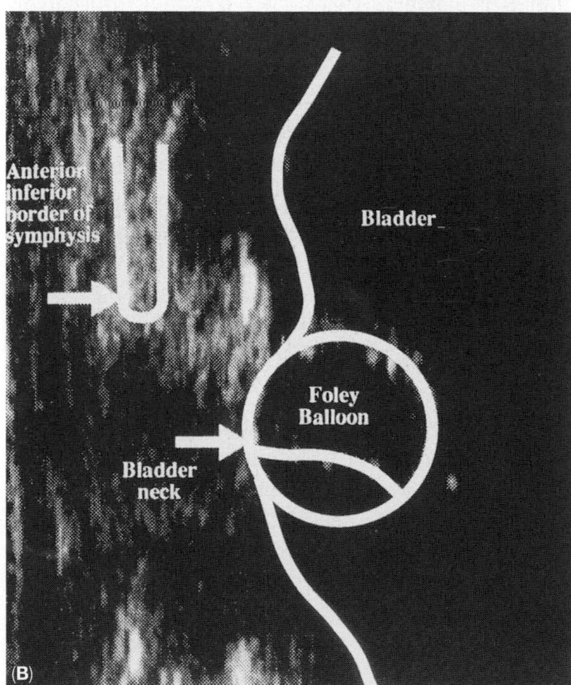

Fig. 14.2 (**A**) A perineal ultrasound scan. This shows the bladder neck at rest. A Foley balloon catheter is in the bladder and the bladder neck taken as the junction between balloon and catheter. The symphysis is seen as two bright parallel echoes. (**B**) The above scan with a line drawing of the findings superimposed over it.

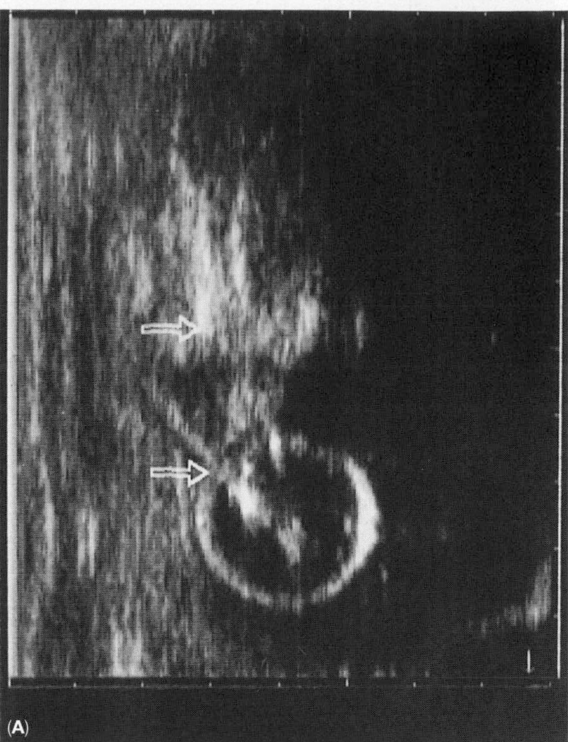

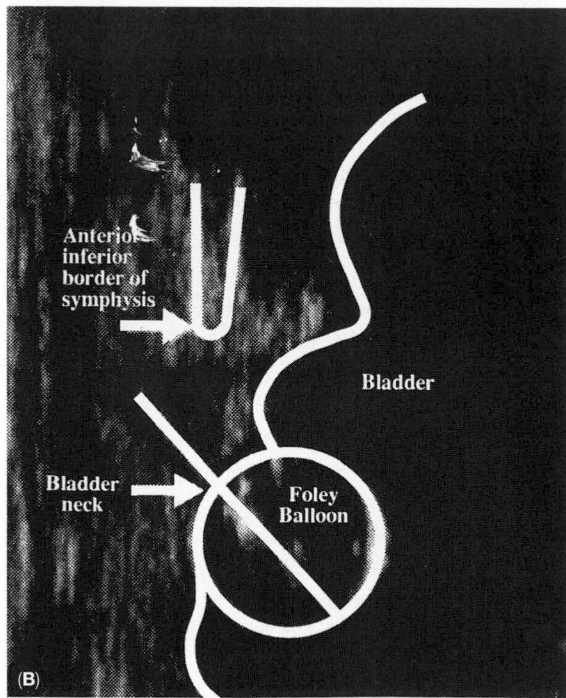

Fig. 14.3 (**A**) This is a perineal scan on the same patient at maximum Valsalva manoeuvre. The change in position of the bladder neck relative to the symphysis is seen. (**B**) The above scan with a line drawing superimposed over it.

or excursion when compared with those who were cured by their operations. Interestingly, those women in whom the Raz procedure failed had much lower bladder necks than those who were cured suggesting failure at elevation. This may have been caused by the cutting through of the sutures as these patients were all elderly. Further work is needed to confirm these findings and to correlate clinical findings with ultrasound results in order to predict surgical success or failure.

Investigation of prolapse

Features of genital wall prolapse such as cystocele, rectocele and vault prolapse can be clearly seen using perineal ultrasound (Fig. 14.4). Using videoultrasonography a dynamic study of the pelvic floor mechanics during the Valsalva and Kegel manoeuvres can be obtained (Creighton et al 1992). It is known that posterior vaginal wall prolapse and its subsequent repair can affect urinary continence and this technique may allow us to clarify the mechanism. Further attempts have been made to standardize measurements of bladder neck and prolapse descent by using a pressure catheter in the rectum to try and standardize cough and Valsalva pressure. This means that the pressure achieved at maximum Valsalva can be measured, although this has not as yet been correlated to clinical and ultrasound findings.

CONCLUSIONS

Ultrasound of the female lower urinary tract correlates well with conventional investigative techniques. Accurate localization of the relationship of the bladder and bladder neck can be seen, although a urethral catheter is often required. At present perineal ultrasonography appears to be the most useful as it is the least likely technique to interfere with bladder neck and urethral function. Ultrasound may potentially be useful in assessing the features of the continent patient as well as assessing surgical results. It may thus be of use in improving our choice of the most appropriate procedure. At present it cannot be used in place of cystometric studies in the choice of surgery as an accurate diagnosis of stress incontinence and the exclusion of detrusor instability is imperative.

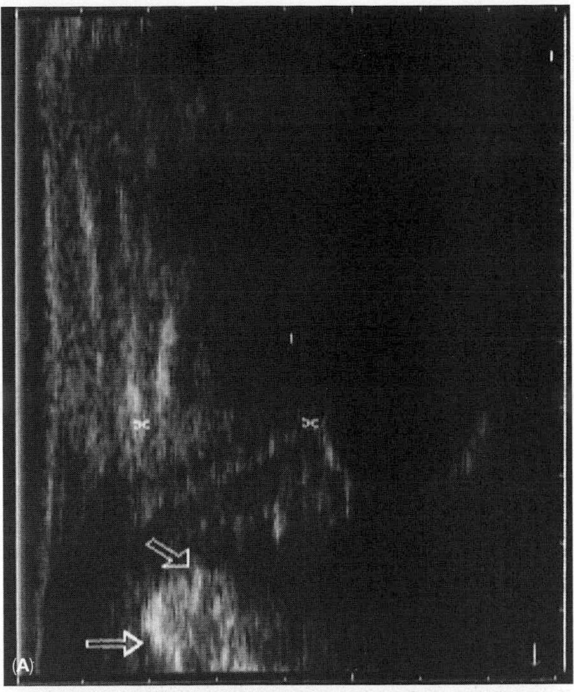

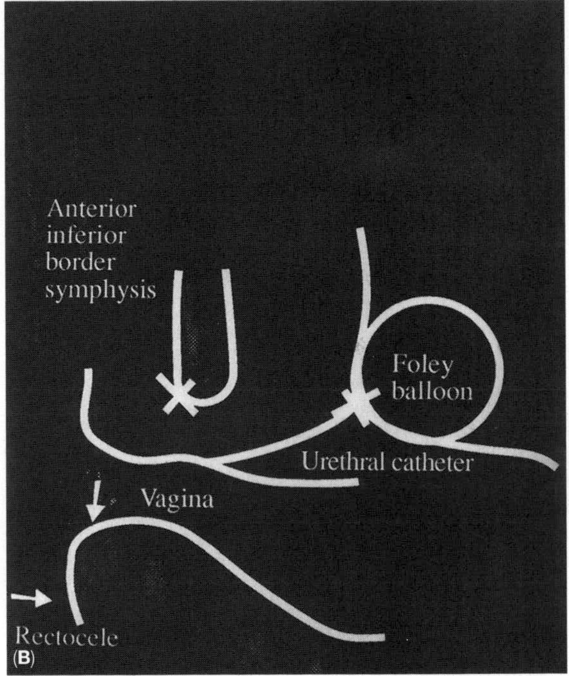

Fig. 14.4 (**A**) A perineal ultrasound scan of a patient with a rectocele after colposuspension. The high position of the bladder neck in relation to the pubic symphysis can be seen and the difference with Fig. 14.2 is clear. The two arrows point to the outline of the rectocele. (**B**) The above scan with a line drawing superimposed over it.

REFERENCES

Beacock C J M, Roberts E E, Rees R W M, Buck A C 1985 Ultrasound assessment of residual urine. A quantitative method. British Journal Urology 57: 410–413

Beco J, Sulu M, Schaaps J P, Lambotte R 1987 Une nouvelle approach des troubles de continence chez la femme: l'echographie urodynamique par voie vaginale Journal de Gynecologie Obstetrique et Biologie de la Reproduction 16: 987–988

Beco J, Leonard D, Lambotted R 1994 Study of the artefacts introduced by linear array transvaginal ultrasound scanning in urodynamics. World Journal of Urology 12(6): 329–332

Benness C J, Tapp A J S, Cardozo L D 1989 Estimation of urinary residual volume in the puerperium by ultrasound. Proceedings of 19th Meeting International Continence Society, Ljubljana

Bergman A, McKenzie C J, Richmond J, Ballard C A, Platt L D 1988 Transrectal ultrasound versus cystography in the evaluation of anatomical stress urinary incontinence. British Journal of Urology 62: 228–234

Bhatia N N, Ostergard D R, McQuown D 1987 Ultrasonography in urinary incontinence. Urology 29: 90–94

Brown M C, Sutherst J R, Murray A 1983 Bladder base dynamics viewed by ultrasound. Proceedings of 13th Meeting International Continence Society, Aachen

Brown M C, Sutherst J R, Murray A, Richmond D H 1985 Potential use of ultrasound in place of x-ray fluoroscopy in urodynamics. British Journal of Urology 57: 88–90

Chapple C R, Helm C W, Blease S, Milroy E J G, Rickards D, Osborne J L 1989. Asymptomatic bladder neck incompetence in nulliparous females. British Journal of Urology 64: 357–359

Creighton S M 1989. Innovative techniques in the investigation and management of female urinary incontinence. M D Thesis, University of London

Creighton S M, Pearce J M, Stanton S L 1992 Perineal videoultrasonography in the assessment of vaginal prolapse. British Journal of Obstetrics and Gynaecology 99: 310–313

Creighton S M, Clark A, Pearce J M, Stanton S L 1994 Bladder neck ultrasound: appearances before and after continence surgery. Ultrasound in Obstetrics and Gynaecology 4: 428–??

De Gonzalez E L, Cosgrove D O, Joseph A E, Murch C, Naik K 1988. The appearances on ultrasound of the female urethral sphincter. British Journal of Radiology 61: 687–690

Ganabathi K, Leach G E, Zimmern P E, Dmochowski R 1994. Experience with the management of urethral diverticulum in 63 women. Journal of Urology 152(5pt1): 1445–52

Gordon D, Pearce J M, Norton P, Stanton S L, 1989. Comparison of ultrasound and lateral chain urethrocystography in the determination of bladder descent. American Journal of Obstetrics and Gynaecology 160: 182–5

Hakenburg O W, Ryall R L, Landlois S L, Marshall V R 1983. The estimation of bladder volume by sonocystography. Journal of Urology 136: 808–12

Haylen B T, Frazer M I, Sutherst J R, West C R 1989. Transvaginal ultrasound in the measurement of bladder volumes in women. British Journal of Urology 63: 149–51

Hodgkinson C P, 1953. Relationships of the female urethra and bladder in urinary stress incontinence. American Journal of Obstetrics and Gynecology 65: 560

Hol M, Van Bolhuis C, Vierhout M E 1995. Vaginal ultrasound studies of bladder neck mobility. British Journal of Obstetrics and Gynaecology 102: 47–53

Holmes JH 1967 Ultrasonic studies of the bladder Journal of Urology 79(4): 654–663

Holmes J H 1971 Ultrasonic studies of bladder filling and contour. In: Hinman JF (ed) Hydrodynamics of Micturition. Charles C Thomas, Illinois

Johnson J D, Lamensdorf H, Hollander I N, Thurman A E 1992. Use of transvaginal endosonography in the evaluation of women with stress urinary incontinence. Journal of Urology 146(2): 421–5

Kiely E A, Hartnell G G, Gibson R N, Gordon Williams 1987. Measurement of bladder volume by real time ultrasound. British Journal of Urology 60: 33–35

Kirschner-Hermans R, Klein H M, Schafer W, Jakse G 1994. Intra-urethral ultrasound in women with stress incontinence. British Journal of Urology 74(3): 31508

Koelbl H, Bernaschek G 1989. A new method for sonographic urethrocystography and simultaneous pressure flow measurements. Obstetrics and Gynecology 74: 417–422

Koelbl H, Bernaschek G, Deutinger J 1990. Assessment of female urinary incontinence by introital sonography. Journal of Clinical Ultrasound 18(4): 370–4

Kohorn E L, Scioscia A L, Genty P, Hubbins J 1986. Ultrasound cystourethrography by perineal scanning for the assessment of female stress urinary incontinence. Obstetrics and Gynecology 68: 269–272

Khullar V, Cardozo L D, Salvatore S, Hill S 1996. Ultrasound: a non-invasive screening test for detrusor instability. British Journal of Obstetrics and Gynaecology 103: 904–908

Nishizawa D, Takadu H, Morita T, Stao S, Tsuchida S 1982. A new synchronous video urodynamics. Tokyo Journal of Experimental Medicine 136: 349–350

Pederson J F, Bartrum R J, Grytter C 1975. Residual urine determination by ultrasound scanning. American Journal of Ròentgenology 125: 474–478

Poston G J, Joseph A E A, Riddle P R 1983. The accuracy of ultrasound in the measurement of changes in bladder volume. British Journal of Ultrasound 55: 361–363

Quinn M J, Beynon J, Mortensen N J McC, Smith P J 1988. Transvaginal endosonography: a new method to study the anatomy of the lower urinary tract in urinary stress incontinence. British Journal of Urology 62: 414–418

Quinn M J, Beynon J, Mortensen N J McC, Smith P J 1989. Vaginal endosonography in the post-operative assessment of colposuspension. British Journal of Urology 63: 295–300

Richmond D H, Sutherst J R 1989a. Clinical application of transrectal ultrasound for the investigation of the incontinent patient. British Journal of Urology 63: 605–609

Richmond D H, Sutherst J R 1989b. Transrectal ultrasound scanning in urinary incontinence: the effect of the probe on Urodynamic parameters. British Journal of Urology 64: 600–603

Richmond D H, Sutherst J R 1989c. Burch colposuspension or sling for stress incontinence? A prospective study using transrectal ultrasound. British Journal of Urology 64: 600–603.

Schaer G N, Koechli O R, Schuessler B, Haller U 1995. Improvement of perineal sonographic bladder neck imaging with ultrasound contrast medium. Obstetrics and Gynecology 86: 950–4

Stamey T A 1983. Endoscopic suspension of the vesical neck. In: Raz S (ed) Female Urology. W B Saunders, Philadelphia, pp 267–268

Stanton S L 1986. In: Stanton S L, Tanagho E A (eds) The Colposuspension in Surgery of Female Incontinence 2nd edn. Springer-Verlag, Berlin, p 96

Wall L L, Peattie A B, Pearce J M, Stanton S L 1994 Bladder neck mobility and the outcome of surgery for genuine stress incontinence. A logistic regression analysis of lateral bead-chain cystoureturograms. Journal of Reproductive Medicine 39 (6): 429–35

Watanabe H, Igari D, Tanahasi Y 1974. Development and application of new equipment for transrectal ultrasonography. Journal of Clinical Ultrasound 2: 91–98

White R D, McQuown D, McCarthy T A, Ostergard D R 1980. Real time ultrasonography in the evaluation of urinary stress incontinence. American Journal of Obstetrics and Gynecology 138: 235–237

Wise B G, Burton G, Cutner A, Cardozo L D 1992. Effect of vaginal probe on lower urinary tract function. British Journal of Urology 80(1): 12–16

Clinical neurophysiology

CLARE J FOWLER

INTRODUCTION

The neurological activity of the muscles and organs of the pelvis is an important aspect of their physiology and any means of assessing this would be valuable. It was with this aim that clinical neurophysiological techniques were introduced to examine pelvic floor function – with some success. However, the principles of clinical neurophysiology are undeniably complicated and an understanding of how to interpret the tests needs some training in the specialty and a knowledge of the uses and limitations of the methods when they are used in general neurology. Clinical neurophysiological investigations have mostly been employed in urogynaecology in well considered research projects but from there the methods have been all too often uncritically applied and a number of misconceptions have crept into the literature. For example, it is wrong to use the pudendal terminal motor latency in a way that implies the test gives information about the possible strength of contraction of muscles of the pelvic floor. The pudendal evoked potential does not assess bladder afferent function, and it is rarely acknowledged that EMG techniques which have been applied to the striated muscles of the pelvic floor tell us more about reinnervation than denervation. In this chapter the principles of clinical neurophysiology will be explained, the clinical value of various tests examined and the basis of some of these common misunderstandings discussed.

ELECTROMYOGRAPHY (EMG)

Electromyography (EMG) is the recording of action current generated by contracting muscle fibres. It is the contraction of the muscle fibres which produces muscle force. This is produced at a molecular level by an energy-requiring reaction between actin and myosin which causes these two filamentous molecules to move over one another.

The chemical reaction is brought about by a rapid depolarization of muscle membrane and it is the depolarizing potentials recorded in the extracellular space that forms the electromyogram. The potentials are generated by depolarization of single muscle fibres but the innervation of muscle is such that a single muscle fibre does not contract on its own but rather in concert with other muscle fibres which are part of the same motor unit, i.e. innervated by the same motor neurone. A clear understanding of the structure and function of the motor unit is fundamental to electromyography.

The motor unit

Figure 15.1 is a schematic diagram of a motor unit. Motor neurones which innervate striated muscle lie in the anterior horn of the spinal cord, their cell bodies are relatively large and their axonal processes correspondingly of large diameter and myelinated to allow rapid conduction of impulses. The motor neurones which innervate the sphincters lie in Onuf's nucleus in the sacral part of the spinal cord. Motor axons leave the spinal cord by the anterior spinal roots and, in the case of the innervation of pelvic structures, travel up to 15 cm within the cauda equina. At the level of the S3,4 foramina in the sacrum the anterior (motor) roots fuse with the posterior (sensory) roots to form spinal nerves. These then fuse in the sacral plexus – a neuronal network in which motor and sensory fibres from different segmental levels combine into peripheral nerves – so that a muscle receives motor innervation from several different nerve roots. In the case of the innervation of the sphincters and pelvic floor, motor axons arise in the S2, 3, 4 spinal segments and travel to the periphery via the pudendal and pelvic nerves.

Within the muscle, the motor axon tapers and then branches to innervate muscle fibres which are scattered throughout the muscle (Fig. 15.1). The innervation of muscle is such that it is unlikely that fibres which are part of the same motor unit will be adjacent to one another. This dispersion of muscle fibres is said to be non-random although the stage of development at which it occurs and the factors determining the arrangement are not known. The number of muscle fibres innervated by an axon is known as the 'innervation ratio' and it is this which determines the possible precision of motor control – the smaller the number of muscle fibres per motor unit, the finer the movement. This is apparent when the innervation ratio of gluteus, which is high, is compared with that of eye muscles, which is low. There is no simple neurophysiological method for estimating this parameter and the number of motor units per muscle is also difficult to estimate by clinical neurophysiological means. The contraction properties of a motor unit depend on the nature of its constituent muscle fibres. Muscle fibres can be classified according to their twitch tension, speed of contraction and histochemical staining properties. Those which are slow twitch and fatigue resistant are classified as Type 1 whereas those with fast-twitch contraction time but which are easily fatiguable are classified as Type 2 fibres. These differences are reflected by histological staining – the fast-twitch, fatiguable fibres stain heavily for glycogen and faintly for oxidative enzymes, while slow-twitch fibres show the reverse. In the pelvic floor and

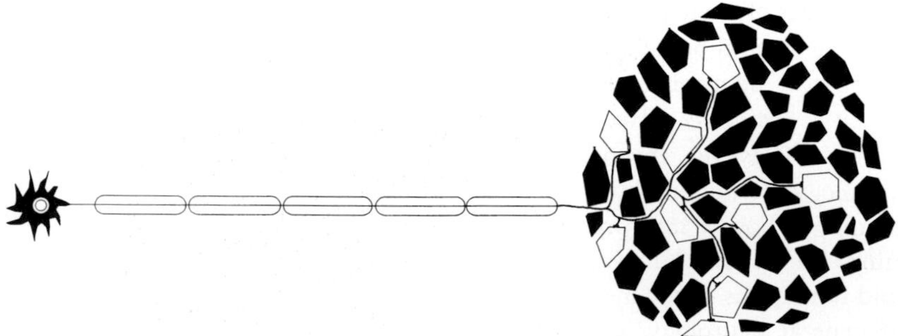

Fig. 15.1 A motor unit is comprised of a single motor neurone, its axon and the muscle fibres it innervates. The motor neurone is located in the anterior horn of the spinal cord and its myelinated axon travels in a peripheral nerve to the muscle. Once within the muscle the axon loses its myelination and branches to innervate muscle fibres distributed throughout the striated muscle, most of which are not adjacent. From Fowler (1995), with permission.

sphincters the muscle fibres are mostly Type 1 although there is some regional variation (Gilpin et al 1989; Heit et al 1996).

EMG recorded by needle electrodes

Electromyographic activity can be recorded distantly using surface electrodes but for better resolution of the signal, an intramuscular electrode is necessary. To facilitate introduction of a wire into muscle tissues, electrodes have been constructed with sharpened tips. Several types of needle electrode have been designed with differing recording characteristics; the type of recording made by each depends upon the size of the non-insulated exposed recording surface of the electrode.

The electrode most commonly used in electromyography is a concentric needle electrode (CNE; Fig. 15.2). This consists of a central insulated platinum wire which is inserted through a steel cannula and the tip ground to give an elliptical area of 580 × 150 μ. This type of electrode has the recording characteristics necessary to record spike or near activity from about 20 muscle fibres. The number of motor units recorded therefore depends both upon the local arrangement of muscle fibres within the motor unit and the level of contraction of the muscle.

Motor units fire tonically at rest in the pelvic floor and so three or four units will be found at the point of insertion using a concentric needle electrode with the subject in a relaxed state (Fig. 15.3A). Using the standard recording facilities available on all modern EMG machines, individual motor units can be captured and their amplitude and duration measured. To facilitate identification of whole motor units and to be certain the late components of complex unit potentials are not due to superimposition of several motor units, it is necessary to capture the same unit repeatedly on an expanded timescale using a trigger and delay line. The trigger device starts the oscilloscope sweep when an incoming signal achieves a particular pre-set value and the delay line has the effect of displaying the triggering signal, not from the moment of triggering, but after the interval some 1–5 ms later. The result is that the triggering potential appears repeatedly in the centre of the oscilloscope screen (Fig. 15.3B).

Characteristics of individual motor units recorded with a CNE

The amplitude of a motor unit is largely determined by the activity of those muscle fibres closest to the recording electrode. Other fibres within 0.5 mm radius of the recording electrode contribute a little to the amplitude but in a normal motor unit there are unlikely to be more than two or three fibres belonging to the same motor unit. Amplitude is highly sensitive to needle position and very minor adjustments of the electrode will result in major changes, e.g. a change in position by 0.5 mm alters the amplitude 10–100-fold. The duration of a motor unit potential is much less sensitive to the exact placement of recording electrodes and it is for this reason that duration is often used as the preferred measurement when assessing motor units.

The duration of a motor unit is the time between the first deflection and the point when the wave form finally returns to the baseline. This will depend on the number of muscle fibres within the motor unit and is little affected by the proximity of the recording electrode to the nearest fibre. The difficulty with this measurement is defining the exact point of return to the baseline (Fig. 15.3B).

The phases of a motor unit potential are defined by the number of times the potential crosses the baseline. A unit that has more than four phases is said to be polyphasic. A related parameter is a ‘turn’ which is defined as a shift in direction of a potential of greater than a specified amplitude.

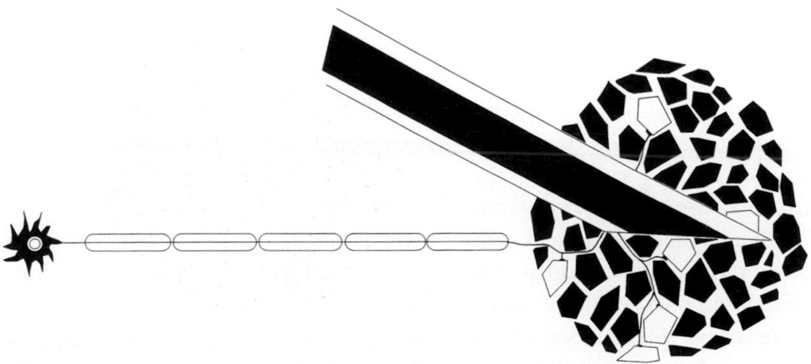

Fig. 15.2 A concentric needle electrode (CNE) recording from a normally innervated motor unit. From Fowler (1995), with permission.

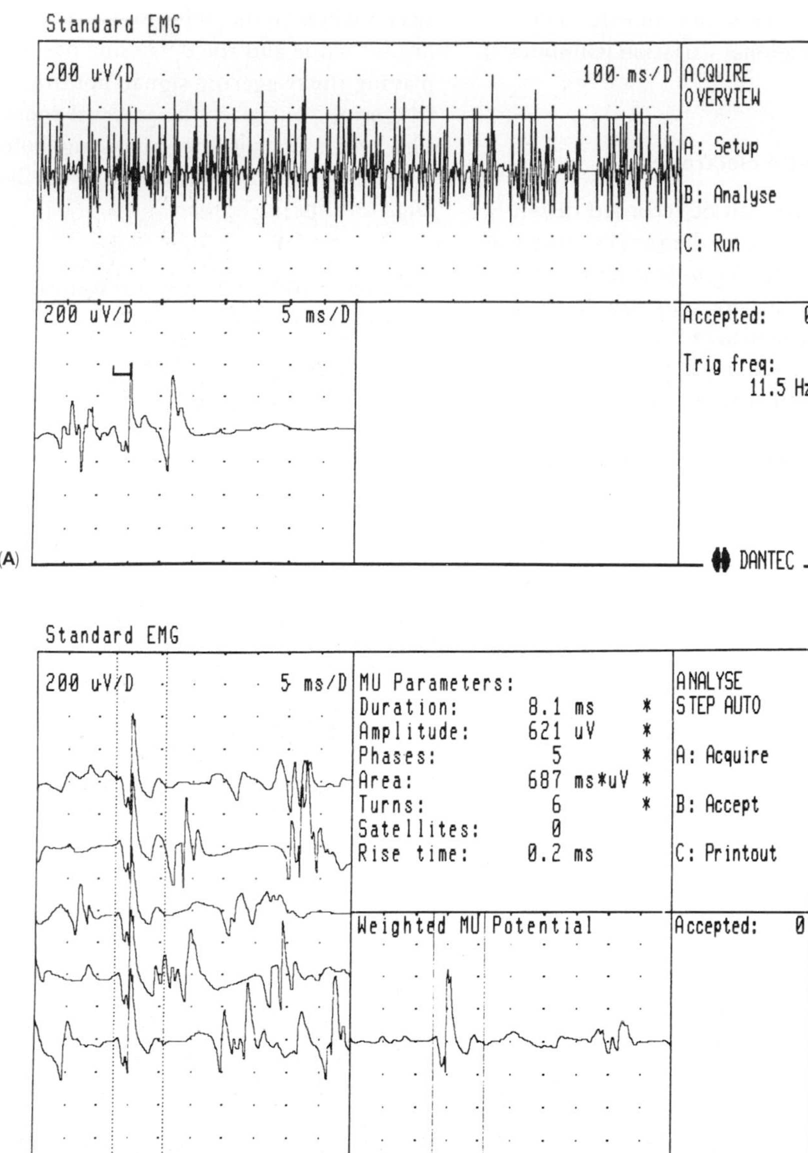

Fig. 15.3 (**A**) The upper panel shows the ongoing tonic activity which can be recorded from the urethral sphincter with a concentric needle electrode over a period of 1 second. The speed of the 'time base' (100 ms/D) is the same as might be used when recording EMG during cystometry or for kinesiological studies. The lower left-hand panel, on a much faster time base (5 ms/D), shows a single motor unit which was of sufficient amplitude to trigger the selection device (transverse line in upper panel and L-shaped device in lower). (**B**) Using the standard trigger and delay line facilities of the EMG machine and with a fast time base (5 ms/D) the individual motor unit seen above has been captured and averaged to give the 'weighted motor unit' potential which can be measured as shown.

Single fibre EMG

The single fibre (SF) needle electrode was developed in Uppsala by Akstedt and Stolberg's group in the 1970s. It has similar external proportions to a concentric needle electrode, being made of a steel cannula 0.5–0.6 mm in diameter with a bevelled tip, but instead of having the recording surface at the tip, a fine insulated platinum or silver wire embedded in epoxy resin is exposed through an aperture on the side, 1–5 mm behind the tip (Fig. 15.4). The platinum wire which forms the recording surface has a diameter of 25 μm and will pick up activity from within a hemispherical volume 300 μm in diameter. This is very much smaller than the volume of muscle tissue from which a concentric needle electrode records, which has an uptake area of 1 mm diameter. Because of the arrangement of muscle fibres in a normal motor unit, a SF needle will record only one to three single muscle fibres from the same motor unit. When recording with a SF EMG needle the amplifier filters are set so that low frequency activity is eliminated and the

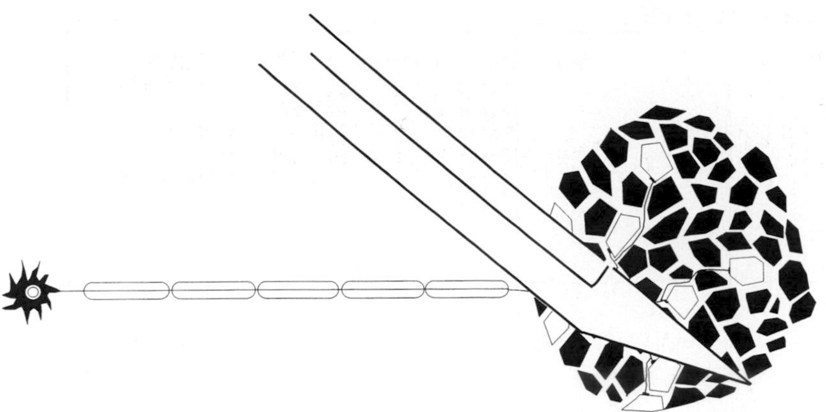

Fig. 15.4 Single fibre needle electrode recording from a normally innervated motor unit. From Fowler (1995), with permission.

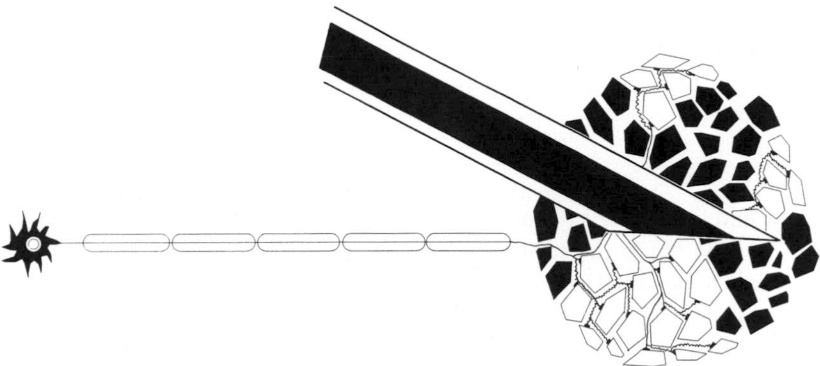

Fig. 15.5 A concentric needle electrode recording from a motor unit which has undergone the process of chronic reinnervation. From Fowler (1995), with permission.

contribution of each muscle fibre appears as a separate positive deflection (Fig. 15.5).

EMG in disease states

EMG changes occur either as a result of disease of the muscle fibres themselves or changes in the arrangement of their innervation. The change that is most commonly looked for is reinnervation. Partial injury to the motor innervation of a muscle, either as the result of disease of the motor neurones or peripheral nerves, will result in loss of innervation of some muscle fibres. Provided there are still some intact motor units within the muscle, surviving motor nerves will sprout and grow out to reinnervate those muscle fibres which have lost their nerve supply (Fig. 15.6). This results in a change in the arrangement of muscle fibres within the unit: whereas in healthy muscle it is unusual for two adjacent muscle fibres to be part of the same motor unit, following reinnervation several muscle fibres all belonging to the same motor unit come to be adjacent to one another.

Early in the process of reinnervation the newly outgrown motor sprouts are thin and therefore conduct slowly, so that the time taken for excitatory impulses to spread through the axonal tree is abnormally prolonged. This is reflected by prolongation of the wave form of the muscle action potential which may have small, late components. Neuromuscular transmission in these newly grown sprouts may also be insecure, so that the motor unit may show 'instability' (Fig. 15.7). In skeletal muscle, with time, and provided there is no further deterioration in innervation, the reinnervating axonal sprouts increase in diameter and thus increase their conduction velocity so that contraction of all parts of the reinnervated motor unit become more synchronous; this has the effect of increasing the amplitude and reducing towards normal the duration of the motor units measured with a CNE. This phenomenon may be different in the sphincter muscles where long duration motor units seem to remain a prominent feature of reinnervated motor units (Palace et al 1997).

Reinnervated motor units recorded with a CNE are prolonged and often polyphasic whereas with a SF electrode multiple potentials are recorded. The 'fibre density' measured with a SF is the mean of the number of potentials recorded at 20 different sampling

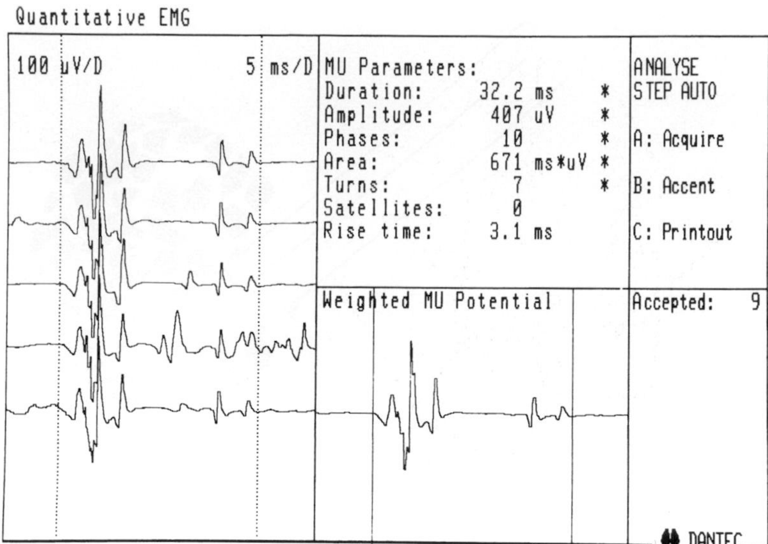

Fig. 15.6 A motor unit captured and recorded as shown in Figure 15.3 but showing extreme changes of chronic reinnervation with multiple phases and a duration of 32.2 ms, compared with the normal motor unit as shown in Figure 15.3 which has a duration of 8.1 ms.

sites within a muscle and in normally innervated muscle this is about 1.5, the figure increasing with reinnervation. An increase in potential duration with a CNE therefore measures the same change as is measured by fibre density with a SF electrode.

Changes in motor units with primary muscle disease

As is evident from the foregoing sections, EMG changes reflect pathological changes in the structure of the motor unit. Changes in EMG due to disease of the muscle fibres are much more subtle and although in skeletal muscle the 'typical' features of myopathy are said to be showers of small, low amplitude polyphasic units recruited at mild effort, such changes have not been reported in the pelvic floor even in patients known to have generalized myopathy (Caress et al 1996).

Little is yet known about what might be expected of an EMG recording from muscle which has been subjected to a severe stretch injury – as occurs during childbirth – but there may well be changes reflecting rupture of individual muscle fibres and injury to small intramuscular nerves.

Abnormal EMG activity at rest

Pelvic floor striated muscle is unlike skeletal muscle in that the motor units of the pelvic floor and sphincters are tonically active and are electrically silent only at the initiation of micturition or defecation. By contrast, skeletal muscle can be made electrically silent provided the subject can relax completely. Following a denervating injury to skeletal muscle, muscle fibres which have lost innervation generate activity known as 'fibrillations'. Finding fibrillations is important to the clinical neurophysiologist examining skeletal muscle for evidence of a root lesion or other denervating pathology, but in the author's experience this type of activity is extremely difficult to identify with any certainty in the sphincters or pelvic floor. The motor units there are smaller than in skeletal muscle and the quiet 'popping' sound of fibrillations heard over the audio system of the EMG machine in an otherwise electrically silent relaxed skeletal muscle is difficult to distinguish from the normal tonic activity of the pelvic floor. The author has only positively identified fibrillations in the sphincters of two patients – both had suffered complete cauda equina lesions and had no surviving motor units.

In skeletal muscle there are other phenomena of similar significance and 'positive sharp waves' are probably generated by the same source as are fibrillations. Also in diseases of the anterior horn cells, 'fasciculations' are often found, which are the result of involuntary contractions of all the muscle fibres of a motor unit; their contraction may be visible through the skin in motor neurone disease. Fasciculations in the pelvic floor have never been reported, even in multiple system atrophy (MSA), a disease which selectively involves the motor neurones which innervate the sphincters and pelvic floor.

However, a spontaneous EMG phenomenon which

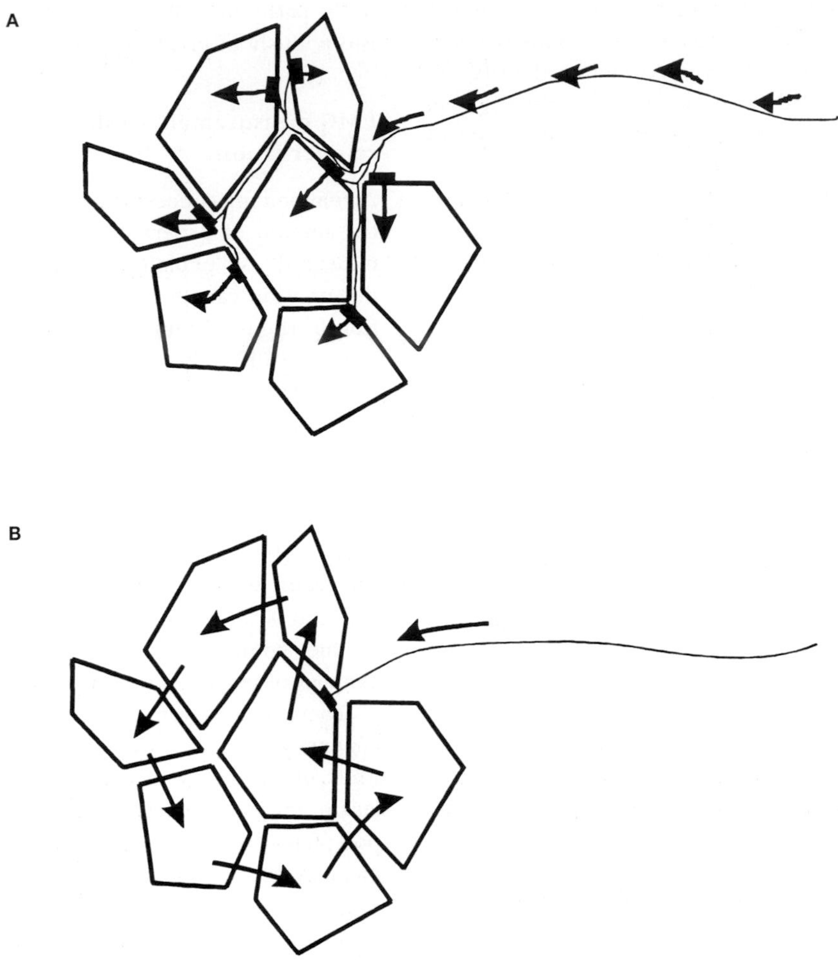

Fig. 15.7 Difference in excitation site giving rise to (**A**) a motor unit showing changes of chronic reinnervation and (**B**) a complex repetitive discharge. An excitatory impulse giving rise to the motor unit which has undergone changes of chronic reinnervation has involved neuromuscular transmission; spread of excitation to give rise to the complex repetitive discharge is by ephaptic transmission, i.e. one muscle fibre to another. The 'jitter' (which is a reflection of time taken by the process of neuromuscular transmission) of the former is great whereas for the latter it is very low. From Fowler (1995), with permission.

is probably of considerable significance and which can be readily recorded from the urethral sphincter and occasionally from the anal sphincter, is complex repetitive discharge activity. This is made up of repetitively firing groups of potentials with so little 'jitter' between the potentials that it is deduced the activity must be due to ephaptic or direct transmission of impulses between muscle fibres (Trontelj & Stolberg 1983; Fowler et al 1985). In skeletal muscle similar activity occurs in various forms of myopathy and occasionally in chronic partial peripheral nerve or root lesions. However, it is commonly found in the striated muscle of the urethral sphincter without any other evidence of neuromuscular disease and it has been hypothesized that it causes impaired relaxation of the muscle and thereby causes obstructed voiding and urinary retention in some young women (Fowler et al 1985).

Specific applications of EMG in urogynaecology kinesiological studies

EMG can be used either to look for changes of reinnervation (from analysis of individual motor units recorded with a CNE or from SF density studies) or can be used as a means of monitoring the activity of a muscle. For some time it was recommended that EMG be recorded as part of cystometry to demonstrate sphincter activity during filling and voiding. Although the best recordings were made by using a CNE in the sphincter or pelvic floor, this inevitably added discomfort to the procedure. The purpose was to demonstrate detrusor sphincter dyssynergia – a disorder where there is a simultaneous contraction of the sphincter with the detrusor muscle. This is a condition which is particularly important to identify following spinal cord trauma in men, although in women upper tract dilatation as a consequence of detrusor sphincter dyssynergia is very much less common. Nevertheless, EMG recording was used during cystometry in women for some time and, because of the discomfort of using needle electrodes, various forms of surface electrode recording were attempted.

Surface electrodes can be placed over the skin of the perineum, a catheter-mounted electrode used to record from the sphincter (Nordling et al 1978), or a vaginal electrode mounted on a sponge (Lose et al 1985) used to record sphincter activity through the anterior vaginal wall. The problem with all these recording methods is that it is difficult to obtain good quality EMG recording as the high frequency components of the signal are attenuated by the tissues between the source generator and recording electrodes, and certainly the more subtle changes described with CNE and SF electrodes are lost.

Recently, using cleverly constructed twisted pair recording electrodes, interesting kinesiological EMG studies have been made of pubococcygeus in nulliparous, continent (Deindl et al 1993) and parous, incontinent women (Deindl et al 1994). The recording electrodes are hooked and inserted through a needle into the muscle on each side. The needle is then removed and the electrodes are retained in the tissue so that prolonged EMG recordings can be made whilst the subject is active in a relatively normal fashion. Bladder filling can be performed, as well as procedures such as coughing and sneezing, and the activity on each side compared.

In nulliparous women, sustained motor unit firing was obtained at most recording sites at rest and during voluntary squeeze, stopping micturition in midstream or coughing, and there was bilateral recruitment of motor units. The precise nature of the recruitment depended on the previous ongoing level of activity (Deindl et al 1993). In parous women with urinary stress incontinence, the length of time for which the women could sustain a voluntary 'squeeze' was considerably shorter than in nulliparous women and, furthermore, asymmetrical and some uncoordinated patterns of levator activation were found in the parous group (Deindl et al 1994). The full explanation of these abnormal reflex responses is not apparent, but they do indicate that the neurological defect which follows childbirth is more complicated than simply one of partial motor denervation, and raise the question as to the role of afferents in determining normal pelvic floor activity. The relevance of these findings to the pathophysiology of genuine stress incontinence is obviously of great interest.

EMG measurement to show changes of reinnervation

A common misconception is that by performing EMG the amount of denervation that has occurred can be measured. As explained in the preceding sections, denervation causes fibrillation activity and a reduction in the total number of motor units, but fibrillations are difficult to identify with certainty in the pelvic floor and, unfortunately, no good method currently exists for estimating the number of motor units. Anyone with practical experience of EMG will be familiar with the fact that the amount of activity that is recorded, i.e. the number of motor units, depends to a large extent on the precise position of the needle within the muscle. Information about denervation is therefore hard to come by but by looking at the configuration of individual motor units, changes of reinnervation may be identified.

There are several conditions in which gross changes of reinnervation may be detected in motor units of the pelvic floor. Following a cauda equina lesion, the motor units are likely to be prolonged and polyphasic (Fowler et al 1984) and similar marked changes are seen in the disease MSA (Palace et al 1997).

MSA is a progressive neurodegenerative disease which is often, particularly in its early stages, mistaken for Parkinson's disease but is poorly responsive to antiparkinsonian treatment. There may, in addition, be autonomic failure causing postural hypotension and cerebellar ataxia causing unsteadiness and clumsiness. Urinary incontinence in both women and men occurs early in this condition, often some years before the onset of obvious neurological features (Beck et al 1994). As part of the neurodegenerative process, loss of motor units occurs in Onuf's nucleus, so that partial but progressive denervation of the sphincter occurs and recorded motor units show changes of reinnervation and become markedly prolonged. Sphincter EMG has been demonstrated to be of value in distinguishing between idiopathic Parkinson's disease and MSA (Eardley et al 1989; Palace et al 1997).

EMG changes in genuine stress incontinence

Because of the suspected role of denervation in the genesis of stress incontinence, EMG techniques have been used to look for the extent of nerve damage following childbirth and in the assessment of women with GSI.

SF EMG was used to measure fibre density in the external anal sphincter and an increase was demonstrated in women with urinary stress incontinence (Anderson 1984). A meticulous study from Manchester looked at the relationship between stress incontinence, genitourinary prolapse and partial denervation of the pelvic floor (Smith et al 1989b). Women with normal urinary control who were parous had an increase in fibre density in pubococcygeus with age which was slightly higher than that of age-matched nulliparous women. Women with stress incontinence without prolapse had much higher fibre densities than comparable age-match control subjects. Fibre density in those with stress incontinence with prolapse and those with prolapse alone were similar and were significantly higher than in asymptomatic women. Thus it was concluded that pubococcygeus is partially denervated and then reinnervated in women with stress incontinence, genital prolapse or both.

Using a CNE to examine pubococcygeus following childbirth, the Manchester group found a significant increase in duration of individual motor units following labour and vaginal delivery (Allen et al 1990). The changes were most marked in women who had urinary incontinence 8 weeks after delivery and who had had a prolonged second stage and given birth to heavier babies.

The EMG changes found in these studies were subtle compared to those that occur following a cauda equina lesion or in MSA. Meticulous care must be taken in any study of GSI which uses EMG of the pelvic floor to define the control group and obtain adequate numbers of motor units from each subject.

Urethral sphincter EMG in women with urinary retention and obstructed voiding

For many years it has been said that isolated urinary retention in young women was due either to psychogenic factors or was the first symptom of onset of multiple sclerosis (Siroky & Krane 1991). However, sphincter EMG in this group has demonstrated that the majority of such patients have complex repetitive discharges and decelerating burst activity in the muscle, which might prevent relaxation at the onset of micturition (Fowler et al 1988). Recorded on an EMG machine, the activity has a very characteristic sound quality which has been likened to underwater recordings of whales. The complex repetitive discharges may be difficult to distinguish from chronically reinnervated motor units except that the jitter of the potentials is very much less (Fowler et al 1985). They produce a rather mechanical sound like a helicopter or motorcycle engine and it is the decelerating bursts which produce the myotonic (or whale-like) sound.

Why this activity should occur is not known, but in the syndrome described by the author it was associated with polycystic ovaries (Fowler et al 1988). The explanation probably lies in some as yet unidentified hormonal abnormality to which the striated muscle is peculiarly sensitive. Loss of stability of membranes within the striated muscle allows ephaptic transmission to manifest as complex repetitive discharges (see Fig. 15.7).

Typically, patients with this syndrome are premenopausal, and the condition has its maximum incidence in women under the age of 30. They present in urinary retention with a bladder capacity in excess of 1 litre without having had previous urgency, which implies that the condition has been partial but asymptomatic for some time and that chronic retention has damaged the afferent innervation of the

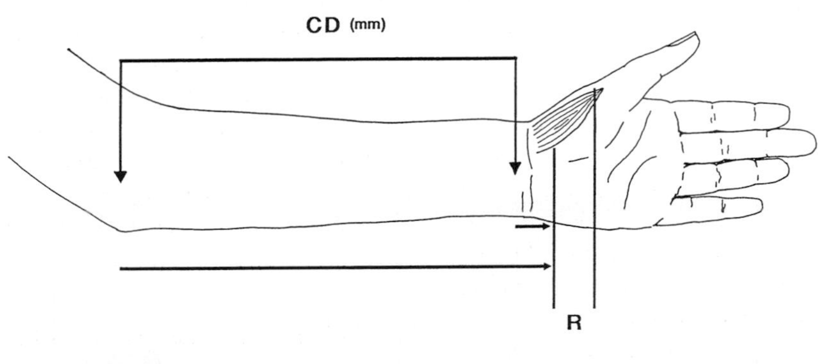

Fig. 15.8 Measurement of motor conduction velocity in the median nerve of the arm. Recordings are made from abductor pollicis brevis in response to stimulation of the nerve at two sites. For calculation of motor conduction velocity, see text. Note the distal site of stimulation to obtain the terminal or distal motor latency (DML). From Fowler (1995), with permission.

bladder, causing loss of the sensation of urgency. The condition may fluctuate and, although it may have a spontaneous onset in some, it can also follow an event such as a general anaesthetic. It is hypothesized that the precipitating event may have an adverse effect on a precariously compromised detrusor muscle and by tipping the balance cause retention. 'Neuromodulation' by sacral nerve stimulation has been the only treatment so far found effective in patients with this disorder, although the mechanism whereby this may work is not yet understood.

Because sphincter EMG will detect both changes of denervation and reinnervation such as occur with a cauda equina lesion, as well as abnormal spontaneous activity, it has been argued that this test is mandatory in women with urinary retention (Fowler & Kirby 1986). It should certainly be carried out before stigmatizing a woman as having 'psychogenic urinary retention'.

NERVE CONDUCTION STUDIES

A fact which surprises many when they first come to learn about nerve conduction studies is that the conduction velocity of a nerve has little bearing on its functional integrity and ability to conduct neural traffic. Nerve conduction velocity is commonly measured in clinical neurophysiology clinics but it is rarely used in the assessment without being considered together with a number of other neurophysiological parameters. Its main use is to identify the presence of either focal or generalized peripheral nerve demyelination, which are the only major causes of slowing.

The conduction velocity of a motor nerve is measured in the following way: surface electrodes are placed over a muscle innervated by that nerve and the nerve is stimulated at two separate points along its length (Fig. 15.8). The recording obtained consists of two compound muscle action potentials of similar shape and amplitude but with different latencies (Fig. 15.9). To calculate motor conduction velocity (MCV), the distance between the two stimulating sites is measured and this value is divided by the conduction time, i.e. the difference in latency between the proximal and distal responses. Latency is measured to the onset of the compound muscle action potential and therefore depends on the conduction velocity of the fastest nerve fibre in the innervating motor nerve. A region of focal demyelination of the nerve such as occurs in the median nerve as it passes through the carpal tunnel produces slowing of conduction and, as shown in Figure 15.9, a prolonged distal motor latency. However, the strength of a muscle's contraction does not depend on the speed of the conduction of the fastest motor fibres but rather on the number of active motor units. Compound muscle action potential amplitude recorded by the surface electrodes gives some indication of this. Unfortunately, amplitude is extremely variable and poorly reproducible because its configuration depends greatly on the precise placement of the recording electrodes relative to the motor end plates. Although elsewhere surface electrodes can be opti-

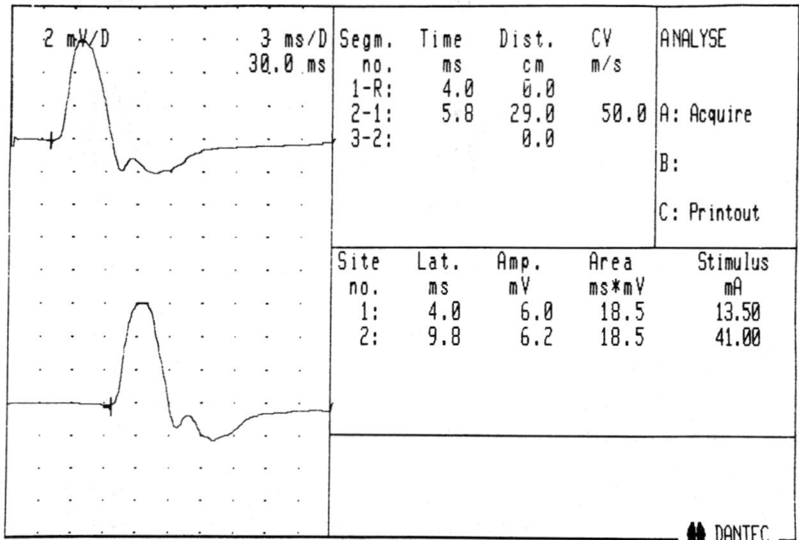

Fig. 15.9 Traces from a patient with carpal tunnel syndrome recorded as shown in Figure 15.8. The upper trace is the response to stimulation of the nerve at the wrist and this is slightly prolonged at 4.0 ms, the normal upper limit being 3.8 ms. MCV is calculated as explained in the text. Note the amplitude of both responses is good, indicating there has not been denervation.

mally positioned, for example over a muscle in the hand, it is almost impossible to be sure where one is recording from with surface electrodes in the pelvic floor (Vodusek 1996).

Following a denervating injury, the amplitude of a compound muscle action potential is likely to be reduced but the motor conduction velocity and therefore latencies may be little affected. This is illustrated in Figure 15.10, which shows the distribution of conduction velocities of the motor units in healthy and denervated muscle. These points are applied to discussion of interpretation of the pudendal terminal motor latency in the following section.

Pudendal terminal motor latency

This measurement was introduced by a group working at St. Mark's Hospital in London who were carrying out research into the mechanism of faecal incontinence (Kiff & Swash 1984). Histochemical studies of pelvic floor musculature had shown changes suggesting the nerve supply to puborectalis and the external anal sphincter had been damaged in patients with idiopathic faecal incontinence (Parks et al 1977) and with this finding the group were led to devise methods of demonstrating neurogenic injury.

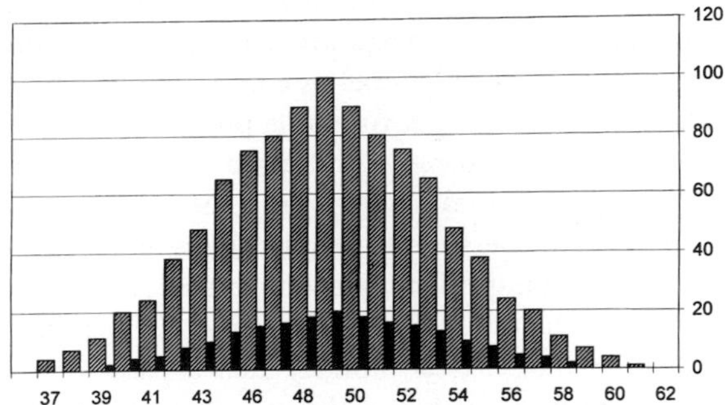

Fig. 15.10 The normal distribution of conduction velocities of motor units in a hypothetical muscle (hatched). Following a denervating injury, 75% of the motor units (black bars are remaining units) are lost, but since this process has not been selective for any particular class of motor unit, the conduction velocity of the fastest motor unit is now 58 when formerly it was 61 m/s.

A stimulating device was constructed which consisted of a rubber finger stall with two bare metal-stimulating electrodes at its tip, and two metal surface electrode-recording plates 4 cm proximally at the base of the finger. A commercial form of this electrode has been sold as the 'St Mark's stimulator' (see Fig. 15.11). The device is mounted on the index finger and inserted into the rectum. Moving the fingertip close to the ischial spine, the site is found at which electrical stimuli to pudendal nerve cause contraction of the sphincter around the finger and a compound muscle action potential can be recorded. Stimulation is then carried out on the opposite side of the pelvis. The branch of the pudendal nerve which innervates the external sphincter is the inferior haemorrhoidal. To record from the perineal branch of the pudendal nerve, recordings are made from the urethral sphincter using a ring electrode mounted on a urethral catheter. Cadaveric studies have shown that the levator ani or pubococcygeus muscle receives innervation direct from sacral nerve roots S2–4 before the formation of the pudendal nerve trunk (Juenemann et al 1988) so that theoretically these muscles should not contract with stimulation of the pudendal nerve at the level of the ischial spine. However, Smith (Smith et al 1989a) and subsequently Allen (Allen et al 1990)

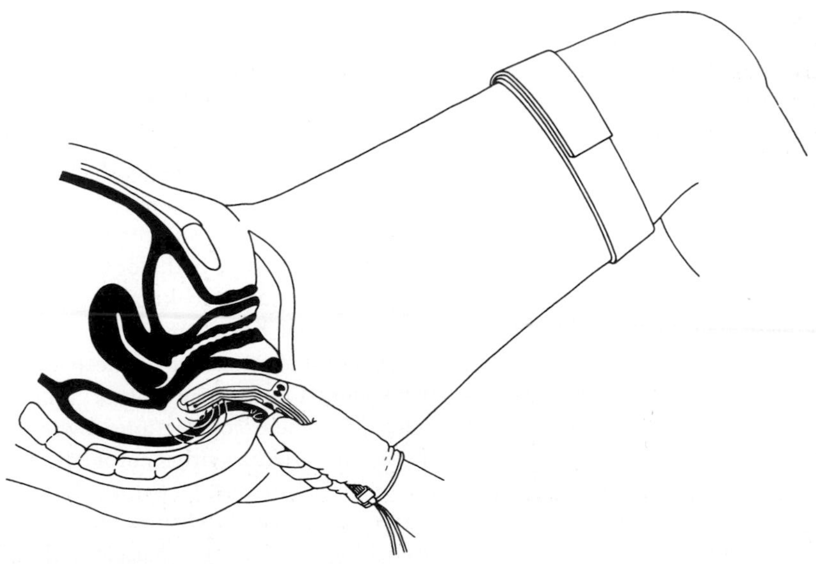

Fig. 15.11 St Mark's stimulator. From Fowler (1995), with permission.

were both able to record the latency of contraction of the pelvic floor stimulating at this point.

The initial studies by the group from St. Mark's showed the perineal latency was abnormally prolonged in patients with urinary stress incontinence (Snooks et al 1985), a finding which was confirmed by the Manchester group (Smith et al 1989a). Working on the hypothesis that the pudendal nerve was stretched and injured during childbirth, several studies have looked at the pudendal or perineal latency immediately postpartum. Although Allen et al (1990) were able to demonstrate, using CNE, that there had been damage to the innervation of pubococcygeus in some women postpartum, they did not find a prolongation of the latency to stimulation of that muscle when women were examined 2 months postpartum. Snooks et al (1984) found a significant increase in the mean pudendal nerve terminal motor latency 48–72 hours after vaginal delivery, but in 60% this had returned to normal 2 months later.

A follow-up study of 14 multiparous women from this group was made 5 years later (Snooks et al 1990) and the mean pudendal motor latency was found to be prolonged on both sides. SF density studies of the anal sphincter were increased and anal manometry showed there had been a reduction in anal canal pressure during maximal squeeze contraction. From this, it was concluded that occult damage to the pudendal innervation of the external anal sphincter had persisted and worsened over the 5-year period and had possibly been exacerbated by abnormal straining patterns of defecation. Although Sultan et al (1993) demonstrated a small (0.1 ms) but statistically significant increase in pudendal nerve latency following vaginal delivery, using anal endosonography they demonstrated a defect of either the internal or external anal sphincter, or both, in 35% of women after vaginal delivery. There was a strong association between these defects and the development of incontinence. Although there was no relation between the change in the pudendal nerve terminal latency and the development of bowel symptoms, or the results of anal manometry, there was an association between abnormal latency and the development of a sphincter defect in primiparous women which was thought to reflect a traumatic cause common to both rather than a causal relation between them. Measurement of the pudendal terminal latency has demonstrated a prolongation in women with pelvic floor prolapse (Smith et al 1989b; Benson & McClellan 1993), with a further lengthening of the latency following vaginal dissection for repair or suspension procedures (Benson & McClellan 1993).

The term 'pudendal neuropathy' is now established in the literature although possibly more used by coloproctologists than urogynaecologists. Those who have written about the pudendal motor latency are careful to avoid claiming that they are making a measurement of denervation of the muscles innervated by the pudendal nerve. However, others less familiar with the theory of clinical neurophysiology tend to equate a prolongation of pudendal motor latency with pelvic floor denervation. This is a mistake (Table 15.1). In general, a prolongation of latency is a poor measure of denervation (see above and Fig. 15.10).

Table 15.1 What is not true.

Prolonged pudendal nerve motor latency = pudendal nerve damage ≠ denervation of pelvic floor

Measurement of the terminal motor latency was introduced because this had proved to be so valuable in identifying carpal tunnel syndrome. However, if the analogy with carpal tunnel is pursued, the conclusion would be that the prolonged latency is indicating a region of focal demyelination in the pudendal nerve distal to the stimulation site. Remember, however, that although demyelination causes slowing it does not produce weakness unless there is a complete conduction block. It is unlikely that a pathological process affecting a nerve so that it causes an increase in latency of less than 1.0 ms over a 5 cm distance could possibly interfere significantly with the timing of reflex responses such as are involved with the recruitment of motor units on coughing or sneezing, i.e. manoeuvres which cause stress incontinence. Furthermore, the cardinal symptoms of carpal tunnel syndrome are pain, with paraesthesiae with weakness and wasting of abductor pollicis brevis occurring only in advanced cases. There is not, therefore, much similarity between the clinical conditions of carpal tunnel syndrome and the disorder which causes weakness of the pelvic floor.

It is true that an abnormality of this latency must indicate some sort of pathology of the pudendal nerve and it is intriguing to know what this might be as there have not been any morphological studies of it yet. The full significance of these findings remains to be explained but it may be that, unlike carpal tunnel syndrome where conduction slowing is in the main trunk, in patients with neurogenic lesions affecting the innervation of the pelvic floor, damage to the nerve occurs distally at sites where the motor nerve is branching within the muscle (Allen et al 1990). Clearly, further work is necessary in this area. In the meantime, it is important that people using this measurement understand its limitations and that, having measured it, they do not assume that if it is abnormal they have demonstrated denervation of the pelvic floor.

SACRAL REFLEXES

The 'sacral reflexes' are reflex contractions of pelvic floor striated musculature in response to a stimulus applied either to the perineum, the genitalia or to the mucosa of the lower urinary tract. The bulbocavernosus (BC), the pudendoanal, the vesicoanal and the anal reflexes are all forms of sacral reflexes. The term 'evoked potentials' has in the past been applied by urologists to the sacral reflexes, but as this term is well established in the clinical neurophysiological literature as referring to responses recorded from the central nervous system, usually by means of signal averaging, it should not be applied to the sacral reflexes. This recommendation has been agreed by the terminology committee of the International Continence Society (Abrams et al 1986).

The early neurourologists elicited the BC reflex as part of their clinical examination of patients with spinal cord injuries. Then a method was described for measuring the latency of the BC reflex, following an electrical stimulation of the dorsal nerve of the penis and recording the response by a needle electrode in the bulbocavernosus muscle. The afferent impulses of the BC reflex are conducted to the sacral cord through the pudendal nerves and the posterior roots. The efferent impulses are also transmitted via the pudendal nerve to the striated pelvic floor muscles. There are often two components to the BC reflex, the first response occurring with a latency of between 24–45 ms and the second at a latency of 60–70 ms. A single fibre EMG study of the reflex has shown that the shortest pathway of the BC reflex is oligosynaptic (Vodusek & Janko 1990) rather than polysynaptic.

In women, electrical stimulation of the dorsal nerves of the clitoris may be similarly used and resulting contractions in the pelvic floor recorded. Recording may be made from the anal or the urethral sphincters, using either a CNE or one of the various surface recording devices described earlier, although the best chance of obtaining a response is with a CNE recording from the anal sphincter (Vodusek 1990a). If this test is performed in the author's laboratory the patient is asked to hold the stimulator over the dorsal nerve of the clitoris herself, thus minimizing any embarrassment and leaving the subject free to remove it if the sensation is uncomfortable. There is considerable variation in the intensity of the stimulus required to elicit the sacral reflexes and sometimes in women it may not be possible to do so at a tolerable intensity – so that little significance can be attached to an absent reflex.

The value of recording the sacral reflexes in patients with suspected neurogenic bladder dysfunction is dubious, the problem being that the test is based on the response of somatic striated muscle to impulses conveyed in large myelinated afferent fibres, whereas bladder function is controlled largely by the autonomic nervous system, whose activity is conveyed in unmyelinated neural activity pathways. There is as yet no electrophysiological test of the parasympathetic innervation of the detrusor.

PUDENDAL EVOKED POTENTIALS

The pudendal evoked potential is recorded from over the sensory cortex using averaging in response to repetitive stimulation of the pudendal nerve. Evoked potentials have been used in clinical neurophysiology laboratories to demonstrate conduction delay within the central nervous system. Before MRI scanning became available, visual evoked potentials were particularly useful in demonstrating optic neuritis in patients with suspected multiple sclerosis. However, although the latency of an evoked potential measures conduction velocity in the central nervous system, it does not test the function of that particular sensory modality. It is possible to have a highly prolonged visual evoked potential in multiple sclerosis with normal visual acuity because, as explained in connection with the peripheral innervation, demyelination need not produce a functional deficit unless there is extreme slowing or complete conduction block. A further limitation of the pudendal evoked potential is related to the same problem that arose with the sacral reflexes; the fibres conveying the afferent information to the cortex are the large myelinated ones because these are the class of fibres which respond first to electrical stimulation, and the unmyelinated bladder afferents which are the functionally important group are not assessed by this means.

Stimulation of the pudendal nerve can be readily performed by asking the patient to hold the stimulator on the dorsal nerve of the clitoris whilst giving repeated stimuli at 2.5 times threshold intensity. The sensory homunculus shows that the genital region is in the inter-hemispheric fissure and so the potential is best recorded using a midline recording electrode placed 2 cm behind a line joining the ears through the crown of the head and referred to a frontal reference electrode. Repeated stimuli produces a typical W shape and it is the latency of the down-going potential, i.e. P40 which is the parameter which is measured (Vodusek 1990b). The latency of the pudendal evoked potential is similar to the tibial evoked potential, which is surprising considering the relative conduction distances, but is thought to be because the pudendal afferents are slower at conducting both in the peripheral nervous system and in the spinal cord (Opsomer et al 1986).

Prolonged pudendal evoked potentials have been demonstrated in patients with spinal cord demyelination in multiple sclerosis (Eardley et al 1991; Rodi et al 1994). A correlation between the presence of an abnormal evoked potential and detrusor hyperreflexia is not surprising, since both phenomena depend on conduction in the spinal cord. However, a recent study suggested that the tibial is more sensitive than the pudendal evoked potential in detecting relevant spinal cord pathology (Rodi et al 1996). Furthermore, a study which looked at the value of the pudendal evoked potential, when investigating urogenital symptoms for detecting relevant neurological disease, found it to be of lesser value than a clinical examination looking for signs of spinal cord disease in the lower limbs, i.e. lower limb hyperreflexia and extensor plantar responses (Delodovici & Fowler 1995). There may, however, be circumstances such as when a patient is complaining of loss of bladder or vaginal sensation that it is reassuring to be able to record a normal pudendal evoked response.

REFERENCES

Abrams P, Blaivas J G, Stanton S L et al 1986 Sixth report on the standardisation of terminology of the lower urinary tract function. World Journal or Urology 4: 2–5

Allen R, Hosker G, Smith A, Warrell D 1990 Pelvic floor damage and childbirth: a neurophysiological study. British Journal of Obstetrics and Gynaecology 97: 770–779

Anderson R 1984 A neurogenic element to urinary genuine stress incontinence. British Journal of Urology 91: 41–45

Beck R O, Betts C D, Fowler C J 1994 Genitourinary dysfunction in multiple system atrophy: clinical features and treatment in 62 cases. Journal of Urology 151: 1336–1341

Benson T, McClellan E 1993 The effect of vaginal dissection on the pudendal nerve. Obstetrics and Gynecology 82: 387–389

Caress J, Kothari M, Bauer S, Shefner J 1996 Urinary dysfunction in Duchenne muscular dystrophy. Muscle and Nerve 19: 819–822

Deindl F M, Vodusek D B, Hesse U, Schussler B 1993 Activity patterns of pubococcygeal muscles in nulliparous continent women. British Journal of Urology 72: 46–51.

Deindl F, Vodusek D, Hesse U, Schussler B 1994 Pelvic floor activity patterns: comparison of nulliparous continent and parous urinary stress incontinent women. A kinesiological EMG study. British Journal of Urology 73: 413–417

Delodovici M L, Fowler C J 1995 Clinical value of the pudendal somatosensory evoked potential. Electroencephalography and Clinical Neurophysiology 96: 509–515.

Eardley I, Nagendran K, Lecky B, Chapple C, Kirby R, Fowler C J 1991 The neurophysiology of the striated urethral sphincter in multiple sclerosis. British Journal of Urology 67: 81–88

Eardley I, Quinn N P, Fowler C J et al 1989 The value of urethral sphincter electromyography in the differential diagnosis of parkinsonism. British Journal of Urology 64: 360–362

Fowler C J, 1995 Nerve conduction studies and EMG sampling. In: Osselton J et al (eds) Clinical Neurophysiology. Butterworth-Heinemann, Oxford, pp 103–138

Fowler C J, Christmas T J, Chapple C R, Fitzmaurice P H, Kirby R S, Jacobs H S 1988 Abnormal electromyographic activity of the urethral sphincter, voiding dysfunction, and polycystic ovaries: a new syndrome? British Journal of Medicine 297: 1436–1438

Fowler C J, Kirby R S 1986 Electromyography of the urethral sphincter in women with urinary retention. Lancet i: 1455–1456

Fowler C J, Kirby R S, Harrison M J G 1985 Decelerating bursts and complex repetitive discharges in the striated muscle of the urethral sphincter associated with urinary retention in women. Journal of Neurology, Neurosurgery and Psychiatry 48: 1004–1009

Fowler C J, Kirby R S, Harrison M J G, Milroy E J G, Turner-Warwick R 1984 Individual motor unit analysis in the diagnosis of disorders of urethral sphincter innervation. Journal of Neurology, Neurosurgery and Psychiatry 47: 637–641

Gilpin S, Gosling J, Smith A, Warrell D 1989 The pathogenesis of genitourinary prolapse and stress incontinence of urine. A histological and histochemical study. British Journal of Obstetrics and Gynaecology 96: 15–23

Heit M, Benson T, Russell B, Brubaker L 1996 Levator ani muscle in women with genitourinary prolapse. Neurourology and Urodynamics 15: 17–29

Juenemann K-P, Lue T, Schmidt R, Tanagho E 1988 Clinical significance of sacral and pudendal nerve anatomy. Journal of Urology 139: 74–80

Kiff E, Swash M 1984 Slowed conduction in the pudendal nerves in idiopathic (neurogenic) faecal incontinence. British Journal of Surgery 71: 614–616

Lose G, Tanko A, Colstrup H, Andersen J T 1985 Urethral sphincter electromyography with vaginal surface electrodes: a comparison with sphincter electromyography recorded via periurethral coaxial anal sphincter needle and perianal surface electrodes. Journal of Urology 133: 815–818

Nordling J, Meyhoff H, Walter S, Andersen J 1978 Urethral electromyography using a new ring electrode. Journal of Urology 120: 571–573

Opsomer R J, Guerit J M, Wese F X, Van Gangh P J 1986 Pudendal cortical somatosensory evoked potentials. Journal of Urology 135: 1216–1218

Palace J, Chandiramani V A, Fowler C J 1997 Value of sphincter EMG in the diagnosis of multiple system atrophy. Muscle and Nerve 20: 1396–1403

Parks A G, Swash M, Urich H 1977 Sphincter denervation in anorectal incontinence and rectal prolapse. Gut 18: 656–665

Rodi Z, Vodusek D, Denislic M 1994 Pudendal nerve versus tibial nerve somatosensory evoked potentials in patients with multiple sclerosis and voiding dysfunction. Neurourology and Urodynamics 13: 362

Rodi Z, Vodusek D, Denislic M 1996 Clinical uro-neurophysiological investigation in multiple sclerosis. European Journal of Neurology 3: 574–580

Siroky M, Krane R 1991 Functional voiding disorders in women. In: Krane R, Siroky M (eds) Clinical Neuro-urology. Little, Brown, Boston, pp 445–457

Smith A, Hosker G, Warrell D 1989a The role of pudendal nerve damage in the aetiology of genuine stress incontinence in women. British Journal of Obstetrics and Gynaecology 96: 29–32

Smith A R B, Hosker G L, Warrell D W 1989b The role of partial denervation of the pelvic floor in aetiology of genitourinary prolapse and stress incontinence of urine. A neurophysiological study. British Journal of Obstetrics and Gynaecology 96: 24–28

Snooks S J, Badenoch D F, Tiptaft R C, Swash M 1985 Perineal nerve damage in genuine stress incontinence. British Journal of Urology 57: 422–426

Snooks S J, Swash M, Mathers S E, Henry M M 1990 Effect of vaginal delivery in the pelvic floor: a 5-year follow-up. British Journal of Surgery 77: 1358–1360

Snooks S J, Swash M, Setchell, M, Henry M M 1984 Injury to the pelvic floor sphincter musculature in childbirth. Lancet ii: 546–555

Sultan A, Kamm M, Hudson C, Thomas J, Bartram C 1993 Anal-sphincter disruption during vaginal delivery. New England Journal of Medicine 329: 1905–1911

Trontelj J, Stolberg E 1983 Bizarre repetitive discharges recorded with single fibre EMG. Journal of Neurology, Neurosurgery, and Psychiatry 46: 310–316

Vodusek D 1990a Pudendal somatosensory evoked potential and bulbocavernosus reflex in women. Electroencephalography and Clinical Neurophysiology 77: 134–136

Vodusek D 1996 Evoked potential testing. Urological Clinics of North America 23: 427–445

Vodusek D B 1990b Pudendal somatosensory evoked potentials. Neurologija 39: 149–155

Vodusek D B, Janko M 1990 The bulbocavernosus reflex. A single motor neuron study. Brain 113: 813–820

SECTION 2
CHAPTER
16

Ambulatory urodynamic monitoring

KAREN BROWN AND PAUL HILTON

INTRODUCTION

The term ambulatory urodynamic monitoring is conventionally applied to the assessment of bladder function by natural fill cystometry whilst the subject is fully ambulant. Its development has overcome some of the limitations of conventional cystometry which is felt to be unphysiological but which is our current 'gold standard' in urodynamic investigation.

Development

Early ambulatory studies as performed by Warrell et al in 1963 used radiotelemetry. A miniaturized radiotransmitter was inserted into the bladder and signals sent to an external receiver. The technique was intended to parallel development of ambulatory monitoring with regard to the gastrointestinal and cardiovascular systems but was slower to gain acceptance, probably because there were problems both with the transmission and reception of signals and with insertion into and the retrieval from the bladder of the transmitter device. Therefore, the technique was largely abandoned. In preference to this, some researchers attempted to use a semi-ambulatory system with very long fluid-filled catheters attached to external transducers and a static recorder. This system was extremely prone to movement artefacts and it was not until around 1990 that it became possible to miniaturize recorders to make them easily portable (Griffiths et al 1989; van Waalwijk van Doorn et al 1991). The popularity of ambulatory monitoring has increased enormously since then and certainly since 1992 there have been several commercially available systems. These are neat and the majority are able to utilize either catheter-mounted microtransducers or fluid-filled catheters. They are, however, expensive.

METHODOLOGY

Equipment

Basic equipment for ambulatory monitoring includes a urethral or suprapubic bladder catheter plus a rectal or a vaginal line as an approximation to intra-abdominal pressure. Although a frequency response of around 4 Hz may be adequate for static cystometry, 10–15 Hz is required to record rapid changes in pressure generated by, for example, coughing or walking during ambulatory monitoring. Whereas fluid-filled catheters with external transducers are most commonly used for static cystometry, catheter-mounted microtransducers are the most popular type of catheter used for ambulatory monitoring. There must be an accurate and easy method for calibrating and sterilizing these catheters and a reliable means of securing them in place for the duration of the test. Most available systems have a channel enabling the collection of data from an electronic nappy. This permits the quantification and qualification of any urine leakage. The portable recording device must be light and compact but with an adequate battery capacity to permit the storage of several hours of urodynamic data. Access to a host computer in order to download the information from the portable device's solid state memory for processing and plotting is also required. The patient is requested to maintain a detailed written diary throughout the investigation and it is useful if some form of event marker is incorporated into the design of the device.

Performing an ambulatory study

The system employed in our own unit is the Urolog system developed by Griffiths et al (1989) (Fig. 16.1).

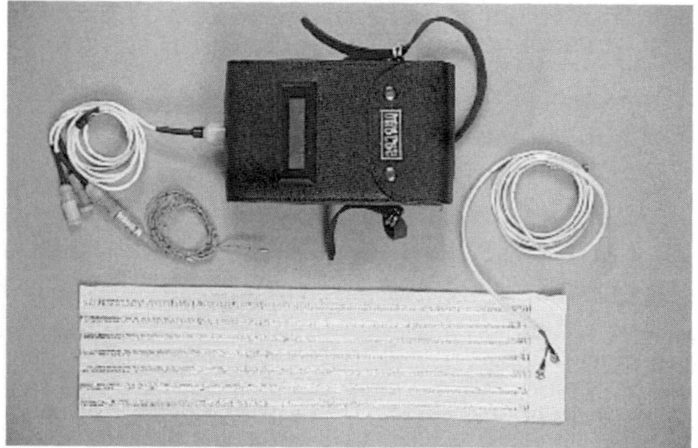

Figure 16.1 Ambulatory monitoring equipment, including the Urolog recording box, a Gaeltec microtransducer and a Urilos electronic nappy. From Heslington (1997), with permission.

Gaeltec 6 F catheter-mounted microtransducers are employed for pressure measurement and the system assimilates data from a Urilos® electronic nappy (James et al 1971). The two microtransducers are calibrated in air and at 30 cm H_2O. The Urilos electronic nappy is also calibrated. The catheters are then sterilized for 20 minutes in glutaraldehyde solution. Whilst the catheters are being sterilized the opportunity is taken to discuss the test in detail with the subjects to ensure that they understand exactly what it entails and what is expected of them. They are instructed to maintain a detailed written diary of events and are also requested to depress an event marker on the recording device at the time of significant events. The catheters are rinsed thoroughly in sterile water and then inserted into the patient. The standard route for the measurement of abdominal pressure is the rectum but in women as long as they have not had previous surgery to significantly shorten the vagina and do not have a marked degree of prolapse, the vaginal route is often more acceptable (James 1978). Whichever route is used, this transducer is protected by a vented fingercot. The catheters are secured with tape and are also maintained in position by asking the subject to wear a pair of elastic pants which have a hole cut into the gusset; these remain in place throughout the test. The Urilos pad is inserted into a second pair of pants which can be removed on voiding. The subject is then asked to ambulate (Fig. 16.2) for around 3 hours, during which time they will undergo periods of rest and daily activities which are likely to provoke symptoms. At some point they are taken through a specific set of provocation tests. The operator checks on the subject periodically to ensure that the lines have not become dislodged and are recording satisfactorily. At the end of the study, the catheters are removed and the recording device attached to a host computer onto which the data is downloaded. Thirty-minute graphic print-outs are obtained from the computer (Fig. 16.3) for analysis. In our centre, analysis is undertaken by hand and takes 15–30 minutes per study. The alternative is to analyse the traces by computer. The disadvantage of this method is that the software is often unable to differentiate abnormal detrusor activity and spontaneous voids or artefact. There is much ongoing work attempting to overcome this problem.

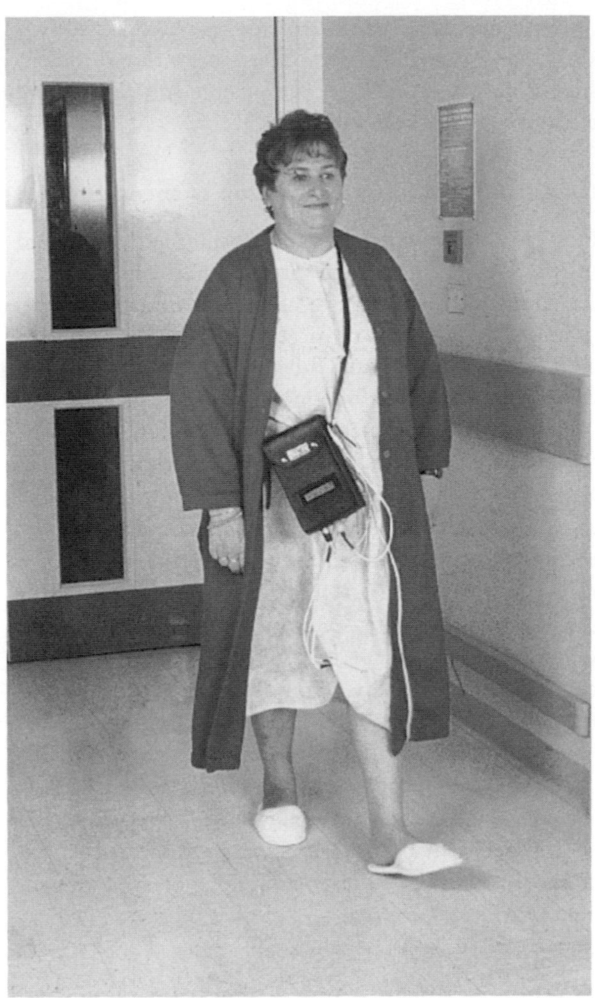

Figure 16.2 A subject ambulating on the ward connected to the Urolog ambulatory urodynamic monitoring device. From Heslington (1997), with permission.

INDICATIONS

Asymptomatic volunteers

Ambulatory monitoring of bladder pressure would seem to be somewhat more physiological than conventional cystometry, and appears to detect a greater number of abnormalities, based on conventional cystometric criteria of normality. It is essential that before a test is introduced into routine clinical practice it is fully evaluated. It is fundamental that normal ranges are established by the study of asymptomatic subjects. There have, however, been only three studies to date which have included female volunteers (Van Waalwijk van Doorn et al 1992a; Robertson et al 1994; Heslington & Hilton 1996a). All of these studies are small and have used different methods of analysis. Despite this, they agreed on several important differences between ambulatory monitoring and conventional cystometry. The incidence of detrusor activity on filling on conventional cystometry ranged from 0 to 18% whereas on ambulatory monitoring the range was 38–69%. The commonly occurring rise in detrusor pressure on filling seen on rapid artificial filling in conventional cystometry was not observed on natural filling, suggesting that this is an artefact induced by rapid filling (Heslington & Hilton 1996a). It was noted in all three of the above studies that voided volumes were lower and voiding pressures higher on ambulatory monitoring than on conventional cystometry. Researchers have suggested that rapid fill conventional cystometry has an adverse effect on detrusor activity

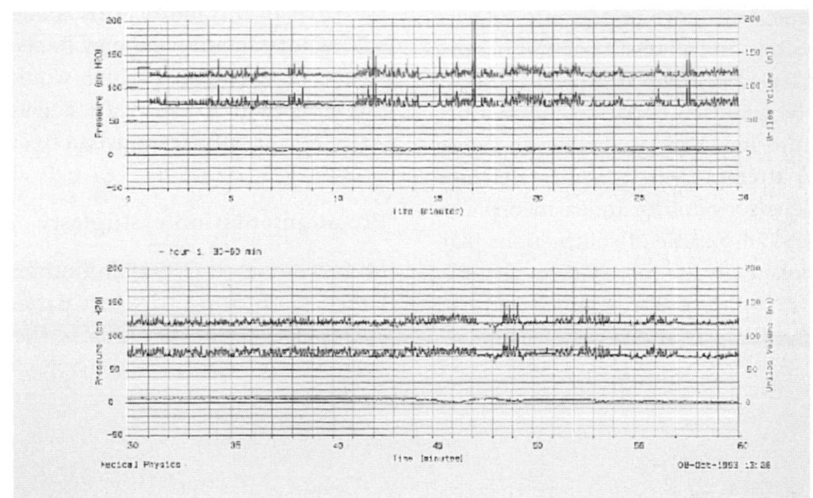

Figure 16.3 An ambulatory monitoring trace showing calibration of the catheters and excellent subtraction of pressures with no artefact. From Heslington (1997), with permission.

and that the parameters on ambulatory monitoring are more physiological.

It must be noted that the above studies did not include simultaneous recording of flow rate data and this means that voiding pressure data must be interpreted with caution. All three papers suspected that the recorded values may be artificially high due to the inclusion of isometric 'after–contraction' pressures as part of the voiding contraction, which seem to be more common on ambulatory monitoring traces than on conventional cystometry recordings. A small series of ambulatory studies by Heslington & Hilton (1996b) would appear to confirm this suspicion. The difficulties in recruiting truly asymptomatic volunteers to ambulatory studies is appreciated but it is evident that, despite the small size of studies to date, differences do exist between the two cystometry techniques. The significance of these differences needs to be further clarified, particularly with reference to symptomatic patient groups.

Mixed symptoms and conventional cystometry

Most clinicians will encounter patients in whom conventional cystometry shows the bladder to be stable despite the patient complaining of often distressing frequency, urgency and/or urge incontinence. Ambulatory monitoring has been used (McInerney et al 1991; van Waalwijk van Doorn et al 1991; Davila et al 1994; Heslington & Hilton 1995a; Cardozo et al 1995) to assess such patients and has shown increased detection of detrusor activity ranging from 40 to 84%. These figures are not dissimilar to those quoted in asymptomatic subjects. This makes interpretation of the findings extremely difficult. Can we regard the activity as significant, and more importantly, do we base treatment decisions on the results of ambulatory monitoring? Many feel that there is a need to find a means to objectively quantify detrusor contractility on ambulatory monitoring. Van Waalwijk van Doorn et al (1991, 1992b) attempted to quantify detrusor overactivity by a detrusor activity index incorporating the frequency and amplitude of contractions. Bailey et al (1989) looked at the percentage unstable filling time using a computer programme but the intra- and inter-individual variations in detrusor contraction characteristics were too great to develop a simple programme for computer recognition of detrusor instability. Further developments in this area are expected in the near future.

Qualification and quantification of incontinence

Conventional cystometry can be combined with a pad test to detect any urinary incontinence. This is crude and does not identify the nature of the leakage, i.e. whether it is stress or urge incontinence. A great advantage of ambulatory urodynamics is that during the test a channel may be included on the recorder to incorporate simultaneous data from an electronic nappy. This was first developed by James et al in Exeter (1971). The pad contains a series of strip electrodes within a dry electrolyte; when fluid leaks onto the pad current flows between the electrodes, and the meter measures change in electrical conductance. It can identify separate episodes of urine leakage and, when recorded concurrently with detrusor pressure, can differentiate between stress and urge incontinence. Others devised temperature devices for identifying urine leakage but the electronic diaper remains the most popular method of measuring urine loss during ambulatory monitoring (Eckford & Abrams 1992). Losses between 0 and 100 ml can be measured but there are not inconsiderable margins of error associated with it.

Monitoring response to treatments for detrusor instability

Ambulatory monitoring has been used to look at the effects of both pharmacotherapy and electrotherapy for detrusor instability. This is one of the areas where ambulatory monitoring may be most useful clinically. Again, this is an area which would benefit from having a method to quantify detrusor overactivity in order to quantify response to treatment.

Pre-augmentation cystoplasty

McInerney et al (1991) and others have used ambulatory monitoring to select patients for 'clam' ileocystoplasty. Whether this is the most appropriate method of selection in light of the findings regarding detrusor activity in asymptomatic individuals is unclear. Sethia et al (1991) and Robertson et al (1991) have used ambulatory monitoring to study detrusor instability in such patients pre- and postoperatively mainly in order to assess the response to the treatment.

Pre-surgery for stress incontinence

Ambulatory monitoring has been used to determine the incidence of urge incontinence and detrusor instability in pre- and postoperative patients undergoing suprapubic bladder neck procedures for genuine stress incontinence proven on conventional cystometry (Heslington & Hilton 1995b). It was felt that ambulatory monitoring might predict the patients who would have problems postoperatively and show whether the presence of detrusor instability preoperatively compromises the results of colposuspension. The conclusions were, however, that the postoperative symptoms and urodynamic state could not be predicted from either preoperative patient symptoms or preoperative ambulatory monitoring findings.

Neurogenic bladder dysfunction

Ambulatory monitoring with its physiological filling has been shown to be particularly useful in the investigation of patients with neurogenic bladder dysfunction. Webb et al (1989) studied a group of patients who had low compliance on conventional cystometry as a result of neurogenic bladder dysfunction. They felt that decreased compliance was unlikely to be the explanation of upper tract dilatation in such patients as, again, the high end fill pressures were not found when the same patients underwent ambulatory urodynamics. They did find, however, that in these patients there was a significantly increased frequency of phasic detrusor activity shown on ambulatory monitoring.

EXAMPLES

Figures 16.4 and 16.5 are examples of ambulatory monitoring traces demonstrating one of the main clinical applications of ambulatory urodynamic monitoring, namely the qualification of urinary incontinence. In Figure 16.4 it can be clearly seen that there is urine loss on coughing, as detected by the Urilos electronic nappy, but no associated detrusor pressure rise. This is genuine stress incontinence. The fall in all three pressures just after the patient coughs is caused by her sitting in order to void. In Figure 16.5 there is again urine loss detected on the Urilos nappy but this is associated with a definite rise in detrusor pressure and the presence of patient symptoms as indicated by her depressing the event marker. This trace, therefore, shows detrusor instability.

THE FUTURE

Advocates predict that ambulatory monitoring will become the new 'gold standard' in urodynamic investigation. Its introduction has caused much excitement and there is no doubt that it detects more abnormalities than conventional cystometry. Present work in the field centres not only on finding new applications but, more importantly, on standardizing the methodology and interpretation of ambulatory studies. Once this is achieved, we will know the full value of the technique and be able to recommend whether it be introduced into routine clinical practice. Several commercial companies have developed systems and are marketing them widely as an adjunct, or alternative, to conventional cystometry. It must be remembered, however, that it is labour intensive and time consuming for both operator and patient. It is also an expensive service to purchase and run, which may limit its use to specialist centres. The most useful applications would appear to be those patients in whom the nature of their incontinence is unclear, those patients in whom conventional cystometry has failed to achieve a diagnosis, and in monitoring the response to various treatments for detrusor instability.

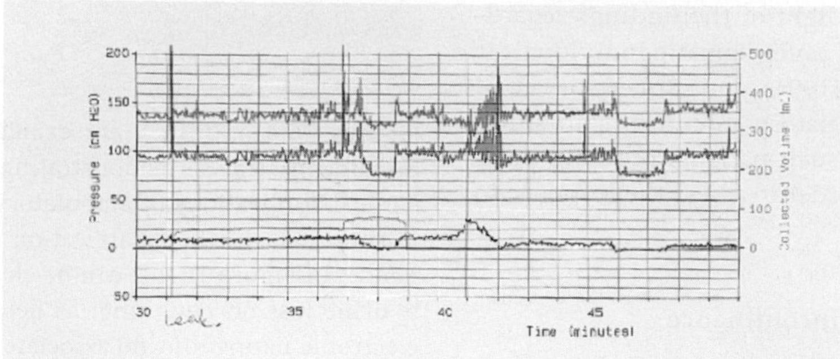

Figure 16.4 An ambulatory monitoring trace showing stress incontinence recorded on the Urilos.

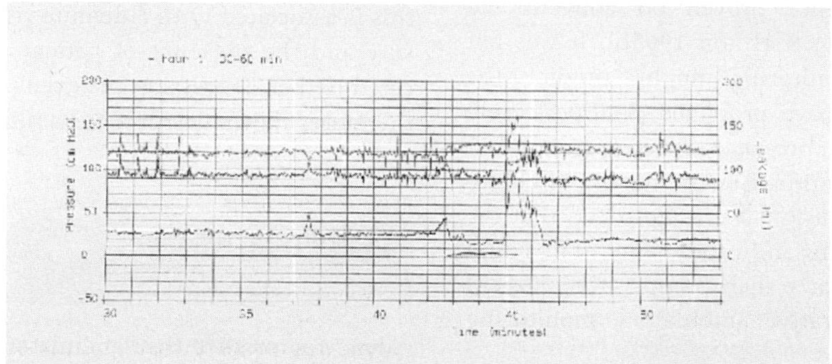

Figure 16.5 An ambulatory monitoring trace showing increased detrusor activity associated with leakage of urine.

REFERENCES

Bailey R, Abrams P, Shepherd A M Bailey D 1989 Development of a micro-computer based system for long-term ambulatory urodynamic monitoring using data-reduction (abstract). Neurourology and Urodynamics 8: 404–405

Cardozo L, Khullar V, Anders K, Hill S 1995 Ambulatory urodynamics: a useful urogynaecological service? (abstract). Proceedings of the 27th British Congress of Obstetrics & Gynaecology 5–7 Jul, Dublin. Royal College of Obstetricians and Gynaecologists, 414

Davila G W 1994 Ambulatory urodynamics in urge incontinence evaluation. International Urogynaecology 5: 25–30

Eckford S D, Abrams P H 1992 A new temperature device to detect incontinent episodes during ambulatory monitoring (abstract). Neurourology and Urodynamics 11: 448–450

Griffiths C J, Assi M S, Styles R A, Ramsden P D, Neal D E 1989 Ambulatory monitoring of bladder and detrusor pressure during natural filling. Journal of Urology 142: 780–784

Heslington K 1997 Ambulatory monitoring – is it an advance? British Journal of Urology 80 (supplement 2): 49–53

Heslington K, Hilton P 1995a The incidence of detrusor instability by ambulatory monitoring in symptomatic females with normal conventional cystometry (abstract). Proceedings of the 25th Annual Meeting of the International Continence Society 17–20 Oct, Sydney, 415–416

Heslington K, Hilton P 1995b The incidence of detrusor instability by ambulatory monitoring and conventional cystometry pre- and post-colposuspension (abstract). Neurourology and Urodynamics 14: 416–417

Heslington K, Hilton P 1996a Ambulatory monitoring and conventional cystometry in asymptomatic female volunteers. British Journal of Obstetrics and Gynaecology 103(5): 434–441

Heslington K, Hilton P 1996b Voiding pressures on ambulatory monitoring and conventional cystometry using fluid filled catheters and microtransducers (abstract). Neurourology and Urodynamics 15: 274–275

James E D, Flack F C, Caldwell K P S, Martin M R 1971 Continuous measurement of urine loss and frequency in incontinent patients. British Journal of Urology 43: 233–237

James E D 1978 The behaviour of the bladder during physical activity. Journal of Urology 50: 387–394

McInerney P D, Harris S A, Pritchard A, Stephenson T P 1991 Night studies for primary diurnal and nocturnal enuresis and preliminary results of the 'clam' ileocystoplasty. British Journal of Urology 67: 42–43

Robertson A S, Davies J B, Webb R J, Neal D E 1991 Bladder augmentation and replacement. Urodynamic and clinical review of 25 patients. British Journal of Urology 68: 590–597

Robertson A S, Griffiths C J, Ramsden P D, Neal D E 1994 Bladder function in healthy volunteers: ambulatory monitoring and conventional urodynamic studies. British Journal of Urology 73: 242–249

Sethia K K, Webb R J, Neal D E 1991 Urodynamic study of ileocystoplasty in the treatment of idiopathic detrusor instability. British Journal of Urology 67: 286–290

van Waalwijk van Doorn E S C, Remmers A, Janknegt R A 1991 Extramural ambulatory urodynamic monitoring during natural filling and normal daily activities: evaluation of 100 patients. Journal of Urology 91: 124–131

van Waalwijk van Doorn E S C, Remmers A, Janknegt R A 1992a Conventional and extramural ambulatory urodynamic testing of the lower urinary tract in female volunteers. Journal of Urology 147: 1319–1326

van Waalwijk van Doorn E S C, Remmers A, Ambergen A W, Janknegt R A 1992b Detrusor activity index a means to quantify detrusor overactivity (abstract). Neurourology and Urodynamics 11: 461–462

Warrell D W, Watson B W, Shelley T 1963 Intravesical pressure measurement in women during movement using a radio-pill and an air-probe. Journal of Obstetrics and Gynaecology of the British Commonwealth 70: 959

Webb R J, Styles R A, Griffiths C J, Ramsden P D, Neal D E 1989 Ambulatory monitoring of bladder pressure in patients with low compliance as a result of neurogenic bladder dysfunction. British Journal of Urology 64: 150–154

Special investigations

L LEWIS WALL AND PHILLIP A BARKSDALE

In addition to standard tests such as cystometry and uroflowmetry, the evaluation of lower urinary tract complaints in women sometimes requires the use of special investigations to obtain additional information. This chapter will describe the use and limits of several specific investigations that clinicians may occasionally find useful: pad tests, the bethanechol chloride supersensitivity test, and the Q-tip test.

PAD TESTING

A quick, inexpensive, and sensitive means of detecting and quantifying urine loss in incontinent patients would be of considerable help in clinical practice. Various forms of pad testing have been devised in an attempt to meet this need, with varying degrees of success. In general, it is easier to detect urine loss than to quantify accurately the degree of incontinence experienced by a patient.

The simplest form of pad test can be carried out by giving the patient a sanitary pad to wear while she undergoes a brief series of exercises (standing up, sitting, stooping, jogging in place, etc.). The pad is then examined to see if it is wet. This provides a quick, standardized way of checking for urine loss. It is useful for corroborating the patient's complaints and for assessing objectively the results of surgery for incontinence. A pad test of this type does not quantify urine loss, and on occasion there may be a question as to whether the wetness on the pad represents urine loss, perspiration, or vaginal discharge (Wall et al 1991).

Dye tests

Giving the patient a drug which changes the colour of the urine is one way around this latter problem. When this is done, discoloration of the pad is taken as evidence of urine loss. Useful substances for dyeing the urine are methylene blue or indigo carmine dye, or phenazopyridine hydrochloride (Pyridium, Parke-Davis). Dye tests by themselves do not allow quantification of urine loss. The results of dye tests should be interpreted with caution. In a controlled study investigating the usefulness of Pyridium in detecting urine loss (Wall et al 1990), 18 women with urodynamically proven genuine stress incontinence were compared with 23 asymptomatic, continent volunteers. After a standardized 1-hour exercise test, all of the patients with genuine stress incontinence had stained pads; however, 11 (52%) of the asymptomatic patients also had stained pads. Analysis of pad weight gain in the two groups showed the former to have a mean weight gain of 16.5 g, while the asymptomatic subjects had a mean weight gain of 0.1 g. This probably indicated that Pyridium-coloured urine which had been passed during normal micturition had stained the periurethral tissues in these women, with subsequent transfer of this discoloration to the pad during the test. Slight staining of a pad during a test of this kind should therefore be interpreted cautiously.

Dye tests can nonetheless be extremely useful when looking for intraoperative damage to the urinary tract, or when searching for a fistula. If cotton-wool swabs are placed in the vagina and the urine is dyed with an appropriate substance, staining of the swabs in the vagina will diagnose the presence of a fistula, especially if the swabs nearest the introitus are not stained. If the bladder is filled with a dye such as methylene blue or indigo carmine, and the patient also is given Pyridium orally, this test can be used to differentiate a vesicovaginal fistula from a ureterovaginal fistula. In the former case, the cotton swabs will be blue; in the latter case, they should be stained orange from the urine coming down through the ureter that has not yet entered the bladder.

Electronic pad tests

Electronic systems for detecting urine leakage have also been devised, including the Exeter 'recording nappy' or Urilos system. This testing system involves the use of a set of strip electrodes embedded in a disposable paper nappy along with a dry electrolyte. When urine is absorbed on the nappy a change in electrical capacitance is induced which is measured by a monitor. This can be converted into millilitres of urine lost by a moving coil meter.

In principle this seems to be an excellent way of detecting and quantifying urine loss (James et al 1971; Caldwell 1974). In practice, however, it has not proved very successful. The system accurately documents urinary leakage and its frequency, but has large errors in the quantification of urine loss (Rowan et al 1976; Stanton & Ritchie 1977; Robinson & Stanton 1981; Eadie et al 1983). The pads with electrodes also are considerably more expensive than ordinary sanitary pads for routine use.

Pad weighing

Another way of assessing incontinence objectively is by measuring the weight gain of a preweighed sanitary pad worn by the patient over a certain period of time. In 1981 Sutherst and colleagues evaluated 50 normal and 100 incontinent women in this manner. These women wore a series of preweighed sanitary pads for 1 hour while engaging in exercise. Normal women had a mean weight gain of less that 1 g in the 1-hour period, and incontinent women had a mean pad weight gain of 12.2 g over the same time. The small pad weight gain in the normal women was thought to represent the effects of vaginal discharge and perspiration, while the pad weight gain of incontinent women was attributed to urinary leakage. The test was recommended as an objective way of screening for urinary incontinence – opinions which have been seconded by others (Walsh & Mills 1981).

To be useful for comparative clinical purposes, pad tests must be reproducible and reliable. Klarskov & Hald (1984) proposed a standardized 60 minute pad test which they felt met these criteria and which has since formed the prototype for most other pad-weighing regimens. In modified form it has been adopted by the International Continence Society as a standardized test (Tables 17.1 and 17.2). Patients started the pad test with a comfortably full bladder. They put on a preweighed sanitary pad and drank 500 ml of sodium-free liquid prior to beginning a standardized activity programme. At the end of the test, the pad was removed, reweighed, and the results recorded. The authors found that the results of tests performed on successive days were highly reproducible and that urine loss expressed as a percentage of bladder vol-

Table 17.1 The one-hour pad test.

1. The test is started without the patient voiding.
2. A preweighed collecting device* is put on and the one-hour test period begins.
3. The patient drinks 500 ml of sodium-free liquid within a short period (max. 15 min), then sits or rests.
4. The patient walks for 30 minutes and climbs stairs equivalent to one flight up and down.
5. During the remaining period the subject performs a standard set of activities:
   a. standing up from sitting 10 times
   b. coughing vigorously 10 times
   c. running in place for 1 minute
   d. bending over to pick up a small object from the floor 5 times
   e. washing hands in running water for 1 minute
6. At the end of the one-hour test period the collecting device is removed and weighed.
7. If the test is regarded as representative the patient voids and the volume is recorded.
8. If the test is not representative it may be repeated, preferably without voiding.

Recommended by the International Continence Society, as discussed at the annual meeting in Bristol, 1987.
* Usually a nappy or pad, which should be worn inside waterproof underpants or have a waterproof backing.

Table 17.2 Classification of pad weight gain.

Less than 1 g	Essentially dry
2–10 g	Slight to moderate loss
10–50 g	Severe urine loss
More than 50 g	Very severe urine loss

Based on the one-hour pad test recommended by the International Continence Society, as discussed at the annual meeting in Bristol, 1987.

ume (voided volume after the test plus the amount of urine lost during the test) was also reproducible. Thirty-eight of 50 patients (76%) felt that the urine loss during the test was representative of their everyday incontinence. The authors have subsequently used this pad test to assess the outcome of patients who have undergone implantation of AMS artificial urinary sphincters, and found that patients' subjective feelings of continence correlated well with the pad-weighing test (Holm-Bentzen et al 1985).

Before embarking on extensive therapy for urinary incontinence – particularly before embarking upon surgery for stress incontinence – it is mandatory to have objective evidence of urine loss. The easiest way to do this is to watch for urine loss during provocative cystometry or during a cough stress test in a patient with a full bladder. Can pad tests be used to replace direct visualization of urine loss from the urethra? How well do they correlate with urine loss visualized indirectly using videocystourethrography (VCU) – a highly reliable study when urine loss is noted, but one that may miss small amounts of urine loss that lie below the threshold at which radiographic visualization can occur? Versi & Cardozo (1986) and Versi et al (1988) found that a positive pad test with a minimum 1.4 g weight gain has a positive predictive value of 89% for urine loss seen on VCU; however, there were false positive and false negative pad tests in these studies when compared with VCU done at maximum cystometric capacity in the erect/oblique position. Stanton & Ritchie (1977) and Hilton & Stanton (1983) have suggested that pad tests can often confirm a patient's complaint of incontinence when VCU is negative. In one study Jorgensen et al (1987) found VCU to have a false negative rate of 50% when compared to a 1-hour weighing test, using a 2 g weight change as diagnostic for incontinence. Since the quantification of urine loss at VCU is purely arbitrary and since no one has yet determined what is the smallest amount of urine loss that can be detected by VCU, it may be that pad tests can pick up small amounts of urine loss which are not seen radiographically.

Bladder volume and the rate of diuresis during the test probably account for many of the discrepancies in the results of pad tests. Lose et al (1986) and Jorgensen et al (1987) both showed substantial intra-individual variations in test results that could be explained by variations in the urine load in the bladder during the test. Using a 40-minute test with the bladder filled to 75% of cystometric capacity, Jakobsen and colleagues (1987) showed substantially greater urine leakage than with a standard 1-hour test performed with an unknown bladder volume. There was a significant correlation between the two tests, but wide intraindividual variations occurred. The authors' opinion was that pad-weighing tests are useful for documenting urinary incontinence and gauging its severity, but the wide within-patient variability limits their usefulness in assessing the outcome of treatment.

In an effort to improve the reliability of pad tests, several authors have proposed extending their duration to 2 hours (Richmond et al 1987) or even to as long as 48 hours (Jakobsen et al 1987; Victor et al 1987). The 48-hour pad test appears to be reliable and gives an indication of the severity of urine loss during a patient's daily routine, but the lack of standardization restricts its usefulness for scientific purposes if weight gain is to be used as the criterion for diagnosis.

Pad tests appear to be reliable in documenting incontinence objectively and they are easy to perform in groups as diverse as geriatric in-patients (Walsh & Mills 1981) and children (Hellstrom et al 1986). A weight gain of 1.0 g or more in a standardized 1-hour test probably represents incontinence. However, different results can be obtained in studying the same group of patients (Christensen et al 1986), and while there is some correlation between tests, intraindividual test variation appears to be substantial enough to make these tests of limited utility in assessing the results of treatment, other than to document whether or not incontinence can still be demonstrated after therapy (Wall et al 1991).

BETHANECHOL CHLORIDE SUPERSENSITIVITY TEST

In 1939 the American physiologist Walter B Cannon proposed a 'law of denervation', which he subsequently developed at some length (Cannon & Rosenblueth 1949). Based upon extensive animal experimentation he stated that when a unit is destroyed in a series of efferent neurones, an increased irritability to chemical agents develops in the isolated structure or structures, the effect being maximal in the part denervated. On this principle and from the observation that structures normally stimulated by acetylcholine become supersensitive to bethanechol chloride when denervated, Lapides and co-workers (1962a, 1962b) developed a test that they used for diagnosing motor or sensory denervation of the bladder:

After initial filling cystometry, the bladder was drained and then refilled with 100 ml of room temperature fluid. The baseline intravesical pressure was recorded. After several control runs to obtain an accurate reading, the patient was given 2.5 mg of bethanechol chloride subcutaneously. Cystometrograms were repeated 10, 20, and 30 minutes after administration of the drug. In normal adults there was an increase in intravesical pressure of 2–5 cm H_2O over baseline values during the test period. Differential blocking studies indicated that the ganglionic synapses and neuromuscular junctions had become supersensitive to bethanechol in patients with motor or sensory paralytic bladders. It was felt that this test was specific and objective for the diagnosis of these conditions. Its accuracy and reliability has since been studied by a number of authors.

Glahn (1970a) investigated the technique in detail after modifying it slightly to use a subcutaneous injection of 0.25 mg carbachol (equivalent to 2.5 mg bethanechol) after filling the bladder with 100 ml of saline and allowing it to accommodate. He found normal bladders usually responded with a pressure rise of less than 15 cm H_2O. Results in the range of 15–20 cm H_2O were felt to be inconclusive, while greater responses indicated denervation with increasing certainty. Glahn's opinion, based on 197 tests in 64 patients, was that a normal test did not always exclude a neurological defect and that the test was only semiquantitative. He found that test results could be affected by bladder volume, integrity of the bladder musculature, emotional stress, and absorption of the drug from the site of the injection site after administration of the drug was advocated to minimize this latter problem. It was felt that the test turned positive at about 2 weeks after the development of a neurological lesion, but not conclusively so until 6–10 weeks later. Supersensitivity was found to decrease with reinnervation. Overall, the test was felt to be reliable and reproducible.

Employing a modified test with gas cystometry, Merrill & Rotta (1974) investigated 102 patients suffering from a variety of conditions. Following an air cystometrogram the authors emptied the bladder and administered 0.035 mg/kg of bethanechol chloride subcutaneously. The cystometrogram was then repeated. All normal patients had a vesical pressure rise of less than 15 cm H_2O. In neurologically abnormal patients, 38% of those with upper motor neurone lesions had positive denervation supersensitivity tests, as did 50% of patients with multiple sclerosis. These results should not be surprising, since upper motor neurone lesions probably can induce denervation in end organs removed from the original lesion and multiple sclerosis can affect either upper or lower motor neurone lesions.

Testing children, using a dose of 0.035 mg/kg of bethanechol chloride, showed the supersensitivity test to be positive in 90% of patients with neuropathic bladder dysfunction (Kass et al 1982). The 10% of patients with false negative tests had been neurologically stable for several years, perhaps implying some degree of reinnervation or decreasing supersensitivity over time. In children with urodynamically normal bladder function, the test was negative in 93%. The false positive tests occurred in children with chronic cystitis or chronic renal failure.

In other studies the test has been found to be positive in hereditary sensory neuropathy (Harris & Benson 1980) and negative in cases of psychogenic urinary retention (Barrett 1978). A comparative study of perineal electromyography and bethanechol chloride supersensitivity testing found the latter to be more sensitive and more specific in corroborating the presence of bladder neuropathy (Pavlakis et al 1983).

Blaivas et al (1980) investigated 33 patients who demonstrated detrusor areflexia during cystometry and claimed a high degree of false negative and false positive tests. All patients underwent a thorough neurological examination. Of 21 patients with a documented neuropathic bladder, 16 (76%) had positive bethanechol denervation supersensitivity tests. Of 12 patients without evidence of a neurological lesion, six had negative tests and six had positive tests. All six patients with positive tests were women with urinary retention of unknown aetiology. All of these patients had normal electromyograms of the external urethral sphincter except for the inability to contract and relax the sphincter on command in five cases, and an absent bulbocavernosus reflex in one patient. However, these data do not exclude the possibility of a focal neurological lesion of the parasympathetic innervation of the bladder (S2–S4) in such patients, a situation similar to that found in patients with bladder dysfunction following radical hysterectomy, where bladder dysfunction appears to correlate well with a positive bethanechol supersensitivity test (Glahn 1970b).

The standard dose for the test is 2.5 mg of bethanechol chloride (0.035 mg/kg) in a 70 kg individual given subcutaneously. Some authors feel that better results are obtained using a dose of 5 mg (Pavlakis et al 1983; Wheeler et al 1988), but over 4 mg of bethanechol chloride given subcutaneously in a normal patient may falsely elevate the intravesical pressure and higher doses should therefore be used carefully (Downie 1984). Bethanechol should be given with caution in patients with asthma or cardiac arrythmias, and atropine should be available to counter its effects if needed.

Overall the data indicate that the bethanechol chloride supersensitivity test is a good way of detecting bladder denervation in patients exhibiting detrusor areflexia at cystometry. A negative supersensitivity test dose not necessarily rule out bladder denervation, but a positive test mandates thorough investigation to eliminate a neurological lesion, as bladder dysfunction may be the only presenting symptom of a more severe neurological process (Sonda et al 1983; Wheeler et al 1988). A positive test should be interpreted cautiously in the presence of infection, azotemia, or emotional distress.

Finally, the denervation supersensitivity test has not been proved useful in determining which patients with voiding disorders might respond to pharmacologic treatment with bethanechol (Melzer 1972; Wein et al 1980). As there is scant evidence to indicate that bethanechol chloride has any clinical efficacy in promoting the return of micturition in patients with voiding difficulties (Finkbeiner 1985), the test cannot be used to help with this vexing problem.

Q-TIP TEST

A simple and inexpensive test for evaluating urethral hypermobility was introduced by Crystle et al (1971). The test involves the insertion of a cotton tipped swab (called a 'Q-tip' in North America, where the test is widely used) into the urethra and measuring the deflection of the shaft of the swab with an orthopaedic goniometer during coughing or Valsalva manoeuvre. Crystle and colleagues stated that the externally measured deflection of the Q-tip shaft was an accurate approximation of the internal descent of the urethra as measured during lateral bead chain cystourethrography. The original authors proposed that the 'Q-tip test' could be used as a substitute for radiographic studies of the bladder neck and urethra in differentiating between patients who had Type I and Type II defects according to Green's old classification of urethral support defects and stress incontinence (Green 1962, 1968).

Green's classification of stress incontinence has long been abandoned by most clinicians and has not been replaced with a generally accepted classification system. Although much has been written about Q-tip testing, generally accepted standards are still lacking, even though most clinicians accept a change in the urethrovesical axis of greater than 30° to be indicative of urethral hypermobility (Wall 1997). Several studies have questioned the reliability of the Q-tip test as a tool for diagnosing stress incontinence. Montz & Stanton (1986) stated that the greatest liability of the Q-tip test was its inability to diagnose detrusor instability or sensory urgency as the aetiology of incontinence. They found that 32% of women with incontinence had a 'positive' Q-tip test associated with pure sensory urgency or pure detrusor instability. They reported that 29% of women with a 'negative' Q-tip test had pure genuine stress incontinence. Montz and Stanton also questioned the need to differentiate between Green's Type I and II defects.

Caputo & Benson (1993) compared Q-tip testing to perineal ultrasound and also found the Q-tip test inaccurate for measuring urethrovesical junction mobility. These authors concluded that the Q-tip test failed to identify patients with urethrovesical hypermobility 75% of the time and falsely diagnosed the presence of urethral hypermobility in 22% of patients. Fantl and colleagues (1986) showed no correlation between urethral axis deviation, as determined by the Q-tip test, and urethral sphincter strength. Handa et al (1995) studied the effect of patient position on proximal urethral mobility and found that of 34 women with a positive supine Q-tip test only 24 (71%) had a positive standing Q-tip test. The authors concluded that patient position has a significant effect on the mobility of the urethrovesical junction. Walters & Diaz (1987) found an association between a positive Q-tip test and the degree of anterior vaginal wall relaxation. They did not, however, find a correlation with a specific urological diagnosis.

Karram & Bhatia (1988) reported on a series of 63 women in an attempt to standardize the Q-tip test technique and determine if bladder fullness or anterior vaginal wall relaxation were significant factors in the test results. They found that bladder fullness did not alter the results. They found no significant differences in the resting or straining angles by Q-tip, but did note that in the absence of vaginal wall relaxation women with genuine stress incontinence had significantly higher maximum straining angles than those with bladder instability. The authors concluded that the Q-tip test, if performed correctly, was an easy, inexpensive and reliable method to quantify bladder neck mobility in incontinent or continent women with or without pelvic relaxation.

Bergman et al (1987) reported that greater than 90% of 69 patients with stress urinary incontinence and no previous surgery had a positive Q-tip test and a 90% sensitivity for the test in this group. They claimed that the test was inexpensive, reliable under certain conditions, and an adequate clinical tool to assess pelvic relaxation. The authors cautioned however, that in patients who had previous anti-incontinence surgery, the Q-tip test was non-contributory.

Bergman et al (1989) reported on the absence of a positive Q-tip test as predictor for failure of retropubic anti-incontinence procedures. These authors stated that a negative Q-tip test was an independent risk factor of surgical failure and that a 'low pressure urethra' was found in four of their 15 patients. The authors state that the Q-tip test is not the final or most sensitive test of support, but that it should be used as a screening tool. They further state that should a negative Q-tip test exist in the presence of stress urinary incontinence then obstructive procedures such as slings should be considered.

Given the lack of consensus regarding the reliability of the Q-tip test, it would be prudent to use it as a screening tool for the presence of urethral hypermobility, but not to use it as the sole criterion for assessing the severity of pelvic organ prolapse or sphincteric strength.

REFERENCES

Barrett D H 1978 Evaluation of psychogenic urinary retention. Journal of Urology 120: 191–192

Bergman A, McCarthy T A, Ballard C A, Yanai J 1987 Role of the Q-tip test in evaluating stress urinary incontinence. Journal of Reproductive Medicine 32: 273–275

Bergman A, Koonings P P, Ballard C A 1989 Negative Q-tip test as a risk factor for failed incontinence surgery in women. Journal of Reproductive Medicine 34: 193–197

Blaivas J G, Labib K B, Michalik S J, Zayed A A 1980 Failure of bethanechol denervation supersensitivity as a diagnostic aid. Journal of Urology 123: 199–201

Caldwell K P S 1974 Clinical use of recording nappy. Urologia Internationalis 29: 172–173

Cannon W B 1939 A law of denervation. American Journal of the Medical Sciences 198: 737–750

Cannon W B, Rosenblueth A 1949 The Supersensitivity of Denervated Structures. Macmillan, New York

Caputo R M, Benson J T 1993 The Q-tip test and urethrovesical junction mobility. Obstetrics and Gynecology 82: 892–896

Christensen S J, Colatrup H, Hertz J B, Fremodt-Moller J 1986 Inter- and intra-departmental variations of the perineal pad weighing test. Neurourology and Urodynamics 5: 23–28

Crystle C D, Charme L S, Copeland W E 1971 Q-tip test in stress urinary incontinence. Obstetrics and Gynecology 38: 313–315

Downie J W 1984 Bethanechol chloride in urology – a discussion of issues. Neurourology and Urodynamics 3: 211–222

Eadie A S, Glen E S, Rowan D 1983 The Urilos recording nappy system. British Journal of Urology 55: 301–303

Fantl J A, Hurt W G, Bump R C, Dunn L J, Choi S C 1986 Urethral axis and sphincteric function. American Journal of Obstetrics and Gynecology 155: 554–558

Finkbeiner A E 1985 Is bethanechol chloride clinically useful in promoting bladder emptying? A literature review. Journal of Urology 134: 443–449

Green T H 1962 Development of a plan for the diagnosis and treatment of urinary stress incontinence. American Journal of Obstetrics and Gynecology 83: 632–648

Green T H 1968 The problem of urinary stress incontinence in the female: an appraisal of its current status. Obstetrical and Gynecological Survey 23: 603–634

Glahn B E 1970a Neurogenic bladder diagnosed pharmacologically on the basis of denervation supersensitivity. Scandanavian Journal of Urology and Nephrology 4: 13–24

Glahn B E 1970b The neurogenic factor in vesical dysfunction following radical hysterectomy for carcinoma of the cervix. Scandanavian Journal of Urology and Nephrology 4: 107–116

Handa V L, Jensen J K, Ostergard D R 1995 The effect of patient position on proximal urethral mobility. Obstetrics and Gynecology 86: 273–276

Harris J D, Benson G S 1980 Positive bethanechol chloride supersensitivity test in hereditary sensory neuropathy. Journal of Urology 124: 923–924

Hellstrom A L, Andersson K, Hjalmas R Jodal U 1986 Pad tests in children with incontinence. Scandinavian Journal of Urology and Nephrology 20: 47–50

Hilton P, Stanton S L 1983 The use of intravaginal oestrogen cream in genuine stress incontinence. British Journal of Gynaecology 90: 940–944

Holm-Bentzen I, Klarskov P, Opsomer R, Maegaard E M, Hald T 1985 Objective assessment of urinary incontinence after successful implantation of the AMS artificial urethral sphincter. Neurourology and Urodynamics 4: 9–13

Jakobsen H, Vedel P, Anderson J T 1987 Objective assessment of urinary incontinence: an evaluation of three different pad-weighing tests. Neurourology and Urodynamics 6: 325–330

James E D, Flack F C, Caldwell K P S, Martin M R 1971 Continuous measurement of urine loss and frequency in incontinent patients. Britist Journal of Urology 43: 233–237

Jorgensen L, Lose G, Andersen J T 1987 One-hour pad-weighing test for objective assessment of female urinary incontinence. Obstetrics and Gynecology 69: 39–42

Karram M M, Bhatia N N 1988 The Q-tip test: standardization of the technique and its interpretation in women with urinary incontinence. Obstetrics and Gynecology 71: 807–811

Kass E J, Rumar S, Roff S A 1982 Bethanechol denervation supersensitivity testing in children. Journal of Urology 127: 75–77

Klarskov P, Hald T 1984 Reproducibility and reliability of urinary incontinence assessment with a 60 min test. Scandinavian Journal of Urology and Nephrology 18: 293–298

Lapides J, Friend C R, Ajemian E, Reus W F 1962a A new test for neurogenic bladder. Journal of Urology 88: 245–247

Lapides J, Friend C R, Ajemian E P, Reus W F 1962b Denervation supersensitivity as a test for neurogenic bladder. Surgery, Gynecology and Obstetrics 114: 241–244

Lose G, Gammelgaard J, Jorgensen T J 1986 The one-hour pad-weighing test: reproducibility and the correlation between the test result, the start volume in the bladder, and the diuresis. Neurourology and Urodynamics 5: 17–21

Melzer M 1972 The urecholine test. Journal of Urology 108: 728–730

Merrill D C, Rotta J 1974 A clinical evaluation of detrusor denervation supersensitivity testing using cystometry. Journal of Urology 111: 27–30

Montz F J, Stanton S L 1986 Q-tip test in female urinary incontinence. Obstetrics and Gynecology 67: 258–260

Pavlakls A J, Siroky M B, Krane R J 1983 Neurogenic detrusor reflexia: correlation of perineal electromyography and bethanechol chloride supersensitivity testing. Journal of Urology 129: 1182–1184

Richmond D H, Sutherst J R, Brown M C 1987 Quantification of urine loss by weighing perineal pads. Observation on the exercise regimen. British Journal of Urology 59: 229–227

Robinson H, Stanton S L 1981 Detection of urinary incontinence. British Journal of Obstetrics and Gynaecology 88: 59–61

Rowan D, Deehan C, Glen E S 1976 Detection of urine loss using the Exeter recording nappy and other similar devices. Urologia Internationalis 31: 70–77

Sonda L P, Kogan B A, Koff S A, Diokno A C 1983 Neurologic disease masquerading as genitourinary abnormality – the role of urodynamics in diagnosis. Journal of Urology 129: 1175–1178

Stanton S L, Ritchie D R 1977 Urilos: the practical detection of urine loss. American Journal of Obstetrics 128: 461–463

Sutherst J, Brown M, Shavor M 1981 Assessing the severity of urinary incontinence in women by weighing perineal pads. Lancet 1: 1128–1130

Versi E, Cardozo L D 1986 Perineal pad weighing versus videographic analysis in genuine stress incontinence. British Journal of Obstetrics and Gynaecology 91: 364–366

Versi E, Cardozo L D, Anand D 1988 The use of pad tests in the investigation of female urinary incontinence. Obstetrics and Gynecology 8: 270–273

Victor A, Larason G, Asbrink A S 1987 A simple patient-administered test of objective quantitation of the symptom of urinary incontinence. Scandinavian Journal of Urology and Nephrology 21: 277–279.

Wall L L 1997 Urinary stress incontinence. In: Rock J A, Thompson J D (eds) TeLinde's Operative Gynecology, 8th edn pp 1087–1134 Lippincott-Raven, Philadelphia

Wall L L, Wang K, Robson I, Stanton S L 1990 The 'Pyridium pad test' for diagnosing urinary incontinence. Journal of Reproductive Medicine 35: 682–684

Wall L L, Couchman G M, McCoy M C 1991 Vaginal discharge as a confounding factor in the diagnosis of urinary incontinence by perineal pad testing. International Urogynecology Journal 2: 219–221

Walsh J B, Mills G L 1981 Measurement of urinary loss in elderly incontinent patients. Lancet 1: 1130–1131

Walters M D, Diaz K 1987 Q-tip test: a study of continent and incontinent women. Obstetrics and Gynecology 70: 208–211

Wein A J, Raezer D M, Malloy T R 1980 Failure of the bethanechol supersensitivity test to predict improved voiding after subcutaneous bethanechol administration. Journal of Urology 123: 202–203

Wheeler J S, Culkin D J, Canniag J R 1988 Positive bethanechol supersensitivity test in neurologically normal patients. Urology 31: 86–89

Clinical conditions

SECTION 3

SECTION 3
CHAPTER

18

Classification of urogynaecological disorders

STUART L STANTON

INTRODUCTION

If the body were divided into specialties by physiology rather than historical or anatomical boundaries, there would be no need to justify urogynaecology. Physiological events and diseases affecting the pelvic organs invariably affect the genital organs, lower urinary tract and lower alimentary system together. This specialty, therefore, is an interface between gynaecologist and urologist and colorectal surgeon.

Studies by Snooks et al (1984a,b), Smith et al (1989) and Sultan et al (1993) show the dramatic effects of vaginal delivery on the pelvic floor, urinary and anal sphincters. Wall & DeLancey (1991) have neatly summarized the case for a holistic approach to pelvic floor disorders involving the three disciplines of gynaecology, urology and colorectal surgery. The American College of Obstetricians and Gynecologists introduced subspecialization into obstetrics and gynaecology and the Royal College of Obstetricians and Gynaecologists followed in 1984. Four subspecialties were created, among them urogynaecology. This comprised congenital anomalies, incontinence, voiding difficulties, urinary fistulae, bladder neuropathy, genital prolapse, urgency and frequency, and urinary infection. By common consent, all upper urinary tract conditions, and neoplasia arising anywhere in the urinary tract, belonged to urology.

To this discipline now should be added the functional abnormalities of the lower bowel, including faecal and flatal incontinence, descending perineum and rectal prolapse, primary and secondary repair of anal sphincter and repair of rectovaginal fistula. These frequently have their origins in childbirth and it is logical to consider an extension of urogynaecology to include these disorders. Many of us now believe in the orientation of urogynaecology towards benign reconstructive pelvic surgery, where a surgeon is trained in urology, gynaecology and colorectal surgery to understand and manage all these conditions. Neoplasia and renal and upper alimentary tract conditions will be excluded unless the surgeon is specifically trained to deal with them.

A number of pelvic floor clinics have been established and demonstrate the benefit of combined expertise in the management of patients, training of surgeons and cross-fertilization for research ideas (Nager et al 1997).

TERMINOLOGY

To provide a common language for clinician and researcher, the International Continence Society (ICS) formed a Standardisation Committee in 1973 to promote standards of terminology of lower urinary tract function. Nine reports have appeared. In 1988 a revised edition was produced (Abrams et al 1988). Further reports include bladder training (Anderson et al 1992), intestinal reservoirs (Thuroff et al 1996); pelvic organ prolapse and pelvic floor dysfunction (Bump et al 1996); pressure flow studies of voiding, urethral resistance and urethral obstruction (Griffiths et al 1997); standardization of outcome studies (Mattiasson et al 1998); outcome measures in adult women (Lose et al 1998); outcome measures in frail older people (Fonda et al 1998) and outcome measures for research into adult males (Nordling et al 1998).

The term 'stress incontinence' was first used by Sir Eardley Holland in 1928 and meant the loss of urine during physical effort. It came to be used not only as a symptom and sign, but also as a diagnostic term. As the pathophysiology of urinary incontinence became more clearly understood, it was apparent that the term 'stress incontinence' was ambiguous as it could be applied to a symptom, a sign and a diagnosis – indeed the symptoms and signs of stress incontinence can be found in most types of incontinence.

Nowadays the term 'stress incontinence' is retained for the symptom of involuntary loss of urine on physical exertion and the sign of urine loss from the urethra immediately on increased abdominal pressure. The term 'genuine stress incontinence' was proposed by the ICS in 1976 to mean 'the condition of involuntary loss of urine when the intravesical pressure exceeds the maximum urethral pressure in the absence of a detrusor contraction' (Bates et al 1976). This condition has a number of synonyms: urethral sphincter incompetence, urethral sphincter weakness, stress urinary incontinence and anatomical stress incontinence. I prefer the term 'urethral sphincter incompetence' because this accurately describes the pathophysiology of this condition. Attempts have been made to subdivide this into hypermobility and intrinsic sphincter defect. The former involves the centre of the bladder neck below the inferior margin of the symphysis and the presence of an open bladder neck and urethra on straining or stress. Intrinsic sphincter defect is defined as an open bladder neck and urethra at rest and in the absence of a detrusor contraction (Blaivas & Olsson 1988). The evidence provided was an unrandomized retrospective analysis of 181 consecutive women, of whom 72 were operated upon using a variety of surgeries. It is far more likely that urethral sphincter incompetence represents a spectrum of pathology that includes hypermobility of the bladder neck, loss of urethral resistance due to muscle trauma or neuropathy, and other factors including collagen deficiency and congenital anomalies such as epispadias.

In a similar way, the term 'dyssynergic detrusor dysfunction' was introduced by Hodgkinson et al in 1963. Other synonyms have followed – urge incontinence, uninhibited bladder and bladder instability/unstable bladder. In 1979 the ICS defined an unstable bladder as one 'shown objectively to contract, spontaneously or on provocation during the filling phase, while the patient is attempting to inhibit micturition.' Unstable symptoms may be asymptomatic and do not necessarily imply a neurological disorder. The contractions are phasic. Another term, 'low compliance', means a gradual increase in detrusor pressure during bladder filling without a subsequent decrease at the end. The term 'detrusor hyperreflexia' is used for phasic uninhibited contraction when there is objective evidence of a relevant neurological disorder. Terms to be avoided include 'hypertonic', 'spastic' and 'automatic'.

CLASSIFICATION

Congenital anomalies

Congenital anomalies effectively cross the boundaries between neurology, colorectal surgery and gynaecology. About one third of abnormal genitalia are associated with upper renal tract anomalies. The main upper tract anomalies that concern the gynaecologist are the pelvic kidney and ectopic ureter, the latter because of unexplained incontinence and the need to know about ectopic ureters during pelvic surgery. The expertise of the gynaecologist is in reconstructive surgery for vaginal anomalies such as those accompanying exstrophy, epispadias, haematocolpos, vaginal atresia and persistent urogenital sinus.

Incontinence

Urinary incontinence forms the major proportion of urogynaecology. It is defined by the ICS as 'an involuntary loss of urine that is objectively demonstrable and a social or hygiene problem.

Incontinence is considered to be involuntary except in two categories of patients. In a child under 3 years of age, control of continence is not yet developed; however, careful observation will show that a normal child is dry between involuntary voids, whereas an incontinent child is wet all the time. The second category of patient is the mentally frail patient who may be incontinent because she has lost her social awareness and consciousness and the appreciation of the need to be dry. The social isolation caused by incontinence is demonstrated by 25% of patients delaying for more than 5 years before seeking advice owing to embarrassment (Norton et al 1988). Ostracization and rejection by relatives may lead to an elderly patient being institutionalized solely because of incontinence; paradoxically, some allegedly 'caring' institutions will not accept an elderly patient if she is incontinent. The challenge today is the management of incontinence in the mentally and physically frail: some 25% of nursing time in institutions may be involved in continence care.

Incontinence may be divided into urethral and extraurethral conditions (Fig. 18.1).

Urethral conditions

1 The commonest form is urethral sphincter incompetence (genuine stress incontinence) which can present from childhood (Ch. 19). This condition has several causes and a range of treatment options exists such as devices, exercises, drugs and surgery.
2 Detrusor instability (Ch. 20). Depending on its cause, this may be divided into neuropathy (hyperreflexia) or non-neuropathic (idiopathic). Some patients with instability and a competent sphincter mechanism may still remain dry. When there is coexistent sphincteric incompetence, the patient may complain of stress and urge incontinence.
3 Urinary retention and overflow (Ch. 24). This may be acute or chronic: the former is usually sudden in onset and may be painful or painless. There may be an obvious cause such as an impacted pelvic mass. Chronic retention, on the other hand, is usually painless and insidious and frequently undetected, so errors in diagnosis are often made. It occurs more commonly in the elderly as a result of neuropathy due to progressive atherosclerosis, diabetes or lumbar spinal canal stenosis.
4 Congenital disorder. Epispadias is usually detected during childhood but occasionally it is not diagnosed until adult life.
5 Miscellaneous. These causes include urethral diverticulum, urinary tract infection and faecal impaction (temporary and commonest in the elderly), drugs, such as α-adrenergic blocking

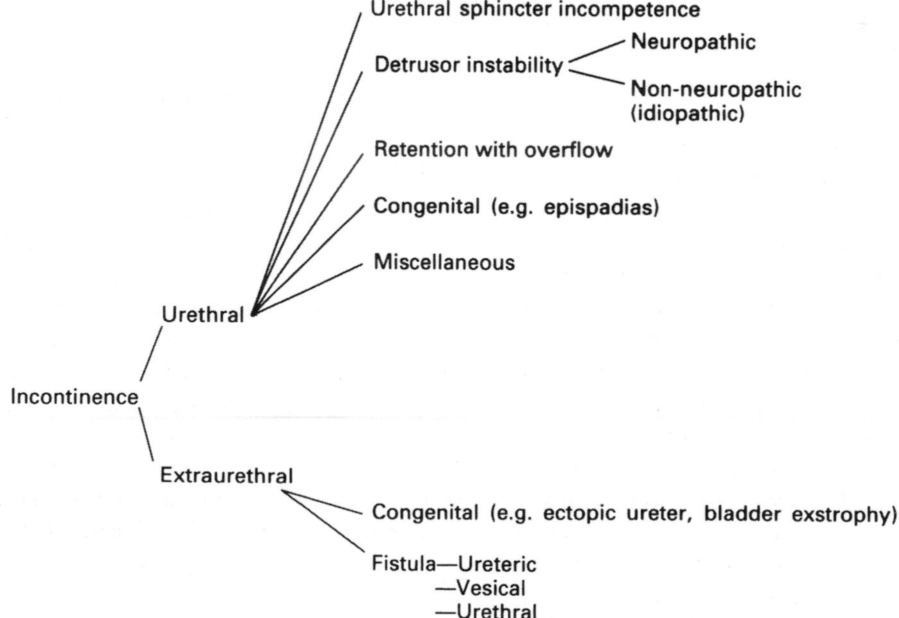

Fig. 18.1 Classification of incontinence.

agents) and functional disorders (dementia). These are rare and the patient should be fully investigated and all other causes excluded before this diagnosis is made. The loss of social awareness of the need to be continent is usually associated with dementia or a space-occupying lesion of the frontal cortex.

Extraurethral conditions

These are distinguished from urethral conditions by the symptom of continuous incontinence. The congenital disorders include ectopic ureter and bladder exstrophy. Urinary fistulae in the developed world are largely iatrogenic, the majority occurring after an abdominal hysterectomy for benign conditions (Ch. 25). Other causes include pelvic carcinoma, and its surgery or radiotherapy. In the developing world, obstetrical causes such as obstructed labour with an impacted vertex are commoner. When the fistula is small, skill and patience are required to detect it.

Voiding difficulties (Ch. 24)

These are uncommon in the female and frequently undiagnosed. Occasionally the upper tract is involved. If untreated, they can lead to recurrent urinary tract infection or chronic retention following otherwise successful bladder neck surgery for incontinence.

Urinary fistulae

These are dealt with at length in Chapter 23.

Bladder neuropathy (Ch. 21)

The neuropathy may principally involve the bladder and urethra or, in the case of a cerebrovascular accident, other systems may be involved requiring close collaboration with a neurologist and a rehabilitation team.

Genital prolapse (Ch. 31)

A genital prolapse may present on its own or be associated with urethral sphincter incompetence or lower bowel disorders such as faecal incontinence.

Urgency and frequency (Ch. 27)

These symptoms can present on their own in the absence of any obvious pathology, or be part of a condition such as urinary tract infection or detrusor instability.

Urinary tract infection (Ch. 29)

This is of common interest to the obstetrician/gynaecologist, urologist and nephrologist and the experience of all may be required for difficult cases. However, the majority of patients are treated by the general practitioner without referral to hospital, even though urinary tract infection may be frequently unproven. Inadequate treatment during pregnancy can lead to acute pyelonephritis and abortion and, if neglected in later life, to chronic pyelonephritis, hypertension and renal failure.

Anorectal conditions (Ch. 38)

These include faecal and flatal incontinence, anal sphincter disruption and its primary and secondary repair, rectal prolapse, rectovaginal fistula and its repair. Some of these can be managed by the urogynaecologist and others will require collaboration with the colorectal surgeon.

This classification is an introduction to urogynaecology. For more specialized reading, a list of selected books is given after the references.

REFERENCES

Abrams P, Blaivas J, Stanton S L, Andersen J 1988 Standardisation of terminology of lower urinary tract function. International Continence Society, Scandinavian Journal of Urology and Nephrology (suppl.) 114: 5–19

Andersen J T, Blaivas J G, Cardozo L, Thüroff J 1992 Lower urinary tract rehabilitation techniques: Seventh Report on the Standardization of Terminology of Lower Urinary Tract Function. Neurourology and Urodynamics 11: 593–603

Bates P, Bradley W, Glen E et al 1976 First report on standardisation of terminology of lower urinary tract function. International Continence Society. British Journal of Urology 48: 39–42

Blaivas J, Olsson C 1988 Stress incontinence: classification and surgical approach. Journal of Urology 139: 727–731

Bump R, Mattiasson A, BØ K et al 1996 Standardisation of terminology of female pelivc organ prolapse and pelvic floor dysfunction. American Journal of Obstetrics and Gynecology 175: 10–17

Fonda D, Resnick N, Colling J et al 1998 Outcome measures for research of lower urinary tract dysfunction in frail older people. Neurourology and Urodynamics 17: 273–281

Griffiths D, Hofner K, van Mastrigt R et al 1997 Standardisation of terminology of lower urinary tract function: pressure flow studies of voiding, urethral resistance and urethral obstruction. Neurourology and Urodynamics 16: 1–18

Hodgkinson C P, Ayers M, Drukker B. 1963 Dyssynergic detrusor dysfunction in the apparently normal female. American Journal of Obstetrics and Gynecology 87: 717–730

Holland E 1928 cited in Jeffcoate T N 1967 Principles of Gynaecology 3rd edn Butterworth, London, p 827

Lose G, Fantl J, Victor A, Walter S, Wells T, Wyman J, Mattiasson A. 1998. Outcome measures for research in adult women with symptoms of lower urinary tract dysfunction. Neurourology and Urodynamics 17: 255–262

Mattiasson A, Djurhuus J, Fonda D, Lose G, Nordling J, Stohrer M. 1998 Standardisation of outcome studies in patients with lower urinary tract dysfunction: a report on general principles from the Standardisation Committee of the International Continence Society. Neurourology and Urodynamics 17: 249–253.

Nager C, Kumar D, Kahn M, Stanton S L 1997 Management of pelvic floor dysfunction. Lancet 350: 1751

Nordling J, Abrams P, Andersen J et al 1998. Outcome measures for research in treatment of adult males with symptoms of lower urinary tract dysfunction. Neurourology and Urodynamics 17: 263–271

Norton P, MacDonald L, Sedgwick P, Stanton S L 1988. Distress and delay associated with urinary incontinence, frequency and urgency in women. British Medical Journal 297: 1187–1189

Smith A, Hosker G, Warrell D 1989 The role of partial denervation of the pelvic floor and the aetiology of genito-urinary prolapse and stress incontinence of urine. A neurophysiological study. British Journal of Obstetrics and Gynaecology 96: 24–28

Snooks S, Swash M, Henry M, Setchell M 1984a. Injury to innervation of pelvic floor sphincter musculature in childbirth. Lancet ii: 546–550

Snooks S Barnes P, Swash M, 1984b Damage to innervation of the voluntary anal and periurethral sphincter musculature in incontinence: an electrophysiological study. Journal of Neurology, Neurosurgery and Psychiatry 47: 1269–1273

Sultan A, Kamm M, Hudson C, Thomas J, Bartram C. 1993 Anal sphincter disruption during vaginal delivery. New England Journal of Medicine 329: 1905–1911

Thüroff J, Mattiasson A, Andersen J et al 1996 The standardization of terminology and assessment of functional characteristics of intestinal urinary reservoirs. British Journal of Urology 78: 516–523

Wall L L, DeLancey J 1991 The politics of prolapse: a revisionist approach to disorders of the pelvic floor in women. Perspectives in Biology and Medicine 34: 489–496

FURTHER READING

Mundy A, Stephenson T, Wein A 1994 Urodynamics: principles, practice and application. 2nd edn. Churchill Livingstone, Edinburgh

Ostergard D, Bent A, 1996 Urogynecology and urodynamics: theory and practice. 4th edn. Williams & Wilkins, Baltimore

Sand P, Ostergard D 1995 Urodynamics and evaluation of female incontinence. Springer-Verlag, London

Stanton S L, Tanagho E 1986 Surgery of female incontinence, 2nd edn. Springer-Verlag, Heidelberg

Wall L, Norton P, DeLancey J 1993 Practical urogynecology. Williams & Wilkins, Baltimore

Walters D, Karram M 1999 Urogynecology and Reconstructive Pelvic Surgery. 2nd edn. Mosby, St. Louis

SECTION 3
CHAPTER

19

Urethral sphincter incompetence

CHARLOTTE CHALIHA AND STUART L STANTON

DEFINITIONS

When a woman coughs and loses urine the condition used to be called stress incontinence, a term coined by Sir Eardley Holland in 1928. Investigations have shown that many conditions can cause stress incontinence and therefore it is preferable to use the term for symptoms and signs only. In 1976, the International Continence Society (ICS) adopted the term 'genuine stress incontinence' (GSI) which was defined as involuntary urethral loss of urine when the intravesical pressure exceeds the maximum urethral pressure in the absence of detrusor activity (Abrams et al 1988). We prefer the term 'urethral sphincter incompetence' (USI) which conveys the pathophysiology more precisely.

We retain the symptom for 'involuntary urine loss on physical effort' and the sign for observation of urine loss from the urethra synchronous with physical exertion.

AETIOLOGY

The mechanism of incontinence is dealt with in Chapter 3. Urethral sphincter incompetence (ISD) is due to two causes – descent of the bladder neck and proximal urethra, and loss of urethral resistance. Frequently the two are combined. In the former there is failure of equal transmission of intra-abdominal pressure to the proximal urethra, leading to reversal of the normal pressure gradient between the bladder and urethra and resulting in a negative urethral closure. Where there is loss of urethral resistance, the resting intraurethral pressure is below the intravesical pressure. The definition of low pressure urethra is where the maximum urethral pressure is less than 20 cm H_20 (Sand et al 1987) or Valsalva leak point pressure is less than 60 cm H_20 (McGuire et al 1993). The factors responsible for this are described below.

Congenital weakness of the bladder neck, e.g. epispadias (Fig. 19.1)

The urethra and bladder neck are imperfectly formed owing to faulty migration and midline fusion of the mesoderm, resulting in a widened bladder neck, a short urethra and defective smooth and striated muscle. The symphysis and clitoris are split. This type of incontinence is usually resistant to conventional bladder neck elevating procedures and is corrected by increasing urethral resistance, i.e. using an artificial urinary sphincter or urethral bulking agent, e.g. collagen.

Congenital weakness from poor pelvic floor support may cause onset of stress incontinence in women in their early teens, which may account for incontinence in 5–10% of young girls (Nemir & Middleton 1954; Thomas et al 1980). Defective collagen formation leading to a reduction in total collagen and decrease in type I collagen have been found in nulliparous women with urethral sphincter incompetence (Keane et al 1992).

Mechanical provocation

Raised intra-abdominal pressure, as seen in obese women and those with chronic respiratory diseases, may lead to stress incontinence. Obesity is more common in premenopausal nulliparous women with stress incontinence compared with parous women with stress incontinence (Creighton et al 1992). Obesity may also predispose women with congenital and developmental weakness of the urethral sphincter mechanism to stress incontinence.

Childbirth

Increasing parity and vaginal delivery are related to an increased risk of stress incontinence (Foldspang et al 1992; Wilson et al 1996). Chaliha et al (1999), in a prospective study of 549 nulliparae found that the prevalence of stress incontinence before, during and after delivery was 3.6%, 43.7% and 14.6% respectively. In a further study of 286 nulliparae who attended for urodynamic investigations in the third trimester the prevalence of genuine stress incontinence was 9.1% and 5.0% in 161 of those who returned at 12 weeks postpartum (Charliha et al 1998). In this group of women the postpartum symptom of stress incontinence was related to a longer active second stage of labour. Delivery may lead to stress incontinence secondary to denervation of the smooth and striated component of the sphincter mechanism and pelvic floor and pubocervical fascia (Snooks et al 1984; Sayer et al 1989) or changes in the urethral support mechanism (Peschers et al 1996).

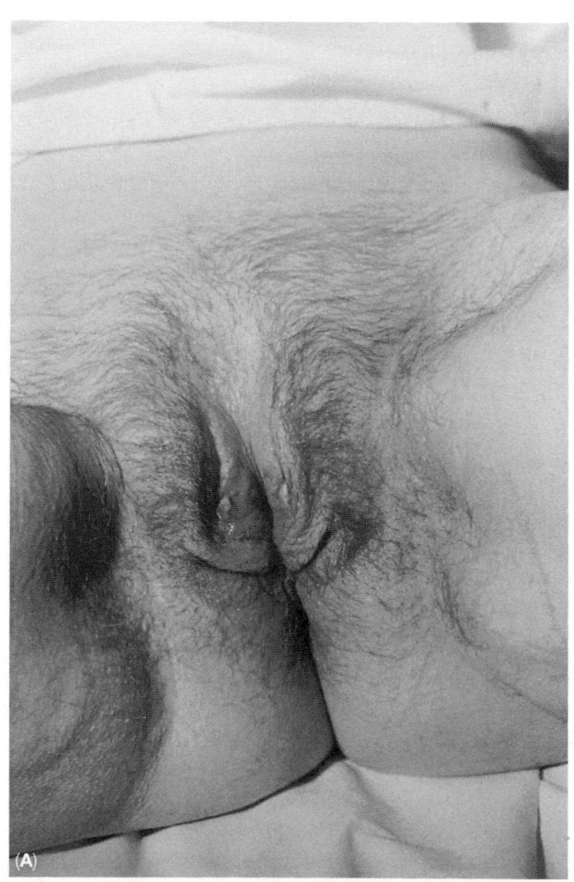
(A)

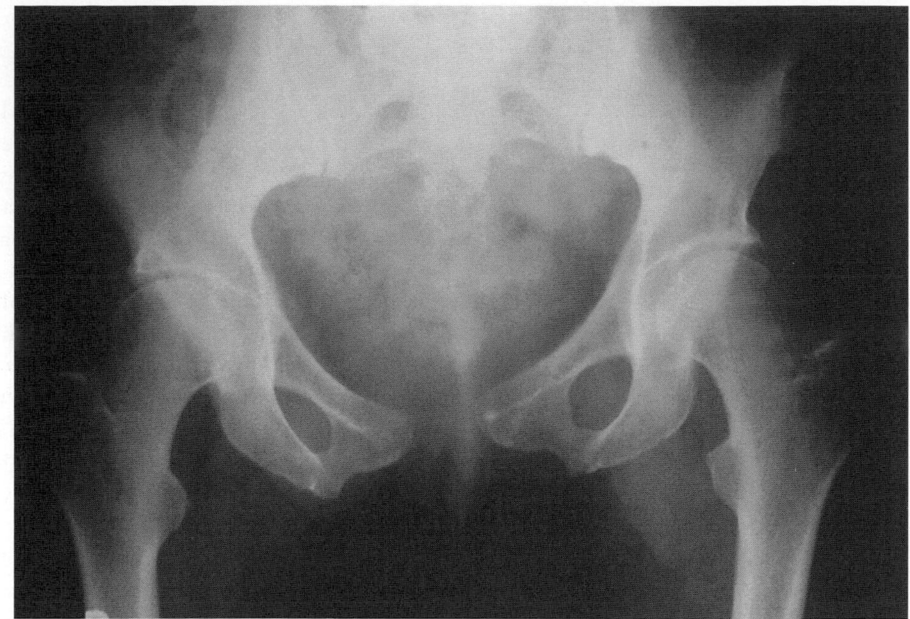

(B)

Fig. 19.1 Epispadias. (**A**) Vulval abnormality. (**B**) Pelvic X-ray showing symphysical separation.

Menopause

Oestrogen deficiency may lead to further weakness of bladder neck supports and loss of hermetic sealing of the urothelium. However, meta-analysis of studies on oestrogen replacement have failed to show any significant improvement in stress incontinence (Fantl et al 1994).

Trauma

This involves fracture of the pelvic ring and symphysial diastasis with avulsion of the bladder neck from its attachment to the back of the symphysis by the pubourethral ligaments (Stanton et al 1981).

Previous surgery

Operations around the bladder neck to correct prolapse or urethral sphincter incompetence may produce recurrent incontinence. The precise mechanisms are unclear but may include damage to the urethral sphincter mechanism and a decrease in urethral resistance and closure pressure, post-surgical fibrosis affecting the urethra and paraurethral tissue, fixation of the urethra to the back of the symphysis with loss of elasticity, and failure to elevate the bladder neck. In a study of 120 women with urodynamically proven genuine stress incontinence, Hilton & Stanton (1983) found that repeat unsuccessful operations were associated with a low urethral pressure.

Drugs

Hypotensive drugs such as prazosin, reserpine, alpha-methyldopa, and phenoxybenzamine act by inhibition of α-1-adrenergic receptors, and are associated with the development of urinary incontinence (Kiruluta & Andrews 1983; Dwyer & Teele 1992). The smooth muscle of the proximal urethra and bladder neck is sympathetically innervated (Awad et al 1976) and α-adrenergic blockade has a relaxant effect of lowering urethral pressure (Anderson et al 1981).

PRESENTATION

Symptoms

The classic symptom of urethral sphincter incompetence is stress incontinence; however, frequency, urge incontinence and incontinence on standing are also complained of by many patients (Cardozo & Stanton 1980) (Fig. 19.2). Usually stress incontinence is worse in the week preceding the menstrual period. Interruption of the urinary stream can be confirmed objectively in about 83% of patients with sphincter incompetence and in 87% of patients with detrusor instability, so this symptom is of no use in differentiating between the two. The patients are usually multiparous. Symptoms commonly occur in pregnancy

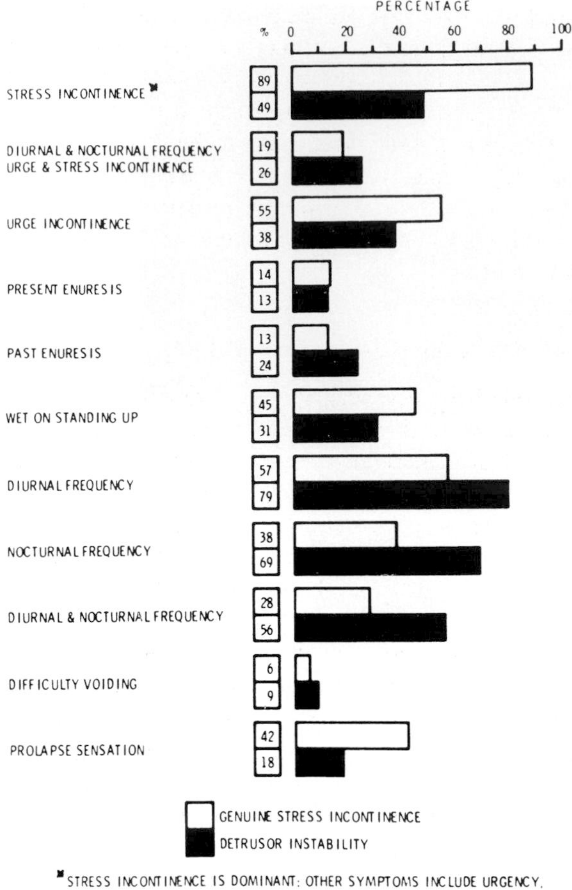

Fig. 19.2 Incidence of symptoms associated with urethral sphincter incompetence and detrusor instability. From Cardozo & Stanton (1980) with permission.

and deteriorate in the postnatal period and in successive pregnancies (Stanton et al 1980; Chaliha 1999).

Signs

There are no special general or neurological features on clinical examination. Epispadias will be readily recognized. Anterior vaginal wall descent (cystourethrocele) will be present in about 50% of women with sphincter incompetence. The vaginal capacity and mobility (indicators of vaginal scarring), need to be assessed as these may be relevant in determining the choice of continence surgery. Other genital prolapse or uterine or ovarian pathology is noted so that surgery for these may be carried out at the same time as continence surgery.

INVESTIGATIONS

The bladder is not a reliable witness. Many clinicians have demonstrated that discrepancy between clinical findings and urodynamic studies (Haylen & Frazer 1987; Ng & Murray 1989). The difficulty lies in the complexity of the history. A combination of stress incontinence, urge incontinence and frequency is more likely to suggest detrusor instability. In a consecutive group of 800 women attending the urodynamic clinic, approximately 50% were diagnosed by urodynamic studies as having urethral sphincter incompetence. Of these only 3% had the symptom and sign of stress incontinence and 1.5% had the sole symptom of stress incontinence (Haylen & Frazer 1987). Of the total group, 85% had urgency, urge incontinence and stress incontinence but only 25% had detrusor instability on testing. It was similar with voiding disorders: 53% had two symptoms suggestive of voiding disorders, which was confirmed in only 10% on testing.

The aims of urodynamic studies are:

1. To confirm the symptoms (e.g. incontinence or voiding difficulty) and their extent
2. To make a diagnosis
3. To detect other abnormalities, e.g. detrusor instability
4. To confirm the cure.

Urodynamic studies are described in Chapters 9, 11, 12, 14, 16 and 17; the following are particularly relevant.

A negative mid-stream urine specimen should precede all urodynamic studies to avoid risk of invasive procedures aggravating urinary tract infection and because the subsequent results will be unreliable.

Cystometry and videocystourethrography (Ch. 9)

The cystometric diagnosis of urinary leakage will indicate the presence of detrusor instability or voiding difficulty; only if detrusor instability is absent is the diagnosis of urethral sphincter incompetence made by exclusion. The combination of cystometry and radiological screening with recording on video tape, together with sound commentary, allows other diagnoses to be made, including the cause of incontinence on standing up, the presence of urethral diverticulum (Fig. 19.3) and occasionally the presence of a urinary fistula (Fig. 19.4). It otherwise adds little to the assessment of straightforward urethral sphincter incompetence (Stanton et al 1986).

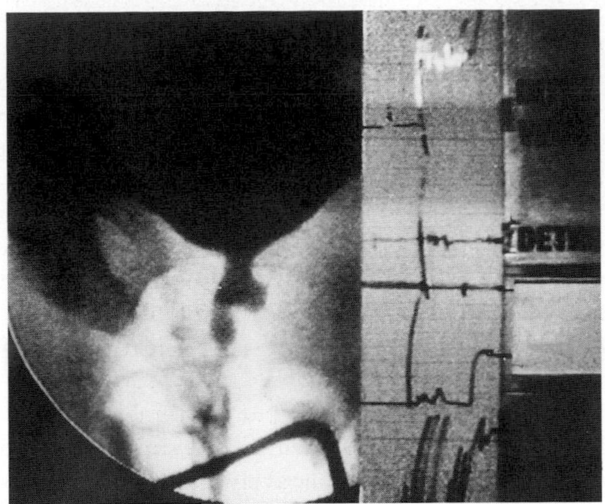

Fig. 19.3 Videocystourethrography showing a urethral diverticulum.

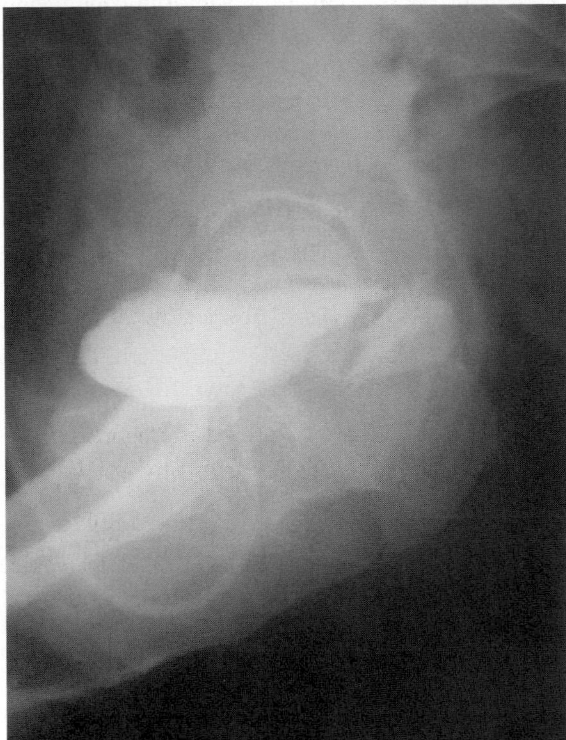

Fig. 19.4 Urinary fistula on videocystourethrography.

Urethral pressure profilometry (Ch. 12)

The role of urethral pressure profilometry (UPP) in the diagnosis of urethral sphincter incompetence remains controversial and undecided. Versi et al (1986) declared that the 'overlap between normal and GSI (USI) was so great as to make accurate diagnosis impossible'. Sand and colleagues (1987) measured the urethral closure pressure and took a cut-off at 20 cm H_2O to detect problems of low-pressure urethra, which they said was a significant feature of failed continence surgery. Hilton (1988) reviewed the concept of the unstable urethra as a cause of sphincter incompetence, and found that a relative change of 30% of maximum urethral closure pressure was the best discriminant to detect this. The main disadvantages of urethral pressure is the relative inflexibility of the catheter, leading to artefact and marked overlap in results between continent and incontinent patients.

Valsalva leak point pressure (VLPP)

The relatively new diagnostic technique may be used to measure urethral resistance to make the diagnosis of intrinsic sphincter deficiency. A pressure less than 60 cm H_20 in the standing position with 150 ml in the bladder has been correlated with intrinsic sphincter deficiency. The test is said to be highly reproducible in approximately 80% of adult women with USI (Bump et al 1995). Compared to UPP, VLPP gives similar results but the test is less expensive and time consuming (Theofrastous et al 1995). However, Alcalay et al (1994) found a high specificity (100%) but poor sensitivity (69%) in the diagnosis of genuine stress incontinence, and poor reliability in the diagnosis of genuine stress incontinence compared to stress UPP variables.

Ultrasonography (Ch. 14)

Ultrasound will detect incomplete bladder emptying, which may cause stress incontinence. It will allow estimation of the position and excursion of the bladder neck, which is relevant to the diagnosis of urethral sphincter incompetence and may help in the analysis of failure of conventional surgery and in the definitive choice of surgery (Creighton et al 1994).

CONSERVATIVE TREATMENT

Conservative and surgical treatment are used depending on the patient's condition and urodynamic diagnosis. Conservative therapy is indicated when:

1 The patient refuses or is undecided about surgery
2 The patient is mentally or physically unfit
3 Childbearing continues
4 There is uncontrolled detrusor instability or voiding difficulty.

Catheters

The continuous indwelling urethral catheter remains a simple or end-stage method of managing urinary incontinence. However, it predisposes to urinary tract infection and may be uncomfortable to wear. For long-term use, suprapubic insertion is preferable and the 'add-a-cath' method of insertion (Bard) using a foley silastic (either a 12 or 16 gauge) is recommended (Lawrence et al 1989) (Fig. 19.5). If there is urethral leakage, urethral closure may be performed.

Pads (Ch. 48)

Absorbent pads are useful when incontinence is mild. The latest are made of gel substance which absorbs many times its volume of water. The pads have a water-repellent backing and absorb urine without it leaking back to the patient's skin (to make it damp) or forward, so making the patient's clothing wet. Good examples are the pads manufactured by Molnlycke, Conveen and Tena.

Exercises

There are a variety of exercises to enhance pelvic floor and tone and control incontinence. These include Kegel exercises and vaginal cones, both of which are discussed below.

Kegel exercises

This is a regimen of regular contractions of the pelvic floor. Tapp et al (1989) found that about 50% of women awaiting surgery were improved by 6 months' physiotherapy alone. Marginally more were improved when faradism was added. Highest success was reported in younger, premenopausal patients with short duration of symptoms, better urethral function during stress and no previous surgery. At least 1 hour of exercise per day is required to show any improvement, which lasts only while the exercises are being carried out. The easiest one to teach is to interrupt the urinary stream and then to practise this technique at other times.

Vaginal cones

These cones were designed by Plevnik (1985), an engineer, as a method of actively and passively exercising the pelvic floor (Fig. 19.6). A cone of graded weight is placed inside the vagina and kept within by pelvic floor contraction. Increasing the cone weight requires increasing strength of the pelvic floor contraction and as the patient knows the weight of the cone she can monitor her own progress. Up to 70% of patients are cured or improved and 90% find it an acceptable method of treatment. Patients should exercise for at least 15 minutes four times a day, and it may be at least 3 months before any benefit is seen.

Devices

There are now several vaginal and urethral devices for stress incontinence. The vaginal devices aim to support the bladder neck during increased abdominal pressure. The Conveen Continence Guard is an arch shaped vaginal device made of polyurethane foam that supports the bladder neck by pressure of two wings. Overall subjective improvement was reported

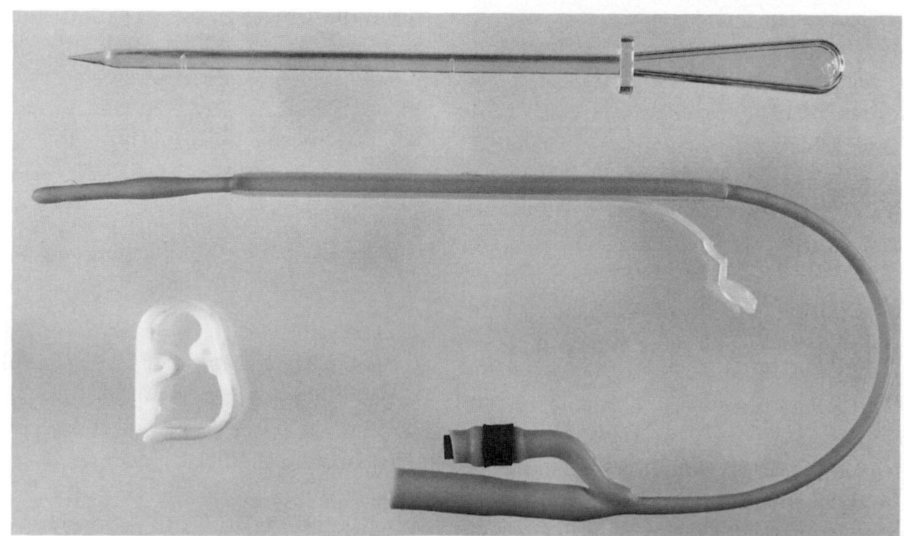

Fig. 19.5 'Add-a-cath' suprapubic catheter (Bard Limited).

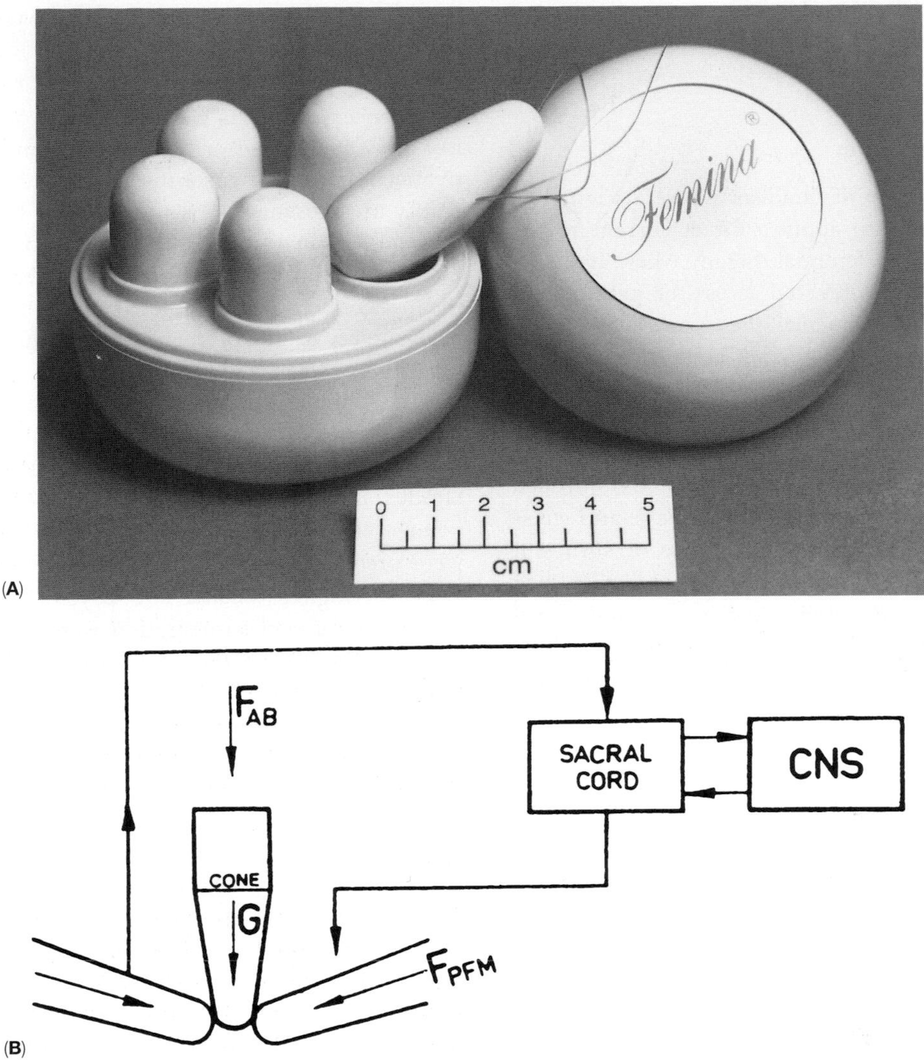

Fig. 19.6 (**A**) Vaginal cones (Colgate Medical). (**B**) Diagrammatic representation of forces on the vaginal cone when in place. G = weight of cone; F_{AB} = force due to abdominal pressure; F_{PFM} = force developed by pelvic floor muscle; CNS = central nervous system.

in 75% and 46% were continent during pad testing after daily use for 4 weeks (Hahn & Milsom, 1996). The device caused some local discomfort in 62% of patients but 72% of these wished to continue use. The Bladder Neck Support Prosthesis used over a period of 12 months provided objective reduction in urinary leakage in 87.5% of women. Complications associated with long-term use include a vaginal serous exudate, vaginal skin abrasion and bacterial cystitis (Foote et al 1996).

Urethral devices, e.g. FemAssist, are placed on the urethral meatus to seal the urethra. It has also been reported as being an effective treatment for women with stress and urge incontinence and does not cause urinary infection. The Reliance Intraurethral Device consists of a tube which is inflated proximal to the bladder neck. Prior to voiding, the balloon is deflated and the device removed. After urinating another device can then be inserted. In a multicentre study of 135 patients treated for 4 months, objective measurement of urinary loss has shown that 80% of subjects were dry and 95% achieved greater than 80% decrease in urinary loss (Staskin et al 1995). Complications with the device included difficulties with insertion, discomfort, haematuria (21%), symptomatic bacteriuria (17%) and misplaced devices (5 patients).

The Autocath 100 is an intraurethral device activated by contracting the lower abdominal muscles. The device remains open until completion of voiding then closes automatically, remaining closed during rises in intra-abdominal pressure. Preliminary results in 24 patients with genuine stress incontinence show a reduction in mean incontinence episodes from 5.53

pre-device insertion to 0.44 after insertion (Wright et al 1996). However, it may cause pain and urinary tract infection and be displaced.

Electrical stimulation

This takes the form of faradism where a vaginal or anal plug is used to apply a direct current to the pelvic floor, or interferential therapy where high frequency voltages are directed across the pelvic floor, generating a low-frequency therapeutic alternating current causing pelvic floor contraction. This method has had variable popularity over the past few years. Daily treatment of 20 minutes over a period of 30 days has been found to be effective (Plevnik et al 1986). In a review of the literature on randomized controlled trials of electrical stimulation to treat urge and stress incontinence, only three studies were of sufficient size for analysis for effect on stress incontinence, and two of these demonstrated a negative and one a positive (20%) effect of cure and 46% improved by pad test. The author concluded that, due to inadequate data regarding the efficacy of electrical stimulation, pelvic floor muscle exercise should be the first choice of treatment for stress incontinence (Bo 1998).

Many of these regimens have not been objectively tested and are often not carried out for an adequate period of time for benefit to be achieved. Berghmans et al (1998) performed a systematic review of randomized trials of physical therapy for stress incontinence. This showed strong evidence that pelvic floor muscle exercises were effective in reducing symptoms of stress incontinence, but limited evidence for the efficacy of high-intensity versus low intensity regimens. There was also no significant evidence that pelvic floor muscle exercise with biofeedback were more effective than biofeedback alone. Electrical stimulation was superior to sham electrostimulation but there was no difference between electrostimulation and other therapies.

More recently Bo & Talseth (1998) compared the effectiveness of pelvic floor exercises, electrical treatment and vaginal cones versus no treatment in a randomized trial in 118 women with genuine stress incontinence. Relief of symptoms was reported by 56% in the pelvic exercise group, 12% in the electrical stimulation group, 7.4% in the cone group and 3.3% in the control group.

SURGICAL TREATMENT

Continence surgery is indicated when conservative measures have failed or the patient wants definitive treatment now. If detrusor instability and voiding difficulty are present, the patient should be cautioned that surgery may make either condition worse and that these conditions should be treated beforehand. If the patient has not completed her family, bladder neck surgery can be performed but should she subsequently conceive and remain dry, an elective caesarean section is advised to avoid further pelvic floor damage.

To be able to predict successful surgery is advantageous. Berglund and colleagues (1997) found that a younger age with a shorter duration of incontinence were predictive factors for success, whilst neuroticism and higher somatic and psychic anxiety and lower level of social integration were common with failures – indicating the need for psychosocial support in this group.

Urge and stress incontinence often coexist. Where the primary symptom is stress incontinence, the patient is more likely to be cured of urge incontinence than those whose primary presenting symptom is urge incontinence (Scotti et al 1998).

Hutchings et al (1998) reviewed 232 patients with stress incontinence operated on by 137 gynaecologists and urologists and analysed patient and health service characteristics for factors associated with a successful outcome. Twenty-two per cent had had previous continence surgery. Reduction in symptom severity and impact were more likely with younger women with little limitation of activities of daily living, without urge or urge incontinence, not grossly obese, non- or only mild comorbidity and who had had preoperative urodynamics. In addition they found that previous continence surgery did not influence outcome. Seventy per cent of patients said they were improved but this was not broken down into primary and secondary results.

Perception of cure is important. Black et al (1997) prospectively studied 442 women undergoing a variety of continence procedures by 137 surgeons. Only 28% said they were cured. Urge incontinence was not considered an adverse factor and preoperative urodynamics had no influence. The surgeon was satisfied with the outcome in 85% of cases. If the patient is to be believed, this study highlights not only a difference in perception of cure but the continuing overall poor results of allowing continence surgery to be carried out by non-specialized centres.

A further meta-analysis by Jarvis (1998) was presented at the first WHO Conference on incontinence (Table 19.1). Jarvis, who had electronically and manually searched journals and the international scientific meeting abstracts, found that many studies did not define or use objective outcome measures, few studies reported beyond one year of follow-up; potentially confounding variables such as age, coexistent gynaecological pathology and severity of incontinence were frequently omitted and very few studies were either randomized or prospective. There needed to be a greater emphasis on detailed quality of life studies for surgeons to be aware of their own success and complications rates.

Aims of surgery

The aims of surgery are to elevate or support the bladder neck or to enhance urethral resistance or both. At the same time, any prolapse should be corrected. The patient should be informed about immediate and late complications, morbidity and success rates. Bladder neck surgery, whether performed for incontinence or prolapse, may have sequelae. The pelvic floor is one unit and surgery in one compartment can adversely affect function and anatomy in another. For example, colposuspension may initiate or cause a rectocele to enlarge, and a sacrocolpopexy or sacrospinous fixation may precipitate urethral sphincter incompetence.

Choice

The choice of surgery is influenced by the following factors.

Clinical features

This takes into account the patient's quality of life, physical fitness and expectations, position of the bladder neck, amount of vaginal scarring as assessed by capacity and mobility on vaginal examination and presence of real, or likelihood of potential prolapse.

Urodynamic data

To confirm whether the prime defect is bladder neck descent or loss of urethral resistance or both, and to detect voiding difficulties and detrusor instability, urodynamic data should be examined.

Characteristics of the operation

The operation may support or elevate the bladder neck or increase urethral resistance or occasionally do both. In addition, the operation may correct or precipitate prolapse, precipitate voiding difficulty or detrusor instability.

The surgeon individualizes the choice and bears in mind the likelihood of side-effects.

Useful operations

Bulking agents

A variety of bulking agents are now commercially available. They act by bulking tissue around the bladder neck and may lengthen the urethra and prevent premature bladder neck opening (Monga & Stanton 1997a). They do not appear to increase urethral resistance, as determined by postoperative peak flow rates and maximum voiding pressures. These agents may

Table 19.1 Meta-analysis of continence surgery.

Procedure	Cure (%)	Complication (%)	Detrusor instability (%)	Void difficulty (%)
Anterior colporrhaphy	37–84	1	8	0
Endoscopic bladder neck suspension	6–43	12	6	6
Marshall-Marchetti-Krantz	75	2.5	11	11
Colposuspension				
– open	69–90	14*	17	10
– laparoscopic	60–80	4	–	–
Paravaginal	72–97	–	–	–
Sling	67	–	17	10
Bulking agents	31–48 (obj.)	–	–	–
Artificial sphincter	92 (subj.)	17	–	–

When possible, the long-term (> 5 years) follow-up results have been used.
*prolapse
From Jarvis (1998), with permission.

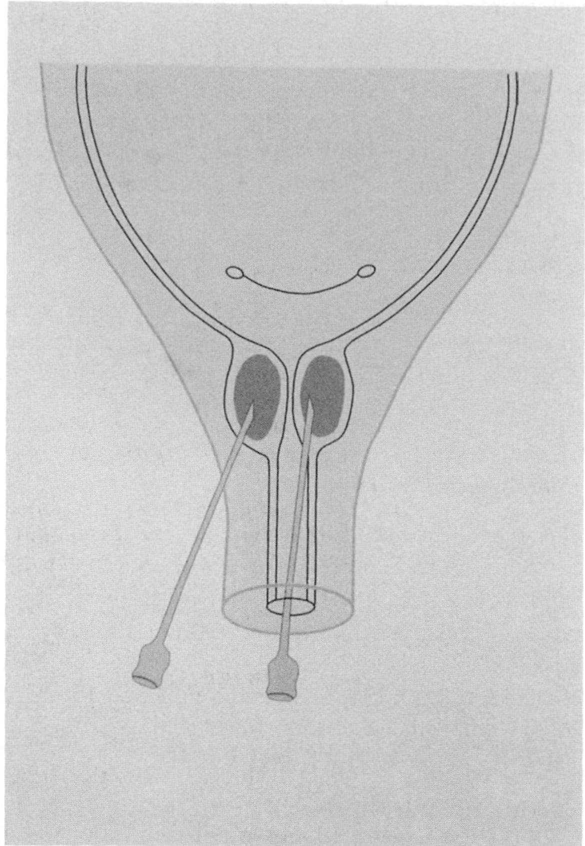

Fig. 19.7 Trans- and periurethral injection routes for bulking agents.

be injected peri- or transurethrally (Fig. 19.7). The advantage of the periurethral route is minimal leak back of bulking agent because of the longer injection route via periurethral tissues. However, there is greater difficulty in placing the agent accurately around the bladder neck compared to the transurethral route, which can be clearly visualized. Nager et al (1998) compared both routes and found no difference in success rate but noted that acute retention was commoner with the periurethral method. Either local or general anaesthesia may be used – more elderly patients prefer a local, and the technique is well established as an out-patient/day-case procedure. Although most used for impaired urethral resistance (instrinsic sphincter defect) success has been reported for hypermobility, probably because of the overlap between the two. The contraindications include acute cystitis and bladder neck or urethral stricture. Various bulking agents are described below.

***Teflon* (polytetrafluorethylene)** was popular in the '60s and '70s but migrated to lung and brain which limited its acceptability thereafter. Short-term effects included dysuria, frequency and perineal discomfort in many patients.

***Collagen* (Contigen: Bard)** is a sterile non-pyrogenic purified form of bovine dermal collagen, cross-linked with glutaraldehyde for stability. It is derived from the North American cow and no case of bovine spongiform encephalopathy has been recorded to date. It is allergenic in about 3% of patients so a skin test is needed 4 weeks before treatment. Typically patients require one to three injection sessions: as the learning curve proceeds a mean of 11 ml of collagen is usually sufficient (Monga et al 1995). Most reports indicate a subjective cure of 2 years of about 70–80% with an objective cure of 50% (Herschorn et al 1996; Cross et al 1998). Similar results are achieved in the elderly (Khullar et al 1997; Stanton & Monga 1997). A reasonable outcome (42% cured and improved) has been found with detrusor instability (Herschorn et al 1996).

***Microparticulate silicone* (Macroplastique – Uroplasty Inc.)** is a solid textured polydimethylsiloxane suspended in a non-silicone carrier gel designed to be encapsulated in fibrin with a particle size between 100 and 300 μm. This should limit its migration, though small particles are susceptible to ingestion by macrophages. It is viscous material and, therefore, needs a geared injection 'gun' with adequate lubrication of the injection needle for easier injection. Success rates appear similar to other injectables. Some concern has been expressed about the long-term use of silicone in younger patients, so careful follow-up is advised (Chaliha & Williams 1995).

Autologous fat must be the cheapest bulking agent but it is the least effective, probably due to variability of absorption.

The main indications for injectables are prior to or a refusal of major surgery because of ill health, incomplete family or further improvement needed for a previous major continence operation.

Marshall-Marchetti-Krantz

This operation has seen some modification since its description in 1949, principally by Symmonds (1972), who opened the bladder for direct visualization of placement of the sutures. This modification, which must have some morbidity, has never been tested. Unabsorbable sutures are placed distal to the bladder neck and then more proximally between periurethral tissues and perichondrium of the symphysis. In a meta-analysis of 56 papers covering 2700 procedures, Mainprize & Drutz (1989) reported a 92% subjective cure rate for a primary procedure. The long-term voiding difficulty and detrusor instability rates are shown in Table 19.1. There is a 2.5–5% instance of osteitis pubis and the operation does not correct a cystocele. There appears to be an insignificant incidence of postoperative prolapse. Colombo et al (1994) compared it to a colposuspension in a randomized control trial, and found the colposuspension to be superior for morbidity, hospital stay, time to resume spontaneous voiding and cure rate.

Tension free vaginal tape (TVT) (Fig. 19.8)

This is one of the most exciting and innovative procedures in the last 20 years of continence surgery. Hitherto, slings had been complicated, inconsistent operations, often with voiding difficulties and leading to erosion of sling materials. The TVT is different for the following reasons:

1 The sling is placed without tension under the mid-urethra
2 The patient is conscious and sling adjustment is made as the patient coughs
3 The operation is under spinal or local anaesthesia and the patient can leave hospital the same or following day
4 No catheter is needed
5 There is no reported increase in postoperative voiding difficulty, urgency or frequency.

The sling was devised by Ulf Ulmsten and Papa Petros and is made of prolene (Polypropylene – Ethicon Inc.) and is covered by a plastic sheath. Either a local anaesthetic of 0.25% of Prylocaine with adrenaline or a spinal anaesthesia is used. A 16 Foley urethral catheter is inserted into the bladder. A vertical incision is made in the anterior vaginal wall 1 cm proximal to the external urethral meatus. The mid-urethra is dissected. The sling is attached at either end to a stout needle and the tip of each is introduced lateral to the mid-urethra, to emerge behind the symphysis pubis, perforating the urogenital diaphragm, rectus sheath and then the suprapubic skin. The bladder neck is deflected by a solid introducer to the opposite side of the needle insertion. This is then repeated on the contralateral side. The catheter is removed, and the patient cystoscoped to exclude a breach of the bladder. The needles are then withdrawn through the suprapubic area and the patient asked to cough. The sling is adjusted without tension but just sufficient to produce continence. The plastic sheath is removed, the sling is trimmed and the wounds closed. The bladder is emptied partially so as to encourage early spontaneous voiding. If retention occurs, in–out catheterization is performed.

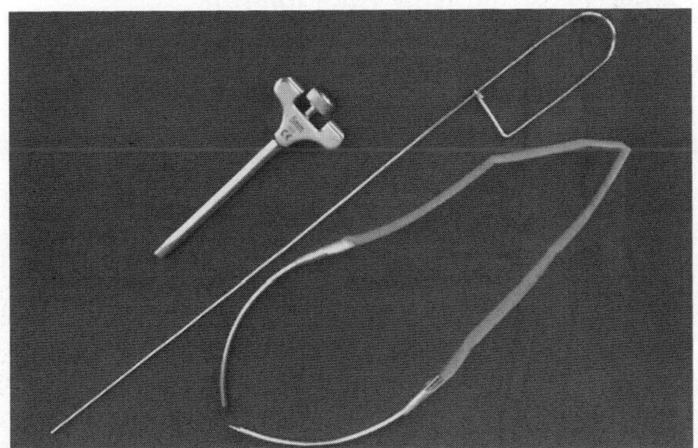

Fig. 19.8 Tension free vaginal tape (Ethicon Ltd) with the two needles, the tape and plastic sheath between them and the introducer.

A multicentre study on 50 women with primary urethral sphincter incompetence showed an objective cure of 86% at 3-year follow-up (Ulmsten et al 1999). The mean operative time was 29 minutes, 90% of patients voided within 24 hours and with insignificant residual volumes and all women were discharged within 24 hours of surgery. There were no surgical complications. There has been no rejection of tape to date. A preoperative urethral pressure profile did not dictate choice of treatment.

The indications are primary surgery without significant cystocele, irrespective of age. Careful selection in the case of secondary surgery is important because of the blind retropubic passage of the tape.

Slings

There are many sling techniques and varieties of sling materials. The latter include:

1 Organic – rectus fascia or fascia lata, porcine dermis and allograft cadaveric fascia
2 Inorganic – PTFE, Silastic bonded to Dacron, Marlex and Prolene.

Inorganic materials are known to have a higher erosion rate (Leach et al 1997). Whilst the sling has often been considered to be a secondary procedure with an objective cure rate of incontinence of about 86% (Jarvis 1994), clinicians increasingly use the sling for primary procedures, particularly where there is a reduced maximum urethral closure pressure (MUCP). Cure rates up to 94% may be obtained (Jarvis 1994) and complications are summarized in Table 19.1.

The sling is well suited to the narrowed scarred vagina and can be used for ISD or hypermobility. The use of bone anchors is a more recent vogue in the mistaken belief that failure is due to detachment of the sling or support from above. Following complications such as local infection and dislodgement, at least one manufacturer has withdrawn these anchors.

Sling complications include:

1 Urinary retention and voiding difficulty. Weinburger & Ostergard (1996) record a mean duration of postoperative catheterization of 10.7 weeks with a 76% cure rate of incontinence. Sling tension was achieved by creating a −5 to +10° bladder neck angle to the horizontal
2 Erosion
3 Urge incontinence with detrusor instability.

The appearance of the TVT would suggest now that the main indication for a sling is secondary surgery, but the technique needs to be refined to minimize the risk of voiding difficulties. The sling is believed to act by maintaining proximal urethral support and increasing the MUCP (Horbach et al 1988).

Colposuspension (Fig. 19.9)

The conventional open colposuspension remains the most popular choice for primary and secondary surgery, justified by its consistent high, short- and long-term success rate (Feyereisl et al 1994; Alcalay et al 1995). Most clinicians follow the classic description of Burch (1961), except for the increased popularity of unabsorbable sutures (Stanton 1986).

The mechanism of the colposuspension is bladder neck elevation and support which raise the pressure transmission ratio to over 100% in the first quadrant of the urethra (Hilton & Stanton 1983). In addition, there is some outlet obstruction. It is sufficient to elevate the paravaginal tissues to come into contact with the pelvic side wall without straining to reach the ileopectineal ligament – which is more likely to induce voiding difficulty, i.e. bowstringing is acceptable.

The indications for the colposuspension include primary and secondary urethral sphincter incompetence with or without a cystourethrocele and in the presence of adequate vaginal mobility and capacity. A low MUCP of < 20 cm H_2O in a woman with previous bladder neck surgery is a contraindication to a colposuspension because it is more likely to fail (Monga & Stanton 1997b). If there is more than a Grade I uterine or vault descent or a rectocele, especially in the presence of a Grade II cystourethrocele, correction is necessary as these are likely to be increased postoperatively (Wiskind et al 1992). Other complications include groin pain, which may be relieved by releasing the stitches on the affected side (Galloway et al 1987). Coexistent detrusor instability and urethral sphincter incompetence are likely to lead to significantly lower success rates for urethral sphincter incompetence and continuation of urge incontinence (Colombo et al 1996). The need to carry out a concomitant total abdominal hysterectomy should not detract from the cure rate, nor will it enhance it (Langer et al 1988).

Laparoscopic colposuspension The history of laparoscopic colposuspension is bedevilled by small studies with subjective outcome measures and inadequate follow-ups. The operation was first described by Vaincaillie in 1991 and by 1999 only two random-

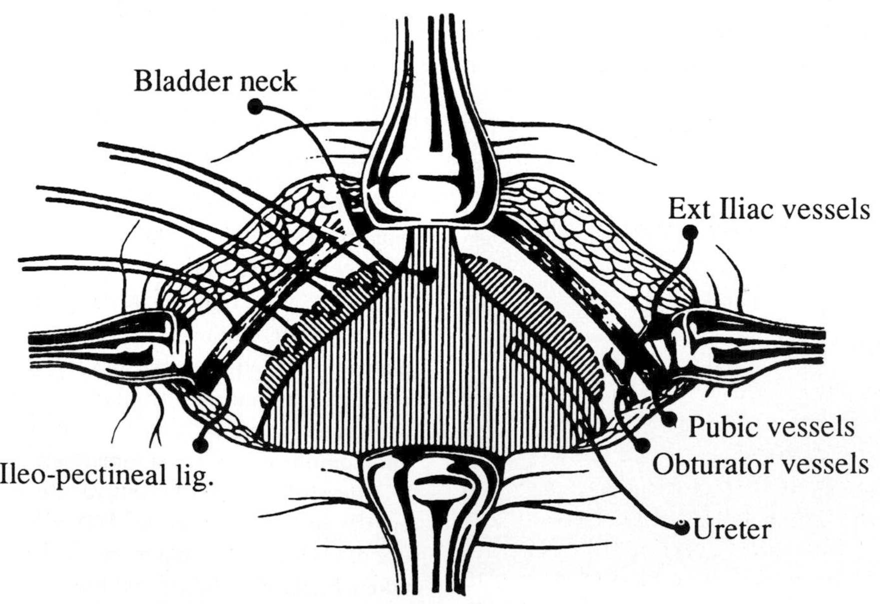

Fig. 19.9 Diagram of colposuspension as seen through a Pfannenstiel incision.

ized control trials had been reported. Most of the studies were described by general gynaecologists without urogynaecological training and often unaware of ICS definitions.

We reviewed 27 studies between 1991 and 1998, involving 1024 patients. Preoperative urodynamics were used in only 18 and postoperatively in only 6. Only 10 studies included patients with previous bladder neck surgery. The mean rate of bladder injury was 3% (0–10%). The conversion rate to open colposuspension was 2% (0–26%). The mean operating time was 92 minutes (30–300). A variety of techniques were described using transperitoneal and extraperitoneal approaches with a variety of sutures – absorbable (7), permanent (17), sutures or mesh (5), or bone anchor (1) or a combination of any of these. Only 5 studies discussed analgesia and only 8 mentioned return to work – both said to be the major advantages of a laparoscopic approach. Not surprisingly, the subjective cure rate varied considerably: 22 studies relied on a subjective assessment with a mean continence rate of 90% (40–100%). Objective outcomes were only used in four studies and gave a mean success rate of 75% (60–89%). One study was published without any results! The mean follow-up time was 19 months (6–36); 7 studies were less than 1 year. Postoperative complications were indifferently described and included prolapse (4 papers), voiding difficulty (6 papers) and detrusor instability (7 papers).

The randomized control trials were by Burton (1997) and Tsung-Hsien Su et al (1997), and adhered to ICS definitions with pre- and postoperative urodynamics. Burton showed a continence rate of 94% for the open and 60% for the laparoscopic procedures at 3 years and Tsung-Hsien Su found a continence rate of 96% for the open and 80% for the laparoscopic at 1-year follow-up.

The future assessments of laparoscopic colposuspension, or indeed any other continence procedure, should involve a randomized control trial with quality of life and objective outcome measures and a follow-up of at least 2 years.

Artificial urinary sphincter

The artificial urinary sphincter was first used in 1973 and has been extensively modified and used since then. Many different models exist and the most reliable and long-standing have been those made by American Medical Systems. The two current models are the AMS 792 which was introduced in 1980 and the AMS 800 which was first used in 1983. The AMS 792 has a separate deactivating valve (Fig. 19.10) whilst the AMS 800 has a deactivating mechanism in the pump (Fig. 19.11). The device is made of medical grade silastic and consists of a hydraulically operated cuff placed around the bladder neck, a reservoir inserted below the sheath and a pump inserted in one

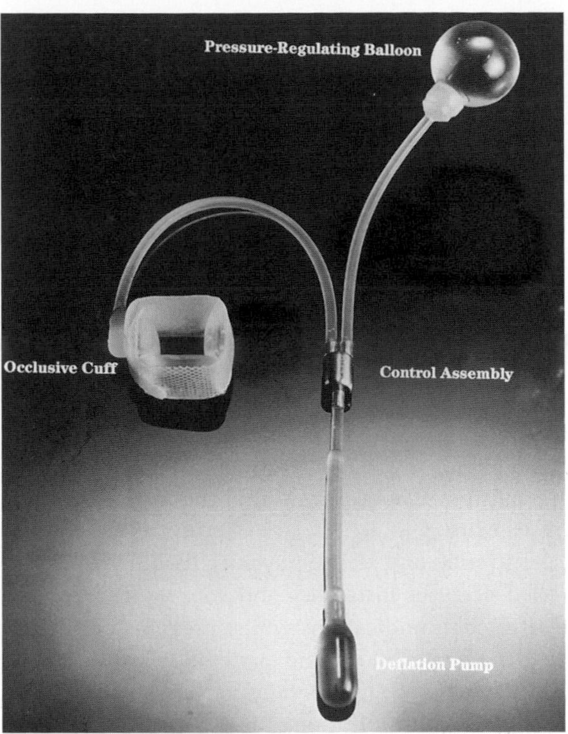

Fig. 19.10 Artificial urinary sphincter 792 (AMS).

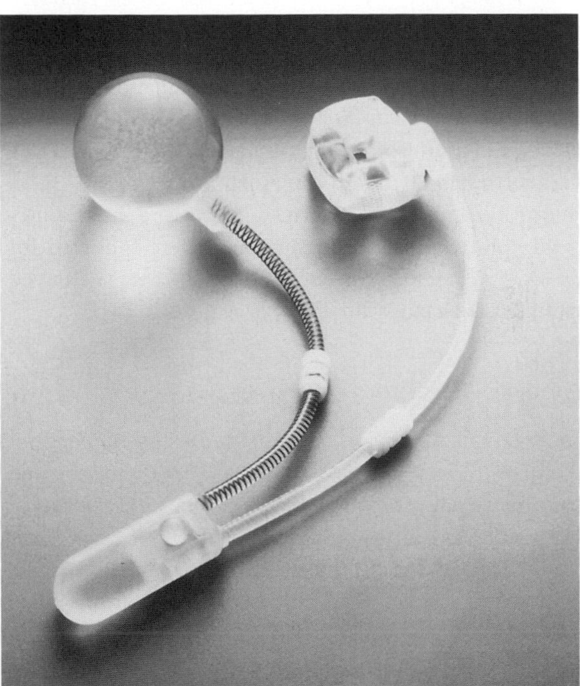
Fig. 19.11 Artificial urinary sphincter 800 (AMS).

or other labium majus. The cuff is made in a variety of sizes to fit the circumference of the urethra. The reservoir is available in three pressure models: 51–60, 61–70, 71–80 cm H_2O. The commonest pressure is between 61–70 cm H_2O. An atrophic or poorly vascularized urethra would need a lower pressure and the patient in whom a low-pressure reservoir has already failed might benefit from a higher pressure reservoir.

The indication is urethral sphincter incompetence in a patient who has failed several conventional continence operations, who has congenital anomalies, e.g. epispadias or exstrophy, and neuropathic bladder disorders with or without bladder augmentation, e.g spina bifida, myelomeningocele, spinal cord injury and multiple sclerosis. Contraindications include local sepsis, urinary infection, lack of motivation and manual dexterity, and severe physical disabilities. Uncontrolled detrusor instability and voiding disorders are relative contraindications whilst previous urethral or bladder neck erosions and patients who have had a radical course of radiotherapy to the pelvis are fairly absolute contraindications. Experience has shown that in these two groups erosion of the cuff is common; this can be reduced by wrapping the urethra with omentum before implanting the cuff.

The results vary with an improvement rate of continence of 60–92%. The five-year reliability of the device is more than 90% but revisional surgery may be needed in up to 32% of patients. The infection rate varies from 0–20% and the erosion rate from 0–30%. In our own series of 38 cases which were mainly urethral sphincter incompetence and were followed for up to 14 years, a continence rate of 60% was achieved (Stanton & Gruenwald 1999).

Paravaginal operation

Paravaginal surgery arose from studies by Richardson et al (1976) and Baden & Walker (1987) who showed the importance of endopelvic fascia as a principal supporting structure within the pelvis, which when torn resulted in stress incontinence and prolapse. Abdominal and vaginal paravaginal operations were devised to repair these defects. Shull & Baden (1989) reported a 97% cure of stress incontinence. However, when Colombo et al (1996) sought to reproduce these results in a randomized control trial with a Burch colposuspension, they only achieved a 72% subjective cure and 61% objective cure of incontinence compared to the 100% subjective and objective cure with a colposuspension. The operations are popular in the United States but less well known in Europe.

Useless operations

Anterior colporrhaphy

Although the anterior colporrhaphy is probably the oldest operation for the correction of stress incontinence and cystourethrocele, systematic reviews have now demonstrated that it is far from perfect, with studies showing continence rate of between 37% (Bergman & Elia 1995) and 65% (Stanton et al 1986). However, there are minimal postoperative complications: voiding disorders are almost non-existent and detrusor instability may only be as high as 8% (Beck et al 1991). There have been no reasonably sized studies of more than 10 years' follow-up.

The main indication today is in the correction of cystourethrocele in a completely dry patient or one who has rare stress incontinence, i.e. once or twice a year.

Endoscopic bladder neck suspension

Since its initial description in 1959 by Pereyra, there have been at least four other eponymous variations (Stamey, Raz, Cobb-Ragde and Gittes). Again systematic reviews have demonstrated that although initially thought to be an excellent minimally invasive operation with minimal side-effects, it only offers a 6–10% continence rate at 10 years (Keveligham & Jarvis 1998; [illegible]lls et al 1996). In addition there are complications including suture pain, sinus formation, detrusor instability and voiding difficulties.

POSTOPERATIVE MANAGEMENT

In the early postoperative phase, suprapubic catheter drainage and early mobilization are almost universal. Later on, avoidance of heavy lifting for 2 months and after that unnecessary heavy lifting for life are sensible.

We clamp the catheter on the second day after surgery and once the evening residual is < 200 ml with voids > 200 ml, we clamp it overnight and remove it the following morning if the same figures are found. Waiting until the residual falls below 100 ml in the presence of normal voiding is tedious and unnecessary.

MANAGEMENT OF RECURRENT INCONTINENCE

The principles of choice of primary and secondary continence surgery are very similar and will be determined by clinical, urodynamic and operative characteristics.

The clinical and urodynamic assessment is carried out; additional investigations such as a urethral pressure profile or Valsalva leak point pressure and ambulatory monitoring are more likely to be used.

The causes include:

1 Persistent urethral sphincter incompetence because the initial procedure was incorrect or inadequately performed or there were poor tissues
2 Appearance of detrusor instability or overflow retention
3 A urinary fistula.

Where a patient is almost cured of her stress incontinence, a urethral bulking agent is an ideal adjunct for further improvement. Further bladder neck elevation may be required using conventional retropubic suspension operations, e.g. colposuspension or a sling. Because of altered anatomy and retropubic fibrosis following primary surgery (particularly retropubic suspensions), the choice of a TVT may be hazardous because of its blind insertion. Where lowered urethral resistance rather than a poorly elevated or supported bladder neck is found, the sling may be more appropriate, but if that has been tried already then an artificial urinary sphincter should be considered. Finally, when all else fails, a continence diversion such as a Mitrofanoff may be used (Woodhouse & MacNeily 1994).

CONCLUSION

The last 10 years have seen clarification of knowledge on the pathophysiology of urethral sphincter incompetence, but there still remains a lag in the development of investigations to determine precisely the cause of incontinence and particularly the measurement of urethral resistance. Audit and evidence-based medicine have led to the abandonment of several operations which have been replaced by exciting new procedures.

Prophylactic measures such as determining the risk profile of women undergoing vaginal surgery to discover which women will benefit from an elective caesarean section, have still to be established. The role of prenatal pelvic floor exercises is still unclear. The potential of genetic modification of collagen which is a basic component of connective tissue, fascia and ligaments, will become more likely.

Professional organizations (such as the American Urogynecologic Society and the International Continence Society), audit and clinical governance and the medico-legal climate and patient expectations are some of the factors which will encourage a more exact application of science to the surgical treatment of incontinence. Practically, it may encourage the referral of secondary surgery to centres that have developed an expertise in this. These centres will need to have a full array of conservative and surgical options.

REFERENCES

Abrams P, Blaivas J G, Stanton S L, Andersen J T 1988 The standardisation of lower urinary tract function. The International Continence Society Committee on Standardisation of Terminology. Scandinavian Journal of Urology and Nephology (suppl.) 114: 5–19

Alcalay M, Griffiths C, Stanton S L 1994 Comparison of valsalva leak point pressure and stress urethral profilometry in the evaluation of genuine stress incontinence. Poster presentation. 24th Annual International Continence Society Meeting. Abstracts pp 39–40

Alcalay M, Monga A, Stanton S L 1995 Burch colposuspension – a 10–20-year follow-up. British Journal of Obstetrics and Gynaecology 81: 281–290

Anderson K E, Ek A, Hedlund H, Mattiasson A 1981 Effects of prazosin on isolated human urethra and in patients with lower motor neuron lesions. Investigative Urology 19: 39–42

Awad S A, Downie J W, Lywood D W, Young R A, Jarzylo S V 1976 Sympathetic activity in the proximal urethra in the patients with urinary obstruction. Journal of Urology 115: 545–547

Baden W, Walker T 1987 Urinary stress incontinence: evolution of the paravaginal repair. Female Patient 12: 89

Beck P, McCormick S, Nordstrom L 1991 A 25 year experience with 519 anterior colporrhaphy procedures. Obstetrics and Gynaecology 78: 1011–1018

Berghmans L C, Hendriks H J, Bo K, Hay-Smith E J, de Bie R A, van Waalwijk van Doorn E S 1998 Conservative treatment of stress urinary incontinence in women: a systematic review of randomized clinical trials. British Journal of Urology 82: 181–191

Berglund A, Eisemann M, Lalos A, Lalos O 1997 Predictive factors of the outcome of primary surgical treatment of stress incontinence in women. Scandinavian Journal of Urology and Nephrology 31: 49–55

Bergman A, Elia G 1995 Three surgical procedures for genuine stress incontinence – a 5 year follow up of a prospective randomised study. American Journal of Obstetrics and Gyneacology 173: 66–71

Black N, Grittiths J, Pope C 1997 Impact of surgery for stress incontinence or morbidity. British Medical Journal 315: 1993–1998

Bo K 1998 Effect of electrical stimulation on stress and urge incontinence. Clinical outcome and practical recommendations based on randomised trials. Acta Obstetrica et Gynecologica Scandinavica 168: 3–11

Bo K, Talseth T 1998 Single blinded randomised controlled trial on the effect of pelvic floor muscle strength training, electrical stimulation, cones or control on severe genuine stress incontinence. Neurourology and Urodynamics 17: 421–422

Bump R C, Elser D M, Theofrastous J P, McClish D K 1995 Valsalva leak point pressures in women with genuine stress incontinence: reproducibility, effect of catheter caliber, and correlations with other measures of urethral resistance. Continence Program for Women Research Group. American Journal of Obstetrics and Gynecology 173: 551–557

Burch J 1961 Urethro–vaginal fixation to Cooper's ligament for correction of stress incontinence, cystocele and prolapse. American Journal of Obstetrics and Gynecology 81: 281–290

Burton G 1997 A 3 year prospective randomised urodynamic study comparing open and laparoscopic colposuspension. Neurourology and Urodynamics 16: 353–354

Cardozo L, Stanton S L 1980 Genuine stress incontinence and detrusor instability: a review of 200 patients. British Journal of Obstetrics and Gynaecology 87: 184–190

Chaliha C, Williams G 1995 Periurethral injection therapy for treatment of urinary incontinence. British Journal of Urology 76: 151–155

Chaliha C, Kalia V, Stanton S L et al 1998 What does pregnancy and delivery do to bladder function? A urodynamic viewpoint. Neurourology and Urodynamics 17: 415–416.

Chaliha C, Kalia V, Stanton S L 1999 Antenatal prediction of postpartum urinary and faecal incontinence. Obstetrics and Gynecology (in press)

Colombo M, Scalambrino S, Maggioni A, Milani R 1994 Burch colposuspension versus modified Marshall-Marchetti-Krantz urethropexy for primary genuine stress incontinence: a prospective randomised control trial. American Journal of Obstetrics and Gynecology 171: 153–159

Colombo N, Milani R, Vitovello D 1996 A randomised comparison of Burch colposuspension and abdominal paravaginal defect repair for female stress urinary incontinence. American Journal of Obstetrics and Gynecology 175: 78–84

Creighton S M, Gillon G, Stanton S L 1992 Aetiological factors in stress urinary incontinence in nulliparous women. Journal of Obstetrics and Gynaecology 12: 130–132

Creighton S M, Clark A, Pearce J M, Stanton S L 1994 Bladder neck ultrasound: appearances before and after continence surgery. Ultrasound in Obstetrics and Gynaecology 4: 428–433

Cross C, English S, Cespedes D, McGuire E 1998 A follow up on transurethral collagen injection therapy for urinary incontinence. Journal of Urology 159: 106–108

Dwyer P L, Teele J S 1992 Prazosin: a neglected cause of genuine stress incontinence. Obstetrics and Gynecology 79: 117–121

Fantl A, Cardozo L, Ekberg J, McClish D 1994 Estrogen therapy in the management of urinary incontinence in postmenopausal women: a meta analysis. Obstetrics and Gynecology 83: 12–18

Feyereisl J, Dreher E, Haenggi W et al 1994 Long term results after Burch colposuspension. American Journal of Obstetrics and Gynecology 171: 697–652

Foldspang A, Lam G W, Elving L 1992 Parity as a correlate of adult female urinary incontinence prevalence. Journal of Epidemiology and Community Health 46: 595–600

Foote A J, Moore K, King J 1996 A prospective study of the long term use of the bladder neck support prosthesis. Neurourology and Urodynamics 15(4): 404–406

Galloway N, Davies N, Stephenson T 1987 The complications of colposuspension. British Journal of Urology 60: 122–124

Hahn I, Milsom I 1996 Treatment of female stress urinary incontinence with a new anatomically shaped vaginal device (Conveen Continence Guard). British Journal of Urology 77: 711–715

Haylen B T, Frazer M I 1987 Is the investigation of stress incontinence really necessary? Neurourology and Urodynamics 6: 188–189

Herschorn S, Steele D, Radonski S 1996 Follow up of intra-urethral collagen for female stress incontinence. Journal of Urology 156: 1305–1309

Hilton P 1988 Unstable urethral pressure: towards a more relevant definition. Neurourology and Urodynamics 6: 411–418

Hilton P, Stanton S L 1983 Urethral pressure measurements by microtransducer: the results in symptom-free women and those with genuine stress incontinence. British Journal of Obstetrics and Gynaecology 90: 919–933

Horbach N, Bianco J, Ostergard D, Bent A, Cornella J 1988 A suburethral sling procedure with polytetrafluorothylene for the treatment of genuine stress incontinence in patients with a low urethral pressure. Obstetrics and Gynecology 71: 648–652

Hutchings A, Griffiths J, Black N 1998 Surgery for stress incontinence: factors associated with a successful outcome. British Journal of Urology 82: 634–641

Jarvis G 1994 Surgery for genuine stress incontinence. British Journal of Obstetrics and Gynaecology 101: 371–374

Jarvis G 1998 The surgery of genuine stress incontinence. Report to the first WHO conference on incontinence, Monaco

Keane D, Sims T, Bailey A, Abrams P 1992 Analysis of pelvic floor electromyography and collagen studies in pre-menopausal nulliparous females with genuine stress incontinence. Neurourology and Urodynamics 11: 308–309

Kevelighan E, Aagaard J, Balasubramaniam B, Jarvis G 1998 The Stamey endoscopic bladder neck suspension: a 10 year follow up study. 28th British Congress Abstracts 47

Khullar V, Cardozo L, Abbott D, Anders K 1997 Gax collagen in the treatment of urinary incontinence in elderly women: a two year follow up. British Journal of Obstetrics and Gynaecology 104: 96–99

Kirulata H G, Andrews K 1983 Urinary incontinence secondary to drugs. Urology 2: 88–90

Langer R, Ron-El R, Neuman M, Herman A, Bukovsky I, Caspi E 1988 Value of simultaneous hysterectomy during Burch colposuspension for urinary stress incontinence. Obstetrics and Gynecology 72: 866–869

Lawrence W, McQuilkin P, Mann D 1989 Suprapubic catheterisation. British Journal of Urology 63: 443

Leach G, Dmochoski R, Appell R, et al 1997 AUA report on surgical management of female stress urinary incontinence. American Urological Association Baltimore

Mainprize T, Drutz H 1989 The MMK procedure – a critical review. Obstetrical and Gynecological Survey 43: 724–729

McGuire E J, Fitzpatrick C C, Wan J et al 1993 Clinical assessment of uretural sphincter function. Journal of Urology 150: 1452–1454

Mills R, Persad R, Ashken M 1996 Long term follow up results with the Stamey operation for stress urinary incontinence of urine. British Journal of Urology 77: 86–88

Monga A, Stanton S L 1997a Urodynamics: prediction, outcome and analysis of mechanism of cure of stress incontinence by periurethral collagen. British Journal of Obstetrics and Gynaecology 104: 158–162

Monga A K, Stanton S L 1997b Predicting outcome of colposuspension – a prospective evaluation. Neurourology and Urodynamics 16: 354–355.

Monga A, Robinson D, Stanton S L 1995 Periurethral collagen injection for genuine stress incontinence: a 2 year follow up. British Journal of Urology 78: 156–160

Nager C, Schulz J, Stanton S L 1998 Bulking agents for genuine stress incontinence: short term results and complications in a randomised comparison of periurethral and transurethral injections. International Urogynecology Journal 10: 76

Nemir A, Middleton R 1954 Stress incontinence in nulliparous women. American Journal of Obstetrics and Gynecology 68: 1166–1168

Ng R, Murray A 1989 Place of routine urodynamics in the management of female GSI. Neurourology and Urodynamics 8: 307–308

Nygaard I E, Thompson F L, Svengalis S L, Albright J P 1994 Urinary incontinence in elite nulliparous athletes. Obstetrics and Gynecology 84: 183–187

Pereyra A 1959 A simplified surgical procedure for the correction of stress urinary incontinence in women. Western Journal of Surgery Obstetrics and Gynecology 67: 223–226

Peschers U, Schaer G, Anthuber C, Delancey J O L, Schuessler B 1996 Changes in vesical neck mobility following vaginal delivery. Obstetrics and Gynecology 88: 1001–1006

Plevnik S 1985 New method for testing and strengthening of pelvic floor muscles. Proceedings of the 15th Annual Meeting of the International Continence Society, London, pp 267–268

Plevnik S, Janez J, Vrtacnik P, Trsinar B, Vodusek D 1986 Short term electrical stimulation: home treatment for urinary incontinence. World Journal of Urology 4: 24–26

Richardson A, Lyon J, Willimans N 1976 A new look at pelvic relaxation. American Journal of Obstetrics and Gynecology 126: 568–575

Sand P K, Boweb L W, Panganiban R, Ostergard D R 1987 The low pressure urethra as a factor in failed retropubic urethropexy Obstetrics and Gynecology 69: 399–402

Sayer T, Dixon J, Hosker G, Warrell D W 1989 A histological study of pubocervical fascia in women with stress incontinence of urine. International Urogynecology Journal 1: 18

Scotti R, Angell G, Flora R, Greston W 1998 Antecedent history as a predictor of surgical cure of urgency symptoms in mixed incontinence. Obstetrics and Gynecology 91: 51–54

Shull B, Baden W 1989 A six year experience with paravaginal defect repair for stress urinary incontinence. American Journal of Obstetrics and Gynecology 161: 432–440

Smith A R B 1991 The aetiology of genuine stress incontinence. Advances in Obstetrics and Gynaecology 1: 3–9

Snooks S J, Swash M, Setchell M, Henry M M 1984 Injury to the innervation of pelvic floor sphincter musculature in childbirth. The Lancet ii: 546–550

Stanton S L 1986 Colposuspension. In: Stanton S L, Tanagho E (eds) Surgery of Female Incontinence, 2nd edn. Springer Verlag, Heidelberg, pp 95–103

Stanton S L, Monga A 1997 Incontinence in elderly women: is periurethral collagen an advance? British Journal of Obstetrics and Gynaecology 104: 154–157

Stanton S L, Gruenwald E (in press) Artificial urinary sphincter for resistant urethral sphincter incompetence in the female. British Journal of Urology

Stanton S L, Cardozo L, Riddle P R 1981 Urological complications of traumatic diastasis of the symphysis pubis in the female. British Journal of Urology 53: 453–454

Stanton S L, Chamberlain G, Holmes D 1986 Randomised study of the anterior repair and colposuspension operation in the control of genuine stress incontinence. Proceedings of the 15th Annual Meeting of the International Continence Society, pp 236–237

Stanton S L, Kerr Wilson R, Harns V G 1980 Incidence of Urological symptoms in normal pregnancy. British Journal of Obstetrics and Gynaecology 87: 897–900

Staskin D, Sant G, Sand P et al 1995 Use of an expandable urethral insert for GSI: longterm results of a multi-center trial. Neurourology and Urodynamics 5: 420–422

Staskin D, Bavendam T, Miller J et al 1980 Prevalence of urinary incontinence. British Medical Journal 281: 1243–1245

Symmonds R 1972 Suprapubic approach to anterior vaginal relaxation and urinary stress incontinence. Clinics in Obstetrics and Gynecology 15: 1107–112

Tapp A, Hills B, Cardozo L 1989 Randomised study comparing pelvic floor physiotherapy with Burch colposuspension. 19th Annual meeting of the International continence Society, Ljubljana. Neurourology and Urodynamics 8: 356–357

Theofrastous J P, Bump R C, Elser D M, Wyman J F, McClish D K 1995 Correlation of urodynamic measures of urethral resistance with clinical measures of incontinence severity in women with pure genuine stress incontinence. The Continence Program for Women Research Group. American Journal of Obstetrics and Gynecology 173: 407–412

Thomas T M, Plymat K, Blannin J, Meade T 1980 Prevalence of urinary incontinence. British Medical Journal 281: 1243–1245

Tsung-Hsien Su, Kuo-Gon Wang, Chin-Yuan Hsu, Hsiao-Jui Wei, Bin-Kuan Hong. 1997 Prospective comparison of laparoscopic and traditional colposuspension in the treatment of genuine stress incontinence. Acta Obstetrica Gynecologica Scandinavica 76: 576–582

Ulmsten U, Johnson P, Rezapour M 1999 A three year follow up of tension free vaginal tape for surgical treatment of stress urinary incontinence. British Journal of Obstetrics and Gynaecology 106: 345–350

Vaincaillie T, Schluessler P 1991 Laparoscopic bladder neck suspension. Journal of Laparoendoscopic Surgery 3: 169–173

Versi E, Cardozo L D, Studd J, Cooper D 1986 Evaluation of urethral pressure profilometry for the diagnosis of genuine stress incontinence. World Journal of Urology 4: 6–9

Weinburger M, Ostergard D 1996 Post operative catheterisation, urinary retention and permanent voiding dysfunction after polytetrafluorethylene suburethral sling placement. Obstetrics and Gynecology 87: 50–54

Wilson P D, Herbison R M, Herbison G P 1996 Obstetric practice and the prevalence of urinary incontinence three months after delivery. British Journal of Obstetrics and Gynaecology 103: 154–161

Wiskind A, Creighton S, Stanton S L 1992 The incidence of genital prolapse after the Burch colposuspension. American Journal of Obstetrics and Gynecology 167: 399–405

Woodhouse C R J, MacNeily A E 1994 The Mitrofanoff principle: expanding upon a versatile technique. British Journal of Urology 74: 447–453

Wright M, Bladou F, Borkowski A et al 1996 Restoring continence with the Autocath 100 in women. Neurourology and Urodynamics 15(4): 401–403

Detrusor instability

SUZIE VENN AND TONY MUNDY

INTRODUCTION

An unstable bladder is defined as 'one that is shown objectively to contract, spontaneously or on provocation, during the filling phase while the patient is attempting to inhibit micturition' (Abrams et al 1988). Put more simply, it is a bladder that contracts when it wants to rather than when its owner wants it to. The result is urgency. The incidence of detrusor instability (DI) is thought to be 10% in the UK (Cardozo 1991). The problem is more common in women, particularly the elderly, but only a small number will seek medical advice.

Detrusor instability can be divided into:

1 Primary idiopathic
2 Secondary to bladder outflow obstruction
3 Neuropathic (now called detrusor hyperreflexia, and considered separate).

AETIOLOGY

There are a number of theories currently postulated to explain DI because the aetiology of DI remains unclear (Chapple & Smith 1994). These include:

1 Postjunctional supersensitivity
2 Altered adrenoceptor function
3 Afferent nerve dysfunction
4 Imbalance of neurotransmitters
5 Primary or acquired myogenic deficit.

These theories are based on two approaches. Male patients with BOO (bladder outflow obstruction) have a higher incidence of DI than their age-matched controls, and following relief of obstruction, the number with DI will return to the age norm (Turner-Warwick 1984). Although there is debate about this statistical method of establishing bladder outflow obstruction as a cause of instability in men, the concept of cause and effect appears to be accepted. Because of this finding, the outlet obstructed animal model has been used to study DI (Jorgensen et al 1983).

The pig model confirmed that DI can be induced by creating bladder neck obstruction and suggested that it could be relieved by removing the obstruction (Sibley 1985; Speakman et al 1991; Brading & Turner 1994). In vivo experiments have shown that detrusor (bladder) muscle fibres from unstable bladders are more sensitive to pharmacological stimulation with acetylcholine and are more sensitive to electrical stimulation than those from stable bladders. The overall pattern of abnormality is one of postjunctional supersensitivity, which characteristically is the result of denervation. Denervation was confirmed by Speakman et al (1987), who also showed evidence that reinnervation occurred after the relief of obstruction. Unfortunately, it has not been possible to demonstrate any significant physiological or morphological difference between stable and unstable obstructed human bladders.

Kinder & Mundy (1987) examined non-obstructed unstable females and found an increased incidence of spontaneous activity in unstable detrusor muscle, noting that this activity was of a greater frequency and amplitude than normal. Unstable detrusor muscle fibres are more responsive to lower frequency stimulation although they are normal at higher frequency. This was thought to be due to a reduction in inhibitory neurotransmitters normally found in the detrusor muscle. This was supported by Gu et al (1983) who found a reduction in the number of VIP or VIP-immunoreactive nerves in unstable detrusor smooth muscle. Subsequent work has confirmed this, and suggested other neuropeptides may also be involved.

Work on geriatric patients with instability due to outflow obstruction (Elbadawi et al 1993) has suggested a reduction in the 'intermediate muscle cell junctions', and replacement by two other junctions resulting in low resistance pathways mediating electrical conduction.

A recent review by Fry & Wu (1998), has suggested that all the changes in cell physiology may result from ischaemia due to reduced blood flow to the detrusor. There is a reduction in blood flow during filling and spontaneous contraction; this is worse with hypertrophy. The contractile changes at a cellular level could be explained by partial denervation due to ischaemia, and exacerbated by the appearance of additional purinergic pathways and alterations in calcium regulation. In addition, improved intracellular coupling would allow any electrical activity to spread more easily. This review brings together a number of the previous theories, and although there are a lot of areas requiring further investigation, it may allow the development of new targeted therapeutic agents and identify causes to prevent development of detrusor instability.

CLINICAL PRESENTATION

Most patients present with urinary frequency, urgency and urge incontinence. The frequency occurs because the unstable contractions usually develop at less than maximum bladder capacity. Urgency occurs because the patient feels that her bladder is about to empty (as indeed it is) and the urge incontinence because the sphincter mechanisms are unable to resist the force of the detrusor contraction. This is either because the sphincter mechanism is intrinsically weak or because attempts to resist the unstable contraction cause discomfort. Some patients have no sensation of detrusor contraction and therefore have insensible incontinence, but this is uncommon. Symptoms are marked when standing or walking and less noticeable at rest, either sitting or lying, but frequently posture and activity make no difference, in which case nocturia may also occur. Patients may have a high threshold for bladder volume before unstable contractions develop and so do not have much in the way of frequency. In these cases, the main symptom is urge. The causes of urgency are:

1 Motor urgency
   (a) Primary detrusor instability
   (b) DI with bladder outflow obstruction
   (c) Neuropathic
2 Sensory urgency
   (a) Lower urinary tract pathology
   (b) Idiopathic
3 Urethral instability.

The distinction between motor and sensory urgency is made on urodynamic testing. Idiopathic bladder hypersensitivity produces characteristic extreme sensitivity on passing a urethral catheter, an early first sensation of filling due to low bladder capacity with no demonstrable detrusor abnormality. This group of patients, although easily recognized, is extremely difficult to treat.

More important diagnostically and therapeutically is the overlap of sensory urgency and DI with normal. It is quite common to find a convincing history that strongly suggests detrusor instability and yet find a normal urodynamic tracing, sometimes on repeated investigation (see 'Ambulatory urodynamics' below). Such an overlap is also seen in patients with the affective disorders and it is recognized that patients with anxiety-depression frequently complain of urge-type symptoms. It has to be said that there are a lot of patients with normal affect who have all the clinical features of an unstable bladder but a normal urodynamic study. These patients tend to respond to bladder retraining techniques but if not are difficult to help.

INVESTIGATIONS

Examination is important, particularly to exclude a neurological condition. It may be necessary to perform a more detailed neurological examination in the light of urodynamic findings.

Urodynamics

A simple flow rate study is often strongly suggestive of the diagnosis of detrusor instability, particularly when taken in conjunction with a strongly suggestive history. A rapidly rising ascending limb of the flow rate study with an early onset of peak flow (Fig. 20.1) is characteristic of the unstable bladder. Having said that, some patients with better control of their sphincters may go rushing to the toilet only to find by the time they get there that the unstable contraction has subsided and that, paradoxically, they have difficulty in emptying.

Definitive urodynamic investigation requires a double-channel subtracted cystometrogram so that subtracted detrusor pressure can be derived to exclude pressure rises due to artefact (Fig. 20.2). About 50% of patients with unstable bladders will show spontaneous detrusor contractile activity during filling: the remainder only show involuntary contractions on provocation. The provocations that are most commonly applied are, firstly, rapid bladder filling, secondly, coughing and thirdly, standing up from lying down. The incidence of response to each of these provocative factors probably varies from unit to unit. In our unit, postural instability is the most commonly observed, but it probably does not matter at all whether the patient has spontaneous instability, cough-induced instability or postural instability. The fact of the matter is they are unstable, although there is some suggestion from sequential studies in children that the usual pattern of development is from spontaneous instability to end-fill instability to postural instability (Borzyskowski & Mundy 1987) and that cough-induced instability is more commonly found in older patients with a more recent onset of symptoms.

The purpose of urodynamic investigation is not just to show the presence or absence of unstable detrusor contractions. In female patients, it is important to exclude associated sphincter weakness incontinence,

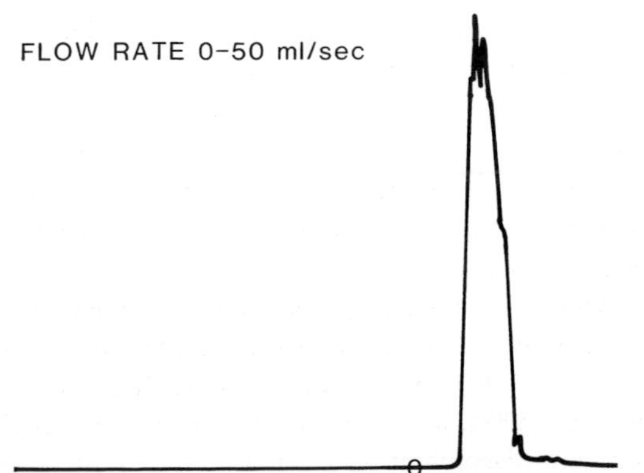

Fig. 20.1 The typical flow pattern of a patient with an unstable bladder. From Mundy & Stephenson (1985).

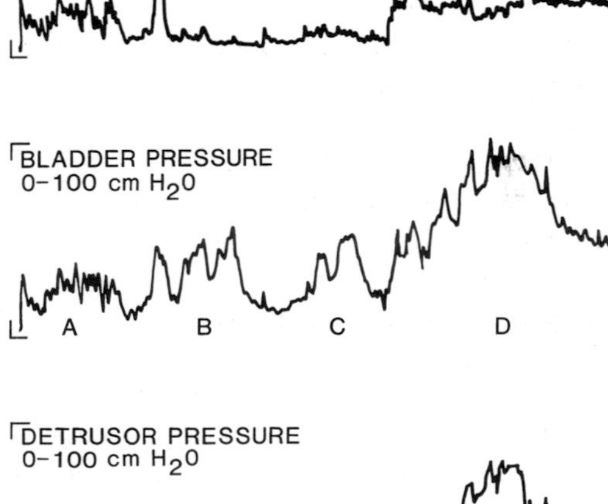

Fig. 20.2 The urodynamic trace of a patient with a very unstable bladder, showing the importance of electronic subtraction to give true detrusor pressure. The pressure changes in the (total) bladder pressure trace at A are entirely due to coughing as shown in the rectal pressure line. The detrusor trace therefore shows no change in pressure. By contrast, at C, the changes in bladder pressure are due to detrusor contraction and the rectal pressure trace therefore shows no significant change. At B, the patient is coughing and this has provoked detrusor instability. There are therefore changes in all three traces but the subtraction allows distinction of the cause in each. At D the patient is (at last) voiding voluntarily. From Mundy & Stephenson (1985).

and in male patients, it is important to exclude associated bladder outflow obstruction, either at the level of the prostate in the elderly or the bladder neck proper in young men. In both sexes, the adequacy or otherwise of bladder emptying is also important to assess because detrusor instability associated with poor bladder emptying is a particularly difficult combination to treat. Most patients have normal bladder compliance and normal urethral relaxation and when abnormalities of these two parameters occur together in association with detrusor instability, it is important to reassess the patient clinically to be sure that a neurological cause has not been overlooked. Usually, however, poor compliance is a response to the rate of bladder filling and sphincteric activity during voiding is more commonly due to nervousness or apprehension.

Ambulatory urodynamics

Ambulatory urodynamics should be considered in patients with a history strongly suggestive of instability, where conventional urodynamics have failed to demonstrate DI. Ambulatory urodynamics demonstated DI where conventional urodynamics had not in 31 patients, in a series of 52 with clinical suspicion of instability (Webb 1991).

Other investigations

These may include urine culture and cytology, and cystoscopy to exclude other causes, and to assess functional bladder capacity of the conscious and anaesthetized patient, to determine how much improvement in bladder function can be achieved.

TREATMENT

The majority of patients with DI are probably dealt with by their family doctor, from whom reassurance will be sought that there is no serious underlying cause. It is important not to overlook the value of this reassurance in an anxious patient. The treatment of DI can be grouped into non-medical, non-surgical; drug therapy; and surgical.

Non-medical, non-surgical

Bladder training

It is important as a first line in the treatment of the unstable bladder to keep the onus of treatment with the patient. Many patients bring along their symptoms to a doctor and hand them over to the doctor. In the first instance, the doctor must hand them back to the patient. This process is glorified with the 'scientific' term 'bladder retraining'. Many patients with minor symptoms from DI can be helped in this way, whereby they are instructed to void at increasing time intervals and to resist the urge to void between times (Frewen 1982), in the hope that improved conscious control will lead to improved subconscious control.

Jarvis (1981) demonstrated an 84% continence rate with in-patient bladder retraining compared with 56% with drug treatment. For patients with frequency and urgency who have a strong enough urethral sphincter mechanism to resist the unstable contraction, this may often be effective on its own. At times, however, an anticholinergic agent may need to be added, at least initially, to help regain bladder control in those with a weak urethral sphincter.

Patients with symptoms of an unstable bladder but a normal urodynamic study do particularly well with this approach, and the improvement is often maintained in the long term (Holmes et al 1983). The results in the other groups are less satisfactory. Patients who have urge incontinence, usually due to an associated sphincter weakness, do not do well with bladder retraining alone and in these patients drug treatment should be routinely added.

Biofeedback

This involves re-education by providing feedback education involving a visual, tactile or auditory signal (Cardozo et al 1978). This method is unlikely to be successful with a weak distal sphincter mechanism, but may have a role with less severe symptoms.

Both the above techniques are very labour intensive. It is pointless to persist if they are not effective, as the patient will lose confidence and it is obviously a waste of paramedical resources.

Electrical stimulation

The principle of peripheral electrical stimulation in idiopathic DI is to stimulate nerve sites in the vaginal or anal areas, to stimulate the urethral musculature to contract and inhibit the detrusor muscle. An 88% improvement or cure has been reported in 48 women with DI, with 77% still successful at one year (Erickson et al 1989). The use of this technique is limited by pain and discomfort.

Drug therapy

Anticholinergics

These are currently the only class of drugs effective in DI. Oxybutynin has for a number of years been the best available. Unfortunately, when given at effective doses, the side-effect of a dry mouth is found intolerable by a large number of patients. Children seem to tolerate the side-effects better. Other alternatives include propantheline, imipramine and others (Steers et al 1996) but it is unusual for these to be beneficial if oxybutynin has failed.

Recently tolterodine, a new anticholinergic, has been licensed. This drug has greater action on the muscarinic receptors in the bladder than the salivary glands. Early results indicate that it is as effective as oxybutynin, but with fewer side-effects (Abrams et al 1998).

Intravesical oxybutynin

Patients unable to tolerate oral oxybutynin can be treated with intermittent clean catheterization and instillation of intravesical oxybutynin. The effects of this treatment have been described (O'Flynn & Thomas 1993). Interestingly, the plasma drug levels are higher than with oral administration, but the side-effects are fewer.

Intravesical capsaicin

The capsaicin-sensitive fibres are on the afferent side of the micturition reflex loop. If these afferent fibres are blocked or desensitized, the reflex contractions are abolished. Capsaicin has been used successfully in detrusor hyperreflexia (Fowler et al 1994) but not in idiopathic DI.

Surgical treatment

Denervation procedures

Over the years there have been numerous attempts at surgical treatment of DI. A number of these have involved techniques aimed at denervating the detrusor muscle. In light of the Oxford group findings (Brading & Turner 1994) that denervation may lead to instability, this approach now seems illogical. However, a number of procedures have been used over the years with some success.

Hydrostatic dilatation This is the simplest approach and involves distending the bladder under general anaesthetic. Initial reports were encouraging but more recent studies have cast doubt on the long-term efficacy of this technique (Lloyd et al 1992).

Bladder transection This consists of full thickness transection of the bladder just above the ureteric bar and orifices, extending around the sides and front wall of the bladder (Mundy 1983). The experience with this technique was gained prior to oxybutynin and two thirds to three quarters of patients showed marked symptomatic improvement, although this was not always mirrored by improvement in objective urodynamic finding, except for functional bladder capacity.

Oxybutynin largely replaced bladder transection, as the same patients responded to both oxybutynin and transection. Its only role was therefore in patients who could not tolerate oxybutynin or did not wish to take the drug long-term.

Infiltration of pelvic plexus with phenol This treatment can be effective and avoids the need for an open operation (Blackford et al 1984). It cannot be used in men due to the high incidence of impotence. There have also been reports of fistula occurring as a result of the procedure, and for this reason it has largely been abandoned (Chapple et al 1991).

Bladder augmentation

For the majority of patients who fail to respond to conservative methods of treatment, augmentation or 'clam' cystoplasty is the only reliable treatment (Mundy & Stephenson 1985).

The principle of a clam cystoplasty is to ignore the detrusor contractile activity, but render it ineffective by transection of the bladder followed by interposition of a gut segment. The surgical details are beyond the scope of this chapter (Mundy 1988, 1993). However, the principle is to split the bladder almost completely from a point a centimetre or two lateral to the bladder neck and a centimetre or two in front of the ureteric orifice on one side, round the maximum coronal circumference of the bladder to a similar point on the other side (Fig. 20.3). The bladder circumference is then measured, a section of ileum of equal length is mobilized at a distance of at least 15 cm, or preferably further, from the ileocaecal valve, to reduce the risk of adverse nutritional and metabolic consequences. The segment of gut is isolated on its vascular pedicle and an enteroanastomosis is performed to restore intestinal continuity. The gut segment is then opened on its antimesenteric border to form a patch and this patch is then sewn into the bisected bladder using a

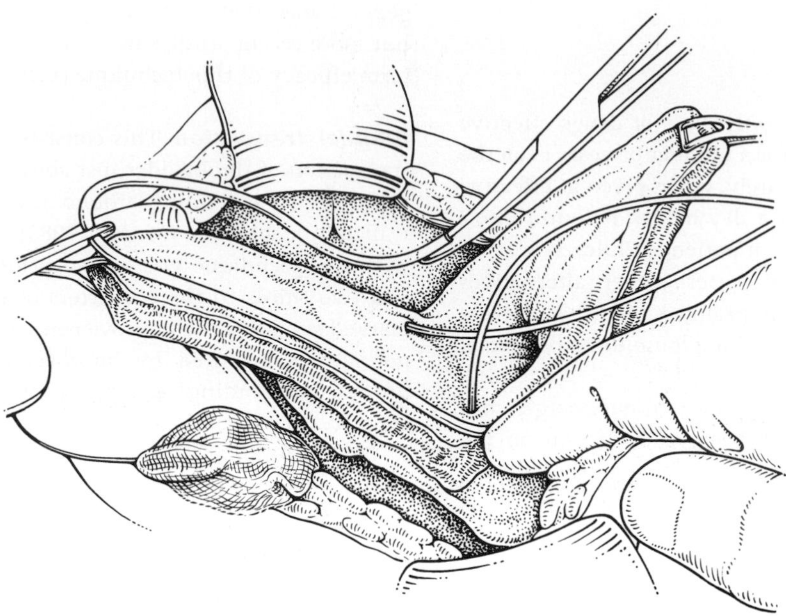

Fig. 20.3 Clam cystoplasty, technique 1. The bladder is opened in the coronal plane; the ureteric orifices have both been catheterized. The maximal bladder circumference is being measured with a length of vinyl tubing to determine the length of the ileal segment to be isolated to form the cystoplasty patch. From Mundy (1988).

running Vicryl stitch (Fig. 20.4). A suprapubic catheter is left in place, brought out through the anterior wall of the bladder, and 10 days later is clamped for a trial of voiding. Once voiding has been re-established, either spontaneously or by intermittent self-catheterization, the suprapubic catheter is removed and the patient discharged home. Follow-up urodynamics are performed at three months to demonstrate the reduction of detrusor contractile activity and to assess voiding efficiency.

The procedure is a major operation with morbidity and potential mortality, so very careful consideration is required before it is undertaken. The patient must persuade the surgeon to perform the operation; not the other way round. Reassessment with urodynamic and psychological and bladder symptom assessment should be performed prior to the operation.

The complications of this procedure are those of any major operation, plus:

1 Failure to empty. The patient must be warned of the possible need to perform clean intermittent self-catheterization (CISC). This is unusual in non-neuropathic DI. Most women have a degree of sphincter weakness which often disappears after a 'clam' but allows the patient to empty. Patients who consider life-long CISC as much of a problem as persistent DI should be dissuaded from further treatment.
2 Fluid and electrolyte disturbance. Because of absorption by the gut segment, a hyperchloraemic acidosis may occur. The resultant compensation may result in demineralization. This has not so far proved to be a problem in adults, but does affect growth in children. Treatment with an adequate dose of bicarbonate is usually all that is required.
3 Stones. Approximately 6% will develop bladder stones any time from 6 months to 8 years postoperatively (Mundy 1993). Those requiring CISC to empty have a much higher incidence.
4 Infections/tumours. Infection on its own is an irritating problem and one that may prove difficult or impossible to eradicate. More common is chronic asymptomatic bacteriuria and the significance of this in the long term is not known. The concern about this is the consequent formation of nitrosamines, which are known to be carcinogenic, and may be responsible for the occasional tumours which have been reported in cystoplasties (Filmer & Spencer 1990).
5 Mucus production. This usually settles, but may cause plugs. Washout with a mucolytic agent may be required. Another alternative is oral ranitidine. With recurrent UTIs, long-term prophylactic antibiotics may be required.
6 Others. Contractile activity of the gut segment is not usually a problem with augmentation cystoplasty. Nutritional (B_{12}) deficiency has not been shown to be significant. Pregnancy is not a

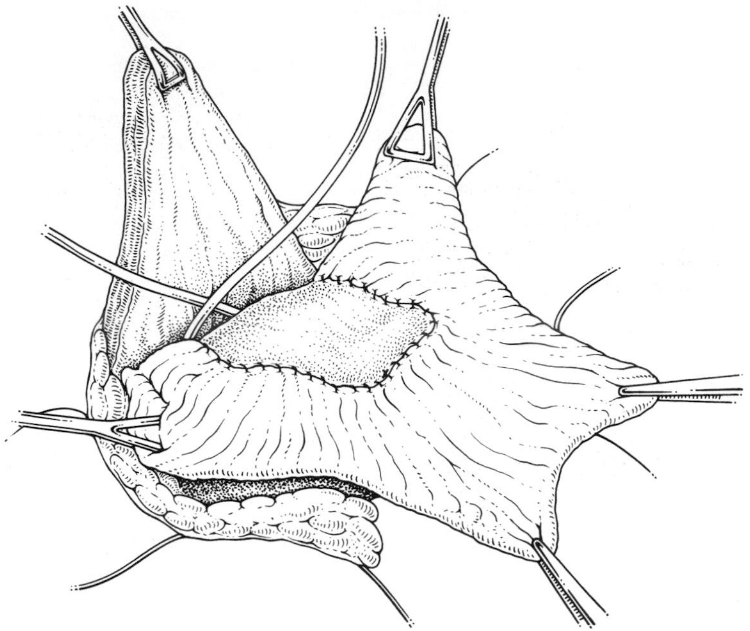

Fig. 20.4 Clam cystoplasty, technique 2. The ileal patch has been sutured to the posterior half of the bladder. From Mundy (1988).

problem with augmentation cystoplasty, but if caesarian section is required the surgeon needs to be aware of the blood supply of the bowel segment to avoid damage. Diarrhoea has recently been shown to be a significant problem in patients undergoing enterocystoplasty (Singh & Thomas 1997) and all patients need to be warned of this risk.

Detrusor myectomy

This procedure, sometimes called auto-augmentation, involves excision of a disc of detrusor muscle from the dome of the bladder, leaving the mucosa intact. Early results are encouraging (Kennelly et al 1994), including increase in bladder capacity and reduction in the frequency of unstable contraction. One-year results in 17 patients with idiopathic DI showed an overall improvement in 12 (Swami 1998). In short, the success rate is lower than with enterocystoplasty but the complications of enterocystoplasty are avoided. Longer-term results are awaited.

Neuromodulation

Sacral neuromodulation of S3 has been explored as a treatment for urge incontinence since the 1980s. A percutaneous electrode is inserted into the S3 foramen. Patients with more than a 50% response are considered suitable for a permanent implant. Neuromodulation is thought to work by activation of the sacral nerve fibres that inhibit parasympathetic motor neurones. Approximately 60% of patients tested are considered suitable for a permanent implantation, and half of these are cured, with a further quarter improved. However, the results at present are short-term, and long-term results are awaited (Ruud Bosch 1998).

REFERENCES

Abrams P H, Blaivas J G, Stanton S L et al 1988 The standardisation of terminology of lower urinary tract function. Scandinavian Journal of Urology Nephrology (suppl.) 114: 5–19

Abrams P H, Freeman R, Anderstrom C, Mattiasson A 1998 Tolterodine, a new antimuscarinic agent: as effective but better tolerated than oxybutynin in patients with an overactive bladder. British Journal of Urology 81: 801–810

Blackford H N, Murray K H A, Stephenson T P, Mundy A R 1984 The results of transvesical infiltration of the pelvic plexus with phenol in 116 patients. British Journal of Urology 56: 647–649

Borzyskowski M, Mundy A R 1987 Videourodynamic assessment of diurnal urinary incontinence. Archives of Diseases in Childhood 62 (2): 128–131

Brading A F, Turner W H 1994 The unstable bladder: towards a common mechanism. British Journal of Urology 73: 3–8

Cardozo L 1991 Urinary incontinence in women: have we anything new to offer? British Medical Bulletin 303: 1453–1456

Cardozo L D, Abrams P H, Stanton S L et al 1978 Idiopathic bladder instability treated by biofeedback. British Journal of Urology 50: 521–523

Chapple C R, Hampson S J, Turner-Warwick R T, Worth P H, 1991 Subtrigonal phenol injection. How safe and effective is it? British Journal of Urology 68 (5): 483–486

Chapple C R, Smith 1993 The pathophysiological changes in the bladder obstructed by benign prostatic hyperplasia. British Journal of Urology 73: 117–123

Elbadawi A, Yalla S V, Reswick N M 1993 Structural basis of geriatric voiding dysfunction detrusor overactivity. Journal of Urology 150: 1668–1680

Erickson B L, Bergman S, Eiknes S H 1989 Maximal electrostimulation of the pelvic floor in female ideopathic detrusor instability and urge incontinence. Neurourology and Urodynamics 8: 219

Filmer R B, Spencer J R 1990 Malignancies in bladder augmentations and intestinal conduits. Journal of Urology 143: 671–678

Fowler C J, Beck R O, Gerrard S et al 1994 Intravesical capsaicin for the treatment of detrusor hyperreflexia. Journal of Neurology Neurosurgery and Psychiatry 57: 169–173

Frewen W K 1982 A reassessment of bladder training in detrusor dysfunction in the female. British Journal of Urology 51: 363–366

Fry C R, Wu C 1998 The cellular basis of bladder instability. British Journal of Urology 81: 1–8

Gu J, Restorick J M, Blank M, Huang W M, Polak J M, Bloom S R, Mundy A R 1983 Vasoactive intestinal polypeptide in normal and unstable bladder. British Journal of Urology 55: 645–647

Holmes D M, Stone A R, Berry P R 1983 Bladder training: three years on. British Journal of Urology 55: 660–664

Jarvis G J 1981 A controlled trial of bladder drill and drug therapy in the management of detrusor instability. British Journal of Urology 53: 565–566

Jorgensen T M, Dijurhuis J C, Jorgensen H S, Sorensen S S 1983 Experimental bladder hyperreflexia in pigs. Urology Research 11: 239–240

Kennelly M J, Gormley G A, McGuire E J 1994 Early clinical experience with adult bladder auto-augmentation. Journal of Urology 152 (2 pt 1): 303–307

Kinder R B, Mundy A R 1987 Pathophysiology of ideopathic detrusor instability and detrusor hyperreflexia. An in vitro study of human detrusor muscle. British Journal of Urology 60: 509–515

Lloyd S N, Lloyds S M, Rogers K et al 1992 Is there still a place for prolonged bladder distension? British Journal of Urology 70: 382–386

Mundy A R 1983 The longterm results of bladder transection for urge incontinence. British Journal of Urology 55: 642–644

Mundy A R 1988 Cystoplasty. In: Mundy A R (ed) Current operative surgery: urology. Baillieire Tindall, London, chap. 11, pp 140–159

Mundy A R 1993 Detrusor instability in urodynamics and reconstructive surgery of the lower urinary tract. Churchill Livingstone, Edinburgh: 107–119

Mundy A R, Stephenson T P 1985 'Clam' ileocystoplasty for treatment of refractory urge incontinence. British Journal of Urology 57: 641–646

O'Flynn K J, Thomas D G 1993 Intravesical instillation of oxybutynin hydrochloride for detrusor hyperreflexia. British Journal of Urology 72: 566–570

Ruud Bosch J L H 1998 Sacral neuromodulation in the treatment of the unstable bladder. Current Opinion in Urology 8: 287–291

Sibley G D 1985 An experimental model of detrusor instability in the obstructed pig. British Journal of Urology 59: 292–298

Singh G, Thomas D G 1997 Bowel problems after enterocystoplasty. British Journal of Urology 79: 328–332

Speakman M J, Brading A F, Gilpin C J, Dixon J S, Gilpin S A, Gosling J A 1987 Bladder outflow obstruction – a cause of denervation supersensitivity. Journal of Urology 138: 1461–1466

Speakman M J, Brading A F, Dixon J S, Gilpin C J, Gosling J A 1991 Cystometric, physiological and morphological studies after relief of bladder obstruction in the rat. British Journal of Urology 68: 243–247

Swami K S, Feneley R C L, Hammonds J C, Abrams P 1998 Detrusor myectomy for detrusor overactivity: a minimum 1-year follow-up. British Journal of Urology 81: 68–72

Steers W D, Barrett D M, Wein A P 1996 Voiding dysfunction: diagnosis, classification and management. In: Gillenwater J Y, Grayhack J T, Howards S S, Duckett J W (eds) Adult and paediatric urology. Year Book Medical Publishers, Chicago; pp 1256–1261

Turner-Warwick R T 1984 Bladder outflow obstruction in the male. In: Mundy A R, Stephenson T P, Wein A J (eds) Urodynamics: principles, practice and applications. Churchill Livingstone, Edinburgh, pp 183–204

Webb R J, Ramsden P D, Neal D E 1991 Ambulatory monitoring and electronic measurement of urinary leakage in the diagnosis of detrusor instability and incontinence. British Journal of Urology 68: 148–152

Neuropathic bladder

ROBERT J KRANE, MIKE B SIROKY AND SANJAY RAZDAN

Neuropathic bladder dysfunction is any disturbance of the function of the vesicourethral unit due to a neurological lesion. This definition excludes voiding disorders resulting from psychogenic causes, anatomical abnormalities, and local causes such as carcinoma, inflammation, radiation or obstruction.

FUNCTIONAL NEUROANATOMY

Urinary continence and voiding involve the coordination of neural events in the peripheral autonomic, somatic, and central nervous systems (CNS). The pontine micturition centre in the brainstem and the sacral reflex centre in the conus medullaris divide the neural control of the lower urinary tract into three segments consisting of: (1) infrasacral (peripheral nerves), (2) suprasacral (spinal cord), and (3) suprapontine or intracranial (Fig. 21.1).

PERIPHERAL INNERVATION

Efferent pathways

These consist of parasympathetic, sympathetic, and somatic nerves. The parasympathetic outflow of the detrusor muscle, which provides the main excitatory influence, originates in the sacral spinal cord, segments S2 to S4, a portion of the spinal cord referred to as the conus medullaris. The conus is situated approximately at the junction of the T12 and L1 vertebral bodies. These preganglionic nerves course along the rectum as the pelvic nerves and synapse

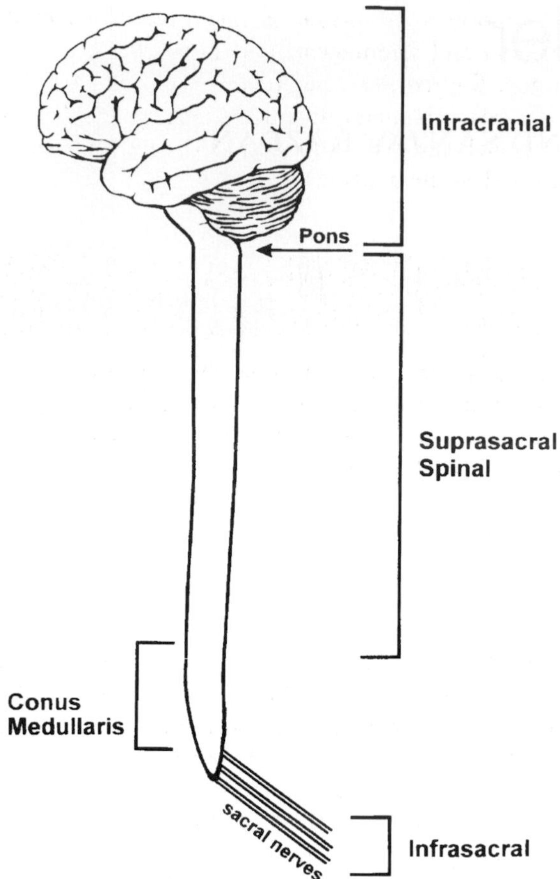

Fig. 21.1 The segmental control of micturition. Lesions within each neuroanatomical region are associated with characteristic voiding dysfunction.

with postganglionic neurones in proximity to the bladder forming the pelvic plexus. The pelvic plexus contains a mixture of parasympathetic and sympathetic fibres. There is abundant cholinergic innervation in the body of the detrusor, with a decreased density in the bladder neck and urethra.

The sympathetic supply to the bladder arises from the thoracolumbar spinal cord. The preganglionic fibres supplying the bladder and urethra originate from spinal cord segments T11 to L2. These preganglionic fibres proceed to synapse on postganglionic neurons in the sympathetic paravertebral chain or hypogastric plexus, and eventually terminate as postganglionic fibres in the bladder. The hypogastric nerve is synonymous with the sympathetic nerve supply of the bladder. There is a sparsity of sympathetic nerves to the body of the detrusor, with a rich adrenergic innervation of the bladder base, bladder neck, and proximal urethra, especially in males (Elbadawi 1982; Gosling et al 1977). The heavy adrenergic distribution at the bladder outlet probably acts to prevent retrograde ejaculation.

The efferent somatic pathways are responsible for the innervation of the striated urethral sphincter (rhabdosphincter) and the pelvic floor musculature through the pudendal nerve. These motor neurones emanate from the S2 to S4 spinal cord segments in proximity to the parasympathetic neurones, from an area termed Onuf's nucleus. Based on the results of animal studies, Elbadawi proposes that the efferent outflow to the human rhabdosphincter consists of somatic and sympathetic components, but its parasympathetic innervation remains to be verified (Elbadawi 1996). Inhibition of this somatic nerve activity during micturition requires supraspinal control, thereby accounting for the failure of external sphincter relaxation in patients with spinal cord lesions (DeGroat 1993).

Afferent pathways

While considerable data exists on the motor innervation of the urinary bladder, much less is known about its sensory function. Afferent fibres have been demonstrated in the pelvic, hypogastric, and pudendal nerves (DeGroat 1993). These sensory neurones have their cell bodies located in the S2 to S4 (parasympathetic and somatic) and T11 and L2 (sympathetic) dorsal root ganglia. Afferent nerves conveying impulses of bladder distension originate in the detrusor muscle and submucosa, and travel in the pelvic nerve. However, mechanoreceptor-linked afferent nerves, which predominate in the submucosa of the bladder base, travel by way of the hypogastric nerve. Nociceptive stimuli are carried in both the pelvic and hypogastric nerves. Afferent nerves from the striated sphincter and urethra, triggered by sensations of temperature, pain, and distension, travel in the pudendal nerve.

CENTRAL NERVOUS CONTROL OF MICTURITION

The neural control of the lower urinary tract may be conceptualized as a system divided into three segments. Each segment is both facilitated and inhibited by influences from higher segments. The peripheral innervation is influenced by the sacral micturition centre which in turn is influenced by the pontine mesencephalic reticular formation (pontine micturition centre; Bhatia & Bradley 1983; DeGroat 1993). Both of these centres are influenced by the cerebral centres. The process of bladder storage and micturition (often misleadingly termed 'the micturition reflex') actually consists of many reflex pathways acting in concert at various levels of the nervous system. Barrington (1921) first referred to micturition as a long route reflex. In other words, the production of a bladder contraction by vesical distension is mediated through the sacral spinal cord, as well as by the pontine micturition centre and higher centres, rather than solely being a segmental sacral cord reflex.

After impulses from the bladder reach the pontine micturition centre (Barrington's centre), they are transmitted to nuclei in the cerebral cortex, hypothalamus, thalamus, and cerebellum. The suprapontine CNS has a net inhibitory effect on micturition (Bhatia & Bradley 1983). The pontine micturition centre is supposed to be the origin of facilitatory impulses in the bladder. It is also responsible for detrusor-striated sphincter coordination during micturition. This organization of the nervous control of micturition has practical clinical consequences. In complete suprasacral spinal cord transection, not only does the detrusor lack inhibition by suprapontine centres, but it also appears to lack facilitation from the pontine micturition centre and thus cannot sustain its contraction. Further, the interaction of the detrusor and the striated urethral sphincter is also affected. Normally, vesical contraction is associated with relaxation of the striated pelvic floor, which occurs before the onset of the bladder contraction. However, in patients with suprasacral cord lesions, impairment of detrusor–sphincter coordination occurs due to dissociation from the pontine micturition centre. In contrast, suprapontine lesions, although resulting in vesical hyperreflexia (due to abolition of suprapontine inhibitory influence), do not disrupt vesicosphincter coordination. Obviously, in certain poorly localized diseases of the central nervous system such as multiple sclerosis, where infrapontine and suprapontine plaques often coexist, a spectrum of abnormalities related to the coordination of the bladder and sphincter may be found (Goldstein et al 1982). Nevertheless, our experience has shown that true vesicosphincter dyssynergia occurs only in cases of spinal cord lesions located above the sacral centre but below the pontine centre.

NEUROPHYSIOLOGY

The micturition cycle may be conceptualized as consisting of two distinct phases: (1) bladder filling, and (2) bladder emptying. The complex interplay of neurones, neurotransmitters, and receptors, in the two phase concept of micturition can be summarized as follows:

Storage phase

The bladder is able to distend progressively to its capacity with minimal increase in the intravesical pressure, a property referred to as compliance (Fig. 21.2). During the initial phase of filling, the viscoelastic properties of the bladder contribute to compliance. However, as filling continues, the next phase of compliance requires relaxation of the smooth muscles of the bladder (Coolsaet 1984). The storage phase of micturition is thus primarily under sympathetic control (Elbadawi 1982). Increased activity in the hypogastric nerve leads to (a) stimulation of β-receptors in the bladder body leading to increased bladder compliance and relaxation, (b) stimulation of α-receptors at the bladder base and urethra leading to increased outlet resistance, and (c) inhibition of parasympathetic transmission leading to decreased detrusor contractility. Storage is further aided by

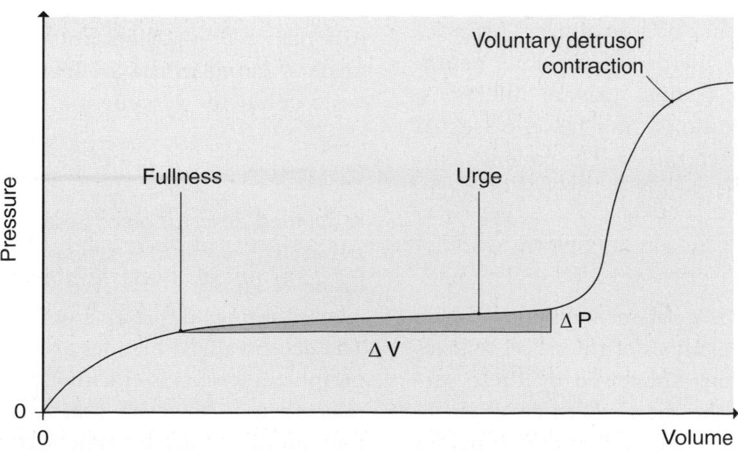

Fig. 21.2 Cystometrogram showing normal bladder compliance.

increased pudendal nerve activity, leading to contraction of the striated sphincter.

Voiding phase

This phase is primarily under parasympathetic control, with modulating influences from brainstem and cortical centres. If the social setting is appropriate, the predominantly inhibitory suprapontine influence is suppressed with activation of the sacral micturition centre (S2–S4). This results in (a) a sustained detrusor contraction mediated through the pelvic nerve, (b) synergistic relaxation of the bladder neck and urethral smooth muscle, and (c) relaxation of the striated urethral sphincter. There is compelling evidence that relaxation of the urethral smooth muscle is mediated by release of nitric oxide (NO) by pelvic nerves (Lee et al 1994; Mevorach et al 1994).

NEUROUROLOGICAL EVALUATION

The patient with known or suspected neuropathic bladder should be assessed in a systematic manner, by using the history, physical examination, and specialized urodynamic tests.

History

This crucial part of the evaluation yields important information if the examiner keeps in mind that the site of a lesion with respect to the neuraxis is what produces characteristic clinical and urodynamic features. Although the nature of the lesion in itself may have little clinical relevance in planning treatment, it may help in predicting the possible site of the neuraxis affected. Thus the neurourological history should focus on identification of aetiologic factors rather than predicting urodynamic abnormalities. The interview should ascertain a history of previous neurological disease, surgery, trauma, urinary infections, incontinence, and medications. Any bowel or sexual dysfunction should be ascertained. The patient's current urological symptoms should be elicited in detail.

Physical examination

Physical examination of the patient with neuropathic bladder should include analysis of the sacral reflexes (S2–S4) and the sensations subserved by these segments. The integrity of the sacral reflex arc is easily tested by the bulbocavernosus reflex and provides significant information regarding detrusor and external sphincter (pudendal nerve) function. The bulbocavernosus reflex is present in almost all normal men and in 70% of normal women. Its absence in a man strongly suggests a sacral cord lesion (Krane & Siroky 1991). This reflex is preserved after complete suprasacral cord transection and, if lost, is the first to return after recovery from spinal shock. The condition of the bladder, whether full (retention) or empty (incontinent), should also be ascertained. Finally, the examiner should evaluate deep tendon reflexes in the lower extremities, clonus, and plantar responses.

Urodynamic tests

Since symptoms of neurogenic bladder are often nonspecific, urodynamic tests assume increasing importance. A reproduction of the patient's symptoms during urodynamic testing is invaluable in improving diagnosis and therapy. However, the correlation between urodynamic tests and symptoms is only about 50% (Katz 1985).

Patients with detrusor areflexia void by abdominal straining. This results in a poor flow, with a sawtooth pattern indicative of an interrupted stream. Stop and start voiding may also be seen in patients with suprasacral cord lesions and vesicosphincter dyssynergia. Despite the aforementioned differences, uroflowmetry alone cannot distinguish between impaired detrusor contractility and outlet pathology (Chancellor et al 1991).

Postvoiding residual urine

Estimation of the postvoiding residual (PVR) urine is the logical next step after the patient has voided during uroflowmetry. An increased PVR generally indicates increased outlet resistance, weak detrusor contractility, or both. With increasing residual urine volumes, the likelihood of impaired detrusor contractility rather than obstruction increases substantially (Ghonheim 1991). Thus, increased postvoid residual urine is found in the areflexic bladder as well as in vesicosphincter dyssynergia.

Cystometry

A detailed description of cystometry and its interpretation is beyond the scope of this discussion (see Krane & Siroky 1991). We will focus on the cystometric findings in patients with a neurogenic bladder. The decentralized bladder as seen in conus and other peripheral lesions is essentially areflexic. It should be remembered, however, that an absent detrusor contraction in the urodynamic setting does not in itself prove areflexia. Corroborative evidence of a neurologic lesion, a history of abdominal straining on micturition, and denervation potentials on a sphincter EMG may help in making the correct diagnosis.

A bethanechol supersensitivity test (BST) may be performed to assess areflexia. This test, originally introduced by Lapides (1962) is based on Cannon's law of denervation, which states that a denervated muscle develops supersensitivity to its natural neurotransmitter. An increase of 15 cm H_2O intravesical pressure over baseline values after subcutaneous injection of 5 mg of bethanechol chloride constitutes a positive BST. Increased salivation and flushing are indicative of an adequate effect of the drug. A positive test strongly suggests neuropathic detrusor areflexia (Pavlakis et al 1983). In recent years significant false positive and negative results have dampened the interest in this test. Furthermore, a positive BST does not mean that a patient with detrusor areflexia will benefit from oral bethanechol chloride therapy. In suprasacral and suprapontine lesions a CMG typically reveals uninhibited detrusor contractions.

Electromyography

Assessment of perineal floor innervation and control is performed by electromyography. Two kinds of information can be obtained from EMG of the perineal muscles. First, determination of the integrity of innervation and the diagnosis of neuropathy, which requires the use of needle electrodes. Second, coordination between the detrusor and the striated sphincter during filling and voiding can be assessed. Perineal EMG cannot determine smooth muscle sphincter activity.

The normal perineal EMG shows a variable level of baseline activity at rest, depending on the patient's state of relaxation. With voluntary contraction, reflex activation, or bladder filling (the guarding reflex), EMG activity increases until a full interference pattern is seen (Siroky 1996). Polyphasic potentials may be observed in the normal EMG but are distinctly rare. Just before the onset of voiding there is a cessation of EMG activity (electrical silence) which is maintained throughout micturition (Fig. 21.3).

Depending on the type and site of the neurological lesion, this normal EMG activity is altered. Infrasacral lesions (sacral cord, cauda equina, or peripheral neuropathy) lead to an absence of activity in the electromyogram. A decreased interference pattern, positive sharp waves, and increased numbers of polyphasic potentials are characteristic. The most prominent feature of complete suprasacral spinal cord lesions is the presence of detrusor sphincter dyssynergia (DSD). DSD is characterized by the presence or persistence of involuntary EMG activity during a detrusor contraction. Incomplete lesions of the spinal cord may, however, be associated with a coordinated sphincter. Patients with suprapontine lesions usually have a completely normal EMG. Bradykinesia and lack of voluntary sphincter control may be profound in patients with Parkinsonism and may lead to incontinence following prostatectomy (Staskin et al 1988). Pseudodyssynergia, characterized by the voluntary contraction of the striated sphincter during detrusor hyperreflexia, may be observed, and should not be misinterpreted as a loss of detrusor–sphincter coordination (Wein & Barrett 1982).

Videourodynamics

The advantage of videourodynamic studies is that they combine the objectivity of urodynamics with the radiographic visualization of the lower urinary tract, thereby leading to more precise description of

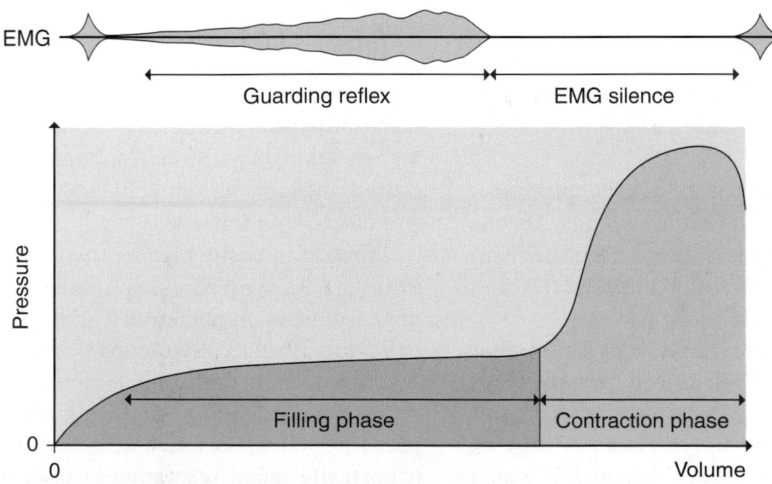

Fig. 21.3 Relationship between perineal floor EMG (top) and cystometrogram (bottom).

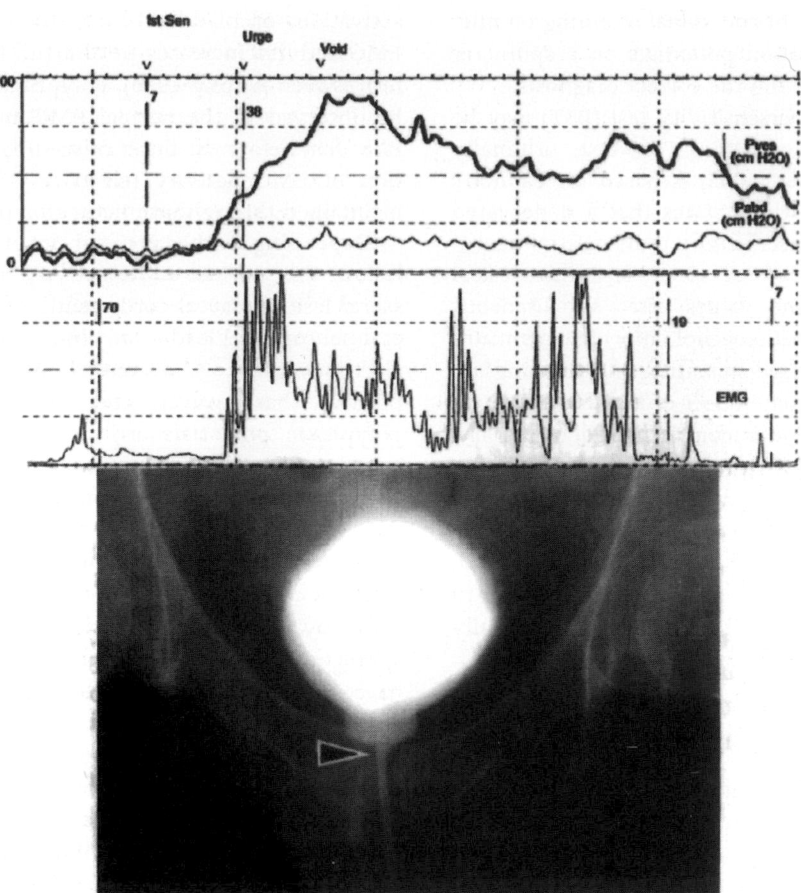

Fig. 21.4 Videourodynamic study in a woman. The voiding cystourethrogram with EMG shows evidence of VSD. Fluoroscopy confirms the site of obstruction at the external urethral sphincter (arrow).

lower urinary tract dysfunction. Patients with neurological diseases and complex detrusor–sphincter dysfunction are best evaluated by videourodynamics. Thus, poor compliance with V–U reflux, detrusor–sphincter dysynergia and pseudodysynergia and areflexia voiding, are best diagnosed by videourodynamics (Fig. 21.4).

CLASSIFICATION AND NOMENCLATURE

Various classification schemes have been proposed, each with its advantages and shortcomings. To one degree or another, current classification schemes concern themselves with abnormal bladder states and concomitant sphincteric dysfunction.

With the use of cystometry, two abnormal bladder states can be diagnosed. Detrusor hyperreflexia is characterized by involuntary detrusor contractions of any pressure, associated with symptoms of urge or leakage occurring during filling cystometry which cannot be consciously suppressed by the patient (Abrams et al 1988). The defining condition of detrusor hyperreflexia is that the patient cannot suppress the detrusor contraction. The volume at which these contractions are provoked is of lesser importance. Detrusor areflexia is defined as the inability to elicit a detrusor contraction during cystometry despite the presence of sensory urgency or discomfort. The presence of detrusor areflexia does not necessarily imply a neurological lesion, since a large number of normal individuals have detrusor areflexia during testing as a result of psychological inhibition. In addition, detrusor areflexia may be a result of myogenic damage caused by long-standing bladder outlet obstruction and chronic retention.

Much akin to the bladder, two abnormal sphincter states are recognized using sphincter electromyography: sphincter hyperactivity and sphincter neuropathy. Normal reflex interactions between the detrusor and the striated urethral sphincter involve increased activity of the sphincter during bladder filling (the guarding reflex). Before a detrusor contraction, there is normally reflex relaxation of both the smooth and striated sphincters. This can be objectively appreciated by an open and funnelled bladder neck on fluoroscopy (smooth muscle sphincter), and decreased EMG activity (striated muscle activity). With striated sphincter hyperactivity there may be no decrease, or an increase in electrical activity during a detrusor contraction. When this is associated with detrusor hyperreflexia, it is called detrusor–sphincter dyssynergia (DSD) (Fig. 21.5). When associated with vesical areflexia, DSD is more accurately called non-relaxing striated sphincter (Fig. 21.6).

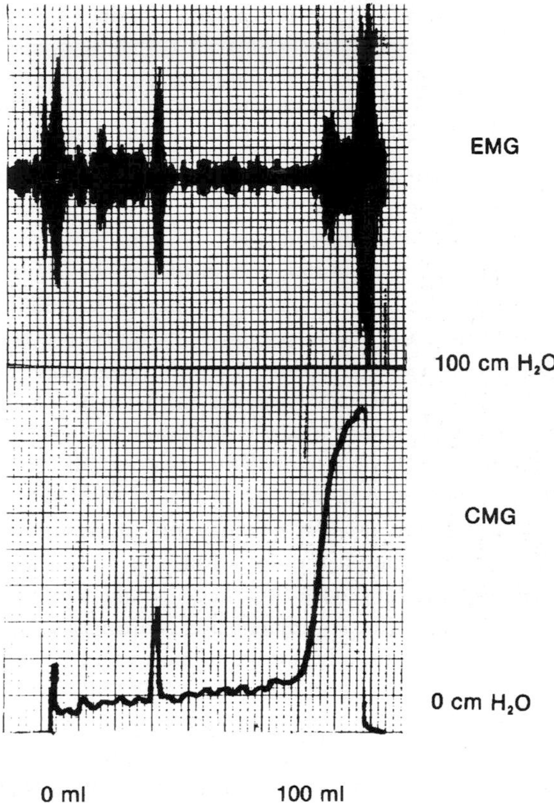

Fig. 21.5 Combined CMG/EMG demonstrating vesicosphincter dyssynergia.

In contrast, sphincter neuropathy is characterized by electromyographic recordings typical of partial or complete denervation. This usually indicates a lesion of the sacral spinal cord, cauda equina, or peripheral nerves. Since, the status of the bladder (hyperreflexic or areflexic) and the sphincter (hyperactive or neuropathic) is primarily responsible for the patient's symptoms, a classification based on these objective parameters would be most clinically useful. Moreover, knowledge of the urodynamic status may have prognostic importance with regard to upper tract deterioration. Thus, treatment for neuropathic bladder should be based on urodynamic findings and not on the level or type of the neurological lesion producing the urodynamic abnormalities.

Although an ideal classification system still eludes us, we have found the urodynamic classification of Krane and Siroky to be objective, and clinically applicable to the diagnosis and management of the neuropathic bladder.

1 Detrusor hyperreflexia
   (a) coordinated sphincters
   (b) striated sphincter dyssynergia
   (c) smooth sphincter dyssynergia
   (d) non-relaxing smooth sphincter

2 Detrusor areflexia
   (a) coordinated sphincters
   (b) non-relaxing striated sphincter
   (c) denervated striated sphincter
   (d) non-relaxing smooth sphincter

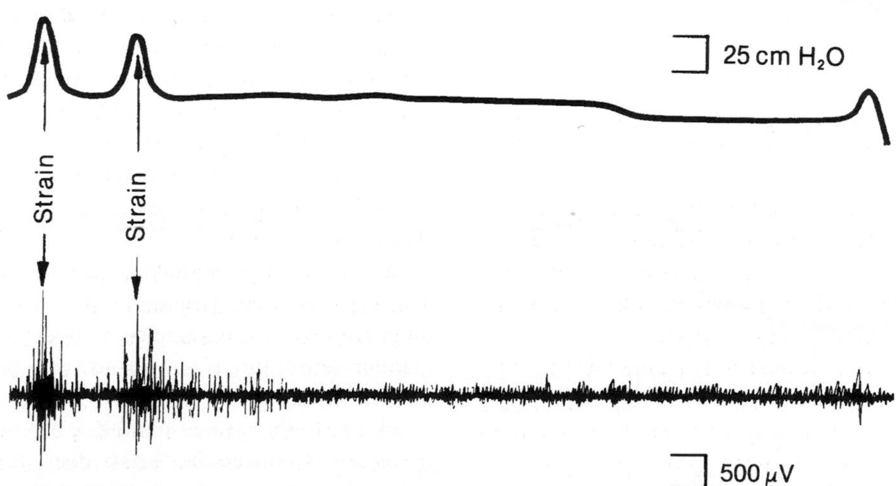

Fig. 21.6 Combined cystometry and sphincter electromyography demonstrating vesical areflexia with non-relaxation of external striated sphincter.

The various detrusor functional abnormalities, in conjunction with any possible sphincter dysfunction, will now be described with an emphasis on urodynamic features and treatment options.

DETRUSOR HYPERREFLEXIA

With coordinated sphincters

This is typically observed in patients with lesions above the pontine micturition centre. Neurological conditions most commonly associated with this finding include cerebrovascular disease (stroke), brain tumours, Parkinson's disease, dementia, multiple sclerosis, Shy–Drager syndrome and normal pressure hydrocephalus. These lesions involve the descending, predominantly inhibitory, supraspinal pathways, but spare the pontine micturition centre, which coordinates detrusor sphincter activity. Thus, detrusor hyperreflexia with sphincter coordination may also occur when the pontine micturition centre is partially separated from the sacral cord by an incomplete spinal cord lesion (herniated intervertebral disc and cervical spondylosis) (Fig. 21.7). The net effect, however, depends on the degree, size, and anatomical location of the lesion.

Following an acute stroke, urinary retention is common and is probably due to 'cerebral shock'. Over a period of time, frequency, urgency, and urge incontinence become the chief complaints. These symptoms usually are due to detrusor hyperreflexia (DH). The bladder has a low threshold and generally contracts at a low volume without warning. Incontinence is further aggravated by any cognitive and language deficits, with patients often voiding in socially inappropriate places (frontal lobe incontinence). The history should specifically enquire about medications as a number of drugs used in patients with intracranial lesions have profound effects on the bladder.

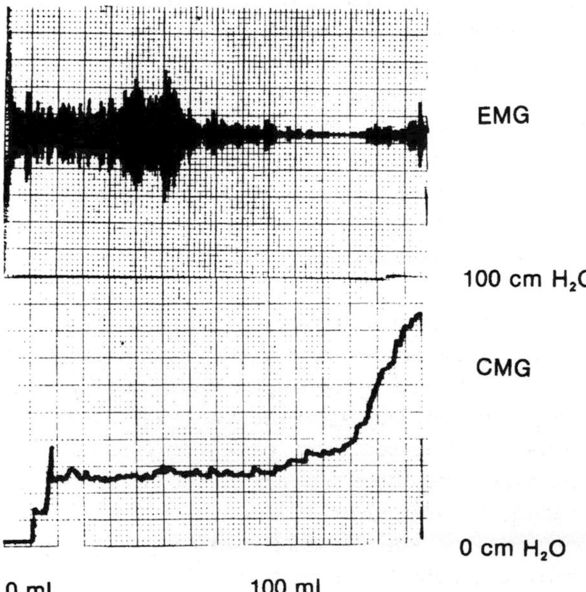

Fig. 21.7 Combined cystometrogram (CMG) and pelvic floor electromyogram (EMG) showing detrusor hyperreflexia with appropriate sphincter relaxation.

Non-neurological causes of irritative voiding, such as urinary tract infection, pelvic irradiation, BPH, and bladder tumour (carcinoma) *in situ* need to be identified prior to urodynamic analysis. Physical examination in patients with detrusor hyperreflexia and coordinated sphincters may reveal hemiplegia, tremor and incoordination. Deep tendon reflexes are brisk and the Babinski sign is positive. The mental status and the level of manual dexterity should be assessed specially if the patient is to be taught self intermittent catheterization. Uroflowmetry may be inconclusive as voided volumes tend to be small. Because of normal sphincter coordination, residual urine is minimal or absent. With marked DH, compliance may be reduced as a result of detrusor hypertrophy and endoscopy may reveal significant trabeculation. Long-standing DH may lead to a small capacity bladder with marked frequency and urgency. Since the sphincters are coordinated, the upper tracts are usually normal in most cases.

With detrusor–sphincter dyssynergia

Under normal circumstances, relaxation of the external urinary sphincter is coordinated with and precedes a detrusor contraction. This synergistic function of the detrusor and striated sphincter is disrupted in patients with complete suprasacral spinal cord injury. Classically due to traumatic spinal cord injury, it may also be seen in cervical spondylosis, transverse myelitis, and the diffuse demyelination of multiple sclerosis. Immediately after a suprasacral cord injury patients demonstrate 'spinal shock', which is characterized by post injury areflexia of skeletal and visceral muscles below the level of injury. The state of spinal shock which may last from 4–8 weeks (occasionally as long as 6 months) results in an areflexic large capacity bladder with absence of bladder sensation. If untreated, this produces overflow incontinence. During the recovery from spinal shock the bulbocavernosus reflex is amongst the first to return, followed by brisk deep tendon reflexes below the lesion, and a positive toe sign. Disruption of the inhibitory and modulatory suprasacral fibres results in reflex detrusor activity. Thus, DH is an almost universal finding in upper motor lesions after the phase of spinal shock has resolved. In a small proportion (5%) of patients with suprasacral lesions, detrusor areflexia persists after recovery from spinal shock possibly due to an occult cord lesion (Light et al 1985).

Further, disruption of fibres from the pons responsible for coordination of detrusor and striated external sphincter activity results in DSD. This DSD is defined by an inappropriate increase in external sphincter activity during an involuntary detrusor contraction. A coordinated sphincter, however, may be seen in incomplete leions. In females, DSD though present, is not of marked clinical importance. These patients usually present with frequency, urgency, and urge incontinence. Bladder sensation is lost in complete lesions.

High residual urine volumes may be due to VSD but another important factor is that patients have detrusor contractions that are unsustained, uncoordinated, and therefore ineffective. DSD induces an elevation in voiding pressure and is particularly detrimental to the upper tracts (Ruutu 1985). The bladder gradually becomes spastic, trabeculated, and of small capacity. Over time, this combination of abnormalities results in ureterovesical obstruction, V–U reflux, stone formation, and eventual upper tract deterioration (Anderson 1983).

With smooth muscle sphincter dyssynergia

Approximately 10–20% of spinal cord injured patients demonstrate DH with dysynergia of the smooth sphincter of the bladder neck (Chancellor et al 1994). This is a difficult diagnosis, which relies on videourodynamics to demonstrate an incompletely open bladder neck during a detrusor contraction. Most often seen in patients with high cord lesions above T-6 level, it may be a constituent of the syndrome of autonomic dysreflexia. This syndrome is characterized by marked hypertension, piloerection, diaphoresis, headache, and flushing in response to bladder or rectal distension. In severe cases cerebral haemorrhage may occur. Reflex bradycardia is the rule. The exact mechanism of autonomic dysreflexia is unclear, although profuse sympathetic discharge due to loss of normal inhibition from higher centres in the brainstem has been implicated. In patients with a history of autonomic dysreflexia, the blood pressure should be continuously monitored during lower urinary tract instrumentation. The crisis is best managed by aborting the procedure and administering sublingual nifedipine. Prophylaxis against autonomic dysreflexia may require chronic α-adrenergic blockade (Chancellor et al 1994).

Treatment

Detrusor hyperreflexia with coordinated sphincters

This is primarily managed medically. The objective of pharmacological therapy is control of the detrusor hypercontractility. Anticholinergics and musculotropic relaxants are of great benefit in this setting. The drug of choice is oxybutynin chloride (Ditropan), a direct smooth muscle relaxant with moderate anticholinergic effects. In an oral dose of 5 mg three or four times a day, it is effective in suppressing DH, increasing bladder volume at first contraction and in increasing total bladder capacity. The dosage should be individually titrated according to the patient's response. Many patients with DH have poor detrusor contractility and oxybutynin may lead to increased postvoid residuals, which may necessitate timed voiding and self intermittent catheterization. Oxybutynin may also be administered intravesically in patients who have an unsatisfactory response or exhibit profound side-effects with oral medication (Kasabian et al 1994). Intravesical therapy is particularly suited to patients on self intermittent catheterization. A slow-release form of oxybutynin (Ditropan XL) is now available for oral use.

Dicyclomine hydrochloride, a musculotropic agent with anticholinergic effects, has been used effectively (20 mg t.i.d.) in patients with DH with an increase in bladder capacity. Flavoxate hydrochloride, another musculotropic agent, however, has been found to have essentially little effect on DH. Imipramine, a tricyclic antidepressant is often used as an adjunct to anticholinergics. The drug decreases bladder contractility and increases outlet resistance in an adult dosage of 25 mg q.i.d. Lower doses are required in the elderly due to profound side-effects, which may include central nervous system and gastrointestinal toxicity.

For most anticholinergic and musculotropic medications, the earliest side-effect is dryness of the mouth, followed by constipation, and finally blurring of vision. Drying of the mouth (xerostomia) is usually the reason most patients withdraw from therapy. Tolterodine, a newer anticholinergic agent, has significantly lower incidence of xerostomia than oxybutynin. The presence of narrow-angle glaucoma is an absolute contraindication to the use of anticholinergics.

When medical therapy fails to abolish DH and control symptoms, non-pharmacological options are employed. These include electrical stimulation, bladder denervation procedures, and augmentation cystoplasty.

Electrical stimulation This modality is used clinically to inhibit an overactive detrusor. Electrical stimulation of the perineal skeletal muscles by intrarectal, intravaginal, or intradural electrodes results in reciprocal bladder inhibition (Vodusek et al 1983). Thus, stimulation of the pudendal afferents leads to contraction of the striated external sphincter, and detrusor inhibition via a pudendal-to-pelvic spinal reflex (Sundin et al 1974). The results of spinal nerve root stimulation in selected patients with DH have been encouraging, with up to 90% cure rates (Koldewijn et al 1994).

Bladder denervation Denervation techniques involve either selective nerve blocks, or transection of the S2–S4 sacral nerve roots which are mainly concerned with bladder contractions. Selective blockade with alcohol or phenol, or sacral rhizotomy, should be considered particularly in spinal cord injured patients with DH that is refractory to other treatment modalities. Superselective sectioning of the S3 anterior spinal root has produced impressive results with minimal side-effects (Lucas et al 1988). Patients are subsequently put on clean intermittent catheterization for the resulting detrusor areflexia. Intradural rhizotomies of all posterior sacral root components from S2 to S5, in combination with implantation of an anterior sacral root stimulator, has produced good results in isolated series of spinal cord injured patients with detrusor hyperreflexia (Koldewijn et al 1994).

Augmentation cystoplasty Enterocystoplasty (clam cystoplasty) using detubularized small bowel has yielded excellent results with a 95% cure rate in refractory DH (Luanghot et al 1991). More recently, detrusor myectomy (autoaugmentation) which entails excision of a strip of detrusor muscle leaving the mucosa intact, has yielded encouraging results with an improvement in the quality of life (Stohrer et al 1995). Further, this procedure can be performed by the laparoscopic route (McDougall et al 1995). These patients may subsequently require self intermittent catheterization for adequate emptying of the bladder.

Detrusor hyperreflexia with detrusor–sphincter dyssynergia

This requires more aggressive treatment to avoid upper tract damage. The treatment of choice in the female patient is the judicious use of anticholinergics in conjunction with intermittent catheterization for bladder drainage. If this treatment is unsuccessful, few options remain aside from chronic indwelling catheters, augmentation cystoplasty, or supravesical diversion. This is in sharp contrast to the situation in male patients, in whom treatment of the external sphincter obstruction by sphincterotomy is successful and condom catheter drainage can be instituted.

In our experience, none of the centrally acting muscle relaxants have a significant effect in relaxing the striated sphincter in patients with DSD. Agents such as dantrolene, diazepam, and baclofen have been used extensively, but results have been disappointing. Sedation, profound muscle weakness, and other side-effects further preclude their use. Recently, intrathecal baclofen has yielded promising results in effectively inhibiting the striated urethral sphincter and abolishing DH, while circumventing the problem of sedation (Steers et al 1992).

Detrusor hyperreflexia with smooth sphincter dyssynergia

This is primarily treated with a combination of an anticholinergic agent with an α-blocker (Prazosin, Terazosin). Krane & Olsson (1973) presented evidence that α-blockers could promote emptying in patients with DH and smooth sphincter dyssynergia. Terazosin (Hytrin) is currently extensively employed to reduce obstruction at the bladder neck due to smooth sphincter dyssynergia. Bladder neck dyssynergia unresponsive to α-blockers can be treated with transurethral bladder neck incision. Extreme caution, however, must be exercised in treating women with a bladder neck incision because of the risk of incontinence.

DETRUSOR AREFLEXIA

Detrusor areflexia is lack of a detrusor contraction resulting from a neurological lesion, usually one of the conus medullaris, cauda equina, or peripheral nerves. Diabetic cystopathy may lead to an areflexic bladder with impaired sensations and increased residual urine. Injury to the pelvic plexus following extirpative pelvic surgery is another cause of detrusor areflexia (Yalla et al 1984). Patients present with a large capacity bladder which is passively overdistended. In late cases, patients present with overflow incontinence as the urge to void is lost. The stream is weak, and the patient voids by suprapubic pressure or abdominal straining. Chronic overdistension eventually leads to myogenic detrusor damage. Examination will reveal absent or decreased cutaneous sensation in the perineum and/or lower extremities and diminished bulbocavernosus reflex, anal sphincter tone, and deep tendon reflexes. A tuft of hair, a lipoma, or a haemangioma over the lower back may be the only evidence of an occult spinal dysraphism presenting as detrusor areflexia. Radiography may confirm a vertebral fracture, spina bifida, or congenital absence of the sacrum.

Striated muscle sphincter

Evidence of denervation of the striated sphincter may be obtained by sphincter electromyography. Immediately after a lower motor neurone injury there is neither voluntary nor reflex activity of the external sphincter. If the injury is complete, fibrillation potentials and positive sharp waves are observed in the resulting muscle. If the neuropathy is incomplete, reinnervation from surviving neurones can take place, producing the characteristic polyphasic potential. During muscle activation, the interference pattern is markedly reduced owing to neuronal loss. More common than a denervated external sphincter is the association of detrusor areflexia with a non-relaxing treated sphincter. Thus, the striated sphincter constitutes a form of obstruction during attempts at voiding by abdominal straining or the Credé's manoeuvre.

Smooth muscle sphincter obstruction

Although a rare occurrence in females, detrusor areflexia may be associated with isolated proximal sphincteric obstruction (Abel et al 1974). Parasympathetic decentralization of the bladder is known to increase the density of α-adrenergic receptors in the bladder (deGroat & Kawatani 1989). This fact is supported by the efficacy of α-blockers in promoting bladder emptying in patients with bladder neck dyssynergia (Olsson et al 1988).

Treatment

In view of the wide variety of sphincter abnormalities that may be found in association with detrusor areflexia, treatment is highly individualized. We will discuss the management options commonly employed to promote bladder emptying.

Self intermittent catheterization Lapides and coworkers are credited for popularizing this modality of treatment in patients with voiding dysfunction. Self intermittent catheterization (SIC) has revolutionized the management of patients with an areflexic bladder who till a few years back were relegated to a life on an indwelling catheter with its attendant complications of infection, sepsis, stones, and carcinoma. Although this method introduces bacteria into the bladder, symptomatic bacteriuria and urinary tract infections are extremely uncommon and easily controlled by suppressive antibiotics. In addition the incidence of bladder stones is significantly less than with any other form of bladder drainage. Further, upper tract deterioration is rare if the bladder pressure in between catheterizations is kept well below 40 cm H_2O (Mcguire et al 1981). A 'clean' technique as opposed to a sterile one is generally adequate for long-term self-catheterization. The technique of SIC in the female without manual or visual impairment takes about an hour. Disposable, inexpensive (Mentor) catheters are readily available commercially. If sphincteric function is preserved and detrusor areflexia is the only problem, SIC is the treatment of choice.

Parasympathomimetic agents The value of bethanecol chloride to promote bladder emptying is at best debatable. Up to 200 mg of bethanecol daily has not proven beneficial in patients with complete areflexia (Wein et al 1996).

α-blockers As discussed earlier, terazosin is being used extensively in patients with evidence of increased outlet resistance at the level of the smooth sphincter (Lepor et al 1992).

Centrally acting muscle relaxants There is no drug that selectively relaxes the striated urethral sphincter. Agents such as dantrolene, baclofen, and diazepam have been used in patients with a non-relaxing striated sphincter. While, baclofen and diazepam act on the central nervous system, dantrolene acts directly on skeletal muscle. Their clinical usefulness is, however, limited because of the troublesome side-effects and muscle weakness.

Surgical therapy This has lost its former preeminence, especially with the advent of self intermittent catheterization. Transurethral incision of the bladder neck is primarily indicated for failure of α-blocker therapy in patients with a non-relaxing smooth sphincter. While recommended in men, its use in women is associated with a disconcerting risk of total incontinence. This unfortunate occurrence would convert a situation easily managed by SIC to one that may require supravesical diversion. In our practice, bladder neck incision does not serve a useful purpose in women with detrusor areflexia. Urethral overdilation to 40 F in women has the same effect as an external sphincterotomy in men. This is, however, rarely performed in women because of the lack of a suitable external collecting device.

Supravesical diversion, though seldom employed, has gained popularity in recent years because of improved techniques of continent diversion. The prime indications for supravesical diversion in women with detrusor areflexia would be: (a) inability to perform self-intermittent catheterization, (b) progressive upper tract deterioration on intermittent catheterization, (c) incontinence following an overzealous incision of the bladder neck.

Complications

Urethral complications An indwelling Foley catheter, if left in place for a prolonged period of time, may be responsible for a urethrovaginal fistula or a periurethral abscess. Fortunately, with the advent of intermittent catheterization, complications involving the urethra are extremely rare.

Bladder complications Infection is by far the commonest complication of the neuropathic bladder. Patients with detrusor areflexia and DSD, conditions associated with increased residual urine, are particularly prone to recurrent infections. Presence of foreign bodies (long-standing catheters and stones) also predispose to infection, and every effort should be made to remove them. The widespread use of clean intermittent catheterization has reduced the incidence of urinary tract infections considerably. Although this methods introduces bacteria into the bladder and bacteriuria is common, the incidence of symptomatic infections of the urinary tract is extremely low. Asymptomatic bacteriuria *per se*, if not associated with vesicoureteral reflux, is of no clinical importance (with the exception of pregnant women) and should not be treated with systemic antibiotics. Symptomatic urinary infections, however should be treated promptly with culture-specific antimicrobial agents.

Bladder calculi occur for the same reasons that tend to cause infections (residual urine and indwelling catheters). Struvite stones due to urea-splitting organisms (Proteus) are particularly common in patients with neuropathic bladders. Skeletal demineralization with its attendant hypercalciuria, as seen in bedridden patients, further encourages stone formation. Again, the use of clean intermittent catheterization has decreased the incidence of this complication, though it may still be encountered in patients with chronic suprapubic tubes.

The increased incidence of squamous cell carcinoma of the bladder in patients with indwelling catheters mandates cystoscopy, and bladder washings at regular intervals.

Vesicoureteral reflux As a cause of upper tract deterioration V–U reflux is potentially a problem in any patient with a neuropathic bladder and high voiding pressures. There is a direct relationship between the voiding pressure and V–U reflux. In one series, an intravesical pressure of >40 cm H_2O during storage was associated with a 68% incidence of V–U reflux, in contrast to no V–U reflux in patients with pressures <40 cm H_2O (McGuire et al 1981). Thus, patients with DH and DSD are particularly prone to the deleterious effects of reflux on renal function. Vesicoureteral reflux is also observed in patients with decreased detrusor compliance and an areflexic bladder. The goal of treatment in patients with a neuropathic bladder and V–U reflux is to maintain a low intravesical pressure and control urinary tract infections. If conservative measures fail, the bladder capacity is adequate, and the upper tracts reasonable, bilateral ureteral reimplantation may be performed. If these criteria cannot be met, a supravesical diversion may be the only way to preserve renal function.

Hydronephrosis Even in the absence of reflux, a neuropathic bladder may impair the drainage of the upper tract, secondary to the development of anatomical or functional obstruction at the ureterovesical junction (Staskin 1991). In addition to high pressure storage (>40 cm H_2O) and extrinsic ureteral compression, anatomical obstruction at the V–U junction due to detrusor hypertrophy may cause hydronephrosis. Thus, patients with suprasacral cord lesions and vesicosphincter dyssynergia, as well as patients with poor bladder compliance should undergo a renal ultrasound to detect hydronephrosis. With modern management, however, this complication is infrequent.

Renal calculi The presence of infection, hydronephrosis, reflux, and hypercalciuria all contribute to the noticeable propensity of patients with neuropathic bladders to form renal calculi. The treatment of renal calculi in the presence of neuropathic bladder does not differ significantly from the usual medical and surgical management of this condition.

SUMMARY

The neuropathic bladder may affect the patient in a wide variety of ways, ranging from inconvenience (frequent urination) and embarrassment (incontinence) to death (renal failure, squamous cell carcinoma). Modern management has greatly decreased the morbidity and mortality of this condition. Such treatment, in turn, rests on accurate identification of the micturition abnormality by appropriate urodynamic techniques.

REFERENCES

Abel B J et al 1974 The neuropathic urethra. Lancet 4: 1229–1230

Abrams P H, Blaivas J G, Stanton S L et al 1988 Standardization of terminology of lower urinary tract function. Neurourology and Urodynarics 7: 403–427

Anderson R U 1983 Urodynamic patterns after acute spinal cord injury: Association with bladder trabeculation in male patients. Journal of Urology 129: 777–779

Barrington F J F 1921 The relation of the hindbrain to micturition. Brain 44: 23 I 1982

Bhatia N N, Bradley W E 1983 Neuroanatomy and physiology: innervation of the urinary tract. In: Raz S (ed) Female Urology. W B Saunders, Philadelphia, pp 12–32

Chancellor M, Blaivas J, Kaplan S et al 1991 Bladder outlet obstruction versus impaired detrusor contractility: the role of uroflow. Journal of Urology 145: 810

Chancellor M B, Erhard M J, Hirsch I H, Staas W E 1994 Prospective evaluation of Terazosin for the treatment of autonomic dysreflexia. Journal of Urology 151: 111–113

Coolsaet B L R A 1984 Cystometry. In: Stanton S L (ed.) Clinical Gynecologic Urology. Mosby, St Louis pp 59–81

de Groat W C 1993 Anatomy and physiology of the lower urinary tract. Urologic Clinics of North America 20(3): 383

de Groat W C, Kawatani M 1989 Reorganization of sympathetic preganglionic connections in cat bladder ganglia following parasympathetic decentralization. Journal of Physiology 409: 431–449

Elbadawi A 1982 Neuromorphologic basis of vesicourethral function. I. Histochemistry, ultrastructure and function of intrinsic nerves of the bladder and urethra. Neurourology and Urodynamics 1: 3–50

Elbadawi A 1996 Functional anatomy of the organs of micturition. Urologic Clinics of North America 23: 177–210

Ghonheim G 1991 Impaired bladder contractility in association with detrusor instability: underestimated occurrence in benign prostatic hyperplasia. Neurourology and Urodynamics 10: 111

Goldstein I, Siroky M B, Sax D S and Krane R J 1982 Neurologic abnormalities in multiple sclerosis. Journal of Urology 128: 541

Gosling J A, Dixon J S, Lendon R G 1977 The autonomic innervation of the human male and female bladder neck and proximal urethra. Journal of Urology 118: 302–305

Kasabian N, Vlachiotis J, Lais A et al 1994 The use of intravesical oxybutynin chloride in patients with detrusor hypertonicity and detrusor hypoerreflexia. Journal of Urology 151: 944–945

Katz G P, Blaivas J G 1985 A diagnostic dilemma: when urodynamic findings differ from clinical impression. Journal of Urology 129: 1170–1174.

Koldewijn E L, Van Kerrebroeck P E, Rosier P F et al 1994 Bladder compliance after posterior sacral root rhizotomies and anterior sacral root stimulation. Journal of Urology 151(4): 955–60

Krane R J, Olsson C 1973 Phenoxybenzamine in neurogenic bladder dysfunction: I. A theory of micturition. Journal of Urology 110: 653–656

Krane R J, Siroky M B 1991 The history and examination in neuro-urology. In Krane and Siroky (ed): Clinical Neuro-urology. Boston, Little, Brown, pp. 275–284

Lapides J 1962 Denervation supersensitivity as a test for neurogenic bladder. Surgery, Gynecology and Obstetrics 114: 241–244

Lee J G, Wein A J, Levin R M 1994 Comparative pharmacology of the male and female rabbit bladder neck and urethra: involvement of nitric oxide. Pharmacology 250–259

Lepor H, Soloway M, Narayan P et al 1992 A multicenter fixed-dose trial of the safety and efficacy of terazosin in the treatment of the symptoms of benign prostatic hyperplasia. Journal of Urology 148: 1467–1474

Light J K, Faganel J, Beric A 1985 Detrusor areflexia in suprasacral spinal cord injuries. Journal of Urology 134: 295–297

Luanghot R, Peng B C, Blaivas J G 1991 Ileocecocystoplasty for the management of refractory neurogenic bladder: surgical techniques and urodynamic results. Journal of Urology 146: 1340–1344

Lucas M G, Thomas D G, Clark S et al 1988 Long-term follow-up of selective sacral neurectomy. British Journal of Urology 61: 218–220.

McDougall E M, Clayman R V et al 1995 Laparoscopic retropubic autoaugmentation of the bladder. Journal of Urology 153: 123–126

McGuire E J, Woodside J R et al 1981 Prognostic value of urodynamic testing in myelodysplastic patients. Journal of Urology 126: 205–209

Mevorach R A, Bogaert G A, Kogan B A 1994 Role of nitric oxide in fetal lower urinary tract function. Journal of Urology 152: 510

Olsson C A, Siroky M B, Krane R J 1977 The phenotolamine test in neurogenic bladder dysfunction. Journal of Urology 117: 481–485

Pavlakis A, Siroky M B, Krane R J 1983 Neurogenic detrusor areflexia: correlation of perineal electromyography and bethanechol supersensitivity testing. Journal of Urology 129: 1182–1184

Ruutu M 1985 Cystometrographic patterns in predicting bladder function after spinal cord injury. Paraplegia 23: 243–252

Siroky M B 1996 Electromyography of the perineal floor. Urologic Clinics of North America 23: 2 pp299–307

Siroky M B, Krane R J 1983 Hydrodynamic significance of flow rate determination. In Hinman F Jr (ed.): Benign Prostatic Hypertrophy. Springer Verlag, New York, p507

Staskin D R 1991 Hydroureteronephrosis after spinal cord injury. Effects of lower urinary tract dysfunction on upper tract anatomy. Urologic Clinics of North America 18: 309–316

Staskin D R, Vardi Y, Siroky M B 1988 Postprostatectomy incontinence in the Parkinsonian patient: The significance of poor voluntary sphincter control. Journal of Urology 140: 117–118

Steers W D, Meyshaler J M, Herrell D et al 1992 Effects of acute and chronic continuous intrathecal baclofen on genitourinary dysfunction in patients with disorders of the spinal cord. Journal of Urology 148: 1849–1855

Stohrer M, Kramer A, Goepel M et al 1995 Bladder autoaugmentation – an alternative for enterocystoplasty: Preliminary results. Neurourology and Urodynamics 14: 11

Sundin T, Carlsson C, Kock N G 1974 Detrusor inhibition induced from mechanical stimulation of the anal region and from electrical stimulation of pudendal nerve afferents. Investigative Urology 11: 374–378

Vodusek D B, Janko M, Lokar J 1983 Direct and reflex responses in perineal muscles on electrical stimulation. Journal of Neurology, Neurosurgery and Psychiatry 46: 67–71

Wein A, Barrett D M 1982 Etiologic possibilities of increased pelvic floor electromyographic activity during cystometry. Journal of Urology 127: 949–952

Wein A J, Barrett D M, Steers W D 1996 Voiding dysfunction: diagnosis, classification, and management. In: Gillenwater et al (eds) Adult and Pediatric Urology. Mosby

Yalla S V, Andriole G 1984 Vesicourethral dysfunction following pelvic ablative surgery. Journal of Urology 132: 503–509

Bladder after radical surgery

ECKHARD PETRI

In 1898 Wertheim first reported the extensive dissection of both ureters and the bladder during abdominal hysterectomy for cervical carcinoma to facilitate the wide removal of paracervical and parametrial tissue. Radiation therapy was applied to the treatment of cervical carcinoma in the early years of this century. Rapid improvement in the radiographic equipment, the clinical use of radium, and the uniformity of dosimetry far outstripped advances in surgery, so that by the late 1920s radiation therapy had replaced surgery in many countries. European, Japanese and American gynaecologists progressed and made their operative techniques more radical in the late 1970s; but follow-up showed a marked increase in complications without improvement of survival rates. Reduced radicality is now recommended, therefore, for earlier stages of cervical carcinoma, generally limited to patients with stage Ib and IIa lesions. In a worldwide attempt to replace surgery by endoscopic procedures, Dargent (1987, 1993) has recommended laparoscopic lymphadenectomy, followed by a vaginal radical hysterectomy (Schauta). There is no follow-up at the present time and caution is recommended: there has only been sampling of pelvic nodes, sexual function of the vagina in young women may be greatly compromised by extreme shortening, and the pelvic floor may be badly damaged by a Schuchardt incision.

Radical hysterectomy requires mobilization of the bladder to allow removal of the upper vagina to ensure an adequate margin of resection. Radical hysterectomy therefore places the bladder at considerable risk. While injury to the urinary tract is rare (Table 22.1), urinary problems continue to be the most significant complications following radical hysterectomy. These postoperative complications include fistulae formation (ureteric and vesicovaginal, see Ch. 23) and bladder dysfunction. The incidence of bladder disturbances following radical pelvic surgery ranges from 16 to 80% in the literature.

With more extensive surgery within the small pelvis, such as abdominoperineal resection or posterior exenteration in selected cases of carcinoma of the cervix, vagina or vulva, a higher incidence of voiding disorders has to be expected.

Table 22.1 Complications after radical pelvic surgery.

Complication	Incidence
Intraoperative lesion to the bladder	3–5%
Intraoperative lesion to the ureter	1–2%
Vesicovaginal fistulae	0.5–3%
Ureterovaginal fistulae	1–13%[†]

[†]Shows the problems and variance in reporting

The literature on urological problems after radical pelvic surgery is numerous. Different indications, different techniques, different forms of pre- or postoperative radiation therapy and different types of postoperative management of the bladder drainage make a comparison of published data almost impossible. Because of changes in surgical techniques (see above) and postoperative regimens, comparison of long-term results is difficult.

PATHOPHYSIOLOGY

The causes of disorders of the lower urinary tract after radical surgery range from calculated injuries to the pelvic nerves and postural changes of the bladder in an empty pelvic cavity to accidental lesions caused by inadequate postoperative bladder drainage and urinary tract infection. The majority of the nerves from the pelvic plexus supplying the bladder pass over and around the vagina. It is therefore apparent that any operation that involves excision of the paracervical and paravaginal web of retroperitoneal tissue will interrupt some portion of the bladder innervation. Some of the fibres pass around the lateral aspect of the vagina; however, it it evident that unless the dissection is carried fairly deep, that is, to include a major segment of the paravaginal portion of the web, complete interruption of the innervation is unlikely. It is also evident that in the operation as usually performed, this is the only site at which the parasympathetic nerves to the bladder enter the field of dissection (Twombly & Landers 1956). Complete interruption of the parasympathetic innervation can take place during abdominoperineal resection of the rectum in posterior exenteration. In these cases an additional lesion of the somatic pudendal nerve may occur.

It has been postulated for a long time that the postoperative phase includes a period of bladder hypertonicity which appears after operation when the catheter is removed. This has been diagnosed from simple, single channel cystometry and it has been suggested that the denervation of the detrusor muscle is responsible. Modern urethro-cystometrograms using microtip transducers have proven that this is an artefact (Asmussen & Miller 1983).

Direct nerve lesions, changes in blood supply, and lymphatic drainage play decisive roles in bladder dysfunction. Removing connective tissue and vessels of the pelvis together with the lymph nodes leads to an interruption of lymphatic drainage. Postoperative oedema and temporary interference with the nervous control results in loss of bladder wall compliance, thus producing overflow incontinence. Given that an adequate 'cancer operation' requires excision of a margin of healthy tissue around the tumor, it is difficult to see how direct damage to the pelvic nerves and plexuses could be completely avoided during radical pelvic surgery. As demonstrated by Mundy (1982) it would appear that the pelvic parasympathetic nerves and the pelvis plexus are far more vulnerable during rectal operations than during uterine surgery. During radical hysterectomy the risk of damage to the pelvic nerves is only small, since the nerves are well posterior and the bulk of the plexus lies below the cardinal ligament. Although this ligament contains some nerve fibres from the plexus, this part of the broad ligament is usually preserved. Only if the cardinal ligaments or an unusually long cuff of the upper vagina is removed, is the field of excision likely to involve the plexus (Petri 1996; Ralph et al 1987, 1988; Table 22.2).

Bilateral oophorectomy in premenopausal women induces typical changes in the mucosa of the bladder, urethra and vagina. An oestrogen deficit results, is known to induce reduction of urethral closure pressure, pressure transmission to the urethra, and alterations in sensibility and contractility of the bladder.

Voiding disorders because of functional outlet obstruction have usually been treated by urethral catheterization, which is a known cause of urethritis and ascending infection. Lack of control of effective voiding, control of residual urine by ultrasound (no desire to void because of the sensory loss) may result in overdistension. Thus the causes of micturition disorders after radical pelvic surgery are multifactorial and comprise: surgical lesions to nerve, vascular, and lymphatic supply; dislocation of the bladder into the wound cavity; and iatrogenic lesions caused by repeated catheterization during the postoperative course.

Table 22.2 Incidence of bladder dysfunction depending on the length of vaginal cuff.

	<2 cm	>2 cm	p
Capacity (ml)	386	399	n.s.
Average flow (ml/s)	12	8	<0.05
Duration (s)	31	55	<0.05
Compliance pathology (%)	38	70	<0.05

From Ralph et al (1988)

INCIDENCE

The great number of surgical modifications, new discussions on lesser or greater radical surgery, radical vaginal techniques still in use and being reinforced by laparoscopists, different forms of preoperative or postoperative radiation therapy and chemotherapy and different types of intraoperative management together with small numbers of patients make objective comparison of the literature difficult.

Differentiation between postoperative data and long-term results is necessary. There are few prospective studies (Seski & Diokno 1977; Christ & Gunselmann 1980; Ralph et al 1987) or control series. Only preoperative assessment of subjective micturition problems together with objective data including urodynamic investigation would be able to bring postoperative problems into correct perspective. Ralph and co-workers (1987) demonstrated that from those women complaining of sphincter incompetence after Wertheim–Meigs procedure (52%) there were only 8% with a *de novo* incontinence, whereas 44% were already leaking before surgery. Additional radiotherapy apparently does not influence bladder symptoms; there is evidence that the shorter the vaginal remnant, the greater the chance of the patient having urinary symptoms. Lewington (1956) demonstrated that 69% of the patients with vaginal length shorter than 4 cm had symptoms in comparison with 21% of patients with a vagina longer than 4 cm. Fraser (1966) found that 73% of patients with a shorter vaginal length were symptomatic. These subjective data were confirmed by Ralph et al (1988) who found a significant decrease of bladder function when the length of the vaginal cuff resected was more than 2 cm (Table 22.2).

If we take the length of postoperative need for bladder drainage as the first sign of damage to the nerve supply, we can demonstrate that with increased radicality of pelvic surgery, the duration of voiding dysfunction increases (Table 22.3).

In a prospective study on 43 patients undergoing a standardized Wertheim–Meigs procedure, Casper & Petri (1993) demonstrated a significant increase in maximal bladder capacity, first sensation and residual together with a marked decrease of flow rates as a sign of a functional outlet obstruction. Functional urethral length, urethral closure pressure at rest and at strain were more or less unchanged (Table 22.4).

Table 22.3 Bladder drainage according to technique.

Technique	
Telinde	8.3 days
Wertheim-Meigs	13.7 days
Schauta	14.7 days
Posterior exenteration	18.5 days

From Petri (1996)

PREVENTION

To reduce the frequency of bladder dysfunction after radical pelvic surgery, and minimize legal problems, detailed preoperative examination of the urinary tract is helpful.

In spite of the possible risks for bladder function, radicality of the procedure has to be decided by the extent of the tumour in order to achieve cure; however, follow-up studies in recent years have shown that there is no decisive benefit in ultraradical procedures like the Latzko, with extensive resection of parametria of paracolpium together with hemicolpectomy. The benefit of the laparoscopical approach for lymphadenectomy, together with the Schauta

Table 22.4 Urodynamic results after radical surgery.

	Preoperative		Postoperative		
Bladder capacity	310+/–65		530+/–120		↑
First sensation	130+/–25		>350	↓	
Flow	32+/–13		14+/–6		↓
Residual	>50	3/48	<50	12/48	↑
			50–100	25/48	
			>100	11/48	
Functional urethra	2.4+/–0.8		2.2+/–0.7		n.s.
Urethral pressure	52+/–21		45+/–19		n.s.
Closure pressure	38/48+		34/48+		n.s.
	10/48–		14/48–		

From Casper & Petri (1993)

procedure with extensive damage to the pelvic floor (Schuchardt incision) and wide resection of paracolpium, must be doubted.

Efficient drainage of wound cavities with peritoneal incisions left open in order to prevent haematomas, lymph cysts and, thus, infection and adhesions plays a decisive role. Bladder drainage is best accomplished with a suprapubic catheter because of:

- Good patient tolerance
- Reduced incidence of urinary infection
- Early return to spontaneous micturition
- Possible control of residual urine without further catheterization
- Avoidance of urethral trauma and discomfort.

In addition, reduction of the incidence of fistula formation seems possible by effective suprapubic drainage (van Nagell et al 1972; Petri & Jonas 1980).

Even after removal of the bladder drainage after supposed sufficient bladder emptying, residual should be controlled by ultrasound in order to prevent overdistension because of the reduced feeling of bladder filling. Should severe voiding disorder persist in spite of this regimen, early urodynamic and endoscopic investigation will enable specific therapy to be adopted.

TREATMENT

We have to differentiate between routine postoperative measures and specific treatment. With standardized surgical technique adapted to the stage of tumour, we have performed more than 450 radical pelvic Wertheim–Meigs procedures with only one vesicovaginal fistula (a stage IIa cervical carcinoma with 21 weeks of gestation) and were able to discharge all patients without a catheter (residual urine in several below 100 ml) between day 8 and day 14. We allow continuous drainage for 5 days, then clamp the suprapubic catheter and ask the patient to void every 3–4 hours, whether or not there is any desire to void.

Indication for the use of physical, medical or surgical action after radical surgery is not determined by the classification of the possible neurological or structural lesion but by subjective complaints and urodynamic and urethrocystoscopic findings.

Adequate emptying of the bladder is a prerequisite of recovery of lower urinary tract function. Loss of sensation for bladder filling and functional outlet obstruction are typical findings that are mostly uninfluenced by pharmacotherapy. Alpha-blockers of the phenoxybenzamine type have severe side-effects (e.g. hypotension) and, hypotonic detrusor being the main cause of obstructed micturition, are of little effect. Cholinergics (e.g. myocholine) have a very short effective half-life and a considerable number of side-effects (including diarrhoea), and are mostly unable to influence the predominant surgical trauma to the bladder wall and the sequelae of tissue reaction to anaemia (ligature of the upper vesical vessels) and the lymph stasis.

In the case of long-lasting obstructed micturition caused by scarification of the bladder neck, or periurethral fibrosis after morphological and urodynamic proof of diagnosis, we perform a bladder neck incision as described by Turner-Warwick et al (1973). We have had a good success rate without serious complications (Petri et al 1978).

The role of physiotherapy (learning relaxation of the pelvic floor and/or induction of a detrusor contraction) and electrostimulation with superficial electrodes is undetermined as yet. Being without serious side-effects, and encouraging the patient to play a more active role in recovery, these techniques are part of our regular postoperative schedule.

Summarizing our strategy in postoperative voiding dysfunction we would like to state that aggressive management of female voiding dysfunction is of little effectiveness. Drugs are largely ineffective, with the exception of hormones (not least because of their psychotropic effect). The logical sequence of events should be: urethrocystoscopy, urodynamic workup, calibration, and (if a suprapubic drainage is not in place) self-catheterization.

In spite of a sometimes definitive loss of sensation of bladder filling within months after surgery, patients learn to feel the distension of the peritoneum covering the bladder as a sign of bladder filling.

POSTERIOR EXENTERATIONS

In selected cases of central tumours of the small pelvis, like squamous cell carcinoma of the cervix, vagina or vulva, melanoma or tumours of the colorectum, posterior exenteration is performed to preserve the bladder and to restrict the psychosocial trauma to a bearable state. In addition, reduction of the extent of surgery should lower morbidity and mortality. Reviewing our long-term survival rate, this seems to be true (70% in comparison with 52% of patients with anterior or total exenteration). However, because of intense denervation and tilting of the

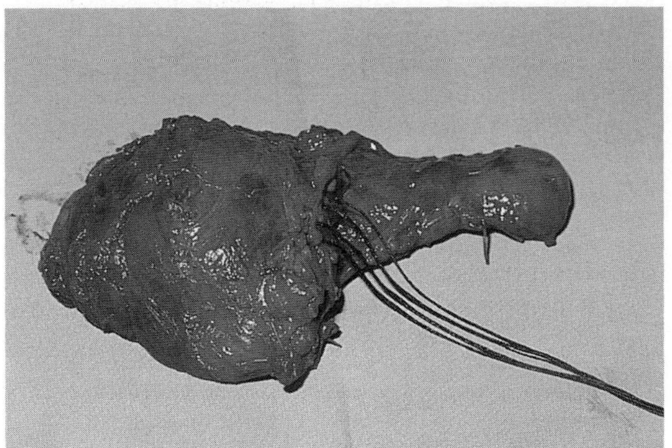

Fig. 22.1 Surgical specimen from posterior exenteration for treatment of squamous cell carcinoma of posterior vaginal wall.

bladder into the empty sacral wound cavity (as in abdominoperineal resection), severe micturition disorders result. Lesions of the pelvic and hypogastric plexuses lead to an atonic bladder with residual urine and complete loss of sensation with additional sphincter incompetence caused by a hypotonic urethra. Despite some incontinence, emptying of the bladder is insufficient and intermittent catheterization or suprapubic drainage is necessary.

In our patients, all forms of bladder training, physiotherapy and electrostimulation, pharmacotherapy and urethral surgery were insufficient. In younger patients with good prognosis for the primary disease, we now recommend total exenteration with a continent pouch diversion (e.g. Mainz pouch; Thüroff et al 1988); we think managing an additional dry stoma is easier to learn and suffer than permanent incontinence, catheterization, and recurrent urinary tract infection (Figs 22.1 and 22.2; Friedberg & Petri 1996).

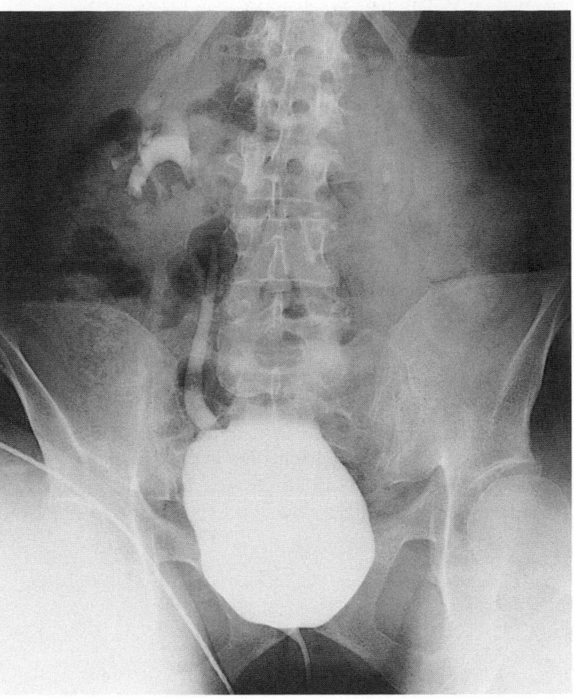

Fig. 22.2 Same patient as Fig 22.1, 1 year postoperatively: voiding cystourethrogram demonstrating residual urine, vesicoureteric reflux and deviation of the bladder neck because of extensive scarring. Clinically this patient had persistent urinary tract infection together with stress incontinence.

SUMMARY

Radical pelvic surgery results in various bladder disturbances because of damage to the pelvic nerves, partial interruption of blood supply, and lymphatic drainage. Dislocation of the bladder into the wound cavity and iatrogenic lesions to the urethra during the postoperative phase augment these disorders. The therapeutic regimen cannot be decided schematically but is influenced by subjective complaints, clinical findings and morphological and urodynamic data. If adequate micturition cannot be established, in spite of suprapubic drainage and adjuvant physiotherapy and electrostimulation, specific drugs, bladder retraining or bladder neck incision may be helpful. With surgical radicality adapted to the stage of tumour there is a decisive reduction in morbidity but, if micturition problems occur, patience is the treatment of choice.

REFERENCES

Asmussen M, Miller A 1983 Clinical Gynaecological Urology. Blackwell Scientific, Oxford

Casper F, Petri E 1993 Urodynamische Befunde nach Radikaloperationen. Archives of Gynecology and Obstetrics 254: 477–478

Christ F, Gunselmann W 1980 Untersuchungen zur Urodynamik von Harnblase und Harnröhre nach Zervixkrebsoperationen. Geburtshilfe und Frauenheilkunde 40: 610–618

Dargent D 1987 A new future for Schauta's operation through a presurgical retroperitoneal pelviscopy. European Journal of Gynaecological Oncology 8: 292–296

Dargent D 1993 Laparoscopic surgery and gynecologic cancer. Current Opinion in Obstetrics and Gynecology 5: 294–300

Fraser A C 1966 The late effects of Wertheim's hysterectomy on the urinary tract. British Journal of Obstetrics and Gynaecology 73: 1002–1007

Friedberg V, Petri E 1996 Möglichkeiten und Grenzen der Exenterationschirurgie. In: Petri E (ed) Gynäkologische Urologie, 2nd edn. Thieme, Stuttgart, New York, pp 119–130
Lewington W 1956 Disturbances of micturition following Wertheim hysterectomy. Journal of Obstetrics and Gynaecology of the British Empire 63: 861–864
Mundy A R 1982 An anatomical explanation for bladder dysfunction following rectal and uterine surgery. British Journal Urology 54: 501–504
Petri E 1996 Bladder dysfunction after intraabdominal or vaginal surgery. In: Bent A, Ostergard D R (eds) Urogynaecology and Urodynamics, 4th edn. Williams & Wilkins, Baltimore.
Petri E, Jonas U 1980 Indikationen der transurethralen und suprapubischen Harnableitung. Urologe (B) 20: 164–165
Petri E, Walz P H, Jonas U 1978 Transurethral bladder neck operation in neurogenic bladder. European Urology 4: 189–191
Ralph G et al 1987 Functionelle Störungen des unteren Harntraktes nach der abdominellen and vaginalen Radikaloperation des Zervixkrebses. Geburtshilfe und Frauenheilkunde 47: 551–554
Ralph G, Tamussino K, Lichtenegger 1988 Urologic complications after radical abdominal hysterectomy for cervical cancer. Bailliere's Clinical Obstetrics and Gynaecology 2: 943–946
Seski J C, Diokno A C 1977 Bladder dysfunction after radical abdominal hysterectomy. American Journal of Obstetrics and Gynaecology 128: 643–651
Thüroff J W, Alken P, Riedmiller H, Jacobi G H, Hohenfellner R 1988 100 cases of MAINZ pouch: continuing experience and evolution. Journal of Urology 140: 293–297
Twombley G H, Landers D 1956 The innervation of the bladder with reference to radical hysterectomy. American Journal of Obstetrics and Gynecology 71: 1291–1300
Turner-Warwick R et al 1973 A urodynamic view of the clinical problems associated with bladder neck dysfunction and its treatment by endoscopic incision. British Journal of Urology 45: 44–59
Van Nagell J R, Penny R M, Roddick J W 1972 Suprapubic bladder drainage following radical hysterectomy. American Journal of Obstetrics and Gynecology 113: 849–850

SECTION 3
CHAPTER
23

Genitourinary fistulae

W GLENN HURT

INTRODUCTION

Throughout history, genitourinary fistulae have been a major cause of morbidity in women. A large vesicovaginal fistula was found in an Egyptian mummy that is estimated to be over 4000 years old (Mahfouz 1960). The same mummy also had a complete perineal laceration. The coexistence of these problems in the same person suggests that both were the result of childbirth. In the developing countries of the world, the leading cause of genitourinary fistulae is still childbirth, but in the developed countries it is pelvic surgery.

Vesicovaginal fistulae were first mentioned in European literature towards the end of the sixteenth century, but there was no mention of cure (Mahfouz 1960). In 1840, John Peter Mettauer, a surgeon in rural Virginia, reported the first successful cure of a vesicovaginal fistula in the United States (Mettauer 1840). In 1852, James Marion Sims, a surgeon in Alabama, acknowledged the cures of Mettauer in Virginia and of Hayward in Massachusetts when he described his own procedure for the treatment of vesicovaginal fistulae (Sims 1852). The cure of vesicovaginal fistulae is recognized as an important milestone in surgery, and because of his contributions in this field Marion Sims became known, on both sides of the Atlantic, as the 'Father of Modern Gynecology'.

CLASSIFICATION

Genitourinary fistulae are usually classified according to organ involvement. 'Simple' fistulae involve two organs; 'complex' fistulae involve three or more organs (Table 23.1). Genitourinary fistulae may be further classified according to aetiology (Table 23.2).

Table 23.1 Anatomical classification of genitourinary fistulae.

Simple fistulae
Urethrovaginal
Vesicovaginal
Ureterovaginal
Vesicouterine
Ureterouterine
Complex fistulae
Vesicoureterovaginal
Vesicoureterouterine
Vesicovaginorectal

Table 23.2 Aetiology of genitourinary fistulae.

Surgical
Obstetrical
Malignant
Radiation
Infection
Foreign body
Traumatic
Spontaneous/idiopathic

AETIOLOGY

The true incidence of genitourinary fistulae in a given population is unknown. Most published reports involve select groups of hospitalized patients. There are many women throughout the world who have genitourinary fistulae but do not seek medical care. And, in the developing countries, there is still a shortage of funds, facilities, and surgeons capable of providing a surgical cure.

Genitourinary fistulae of obstetrical origin usually occur for two reasons: (a) obstructed labour causes pressure necrosis and slough of the bladder and sometimes the urethra, and (b) traumatic injury of the bladder and urethra at the time of delivery. In developing countries, the incidence of genitourinary fistulae secondary to infection, malignancy, and surgery is much less frequent.

In developed countries, most genitourinary fistulae are due to pelvic surgery, malignancy, or radiation therapy. Obstetrical fistulae are more likely to be the result of forceps delivery, caesarean section, or peripartum hysterectomy.

In the United States, vesicovaginal fistulae are about five times more common than ureterovaginal fistulae (Lee et al 1988). Seventy per cent of vesicovaginal fistulae result from either an abdominal or vaginal hysterectomy (Lee et al 1988) which in most cases was performed for a benign condition. Genitourinary fistulae are less often associated with radical pelvic surgery or radiation therapy for malignant conditions. Occasionally, a vesicovaginal fistula will develop following cervical conization, anterior colporrhaphy, a urinary continence procedure, bladder neck resection, or other lower urinary tract or bowel surgery. Infrequent non-surgical causes of vesicovaginal fistulae include pelvic infections, bladder stones, foreign bodies or neglected pessaries, sexual intercourse, and pelvic trauma.

Urethrovaginal fistulae may develop following traumatic instrumentation of the urethra, urethral diverticulectomy, or anterior colporrhaphy. Ureterovaginal fistulae are more often a complication of pelvic surgery or radiation therapy than the result of obstetrical trauma. They may develop following urological procedures such as partial cystectomy, ureterectomy, and operations for the removal of calculi.

SYMPTOMS AND SIGNS

Women with vesicovaginal and ureterovaginal fistulae often complain of uncontrollable and continuous leakage of urine from the vagina. Some fistulae, because of their small size, the pattern of their tract, or the location of their openings, will leak only intermittently. Women who have a urethrovaginal fistula that is located away from the bladder neck may have a problem with their urinary stream but experience no significant urinary incontinence. When there is uncontrollable leakage of urine, in addition to wetness, there is the offensive ammoniacal odour of urine, and the likelihood of developing vulvovaginitis due to irritation by urine and the use of absorbent protective pads and undergarments.

The presence of a urinary tract infection or a vaginal infection will intensify the discomfort. The well-oestrogenized vagina is less likely than the hypo-oestrogenic vagina to be irritated by urine. Likewise, genitourinary fistulae associated with cellulitis or malignancy or those occurring in previously radiated tissues are more likely to have more intense symptomatology. It is extremely important to diagnose and treat all associated infections and to give oestrogen to hypo-oestrogenic women, unless there is some contraindication to its use.

DIAGNOSIS

A complaint of urinary incontinence in a clinical setting of recent pelvic surgery, pelvic malignancy, pelvic radiation, and childbirth should increase the diagnostician's suspicion of a fistula. On pelvic examination, if a woman has a collection of urine in her vagina, she should be suspected of having a genitourinary fistula.

The vaginal opening of most vesicovaginal fistulae is obvious. At the time of vaginal examination, urine will usually be seen to be leaking through the fistula into the vagina. Small fistulae may be more difficult to see on routine inspection of the vagina. This may be due to the size or location of the fistula, the route of the fistulous tract, or the fact that the fistula is obscured or obstructed by vaginal pressure or instrumentation.

It is helpful to know the location of the various components of the lower urinary tract with respect to the vaginal canal (Fig. 23.1). Simple urethrovaginal fistulae should be located in the distal third of the anterior vaginal wall; simple vesicovaginal fistulae usually involve the upper two thirds of the anterior vaginal wall and, more commonly, the anterior portion of the vaginal apex. Simple ureterovaginal fistulae usually drain into the vaginal apex, and vesicouterine fistulae drain through the cervix. The drainage of complex fistulae is more unpredictable. A detailed preoperative diagnostic examination is a critical and essential part of the care of a patient with a genitourinary fistula. Several diagnostic procedures may be indicated (Hurt 1996).

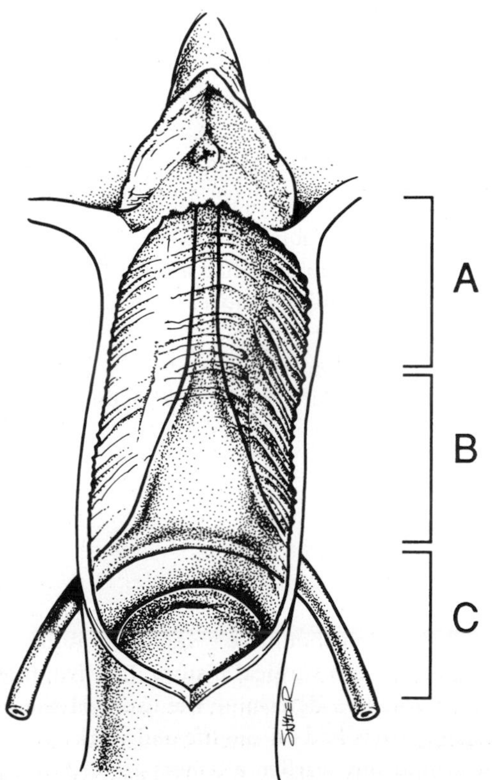

Fig. 23.1 Location of lower urinary tract structures outside the anterior vaginal wall. Note the location of the urethra, trigone, ureters, and base of the bladder with respect to the lower third (A), middle third (B), and upper third (C) of the vagina. Most post-hysterectomy vesicovaginal fistulae are located above the trigone. From Hurt (1996), with permission.

Intravesical dye test

The presence of a vesicovaginal fistula is usually confirmed by inserting either a straight or a balloon catheter through the urethra into the bladder and filling the bladder with a sterile solution containing a dye such as indigo carmine or methylene blue. Concomitant examination of the anterior vaginal wall and vaginal apex with a Sims vaginal speculum to retract the posterior vaginal wall documents the presence of a fistula and determines the location of its entry into the vagina (Fig. 23.2). Failure to distend the bladder adequately, or application of too much tension on the walls of the vagina, may prevent leakage of the distending solution through some small vesicovaginal fistulae.

Vaginal tampon test

Moir's 'tampon' or 'cotton ball' test is used to determine the type and location of small genitourinary fistulae within the vaginal canal (Moir 1973). The vagina is inspected and cleansed of secretions. Three or four tampons or large cotton balls are placed one after the other throughout the length of the vagina. A urethral catheter is used to fill the bladder with a sterile solution containing a dye such as indigo carmine or methylene blue. The catheter is removed and the patient is requested to ambulate and perform Valsalva manoeuvres. If the last cotton ball placed in the lower vagina is the only blue one found when she is reexamined in the lithotomy position, it can be assumed that the leakage is from the external urethral meatus. This leakage could be evidence of stress urinary incontinence, an unstable bladder, or a urethrovaginal fistula. Wet, blue cotton balls in the upper vagina suggest a vesicovaginal fistula. Cotton balls in the vaginal apex that are wet but not blue suggest a ureterovaginal fistula. Complex fistulae interfere with the diagnostic potential of the tampon or cotton ball test.

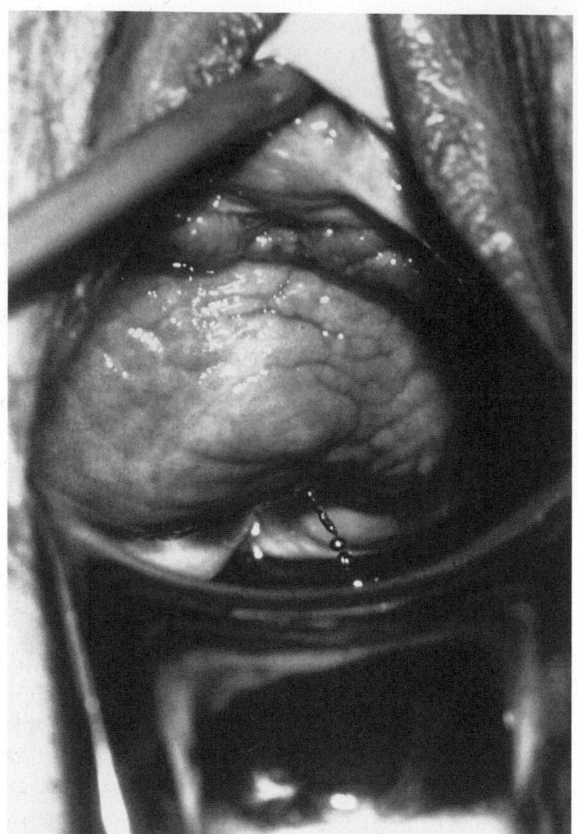

Fig. 23.2 Vesicovaginal fistula as demonstrated by the intravesical dye test. From Hurt (1996), with permission.

Flat tyre test

The patient, after voiding, is placed in the knee–chest position. A clear irrigation solution such as water or saline is used to fill the vagina to as high a level as possible, covering the anterior vaginal wall and filling the vaginal fornices. A catheter or cystoscope sheath is then placed transurethrally into the bladder to slowly fill it by the controlled instillation of an appropriate gas. The origin of escaping small gas bubbles through the liquid contained within the vagina determines the location of the vesicovaginal fistula.

Urograms

Voiding cystourethrograms can be used to document fistulae. Intravenous or bulb retrograde urograms are important diagnostic procedures when there is any likelihood that there is ureteric involvement by the fistula. Urograms are used for determining bilateral renal function, for documenting ureteral patency, for diagnosing complex ureterovesicovaginal fistulae, and for determining the presence of rare congenital abnormalities such as an ectopic ureteric opening.

Cystourethroscopy

Cystourethroscopy is performed to determine the number, size, and location of vesicovaginal fistulae and to reveal the anatomical relationship of vesicovaginal fistulae to the ureteric openings, trigone, and bladder neck. Cystoscopy can assess the inflammatory response of the bladder and can be used for removing sutures and foreign bodies. If cystoscopy in the lithotomy position is impossible because of the size of the fistula, the patient may be placed in the knee–chest position and air may be used as the distending medium. Intravenous injection of 5 cc of indigo carmine or methylene blue at the time of cystoscopy will cause the kidneys to excrete blue urine and will determine bilateral renal function and help locate both ureteric orifices, which are sometimes difficult to see because of tissue reaction and anatomical distortion. At the time of cystoscopy there may be an indication for the passage of ureteral catheters to determine the integrity of a ureter, possible involvement with a vesicovaginal fistula, for the drainage of a kidney, or as an aid to surgery. It is often necessary to repeat cystoscopy during the preoperative period to evaluate the condition of the tissues around the fistula and to determine a suitable time for fistula surgery.

Hysterograms

Hysterograms or hysteroscopy may be useful in diagnosing complex vesicovaginal fistulae involving the uterine cavity. All abnormal tissues within the bladder of patients who have had a pelvic malignancy or whose clinical findings suggest a malignancy should undergo biopsy for possible recurrence or the development of malignancy, and all tissues excised at the time of fistula closure should be examined by a surgical pathologist.

PREOPERATIVE CARE

Special attention should be given to obtaining a complete medical and surgical history. Incisive questions must be asked to determine the cause of the fistula, the effect it has had on the life and work of the individual, and any earlier attempts towards diagnosis and cure.

A general physical examination should be performed to determine the presence and severity of any medical or psychological conditions that might affect the patient's ability to care for herself, to withstand surgery, and to heal her fistula. Detailed examination of the vagina, bladder, and rectum complete with endoscopy should be made initially and repeated as necessary. The examination should determine the anatomical location of and the organs affected by the fistula, the condition of all surrounding tissues, the status of the remaining genital organs, the status of the pelvic support system, and any changes resulting from prior operative procedures.

Basic laboratory studies should include a complete haemogram, blood and electrolyte studies, renal function tests, and a urine culture of the best possible catheterized or voided urine specimen. Additional bacteriologic, serologic, or cytologic studies should be performed according to the patient's history and physical findings. All laboratory studies should be repeated as indicated to determine that renal function is optimum, that there is no evidence of local or systemic infection, and that a chronic illness such as diabetes is well controlled. It is important to remove any bladder calculi or non-absorbable suture material and to clear the patient of any urinary tract or vaginal infection.

Some small, fresh vesicovaginal fistulae not associated with a malignancy or radiation therapy may spontaneously close if the urine can be diverted within several days of their occurrence. In selected cases, it is reasonable to use an indwelling bladder catheter for 4–6 weeks to see whether spontaneous healing will occur (Waaldijk 1994). Urinary diversion is less likely to permit healing and spontaneous closure of a vesicovaginal fistula if the fistulous tract is well epithelized.

For years, the standard procedure has been to delay the repair of vesicovaginal fistulae that are the result of obstetric and surgical injuries for 3–6 months and to delay the repair of radiation-induced fistulae for up to one year. Recently, an effort has been made to relieve the patients of their misery by undertaking earlier repair of fistulae (Moriel et al 1993; Blaivas et al 1995). Some vesicovaginal fistulae that are diagnosed within 24–48 hours of surgical injury can be repaired immediately; however, when an inflammatory response, infection, or tissue necrosis is present, it is best to delay an attempt at closure until these problems are corrected.

Because the vagina and bladder are both oestrogen-sensitive organs, it is reasonable to begin oestrogen replacement therapy in hypo-oestrogenic women awaiting fistula surgery in an effort to improve the blood supply and the pliability and integrity of the pelvic tissues.

The timing of fistula repair depends on the cause of the fistula, its size, its location, and the quality of the tissues involved. In general, fistulae following surgical injury may be closed earlier than those following obstetrical injury; fistulae following radiation injury require a longer waiting period to allow the long-term vascular effects of the radiation therapy to occur. The first attempt at repair is the one most likely to result in cure. Therefore, even though the procedure is elective and rapid repair may be urgent for the patient, the precise timing of the surgery must be left to the judgement of the operating surgeon.

Bladder catheters should not be used at least a week before fistula surgery to help clear the bladder

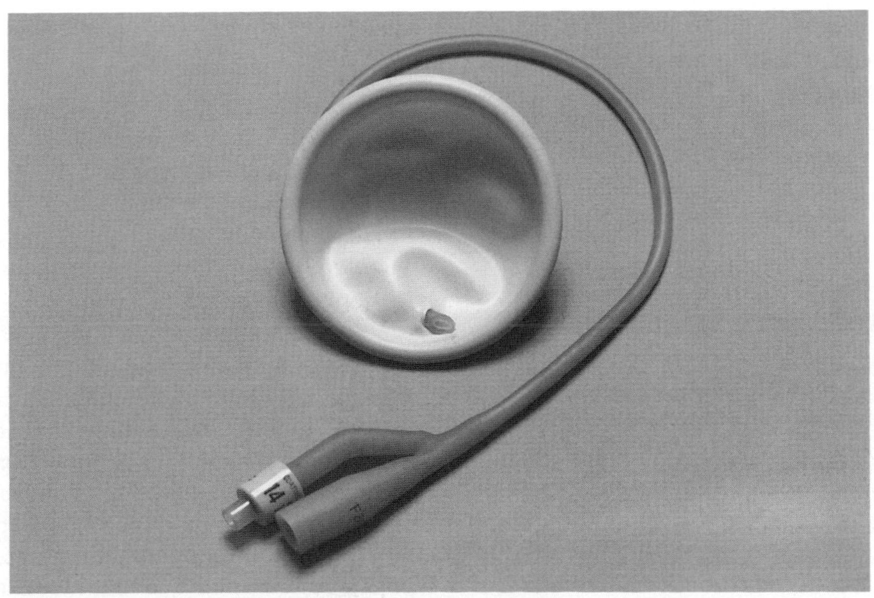

Fig. 23.3 Vaginal urinary drainage device fashioned from a contraceptive diaphragm and urethral catheter. From Hurt (1992), with permission.

of infection and reduce inflammation. Patients should be advised to use hyperabsorbent pads to collect their urine and to keep it away from the perineal tissues. To improve patient comfort, a vaginal urinary drainage device can be constructed by using a contraceptive diaphragm and urethral catheter (Fig. 23.3).

NON-SURGICAL MANAGEMENT

As previously stated, some small, fresh genitourinary fistulae will heal spontaneously if urine is diverted from the fistulous tract. Cystoscopic fulguration of the fistulous tract and subsequent bladder drainage have successfully cured some vesicovaginal fistulae with a diameter of less than 3 mm (Stovsky et al 1994). If this type of therapy is undertaken, the electrical current should be used to disrupt only the epithelium of the tract. Thermal injury to the adjacent tissues may actually cause the fistula to enlarge.

SURGICAL MANAGEMENT

The basic surgical principles involved in treating genitourinary fistulae are listed in Table 23.3.

Urethrovaginal fistulae

Urethrovaginal fistulae may be more difficult to cure than vesicovaginal fistulae. The treatment of urethrovaginal fistulae has to be individualized depending upon the size, location, and degree of involvement of the urethral continence mechanism. It is often difficult to repair a significant urethral defect and assure postoperative urinary continence. The latter condition may require a second operation.

Simple urethrovaginal fistulae that do not involve the continence mechanism of the proximal urethra may be repaired by excision of the vaginal end of the fistulous tract and a layered closure of the urethral muscularis with adsorbable suture (e.g. 4–0 chromic catgut), and of the fibromuscular wall of the vagina and the vaginal epithelium with delayed absorbable suture (e.g. 3–0 or 4–0 polyglactin or polyglycolic acid). It is often desirable to add depth to the closure by the interposition of a well-vascularized pedicle of fatty tissue (Martius' labial fat pad). If no tissue is brought in to add depth to the closure of a urethrovaginal fistula, it is important to mobilize the final layer of the vaginal wall in a manner that will allow it to cover subjacent suture lines and not have its suture line superimposed upon them.

Table 23.3 Surgical principles for genitourinary fistula closure.

Clear all infections of urinary tract and vagina; prescribe prophylactic perioperative antibiotics
Good exposure of operative field
Good light source and suction
Wide mobilization of tissue layers around fistula
Meticulous haemostasis
Invert urothelium and adjacent submucosa
Layered, tension-free closure
Augmentation of repair by use of homologous tissues, if indicated (labial fat pad, peritoneal flap, omentum, myocutaneous flap, etc.)
Adequate urine drainage
Recommend a period of 'pelvic rest'

Vesicovaginal fistulae

Vesicovaginal fistulae are by far the most common genitourinary fistula encountered in the developed countries of the world. Most occur as the result of gynaecologic surgery performed for a benign condition. If such a fistula is diagnosed within the first 48 hours following surgery, and if there is no significant inflammatory response or necrosis about the fistula, immediate reoperation and repair should be considered. Vesicovaginal fistulae that have an associated inflammatory response should be treated by continuous bladder catheter drainage. Some can be expected to heal spontaneously (Stovsky et al 1994). If a vesicovaginal fistula does not close after four to six weeks of continuous bladder drainage, it is unlikely to do so.

Latzko procedure

Most simple vesicovaginal fistulae seen following a hysterectomy for benign disease are small and are located in the vaginal apex, at or just above the interureteric ridge (Mercier's bar). This particular type of fistula can be treated soon after it occurs and with greater than 90% success by the Latzko procedure (Latzko 1942). The Latzko procedure (Fig. 23.4) is performed with the patient in the full lithotomy position. The vaginal epithelium about the vaginal opening of the fistula may be separated from the fibromuscular wall of the bladder by hydrodissection, employing either sterile saline or a dilute solution of a vasoconstrictive agent (e.g. Pitressin, neosynephrine, or epinephrine). A superficial circular incision is made through the vaginal epithelium 1–2 cm outside the opening of the fistula. This circle is then divided into four quadrants around the opening of the fistula. With great care, all of the vaginal

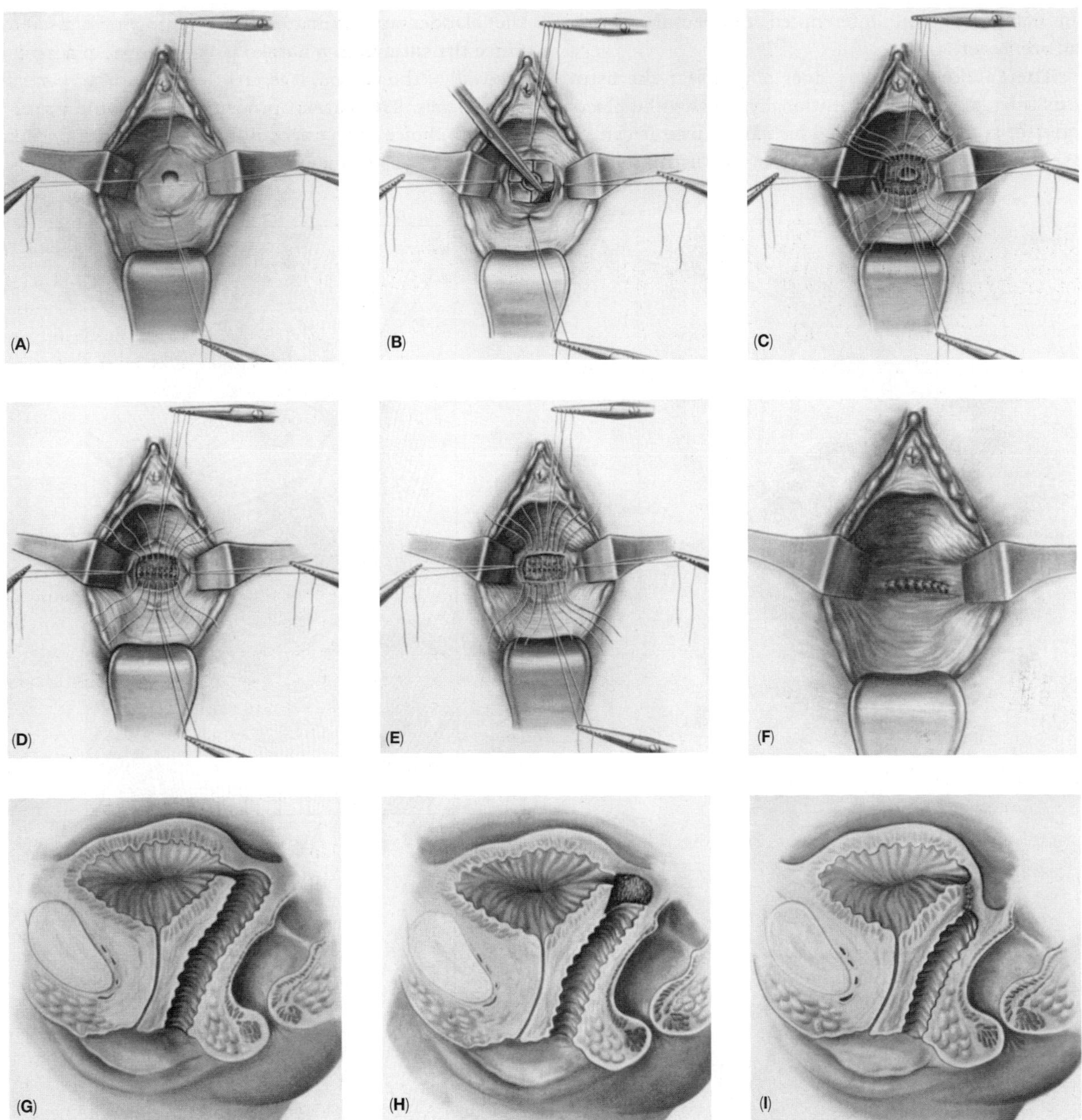

Fig. 23.4 Latzko procedure for vesicovaginal fistula repair. (**A**) Typical post-hysterectomy vaginal vault fistula. (**B**) Incision of vaginal epithelium about the fistula and the beginning of removal of vaginal epithelium. (**C**) The first layer approximates the vaginal wall over the fistula and inverts the fistulous tract. (**D**) The second suture layer approximates the vaginal wall over the first suture layer. (**E**) The third suture layer approximates the vaginal epithelium. (**F**) Closed site of the vesicovaginal fistula. (**G**) Location of a typical post-hysterectomy vesicovaginal fistula in the anterior apex of the vaginal vault. (**H**) Vaginal apex with vaginal epithelium removed from around the vesicovaginal fistula's entry into the vagina. (**I**) Completed Latzko partial colpocleisis. From Falk & Bunkin (1951), with permission.

epithelium is dissected off the fibromuscular wall of the vagina within the area of dissection. When this has been accomplished, the fibromuscular wall of the bladder is approximated over the fistulous opening using absorbable interrupted sutures (e.g. 3–0 or 4–0 chromic). Subsequently, the first layer of the closure is oversewn using interrupted delayed-absorbable imbricating sutures (3–0 or 4–0 polyglactin or polyglycolic acid) in the adjacent fibromuscular wall of the bladder. At this point, the closure is tested for watertightness by the instillation of 250–300 ml of a sterile solution (e.g. milk or a dilute solution of indigo carmine or methylene blue) into the bladder. If leakage occurs, interrupted sutures are placed to make the closure watertight. When this has been accomplished, the vaginal epithelium is approximated with the same type of interrupted delayed-absorbable suture material.

The Latzko procedure does not dissect the fistulous tract, nor does it intentionally involve the placement of sutures in the bladder muscularis. It can be used even though the opening of the fistula within the bladder approximates the opening of a ureter. Since the sutures in a Latzko procedure are placed in the wall of the vagina, it is, in effect, an apical, partial colpocleisis. The Latzko procedure is not the procedure of choice for vesicovaginal fistulae that do not involve the vaginal vault.

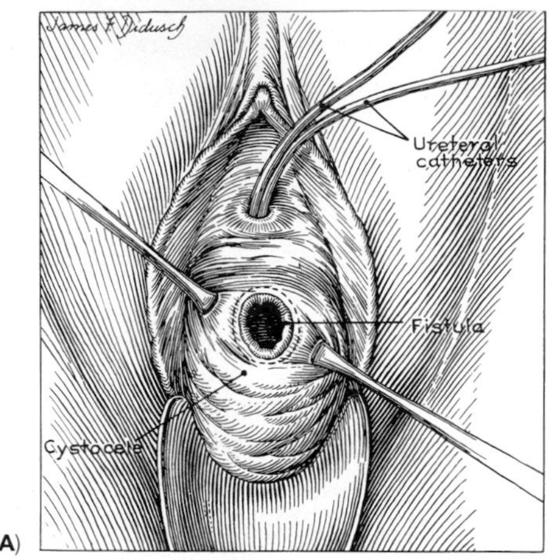

(A)

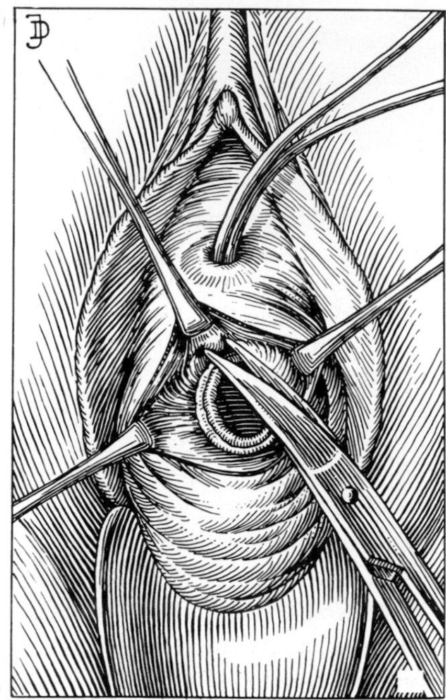
(B)

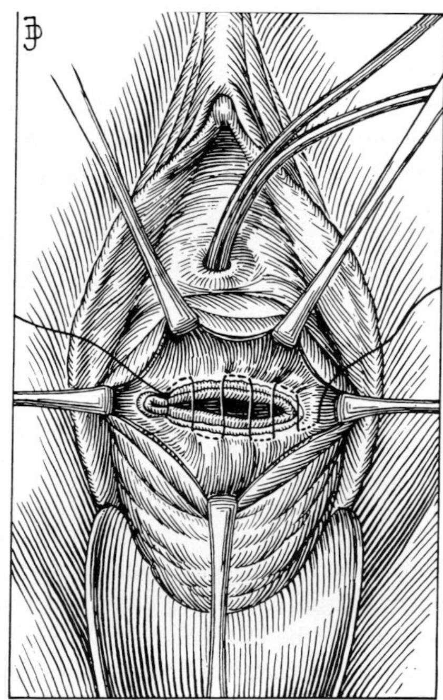
(C)

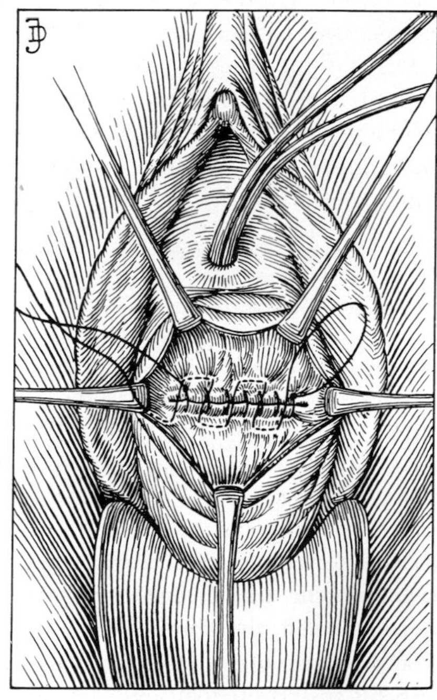
(D)

Fig. 23.5 Vaginal layered closure of simple vesicovaginal fistula. (**A**) Ureteral catheters are in place and the location of the incision around the fistulous opening is indicated by a dotted line. (**B**) Vaginal epithelium is mobilized around the fistula. (**C**) The first suture line of absorbable suture is placed, with the urothelium inverted into the bladder. (**D**) The second suture line inverts the first. Excess vaginal mucosa is trimmed and approximated with interrupted sutures. From Rock & Thompson (1997), with permission.

Layered vaginal repair

Vesicovaginal fistulae that do not involve the vaginal apex are best treated by a layered dissection and closure of the vaginal wall (Fig. 23.5). In the past, a lot of attention has been give to dissection and removal of the entire fistulous tract. When this is done, the surgeon must be careful that the dissection does not enlarge the fistula and place its submucosal closure under significant tension. It is often preferable to leave the fistulous opening into the bladder and to preserve its fibrotic ring. In doing so, the fistula is not enlarged, bleeding is minimized, and the tissue about the opening is more easily sutured in a way that will invert the mucosa into the lumen of the bladder. Following the closure of the opening into the bladder with interrupted absorbable suture material (3–0 or 4–0 chromic catgut), a layered closure of the bladder muscularis and subsequently of the fibromuscular wall of the vagina is performed with delayed-absorbable sutures (3–0 or 4–0 polyglactin or polyglycolic acid). At this point the closure should be tested for watertightness. The cut edges of the vaginal epithelium are then approximated with interrupted delayed-absorbable suture material. It would be preferable to close the vaginal epithelium by mobilizing a flap that would cover the repair without the superimposition of suture lines. It is more important, however, to effect a tension-free closure throughout.

The surgeon who repairs a vesicovaginal fistula should be aware of the possible involvement of one or both ureters, making it a complex fistula. Such involvement also requires surgical correction of the ureteric defect. Intravenous dye (e.g. indigo carmine or methylene blue, 5 ml) can be administered and cystoscopy performed to test the kidney and ureteral function following the repair of a vesicovaginal fistula.

Abdominal repair

This approach is recommended for complex fistulae. It may be the procedure of choice for radiation-induced fistulae since it allows placement of a portion of the omentum to separate the repairs of the bladder and the vagina. The vesicovaginal component of the fistula is often approached by a sagittal cystotomy to the site of the fistula (Fig. 23.6). The fistulous tract is excised and the vesicovaginal septum is widely dissected. The opening into the vagina is closed with two layers of delayed-absorbable sutures (3–0 polyglactin or polyglycolic acid). The incision in the bladder is repaired in three layers using absorbable suture (3–0 chromic) to approximate the submucosa and two layers of delayed-absorbable

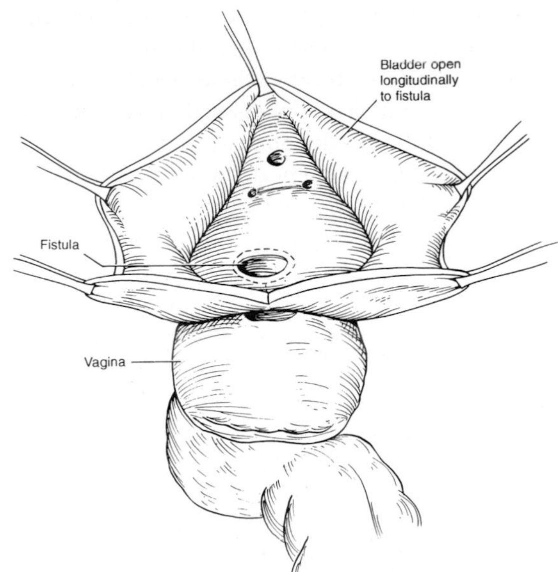

Fig. 23.6 Abdominal closure of vesicovaginal fistula. A sagittal cystotomy has been performed. The fistulous tract will be excised, the rectovaginal septum dissected, and layered closures performed. From Saclarides & Fenner (1996) with permission.

suture (3–0 polyglactin or polyglycolic acid) to imbricate the adjacent muscularis. A pedicle of omentum is mobilized and sutured between the vaginal and the bladder defect repairs. If other organs are involved in the fistula, their individual defects must be individually managed.

Ureterovaginal fistulae

Most ureterovaginal fistulae involve the distal 4–5 cm of one or both ureters. Such fistulae are most easily repaired by a reimplantation procedure known as ureteroneocystotomy. When the upper ureter is involved and there is a viable lower ureteric segment, the ureteric defect may be repaired by ureteroureterostomy.

Ureteroneocystotomy

This is usually an abdominal procedure. If there is a distal ureteric stump, it should be ligated with permanent suture material. The dome of the bladder is opened and the bladder wall is incised at a location that will allow tension-free entry of the distal end of the involved ureter. The end of the ureter is spatulated bilaterally within the bladder and each flap is secured to the bladder mucosa with interrupted absorbable suture (3–0 chromic catgut). The adventitia of the ureter is secured to the outside bladder wall with several fine interrupted delayed-absorbable or permanent sutures. It is very important that there be no tension on any ureteric anastomosis. If this is likely, it can be overcome by mobilizing the bladder upwards after detachment of the dome of the bladder from the retrosymphysis by dissection of the space of Retzius, by suturing the dome of the bladder to the psoas muscle (psoas hitch), or by creating a bladder tube (Boari flap) into which the distal end of the ureter is sewn.

Ureteroureterostomy

This is an abdominal procedure that involves the joining of the two ends of a transected ureter. If there is a damaged ureteric segment, it should be completely excised. The cut ends of the ureter may be spatulated to increase the diameter of the closure and to help prevent postoperative stenosis. The ureteric anastomosis should be performed over a stenting catheter using fine interrupted-absorbable or delayed-absorbable sutures. Again, it is important to emphasize that there should never be tension on a ureteric anastomosis.

Ureteric anastomoses should have a negative pressure drain placed within the operative site but not in direct contact with the anastomosis. This drain should be brought out of the pelvis, extraperitoneally, and exit the skin through its own separate abdominal wall incision. The purpose of the drain is to remove any blood, serum, lymph, or urine that may collect about the ureteric anastomosis.

Complex genitourinary fistulae

A discussion of the treatment of the various complex forms of genitourinary fistulae is beyond the scope of this chapter. The care of such fistulae has to be individualized depending upon aetiology, location, size, organ involvement, and the association with malignancy or a history of radiation therapy. Most complex fistulae will be repaired by an abdominal approach (Moriel et al 1993). The surgeon is encouraged to use peritoneal or omental flaps to separate the individual repairs that may involve the lower urinary tract, vagina, and bowel.

POSTOPERATIVE CARE

During the immediate postoperative period the surgeon should be most concerned about bleeding, infection, and urinary tract drainage. Bleeding into the operative site can result in haematoma formation and the disruption of the repair. It may also predispose to infection and the development of an abscess. Bleeding into the bladder can interfere with bladder drainage. Meticulous haemostasis is one of the hallmarks of a successful repair.

Perioperative 'prophylactic' antibiotics are recommended for genitourinary fistula repair. Postoperatively, the need to continue antibiotic therapy must be left to the judgement of the surgeon. Symptomatic urinary tract infections and any infection of the operative site must be treated aggressively according to its microbiology. Patients should also be examined for vaginal infections and, if present, these should be treated.

It is important to provide adequate urinary drainage. Most surgeons will place a suprapubic bladder catheter during surgery and use it for postoperative bladder drainage. The incidence of urinary tract infections will be reduced if the catheter is connected to a closed drainage system. When operating upon the ureter, the need for ureteral stents and catheters is very much dependent upon the operative procedure and the experience of the surgeon. It is best to place a negative pressure silicone drain (e.g. Jackson-Pratt) to the operative site of a ureteric anastomosis to help prevent the formation of a haematoma or urinoma.

The timing of removal of all drains, stents, and catheters should be based upon the operative procedure, tissue conditions, and the surgeon's judgement. Postoperative intravenous urograms or cystograms may be indicated to determine urinary tract function and the integrity of the repair.

COMPLICATIONS

Immediate complications of genitourinary fistula repair include bleeding, infection, and urinary leakage. Any of these complications may cause operative failure. Long-term complications include stress urinary incontinence, detrusor instability incontinence, or incontinence due to a recurrent genitourinary fistula. Ureteral stenosis may jeopardize renal function and, if bilateral, may be life-threatening.

RESULTS

One of the most controversial aspects of genitourinary fistula surgery has to do with the time of the repair. Since it is the first surgical procedure that is most likely to cure the fistula, timing is of utmost

Table 23.4 Literature summary on cure of vesicovaginal fistulae From Blaivas et al (1995), with permission.

Reference	No.	No. success (%)	Timing of repair	Approach
Collins et al	24[a]	16 (67)	20 early (< 8 wks) 4 late (>4 mos)	24 vaginal
Eisen et al	29[a]	26 (90)	Late (>3 mos)	29 abdominal
Persky et al	7[a]	6 (86)	Early (<10 wks)	6 abdominal 1 vaginal
Tancer (1980)	45[a]	42 (93)	Late (8–16 wks)	43 vaginal 1 abdominal 1 spontaneous closure
Wein et al	34[a]	30 (88)	Late (>3 mos)	34 abdominal
Keetel & Laube	168[a]	158 (94)	Late (3–4 mos)	156 vaginal 6 abdominal 6 abdominal and vaginal
Bissada & McDonald	7[a]	7 (100)		7 abdominal
Cruikshank	11	11 (100)	Early (10–35 days)	9 vaginal 1 abdominal 1 abdominal and vaginal
Lee et al	182[a]	178 (98)	15 early (<8 wks) 167 late (>8 wks)	15 vaginal 130 vaginal 37 abdominal
Elkins et al	23[a]	21 (91)	Late (2–3 mos)	23 vaginal
Wang & Hadley	16	15 (94)	7 early (<3 mos) 9 late (>3 mos)	16 vaginal
Blandy et al	25	25 (100)	12 early (<6 wks) 13 late (>6 wks)	25 abdominal
O'Conor	77	70 (91)	Late (2–3 mos)	77 abdominal
Raz et al	19	16 (84)	Late (2–3 mos)	19 vaginal
Blaivas et al	24	23 (96)	14 early (<12 wks) 10 late (>12 wks)	8 vaginal 5 abdominal 1 spontaneous closure 7 vaginal 3 abdominal

[a]Indicates obstetrical and radiation-induced fistulae.

importance. There is no consensus in surgical literature as to what constitutes the timing of an early repair versus a late repair. Recent experience has shown that, once the local inflammatory response has subsided, there is no benefit from delaying surgery if the surgeon is experienced in fistula repair (Moriel et al 1993; Blaivas et al 1995). Recent surgical literature documents the fact that most gynaecologists and an increasing number of urologists are repairing the majority of vesicovaginal fistulae vaginally (Blaivas et al 1995). Currently, the abdominal approach is being used primarily for complex genitourinary fistulae involving other pelvic organs (e.g. uterus, bowel), ureteric fistulae, and some radiation fistulae. Results of previous series of vesicovaginal fistula repairs, indicating timing of repair and surgical approach, are given in Table 23.4.

REFERENCES

Bissada N K, McDonald D 1983 Management of giant vesicovaginal and vesicourethrovaginal fistulas. Journal of Urology 130: 1073–1075

Blandy J P, Badenoch D F, Fowler C G, Jenkins B J, Thomas N W M 1991 Early repair of iatrogenic injury to the ureter or bladder after gynecological surgery. Journal of Urology 146: 761–765

Blaivas J G, Heritz D M, Romanzi L J 1995 Early versus late repair of vesicovaginal fistulas: vaginal and abdominal approaches. Journal of Urology 153: 1110–1113

Collins C G, Pent D, Jones F B 1960 Results of early repair of vesicovaginal fistulas with preliminary cortisone treatment. American Journal of Obstetrics and Gynecology 60: 1005–1009

Cruikshank S H 1988 Early closure of posthysterectomy vesicovaginal fistulas. Southern Medical Journal 81: 1525–1528

Eisen M, Jurkovic K, Altwein J E, Schreiter F, Hohenfellner R 1974 Management of vesicovaginal fistulas with peritoneal flap interposition. Journal of Urology 112: 195–198

Elkins T E, DeLancey J O, McGuire E J 1990 The use of modified Martius graft as an adjunctive technique in vesicovaginal and rectovaginal fistula repair. Obstetrics and Gynecology 75: 727–733

Falk H C, Bunkin I A 1951 The management of vesicovaginal fistula following abdominal total hysterectomy. Surgery, Gynecology, and Obstetrics (now known as the Journal of the American College of Surgeons) 93: 404–410

Fichtner J, Voges G, Steinbach F, Hohenfellner R 1993 Ureterovesicovaginal fistulas. Surgery, Gynecology, and Obstetrics 176: 571–574

Hurt W G 1992 Urogynecologic Surgery. Lippincott-Raven, Philadelphia.

Hurt W G 1996 Vesicovaginal fistulas. In: Advances in Obstetrics and Gynecology Volume 3, Mosby Year Book, St Louis pp 179–201

Keetel W C, Laube D W 1982 Vaginal repair of vesicovaginal and urethrovaginal fistulas. In: Buchsbaum H J, Schmidt J D Gynecologic and Obstetric Urology, 2nd edn. W B Saunders, Philadelphia, chap. 21, pp 318–326

Latzko W 1942 Postoperative vesicovaginal fistulas: genesis and therapy. American Journal of Surgery 58: 211–228

Lee R A, Simmonds R E, Williams T O 1988 Current status of genitourinary fistula. Obstetrics and Gynecology 72: 313–319

Mahfouz N 1960 Genitourinary fistula – general survey. In: Youssef A F (ed) Gynecological Urology. Thomas, Springfield, Illinois pp 137–161

Mettauer J P 1840 Vesico-vaginal fistula. Boston Medical Journal 22: 154–155

Moir J C 1973 Vesico-vaginal fistulae as seen in Britain. Journal of Obstetrics and Gynaecology of the British Commonwealth 80: 598–601

Moriel E Z, Meirow D, Zilberman M, Farkas A 1993 Experience with the immediate treatment of iatrogenic bladder injuries and the repair of complex vesicovaginal fistulas by the transvesical approach. Archives of Gynecology and Obstetrics 253: 127–130

O'Conor V J Jr 1991 Transperitoneal transvesical repair of vesicovaginal fistula with omental interposition. American Urological Association Update Series, vol. 10, lesson 13

Persky L, Herman G, Guerrier K 1979 Nondelay in vesicovaginal fistula repair. Urology 13: 273–275

Raz S, Bregg K J, Nitti W, Sussman E 1993 Transvaginal repair of vesicovaginal fistula using a peritoneal flap. Journal of Urology 150: 56–59

Rock J A, Thompson J D 1997 TeLinde's Operative Gynecology 8th edn. Lippincott-Raven, Philadelphia, p. 1191

Saclarides T J, Fenner D E 1996 Urinary tract fistulas. In: Brubaker L T, Saclarides T J (eds) The Female Pelvic Floor – disorders of function and support. F A Davis, Philadelphia, p. 186

Sims J M 1852 On the treatment of vesico-vaginal fistula. American Journal of Medical Science 23: 59–82

Stovsky J D, Ignatoff J M, Blum M D, Nanninga J B, O'Conor V J, Kursh E D 1994 Use of electrocoagulation in the treatment of vesicovaginal fistulas. Journal of Urology 152: 1443–1444

Tancer M L 1980 The post-total hysterectomy (vault) vesicovaginal fistula. Journal of Urology 123: 839–840

Tancer M L 1992 Observations on the prevention and management of vesicovaginal fistula after total hysterectomy. Surgery, Gynecology, and Obstetrics 175: 501–506

Tancer M L 1993 A report of thirty-four instances of urethrovaginal and bladder neck fistulas. Surgery, Gynecology, and Obstetrics 177: 77–80

Waaldijk K 1994 The immediate surgical management of fresh obstetrics fistulas with catheter and/or early closure. International Journal of Gynaecology and Obstetrics 45: 11–16

Wang Y, Hadley H R 1990 Nondelayed transvaginal repair of high lying vesicovaginal fistula. Journal of Urology 144: 34–36

Wein A J, Malloy T R, Carpiniello V L, Greenberg S H, Murphy J 1980 Repair of vesicovaginal fistula by a suprapubic transvesical approach. Surgery, Gynecology, and Obstetrics 150: 57–60

Voiding difficulties and retention

P JULIAN R SHAH AND PROKAR DASGUPTA

INTRODUCTION

Normal voiding takes place by initiation of bladder contraction with simultaneous relaxation of the bladder neck and urethra. The act of micturition is determined by a number of separate factors: control from higher centres, the sacral reflex arc, the innervation of the bladder muscle and sphincter mechanisms, the outflow resistance and the speed of contraction of the detrusor muscle fibres. If there are abnormalities present in any part of this complex mechanism, a voiding disorder may develop.

Voiding disorders in women are common but too often go unrecognized until the patient presents with symptoms which are troublesome, such as recurrent urinary tract infection or incontinence. Difficulty with micturition may not be as noticeable to the patient, as she may not be aware of the rate of a change in the rate of urine flow. Competitive voiding, which is a natural accompaniment of male development, is not found in the female! Normal voiding is accomplished without straining. However, some normal women occasionally void by straining. Increases in flow rate may be achieved by a rise in intra-abdominal pressure in the female because of the lower outflow resistance within the short female urethra. Female voiding occurs at a higher flow rate and at a lower voiding pressure than in the male. It is not unusual to observe, during videocystometry, rapid and efficient voiding taking place with no rise in intravesical pressure. This phenomenon is not due to the fact that the urine 'just falls out', as is sometimes said, but because a very low resistance requires a very low pressure to overcome it. If these bladders are observed during voiding on videocystometry they can be seen to be contracting very efficiently. The speed of contraction of these low-pressure bladders is normal, the tension in the bladder muscle fibres is low and thus the voiding pressure is low. These low-pressure bladders tend to have little reserve and are more prone to develop voiding difficulty if the outflow resistance is increased. The majority of patients with low pressure but efficient voiding who have surgery for stress incontinence may have initial difficulty with voiding demonstrated by incomplete bladder emptying. In some, this may be asymptomatic. Almost all of these bladders return to satisfactory emptying within a month after surgery.

DEFINITIONS

It is worthwhile having a simple definition for each of the commonly encountered voiding disorders, which will ensure that all clinicians refer to the same conditions with the same terminology (see Table 24.1).

Acute retention is the sudden onset of the inability to void. This may be either painful (where neurology is normal) or painless (where abnormal neurology is present). Acute retention usually occurs over a period of 4–6 hours but may be present for longer periods. A volume equal to or greater than normal capacity is removed by catheterization (usually 500 ml or more).

Chronic retention is difficult to define, as different clinicians may have different opinions as to its nature. It is worthwhile remembering that normal bladders do not retain residual urine (Shah et al 1981). It is quite logical to consider that retained residual volume of 50 ml must be associated with a voiding dysfunction. Though this may be true, a generally acceptable definition of chronic retention is not available. One possible definition is that chronic retention is present when the bladder constantly retains a volume equal to its normal capacity (e.g. approximately 500 ml), is painlessly enlarged and usually palpable. Bladders that do not normally empty completely and leave any residual urine on a regular basis are abnormal

Table 24.1 Classification of voiding difficulties and retention.

Condition	Symptom	Urodynamic data
Asymptomatic voiding difficulty	Frequency Urgency due to urinary infection or infection or no symptoms	Obstructed flow Elevated, normal or reduced voiding pressure ± Residual urine or large bladder capacity with low pressure voiding
Symptomatic voiding difficulty	Poor stream Incomplete emptying Straining Frequency	Flow < 15 ml/s Elevated voiding pressure >50 cm H_2O ± Residual urine
Acute retention	Painful or painless Sudden onset	Residual urine
Chronic retention	Reduced sensation Hesitancy Straining to void Frequency, nocturia Urgency, incontinence Urinary tract infection	Flow < 15 ml/s Residual urine High pressure or low pressure voiding
Acute-on-chronic retention	Painful or painless Sudden onset History of chronic retention Incontinence	Residual urine

and the definition of chronic retention is one of degree. Chronic retention may be a cause of urinary incontinence because of overflow and may occur without any known aetiology (Deane & Worth 1985).

Many patients may have a voiding disorder of which they are unaware. Even the presence of severe abnormalities of bladder emptying may be accepted as normal for an individual if there is no means of comparison. This is more likely in women, for reasons already stated. The likely sequence of events in a patient with urethral obstruction will be that of raised intravesical pressure with normal flow to be followed by raised intravesical pressure and reduced flow and eventually that of bladder 'decompensation' with low pressure/low flow voiding and residual urine. As many as 14% of women who presented to a urodynamic clinic with bladder symptoms were shown to have voiding disorders (Stanton et al 1983).

Table 24.2 Causes of voiding difficulties and retention.

1. Neurological disease
   - As a result of spinal injury – spinal shock phase
   - Upper motor neurone lesion – spinal injury, multiple sclerosis
   - Lower motor neurone lesion – spinal injury
   - Autonomic lesion
2. Pharmacological
   - Tricyclic antidepressants
   - Anticholinergic agents
   - Adrenergic agents
   - Ganglion blocking agents
   - Epidural anaesthesia
3. Acute inflammation
   - Acute urethritis
   - Acute cystitis
   - Acute vulvovaginitis
   - Acute anogenital infection (including herpes)
4. Obstruction
   - Distal urethral stenosis
   - Acute urethral oedema of surgery
   - Chronic urethral stenosis
   - Foreign body or calculus in the urethra
   - Impacted pelvic mass – retroverted gravid uterus
     - – haematocolpos
     - – uterine fibroid
     - – ovarian cyst
     - – faecal impaction
   - Urethral distortion with cystocele
   - Ectopic ureterocele
   - Uterine prolapse
   - Leiomyoma of the bladder
5. Endocrine
   - Hypothyroidism
   - Diabetic neuropathy
6. Overdistension
7. Psychogenic
   - Anxiety or depressive illness
   - Hysteria
8. Iatrogenic
   - After transtrigonal phenol injections
   - After surgery for stress incontinence
   - After anal surgery
   - After hysterectomy
9. Failure of relaxation of external urethral sphincter
10. Detrusor myopathy
11. Idiopathic

AETIOLOGY AND PATHOPHYSIOLOGY

There are many causes of voiding disorders in women. Abnormalities of voiding function may be due to interruption of the normal voiding reflex which occurs in neurological disease, failure of detrusor contraction or to an abnormality of urethral function. Habit and psychological factors may also be involved. The many causes of voiding dysfunction are listed in Table 24.2.

Neurological disorders

Lesions in the nervous system tend to produce specific types of voiding abnormality. Lesions in the brain which affect voiding function may occur in the frontal lobes, internal capsule, reticular formation of the pons and cerebellum. These abnormalities will tend to vary according to the severity of the lesion, the age of the patient and whether dementia forms part of the neurological process. Voiding disorders that are associated with confusional states in the elderly often right themselves once the confusional state is corrected. Urinary retention may result from acute lesions such as cerebrovascular accidents, whereas more chronic lesions such as multiple sclerosis and Parkinson's disease may be associated with detrusor hyperreflexia and its consequences of urinary frequency, urgency and incontinence.

Lesions in the spinal cord may be caused by trauma, tumours, prolapse of an intervertebral disc or spina bifida. If the lesion is above the sacral parasympathetic reflex arc, after a period of spinal shock (which occurs after acute spinal cord insult), the bladder becomes autonomous and its urodynamic dysfunction is represented by hyperreflexic detrusor behaviour combined with detrusor sphincter dyssynergia. This combination almost invariably leads to urinary incontinence in women, often combined with the retention of varying degrees of residual urine due to the uncoordinated relationship between detrusor and sphincter function.

Lesions which occur below the reflex arc, at or below the level of the outlet of the sacral roots, tend to produce bladder acontractility. This type of bladder dysfunction produces a bladder that does not contract (acontractile), with an associated non-relaxing sphincter mechanism. These patients tend to void by straining, often leaving a residual urine, though incontinence may be a feature due to chronic retention with overflow.

Pelvic plexus injuries occur as a result of damage to the pelvic plexus nerves during surgical procedures in the pelvis, such as abdominoperineal excision of the rectum or radical hysterectomy. The neurological lesion may be incomplete and produces a disorder of bladder function which is unpredictable. A bladder with reduced compliance, urinary incontinence and incomplete emptying may result.

A pelvic nerve injury may also rarely follow the transtrigonal injection of the pelvic plexus nerves with phenol for the treatment of detrusor instability (Cox & Worth 1984).

Pharmacological causes

The use of anticholinergic agents, of which there are now many, in general may cause voiding dysfunction. The most commonly prescribed agents are atropine (used in premedication), probanthines, oxybutynin, imipramine and other tricyclic antidepressants. All these agents have potent anticholinergic effects which reduce the power of bladder contraction. If used for the treatment of detrusor instability or detrusor hyperreflexia they usually produce beneficial reduction in voiding frequency and incontinence. However, if used in the presence of undiagnosed detrusor hypofunction, these agents may be responsible for the weakening of detrusor power and varying degrees of retention. In spinal injury units, anticholinergic agents are used to produce retention so that continence may result. Bladder drainage is then achieved by intermittent catheterization.

Ganglion blocking agents produce similar effects to the anticholinergic drugs, whilst alpha-stimulants increase outflow resistance and consequent voiding dysfunction.

Epidural anaesthesia may produce temporary retention by interruption of the reflex arc. A recent study using a Female Urinary Symptoms Questionnaire has shown that epidural anaesthesia during labour increases the risk of subsequent urinary symptoms in primiparous women, particularly when associated with a prolonged second stage (Jackson et al 1995).

Acute inflammation

Acute inflammation of the urethra, vulva, vagina or bladder may be associated with urinary retention or abnormalities of bladder emptying with frequency of micturition, obstructed flow and incomplete bladder emptying. If the acute inflammatory process produces urethral oedema this will increase the outflow resistance.

Genital herpes affecting the anogenital region (Oates & Greenhouse 1978), the cervix or vulva (Hemrika et al 1986; Ryttov et al 1985) can cause acute urinary retention. The urinary effects are thought to be due to central nervous involvement with the likeliest lesion being a lumbosacral meningomyelitis. However, any painful vulvovaginal lesion may contribute to voiding dysfunction.

Obstruction

Bladder outflow obstruction in the normal woman is usually a consequence of failure of relaxation of the urethral sphincter mechanism. In the patient with a neurogenic bladder, this tends to be due to detrusor sphincter dyssynergia.

Urethral stenosis in women is uncommon and is usually the result of scarring following chronic urethral inflammation, in association with surgery around the urethra, or as a consequence of instrumentation. Typically, the condition occurs in the postmenopausal patient and there is no obvious aetiology. Occasionally a urethral caruncle may be associated with urethral stenosis, or its surgical treatment may cause stenosis. The diagnosis of urethral stenosis is made at the time of urethral catheterization, cystometry or cystography, or at endoscopy to diagnose voiding difficulty. Urethral stenosis is treated by urethral dilatation, either by means of graduated urethral dilators or the Otis urethrotome. Other causes of urethral obstruction include urethral oedema secondary to premenstrual fluid retention and foreign bodies within the urethra, including urethral calculi.

Impaction of a retroverted gravid uterus, uterine fibroids and ovarian cysts may all cause retention of urine. A haematocolpos may also cause retention if impacted in the pelvis. An ectopic ureterocele may be a rare cause of voiding dysfunction in children.

A large cystocele with descent of the bladder neck may cause urethral distortion or 'kinking' which may produce a functional obstruction. Repair of the cystocele may then be all that is necessary to restore the normal continuity of the urethra and normal voiding. This underlines the importance of vaginal examination in all patients with voiding difficulties.

Surgery for stress incontinence is associated with abnormalities of bladder emptying. Although repositioning of the bladder neck into an intra-abdominal environment is the primary aim of the modern surgical treatment of stress incontinence in women, there is sufficient evidence to suggest that voiding difficulty is a consequence of both vaginal and abdominal procedures due to an obstructive effect (Copcoat et al 1987). The Burch colposuspension produces a high lift to the bladder neck. It should be expected that these patients may experience voiding problems after surgery (Walter et al 1982; Lose et al 1987). Those patients with preoperative low pressure voiding are particularly likely to run into difficulty with bladder emptying in the early postoperative phase. All but a small percentage of these patients will recover normal bladder emptying but usually with reduced flow rates.

As well as those iatrogenic causes mentioned above which may be partly or entirely responsible for voiding dysfunction, anal surgery (Lyngdorf et al 1986) and other factors listed in Table 24.2 may be involved and should be carefully considered in the aetiology if the primary cause is not immediately obvious.

The hypersensitive female urethra

There is a group of women patients with the symptoms of frequency, nocturia and urgency who, when undergoing urodynamic investigations, are found at the time of catheterization to have exquisitely sensitive urethras (Shah et al 1983). The results of urodynamic study in these patients reveals a lower incidence of detrusor instability and a high incidence of obstructed voiding when compared with a similar group of patients with the same symptoms but normal urethras (Table 24.3). The hypersensitive urethra probably represents an inflammatory condition of unknown aetiology which gives rise to the symptoms mentioned. Urethral dilatation using the Otis urethrotome appears to provide some of these patients with relief. A cause for the inflammatory process should be sought.

Overdistension

Bladder overdistension should never be overlooked as a cause of voiding disturbance. After surgical procedures such as hysterectomy, or during delivery, any retention should be relieved immediately. A single episode of urinary retention of several hours can result in a hypo-or acontractile bladder. This should sound a note of caution. Ignoring the patient's symptoms is not acceptable as the patient is usually correct. If the retention is relieved quickly the patient is very grateful and a long-term voiding problem can be avoided. The patient may void in a hot bath or shower which does assist pelvic floor and general relaxation but if the bladder is significantly overdistended this may not be successful. Drugs to stimulate bladder contraction such as bethanecol (Shah 1990) and Ubretid are usually unsuccessful and carry their own risks and side-effects.

It is well recognized that irreversible detrusor damage due to laying down of collagen can occur following postoperative overdistension of the bladder (Hinman 1976). Massive leg oedema as a result of an overdistended bladder causing venous obstruction has been reported (Mulcahy & Bivins 1979) and vesical necrosis may occur in the most severe cases (Khan et al 1982). Overdistension may contribute to changes in lactic dehydrogenase isoenzyme patterns (Newman et al 1984) and animal experiments have shown a significant increase in thymidine labelling of the urothelial basal cells, which supports the theory that the urothelium is probably the initial site of the proliferative response of the bladder to outlet obstruction (Tong et al 1992). An increase in intravesical pressure leads to weakening of the bladder wall, and vesical infarction due to ischaemic changes can follow (Haddad et al 1994).

Table 24.3 Urodynamic diagnoses in women with a hypersensitive urethra and the symptoms of frequency, nocturia and urgency of micturition.

Urodynamic diagnosis n=	Hypersensitive urethral state 50	Normal urethra 50
Detrusor instability	14 (28%)	36 (72%)
Normal detrusor function	36 (72%)	14 (28%)
Obstructed	15 (30%)	6 (12%)
Stress incontinence	15 (30%)	12 (24%)

$p<0.05$

Psychogenic retention

This diagnosis should only be made when, after a careful process of exclusion, no abnormalities have been discovered. The occasional late neurological abnormality may turn up in an initially apparently normal patient. A careful history and examination are necessary along with a neurological examination performed by a neurologist. The majority of patients suffering from psychogenic retention of urine are women aged between 15 and 45 years. There is usually a relationship between the onset of the retention and a stressful event such as childbirth, marital discord, surgical treatment or rape. Hysteria, depression, and schizophrenia may all be causes of this problem. However, once a psychiatric diagnosis is made, the treatment remains the same as in other patients. Return to normal voiding function may be expected in the majority (Barrett 1978), though the use of clean intermittent catheterization is satisfactory management.

Sphincter dysfunction in women

Electromyography (EMG) has been found to be particularly useful in this group of patients. If urethral sphincter EMG is performed, distinct sounds which are likened to the underwater recordings of ocean cetacea can be heard. Complex repetitive discharges along with decelerating bursts are responsible for these characteristic 'whale noises' (Fowler & Kirby 1985). This is a primary disorder of the urethral sphincter in the absence of any other neurological or urological abnormality and vesical hypo-or acontractility seems to be secondary to the failure of the sphincter to relax. In the syndrome described by Fowler et al, this disorder of the external urethral sphincter was found to be associated with polycystic ovaries (Fowler et al 1988).

Detrusor myopathy

The histological features of this curious entity were described in chronic abacterial cystitis by Holm-Bentzen et al in 1985. A few of the patients having this condition were in urinary retention. Detrusor muscle cell degeneration, fatty replacement, hydropic cytoplasm, perinuclear vacuolization, karyopyknosis and karyorrhexis were noted and electron microscopic studies showed a decrease in myofibrillar mass and cytoplasmic density of some detrusor cells along with formation of cytoplasmic vacuoles (Holm-Bentzen et al 1985). More recently, lipid inclusion bodies in the detrusor have been reported as a form of primary myopathy causing urinary retention (Martin et al 1993). This disorder needs to be studied further and could provide the basis for interesting research in the future.

PRESENTATION

Symptoms

Many women are infrequent voiders. That is to say that they may void only once or twice a day. Some patients with disorders of voiding function may not be aware that they have a problem until they develop urinary tract infection or retention. Bladder inflammation is common in the female, occurring in childhood in association with abnormalities of the urinary tract, in young adult life in association with sexual intercourse, in middle age with the menopause, and in the elderly in association with urinary tract pathology such as tumours, calculi and chronic inflammation. The young adult patient should be questioned about voiding difficulty if infection occurs. A free flow rate will generally exclude an obstructive problem.

Lower urinary tract infection in an older woman should be investigated more completely as abnormalities of bladder function are more likely.

Women will admit to the symptom of poor stream. Straining to void is associated with reduced contractility of the detrusor. A feeling of incomplete emptying may be associated with retained residual urine. Urinary frequency may occur, with chronic retention leading to urinary incontinence as an overflow phenomenon, although this is uncommon in women.

A general history with particular reference to past medical and surgical treatment is very important, as many voiding problems stem from or are temporarily related to previous pelvic and abdominal surgery and childbirth. A drug history should also be obtained.

Signs

Examination of the urinary tract is often felt to be unrewarding. It is all the more important, therefore, that a careful general, abdominal and pelvic examination should be undertaken. The kidneys should be carefully palpated. Abdominal masses should be noted. It is not always easy to palpate the full bladder during abdominal examination. Bimanual examination will often confirm one's suspicions of bladder fullness, as the bladder may be more easily palpable. Gentle percussion in the suprapubic region will reveal the characteristic dullness which is present when the bladder is full or when other pelvic masses are present.

The importance of clinical examination cannot be overemphasized and this particularly applies to the wheelchair-bound patient who is particularly difficult to examine because of immobility and deformity. When examining this group of patients one often discovers the most severe abnormalities.

The urethra should be examined for its appearance, position and tenderness. Urethral tenderness can be assessed by its compression against the back of the pubic symphysis. The normal female urethra is not tender. The vulva and vagina should be observed for signs of hormonal withdrawal and inflammation, for prolapse and scarring in association with childbirth and previous surgery. A careful bimanual examination should also be made.

A general neurological examination should be performed, though if a neurological abnormality is suspected, a neurologist's opinion should be sought. The patient's general demeanour should also be observed.

INVESTIGATION

The patient should be investigated according to the suspected abnormality. As these patients' symptoms are related to the lower urinary tract, it is quite unnecessary to perform urography. The simplest tests available are a flow rate, abdominal radiograph (to look for calcification and soft tissue masses) and pelvic and, if appropriate, renal ultrasonography. The demonstration of a reduced flow and a residual urine on bladder ultrasound will confirm a diagnosis of voiding difficulty and the next step will be to perform urodynamic studies.

The frequency/volume voided chart or urinary diary

If the patient is referred with a voiding problem, useful information will be obtained by asking the patient to keep a urinary diary for one week prior to attending for consultation. A standard diary sheet should be sent to the patient with the out-patient appointment and the patient given instructions on how to fill it in. Even the most elderly patient will not find this task difficult. These charts are also valuable later for the assessment of the response to therapy (Giesy 1986).

Infrequent voiding

Normal voiding frequency, generally accepted as less than seven times daily, is determined by fluid intake, habit, anxiety and stress, and the presence of abnormalities of bladder function which may be motor or sensory. Infrequent voiding, i.e. the passing of urine less than two or three times a day with a normal fluid intake is abnormal. Patients who void infrequently should be investigated at least with a frequency/intake output/volume voided chart and, based upon the information obtained, advised about their normal requirements of intake and the frequency of voiding. Infrequent voiders should be recommended to void every 3–4 hours during the day. Infrequent voiding with normal bladder volumes should not lead to long-term bladder harm.

The flow rate

The free urine flow rate is the simplest and possibly most useful urodynamic investigation, particularly because it is non-invasive. The flow machine should be kept in a private area, preferably a toilet, so that the patient may void in privacy. This reduces the erroneous flows that may be seen when the patient is inhibited or embarrassed.

A series of flow rates obtained on a single day with bladder volumes greater than 200 ml demonstrates the benefit of the flow rate clinic. A single flow rate is not sufficient for providing a true indication of flow and three consecutive flow rates should be obtained. The patient should be asked to void when full but not to hold on too long. Flow rates should be obtained with voided volumes of 200 ml or more, though flow rate values will fall within the normal range (in normal women) when small volumes are passed (Fig. 24.1). If the volume voided is persistently small the pattern of the flow curve should be examined

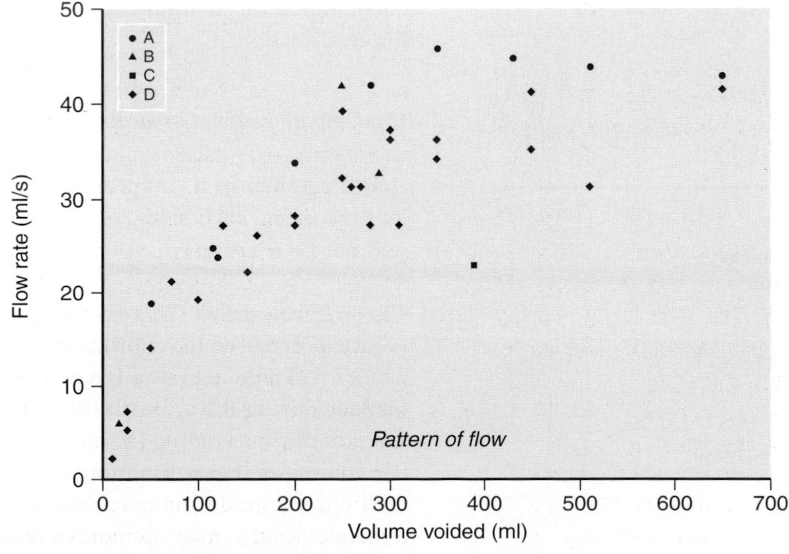

Fig. 24.1 Flow rates in normal women according to volumes voided.

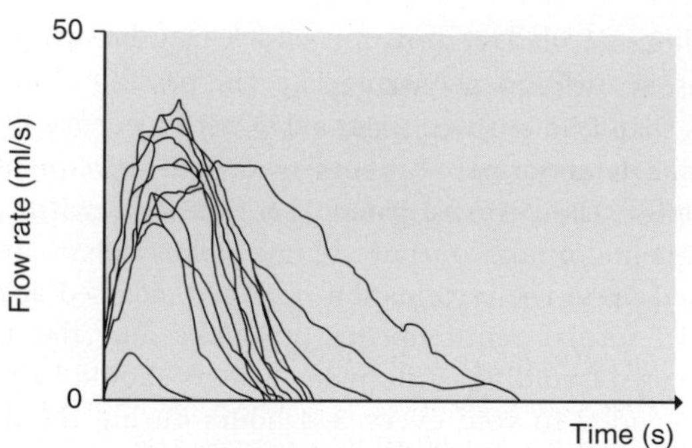

Fig. 24.2 Flow rates at different volumes in a normal woman to demonstrate the uniformity of the flow curves except where bladder volumes are either very small or very large.

carefully. If the volume voided is less than 200 ml, an artificially low flow rate may be recorded and give rise to misinterpretation. The superimposition of a number of flow curves in the same patient demonstrate that, except when the volumes are very small or very large, the flow curves are very similar (Fig. 24.2).

A normal flow rate is seen in Figure 24.3. Examples of abnormal flow patterns are shown in Figures 24.4 and 24.5. The normal flow rate depends upon: (a) volume voided, and (b) age. As ageing progresses the flow rate values tend to fall. Abrams & Torrens (1979) quote the following lower limits for flow rate at different ages:

under 50 years: >25 ml/s
over 50 years: > 18 ml/s

Obstructed voiding may occur even in the presence of normal flowmetry. This is because the bladder

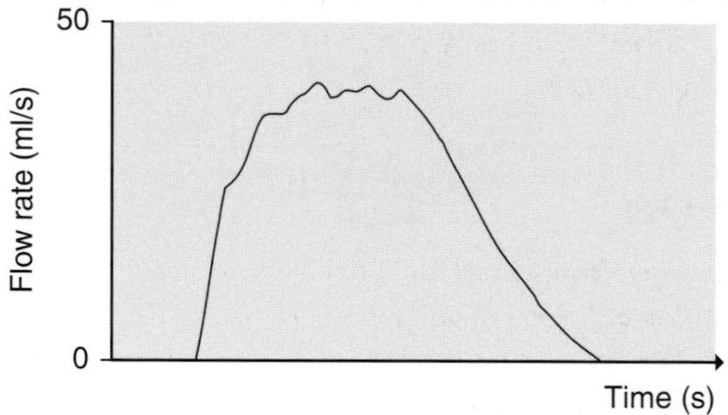

Fig. 24.3 Normal flow rate in a woman.

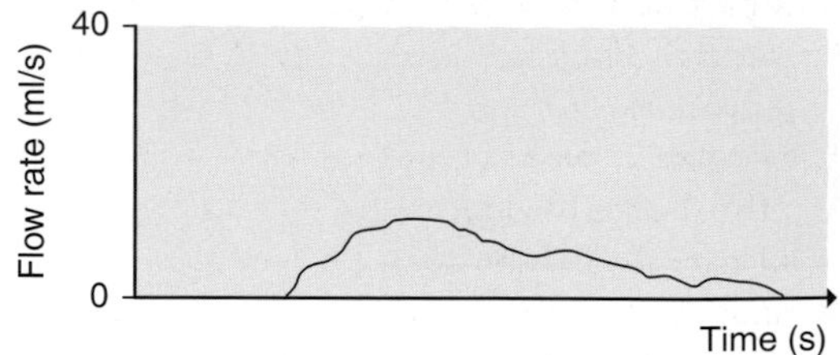

Fig. 24.4 Low flow due to outflow obstruction.

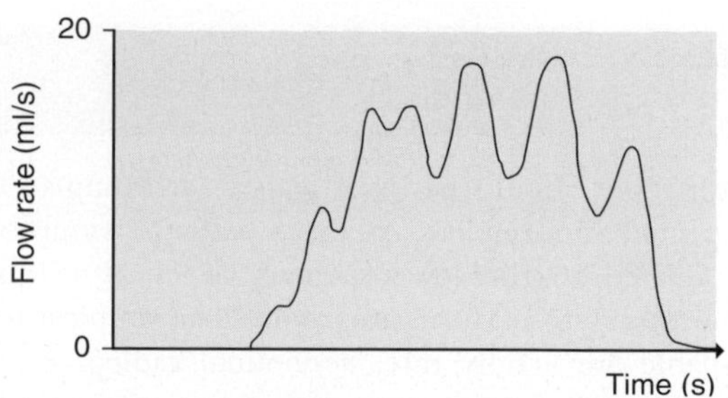

Fig. 24.5 Intermittent flow associated with hypocontractile detrusor function and straining to void.

has been able to compensate through an increase in the force of contraction associated with a rise in voiding pressure. In these patients it is important to listen carefully to the symptom complex and if obstructed voiding is present, in spite of normal flowmetry, urodynamic evaluation is indicated.

Cystometry

Filling and voiding cystometry may be all that is necessary for the majority of patients; however, combined synchronous videocystometry is preferable where available. Videocystometry enables radiological examination of the voiding process and will provide information about the bladder appearance – the presence or absence of trabeculation, diverticula and reflux, and the behaviour of the bladder neck and urethral mechanisms. External striated sphincter function should be carefully examined during videocystometry. Abnormalities of sphincter function are seen in some normal patients who have inhibited voiding and in neurogenic disorders where detrusor sphincter dyssynergia gives rise to obstructed voiding. Table 24.4 describes the features which may be encountered in the urodynamic investigation of voiding dysfunction.

Urodynamic findings according to the disorder

Acute retention If the primary cause is known and its treatment successful, urodynamic investigation will not be necessary.

Chronic retention This may be due to a complete failure of detrusor function. If this is the case, urodynamics will demonstrate a large capacity, low pressure bladder during filling, with little or no detrusor contraction during voiding (acontractile or hypocontractile voiding detrusor function).

If chronic retention is related to obstruction, urodynamic study may demonstrate a high voiding detrusor pressure, low flow rate and may be with or

Table 24.4 Urodynamic features of voiding disorders. (Residual urine >50 ml)

First sensation may be greatly reduced or delayed; may be associated with early first sensation and urgency in upper motor neurone lesions
Capacity reduced with hyperreflexic bladder dysfunction; increased with acontractile bladders
End-filling detrusor pressure and compliance usually normal except in association with upper motor neurone hyperreflexic bladders or chronic bladder fibrosis
Isometric pressure (p_{iso}). The additional detrusor pressure rise seen at the point of maximum detrusor pressure during voiding when voiding is suddenly stopped. The p_{iso} tends to relate to detrusor reserve. In patients with low pressure voiding the p_{iso} may be non-existent. Patients with low isometric pressures, low voiding pressures (unpublished observation) and low preoperative maximum urethral closure pressures (Karram et al 1992) tend to be those who take longer to recover normal bladder emptying after surgery for stress incontinence
Maximum voiding pressure. Voiding pressure is raised above the female upper limit of accepted normality (50 cm H_2O) where obstruction is present. Voiding pressure may be low or non-existent where detrusor failure is present

without residual urine. If, however, it is related to neurological disease, the retention of residual urine is either due to a lower motor neurone lesion with detrusor acontractility or to obstructed detrusor hyperreflexia (detrusor sphincter dyssynergia). Practically the only women patients who develop upper urinary tract dilatation in association with abnormalities of bladder function are those with neurogenic bladder disorders, with high pressure contractions, detrusor sphincter dyssynergia and residual urine under pressure due to poor bladder compliance.

Disorders of voiding function For obstructed voiding, flow rate and post-micturition bladder ultrasound should be carried out initially, followed by videocystometry to confirm the site of obstruction.

Electromyography (EMG)

Sphincter EMG requires special equipment and considerable experience in its use and interpretation. That is not to say that it should not be employed in the special circumstances in which it is useful, i.e. pelvic floor denervation or suspected but unproven neuropathy.

The EMG may be performed either by a concentric needle placed into the distal urethral or external anal sphincter or by means of a plug electrode. Careful attention to the sounds emitted during the test is as important as the actual recording of the motor unit potentials themselves. Multiphasic motor unit potentials are associated with denervation. Reflex latency times may also be assessed using the EMG and are recommended in patients with unexplained acute retention of urine in whom a neurological abnormality may be present (Fidas et al 1987).

Sphincter EMG is particularly useful in the diagnosis of two specific conditions:

1. External sphincter dysfunction in women: failure of adequate relaxation of the sphincter can be detected by recording 'whale noises' on concentric needle EMG. These are due to complex repetitive discharges with decelerating bursts.
2. Multiple system atrophy: this condition, which mimics Parkinson's disease, is characterized by an atrophy of cells in the Onuf's nucleus in the sacral cord. The mean duration of the motor units as recorded from the anal sphincter is more than 10.0 ms and >20% of the units are of prolonged duration. The prognosis in multiple system atrophy as compared to Parkinson's disease is much worse and it is important to differentiate between these two conditions.

Radiology

Radiological investigations should include a plain abdominal radiograph and, where necessary, a bladder and upper urinary tract ultrasound scan. Ultrasonography of the pelvic organs may also be helpful in displaying uterine enlargement and ovarian abnormalities. Videocystometry should be used as suggested above. An intravenous urogram is not a dynamic investigation and should not be necessary except where the anatomy of the urinary tract needs to be delineated.

Endoscopy

Endoscopy should not be used as a means of diagnosing abnormalities of detrusor function. Obstruction, except for the presence of urethral stenosis, cannot be diagnosed at endoscopy. Endoscopy is necessary for the diagnosis of suspected intravesical abnormalities such as tumours, foreign bodies and stones. It is also used as part of a treatment regime, i.e. in association with urethral dilatation, Otis urethrotomy or repositioning procedures.

Trabeculation which is seen at cystoscopy is common in the female bladder. The very thin female bladder wall may look trabeculated when overdistended. Trabeculation and diverticula are more likely to be associated with detrusor instability than with obstruction (Shah et al 1981).

Trabeculation

Bladder smooth muscle bundles are arranged in a criss-cross or decussating fashion and when affected by hypertrophy are known as trabeculation. Trabeculation may be seen at cystoscopy in the female bladder and in its milder forms may be a part of the range of normal bladder appearances, particularly when the bladder is overdistended.

Trabeculation, however, is generally a sign of developing smooth muscle hypertrophy and its degree varies from very mild to very gross and represents exercise hypertrophy of the smooth muscle bundles. In the late phase of trabeculation the muscle fibres become replaced by connective tissue. It may be seen at cystoscopy or on radiological investigations of the bladder, such as urography or cystography. Trabeculation may be caused by outflow obstruction following urethral stenosis or external sphincter dyssynergia in neurogenic bladder disorders following spinal injury or spina bifida or as a result of detrusor instability. If trabeculation is seen during investigation, detrusor instability and hyperreflexia are more common causes than obstruction, and this applies both to male and female patients (Shah et al 1981). Gross trabeculation is less common in the female with neurogenic bladder than in the male because the outflow resistance is lower and thus the recurrent effects of isometric detrusor contractions are less marked.

TREATMENT

Prophylactic measures

Many voiding difficulties may be avoided by the early recognition of potential problems. Therefore, if urinary retention is suspected or imminent after surgical procedures, the early use of bladder catheterization before bladder overdistension has occurred will prevent many long-term bladder problems. If a patient complains of voiding difficulty after surgery, or cannot void, the institution of a programme of intermittent catheterization until the time of recovery of bladder function is recommended. If the patient will not accept this regime and voiding problems are likely to be prolonged, a suprapubic catheter is recommended.

Difficulty with resuming normal micturition after surgical treatment may occur in over 60% of patients undergoing surgery for stress incontinence (slings, colposuspension and endoscopic bladder neck suspension), and in 45% of patients undergoing radical pelvic surgery (for gynaecological malignancy or after rectal surgery) (Fraser 1966; Smith et al 1969) and after epidural anaesthesia for childbirth or gynaecological procedures. Indwelling catheters should therefore be used prophylactically after any surgical procedure which may, through a direct or indirect effect, be associated with voiding problems. If the catheter is to be placed for only a short period of time, a urethral catheter of small calibre (e.g. 14 Fr) should be used. However, if a catheter is required for longer periods or if trials of voiding and assessment of bladder emptying by measurement of residual urine are necessary, a self-retaining suprapubic catheter is preferable.

A clear explanation of the possibility of voiding difficulty should be given to all patients who are to undergo any surgery which carries this risk. Those patients who express dissatisfaction with surgical outcome are those who have not received an adequate preoperative explanation of the potential problems. It is also very helpful, where indicated, to teach the woman patient the art of self-catheterization preoperatively. If it is not needed later, the patient is very pleased; if it is found necessary, the patient is not aggrieved.

The process of intermittent catheterization should be a part of the training of both medical and nursing staff involved in the management of these patients.

Intermittent self-catheterization

Intermittent self-catheterization was first described by Guttman & Frankel in 1966 for the management of incomplete bladder emptying in the spinal injured patient. Intermittent catheterization has revolutionized the management of disorders of voiding and enables many women to lead normal lives with efficient bladder emptying, freed from the constraints of struggles with voiding which may involve considerable discomfort, distress and time. It is not unusual to find that a patient with voiding difficulty due to acontractile bladder function may spend several hours a day on the toilet in the act of voiding. This particularly applies to patients following spinal injury.

The value of intermittent catheterization as a routine form of bladder management cannot be overemphasized. Education of medical and nursing personnel about the value of this technique is still required to overcome the many barriers that do exist to its use. Patients will take to intermittent catheterization with ease, provided they are properly counselled by clinicians or nursing staff committed to its use.

Sterile intermittent catheterization (SIC)

This method of catheterization is performed under aseptic conditions, usually by medical or nursing staff in the setting of a hospital or clinic. It is generally used for the management of inefficient bladder emptying in patients with neurogenic bladders or following surgery for stress incontinence (it is current practice in the United States to teach patients to use intermittent catheterization after surgery for stress incontinence so that they may be discharged home early after surgery, continuing to use CISC until bladder emptying is efficient). On each occasion a catheter is passed using full aseptic principles. The catheter is discarded after a single use, as is usual in a hospital setting.

SIC is correct in a hospital setting where resistant micro-organisms are present and cross-contamination is possible. However, the use of a sterile technique is inappropriate in everyday life, being too time-consuming and unnecessarily wasteful of resources. Therefore, in the community, clean intermittent catheterization is the norm.

Clean intermittent catheterization (CIC)

This method, also known as clean intermittent self-catheterization (CISC) (Lapides et al 1972; Murray et al 1984) is performed by the patient or by a care attendant, nurse or relative when the patient is unable to do this for him/herself. This technique is designed for patient use in an everyday setting. The patient is taught how to insert a fine-bore catheter into the bladder using a clean rather than sterile technique. It is important to emphasize to the patient that CISC is not harmful and that it may be performed five or six times a day without causing urethral injury if correctly used. A common misconception is that a disposable catheter should be used on each occasion. This is quite unnecessary and wasteful. A single plastic catheter of small calibre (10, 12 or 14 Ch) may be used over and over again and should be made to last for at least a week. Most patients may keep a catheter in use for 4 weeks. It is important to advise the patient to wash the catheter carefully after each use, store in a clean polythene bag in-between times, but not to immerse the catheter in antiseptic overnight (Milton is not recommended, since infection rates appear to be increased with this technique).

The patient is taught by a nurse trained in the technique. It may be necessary for the patient to use a mirror to guide catheter insertion in the first place. Once they become familiar with their anatomy, most patients manage catheterization without difficulty by feel alone. Hydrophilic-covered catheters (Lofric®, Easycath®) which when wetted become slippery are both popular and effective for patients using CISC.

Pharmacological treatment of voiding disorders

Drugs which have been used to improve detrusor function include bethanecol chloride, distigmine bromide (Cameron 1966) and intravesical prostaglandin E2 and F2 (Bultitude et al 1976; Delaere et al 1981). These drugs have been widely used but recently appear to be losing popularity. The authors' view is that none of these drugs have been conclusively shown to be of any long-term benefit and much of the published data are conflicting. It is important to realize that if the bladder does not contract, nothing will make it do so except perhaps direct nerve-root stimulation.

Alpha-adrenergic blocking agents are useful in men with urodynamically proven bladder neck obstruction. This condition is exceedingly rare in women and thus these agents which include phenoxybenzamine, prazosin and indoramin find little place in the management of outflow obstruction in women. The occasional patient who has a neurologically induced voiding disorder may have improved bladder emptying with α-adrenergic blockade.

Postoperative voiding problems may be improved by a small dose of an anxiolytic such as diazepam (Stanton & Cardozo 1979).

Surgical management

Urethral dilatation

If outflow obstruction is due to urethral stenosis, urethral dilatation will help to relieve the symptoms (Worth 1986). Provided there is adequate external sphincter function, a generous urethral dilatation with Hegar's sounds may be performed without causing incontinence. Alternatively, an Otis urethrotome may be employed. Dilatation up to 45 Ch may be performed without causing incontinence in the normal woman. It seems illogical to employ the cutting blade as it does not appear to contribute to the results and increases urethral bleeding and patient discomfort.

Urethral calibration is very rarely used nowadays for the assessment of urethral diameter (Farrar & Turner-Warwick 1979). Urethral obstruction is either stenotic or functional. If urethral stenosis is present, it is helped by dilatation but will be likely to recur, as it does in men, when healing of the dilated area causes scarring. Patient self-dilatation with a wide-bore catheter may be of use in these patients after initial surgical overdilatation. If urethral obstruction is functional, dilatation will provide a longer-lasting response and is helped if the primary cause of the problem is discovered and remedied.

Bladder neck incision

The place of bladder neck incision in patients with 'outflow obstruction' is a contentious issue. Bladder neck obstruction in women is rare. Continence in some patients is often entirely or largely based upon a normally functioning bladder neck mechanism. Unless a diagnosis of bladder neck obstruction is confirmed by pressure/flow videourodynamics, bladder neck incision should never be performed.

Alternatives to intermittent catheterization and future trends

Alternatives to clean intermittent self-catheterization (CISC) are continually being searched for. Electrostimulation of the bladder neck (Moore et al 1993) has been tried recently, as has sacral nerve root stimulation (Elabaddy et al 1994). The latter involves a two-stage procedure, with the initial phase being a percutaneous nerve evaluation of the S3 root using a temporary electrode inserted under local anaesthetic. Permanent implantation of a sacral nerve root stimulator is carried out as the second phase in patients demonstrating at least 50% improvement in their voiding symptoms after the placement of the temporary lead. This technique of neuromodulation has shown promise in treating selected patients in retention as well as those suffering from dysfunctional voiding resistant to other conservative means of treatment. Its exact mechanism of action is as yet unclear but research into this is in progress.

Partial cystectomy has been performed for treating the myogenic decompensated bladder with excessive residual urine (Klarskov et al 1987). However, the results are disappointing and cystoreduction is not associated with a return to normal voiding function. A select group of patients, especially those with spina bifida, benefit from urinary diversion using the Mitrofanoff principle. Substitution sigmoid colocystoplasty has been suggested as an option in patients who are unhappy to perform CISC (Taguchi 1987). The 'vesical cap' operation which involves strengthening the acontractile detrusor by ileal seromuscular patch grafts has been successfully used in animal as well as human experiments (Marz et al 1992). Latissimus dorsi myoplasty has recently been used in dog experiments and the results are encouraging (Von Heyden et al 1994). It works on the principle of using skeletal muscle contraction to facilitate bladder emptying. The transposed muscle can evacuate up to 50% of a bladder-like reservoir; however, a residual volume of 50% still necessitates the use of intermittent catheterization.

A new intraurethral prosthesis containing a small valve and pump, controlled by a battery-operated remote control unit has recently been reported as being effective in chronic female urinary retention due to acontractile detrusor (Monga et al 1996).

SPECIFIC CONDITIONS

Asymptomatic voiding disorder

No active treatment is necessary if a voiding disorder is present without symptoms. If urinary tract infection occurs with residual urine, urethral dilatation may help; if not, daily intermittent catheterization will remove the residual and reduce the incidence of infection. These patients should be investigated by urodynamic studies. An occasional patient with a neurogenic bladder disorder may not complain of a voiding problem but may have a thick-walled, high-pressure bladder with dilated upper urinary tracts.

Symptomatic voiding disorder

The treatment of each problem is according to the particular features that are provided by clinical investigation.

Acute retention of urine

The insertion of a small-calibre urethral catheter with drainage of the retained urine may be all that is necessary to permanently relieve this problem. Early intervention by catheterization is highly recommended where acute retention presents. It is quite illogical to wait for a trial of drugs, hot baths, etc., as the single passage of a small urethral catheter will often relieve the problem in the majority of patients. Where the retention persists in spite of intermittent catheter drainage, the cause of the retention should be strenuously sought.

Chronic retention of urine

Some patients with chronic voiding disorders may never empty their bladders efficiently, always leaving residual urine. If the residual urine is relatively small and under low pressure, does not produce infection or voiding symptoms, then it may safely be left. No harm should come from the presence of asymptomatic residual urine. If problems arise as a result of residual urine, a regimen of intermittent catheterization should be introduced. Voiding efficiency does recover dramatically in many patients who have a surgical cause for their voiding difficulty (e.g. after surgery for stress incontinence). Their voiding pressures increase in response to the change in outflow resistance and residual urines almost invariably fall to nothing within a few days or weeks.

Those bladders that never recover normal function in spite of intermittent catheterization are best managed with this technique indefinitely. Some clinicians do use either urethral dilatation or bladder neck incision for this condition but it is not considered appropriate in the authors' view.

Rarely, a patient with chronic retention will not tolerate the regime of intermittent catheterization (usually for psychological reasons). A surface urinary diversion may be the only option open to this patient.

Neurological disorders

Neurological disorders will either produce problems with bladder emptying or urinary incontinence or both. The abnormality should be investigated appropriately in all patients with a neurological aetiology; the simplest of these is a flow and ultrasound residual to measure bladder emptying. Only a few patients need to have cystometrys. If failure of bladder emptying is the primary problem, intermittent catheterization is the ideal. This form of management is dependent upon the ability and motivation of the patient or the presence of carers. In patients with detrusor hyperreflexia and incomplete bladder emptying, intermittent catheterization can be effectively combined with an oral anticholinergic like oxybutynin. If the patient is unable to self-catheterize, or this form of management is socially unacceptable (for many reasons), an indwelling catheter may be the last line of management. An indwelling urethral catheter that is chosen for long-term management should be of small calibre, changed regularly, positioned properly and have long-term medical supervision. All this is necessary to avoid the problems of catheter rejection, infection, stones and urethral destruction which are frequently caused by neglected catheter management. A suprapubic catheter is always more acceptable than an indwelling urethral catheter. The solution in those patients with urethral destruction due to an indwelling catheter is surgical urethral closure and permanent suprapubic catheter drainage.

CONCLUSION

Consider the patient's symptoms and voiding disorders will be detected early. They can then be treated appropriately. Acute retention should never be overlooked or trivialized. The patient is usually right. Surgical treatment of voiding disorders is usually the last resort after urodynamic investigation and conservative measures have been tried.

REFERENCES

Abrams P H, Torrens M 1979 Urine flow studies. Symposium on Clinical Urodynamics. Urology Clinics of North America 6: 71–79

Barrett D M 1978 Evaluation of psychogenic urinary retention. Journal of Urology 120: 191–192

Bultitude M I, Hills N H, Shuttleworth K E D 1976 Clinical and experimental studies on the action of prostaglandins and their synthesis inhibitors on detrusor muscle in vitro and in vivo. British Journal of Urology 48: 631–637

Cameron M D 1966 Distigmine bromide (Ubretid) in the prevention of post-operative retention of urine. Journal of Obstetrics and Gynaecology of the British Commonwealth 73: 847–848

Coptcoat M J, Shah P J R, Cumming J et al 1987 How does bladder function change in the early period after surgical alteration in outflow resistance? Preliminary communication. Journal of the Royal Society of Medicine 80: 753–754

Cox R, Worth P H L 1984 Chronic retention after extratrigonal phenol injection for bladder instability. British Journal of Urology 58: 229–230

Deane A M, Worth P H L (1985) Female chronic urinary retention. British Journal of Urology 57: 24–6

Delaere K P J, Thomas C M G, Moonen W A, Debryune F M J 1981 The value of intravesical prostaglandin E2 and F2 in women with abnormalities of bladder emptying. British Journal of Urology 53: 306–9

Elabbady A A, Hassouna M M, Elhilahi M M 1994 Neural stimulation for chronic voiding dysfunctions. Journal of Urology 152: 1–5

Farrar D, Turner-Warwick R T 1979 Outflow obstruction in the female. Symposium on Clinical Urodynamics. Urology Clinics of North America 6: 217–25

Fidas A, Galloway N T M, Varma J et al 1987 Sacral reflex latency in acute retention in female patients. British Journal of Urology 59: 311–3

Fowler C J, Christmas T J, Chapple C R et al 1988 Abnormal electromyographic activity of the urethral sphincter, voiding dysfunction, and polycystic ovaries: a new syndrome? British Medical Journal 297: 1436–8

Fowler C J, Kirby R S 1985 Abnormal electromyographic activity (decelerating burst and complex repetitive discharges) in the striated muscle of the urethral sphincter in 5 women in urinary retention. British Journal of Urology 57: 67–70

Fraser A C 1966 The late effects of Wertheim's hysterectomy on the urinary tract. Journal of Obstetrics and Gynaecology of the British Commonwealth 73: 1002–7

Giesy J D 1986 Voiding problems in women. Postgraduate Medicine 79: 271–8

Guttmann L, Frankel H 1966 The value of intermittent catheterisation in the early management of traumatic paraplegia and tetraplegia. Paraplegia 4: 63–84

Haddad F S, Pense S, Christenson S 1994 Spontaneous intraperitoneal rupture of the bladder. Journal Medical Libanais 42: 149–54

Hemrika D J, Schutte M F, Bleker O P 1986 Elsberg syndrome: a neurologic basis for acute urinary retention in patients with genital herpes. Obstetrics and Gynecology 68: 37S–39S

Hinman F 1976 Postoperative overdistention of the bladder. Surgery Gynecology and Obstetrics 142: 901–2

Holm-Bentzen M, Larsen S, Hainau B, Hald T 1985 Non-obstructive detrusor myopathy in a group of patients with chronic abacterial cystitis. Scandinavian Journal of Urology and Nephrology 124: 1015–7

Jackson S, Barry C, Davies G et al 1995 Duration of second stage of labour and epidural anaesthesia: effect on subsequent urinary symptoms in primiparous women. Neurourology and Urodynamics 14: 498–9

Karram M M, Angel O, Koonings P et al 1992 The modified Pereyra procedure: a clinical and urodynamic review. British Journal of Obstetrics and Gynaecology 99: 655–8

Khan A U, Stern J M, Posalaky Z 1982 Vesical necrosis associated with acute bladder overdistention. Urology 19: 197–9

Klarskov P, Anderson J T, Asmussen C F et al 1987 Acute urinary retention in women: a prospective study of 18 consecutive cases. Scandinavian Journal of Urology and Nephrology 21: 29–31

Lapides J, Diokno C, Silber S J, Lowe B S 1972 Clean intermittent self catheterisation in the treatment of urinary tract disease. Journal of Urology 107: 458–61

Lose G, Jorgensen L, Mortensen S O et al 1987 Voiding difficulties after colposuspension. Obstetrics and Gynecology 69: 33–8

Lyngdorf R, Frimodt-Moller C, Jeppesen N 1986 Voiding disturbances following anal surgery. Urologia Internationalis 41, 67–9

Martin J E, Sobeh M, Swash C, Nickols C et al 1993 Detrusor myopathy: a cause of detrusor weakness with retention. British Journal of Urology 71: 235–6

Monga A K, Beyar M, Nativ O, Stanton S L 1996 A new intraurethral sphincter prosthesis for retention: preliminary clinical results. Neurourology and Urodynamics 15, 406–7

Moore K N, Griffiths D J, Metcalfe J B, McCracken, P N 1993 Electrostimulation of the bladder neck in acontractile bladder: two case reports. Urology Nursing 13, 113–5

Mraz J, Michek J, Sutory M, Zerhau P 1992 Surgical treatment of the atonic bladder ('vesical cap'). Urology Research 20, 241–5

Mulcahy, J J, Bivins, B A 1979 Leg edema as complication of bladder overdistention. Urology 13, 546–7

Murray, K, Lewis P, Blannin J, Shepherd A 1984 Clean intermittent selfcatheterisation in the management of adult lower urinary tract dysfunction. British Journal of Urology 56, 379–80

Newman E, Ibrahim G, Price M 1984 Urine lactic dehydrogenase – an aid in the management of patients with spinal cord injury. International Rehabilitative Medicine 6, 170–2

Oates J K, Greenhouse P R D H 1978 Retention of urine in anogenital herpetic infection. Lancet 1, 691–2

Ryttov N, Aagaard J, Hertz J 1985 Retention of urine in genital herpetic infection. Urologia Internationalis 40, 22–4

Shah P J R, Whiteside C G, Milroy, E J G, Turner-Warwick, R T 1981 Radiological trabeculation for the male bladder – a clinical and urodynamic assessment. British Journal of Urology 53: 567–70

Shah P J R, Whiteside C G, Milroy E J G, Turner-Warwick, R T 1983 The hypersensitive female urethra – a catheter diagnosis? Proceeding of the XIIIth Annual Meeting of the International Continence Society, pp 202–3

Shah, P J R 1990 Bethanecol chloride. In: Dollery (ed) Therapeutics Drugs. Churchill Livingstone, Edinburgh

Smith P H, Turnbull G A, Currie D W, Peel K R 1969 The urological complications of Wertheim's hysterectomy. British Journal of Urology 41: 685–8

Stanton S L, Cardozo L D 1979 A comparison of vaginal and suprapubic surgery in the correction of incontinence due to urethral sphincter incompetence. British Journal of Urology 51: 497–9

Stanton S L, Ozsoy C Hilton P 1983 Voiding difficulties in the female: prevalence, clinical and urodynamic review. Obstetrics and Gynecology 61: 144–7

Taguchi Y 1987 Augmentation and replacement sigmoid colocystoplasty. A review of 10 patients. British Journal of Urology 60: 231–5

Tong Y C, Monson F C, Erika B, Levin R M 1992 Effects of acute in vitro overdistension of the rabbit urinary bladder on DNA synthesis. Journal of Urology 148: 1347–50

Von Heyden B, Anthony J, Kaula N et al 1994 The latissimus dorsi muscle for detrusor assistance: functional recovery after nerve division and repair. Journal of Urology 151: 1081–7

Walter S, Olesen K P, Hald T et al 1982 Urodynamic evaluation after vaginal repair and colposuspension. British Journal of Urology 54: 377–80

Worth P H L 1986 Urethrotomy. In: Stanton S L, Tanagho E A (eds) Surgery for Female Incontinence, 2nd edn. Springer-Verlag, London and Berlin, pp 185–191

Urinary tract and benign and malignant disease

CHRISTIAN G BARNICK AND LINDA D CARDOZO

INTRODUCTION

The urinary and genital systems develop from a common intermediate mesodermal ridge and initially the excretory ducts of both systems enter a common cavity, the cloaca. Throughout life the lower urinary tract and the genital organs lie in close anatomical proximity, thus benign and malignant disorders of the genital tract may involve the ureters, bladder or urethra. This involvement may be due to direct invasion of the lower urinary tract or to compression by an enlarging pelvic tumour. The lower urinary tract may in addition be affected by treatment of gynaecological disease, especially if this involves pelvic surgery.

It is therefore important to consider the possibility of a gynaecological cause whenever investigating urinary symptoms and to be aware of the possibility of lower urinary tract involvement by gynaecological disease in order to minimize the risks of intraoperative trauma or postoperative complications.

GYNAECOLOGICAL CANCER

Urinary dysfunction can occur secondary to the malignancy but is seen more commonly as a consequence of treatment which may involve surgery, radiotherapy or chemotherapy. It is usually the primary disease that is responsible for the symptoms, although metastatic spread may occasionally be the cause. Lower urinary tract involvement is important in the staging of genital tract tumours and has grave prognostic implications.

CARCINOMA OF THE CERVIX

Cervical cancer kills 2500 young women each year in the UK. The lower urinary tract is in direct apposition to the cervix and paracervical fascia and lymphatics and carcinoma may produce significant urological morbidity.

Carcinoma of the cervix spreads chiefly in two ways: by direct extension into surrounding tissues and via the lymphatics to the regional lymph nodes. Extension inferiorly may involve the vaginal fornices and the rest of the vagina, whence it extends to involve the bladder and urethra anteriorly or the rectum posteriorly. The most common pathway of spread is unilateral or bilateral extension into the parametrium towards the pelvic side wall, which may cause unilateral or bilateral ureteric obstruction and progressive loss of renal function.

Tumour dissemination into the lymphatic network occurs by direct invasion and embolization (Fig. 25.1). The incidence of lymph node metastases is influenced by tumour size (Piver & Chung 1975) and stromal invasion (Gauthier et al 1985); further spread within this system appears to be quite orderly. The first nodes to be involved are usually the parametrial nodes, situated at the intersection of the uterine artery and the ureter. From there, spread occurs to involve the following, usually in order: obturator nodes, surrounding the obturator vessels and nerves, the internal and external iliac nodes, the common iliac nodes and finally the para-aortic nodes. The ureter may become obstructed by enlarged lymph nodes as it enters the true pelvis at the bifurcation of the common iliac vessels over the sacroiliac joint, or during its course along the pelvic side wall and in the base of the broad ligament (see also Fig. 10.8).

The majority of women with urinary tract involvement by cervical cancer do not have urinary symptoms. Ureteric obstruction may cause flank pain, fever or evidence of renal failure but is often asymptomatic if unilateral. If the bladder is compressed there may be symptoms of urgency and frequency, and direct invasion into the bladder may cause haematuria or, in advanced disease, symptoms due to a urinary fistula or urethral obstruction. Because of the significance of urinary tract involvement, both to the treatment and subsequent prognosis of carcinoma of the cervix, routine assessment of urinary tract involvement should be carried out in all cases of invasive cervical carcinoma.

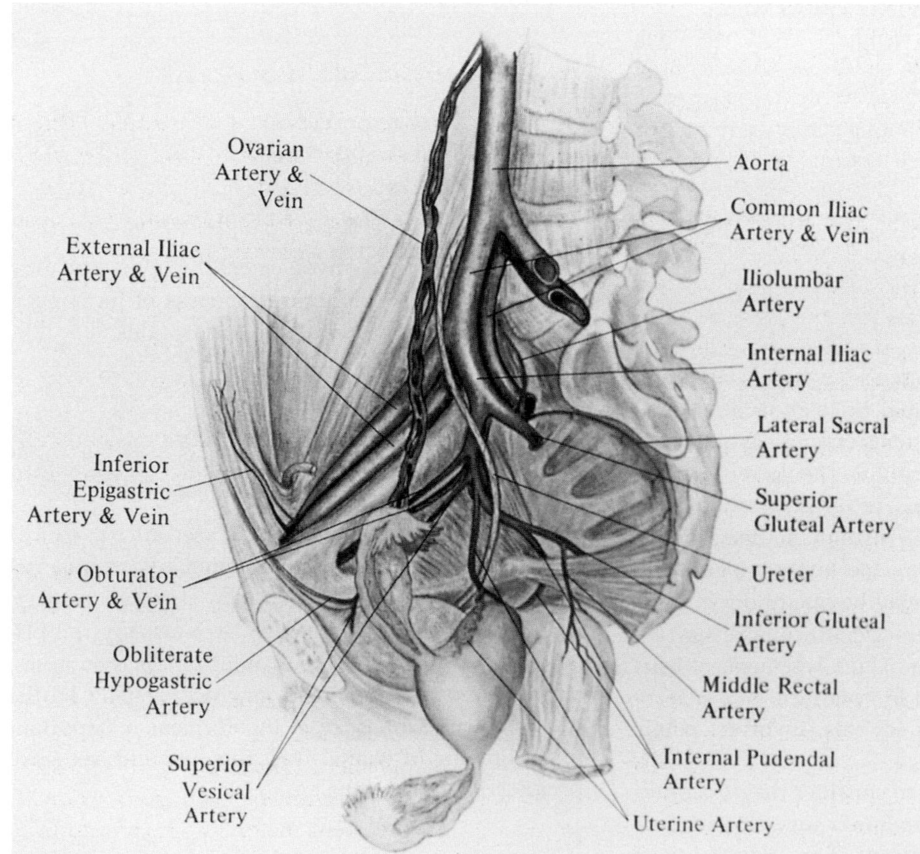

Fig. 25.1 Common pattern of arterial and venous supply to the pelvis. From Masterson (1986), with permission.

The incidence and prognostic significance of urinary tract involvement in cervical carcinoma is partly dependent on whether the tumour is primary or recurrent.

Primary cervical cancer

The commonest single cause of death in women with carcinoma of the cervix is urinary obstruction, which is responsible in at least 50% of cases (Henriksen 1949). The ureter usually becomes obstructed at the ureterovesical junction as a result of extrinsic compression, rather than invasion of the ureter, which is relatively rare (van Nagell et al 1978). This ureteric compression may be caused by the central tumour or by metastatic deposits in pelvic lymph nodes (van Nagell et al 1982).

In 1950 Aldridge and Mason studied 458 patients of which 333 had intravenous urography (IVU) performed prior to treatment. Of the patients tested, 219 were found to have a normal IVU, while 115 (34.5%) had abnormalities thought to be related to the carcinoma. In the group with an abnormal IVU, the overall survival rate was only 16%, compared to 62% in the group with a normal IVU. Since then, many authors have studied the incidence and prognostic significance of urinary tract involvement by invasive cervical cancer (Burns et al 1960; Barber et al 1963; Kottmeier 1964; Bosch et al 1973). In these studies, involving a total of 3935 patients, the incidence of urinary tract involvement in all stages of disease was found to vary between 19.1% and 34.5%, with an overall incidence of 23.2%.

The 5-year survival rates for patients with or without ureteric obstruction were compared. In patients without ureteric obstruction, the survival rates were found to vary between 22% and 62%, with an overall average of 50%. In patients with ureteric obstruction, the survival rates varied between 8.8% and 24%, with an average of 14%.

Ureteral obstruction has therefore been shown to be of grave prognostic significance, and this finding implies advanced stage group (IIIB) disease. It is therefore essential that the urinary tract is evaluated preoperatively in all women with cervical cancer. This may require an IVU although abdominal ultrasound, CT scanning or MRI may be used as alternatives (Fig. 25.2).

Bladder involvement by carcinoma of the cervix is much less common and implies Stage IV disease. The presence of bullous oedema or a growth bulging into the bladder, seen at cystoscopy, does not allow allocation of a case to Stage IV unless bladder invasion is proved by histological examination of a biopsy.

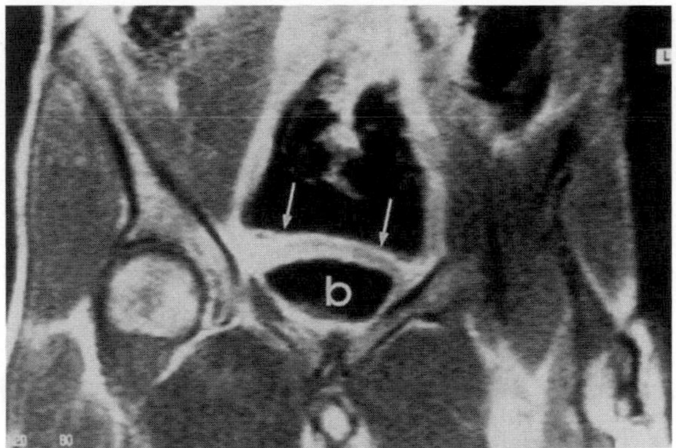

Fig. 25.2 Bladder invasion by rectal carcinoma: coronal immediate postgadolinium SGE. From Semelka et al (1997), with permission.

The vast majority of these patients are incurable, not because of their central disease, but because they already have distant metastases, and the overall 5-year survival rate is only about 11% (Million et al 1972).

In patients who are allocated to the Stage IV group because of bladder invasion alone, the 5-year survival rate following treatment with anterior pelvic exenteration and/or radiotherapy is about 30%. However, this group represents less than 2% of all Stage IV carcinomas of the cervix (Million et al 1972).

Recurrent cervical carcinoma

The diagnosis of recurrent cervical carcinoma is often difficult. The reason for this is that following treatment it may be difficult to distinguish between recurrent disease, radiotherapy reaction and postoperative scarring or adhesions. Unfortunately, urinary tract involvement again carries a poor prognosis. In patients with obstructive uropathy there are no survivors at 5 years, compared to about 40% overall 5-year survival for recurrent disease (Halpin et al 1972; Van Dyke & van Nagell 1975). Bladder involvement has also been shown to decrease the 5-year survival rate (Spratt et al 1973) and is related to the incidence of lymph node metastasis.

The importance of an abnormal IVU and cystoscopy has already been discussed, and these remain the standard for the assessment of urinary tract involvement.

CT scanning has been quite extensively studied but unfortunately the results are not very encouraging, particularly as there is still difficulty in assessing parametrial involvement. However, it may demonstrate loss of the periureteral fat plane, due to parametrial involvement before hydronephrosis is present (Vick et al 1984). Involvement of the bladder is characterized by nodular indentations along the posterior bladder wall or intraluminal tumour mass. An earlier sign is loss of the posterior perivesical fat plane; however it may still prove difficult to distinguish between bladder invasion and external compression, so cystoscopy and biopsy remain necessary.

Reports on the use of MRI have been encouraging. They have shown that MRI findings correlate better with the surgical pathology than either clinical evaluation or CT scanning (Rubens et al 1988).

Reports using transvaginal ultrasound assessment of bladder invasion suggest that, in skilled hands, this may offer similar accuracy to CT and MRI and that it is useful for detecting invasion of the bladder wall by cervical cancer (Iwamoto et al 1994).

ENDOMETRIAL, VAGINAL AND VULVAL CANCER

Endometrial cancer

This is the commonest gynaecological cancer. Involvement of the lower urinary tract is dependent on tumour size, differentiation and invasion. Tumour differentiation is graded from I to III. The less differentiated tumours more commonly invade the myometrium and thus are more likely to extend to the serosal surface and to involve adjacent organs. Invasion is seen in approximately 5% of well differentiated tumours (Grade I) as compared to 30% of poorly differentiated tumours (Grade III). This invasion is directly related to the incidence of pelvic lymph node metastases and has a negative impact on survival (Creasman et al 1976). Other factors such as tumour size influence tumour dissemination but the lower urinary tract is not involved as commonly as in cervical carcinoma. This can be accounted for by the greater distance between the uterine fundus and the bladder and ureters, and because uterine carcinoma does not extend beyond the confines of the uterus as rapidly as does a cervical lesion. Carcinoma involving the isthmus of the uterus may spread laterally into the parametrium and in advanced cases as far as the pelvic side wall. When such invasion occurs, similar ureteric compression to that found in carcinoma of the cervix may occur, leading to hydronephrosis and renal damage. The ureter may also become compressed or displaced by metastatic inguinal or para-aortic lymph nodes.

Bladder involvement by endometrial carcinoma is rare and usually only occurs in advanced disease, but where the tumour has spread onto the anterior vaginal wall the proximal urethra is not uncommonly involved. The distal urethra may also be affected by a satellite lesion in the lower third of the anterior vaginal wall, which is often seen in association with upper vaginal spread of the disease. Urethral obstruction is usually suspected on clinical grounds and may be confirmed by urethroscopy.

Vaginal and vulval carcinoma

Vulval carcinoma accounts for approximately 5% of all genital cancers and vaginal cancer is even rarer. In both tumours, lower urinary tract involvement occurs in advanced Stage IV disease. Urinary symptoms may occur but patients will usually present prior to this with other symptoms such as a mass causing discharge or pain or bleeding.

COMPLICATIONS FOLLOWING THE TREATMENT OF GYNAECOLOGICAL CANCER

Urinary tract complications following the treatment of gynaecological cancer arise mostly as a result of surgery and radiotherapy, or a combination of the two, and are dealt with in some detail in Chapter 22 but are worthy of a further mention in this chapter as they are so common. Urological problems develop in over 25% of women treated for carcinoma of the cervix. Many of these reported complications are relatively minor but approximately 7% have major complications which are likely to be long-term as a large proportion of these women have no evidence of active disease (Jones et al 1984).

In the past, ureterovaginal and vesicovaginal fistulae have been the most important urological complications (Meigs 1951) (see also Ch. 23), but now that their postoperative incidence has been reduced to less than 1% in most centres (Lerner et al 1980; Larson et al 1987) they have been superseded in importance by disorders of micturition.

Surgery for early stage carcinoma of the cervix has a 5-year cure rate of over 85% in selected populations, the mainstay of surgical management being the Wertheims hysterectomy (Wertheim 1912). Permanent bladder dysfunction is the most unpleasant and least well tolerated side-effect of this procedure.

This relationship between radical pelvic surgery and lower urinary tract dysfunction has been studied by several authors. Kadar et al (1983) found that about 50% of patients will develop some form of urinary abnormality following surgery, although for most this presents only minor difficulties.

The frequency of urinary incontinence has been found to vary between 11% and 28% (Lewington

1956; Forney 1980), this being severe in at least 5% of patients. It is thought to occur partly due to damage of the nerve supply to the bladder and urethra. This damage may occur when the cardinal and uterosacral ligaments are divided and may relate to the radicality of the surgery performed (Forney 1980), although this has been questioned (Photopoulos & Vander Zwaag 1991).

The relationship between the radicality of the surgery performed and pre- and postoperative urodynamic findings has been studied by Debus-Thiede et al (1993). They suggest that within the variations of radical hysterectomy of medium radicality (Wagner-Wertheim procedure), the urodynamic findings are not strikingly affected by the length of vaginal cuff or the length of resected parametrial tissue. This contradicts an earlier long-term follow-up study (1–15 years) by Ralph et al (1991) showing that impaired bladder sensation, bacteriuria and residual urine are significantly more common following more radical surgery. Seski & Diokno (1977) suggest that postoperative oedema, haematoma and scar formation may be contributing factors, but that partial parasympathetic denervation leading to detrusor hypotonia, together with decreased sensation, are the fundamental problems.

It may also be the case that if postoperative bladder care is inadequate, then asymptomatic overdistension of the bladder may occur, leading to decompensation and permanenent voiding difficulties. This does not seem to be affected by radiotherapy (Kadar et al 1983). Appropriate postoperative bladder care will expedite the return to normal function (Green et al 1962; Glahn 1970), and takes the form of continuous bladder drainage, preferably suprapubic, for at least 8 days postoperatively or until normal voiding function returns. If necessary, this can be replaced by clean intermittent self-catheterization in the medium term until the resumption of normal voiding.

The primary treatment of vulval carcinoma is vulvectomy and hyprodenectomy. The tumour is often situated anteriorly, close to the urethra which may need to be partially removed in order to obtain adequate excision margins. Misdirection or spraying of the urinary stream is the most common complaint and is found in 17% (Culame 1980) to 65% (Reid et al 1990).

Urethral function may also be compromised by this procedure and genuine stress incontinence may occur. Reid et al (1990) in a study of 21 women, pre- and postoperatively, showed that the distal urethral pressure is reduced following surgery and that there is also a reduction in urethral length, although this is not significant.

Currently there is a trend towards less radical vulvectomy with individualization of patient care. It is suggested that this will lead to fewer urinary complications (Burke et al 1990).

Radiotherapy for gynaecological cancer inevitably affects the lower urinary tract because of the anatomical position of the ureter and the bladder in relation to the uterus and cervix. The degree of damage is dose-dependent and can thus be reduced by careful placement of the radioactive source. Symptoms are acute or chronic. Acute symptoms are usually irritative: frequency, urgency, cystitis and haematuria, whilst chronic symptoms are related to decreased bladder compliance and decreased bladder capacity.

Biopsy specimens of ureter and bladder from patients who have received pelvic irradiation have shown histopathologically distinct early and late changes. These include submucosal inflammation, fibrosis, epithelial damage, interstitial haemorrhage, ureteritis, squamous metaplasia and perineural inflammation (Suresh et al 1993).

Urinary tract infection is often concurrent in women suffering from radiation trauma. Women should therefore be screened for this and given appropriate treatment. Unfortunately, conventional therapy in the form of anticholinergic medication is ineffective in curing these irritative symptoms and, as a last resort, a urinary diversion may be required.

Urinary fistulae occur in less than 5% of women following radiotherapy and are related to tumour recurrence in 50% (Cushing et al 1968). Treatment is usually conservative, with long-term bladder drainage and antibiotics. Using this treatment, some fistulae will resolve, although primary repair or, more usually, urinary diversion may be required.

BENIGN GYNAECOLOGICAL DISEASE

Fibroids

Uterine fibroids are the commonest tumour in the human female. They are present at necropsy in approximately 20% of all women and are more common during the reproductive years. They arise from the smooth muscle of the uterus but may also rarely occur anywhere within the genital tract, including the bladder (Goluboff et al 1994). Although they are known to be hormone-sensitive, their exact aetiology remains uncertain.

Macroscopically the appearance is of a firm, round tumour with a smooth surface, situated in the uterine wall (Fig. 25.3). In this position they are called

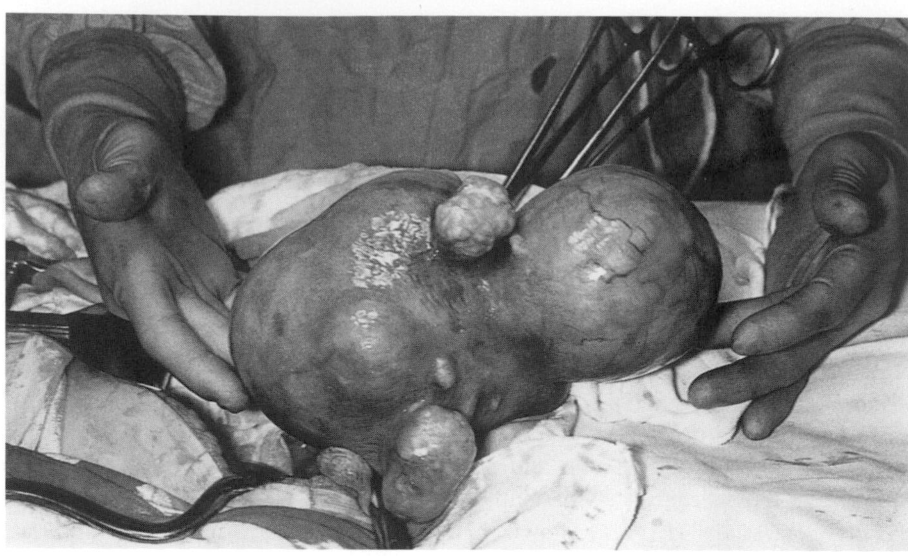

Fig. 25.3 Multiple fibromyomata seen at abdominal hysterectomy. The tumours were subserosal, intramural and submucosal. From Beischer and MacKay (1981), with permission.

intramural; however, they may also be subserous, submucous or intraligamentary. Subserous fibroids may become pedunculated, and submucous fibroids polypoidal. Rarely, pedunculated fibroids may become parasitic. When such a parasitic leiomyoma occurs in relation to the ureter, ureteral obstruction may occur (Zaiton 1986).

The incidence of urinary complications is related to the size, position and mobility of the tumour. Fibroids normally have a smooth surface and are mobile; however, they can become fixed in position if associated with other pelvic pathology such as pelvic inflammatory disease or endometriosis. These cause fibrosis and adhesions and are thus more likely to cause ureteral obstruction (Long & Montgomery 1950).

Adjacent organs become compressed as the fibroids enlarge within the pelvis. The urinary bladder is particularly susceptible to this as it is closely approximated to the front of the uterus (Fig. 25.4). Usually this compression causes distorsion of the bladder, giving rise to the symptom of urinary frequency.

Evidence obtained by shrinking tumour size using LHRH analogues shows that not all urinary symptoms are related to the size of the fibroids. Langer et al (1990) showed that a 55% reduction in the size of large fibroids reduced the symptoms of diurnal frequency, nocturia and urinary urgency, but did not affect symptoms of urge or stress incontinence.

Fibroids may become large enough to fill the whole of the abdominal cavity. Even in such cases, it is unusual for the ureter to be significantly obstructed. This is probably because fibroids are usually mobile irrespective of their size, and as they are firm they do not mould well to the shape of the pelvis. The extraperitoneal position of the ureter also protects it from external compression.

Ureteral obstruction, when it occurs, is usually at the level of the pelvic brim and is more common on the right side than the left. This is thought to be because of the difference in the anatomy of the two sides, especially the protection afforded to the left ureter by the sigmoid colon. In all reported series, ureteral compression is more common in tumours large enough to be palpable above the pelvic brim (Kretschmer & Kanter 1937; Chamberlin & Pain 1944; Long & Montgomery 1950). In these studies, some degree of ureteral obstruction in the presence of large fibroids (above the pelvic brim) was found in between 66.6% and 72.5% of cases. More recently, these figures have been disputed: Buchsbaum & Schmidt

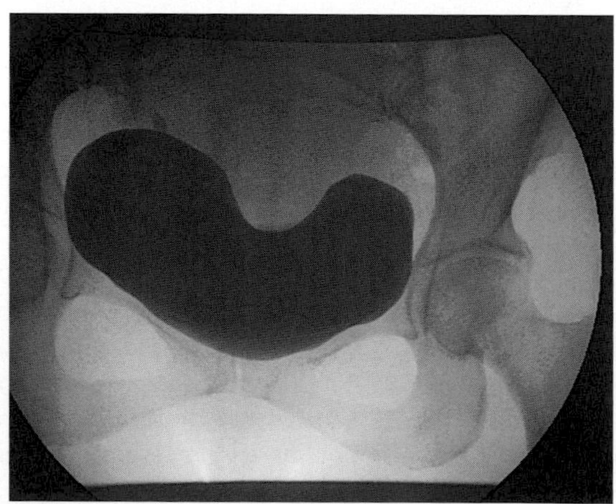

Fig. 25.4 X-ray of fibroids indenting bladder.

(1982) found significant ureteral obstruction in only 9 of 598 patients with fibroids of all sizes.

It is not only the size, but also the position, of the fibroids that is important in causing symptoms. The bladder may become lifted by low-lying fibroids and the urethra may be distorted or obstructed leading to symptoms of voiding difficulty, poor stream and incomplete emptying, or even acute urinary retention. Intraligamentary fibroids, situated between the leaves of the broad ligament, are relatively fixed, and because of their position, enlargement is more likely to cause ureteral displacement and obstruction (Chamberlin & Pain 1944).

When fibroids are found in association with other pelvic pathology such as pelvic inflammatory disease or endometriosis, which cause fibrosis and adhesions, they become relatively fixed and are thus more likely to cause ureteral obstruction (Long & Montgomery 1950).

In summary, fibroids often cause symptoms by a mass effect on the bladder and may cause some degree of ureteric obstruction. This ureteral obstruction and dilatation does not usually lead to permanent renal damage and once the pelvic mass has been removed the radiographic changes rapidly revert to normal. Care should be taken, especially when removing intraligamentous tumours, not to damage the lower urinary tract, as the course of the ureter may be greatly deviated from its normal position.

Pelvic inflammatory disease

Pelvic inflammatory disease (PID) is an extremely common gynaecological problem, responsible for a large proportion of all admissions to acute gynaecological wards. It is particularly common in developing countries, but its incidence in the Western world has increased dramatically over the last two decades.

Infection starts in the lower genital tract and, if untreated, ascends to involve the fallopian tubes. The epithelium is damaged and cilial motility is lost, leading to a build-up of inflammatory exudate (pus). Initially the fimbrial end of the tube remains patent and pus may enter the peritoneal cavity. Here it causes severe inflammation and becomes walled off by bowel, ovary and omentum to form a tubo-ovarian abscess. If the fimbrial end of the tube becomes sealed off, then pus accumulates within the fallopian tube to form a pyosalpinx.

During its course through the pelvis, the ureter lies in contact with the peritoneum of the pouch of Douglas and then travels forwards and medially, in the loose areolar tissue of the parametrium, into the bladder. It is therefore situated in a prime site for involvement by the inflammatory process of PID.

The ureter may become inflamed and this may lead to impaired peristalsis and urinary stasis (Long & Montgomery 1950). In addition, locally released bacterial toxins may also cause paralysis and atony of the ureter. Antibiotic therapy may resolve this inflammation but permanent stricture formation can occur.

Despite these potential mechanisms of ureteric involvement, it is relatively rare to find urinary tract complications in this condition. Even when a fixed pelvic abscess with extensive adhesions has developed, the incidence of ureteric complication varies widely in the available reports. It is believed that urinary tract obstruction does not occur even in extensive pelvic infection, although Long & Montgomery (1950) found dilatation of the upper urinary tract in 49.9%, and an abnormal delay in drainage in a further 9% of patients with extensive pelvic inflammatory disease.

Pelvic abscesses, especially those secondary to surgery or the intrauterine contraceptive device, may rarely drain into the bladder by the formation of a fistula. This is characterized by the passage of thick purulent material in the urine, with a simultaneous reduction in size of the pelvic mass and a reduction in the severity of symptoms (Altman 1972; London & Burkman 1979). Spontaneous closure of the fistula usually occurs, on appropriate antibiotic therapy, once the abscess has drained.

Benign and malignant ovarian neoplasia

Ovarian neoplasia, benign or malignant, exert a very similar effect on the lower urinary tract to that of fibroids. Thus most of the effects are pressure effects on the bladder, giving rise to symptoms of frequency and urgency, or on the ureter, leading to ureteric obstruction. It is rare to find direct invasion into the bladder, even in advanced stages of malignant ovarian tumours (Fig. 25.5).

Ureteric obstruction is more likely to occur in ovarian tumours, as compared to fibroids, because they tend to be cystic and mould to the contours of the pelvis more readily than do leiomyomata. The incidence of ureteric obstruction by large ovarian neoplasms is between 40% and 81.8%. It has been found to be slightly commoner in malignant (69.2%) than benign (57.8%) tumours.

The site of ureteric obstruction is related to the size, consistency and shape of the tumour and usually occurs, at the pelvic brim, on the side from which the tumour originates (Long & Montgomery 1950). Malignant ovarian tumours may also metastasize to

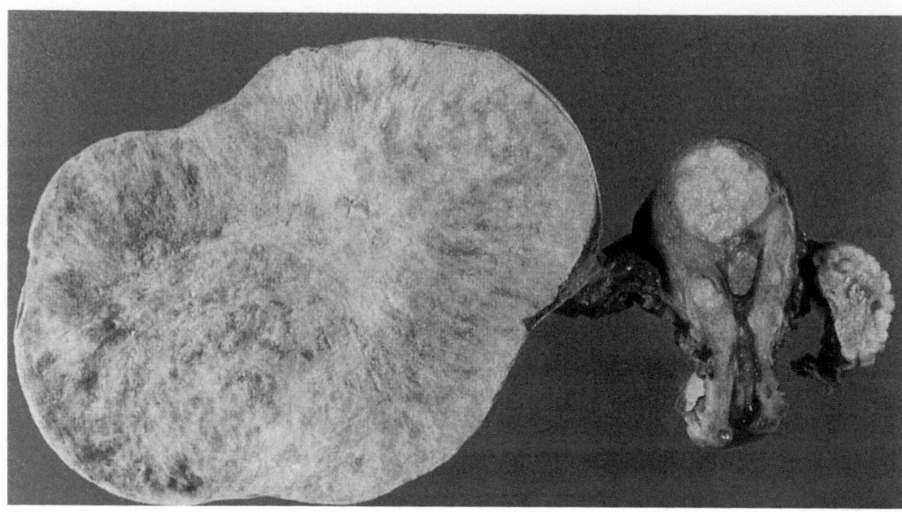

Fig. 25.5 Large Theca cell tumour of the ovary (830 grams). The uterus contains intramural and subserous fibromyomata. From Beischer and MacKay (1981), with permission.

regional lymph nodes, leading to further displacement and obstruction of the ureters. This is particularly likely to occur when the common iliac lymph nodes become enlarged. Usually, ureteric function will return to normal once the tumour has been excised (Morrison 1960).

Cytoreduction and maximum surgical resection have been shown to increase mean survival in patients with ovarian cancer and sometimes it is necessary to open the bladder or remove part of the ureter or bladder to achieve this. It has been suggested that a routine cystotomy may facilitate optimal resection of adherent bladder tumours (Ben-Baruch et al 1991). Unfortunately, in women with advanced ovarian cancer invading the lower urinary tract, optimal cytoreduction is only possible in around 60% of patients and the mean survival is approximately 15 months (Malviya et al 1989).

Ovarian remnant syndrome

The ovarian remnant syndrome is an unusual complication of oophorectomy in which remnants of the ovary, left behind after surgery, or embryological remnants within the pelvis, become functional and/or cystic, giving rise to pain with or without a pelvic mass.

It occurs following 'difficult' oophorectomy in conditions such as endometriosis and pelvic inflammatory disease, when the ovary is embedded in dense adhesions (Symmonds & Pettit 1979). The diagnosis is suggested by premenopausal levels of oestradiol and gonadotrophins and is confirmed by surgery and pathological studies which demonstrate the presence of ovarian tissue where there should be none.

The ovarian remnant is usually a complex of corpus luteum cysts and dense fibrous tissue. It is situated on the lateral pelvic side wall and may obstruct the ureter at this site. Several reports of this condition involving the ureter have been published (Kaufmann 1962; Horowitz & Elguezabal 1966; Major 1968; Scully et al 1979).

Medical treatment to suppress ovarian function may be considered in women without ureteric involvement. Surgical removal of the ovarian remnant and surrounding fibrous tissue is difficult, particularly because of the proximity of the ureter. In order to avoid surgical trauma to the ureter during the procedure it must be identified and mobilized. This is best performed by the placement of an indwelling retrograde ureteral catheter prior to the operation (Berek et al 1979). Medical stimulation with hMG may further assist identification of the ovarian remnant at the time of surgery (Kaminski et al 1990).

Endometriosis

Endometriosis is an extremely common gynaecological condition most often seen in the late reproductive years in nulliparous women. In this condition, tissue similar to normal endometrium is found in sites other than the lining of the uterine cavity. Numerous theories have been suggested to account for this phenomenon and it seems that no one theory will explain all forms of the disease. The three most commonly accepted are: the implantation theory via retrograde menstruation, the coelomic metaplasia theory and the lymphatic and vascular dissemination theory.

Endometriosis of the urinary tract is rare but most commonly involves the urinary bladder followed by the ureters (Abeshouse & Abeshouse 1960). The urethra is very rarely involved, but occasionally a nodule may be seen at the urethral meatus which increases in size at the time of menstruation.

The true incidence of urinary complications is not known as not all sufferers are fully urologically investigated; however a study of 720 patients by Ball & Platt (1962) found that 34 had major urological complications. These findings and those of other authors (Kerr 1966; Thomsen & Schroder 1987) would suggest that it is important to consider urinary tract involvement in all cases of severe endometriosis and that a routine IVU or ultrasound follow-up may be required following treatment (Miller & Morgan 1990).

Vesical endometriosis may occur as a manifestation of a generalized pelvic disease or as a result of iatrogenic dissemination, most commonly after caesarean section (Vercellini et al 1996). The bladder involvement may be epithelial or full thickness thus forming an endometrioma which is visible on the epithelial surface (Fig. 25.6). Frequency, urgency, dysuria, suprapubic pain or 'bladder irritation' are reported in approximately 80% of patients, and haematuria in about 30%. The symptoms may be aggravated in the second half of the cycle and during menstruation (Aldridge et al 1985).

The severity of the symptoms is related more to the size of the lesion, which may exceed 8 cm, than to its location. A lesion near the relatively fixed trigone is not disturbed as much by bladder filling and emptying, and therefore produces less pain than a lesion in the relatively mobile fundus.

In about half the cases a bladder mass can be palpated (Makar et al 1993); however it is unusual for the bladder to be the only site of endometriosis. Bimanual examination may reveal a retroverted uterus fixed in the pouch of Douglas, involvement of the uterosacral ligaments and cysts on the ovaries adherent to the broad ligament or pelvic side wall (Kane & Drouin 1985) (Fig. 25.7).

If the latter is suspected, a cystoscopic examination is mandatory. The findings vary with the size and location of the lesion: a sub-epithelial lesion may only be seen as bullous oedema, whereas an epithelial lesion will be seen as a bluish nodule, if the epithelium is intact, or as an ulcer if it is breached. The ectopic endometrium causes an inflammatory reaction in the surrounding tissue, marked by reddening, congestion and oedema (Ball & Platt 1962). A biopsy should be taken under direct vision to differentiate the lesion from a primary neoplasm, or metastatic disease in the bladder from other pelvic organs.

The management may be conservative or surgical, depending on such factors as the severity of the disease, age or the desire for future pregnancies. Surgical therapy still seems to offer the best results (Moore et al 1979) and involves excision of the endometrioma (segmental cystectomy) combined with a total abdominal hysterectomy and bilateral salpingo-oophorectomy (Foster et al 1987).

If the patient wishes to have more children, a more conservative approach is indicated. Nehzat & Nehzat (1993) report the use of laparoscopic segmental bladder resection rather than open surgery, while various non-surgical treatments such as continuous progestogens, the combined oral contraceptive pill, Danazol and GRH analogues have been tried with some degree of success (Ball & Platt 1962; Lavelle et al 1976).

Ureteral involvement by endometriosis is a well-known but very uncommon finding; to date more than 100 cases have been reported in the literature. Endometriosis involving the ureter is not a completely

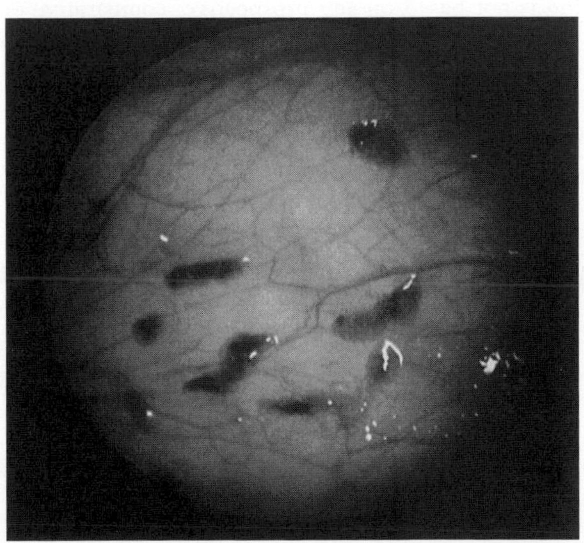

Fig. 25.6 Multiple superficial vesicles in a patient with biopsy proven endometriosis. From Shaw (1993), with permission.

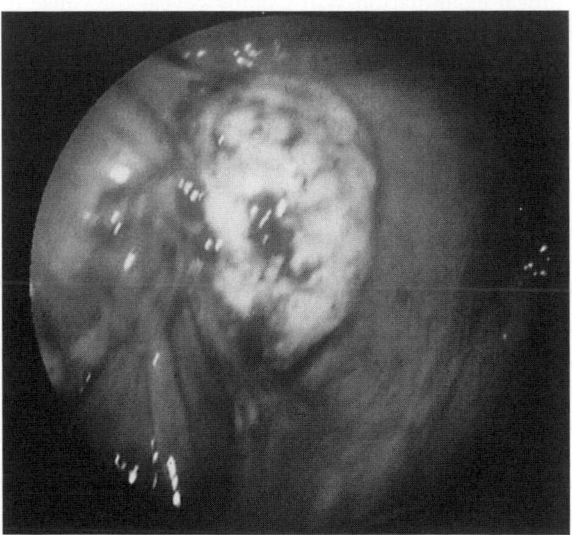

Fig. 25.7 Multiple superficial deposits of endometriosis on the posterior aspect of the right ovary. From Shaw (1993), with permission.

benign condition; about 25% of kidneys are lost when endometriosis obstructs the ureter (Stanley et al 1965; Kerr 1966; Moore et al 1979). If bilateral obstruction occurs this may lead to endstage renal failure (Mourin-Jouret et al 1987). Obstruction may occur when there is extensive endometriosis, but can also complicate relatively minimal disease, particularly when it involves the uterosacral ligaments (Moore et al 1979).

The ureter may be involved in two ways, extrinsic or intrinsic. In extrinsic involvement the ureter becomes compressed by endometriosis originating at another site, e.g. the broad ligament or ovary. Intrinsic involvement implies that there is endometriosis within the ureteral wall itself, usually in the muscularis, causing significant narrowing of the lumen. This is much rarer than extrinsic involvement.

Urinary symptoms are caused either by haemorrhage or ureteric obstruction, which leads to hydroureter, hydronephrosis and, in time, obstructive nephropathy. In most instances, ureteral obstruction occurs insidiously with few symptoms and may progress relatively asymptomatically to cause renal failure (Gourdie & Rogers 1986). Symptoms such as loin pain, oliguria and haematuria may be cyclical or may mimic ureterolithiasis (Traub et al 1976), especially when they are caused by an endometriotic ureteral nodule. More commonly, however, the symptoms are caused by ureteral compression or stricture, and are steadily progressive, mimicking urological problems following obstructive disease from other causes.

As with the bladder, it is uncommon for the ureter alone to be involved by endometriosis, although this has been reported (Bulkley et al 1965), and therefore clinical examination will usually reveal the cause of the obstruction.

Cystoscopy is normally unrewarding, although bleeding from the terminal ureter may be seen if cystoscopy is performed during menstruation. The passage of ureteral catheters is not particularly helpful when performed as a single examination, but if performed at different times during the menstrual cycle may reveal varying degrees of obstruction. Intravenous urography, too, may show obstruction of the ureter but again may have to be performed at different times in the cycle if the obstruction is partial. At laparotomy, frozen section may be required to make the correct diagnosis.

Extrinsic endometriosis involving the ureter is managed by surgical removal of the endometriosis, thereby releasing the ureter from the constricting mass. A portion of the ureter will only need to be removed if there is intrinsic involvement of the ureteric wall by an endometrioma. Radical surgery for the endometriosis, particularly bilateral salpingo-oophorectomy, seems to improve the long-term prognosis (Kerr 1966; Langmade 1975).

More recently, laparoscopic surgical techniques have been used to treat pelvic endometriosis, the principle therapy being laser ablation of the endometriotic deposits. Unfortunately, ureteral injury can occur even when using the CO2 laser and hydrodisection techniques and it is therefore extremely important that this is performed only by experienced laparoscopists (Bakri et al 1994). Laparoscopically assisted hysterectomy has also been employed successfully in the treatment of severe endometriosis with apparently 'acceptable rates' of bowel and ureteric injury. The mean operating time with this technique remains high, at over 3 hours, even in experienced hands (Davis et al 1993).

Conservative measures are the same as for bladder endometriosis and when used as a first-line treatment may relieve ureteric obstruction, as long as this is not caused by a secondary inflammatory stricture (Lavelle et al 1976; Watanabe et al 1989). They should be considered in all cases following surgical treatment.

Complications of 'simple hysterectomy'

Hanley (1969), in an anecdotal report, suggested an association between urinary symptoms and total hysterectomy. As a consequence it has been widely accepted that hysterectomy may cause debilitating bladder symptoms. In his report of many years of clinical experience he comments that such symptoms are more common following total rather than subtotal hysterectomy, though he freely admits that this feeling is not based on any prospective, comparative or controlled study. In addition, no attempt was made to obtain a record of preoperative urinary symptoms in women undergoing hysterectomy, nor did he give any analysis of the indications for the operation. However, a large proportion of hysterectomies are performed in perimenopausal women in whom there is a high prevalence of lower urinary tract dysfunction. Thus a number of prospective studies have been performed in which pre- and postoperative urinary symptoms have been evaluated.

Jequier (1976) studied urinary symptoms preoperatively, at 6 weeks and 6 months postoperatively, in 104 women undergoing total abdominal hysterectomy. She found that 62% were symptomatic preoperatively and 50% postoperatively, with frequency and urgency of micturition being the commonest symptoms.

More recently, studies have been performed comparing pre- and postoperative urodynamic data and urinary symptoms. Parys et al (1989), in a study of 42 women, found a significant increase in urinary symptoms after hysterectomy and a new urodynamic abnormality in 14 women. Genuine stress incontinence was found in 5, detrusor instability in 2 and urethral obstruction in 3. In addition, he found a significant increase in sacral reflex latencies postoperatively, suggesting a possible neurological cause for these. In a later study (Parys et al 1989) he concluded that there was a significant increase in the subjective and objective incidence of vesicourethral dysfunction. This study could, however, be criticized for including women having vaginal or abdominal hysterectomies and it is of interest that there was no change in any of the urethral pressure profile data.

Griffith-Jones et al (1991) failed to show any increase in urinary symptoms after hysterectomy. In an elegant study he compared urinary symptoms before and after hysterectomy with symptoms prior to and after dilatation and curettage. No urinary symptom was found more commonly after hysterectomy than after curettage. Similarly, Langer et al (1989) found that in a small highly selected group of women who were premenopausal and had no urinary symptoms prior to hysterectomy, there were no new symptoms of frequency, nocturia, urgency, urge incontinence or stress incontinence at 4 weeks or 4 months postoperatively ($n = 16$).

In summary, urinary symptoms are often reported as having occurred since hysterectomy but in many instances the symptoms predate the operation, although some women may develop problems de novo.

It has been suggested that subtotal hysterectomy should be performed in preference to total hysterectomy, and that this may minimize the chances of causing bladder dysfunction by limiting bladder dissection at the time of the procedure. To date, there have been no large randomized controlled studies to investigate this hypothesis, while there are anecdotal reports of bladder dysfunction following subtotal hysterectomy (Lose 1995).

Direct surgical trauma to the bladder or ureters may occur during bladder dissection, securing of the uterine pedicles and uterosacral ligaments and vaginal cuff closure (Fig. 25.8). It is not the remit of this chapter to discuss this in detail, although there has recently been renewed interest in this complication, particularly as it appears to occur relatively commonly during the 'learning curve' associated with minimal access surgery and laparoscopically assisted vaginal hysterectomy (Kadar & Lemmerling 1994).

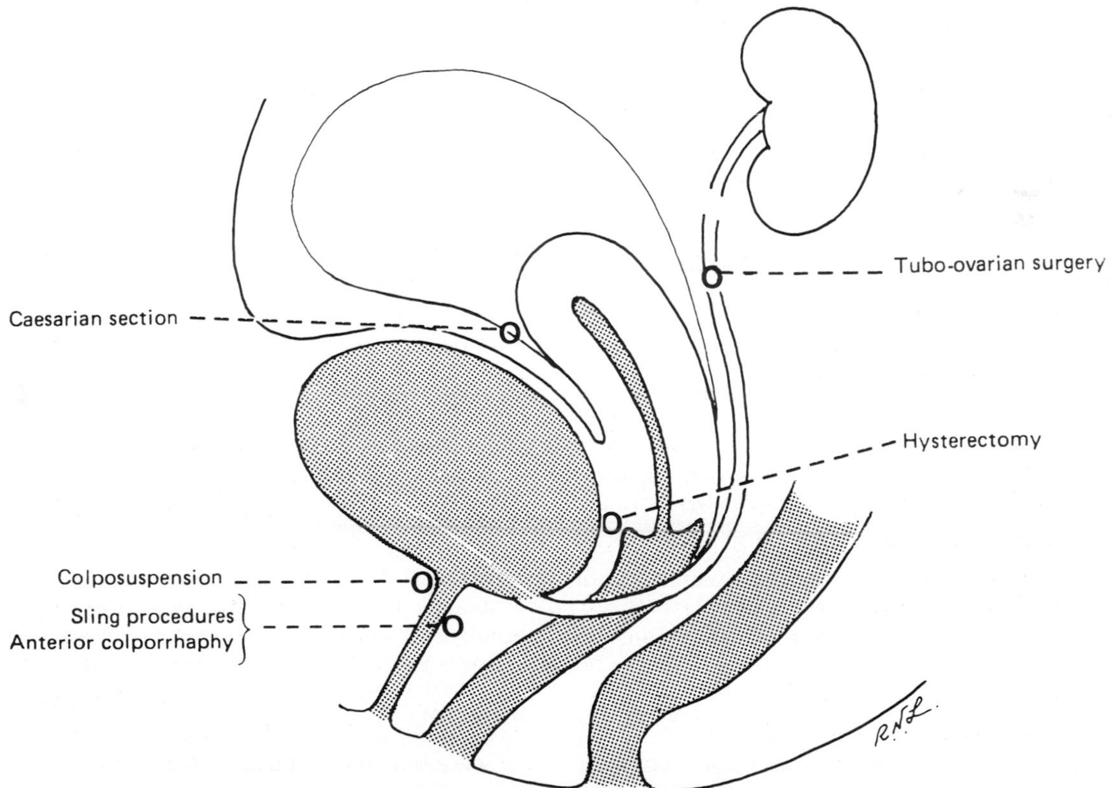

Fig. 25.8 The commonest sites and causes of urological injury during the gynaecological surgery. From Mundy (1987), with permission.

CONCLUSION

The genital and urinary tract are close embryologically and anatomically. It should therefore not come as a surprise that gynaecological disease often has urinary tract sequelae. Thus it is imperative that those who treat gynaecological conditions are aware of possible lower urinary tract involvement by the disease process and the possible damage that may occur as a result of treatment. Similarly, urologists must consider the possibility of an underlying gynaecological disease process when investigating and treating lower urinary tract dysfunction.

REFERENCES

Abeshouse B S, Abeshouse G 1960 Endometriosis of the urinary tract: a review of the literature. Journal of the International College of Surgeons 83: 100–102

Aldridge C W, Mason J T 1950 Ureteral obstruction in carcinoma of the cervix. American Journal of Obstetrics and Gynecology 60: 1272–1280

Aldridge K W, Burns J R, Singh B 1985 Vesical endometriosis: a review and two case reports. Journal of Urology 134: 539–541

Altman L C 1972 Ovarian abscess and vaginal fistula. Obstetrics and Gynecology 40: 321–322

Bakri Y N, Sundin T, Mans M 1994 Acta Obstetrica et Gynecologica Scandinavica 73(8): 665–667

Ball T L, Platt M A 1962 Urological complications of endometriosis. American Journal of Obstetrics and Gynecology 84: 1516–1521

Barber H R K, Roberts S, Brunschwig A 1963 Prognostic significance of preoperative non-visualising kidney in patients receiving pelvic exenteration. Cancer 16: 1614–1615

Beischer N A, MacKay E V 1981 Colour Atlas of Gynaecology. W B Saunders, Artamon

Ben-Baruch G, Schiff E, Sivan E, Menczer J 1991 Cystotomy – for facilitation of optimal resection of adherent pelvic tumors. Gynecologic Oncology 41(2): 139–140

Berek J S, Darney P D, Lopkin C et al 1979 Avoiding ureteral damage in pelvic surgery for ovarian remnant syndrome. American Journal of Obstetrics and Gynecology 15: 221–222

Bosch A, Frias Z, de Valda G G. 1973 Prognostic significance of ureteral obstruction in carcinoma of the cervix uteri. Acta Radiologica 12: 47–50

Buchsbaum H, Schmidt J 1982 Gynecological and Obstetric Urology, 2nd edn. W B Saunders Philadelphia Chap. 26, p 397

Bulkley G J, Carrow L A, Estensen R D 1965 Endometriosis of the ureter. Journal of Urology 93: 139–143

Burke T W, Stringer A, Gerhenson D M et al 1990 Radical wide excision and selective inguinal node dissection for squamous cell carcinoma of the vulva. Gynecologic Oncology 38: 328–331

Burns B C, Everett H S, Brack C B 1960 Value of urologic study in the management of carcinoma of the cervix. American Journal of Obstetrics and Gynecology 80: 997–1004

Chamberlin G W, Pain F L 1944 Urinary tract changes with benign pelvic tumours. Radiology 42: 117–120

Creasman W T, Boronow R C, Morrow C P et al 1976 Adenocarcinoma of the endometrium: its metastatic lymph node potential. Gynecologic Oncology 4: 239–243

Culame R J 1980 Pelvic relaxation as a complication of the radical vulvectomy. Obstetrics and Gynecology 55: 716–718

Cushing R M, Tovell H M M, Liegner L M 1968 Major urological complications following radium and x-ray therapy for cervical carcinoma of the cervix. American Journal of Obstetrics and Gynecology 101: 750–754

Davis G D, Wolgamott G, Moon J 1993 Laparoscopically assisted vaginal hysterectomy as definitive therapy for stage III and IV endometriosis. Journal of Reproductive Medicine 38(8): 577–581

Debus-Thiede G, Maassen V, Dimpfl T, Klosterhalfen T, Kindermann G 1993 Late disorders of bladder function after Wertheim operation – an analysis of urodynamic parameters with reference to surgical radicality. Geburtshilfe und Frauenheilkunde 53(8): 525–531

Forney J P 1980 The effect of radical hysterectomy on bladder physiology. American Journal of Obstetrics and Gynecology 138: 374–382

Foster R S, Rink R C, Mulcahy J J 1987 Vesical endometriosis: medical or surgical treatment. Urology 29(1): 64–65

Gauthier P, Gore I, Singleton H M 1985 Identification of histopathologic risk groups in stage Ib squamous cell carcinoma of the cervix. Obstetrics and Gynecology 66: 569–575

Glahn B E 1970 The neurogenic factor in vesical dysfunction following radical hysterectomy for carcinoma of the cervix. Scandinavian Journal of Urology and Nephrology. 4: 107–111

Goluboff E T, O'Toole K, Sawczuk I S 1994 Leiomyoma of bladder: report of case and review of literature. Urology 43(2): 238–241

Gourdie R W, Rogers C N 1986 Bilateral ureteric obstruction due to endometriosis presenting with cyclical hypertension and cyclical oliguria. British Journal of Urology 58: 224

Green T H, Meigs J V, Ulfelder H et al 1962 Urological complications of radical Wertheim hysterectomy: incidence, etiology, management and prevention. Obstetrics and Gynecology 20: 293–312

Griffith-Jones, Jarvis G J, McNamara H M 1991 Adverse urinary symptoms after total abdominal hysterectomy – fact or fiction? British Journal of Urology 67: 295–297

Hanley H G. 1969 The late urological complications of total hysterectomy. British Journal of Urology 41: 682–684

Halpin T F, Frick H C III, Munell E W 1972 Critical points of failure in the therapy of cancer of the cervix: a reappraisal. American Journal of Obstetrics and Gynecology 114: 755–758

Henriksen E 1949 The lymphatic spread of carcinoma of the cervix and of the body of the uterus. American Journal of Obstetrics and Gynecology 58: 924–927

Horowitz M I, Elguezabal A 1966 Obstruction of the ureter by a recent corpus luteum located in the retroperitoneum: report of two cases. Journal of Urology 95: 706–710

Iwamoto K, Kigawa J, Minagawa Y, Miura H, Terakawa N 1994 Transvaginal ultrasonographic diagnosis of bladder-wall invasion in patients with cervical cancer. Obstetrics and Gynecology 83(2): 217–219

Jequier A M 1976 Urinary symptoms and total hysterectomy. British Journal of Urology 48: 437–441

Jones C R, Woodhouse C R J, Hendry W F 1984 Urological problems following treatment of carcinoma of the cervix. British Journal of Urology 56: 609–613

Kadar N, Saliba N, Nelson J H 1983 The frequency, causes and prevention of severe urinary dysfunction after radical hysterectomy. British Journal of Obstetrics and Gynaecology 90: 858–863

Kadar N, Lemmerling L 1994 Urinary tract injuries during laparoscopically assisted hysterectomy: causes and prevention. American Journal of Obstetrics and Gynecology. 170: 47–48

Kaminski P F, Sorosky J I, Mandell M J et al 1990 Clomiphene citrate stimulation as an adjunct in locating ovarian tissue in ovarian remnant syndrome. Obstetrics and Gynecology 76: 924–928

Kane C, Drouin P 1985 American Journal of Obstetrics and Gynecology 151(2): 207–211

Kaufman J J 1962 Unusual causes of extrinsic ureteral obstruction, part II. Journal of Urology 87: 328–332

Kerr W S 1966 Endometriosis involving the urinary tract. Clinics in Obstetrics and Gynecology 9: 331–335

Kottmeier H L 1964 Surgical and radiation treatment of carcinoma of the uterine cervix. Acta Obstetrica et Gynecologica Scandinavica 43 (suppl. 12): 1

Kretschmer H L, Kanter A E 1937 The effect of certain gynecological lesions on the upper urinary tract. Journal of the American Medical Association 14: 1097–2003

Langer R, Neuman M, Rou-El R, Golan A, Bukovsky I, Caspi E 1989. The effect of TAH on bladder function in asymptomatic women. Obstetrics and Gynecology 74: 205–207

Langer R, Golan A, Neuman M et al 1990 The effect of large uterine fibroids on urinary bladder function and symptoms. American Journal of Obstetrics and Gynecology. 163: 1139–1141

Langmade C F 1975 Pelvic endometriosis and ureteral obstruction. American Journal of Obstetrics and Gynecology 122 (4): 463–469

Larson D M, Malone J M, Copeland L J et al 1987 Ureteral assessment after radical hysterectomy. Obstetrics and Gynecology 69: 612–614

Lavelle K J, Melman A W, Cleary R E 1976 Ureteral obstruction owing to endometriosis: reversal with synthetic progestin. Journal of Urology 116: 665–666

Lerner H M, Jones H W, Hill E C 1980 Radical surgery for the treatment of early invasive cervical carcinoma (Stage IB): review of 15 years' experience. Obstetrics and Gynecology 56: 413–418

Lewington W 1956 Disturbances of micturition following Wertheim hysterectomy. Journal of Obstetrics and Gynaecology of the British Empire 63: 861–864

London A M, Burkman R T 1979 Tuboovarian abscess with associated rupture and fistula formation into the urinary bladder: report of two cases. American Journal of Obstetrics and Gynecology 135: 1113–1134

Long J P, Montgomery J B 1950 The incidence of ureteral obstruction in benign and malignant gynecologic lesions. American Journal of Obstetrics and Gynecology 59: 552–562

Lose G 1995 Persistent postoperative urinary retention treated with transurethral intravesical electrostimulation. Acta Obstetrica et Gynecologica Scandinavica 74(10): 842–845

Major F J 1968 Retained ovarian remnant causing ureteral obstruction. Obstetrics and Gynecology 32: 748–750

Makar A P, Wauters H A, van Dijck H H, van de Looverbosch R L, de Schrijver D H 1993 Vesical endometriosis: value of laparoscopy. British Journal of Urology 72(1): 115

Malviya V K, Malone J M Jr, Deppe G 1989 Advanced ovarian cancer: urinary tract resection as a part of cytoreductive surgery. European Journal of Gynaecological Oncology 10(2): 69–72

Masterson B J 1986 Manual of Gynecologic Surgery, 2nd edn. Springer Verlag, New York.

Meigs J V 1951 Radical hysterectomy with bilateral lymph node dissections. A report of 100 women operated on five or more years ago. American Journal of Obstetrics and Gynecology 62: 854–858

Miller M A, Morgan R J 1990 Bilateral ureteric obstruction due to endometriosis resulting in unilateral loss of renal function. British Journal of Urology 65(4): 421

Million R R, Rutledge F, Fletcher G H 1972 Stage IV carcinoma of the cervix with bladder invasion. American Journal of Obstetrics and Gynecology 113: 239–246

Moore J G, Hibbard L T, Growden W A et al 1979 Urinary tract endometriosis: Enigmas in diagnosis and management. American Journal of Obstetrics and Gynecology 134(2): 162–172

Morrison J K. 1960 The ureter and hysterectomy. Including the effects of certain gynaecological conditions on the urinary tract. Journal of Obstetrics and Gynaecology of the British Empire 67: 66–72

Mourin-Jouret A, Squifflet J P, Cosyns J P, Pirson Y, Alexandre G P 1987 Bilateral ureteral endometriosis with end stage renal failure. Urology 29(3): 302–306

Mundy A R 1987 Urological injury and how to cope. In: Stanton S L, Principles of Gynaecological Surgery, Springer Verlag, Berlin.

Nehzat C R, Nehzat F R 1993 Laparoscopic segmental bladder resection for endometriosis: a report of two cases. Obstetrics and Gynecology 81, 5(2): 882–884

Parys B T, Haylen B T, Hutton J L, Parsons K F 1989 The effects of simple hysterectomy on vesicourethral function. British Journal of Urology 64: 594–599

Photopoulos G J, Vander Zwaag R 1991 Class II hysterectomy shows less morbidity and good treatment efficacy compared to class III. Gynecologic Oncology 40: 21–25

Piver M S, Chung W S 1975 Prognostic significance of cervical lesion size and pelvic lymph node metastasis in cervical carcinoma. Obstetrics and Gynecology 46: 507–510

Ralph G, Winter R, Michelitsch L, Tamussino K 1991 Radicality of parametrial resection and dysfunction of the lower urinary tract after radical hysterectomy. European Journal of Gynaecological Oncology 12(1): 27–30

Reid G C, DeLancey J O L, Hopkins M P et al 1990 Urinary incontinence following radical vulvectomy. Obstetrics and Gynecology 75: 852–854

Rubens D, Thornbury J R, Angel C et al 1988 Comparison of clinical, M R, and pathological staging. American Journal of Roentgenology 150: 135–138

Scully R E, Galdabini J J, McNeely B V 1979 Case records of the Massachusetts General Hospital. Case 48–1979. New England Journal of Medicine 301: 1228–1232

Semelka R C, Ascher S M, Reinhold C 1997 MRI of the Abdomen and Pelvis. Wiley-Liss, New York.

Seski J C, Diokno A C 1977 Bladder dysfunction after radical abdominal hysterectomy. American Journal of Obstetrics and Gynecology 128: 643–648

Shaw R W 1993 An Atlas of Endometriosis. The Parthenon Publishing Group, Carnforth.

Spratt J S, Butcher H R Jr, Bricker E M 1973 Exenterative surgery of the pelvis. W B Saunders, Philadelphia, p. 49
Stanley K E Jr, Utz D C, Dockerty M B 1965 Clinically significant endometriosis of the urinary tract. Surgery, Gynecology and Obstetrics 120: 491–493
Suresh U R, Smith V J, Lupton E W, Haboubi N Y 1993 Radiation disease of the urinary tract: histological features of 18 cases. Journal of Clinical Pathology. 46(3): 228–231
Symmonds R E, Pettit P D M 1979 Ovarian remnant syndrome. Obstetrics and Gynecology 54: 174–177
Thomsen H, Schroder H M 1987 Simultaneous external and internal endometriosis of the ureter. Case report. Scandinavian Journal of Urology and Nephrology
Traub Y M, Fischelovitch J, Neri A et al 1976 Endometriosis mimicking ureterolithiasis. British Journal of Urology 48: 27–30
van Dyke A H, van Nagell J R Jr 1975 The prognostic significance of ureteral obstruction in patients with recurrent carcinoma of the cervix uteri. Surgery, Gynecology and Obstetrics 141: 371–373
van Nagell J R Jr, Donaldson E S, Wood E G et al 1978 The significance of vascular invasion and lymphocytic infiltration in invasive carcinoma of the cervix. Cancer 41: 228–234
van Nagell J R Jr, Donaldson E S, Gay E R 1982 Urinary tract involvement by invasive cancer. In: Buchsbaum, Schmidt (eds) Gynaecologic and Obstetric Urology. WB Saunders, Philadelphia
Vercellini P, Meschia M, De Giorgi O, Panazza S, Cortesi I, Crosignani P G. 1996 Bladder detrusor endometriosis: clinical and pathogenic implications. Journal of Urology 155(1): 84–86
Vick C W, Walsh J W, Wheelock J B et al 1984 CT of the normal and abnormal parametria in cervical cancer. American Journal of Roentgenology 143: 597–603
Watanabe T, Minakata S, Kitagawa M 1989 Two cases of ureteral endometriosis. Acta Urologica Japonica 35(2): 315–321
Wertheim E 1912 The extended abdominal operation for carcinoma uteri. American Journal of Obstetrics and Gynecology 66: 169–173
Zaiton M M 1986 Retroperitoneal parasitic leiomyoma causing unilateral ureteral obstruction. Journal of Urology 135: 130–131

SECTION 3
CHAPTER

26

Congenital abnormalities

PETER H L WORTH AND SHEILA L B DUNCAN

Part One: Urological aspects

Part Two: Gynaecological aspects

Part One:Urological aspects

Peter H L Worth

The development of the kidney and the ureter is a complex matter, and it is not therefore surprising that there are many congenital abnormalities. It is always difficult to be certain of the true incidence of congenital anomalies of the urinary tract, because they tend to be associated with a high incidence of disease. Finding a congenital abnormality does not necessarily mean it is the cause of the particular symptom; for instance, not infrequently, one finds duplicated system on a contralateral side to the patient's pain. Since abnormal genitalia are said to be associated with upper tract anomalies in one third of cases, it is sensible to image the upper tracts before carrying out gynaecological surgery.

CONDITIONS ASSOCIATED WITH ABNORMAL KIDNEY POSITION OR FUSION

Pelvic kidney

The incidence of a pelvic kidney is about 1 in 800, but in 1 in 2000 it may be the only kidney. It may present as a pelvic mass on vaginal examination, and is a rare cause of obstruction in labour. A solitary pelvic kidney often has multiple blood vessels and may cause hypertension. It may be missed on routine intravenous urography because the calyces overlie the sacrum and the contrast may merge imperceptibly with the bone. If the diagnosis of pelvic kidney is not entertained, serious problems can be encountered if a laparotomy is undertaken. No attempt should ever be made to remove a pelvic kidney without having full information about the contralateral kidney (Fig. 26.1).

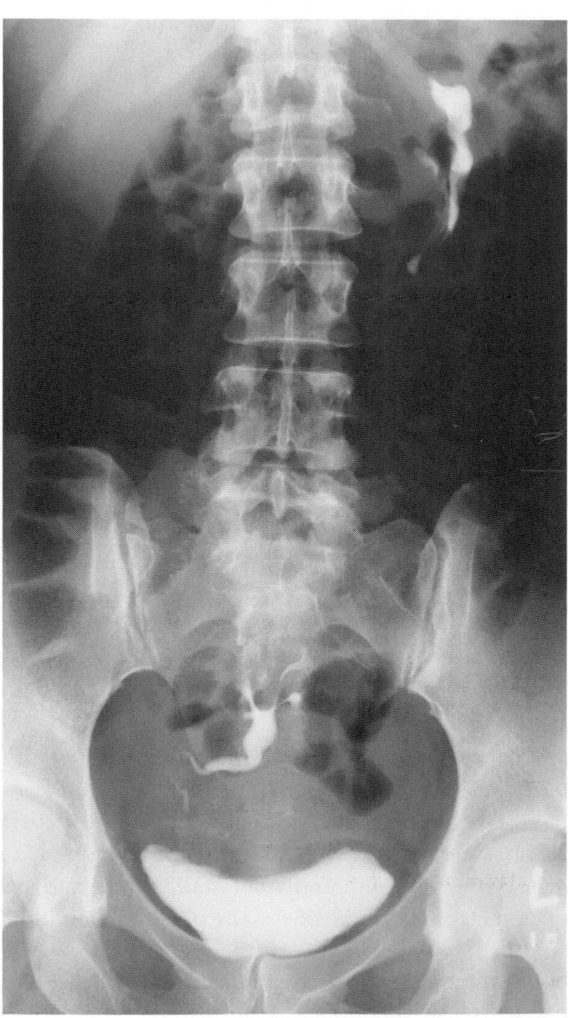

Fig. 26.1 Pelvic kidney. Note the left kidney is also malrotated.

Crossed ectopia

Crossed ectopia has an incidence of about 1 in 2000. The kidney may be in close proximity or fused with the opposite kidney. The ureter usually opens in the normal position (Fig. 26.2). This kidney as with other forms of ectopia may be more easily palpable, therefore the investigation of any abdominal mass should include an ultrasound or intravenous urogram (IVU). No specific treatment is indicated unless there is obstruction or infection.

Horseshoe kidney

The incidence of horseshoe kidney is approximately 1 in 6000. These kidneys are usually fused across their lower poles, and may therefore be easily palpable. It is often associated with other congenital abnormalities, especially cardiac problems. It also has a high incidence of urological problems; for instance, pelviureteric junction obstruction which may be accompanied by pain and urinary infection. The intravenous urogram is characteristic with malrotation of both kidneys and the lower calyx usually lying medial to the ureter (Fig. 26.3). When surgery is required, there is nothing to be gained by dividing the bridge

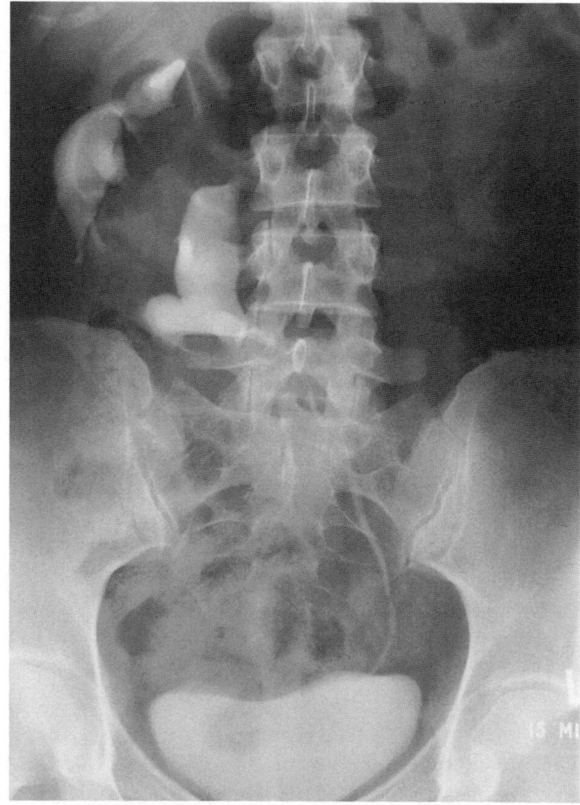

Fig. 26.2 Crossed ectopia. Note the ureter from the lower kidney crossing to the left side.

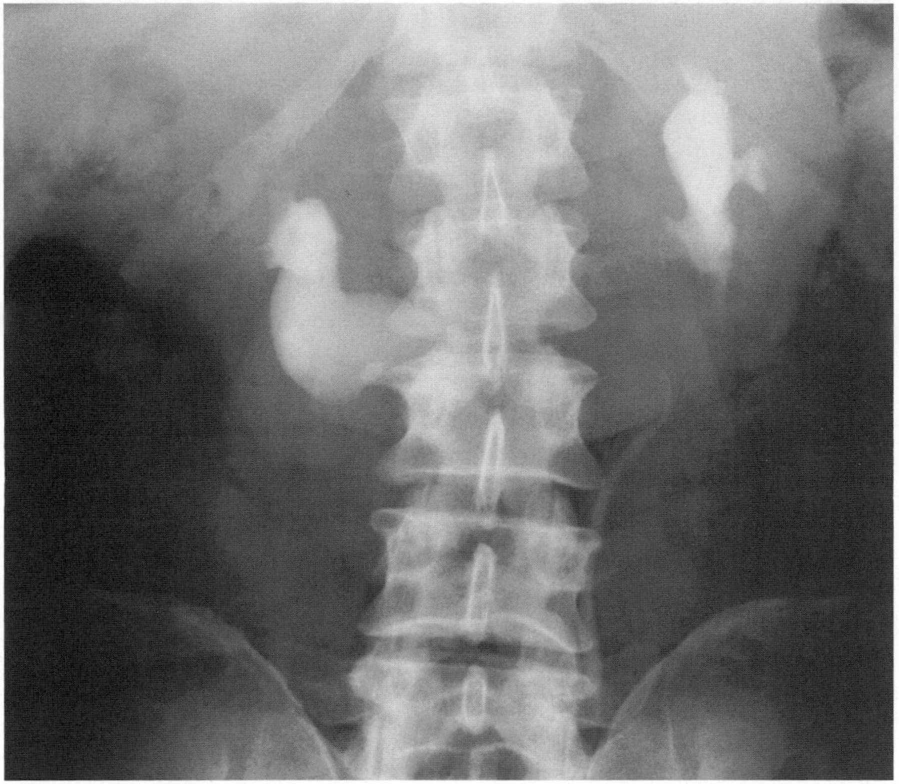

Fig. 26.3 Horseshoe kidney.

because these kidneys often have multiple blood vessels and the kidneys will not fall back into their normal position if the bridge is divided.

RENAL MASS

Although there are many causes of renal enlargement, there are two that need to be discussed.

Hydronephrosis

Hydronephrosis is commonly secondary to pelviureteric junction obstruction and is caused by an abnormality at the pelviureteric junction that fails to allow propulsion of urine down the ureter. A similar abnormality may be found at the lower end of the ureter – achalasia of the ureter or megaureter. In this situation, both the ureter and pelvis are dilated but rarely is the kidney palpable. As a result of the obstruction at the pelviureteric junction, the pelvis and calyces enlarge and in some cases may contain more than a litre of urine. In 10% of cases the condition is bilateral. The severity of the obstruction will dictate at what age the individual becomes symptomatic. Vague loin pain, intermittent in nature and often worse at night is often common. The pain may be precipitated by a big fluid load. If infection develops in the presence of this obstruction, the patient may be quite ill, with a high fever associated with abdominal pain and vomiting; it is certainly a condition to be considered in a pregnant patient with severe loin pain.

The ultrasound will show dilated calyces and pelvis. An IVU which is performed with the patient dehydrated, may not always demonstrate the problem. Where there is a strong suspicion that the diagnosis has been missed, the IVU should be repeated with the patient hydrated following the injection of contrast medium and also given diuretic by injection (Fig. 26.4). This may cause the pelvis to distend and cause the patient pain. A diuretic renogram is a better way of demonstrating obstruction and also shows how much impairment there is of renal function (Fig. 26.5). In equivocal cases of obstruction it may be necessary to puncture the kidney and perfuse it with saline at 10 ml per minute and measure the intrapelvic pressure which should not exceed 15 cm H_20 (Whitaker test; Whitaker 1979).

Treatment is by some form of pyeloplasty which either removes the obstruction, such as the Anderson–Hynes procedure, or opens it out, such as the Culp procedure. It may also be possible to do an

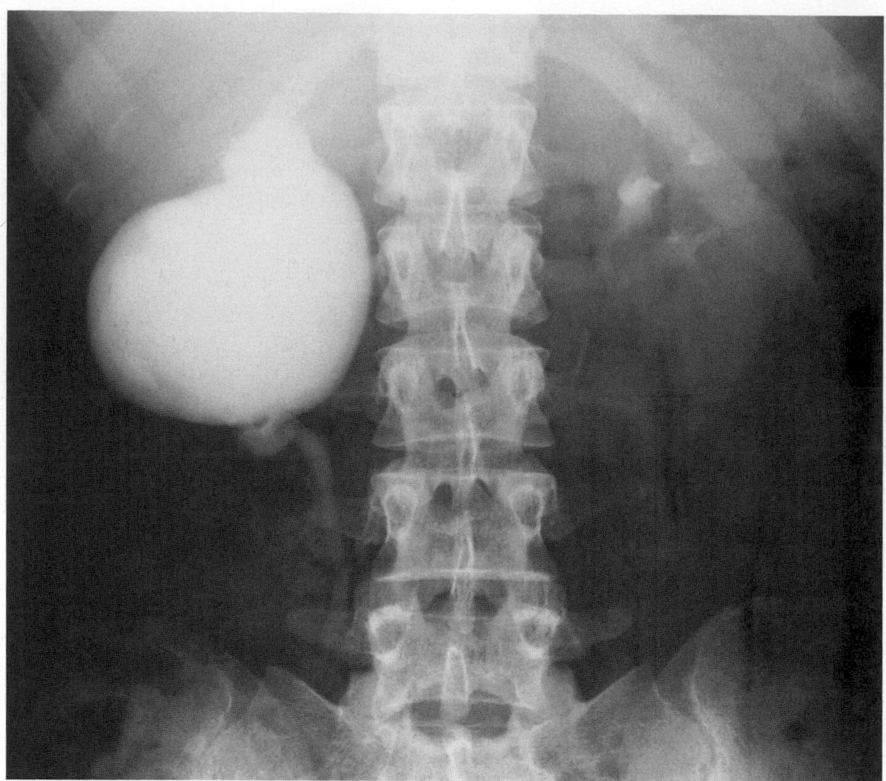

Fig. 26.4 Pelviureteric junction obstruction.

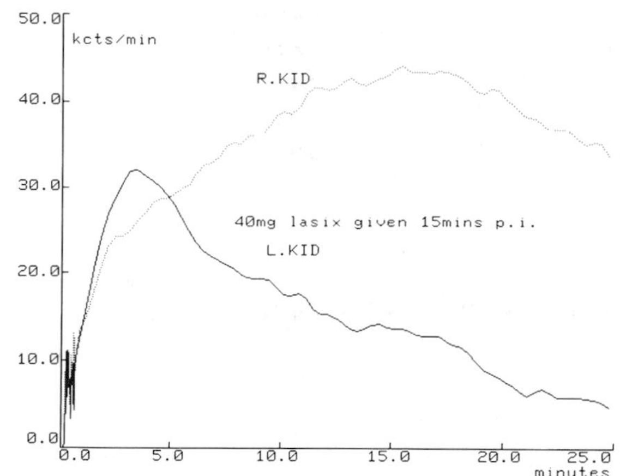

Fig. 26.5 Isotope renogram. Note a slowly rising curve due to obstruction.

endoscopic pyelolysis through a percutaneous track or balloon dilatation of the pelviureteric junction. Nephrectomy is rarely necessary, but close follow-up of the remaining kidney is necessary if it is carried out. This is because a subclinical obstruction of the pelviureteric junction may become real, since the remaining kidney has to cope with an increased urine output. An obstructed kidney loses its concentrating ability, therefore its removal will more than double the urine output of the remaining kidney.

Polycystic disease

Polycystic disease is an important condition in women. There are two types: first, there is the congenital variety, which may interfere with labour and cause problems, not only to the fetus but also to the mother; and second there is the adult, inherited form of the disease (Fig. 26.6). The latter may not appear until middle age, which is usually after childbearing and one cannot give a guarantee to an individual, even in the presence of a normal IVU that she will not manifest the condition. However, ultrasound is more accurate and small cysts may be picked up before anything is obvious on urography. It is therefore recommended that young children of patients with polycystic disease are studied by ultrasound. More severe forms manifest themselves earlier, and pregnancy may be contraindicated because of impaired renal function. Associated hepatic and pancreatic cysts may also be present.

The congenital variety is autosomal recessive, and the adult form is autosomal dominant. There is an abnormality of the development of the collecting ducts and tubules, which also fail to fuse. In adults, 95% are bilateral; therefore the findings of bilateral renal swellings should suggest the diagnosis. Patients often have bouts of pain, infection and haematuria and may be hypertensive.

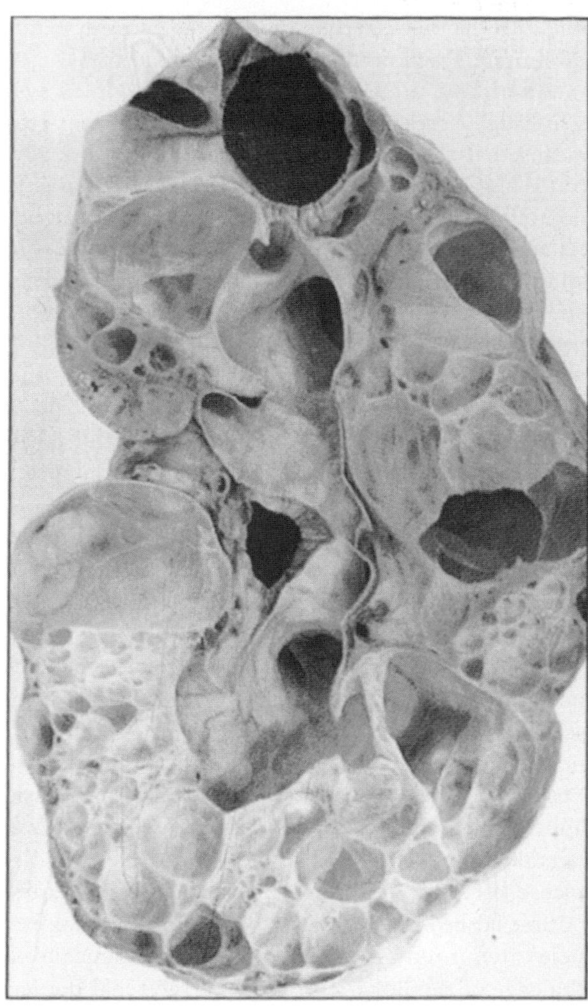

Fig. 26.6 Polycystic kidney.

The disease is readily diagnosed on the basis of radiological investigation, but must be distinguished from other forms of cystic disease, which may also be bilateral. Until the patient is symptomatic or uraemic, no specific treatment is necessary. Life expectancy is usually 5–10 years after the diagnosis has been made, but patients are usually considered for transplantation. Unlike other patients with renal failure, erythropoietin production ensures that they are not anaemic, and therefore at least one kidney should be preserved until the time of transplantation.

EXSTROPHY

Bladder exstrophy occurs in 1 in 30 000 births, with a 3:1 male predominance. It is rarely familial but I have seen a child with exstrophy whose mother had severe epispadias.

Under the broad heading of bladder exstrophy there are several conditions: 60% are classic exstrophy; 30% epispadias and 10% include cloacal anomalies. Female epispadias can be difficult to identify and occasionally the only urological problem is an incompetent bladder neck which would be picked up on an IVU when a slightly wide symphysis with contrast in the proximal urethra will be seen. In these patients the umbilicus may be very flat and the recti divaricate to the split symphysis. In the classic form the clitoris is bifid and the vagina may be narrowed and tilted anteriorly.

The aim of surgery in these cases should be to achieve continence with a satisfactory capacity with the preservation of the upper tracts. Probably 75% of children can be reconstructed satisfactorily. The surgery is very complex and should be undertaken by a specialist paediatric urologist. The policy now is to operate within the first 24 hours if practical. The first operation involves closing the bladder and abdominal wall without any formal attempt being made to reconstruct the bladder neck. It may be necessary to do an osteotomy on the inominate bones to help the approximation of the recti and abdominal wall. It is to be hoped that this primary procedure will produce some continence and allow the bladder volume to increase. Previously when surgery was delayed, the bladder mucosa became hyperplastic and the bladder muscle fibrotic.

Two to three years later a formal bladder neck construction, such as a Young–Dees procedure is undertaken together with urethral reconstruction. It is also necessary to reimplant the ureters because there is likely to be reflux. If this surgery fails to produce continence, so that the bladder capacity is poor, bladder enhancement is carried out at the age of 5–6 years. If further bladder neck surgery is considered impossible, then an artificial urinary sphincter may also be used to produce continence, but it may be necessary to empty the bladder by clean intermittent self catheterization. No formal attempt needs to be made to improve the cosmetic appearance of the vulva or clitoris, but if the vaginal opening is too small, it should be enlarged.

Urine diversion is avoided in exstrophy, as it is in other conditions in children, such as spina bifida and neuropathic bladders. The reason for this is that ileal conduits – the preferred diversion in children – lead to a diminution in renal function in the long term. This probably relates from an increased pressure in the conduit secondary to stomal stenosis, which is a common problem in children and which produces reflux up the ureters. Even if non-refluxing ureteroileal anastomoses have been done, the increase in pressure in the conduit will result in increased pressure in the upper tracts. Any child with a conduit has to be very carefully followed up and it is important to measure the residual volume in the conduit at each out-patient visit. It should be less than 10 ml.

Ureterosigmoidostomy is rarely done nowadays because of the long-term damage to the upper tracts. Children with exstrophy may also have rectal problems and lack anal continence, making this type of diversion more unsatisfactory. Long-term survival without upper tract problems predisposes patients to a 5% risk of bowel cancer, developing at the site of ureteric implantation after 20 years – this is the result of interaction of bowel flora, amines and urinary nitrates (see Ch. 45 on urinary diversion).

There is no evidence to suggest that a colonic conduit gives any better long-term results than an ileal conduit, and the incidence of ureterointestinal anastomotic problems appears to be much higher. Appliance-free continent diversions are becoming more popular but are technically more difficult to do. They include the Kock pouch principle, when a non-refluxing valve of small bowel is invaginated into a small or large bowel reservoir. Alternatively the Mitrofanoff procedure can be used where a segment of ureter, the appendix or small bowel, is adapted for catheterization of a bladder augmented with bowel.

URETERIC DUPLICATION

Degrees of duplication vary from a bifid pelvis to a completely double ureter opening separately into the bladder. Duplication occurs as a result of premature division of the metanephric bud and is relatively common. It may be asymptomatic and certainly it should not be assumed that it is responsible for symptoms just because it is found. Incomplete duplication may cause pyelonephritis by means of the so-called yo-yo phenomenon, where reflux occurs from one ureter to the other because of a slightly abnormal segment just below where they join. In complete duplication it is usually the lower pole ureter with the higher insertion that it is likely to reflux, because it has the shorter course through the bladder wall; therefore it is the lower pole that may be scarred.

An ectopic ureter may be single or part of a duplex system. The single ectopic ureter will result in incontinence, because the bladder neck and trigone are usually deficient. This can usually be seen on an IVU with low insertions of the ureter and a wide open bladder neck. Treatment is difficult because not only will bladder neck reconstruction be necessary, but both ureters will need to be reimplanted.

An ectopic ureter that is part of that duplex system usually presents as dribbling incontinence. This means that the patient passes urine quite normally, but is always a little damp in between times. Patients do not always admit to this symptom and the diagnosis may then be difficult. One woman I saw only admitted to the symptom after her daughter had been cured of her incontinence by removal of an ectopic ureter. Some patients are not affected by dribbling incontinence until they are in their late teens, and sometimes their initial symptom is a kidney infection with the onset of sexual intercourse, or they may notice a watery vaginal discharge. This late appearance of symptoms may be a result of the fact that the terminal part of the ureter is intimately related to the bladder neck muscle, and if the ureter opens into the urethra, the distal mechanism may have sufficient strength to control the leakage.

These ureters may open anywhere from the bladder neck down to the urethral orifice, or in the perineal skin or in the vagina, and the opening may be very difficult to identify. It is not essential to find the opening, but it is helpful to do so. The IVU has a classic appearance, with the lower part of the kidney lying laterally and the pelvis flattened and the ureter displaced laterally (Fig. 26.7). It may be possible to see the outline of the kidney and the 'give-away' (if the upper pole calyx is not visualized) is the long distance from the edge of the uppermost calyx to the renal border. With high dose tomography some excretion may be seen. Occasionally the IVU may look normal. If a duplex system is obvious or suspected on one side, the other kidney should be carefully inspected in case there is a similar problem that is not obvious.

As already mentioned it may be difficult to identify the ectopic ureter, even if the urine is stained with a dye. A catheter can be inserted into the ectopic ureter under direct vision and contrast injected (Fig. 26.8). Simultaneously a catheter can be put into the other ureter through a cystoscope and X-rays taken after contrast is injected. Sometimes the opening is big and in the urethra, so that a urethral catheter may enter it rather than go into the bladder.

Treatment involves removing that part of the kidney draining into the ectopic ureter. The kidney usually has more than one artery and vein; therefore the abnormal ureter should be carefully freed from the lower pole ureter, the branch of the renal artery going to the apex of the kidney should be isolated and tied, and an upper pole partial nephrectomy performed. Usually the portion of kidney that has to be removed is quite small and often dysplastic. A separate inci-

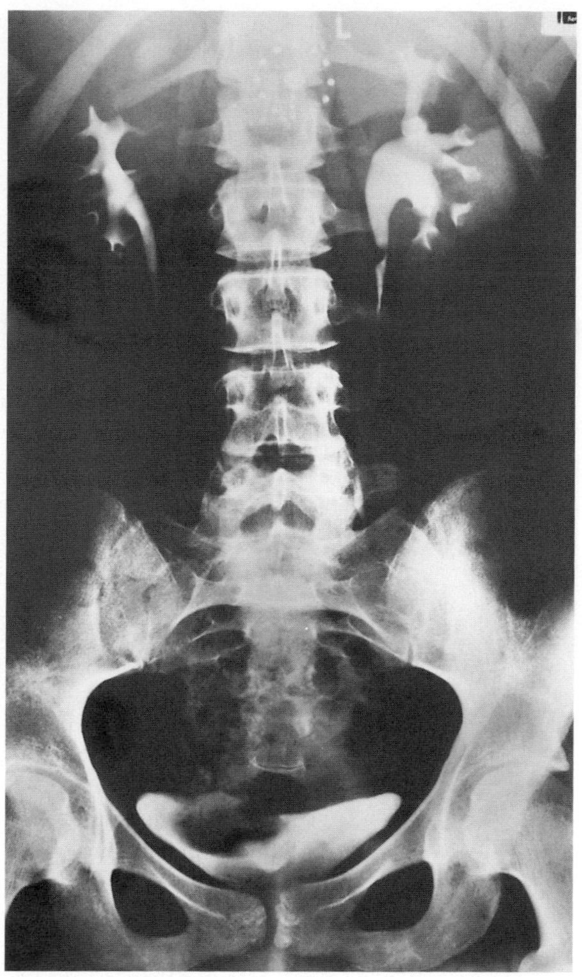

Fig. 26.7 Ectopic ureter. Note the lower moiety of the right kidney displaced laterally. There is also some contrast in the upper calyx above the 12th rib.

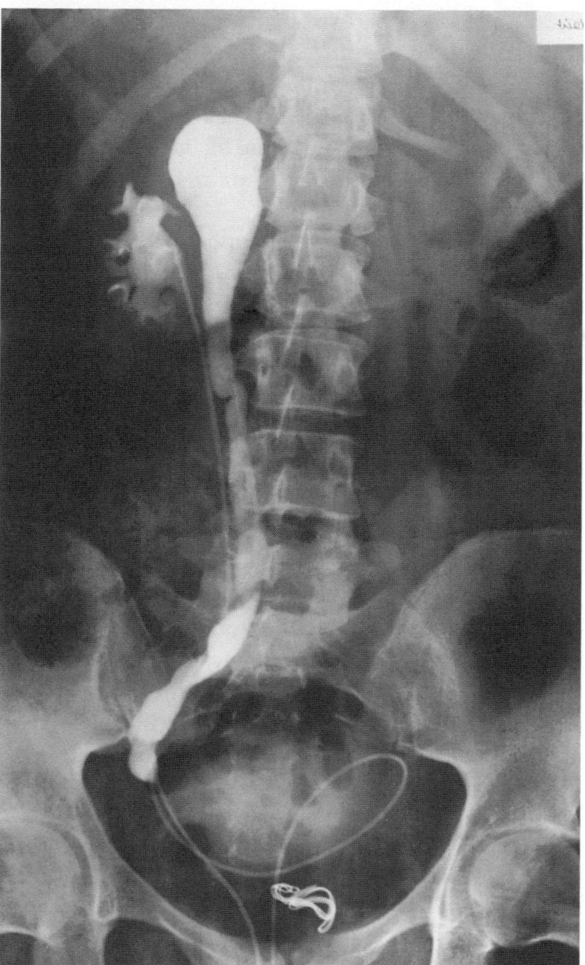

Fig. 26.8 Ectopic ureter. A ureterogram showing the upper moiety and dilated ureter. The opening was adjacent to the urethral orifice.

sion must be made to explore the lower end. As the ureters get near the bladder they run in the same sheath, so that the normal ureter can be easily damaged. The ectopic ureter is intimately connected to the muscle at the base of the bladder and bladder neck, and it should be divided as low as possible. The stump needs to be removed at a later date only if the patient develops problems from it. If it is connected to the urethra, reflux may occur into it and the patient may get recurrent infection or still have some incontinence. Removal of this lower segment may be quite difficult.

URETEROCELE

A ureterocele is an out pouching of the distal ureter into the bladder causing obstruction. It may be single and orthotopic, but in 75% of cases it is associated with duplication. The complex ones will usually be symptomatic in young children, but occasionally they may not be detected until the late teens.

A ureterocele may cause a variety of symptoms. If large, it may cause incomplete bladder emptying and in young girls it may present as a lesion at the external urethral orifice. The ureterocele may obstruct its own ureter (it is the upper part of the kidney that is obstructed), but in addition, because of dilatation, the ipsilateral ureter may be either obstructed or develop reflux. The contralateral ureter may also be obstructed.

The diagnosis of a ureterocele is made by means of an IVU and micturating cystography. High quality ultrasound may also identify a duplicated kidney. If the function in the affected portion is very poor, details may be seen on the intravenous urogram only after the use of large doses of contrast and delayed films. The position of the remaining calyces of the middle and lower part are characteristically displaced as in an ectopic ureter. As mentioned in the preceding clinical presentation there may be changes in the contralateral kidney as well. The ureterocele may be seen as a negative shadow in the bladder. If the ureterocele is compressible or has ruptured, the cystogram will show reflux.

Treatment depends on a number of factors: in a young child presenting in a very toxic state the diagnosis may be made by ultrasound (Fig. 26.9). The infected, obstructed upper part of the kidney should be drained by percutaneous methods and definitive surgery deferred until the clinical state improves. If the function is poor, it is usually necessary to do a heminephroureterectomy. If the ureterocele is complex, it will usually be necessary to consider reimplantation of the remaining ipsilateral ureter and there may be a lot of reconstruction to do to the bladder wall where the ureterocele lay. If the ureterocele extends below the bladder neck, it may be a formidable undertaking. Single orthotopic ureterocele should be treated only if there is obstruction, with or without infection. Simple endoscopic uncapping is likely to lead to reflux so that primary reimplantation is probably indicated.

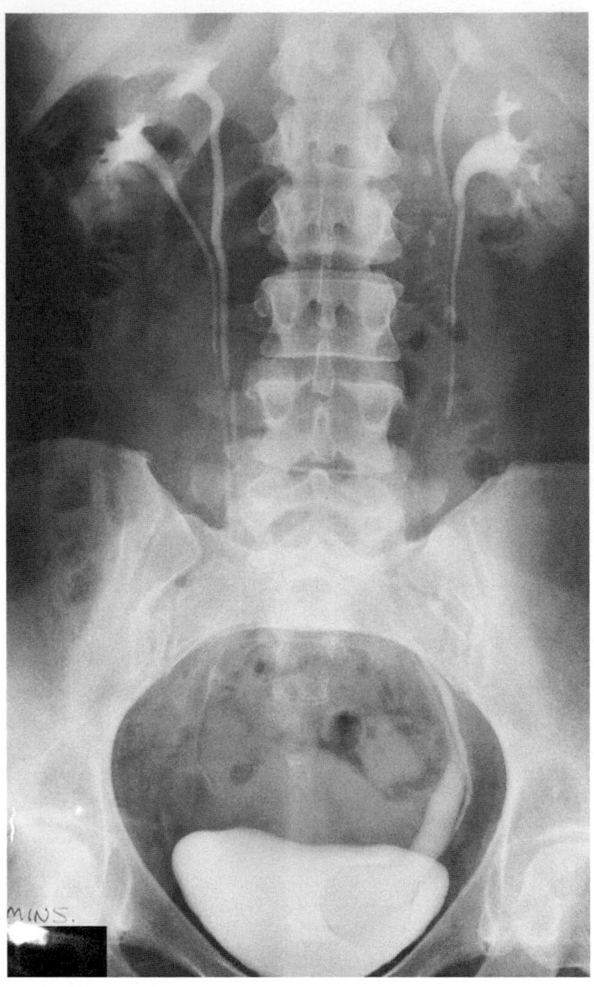

Fig. 26.9 Ureterocele. Note it is the upper ureter that has the ureterocele.

Part Two: Gynaecological aspects

Sheila L B Duncan

GENERAL CONSIDERATIONS

Genital tract anomalies tend to consist of some degree of failure of fusion of the uterus, cervix or vagina, or some disorder of canalization. Associated urinary anomalies can be important in diagnosis as well as management. Despite many variations there are systematic associations. A urinary abnormality is very likely when there is asymmetry and absence or imperfect development of one side of the müllerian system but less likely where there is symmetrical fusion yet failure of canalization, e.g. an obstructed vagina. When there is a single kidney there is a high likelihood of a genital anomaly. Recognition of a single kidney may be made in the fetus or child nowadays and should prompt surveillance at puberty. Abnormalities of the genital and urinary systems may involve multisystem maldevelopment affecting especially the spine or bowel. Estimates of the incidence of various anomalies are poor since this depends on the range and severity of the conditions that are counted and the age group of ascertainment. External or more severe anomalies are noted in the neonate but the child may not survive to be counted at a later age. Around puberty, conditions affecting menstruation may be diagnosed but others, notably uterine malformations, may be diagnosed in pregnancy, during gynaecological investigations or not at all. Only conditions requiring gynaecological care are considered here and these involve fewer than 1% of women. It should, however, be remembered that when anomalies of the genital tract complicate pregnancy the urinary system should be considered.

The gynaecologist tends to be involved after puberty but it is helpful to combine with the paediatric surgeon in the management in infancy of anomalies that affect the genital tract. Study of the original anatomy enhances understanding of the problems at puberty or later, especially where further reconstructive surgery becomes necessary. Such liaison should encourage more thorough investigation of both the genital and urinary systems where an anomaly of one is found. Despite awareness of the numerous associations, it is discouraging to note that in a follow-up study of the treatment of imperforate anus and of associated urinary problems there was very little genital information (Fleming et al 1986). Equally, before operating on any patient known to have a genital tract anomaly it is essential to ascertain the number and position of kidneys and ureters.

OBSTRUCTION

Hydrocolpos

A fluid or mucus collection in the vagina may extend to the uterus and tubes. It may present in the neonate, be diagnosed in the fetus or may even obstruct delivery; the condition is rare but is an important cause of abdominal distension in the neonate. The exact cause may vary. There may be a thin membrane at or just above the level of the hymen, with a bulging mass between the labia. A vaginal collection may be small but may obstruct the urethra and the abdominal swelling may be mainly bladder. In other instances the hydrocolpos may contain urine from a high entry of the urethra into a fully or partially obstructed lower vagina. A high transverse vaginal obstruction where the lower vagina looks normal may confound diagnosis.

Ultrasound is the most useful initial investigation, followed by careful exploration, endoscopy and sometimes instillation of contrast. Correct diagnosis is important to avoid an unnecessary laparotomy or even removal of the uterus and vagina. If the bowel is involved then other considerations arise but the primary management is relief of obstruction. Incision of an obstructing membrane after identification of the urethral meatus may be all that is required. Where the obstruction is higher there may be more difficulty in drainage but a catheter in the bladder and a probe in the rectum may enable sufficient dissection to reach the fluid collection and achieve drainage. Occasionally laparotomy and a 'pull-through' procedure are required. Morbidity and prognosis depend on the presence of associated anomalies. There is a high incidence of urinary or associated bowel anomalies in cases diagnosed in infancy and a good account of the pathogenesis and management of this condition is given by Hahn-Pedersen and colleagues (1984).

Haematocolpos

After the neonatal period, vaginal obstruction is unlikely to present until the pubertal surge of oestrogens promotes, first a mucoid collection and then retained menses. The thickness and level of the obstructing tissue is variable as the canalization of the solid stage of the müllerian system may fail at any distance from the urogenital sinus and a thin or a thick septum, or a long segment of atresia may result. There are many variations of the vagina and hymen causing symptoms but only conditions with obstruction to menses are considered here. A low obstruction presenting at puberty is more likely to be an isolated abnormality. The incidence of haematocolpos is estimated to be about 1 in 4000 teenage girls with the majority being a low (though usually suprahymenal) obstruction. A high obstruction is less common, is usually at the level of the upper and middle third of the vagina and the lower vagina may be patent or absent. Presentation is usually:

- A teenage girl with primary amenorrhoea
- Well developed secondary sexual characters
- Recurrent (but not usually monthly) episodes of lower abdominal pain
- A lower abdominal mass
- Urinary retention.

Diagnosis

Where there is a bulging membrane the diagnosis is obvious. However, at an earlier stage or a higher obstruction the physical signs may be less obvious and awareness of the condition in all those caring for teenage girls is important because the first contact is liable to be made with a doctor who has never previously encountered the condition. Delay may be harmful.

The diagnosis is even more important when the obstruction is higher and is especially difficult when there is a normal lower vagina (Fig. 26.10). In a high obstruction:

- There may be less abdominal distension and more pain because of retrograde menstruation or haematosalpinx
- Ultrasound examination is usually diagnostic (Fig. 26.11). This should be offered early in any girl with primary amenorrhoea and new lower abdominal pain or urinary symptoms.

Obvious differential diagnoses include appendicitis, urinary tract infection, pregnancy and genital tract infection. A familial element may exist in some cases.

Management

A low obstruction requires an adequate cruciate incision of the obstructing membrane to permit free drainage. Even this apparently simple procedure requires care to avoid stenosis or unnecessary fibrosis (Duncan 1996). Laparoscopy after one or more menstrual flows will diagnose or exclude endometriosis or other abnormality of the upper vaginal tract. The urinary tract anatomy should be clarified. Vaginal atresia is much more difficult. As in the neonate, it is sometimes possible to reach the collection from the perineum with a catheter in the bladder and a probe in the rectum. The vaginal epithelium should be reflected laterally and conserved. Dissection to reach the collection may be more difficult than it appears, and if access is not readily obtained it may be better to proceed to laparotomy and define the upper vagina. Mobilization is easier in the distended vagina and should be done before colpotomy. Whether this is done from below or above, the aim is to free the upper distended vaginal edges enough to bring down to meet the edges of the original vaginal incision. Where there has been a substantial gap this is difficult, and the contraction of the upper vagina after drainage is remarkable. Haematosalpinges and/or endometriosis require identification.

There are various procedures to try to maintain long-term patency as well as immediate drainage (Edmonds 1994). Free drainage is essential, even if menstruation is suppressed and some form of hollow vaginal mould is required. A mould that impinges on the perineum may not be tolerated. An inflatable (e.g. endotracheal) tube with the inflated portion at the level of the stenosed area may be useful and the central tube can be cut to an appropriate length with the lumen providing drainage. The inflatable collar can be deflated for removal. Some girls can insert an appropriate vaginal mould at night. Restenosis is liable to occur until regular sexual activity is established. Where there is no lower vagina the management is even more difficult. Labial and perineal skin can be used to form a lower vagina but much ingenuity may be required to maintain patency.

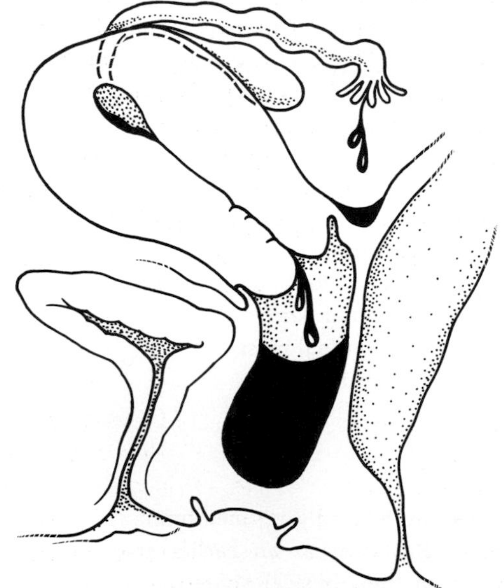

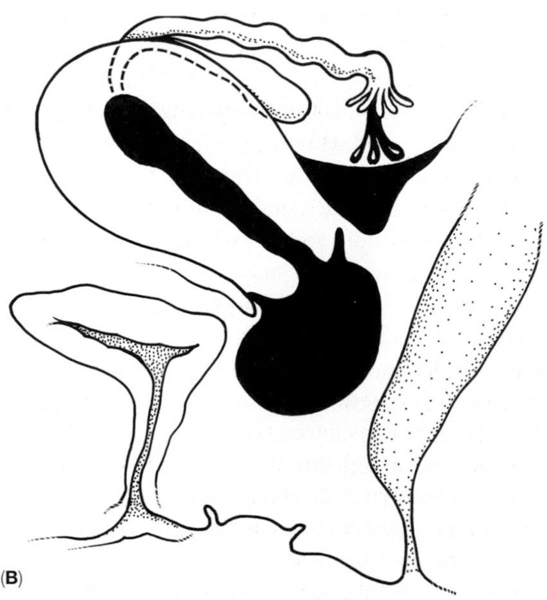

Fig. 26.10 Diagram of haematocolpos due to (**A**) low (**B**) high obstruction. Note haematometra and greater tendency to backflow in (**B**).

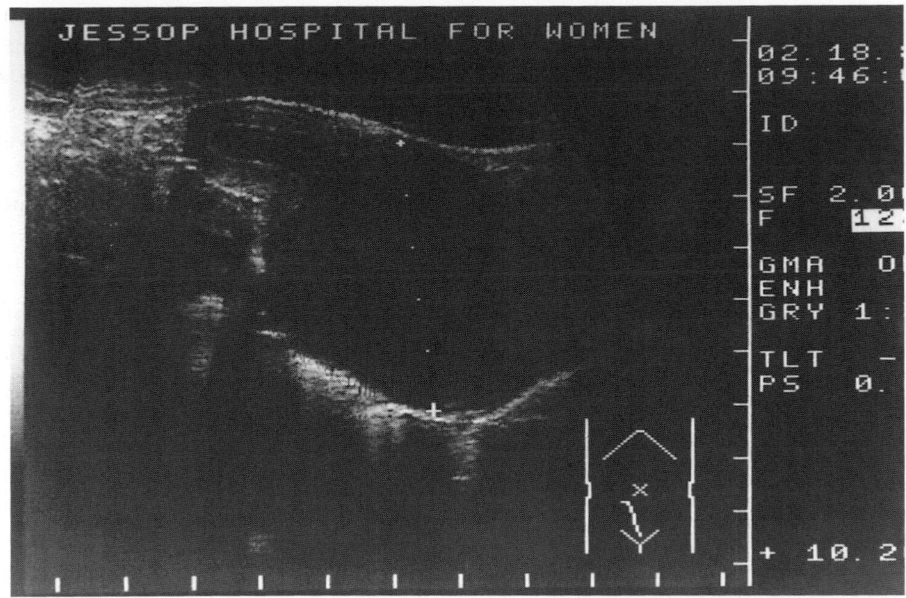

Fig. 26.11 Scan of haematocolpos due to atresia of mid vagina. There is a small haematometra (left of picture).

Unilateral haematocolpos

When only part of the genital tract is obstructed, diagnosis is difficult because of the concomitant menstruation and is usually made later than in complete haematocolpos. Unilateral haematocolpos in a uterus didelphys with an occluded hemivagina and absence of the ipsilateral kidney is a well-recognized entity (Stassart et al 1992; Duncan 1997). Awareness of the condition enables recognition when the clinical features fit:

- The condition has been reported more often with the obstruction on the right side and the features are thus easily confused with appendicitis.
- The occluded hemivagina varies in size but has less capacity than a single vagina and retrograde tubal spill, with or without haematosalpinx is especially likely.
- Presentation is usually recurrent episodes of unilateral pain in a teenage girl, 1 or 2 years after menarche.
- Abdominal mass or tenderness are unusual.
- There may be a cystic swelling below the uterus and behind the bladder, identified either rectally or vaginally, but a small cystic collection high in the vaginal fornix may easily be missed.
- Ultrasound reveals a fluid collection unilaterally behind the bladder and may reveal a distended uterine horn or tube. Identification of two uterine horns may be difficult.
- The kidney on the side of the cystic swelling is missing.

Mistaken suspicion of an appendicitis or an ovarian cyst may lead to laparotomy. Retrograde bleeding, a distended tube or hemiuterus may be identified. Even then, differentiation from an occluded rudimentary horn may be difficult.

The appropriate management is incision of the occluded vagina from below with wide excision of the septum which is often very thick (Fig. 26.12). Ultrasound after drainage may clarify the anatomy. There is usually a uterus didelphys, each half with its own cervix but a connection between the cavities may exist. It is wise to look again after one or two periods to ensure optimum excision of the septum and accessibility of the cervix on the originally occluded side. If this is not done the initial opening may close over. It may be helpful to carry out laparoscopy to document the exact shape of the uterus and to recognize haematosalpinx or endometriosis. Occasionally a poorly functioning rudimentary horn may require removal. Any surgery in such cases should be with awareness of the exact location of the single kidney.

Absence of the cervix

Congenital absence of the cervix is rare and serious, since retrograde spill or haematosalpinx occurs early. The body of the uterus may be normal or didelphic. The lower lined end of the uterus may be connected to the vagina by a fibrous cord but there is no structure of a cervix and no upper vagina. There may be no lower vagina or a small pouch. Presentation is with

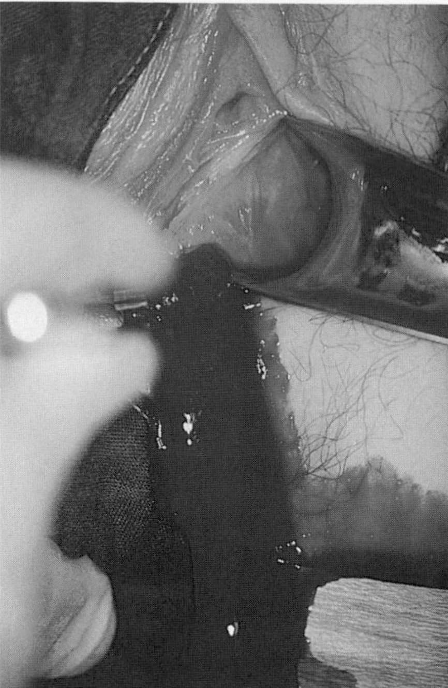

Fig. 26.12 Drainage of unilateral haematocolpos. The urethra is visible anteriorly and the speculum is in the left, normal hemivagina.

recurrent abdominal pain with amenorrhoea in a teenage girl soon after the expected menarche. There may be other malformations including the renal tract. Ultrasound, MR imaging or laparoscopy may be necessary to clarify the precise diagnosis. Functioning endometrium in a rudimentary horn has to be differentiated. Attempts to create a channel around a stent, as an alternative to hysterectomy, has sometimes been successful, although obstruction to outflow and adnexal infection constitute a substantial risk. There has been an evolution in possible techniques for this condition (Edmonds 1993) and successful pregnancy following reconstructive surgery has been reported. Where there is only a rudimentary horn or bilateral rudimentary horns with functioning endometrial tissue, the management is usually surgical removal, although attempts are being made at reconstruction.

MÜLLERIAN AGENESIS

Absence of all or most of the genital tract occurs in several types of congenital anomaly including some forms of male pseudohermaphrodism. The more common form is müllerian agenesis which has several features:

- Presents in teens with primary amenorrhoea and developed sex characteristics
- Absence of the vagina and either complete absence of the uterus, or small fallopian tubes with a remnant of müllerian tissue often lateral in the pelvis
- Normal ovarian function but ovaries unusually high and lateral
- The incidence is estimated to be about 1 in 10 000 female births but this is probably an underestimate as ascertainment may be very late.

The condition is second only to gonadal failure as a cause of amenorrhoea in a girl with well developed secondary sex characteristics. The incidence of urethral or renal anomalies varies from about 15% in the otherwise uncomplicated case to over 80% in a girl with bowel and skeletal anomalies (Duncan et al 1979). The ureterorenal abnormalities include agenesis of one kidney or ectopia, fusion abnormalities, horseshoe kidney, duplication of ureters and ureteroceles.

Myometrial remnants are most likely to be found when there is normal bilateral renal development. If there is no kidney, there is usually no uterine remnant on the ipsilateral side (Smith 1983). The aetiology of the condition is not clear and is probably not single. Apparent familial clustering may represent biased reporting. A genetic element is suspected and may be better elucidated in future when girls with this condition have genetic offspring by surrogacy.

Diagnosis

Absence of the vagina in the prepubertal girl can be confused with labial adhesions and differentiation is obviously vital. Adherent labia obscure the hymen and urethral meatus and present a very characteristic appearance (Fig. 26.13). In vaginal agenesis, the urethral meatus is visible with normal formation of separate labia. Inspection of the vulva may be misleading because of a small vaginal pouch from the original urogenital sinus or from attempts at coitus. There may even be a clear hymenal opening. Passage of a lubricated sound (e.g. about Hagar size 6) will identify the length of the vagina and is much more considerate than digital examination. Ultrasound examination is important but requires care in interpretation since:

- A vestigial uterus may be apparent on ultrasound but be uncanalized
- Normal ovaries may be missed because of unduly lateral position
- Ultrasound appearances are more difficult to interpret without a vagina.

If there are abdominal symptoms or a visible structure on ultrasound, it is important to establish whether

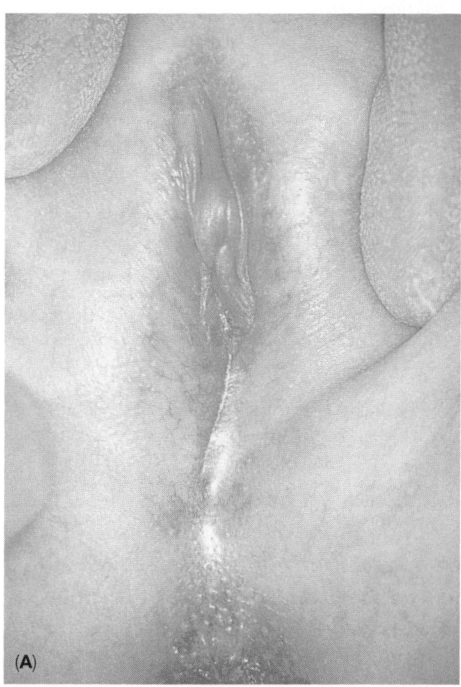

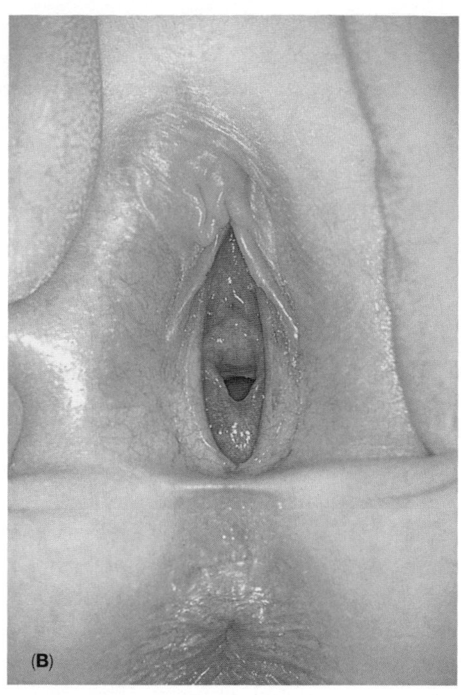

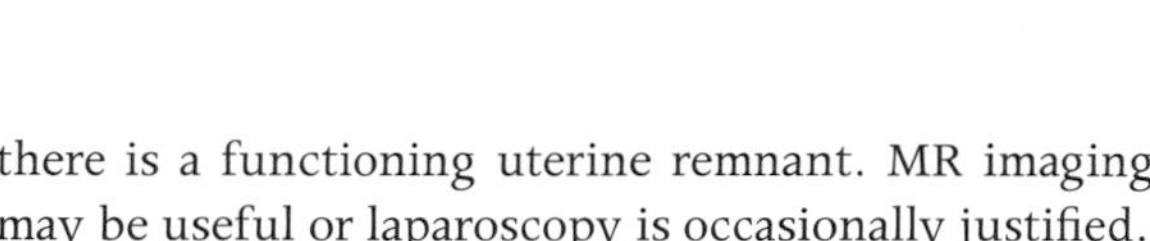

Fig. 26.13 Labial adhesions (**A**) before and (**B**) after separation.

there is a functioning uterine remnant. MR imaging may be useful or laparoscopy is occasionally justified.

Management

This includes sensitive handling of the psychological aspects. It is essential to identify any abnormality of the urinary system before considering any surgery, even laparoscopy. Abnormalities of the urinary system may complicate management but even a pelvic kidney need not preclude the formation of a functioning vagina. Provided there is no uterine function it is usually best to await interest in sexual activity before attending to the vagina but this varies as many teenage girls are eager to achieve some sort of normalization of their vagina soon after they are aware of their condition.

There are many techniques for trying to achieve a vagina for coitus. The initial vaginal 'pit' may range from a very hypoplastic vulva to a small existing lower vagina. In most instances the initial treatment should be conservative and involves dilatation techniques. The degree of vaginal distension in a well motivated patient with good tissues can be remarkable. Even with rigid or hypoplastic tissues dilatation is a useful adjunct, before and after any necessary surgery. There have been many modifications of the Frank dilatation technique over the last half century and a very effective regimen was described by a bicycle seat modification (Ingram 1981). Where this is not successful there are many possible surgical techniques, mainly based on dissection of an appropriate space and a skin or amnion inlay (for description and references see Edmonds 1994). In younger children where a conduit is necessary, or where there are other anomalies requiring correction, a range of other techniques including sigmoid, peritoneal or bladder grafts are possible (for references see Martinez-Mora et al 1992). Patience, ingenuity, and motivation are required and achievement of a functional vagina is vastly accelerated by a heterosexual relationship. The psychological boost when coitus is achieved is dramatic.

DEFECTIVE LOWER UROGENITAL DEVELOPMENT

Persistent cloaca

Persistence of a single perineal opening for the urinary, genital and bowel systems results in complex problems. The condition arises from failure of the urorectal fold to separate the rectum from the urovaginal canal. There is a wide range of anatomical possibilities with various levels and sites of union. These range from a low convergence of the three systems with the basic structure of each present, to a high confluence with absence of the urethra, vagina and rectum. There may be duplication of the vagina with or without some uterine abnormality. There are often other abnormalities. The condition is rare and a collected series of 35 cases provides useful generalizations and evidence of good functional results with careful planning (Hendren 1982). Obstruction is a major problem and the genital aspect must be considered in the childhood management to ensure good vaginal drainage. Otherwise, extensive endometriosis and/or intraperitoneal adhesions can occur. The initial priority is to achieve adequate drainage of all three systems with urinary and bowel continence and a functioning vagina. The options and problems are well covered in paediatric surgical texts (Colodny 1985). The anus usually requires resiting more posteriorly and perineal skin flaps may be used to create a vaginal opening. Most of the urogenital sinus may be required to construct a urethra. Careful planning is required and fewer comprehensive procedures are recommended (Hendren 1982) to avoid distortion and scarring from repeated surgery. The necessity to ensure function of the urinary and bowel systems at an early age may eclipse provision of an adequate vagina. The planning for this should be built in from the start but revision after pubertal development may be required.

EXSTROPHY

Bladder

Unlike some of the other congenital anomalies, this condition is not an arrest of normal development. There is no stage of normal embryogenesis which resembles it. Whatever the precise cause, the mechanism is failure of mesodermal invasion of the cloacal membrane. There is a range of severity:

- A single or horseshoe kidney, although there may be no upper renal abnormality
- The bladder surface area varies
- Absence of the anterior pelvic girdle, and of the lower abdominal wall
- Genital tract may be unfused or incompletely so, but is usually functional
- Vaginal stenosis or atresia.

Urological problems include infection, vesicourethral reflux or outflow obstruction. The exstrophic bladder is abnormal and subject to squamous metaplasia and adenocarcinoma. The musculature of the pelvic floor is disorganized because of the more lateral attachment to the pubis.

The incidence of bladder exstrophy is estimated to be between 1 in 10 000 and 1 in 50 000 newborns, more in boys than girls and is therefore about 1 in 100 000 female births. Care may involve many professionals over a long period and should be concentrated in a major centre. There are many surgical options (see Johnston 1982) to effect closure of the bladder and repair of the anterior defect with the aim of achieving an acceptable cosmetic effect and a functioning urinary bladder neck, although diversion of the urinary system into an ileal bladder may be necessary. The gynaecologist is apt to be involved where there is vaginal stenosis or a genital abnormality affecting drainage. Prolapse of the genital tract, especially the anterior vagina, is common due to poor pelvic musculature. Management of pregnancy depends on the measures taken to achieve urinary continence. There may be less resistance of the genital tract to delivery but this should not be allowed to damage a good urinary repair.

Epispadias

This represents the milder end of the exstrophy spectrum. The term is used when there is a ventral defect in the urethra and bladder neck. Characteristically, in the female there is:

- Separation of the pubic bones
- A bifid clitoris
- Anterior separation of the labia majora and minora
- A wide, open and incompetent bladder neck
- A short, patulous urethra.

The clinical problem arises when there is incontinence because of the bladder neck defect and this may be severe. There may be vesicoureteral reflux and subsequent hydronephrosis. As an isolated defect the condition is even less common than bladder exstrophy and is commoner in males than females by a ratio of 3:1 (Saltzman et al 1985), but this may be an underestimate because only severe cases are included. Collected series which include female cases give a useful insight (Kramer & Kelalis 1982; Saltzman et al 1985). There has been evolution of the techniques for repair, best effected between the ages of 3 and 5, the aim being to achieve a competent bladder neck and urethra, often using a mucosal strip of bladder. The increased bladder capacity, and improved bone structure and musculature around the time of puberty may help continence. In a few severe cases persistent reflux and hydronephrosis may necessitate diversion

(Saltzman et al 1985). There are no particular obstetric difficulties other than the need to avoid disturbing the previous surgery. Encouragingly, in Saltzman's series no siblings had the condition and no sufferer had a child with it.

Cloacal exstrophy (vesicointestinal fissure)

This is the most severe variant of this defect. There is, usually, in girls:

- Omphalocele
- Exstrophy of ununited bladder segments
- A central bowel field between the bladder segments
- Imperforate anus
- Foreshortened hindgut
- Orthopaedic deformities
- An unfused genital tract with bifid clitoris.

The surgical challenge in the neonate is formidable (Johnston 1982) but survival beyond puberty is now occurring. The intrinsic genital problems are compounded by the reconstructive surgery and are individual by puberty. Even in the neonate the openings of the duplex vagina may be sagittal, widely separated or obstructed. When menstruation occurs, obstruction may require relief. It may be possible to unite the vaginas and fashion an acceptable introitus or it may be necessary to remove one side. Close liaison between paediatric surgeon and gynaecologist is required, preferably from an early stage, and there is not yet adequate follow-up into adult life and evaluation of possible pregnancy.

ABNORMAL FUSION AND VIRILIZATION

Persistent urogenital sinus

This term is used when there is a common channel for the lower vagina and urethra. It is a normal stage of development in the female fetus. Since a common genitourinary channel is the basic arrangement in the mature male infant, some degree of persistent urogenital sinus is an inevitable result of masculinization of a female fetus. It is not a single entity and masculinization is not an essential feature, since failure of caudal movement and development of the lower vagina also results in a common channel. A normal rectum differentiates the condition from a cloacal defect, although many of the problems are similar. It is more common than a cloacal defect since the condition includes cases of intersex in infants brought up as females and girls with adrenogenital syndrome.

Diagnosis of the more severe degrees is made in infancy and initial, often definitive, surgery may be carried out then. The topic has suffered relative neglect in the gynaecological literature but is relevant to the gynaecologist because:

- In some instances a diagnosis may not be made until puberty
- The oestrogen effects of puberty may have been awaited before surgery
- Revision surgery to achieve coitus may be necessary.

The disorder has a wide spectrum and there may or may not have been masculinizing influences. The anatomy may range from incomplete male development with a phallus to female anatomy with deficiency of vaginal tissue. Subdivision into identifiable anatomical groups, based on clinical experience has been proposed (Williams & Bloomberg 1976). Grouping based on the level of confluence of the systems, the presence of virilized features, stenosis or obstruction can be expressed in gynaecological terms (Fig. 26.14).

Hypospadias

This term is used when the urethral meatus is abnormally proximal. Wide variation normally means that minor degrees do not warrant diagnosis. The incidence therefore is uncertain but the condition is certainly commoner than anterior defects. There may be associated vaginal or uterine anomalies.

Stenosis of the meatus in the neonate may cause obstruction and require dilatation. After infancy, a clinically important degree of hypospadias is associated with sphincter deficiency and incontinence. The basic principle of repair is a U-shaped urethroplasty, using vaginal tissue. The urethra must be long enough to prevent urine collecting in the vagina and inward rotation of a labial flap may be required (Williams & Bloomberg 1976).

Vaginoplasty

Where the problem with a urogenital sinus is undue narrowing of the introitus, the basic surgical aim is reduction of the clitoris if required, separation and, if necessary, reduction of the labioscrotal folds and formation of a vagina adequate to allow menstruation and for coitus. The timing of surgical procedures will depend on the degree of fusion and the appearance. In the intersex condition at birth, diagnosis, gender assignment and medical control of adrenogenital

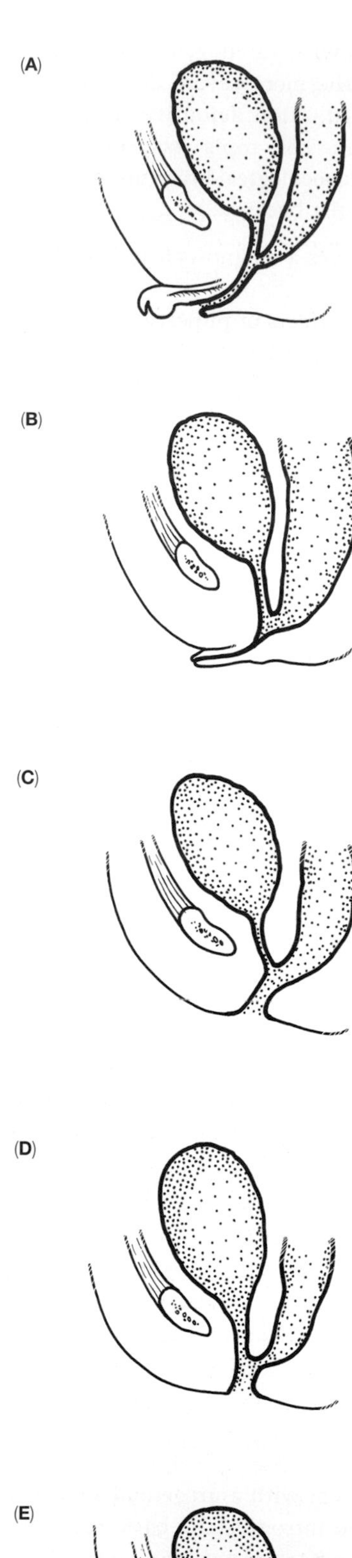

Fig. 26.14 Diagram of the anatomy of the urogenital sinus. (**A**) Virilization of female fetus as occurs in variable degree in adrenogenital syndrome and intersex states. (**B**) Vulvar obstruction without virilization – may present in infancy with hydrocolpos. (**C**) High opening of urethral meatus – female hypospadias. (**D**) Lower vaginal atresia with a wide urethra – often with deficiency of the bladder neck. (**E**) Urovaginal confluence with absence of bladder neck – child is incontinent. Surgery must take account of adequacy of vagina. After Williams & Bloomberg (1976), with permission.

syndrome are priorities. Diagnostic assessment will usually include identification of the level of entry of the vagina into the urethra or urogenital sinus by contrast techniques and/or endoscopy.

In infancy the first necessity is to ensure adequate urethral drainage and reduce an enlarged clitoris to enable acceptance of the child in the female role. If the vaginal entry is very low a flap vaginoplasty may be adequate (for references see Perlmutter & Reitelman 1992). Where fusion is more severe and the insertion of the vagina high the alternatives are a 'pull-through' procedure in childhood or deferment of reconstructive surgery until after puberty. There may be absence of the uterus or presence of a hemiuterus. In adrenogenital syndrome the uterus and cervix are usually normal and there is not usually any obstruction to menstrual flow, although amenorrhoea may occur despite good replacement treatment. Surgical considerations are only one aspect of the complex management of girls with intersex or adrenogenital conditions.

The gynaecologist, therefore, is liable to be faced with vaginal reconstruction around or after puberty associated with:

- Virilization which occurs or is first diagnosed around puberty
- High entry of the vagina into the urogenital sinus
- Previous surgery requiring revision of the introitus and vagina.

Before planning vaginoplasty it is essential to define the precise level of the vaginal insertion and the calibre and length of the vagina. This can be done, usually under anaesthesia, by insertion of a Foley catheter into the bladder and instillation of contrast medium by a simple catheter inserted posteriorly. Where the upper vagina is of normal calibre there is a characteristic lozenge-shaped outline (Fig. 26.15). Where the vaginal opening is very narrow and close to or above the external sphincter mechanism it may be necessary to use endoscopy to insert a catheter into the high narrow junction (Fig. 26.16).

Where the insertion is low with an adequate upper

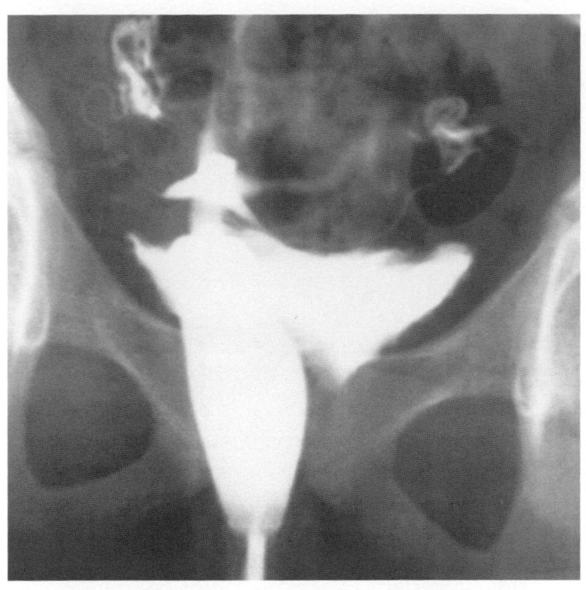

Fig. 26.15 Sinogram of urogenital sinus in adrenogenital syndrome. Contrast in vagina has outlined the uterus and tubes.

(A)

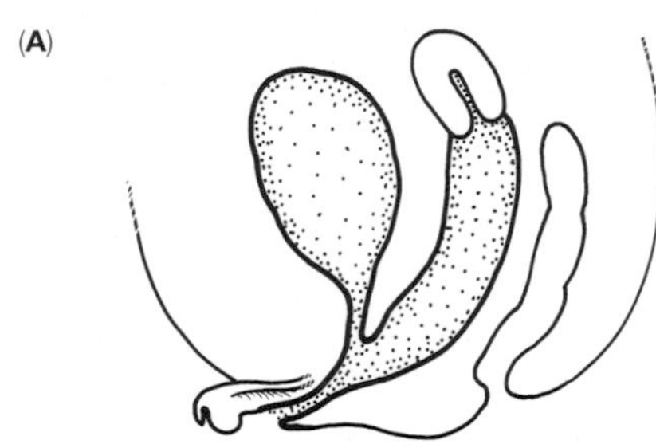

(B)

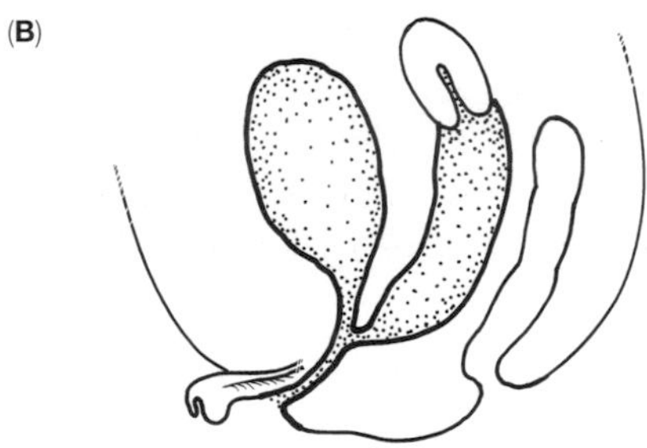

Fig. 26.16 Diagram of (**A**) low and (**B**) high entry of vagina in adrenogenital syndrome.

vagina, reconstruction using a flap of perineal skin, based posteriorly, can be used to provide skin cover for the otherwise too short posterior vaginal wall (Fig. 26.17). Bulky labioscrotal folds are an advantage and can be used posterolaterally to complete the skin cover. This technique has been refined and developed over the last 30 years (Fortunoff et al 1964; Edmonds 1994). Where access to the upper vagina is very long and narrow, reconstruction is much more difficult. The main technique is a 'pull-through' procedure into a new perineal orifice or a vaginal reconstruction procedure as for haematocolpos with vaginal atresia. A good account of these techniques is provided by Donahoe and Hendren (1984) and summarized by Perlmutter and Reitelman (1992). Further recent techniques include very elegant procedures to feminize the vagina and perineum in infancy, using redundant clitoral tissue (Passerini-Glazel 1994). This gives a pleasing result in the child and the consequences in terms of differential growth through childhood and puberty are awaited with interest.

Where there has been an androgen stimulus and scrotal fusion, the tissues are very sturdy and comparatively unyielding, and much difficulty may be encountered in maintaining patency at the anastomosis and adequacy for coitus. Results have been disappointing with respect to later sexual activity, especially in women with salt-losing congenital adrenal hyperplasia. This may owe as much to a disturbed body image and indifference to sexuality as to the vaginal anatomy (Kuhnle et al 1995). The gynaecologist is working half a generation behind the neonatal surgeon and improved techniques in the recent past may yield better results in the foreseeable future.

Clitoral reduction

Anomalies with a masculinizing component may lead to a need for removal or reduction of an enlarged clitoris. Infancy treatments are generally carried out by the paediatric surgeon. However, an indication may arise at or after puberty, even when the reason has been congenital:

- A clitoris only slightly enlarged in infancy (e.g. in congenital adrenal hyperplasia) may grow considerably around the time of puberty.
- In conditions such as partial androgen insensitivity or other forms of male pseudohermaphrodism, the pubertal surge of testicular activity may cause clitoral enlargement.
- The puberty oestrogens may provoke embarrassing enlargement in a clitoris which was slightly enlarged *in utero* (e.g. after ingestion of maternal androgens), but subsequently regressed in childhood.

Reduction of an enlarged clitoris may be appropriately carried out at the time of another procedure such as vaginal enlargement or removal of inappropriate (e.g.

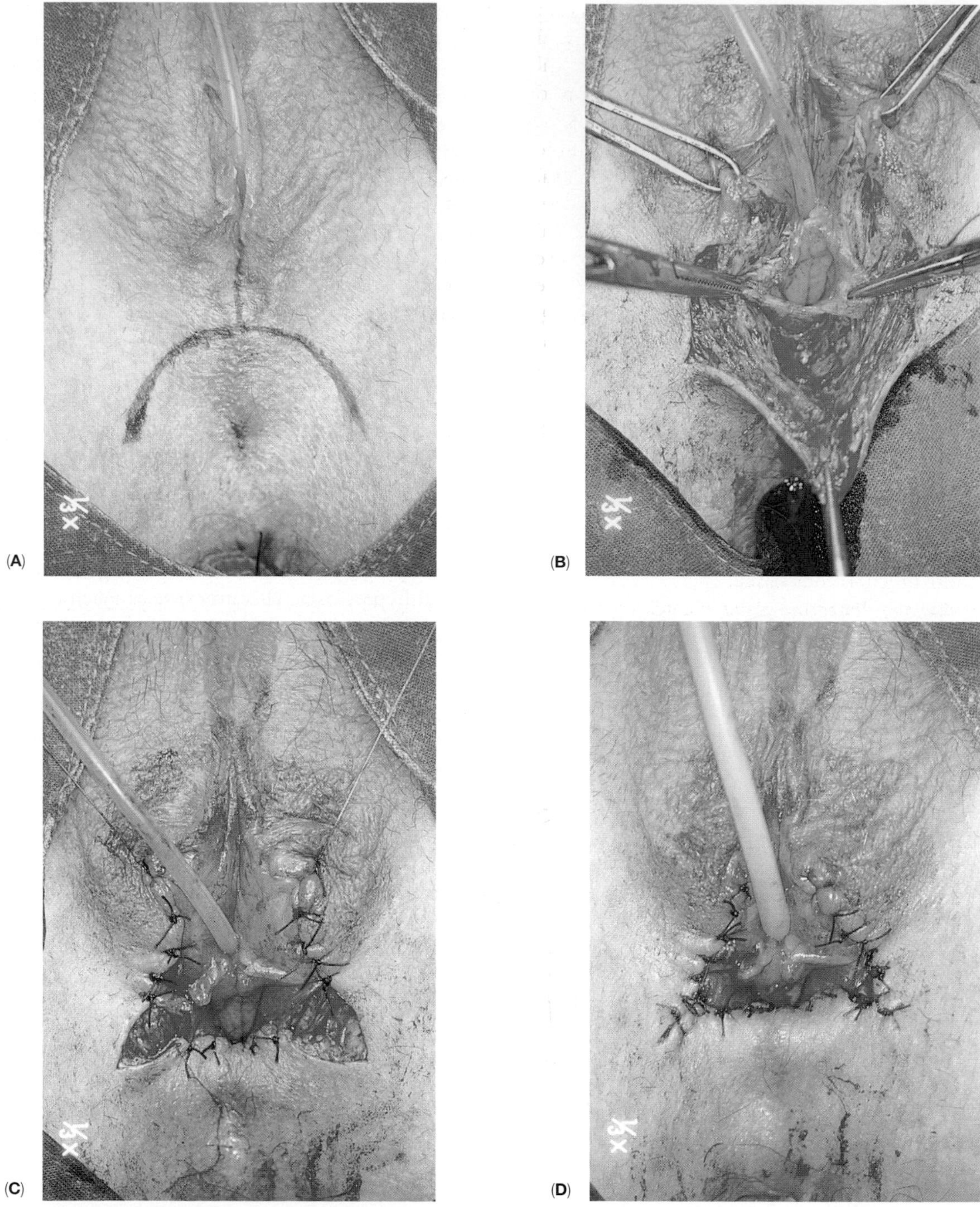

Fig. 26.17 (**A**) Flap vaginoplasty – outline of skin incisions. (**B**) Exposed tissues after raising posterior perineal flap and dividing perineal muscles and lower vagina. (**C**) Apex of posterior perineal incision has been sutured to opened posterior vagina. (**D**) Lateral incisions closed.

XY) gonads and it may be appropriate for the urogynaecologist to perform clitoral reduction. There are several possible techniques. Those involved in complete, simultaneous reconstruction (Hinman 1989; Perlmutter & Reitelman 1992) are less relevent to the gynaecologist faced with only a relative degree of enlargement or a previously treated girl. Essentially, clitoral reduction involves a procedure to remove, recess, reduce or resect the shaft.

Clitoridectomy This procedure is comparatively easy and definitive but is unnecessarily radical.

Clitoral recession This alternative to amputation (Lattimer 1961) involves dissection of the clitoral shaft and relocation of the glans closer to the urethral meatus. A modification, described by Randolph and Hung (1970) reduces the clitoris and foreskin but retains the anatomical position and essential pubic contours. It is not a popular method in the neonatal period (Spence & Allen 1973) because of residual size, subsequent unpredictable growth and later painful enlargement. It can be satisfactory, however, in the adolescent girl where the shaft is not too large, the growth completed and especially in situations (e.g. partial androgen insensitivity or testicular biosynthetic defects) where the androgenic stimulus has been or is going to be removed.

Essentials of the technique are as follows (Fig. 26.18):

- An incision in the coronal sulcus is extended laterally to join an elliptical incision over the mons, removing some of the bulky, redundant skin and subcutaneous tissue.
- Following the dissection plane of Buck's fascia, most of the shaft and the suspensory ligament are exposed.
- The ligament is divided, thus freeing the clitoris beneath the pubic angle.
- Provided the shaft is not too long (in which event resection should be used), the fascia of the shaft is sutured to the periosteum of the lower border of the pubis.
- As these sutures are tied, the clitoral shaft is 'recessed' beneath the pubis.
- The mons veneris is reconstructed to cover the recessed clitoris and some lateral skin from the prepuce brought posteriorly to form or augment the labia minora.

Clitoral resection An alternative technique involves resection of the mid-shaft with suture of the glans to the proximal shaft. There are various modifications of the technique originally proposed by Spence and Allen (1973). The procedure is more invasive than recession but is superior where the shaft is long or the glans is large. Subsequent modification (Kogan et al 1983) emphasizes the superiority of a ventral approach, with dissection and intact preservation of the neurovascular supply. Reduction of the shaft and glans can be individual. This technique has mainly

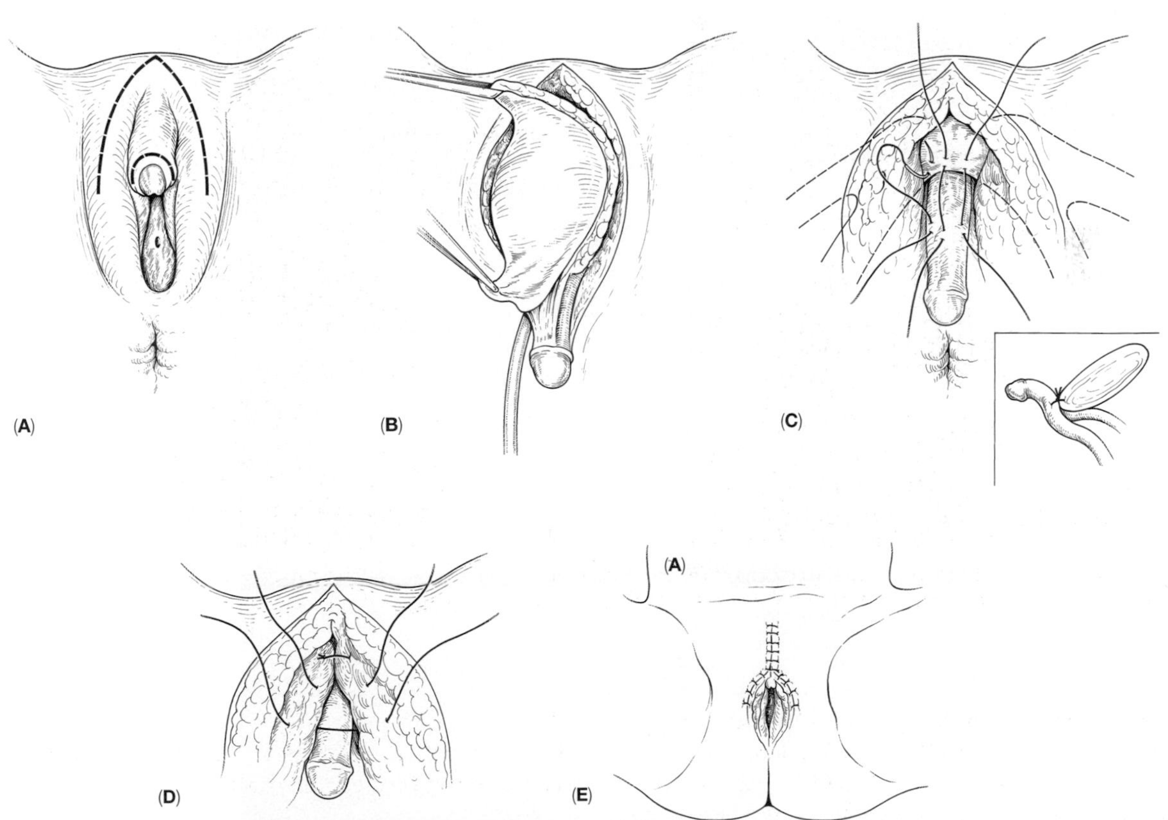

Fig. 26.18 Clitoral recession: **(A)** incision in coronal sulcus and over symphysics; **(B)** exposure of suspensory ligament before division; **(C)** suturing of shaft to under surface of pubis; **(D)** use of mons fat to cover recessed shaft; **(E)** appearance of recessed clitoris.

been developed and described in relation to early childhood but is also satisfactory in the adolescent or adult.

ASSOCIATED URINARY TRACT ANOMALIES

Pelvic kidney

A pelvic kidney may or may not be the only kidney. Its importance to the gynaecologist lies in its capacity for diagnostic confusion and vulnerability to surgical damage (e.g. laparoscopy). When there is a single pelvic kidney, a genital anomaly is likely and should be sought. There is a well recognized association with vaginal agenesis and with other, notably vertebral, anomalies. A specific combination of müllerian duct aplasia, renal aplasia and cervicothoracic somite syplasia – the MURCS association – has been described (Duncan et al 1979). Where there is known to be a pelvic kidney it is essential to define the anatomy and precise direction of the ureter before any surgery to the genital tract (Fig. 26.19).

Ectopic ureter

An ectopic ureter may be the sole drainage from a kidney or part of a duplex system. It may be unilateral or bilateral and may open outside the urinary tract. Its importance to the gynaecologist occurs when it opens onto the genital tract, although a urethral opening may also cause diagnostic confusion. The commonest single site of opening into the genital tract is the vestibule; the vagina is next commonest and opening into the uterus or cervix occurs rarely (Gray & Skanalakis 1972). An opening into the uterus or cervix is very likely to be associated with an abnormality of the genital tract. The symptoms depend on the site of entry and functional activity of the relevant kidney or portion of kidney. There may be ureteral obstruction and the presentation may be one of continuous or intermittent incontinence yet with normal voiding. Diagnosis depends on careful urological investigation. Management depends on the functional capacity of the rest of the urinary system and especially on whether the ectopic ureter is the sole outlet for that kidney or is part of a duplex system. When diagnosed beyond childhood, the ectopic ureter is more likely to be part of a duplex system and the ectopic ureter gen-

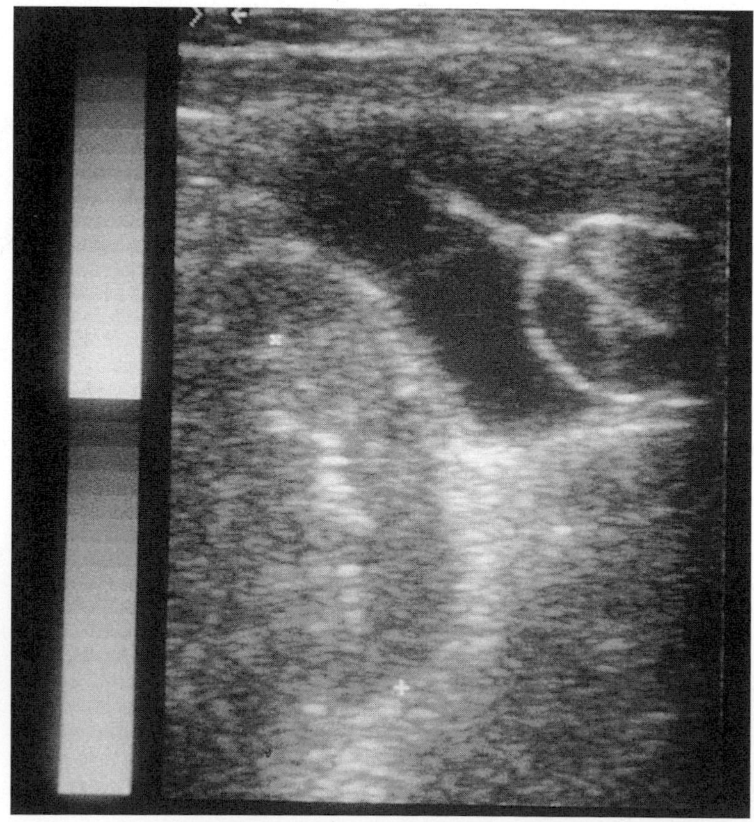

Fig. 26.19 Pelvic kidney (single) lying close to bladder (Foley catheter *in situ*). Posterior to bladder, on right of picture, upper outline of a mould for construction of a neovagina is seen.

erally drains the upper renal segment. The function of the relevant kidney portion will determine whether reimplantation into the bladder or removal of the kidney segment and ureter is best.

Ectopic ureterocele

A cystic dilatation of the distal portion of an ectopic ureter may prolapse into the bladder, urethra or both. It may occur at any age but is especially seen in children and in older women. The main problem for the gynaecologist lies in diagnosis when there is protrusion into or beyond the urethra. It tends to bulge and obstruct the meatus and its prolapse may be intermittent and confusing. Diagnosis depends on identification of the relationship to the meatus and recognition of the mucosal lining. It must be differentiated from:

- Imperforate hymen or rhabdomyosarcoma, in the child
- Urethral prolapse
- Uterovaginal prolapse
- Paraurethral cyst
- Warts
- Urethral or vaginal carcinoma, in the older woman.

A filling defect in the bladder on excretory urography is an important diagnostic sign, especially in the child where it may be from a single kidney and urinary symptoms tend to arise before prolapse. Beyond childhood, the prolapsing ureterocele is likely to be from part of a duplex system. Management will depend on age, kidney function and other abnormality and may involve excision of the upper renal segment and involved ureter, although conservative measures using transurethral incision and cautery may be used, especially where there is a single ureter. Ureteric reflux with conservative measures is common (Caldamone et al 1984).

CONCLUSION

This overview has necessarily been selective. Photographs of unusual conditions can be found in larger textbooks or in early descriptions of a condition. For operative procedures recent reviews provide an update of techniques but much may be learned from the original descriptions of procedures where relevant embryological, anatomical and surgical details are given.

ACKNOWLEDGEMENT

I should like to acknowledge the help of Mr Patrick Elliot, Medical Artist, Royal Hallamshire Hospital, Sheffield, with the line drawings.

REFERENCES

Caldamone A A, Snyder H M C, Duckett J W 1984 Ureteroceles in children: Follow up of management with upper tract approach. Journal of Urology 131: 1130–1132

Colodny A H 1985 Disorders of the female genitalia. In: Kelalis P P, King R L, Belman A B (eds) Clinical Pediatric Urology, 2nd edn. Saunders, Philadelphia, pp 888–903

Donahoe P K, Hendren W H 1984 Perineal reconstruction in ambiguous genitalia infants raised as females. Annals of Surgery 200: 363–371

Duncan P A, Shapiro L R, Stangel J J, Klein R M, Addonizio J C 1979 The MURCS association: Mullerian duct aplasia, renal aplasia and cervicothoracic somite dysplasia. Journal of Paediatrics 95: 399–402

Duncan S L B 1996 Treatment of imperforate hymen should be appropriate. Current Obstetrics and Gynaecology 6: 165–167

Duncan S L B 1997 Embryology of the female genital tract: its genetic defects and congenital anomalies. In: Shaw R, Soutter P, Stanton S (eds) Gynaecology, 2nd edn. Churchill Livingstone, Edinburgh, pp 3–22

Edmonds D K 1993 Surgical management of congenital abnormalities. In: Studd J, Jardine Brown C (eds) The Yearbook of the Royal College of Obstetricians and Gynaecologists, RCOG Press, London, pp 43–53

Edmonds D K 1994 Sexual developmental anomalies and their reconstruction: upper and lower tracts. In: Sanfillipo J S, Muram D, Lee P A, Dewhurst J (eds) Pediatric and Adolescent Gynaecology. Saunders, Philadelphia, pp 535–566

Fleming S E, Hall R, Gysler M, McLorie G A 1986 Imperforate anus in females: Frequency of genital tract involvement, incidence of associated anomalies and functional outcome. Journal of Paediatric Surgery 21: 146–150

Fortunoff S, Lattimer J K, Edson M 1964 Vaginoplasty technique for female pseudohermaphrodites. Surgery, Gynaecology and Obstetrics 118: 545–548

Gray S W, Skandalakis J E 1972 The female reproductive tract. In: Gray S W, Skandalakis J E Embryology for Surgeons. Saunders, Philadelphia

Hahn-Pedersen J, Kvist N, Nielson O H 1984 Hydrometrocolpos: Current views on pathogenesis and management. American Journal of Obstetrics and Gynaecology 132: 537–540

Hendren W H 1982 Further experience in reconstructive surgery for cloacal anomalies. Journal of Paediatric Surgery 17: 695–717

Hinman F 1989 Atlas of Urological Surgery. Saunders, Philadelphia, pp 93–100

Ingram J M 1981 The bicycle seat stool in the treatment of

vaginal agenesis and stenosis: a preliminary report. American Journal of Obstetrics and Gynaecology 140: 867–871

Johnston J H 1982 Extrophies. In: Innes Williams D, Johnston J H (eds) Paediatric Urology, 2nd edn. Butterworth, London, pp 299–316

Kogan S J, Smey P, Levitt S B 1983 Subtunical total reduction clitoroplasy: a safe modification of existing techniques. Journal of Urology 130: 746–748

Kramer S A, Kelalis P P 1982 Assessment of urinary continence in epispadias. Review of 94 patients. Journal of Urology 128: 290–293

Kuhnle U, Bullinger M, Schwarz H P 1995 The quality of life in adult female patients with congenital adrenal hyperplasia: a comprehensive study of the impact of genital malformations and chronic disease on female patients life. European Journal of Paediatrics 154: 708–716

Lattimer J K 1961 Relocation and recession of the enlarged clitoris with preservation of the glans: an alternative to amputation. Journal of Urology 86: 113–116

Martinez-Mora J, Isnard R, Castellvi A and Lopez Ortiz P 1992 Neovagina in vaginal agenesis: surgical methods and long-term results. Journal of Pediatric Surgery 27: 10–14

Passerini-Glazel G 1994 Combined cliteroplasty and vaginoplasty. In: Hinman Jr F (ed) Atlas of Pediatric Urologic Surgery. Saunders, Philadelphia, pp 644–648

Perlmutter A D and Reitelman C 1992 Surgical management of intersexuality. In: Walsh P C, Retik A B, Stanley T A, Vaughan E D (eds). Campell's Urology, 6th edn. W B Saunders, Philadelphia, pp 1951–1966

Randolph J G, Hung W 1970 Reduction clitoroplasty in females with hypertrophied clitoris. Journal of Paediatric Surgery 5: 224–231

Saltzman B, Mininberg D T, Muecke E C 1985 Epispadias: Contending with continence. Urology 26: 256–264

Smith M R 1983 Vaginal aplasia: Therapeutic options. American Journal of Obstetrics and Gynaecology 146: 488–494

Spence H M, Allen T D 1973 Genital reconstruction in the female with the adrenogenital syndrome. British Journal of Urology 45: 1216–130

Stassart J P, Nagel T C, Prem K A, Phipps W R 1992 Uterus didephys, obstructed hemivagina and ipsilateral renal agenesis: the University of Minnesota experience. Fertility and Sterility 57: 756–761

Whitaker R H 1979 An evaluation of 170 diagnostic pressure flow studies of the upper urinary tract. Journal of Urology 121: 602–604

Williams D I, Bloomberg 1976 Urogenital sinus in the female child. Journal of Pediatric Surgery 11: 51–56

FURTHER READING

Walsh P C, Retik A B, Darracott Vaughan E, Wein A J (eds) 1997 Campbell's Urology, 7th edn. W B Saunders, Philadelphia

Bauer S B Chapter 58: Anomalies of the kidney and ureteropelvic junction. pp 1708–1755

Glassberg K I Chapter 59: Renal dysplasia and cystic disease of the kidney. pp 1757–1813

Schlussel R N, Retik A B Chapter 60: Anomalies of the ureter. pp 1814–1853

SECTION 3
CHAPTER

27

Urinary frequency and urgency

LINDA D CARDOZO

INTRODUCTION

Urinary frequency and urgency are common symptoms in women of all ages which may occur in isolation or in conjunction with other symptoms such as urinary incontinence or dysuria. The combination of urinary frequency, nocturia, urgency and urge incontinence is commonly referred to as 'the urge syndrome' as urgency is often the cardinal symptom (McGuire 1985). The many different underlying causes of these symptoms sometimes make it difficult to target investigations appropriately, and it is frustrating when the results of all reasonable tests prove negative. For many women, the unsatisfactory result of complex invasive investigations fails to provide a diagnosis and treatment has to be aimed at the symptoms rather than an underlying cause. However, as in all other areas of urogynaecology, quality of life is of paramount importance and we must therefore try to individualize our management of 'the urge syndrome'.

DEFINITIONS

Diurnal frequency is the passage of urine every two hours or more than seven times during the day.

Nocturia is interruption of sleep more than once each night because of the need to micturate. It is common to void during the night when sleep is disturbed for other reasons – e.g. insomnia or lactation – but this does not constitute nocturia.

Urgency is a strong and sudden desire to void which, if not relieved immediately, may lead to urge incontinence.

Urge incontinence is involuntary leakage of urine, usually preceded by urgency.

PREVALENCE

Frequency and urgency are common. It is unusual for urgency to occur alone because once it is present it almost invariably leads to frequency in order to avoid urge incontinence, or to relieve the unpleasant symptom which may be interpreted as pain.

In an epidemiological study Bungay et al (1980) assessed the prevalence of various symptoms in 1120 women and 510 men, aged between 30 and 65 years. They found that approximately 20% of women admitted to frequency and that this did not significantly alter with age. However, less than 10% of men below the age of 50 years complained of frequency but above that age there was a marked increase in the incidence of urinary frequency. Urgency showed a similar pattern: about 15% of women reported this symptom irrespective of age, whereas few men under the age of 50 years had urgency; but nearly 30% of men complained of urgency by the age of 65 years. It is interesting to note that in this study there was no specific increase in the prevalence of frequency or urgency of micturition amongst women in their peri- or postmenopausal years.

The number of nighttime voids increases after the age of approximately 60 years, and in general one nighttime void can be added for each decade past that age, so that it would not be considered abnormal for an 85-year-old to void four times a night.

CAUSES

There are many different causes of urinary frequency and urgency. The more common of these are listed in Table 27.1.

Table 27.1 Common causes of frequency and urgency of micturition.

Psychosocial	Excessive drinking
	Habit
	Anxiety
Urological	Urinary tract infection
	Detrusor instability (hyperreflexia)
	Small capacity bladder
	Interstitial cystitis
	Chronic follicular cystitis
	Chronic urinary retention/residual
	Genuine stress incontinence
	Bladder neoplasm
	Carcinoma *in situ*
	Tuberculosis
	Bladder calculus
	Urethral syndrome
	Urethritis
	Urethral diverticulum
Gynaecological	Pregnancy
	Cystocele
	Pelvic mass, e.g. fibroids
	Previous pelvic surgery
	Radiation cystitis/fibrosis
	Urethral caruncle
	Postmenopausal urogenital atrophy
Sexual	Coitus
	Genital warts
	Sexually transmitted diseases
Medical	Diuretic therapy
	Upper motor neurone lesion
	Impaired renal function
	Congestive cardiac failure (nocturia)
	Hypokalaemia
Endocrine	Diabetes mellitus
	Diabetes insipidus
	Hypothyroidism

PRESENTATION

History

Many of the more common disorders which cause the symptoms of frequency and urgency can be excluded by a thorough history. This should include documentation of the patient's specific complaint and any additional urological symptoms, especially stress incontinence, dysuria or voiding difficulties such as straining to void, poor stream or incomplete emptying. A past history of recurrent urinary tract infections, childhood enuresis beyond school age, or episodes of acute urinary retention may be relevant.

The gynaecological history should include symptoms of prolapse, abnormal vaginal discharge or the possibility of sexually transmitted diseases, as well as details of the menstrual cycle or the menopause if they are related to the urological symptoms. A woman in her reproductive years should be asked whether she could be pregnant. Previous pelvic surgery or trauma or pelvic irradiation involving the lower urinary tract are also important factors.

Neurological symptoms including leg weakness, paraesthesia, faecal soiling or backache may indicate a neuropathy which could also be responsible for the symptoms of frequency and urgency.

Details of the patient's drinking and voiding habits should be recorded and she should be questioned about any concurrent medical disorders such as renal disease or congestive cardiac failure, or endocrine problems including diabetes or hypothyroidism. In particular, it is important to know whether she has any current or past psychiatric problems. A drug history is relevant because diuretics will cause frequency of micturition and in an elderly woman may precipitate urge incontinence.

Clinical examination

A brief general examination may reveal anxiety as an underlying cause. If the patient appears unwell then her renal function should be checked and if she is abnormally slow or has other manifestations of hypothyroidism it is important to check her thyroid function.

Inspection of the vulva may reveal a heavy vaginal discharge or excoriation, in which case swabs should be taken and the possibility of urinary incontinence considered. Vulval warts or a urethral caruncle will also be obvious if present. In a postmenopausal woman, signs of vulval atrophy should be noted. Pelvic examination is important and will reveal a cystocele, confirm pregnancy or diagnose a pelvic mass. In addition, it is usually possible to detect a urinary residual on bimanual examination if more than 200 ml is present in the bladder.

A simple neurological examination should be performed to detect nystagmus, change in balance and lower limb reflexes, power and sensation. Particular reference is made to the second, third and fourth sacral nerves. If a neuropathy is suspected the patient should be referred to a neurologist.

INVESTIGATIONS

General

Before expensive and time-consuming investigations are undertaken, certain simple causes can be excluded. A urinary or serum Beta-HCG will diagnose pregnancy. Women with an abnormal vaginal discharge, a history of sexually transmitted diseases or obvious vulval excoriation should have vaginal, cervical and urethral swabs sent for culture. *Chlamydia* may be a causative organism; this requires a special culture medium for its detection.

Women with a history of haematuria and loin or groin pain, in whom a urinary tract infection cannot be identified, should be sent for intravenous urography and cystoscopy and referred to a urologist. If impaired renal function is suspected, serum urea and electrolyte concentrations, creatinine clearance and urine osmolarity should be estimated. If there is clinical suspicion of an underlying medical condition the appropriate investigations should be instigated, e.g. thyroid function tests, a glucose tolerance test, or an electrocardiograph.

Urine culture

One of the commonest causes of frequency and urgency of micturition is lower urinary tract infection – either cystitis or urethritis. When difficulty is encountered obtaining an uncontaminated midstream specimen of urine, suprapubic aspiration should be employed. If symptoms are strongly suggestive of an infection but results of culture are repeatedly negative, three early morning specimens should be sent for testing for acid-fast bacilli. Fastidious organisms such as *mycoplasma homonis* and *ureaplasma urealyticum* will not be picked up on routine culture and should be specifically looked for. These organisms are becoming increasingly common and may be the cause of long-standing symptoms which have failed to respond to conventional antibiotic therapy.

Frequency volume charts

Frequency of micturition often occurs in women who have a normal bladder capacity. The most common reason for this is excessive fluid intake, which can easily be determined using a frequency volume chart (urinary diary). The patient is instructed to measure the volume of all her standard drinking utensils and for five days she is asked to chart everything she drinks and the volume she voids at the appropriate times on her chart. A typical frequency volume chart is shown in Figure 27.1.

For some women who void frequently through habit or because they are anxious that they might be incontinent if they do not always have a relatively empty bladder, a frequency volume chart may be therapeutic. Most people void a much larger volume when they wake in the morning than at any other time of day and once they realize this and it has been

	Day 1			Day 2			Day 3			Day 4			Day 5		
Time	In	Out	W	In	Out	W	In	Out	W	In	Out	W	In	Out	W
6.00 am							200								
7.00 am								150						300	
8.00 am	200	350		200	250		200								
8.30 am	100										350		200		
9.00 am										400	50		200	150	
10.00 am	200				75										
10.45 am		50													
11.00 am								50		200					
12.00 pm				200	60		200				50			50	
1.00 pm	200	100						25					200		
2.00 pm				200	60					200	100			175	
3.00 pm	100				100					100					
4.00 pm		75					200	100					50	100	
5.00 pm				50	150			300							
5.30 pm	100									100					
6.00 pm											100				
6.15 pm		150											40		
7.00 pm		100			50									100	
8.00 pm							200	175		200	150				
9.00 pm		250			100					150			50	100	
10.00 pm	200				50		200				100				
11.00 pm		200						325			100			150	
11.30 pm		100													
12.00 am							100								
1.00 am															
1.30 am		100		100	50						100				
2.00 am								50							
3.00 am		75													
4.00 am					150										
5.00 am											150			200	

Fig. 27.1 Frequency volume chart completed for five consecutive days showing small urinary volumes voided frequently with a normal (or even reduced) fluid intake. (W = Wet.)

explained to them that their bladder sensation is unreliable these women may be reassured and find it easier to void less often.

Cystourethroscopy

Unless there is an obvious cause for the symptoms of urgency and frequency, endoscopy should be undertaken. Use of the flexible cystoscope and urethroscope enable both cystoscopy and urethroscopy to be undertaken without a general anaesthetic. However, it is not possible to take adequate biopsies in this way and therefore a day-case procedure using a general anaesthetic may be preferable.

At cystourethroscopy the residual urine volume should be noted (normally less than 50 ml) and the bladder capacity (normally 400–800 ml) should be recorded. True small capacity bladders are rare, but may be caused by interstitial cystitis which is classically diagnosed by the appearance of small haemorrhagic patches appearing during bladder filling (especially second fill) followed by the development of shallow, irregular, linear ulcers in the vault of the bladder. The bladder should also be inspected for trabeculation, diverticulae and mucosal injections. A neoplasm may be seen as a papilloma, or a calculus may be present. Urethroscopy will exclude urethritis or a urethral diverticulum.

Imaging

Radiology

A plain abdominal X-ray (KUB) is useful to diagnose a calculus and in cases of a significant urinary residual an X-ray of the lumbosacral spine should be obtained. Intravenous urography is still preferable to ultrasound when there is haematuria in the absence of a urinary tract infection, or when recurrent urinary tract infections fail to respond to treatment. Cystourethrography can be used to diagnose a bladder or urethral diverticulum but is of more use when combined with pressure flow studies in the form of videocystourethrography.

Ultrasound

Transabdominal ultrasound can be used to estimate a urinary residual volume and may occasionally identify an abnormality within the bladder. Transperineal, introital or vaginal ultrasound can be employed to measure bladder wall thickness as a screening test for detrusor instability (Khullar et al 1996).

Urodynamics

For women with incontinence in addition to frequency with or without urgency, it is best to organize urodynamic studies prior to cystourethroscopy, as the latter is usually unrewarding.

Cystometry

Subtracted cystometry detects detrusor instability which is a major cause of urgency and frequency. Low compliance may be difficult to interpret but can be caused by bladder fibrosis following radiation cystitis, or may be the end result of long-standing detrusor instability. Chronic retention of urine with an atonic bladder can be diagnosed on cystometry and this may lead to frequency or recurrent urinary tract infections. Sensory urgency can be diagnosed on cystometry by an early first sensation associated with a sensation of urgency during bladder filling and a reduced functional bladder capacity. Videocystourethrography with pressure and flow studies is useful if there is concomitant incontinence of urine because in the majority of cases it enables the cause to be determined. It also shows vesicoureteric reflux, trabeculation of the bladder, and urethral diverticulae.

Ambulatory monitoring

Conventional laboratory urodynamics have been shown to have a relatively low sensitivity for the diagnosis of detrusor instability (Webb et al 1991). Long-term ambulatory monitoring has recently been advocated because of its higher 'pick up' rate of 'abnormal detrusor activity'. However, there are still concerns regarding the diagnostic accuracy of ambulatory urodynamics, as normal ranges have not yet been defined and it is possible that artifacts may arise (Heslington & Hilton 1996). Ambulatory urodynamics provide a useful additional investigation in cases where symptoms persist despite normal laboratory urodynamic results, but at present this technique is still employed mainly as a research tool and has not been fully adopted into routine clinical practice.

Urethral pressure profilometry

The clinical significance of 'urethral instability' is still uncertain. Complete loss of urethral closure pressure (urethral relaxation) will cause incontinence (Kulseng-Hanssen 1983; Sand et al 1986), and the International Continence Society has defined urethral instability as an involuntary fall in intraurethral pressure in the absence of detrusor activity resulting in the leakage of urine (ICS 1981). However, many authors have used lesser, arbitrary, values to define urethral instability (Ulmsten et al 1982; Herbert & Ostergard 1982; Kulseng-Hanssen 1983). Fluctuations in urethral pressure which exceed one third of the maximum urethral pressure should probably be regarded as abnormal (Versi & Cardozo 1985). However, 16% of a cohort of healthy female volunteers without urological complaints have been shown to have urethral pressure variations greater than one third of their maximum urethral pressure (Tapp et al 1988), so although urethral pressure profilometry may be 'abnormal' in women with frequency and/ or urgency of micturition this is not of clinical significance.

Urethral electric conductance

Bladder neck electric conductance has been used in the assessment of women with urgency. First described by Plevnik et al (1985) this test utilizes a 7-French probe with two gold-plated brass electrodes, 1 mm in width, mounted 1 mm apart on a flexible silicone tube. A constant sinusoidal voltage with an amplitude of 20 mV peak to peak and frequency of 50 kHz is applied to the electrodes and the amplitude of the current between them measured. Holmes et al (1985) showed that any change in bladder neck electric conductivity greater than 13 MA was associated with the symptom of urgency and entry of fluid into the proximal urethra, whereas there was no such correlation with the symptom of stress incontinence. Peattie et al (1987) assessed sensory urge incontinence using bladder neck electric conductance and found a much greater maximum deflection in those women as compared to normal controls. However, this test has not gained popularity in the clinical management of women with urgency and urge incontinence.

NEGATIVE FINDINGS

In a large proportion of cases no obvious cause will be found for the symptoms of frequency and urgency. Some women with negative findings void frequently through habit, which usually develops following an acute urinary tract infection or an episode of incontinence. Alternatively, the bad habit may have been present since childhood, especially if one parent voids frequently; it is interesting that often several members of the same family from different generations suffer from similar urinary complaints.

TREATMENT

General

If an underlying cause can be identified this should be treated first. It is often difficult to treat patients in whom there is no obvious organic disease. Women with urgency and frequency should be advised to limit their fluid intake to a litre or a litre and a half per day and avoid drinking at times when their frequency causes the most embarrassment. Certain drinks, such as tea, coffee and other caffeine-containing fluids, as well as alcohol, precipitate frequency, especially nocturia, in some individuals and should therefore be avoided. Sometimes women are helped by a urinary diary (frequency volume chart) alone.

Habit re-training

Habit re-training (bladder drill) is useful for women without organic disease and can be undertaken by patients at home (Frewen 1982). They are advised to void by the clock and each week to increase the length of time between voiding until the time interval is socially acceptable. For those who cannot manage this at home, in-patient bladder drill has been used (Jarvis 1981). However, Holmes et al (1983) found the best long-term results for bladder training in the management of 'the urge syndrome' were achieved in women with stable bladders prior to treatment. As habit re-training is associated with no side-effects or complications, it may be worth trying in the first instance and can always be used in conjunction with other types of treatment.

Drug therapy

Drug therapy for frequency and urgency and detrusor instability are similar; however, the responses can be variable. The drugs are anticholinergic, musculotrophic, antidiuretic hormone analogues, quarternary amines and calcium channel blockers.

Propantheline hydrochloride 30-60 mg three or four times daily may help women with frequency. If anxiety, nocturia or both are problems then imipramine 50 mg twice daily should be tried, but if this causes tiredness during the day then a combination of propantheline during the day and imipramine at night can be tried.

Desmopressin (synthetic vasopressin analogue) is useful in patients who complain of nocturia alone (Hilton & Stanton 1982). It is available as a 200 microgram tablet, to be taken at night. Hypertension and ischaemic heart disease should be excluded before desmopressin is prescribed. Obviously this drug cannot be used simultaneously to alleviate diurnal frequency.

If urgency or urge incontinence co-exist with frequency then oxybutynin hydrochloride 2.5 mg twice daily to 5 mg three times daily should be tried. It may be helpful in relieving symptoms but has the well recognized unpleasant side-effect of a dry mouth when an effective dose is prescribed. A controlled release preparation is also available at a starting dose of 5 mg a day and has been shown to be as effective as the immediate release preparation in patients with urinary urge incontinence or mixed urinary incontinence with an urge component (Gleason et al 1998).

As the use of oxybutynin is often limited by its anticholinergic side-effects, a rectal preparation has been used and found to be associated with fewer side-effects (Delaere and Branje 1998).

Tolterodine is a new muscarinic antagonist and is more selective for the bladder with fewer salivary gland side-effects, in comparison with previous anticholinergics. At a dose of 2 mg twice daily it is efficacious for the management of frequency and urge incontinence and has a lower incidence of side-effects compared to other anticholinergic agents (Millard et al 1997; Drutz et al 1998). This may be particularly useful in the elderly patient where tolterodine has been shown to be safe and efficacious at the 1 mg and 2 mg twice daily dose.

Trospium chloride is a quaternary amine with both anticholinergic and antispasmodic activity. It is prescribed at a dose of 20 mg twice daily and is effective for motor urge incontinence and is well tolerated (Alloussi et al 1998; Chaliha et al 1999).

The combination of anticholinergic and calcium antagonist properties is an acceptable approach and and is available as propiverine hydrochloride. The recommended dose is 15 mg two to three times daily. In a multicentre study of 50 patients with urgency and urge incontinence, propiverine hydrochloride 30–45 mg daily led to an increase in bladder capacity, decrease in bladder pressure and an increase in compliance. During the treatment period the incidence of adverse side-effects decreased and the overall acceptability increased (Mazur et al 1994).

SPECIAL CONDITIONS

Urethral syndrome

The urethral syndrome is a common cause of frequency together with urgency and/or dysuria. It is defined as recurrent episodes of frequent painful micturition not associated with any abnormality of the female lower urinary tract. This is a broad definition which has been used to include urinary infection and urethral hypersensitivity (Powell et al 1981). The urethral syndrome may occur at any age and it is important that an organic cause be excluded before the diagnosis is made.

There are believed to be two basic causative factors – bacterial and urethral. The bacterial element has always been thought to be caused by migration of *Escherichia coli* across the urethra for which Smith (1981) recommended perineal hygiene, especially after sexual intercourse. In the case of an acute attack he (and other authorities) suggest a high fluid intake combined with bicarbonate of soda to alter the pH of the urine and short courses of antibiotics such as co-trimoxazole (Septrin) or nitrofurantoin (Furadantin). More recently, Norfloxacin (a quinalone) has been advocated. Prolonged low-dose chemotherapy is sometimes necessary for relapsing or chronic cases.

Stamm et al (1981) found that 71% of young women with the urethral syndrome had abnormal pyuria (defined as eight or more leucocytes per mm^3 of mid-stream urine), and 88% of these had a lower urinary tract infection with $<10^5$ coliforms, *Staphylococci* or *Chlamydia trachomatis*. In a randomized controlled double-blind trial of doxycycline and placebo they found that doxycycline was significantly more effective than placebo in eradicating urinary symptoms, pyuria and infecting micro-organisms. They did not recommend antibiotic therapy for women with the acute urethral syndrome without pyuria. These results stress the need for repeated culture and sensitivity of clean specimens of urine. Nowadays fastidious organisms, including *ureaplasma urealyticum* and *mycoplasma hominis*, are becoming increasingly prevalent and need to be treated for at least three months with low-dose doxycycline or ofloxacin in order to effect a cure.

Various surgical methods of treatment have been tried for resistant cases of the urethral syndrome. Urethral dilatation is often employed but there is no rationale behind its use, since it is rare to find outflow obstruction in these patients. Similarly, urethrotomy is sometimes performed; however, it is not indicated and may cause incontinence. Rees et al (1975) found that less than 8% of 156 women with the urethral syndrome had outflow obstruction and that the results of urethral dilatation or internal urethrotomy were no better than medication alone.

Selective sacral cryoneurolysis has been used to treat patients with a hypersensitive bladder (Awad et al 1987). Although the mean duration of effect was only five months, the technique is relatively simple and can be repeated as necessary. This technique has not gained widespread use.

Interstitial cystitis

Interstitial cystitis is a chronic inflammatory condition of the lamina propria of the bladder wall which is ill-defined and poorly understood. It was first recognized by Nitze in 1908 and subsequently by Hunner (1915) after whom the characteristic ulcerating lesion is named. In 1958 Simmons & Bruce described an increased number of mast cells in the lamina propria of the bladder in patients with symptoms of interstitial cystitis.

Pain is the presenting complaint in over 70% of patients (Koziol 1994). It is usually suprapubic, although urethritis, loin pain and dyspareunia are also frequently encountered. A long history of a combination of irritative urinary symptoms in the absence of proven infection is often present. Many women have previously undergone hysterectomy but this may reflect desperate attempts on the part of the doctor to relieve the patients' pain. Clinical examination is usually unrewarding but sensory urgency is nearly always diagnosed on cystometry. Cystoscopy with bladder biopsy must be undertaken to confirm the diagnosis. Characteristic cystoscopic findings include petechial haemorrhages on distension with haematuria on second fill, reduced bladder capacity, but uncommonly (5–20%) ulceration. Unfortunately, there is considerable confusion over the diagnostic parameters commonly employed. Hanno (1994) states that the bladder capacity must not exceed 350 ml, whereas Messing & Stamey (1978) demonstrated that the bladder capacity differed significantly between cystoscopies with local or no anaesthetic, and those performed under general anaesthesia, concluding that bladder volumes were not a useful guide to diagnosis.

The National Institute of Arthritis, Diabetes, Digestive and Kidney Diseases (NIADDK) established consensus criteria for a diagnosis in 1987 (Gillenwater & Wein 1988). They concluded that to be diagnosed with interstitial cystitis patients must have either glomerulations on cystoscopic examination or a classic Hunner's ulcer and they must have either bladder pain or urinary urgency. Table 27.2 lists the criteria which exclude a diagnosis of interstitial cystitis.

Table 27.2 Criteria for excluding the diagnosis of interstitial cystitis.

Bladder capacity >350 ml on awake cystometry.
Absence of an intense desire to void at 150 ml with a medium filling rate (30–100 ml/min).
Demonstration of phasic involuntary bladder contractions on cystometry.
Symptomatology of less than 9 months duration.
Absence of nocturia.
Symptoms relieved by antimicrobials, urinary antiseptics, anticholinergics or antispasmodics.
Urinary diurnal frequency <9 times.
A diagnosis of bacterial cystitis within 3 months.
Bladder calculi.
Active genital herpes.
Gynaecological malignancy.
Urethral diverticulum.
Chemical cystitis.
Tuberculosis.
Radiation cystitis.
Bladder tumours.
Vaginitis.
Age <18 years.

Interstitial cystitis is most prevalent amongst Caucasian women between the ages of 40 and 60 years with 30–500 cases per 100 000 women (Jones & Nyberg 1997). The condition usually has an initial rapid progression followed by stabilization regardless of treatment. These features are consistent with many autoimmune diseases. An association with Sjögren's syndrome has been demonstrated by Van der Merwe et al (1993). In addition, Mattila et al (1983) have shown raised levels of complement C3 and eosinophil cationic protein. This has led to the therapeutic use of heparin which is known to reduce the concentration of the latter. Views regarding the efficacy of this treatment are contentious (Lose et al 1983; Steinert et al 1994).

There is an association between interstitial cystitis and the irritable bowel syndrome raising a suspicion of a psychosomatic component (Koziol 1994).

There is still no consensus on the role of mast cells or their usefulness as a diagnostic criterion in interstitial cystitis. MacDermott et al (1991) found no statistical correlation between the severity of histological findings at diagnosis and the eventual outcome of the disease. However, two studies have investigated the degranulation of mast cells and both have shown increased degranulation in patients suffering from interstitial cystitis (Lynes et al 1987; Christmas & Rode 1991).

A failure of the protective function of the mucosal glycosaminoglycan layer of the bladder allowing infective agents to attack the underlying epithelium has been proposed by Parsons et al (1980), who later postulated that patients with interstitial cystitis have an abnormal sensitivity to intravesical potassium. Sodium pentosanpolysulphate is believed to decrease bladder wall permeability and this has been used with some success in the treatment of interstitial cystitis.

Treatment

As it is likely that interstitial cystitis is the final common pathway of a multifactorial disease process, it is not surprising that many different treatments have been proposed. Anti-inflammatory agents, both nonsteroidal and steroidal, have been used, with initial success rates up to 70%. Azathioprine, sodium chromoglycate and chloroquine have all been effective in some cases, however none has become an established form of treatment. Antihistamines have been employed in an attempt to stabilize or counteract the effect of the increased number of mast cells (Seshadri et al 1994). Heparin 8 and sodium pentosanpolysulphate, which works in a similar way to heparin, have also been employed with success rates ranging from 27 to 83% (Mulholland et al 1990; Parsons et al 1993).

Alternatively, an infective hypothesis has been proposed and long-term antibiotics have been prescribed. Norfloxacin 400 mg at night for three months is a commonly used regimen. Alternatively, a bladder antiseptic, such as hexamine hippurate 1 g twice a day for three months, may be used.

Dimethylsulphone (DMSO) has been instilled into the bladder with some success although it does not appear to give long-term benefit and there are concerns that it may be carcinogenic. Other treatments include local anaesthetics, calcium channel blockers and tricyclic antidepressants. Recent reports of randomized placebo controlled trials in the treatment of interstitial cystitis have demonstrated significant beneficial effect (generally double the response rate of placebo) with oral L-arginine, a nitric oxide synthase inhibitor (Smith et al 1998), intravesical TICE Bacille Calmette-Geurin (BCG) (Peters et al 1997) and intravesical pentosanpolysulfate sodium (Bade et al 1996). Open label trials of the oral histamine antagonists hydroxyzine (Theoharides & Sant 1997), and intravesical hyaluronic acid (Morales et al 1997) have also demonstrated some efficacy and the results of randomized trials are awaited.

Bladder distension has been used as a treatment for sensory bladder disorders and although short-term benefit has been achieved there is no evidence of long-term cure. In addition, repeated distensions may lead to an exacerbation of symptoms. Denervation procedures have been tried as well as phenol injections (which are now no longer employed) and more recently, laser ablation of the vesicoureteric plexuses (Gillespie 1994). As a last resort there is still a place for substitution cystoplasty or urinary diversion in severely affected patients but augmentation cystoplasty is rarely effective as pain continues to be a problem.

Many patients do benefit from simple measures such as the avoidance of caffeine-containing compounds including tea, coffee and 'cola'-type soft drinks as well as the withdrawal of alcohol from their diet. There are some patients for whom transcutaneous electrical nerve stimulation (Fall & Lindstrom 1994) and/or acupuncture (Geirsson et al 1993) may provide adjunctive help but rarely provide a complete cure.

The majority of women with a diagnosis of interstitial cystitis find that they are subject to spontaneous remissions and exacerbations and eventually develop a set of coping strategies to help with their problems when they are worse. Self-care regimens, together with treatment of chronic pain, anxiety and depression are often more effective than a supposedly focused remedy. It is not unusual for all the therapies mentioned here to be utilized in the same patient at some time or another before eventually the condition abates spontaneously, the woman learns to live with her symptoms, or a urinary diversion is undertaken (Toozs-Hobson et al 1996).

Sexual problems

Many women develop an urgent desire to pass urine during or immediately after sexual intercourse. This is thought to be caused by the rigid nulliparous perineum which allows irritation of the posterior bladder wall to occur during repeated penile thrusting. The postcoital dysuria which ensues is known as 'honeymoon cystitis' and may be followed by a urinary tract infection. Many studies have shown that contraceptive diaphragms may lead to bouts of frequency, urgency and dysuria, and urinary tract infections are common in women using these (Vessey et al 1987; Hooton et al 1996). Despite this, many women continue to use this method of contraception, although it would obviously be wise for an alternative to be sought.

The common symptoms of frequency and urgency associated with sexual intercourse can often be helped by simple measures such as perineal hygiene, change of coital technique, voiding after sexual intercourse with a fluid pre-load beforehand. For postmenopausal women, failure of adequate lubrication during intercourse may be a problem, so a lubricant gel or oestrogen replacement should be prescribed.

Some women who associate attacks of the urethral syndrome with sexual intercourse have their urethral meatus far back along the anterior vaginal wall, where it is vulnerable to trauma during coitus. Symptoms in such women may be relieved by a urethrovaginoplasty with freeing and advancement of the urethra or urethrolysis.

Urogenital atrophy

The symptoms of frequency and urgency of micturition may develop for the first time at or after the menopause. Oestrogens, prescribed orally, parenterally or locally to the vagina may alleviate the symptoms. Prolonged unopposed oestrogen replacement therapy may, however, lead to cystic glandular hyperplasia of the endometrium or even adenocarcinoma, so a progestogen should be given for 10–13 days each month in women with a uterus.

For women who have undergone a hysterectomy, treatment options are almost infinite with many different tablets, patches and implants to choose from.

However, for women with a uterus who do not wish to suffer withdrawal bleeds, it is more acceptable to prescribe local oestrogen therapy which does not increase the serum oestrone or oestradiol. This can be achieved using oestriol pessaries (losif 1992), sustained-release low dose 17-Beta oestradiol vaginal tablets (Eriksen & Rasmussen 1992), or an oestradiol releasing vaginal ring (Smith et al 1993).

CONCLUSIONS

Frequency and urgency of micturition are only symptoms which may be caused by many different diseases. It is often helpful to adopt an algorithmic approach to the management of patients with these complaints (Cardozo 1986). After organic pathology has been excluded there remains a group of women whose symptoms are psychosomatic and who will benefit from a psychiatric referral. For the rest treatment must, unfortunately, be empirical and there will undoubtedly be a proportion of sufferers resistant to all current available therapy.

REFERENCES

Alloussi S, Laval K, Eckert R, et al 1998 Trospium chloride in patients with motor urge syndrome (detrusor instability): a double blind, randomised, multicentre, placebo-controlled study. Journal of Clinical Research 1: 439-451

Awad S A, Acker K L, Flood H D, Clarke J C 1987 Selective sacral cryoneurolysis in the treatment of patients with detrusor stability/hyperreflexia and hypersensitive bladder. Neurourology and Urodynamics 6(3): 263–264

Bade J J, Laseur M, Nieuwenburg A et al 1996 A placebo-controlled study of intravesical pentosanpolysulfate for the treatment of interstitial cystitis. British Journal of Urology 79: 168-171

Bungay G, Vessey M P, McPherson C K 1980 Study of symptoms in middle life with special reference to the menopause. British Medical Journal 281: 181–183

Cardozo L D 1986 Urinary frequency and urgency. British Medical Journal 293: 1419–1423

Chaliha C, Halaska M, Stanton SL 1999 Efficacy and tolerability of Trospium chloride for detrusor instability; a dose ranging study. British Journal of Urology (submitted)

Christmas T J, Rode J 1991 Characteristics of mast cells in normal bladder, bacterial cystitis and interstitial cystitis. British Journal of Urology 68: 473–478

Delaere K P J, Branje J P 1998 Rectal administration of oxybutinin in the treatment of detrusor instability: preliminary promising results of a pilot study. Neurourology and Urodynamics 17(4): 317

Drutz HP, Appell RA, Gleason D, Klinberg I, Radomsny S 1998 Long term treatment with tolterodine in patients with overactive bladder. Neurourology and Urodynamics 17(4): 319-320

Eriksen P S, Rasmussen H 1992 Low-dose 17-estradiol vaginal tablets in the treatment of atrophic vaginitis: a double blind placebo controlled study. European Journal Obstetrics Gynaecology and Reproductive Biology 44: 137–144

Fall M, Lindstrom S 1994 Transcutaneous electrical nerve stimulation in classic and nonulcer interstitial cystitis. Urology Clinics of North America 21: 131–139

Frewen W K 1982 Bladder training in general practice. Practitioner. 226: 1874–1879

Geirsson G, Wang Y H, Lindstrom S, Fall M 1993 Traditional acupuncture and electrical stimulation of the posterior tibial nerve: a trial in chronic interstitial cystitis. Scandinavian Journal of Urology and Nephrology 27: 67–70

Gillenwater J Y, Wein A J 1988 Summary of the National Institute of Arthritis, Diabetes, Digestive and Kidney Diseases workshop on interstitial cystitis. Journal of Urology 140: 203–206

Gillespie L 1994 Destruction of the vesicoureteric plexus for the treatment of hypersensitive bladder disorders. British Journal of Urology 74: 40–43

Gleason DM, for the Oxybutinin XL study group 1998 Evaluation of efficacy, safety, dose conversion of a once-a-day controlled release oxybutinin chloride formulation for urge urinary incontinence. Neurourology and Urodynamics 17(4): 318-319

Hanno P 1994 Diagnosis of interstitial cystitis. Urology Clinics of North America 21: 63–66

Herbert D B, Ostergard D R 1982 Vesical instability: Urodynamic parameters by microtip transducer catheters. Obstetrics and Gynecology 60: 331–337

Heslington, Hilton 1996 Ambulatory urodynamic monitoring British Journal of Obstetrics and Gynecology 103: 393–399

Hilton P, Stanton S L 1982 Use of desmopressin for nocturia in the female. British Journal of Urology 54: 252–255

Holmes D M, Plevnik S, Stanton S L 1985 Bladder neck electric conductance (BNEC) tests in the investigation and treatment of sensory urgency and detrusor instability. Proceedings of the 15th Annual meeting of the International Continence Society, London, pp 96–97

Holmes D M, Stone A R, Bary P R, Richards C J, Stephenson T P 1983 Bladder training – 3 years on. British Journal of Urology 55: 660–664

Hooton T M, Scholes D, Hughes J P et al 1996 A prospective study of risk factors for symptomatic urinary tract infection in young women. New England Journal of Medicine 335(7): 468–474

Hunner G L 1915 A rare type of bladder ulcer in women: report of cases. Boston Medical and Surgical Journal 172: 660–664

International Continence Society 1981. Fourth report on the standardisation of the terminology of lower urinary tract function. British Journal of Urology 53: 333–335

Iosif C S 1992 Effects of protracted administration of oestriol on the genitourinary tract in postmenopausal women. Archives of Gynecology 251: 115–120

Jarvis G 1981 The management of urinary incontinence due to vesical sensory urgency by bladder drill. Proceedings of the 11th Meeting of the International Continence Society, Lund. 123–124

Jones CA, Nyberg L 1997 Epidemiology of interstitial cystitis. Urology 49 (supl 5A):2-9

Khullar V, Cardozo L D, Salvatore S, Hill S 1996 Ultrasound: a non-invasive screening test for detrusor instability. British Journal of Obstetrics and Gynaecology 103: 904–908

Koziol J A 1994 Epidemiology of interstitial cystitis. Urology Clinics of North America 21: 7–20

Kulseng-Hanssen S 1983 Prevalence and pattern of unstable urethral pressure in 174 gynecologic patients referred for urodynamic investigation. American Journal of Obstetrics and Gynecology 146: 895–900

Lose G, Frandsen B, Johensgard J C, Jespersen J, Astrup T 1983 Chronic interstitial cystitis: increased levels of eosinophil cationic protein in serum and urine and ameliorating effect of subcutaneous heparin. Scandinavian Journal of Urology and Nephrology 17: 159

Lynes W L, Flynn L D, Shortliffe M L, Zipser R, Roberts J, Stamey T A 1987 Mast cell involvement in interstitial cystitis? British Journal of Urology 67: 44–47

MacDermott J P, Charpied G C, Tesluk H, Stone A R 1991 Can histological assessment predict the outcome in interstitial cystitis? British Journal of Urology 67: 44–47

Mattila J, Harmoninen A, Hallstrom O 1983 Serum immunoglobulin and complement alterations in interstitial cystitis. European Urology 9: 350

Mazur D, Alkan R 1994 Tolerance and efficacy of long-term therapy with propiverine chloride for symptoms of urgency and urge incontinence - a multicentre study. Kontinenz 3: 74-78

McGuire E J 1985 Clinical evaluation of the lower urinary tract. Clinics in Obstetrics and Gynecology 12: 311–317

Messing E D, Stamey T A 1978 Interstitial cystitis: early diagnosis, pathology and treatment. Urology 12: 381–391

Millard R, Moore K, Dwyer P, Tuttle J 1997 Treatment of detrusor instability. Neurourology and Urodynamics 16: 343–344

Morales A, Emerson I, Nickel J C 1997 Intravesical hyaluronic acid in the treatment of refractory institial cystitis. Urology 49(suppl 5A): 111-113

Mulholland S G, Hanno P, Parsons C L, Sant G R, Staskin D R 1990 Pentosan polysulfate sodium for therapy of interstitial cystitis. A double-blind placebo-controlled clinical study. Urology. 35: 552–558

Nitze M 1908 Lehrbuch der Cystoskopie: ihre Technik und Klinische Bedeutung. JE Bergman, Berlin, pp 205–210

Parsons C L, Schmidt J D, Pollen J Y 1983 Successful treatment of interstitial cystitis with sodium pentosanpolysulphate. Journal of Urology 130: 51

Parsons C L, Stauffer C, Schmidt J D 1980 Bladder surface glycosaminoglycans: an efficient mechanism of environmental adaptation. Science 208: 605

Parsons C L, Stein P C, Bidair M, Lebow D 1994 Abnormal sensitivity to intravesical potassium in interstitial cystitis and radiation cystitis. Neurourology and Urodynamics 13: 515–520

Peattie A B, Plevnik S, Stanton S L 1987 Assessment and treatment of sensory urge incontinence using the bladder neck electric conductance (BNEC) test. Neurourology and Urodynamics 6(3): 265–266

Peters K, Diokno A, Steinert B et al 1997 The efficacy of intravesical Tice strain Bacillus Calmette-Geurin in the treatment of interstitial cystitis: A double-blind, prospective, placebo-controlled trial. Journal of Urology 157: 2090-2094

Plevnik S, Holmes D M, James J, Mundy A R, Vrtacnik P 1985 Urethral electric conductance (UEC) – A new parameter for evaluation of urethral and bladder function: methodology of the assessment of its clinical potential. Proceedings of 15th Annual Meeting of the International Continence Society, London, pp 90–91

Powell P H, George N, Smith P, Fenery R C L 1981 The hypersensitive female urethra – a cause of recurrent frequency and dysuria. Proceedings of the 11th Annual Meeting of the International Continence Society, London pp 81–82

Rees D L, Whitfield H N, Islam A K, Doyle P T, Mayo M E, Wickham J E 1975 Urodynamic findings in the adult female with frequency and dysuria. British Journal of Urology. 47: 853–860

Sand P K, Bowen L W, Ostergard D R 1986 Uninhibited urethral relaxation: an unusual cause of incontinence. Obstetrics and Gynecology 68: 645–648

Seshadri P, Emerson L, Morales A 1994 Cimetidine in the treatment of interstitial cystitis with intravesical heparin. British Journal of Urology 73: 504–507

Simmons J L, Bruce P L 1958 On the use of an antihistamine in the treatment of interstitial cystitis. American Surgery 24: 6564–6667

Smith P J, Heimer G, Lindskog M, Ulmsten U. 1993 Oestradiol releasing vaginal ring for treatment of postmenopausal urogenital atrophy. Maturitas 16: 145–154

Smith P J. 1981 The urethral syndrome. In: Fisher A M, Gordon H (eds) Gynaecological enigmata. Clinical Obstetrics and Gynaecology 8(1): 161–172

Smith S 1997 L-arginine treatment. Paper presented at Ninth National ICA Meeting, Washington, DC

Stamm W E, Running K, McKevitt M, Counts G W, Turck M, Holmes K K 1981 Treatment of the acute urethral syndrome. New England Journal of Medicine 304(16): 956–958

Steinert B W, Diokno A C, Robinson J E, Mitchell B A 1994 Complement C3, Eosinophil cationic protein and symptom evaluation in interstitial cystitis. British Journal of Urology 151: 350–354

Tapp A J S, Cardozo L D, Versi E, Studd J W W 1988 The prevalence of variation of resting urethral pressure in women and its association with lower urinary tract function. British Journal of Urology 61: 314–317

Theoharides T C, Sant G R 1997 Hydroxyzine therapy for interstitial cystitis. Urology 49(suppl 5A): 108-110

Toozs-Hobson P, Gleeson C, Cardozo L D 1996 Interstitial cystitis – still an enigma after 80 years. British Journal of Obstetrics and Gynaecology 103: 621–624

Ulmsten U, Henriksson L, Iosif S 1982 The unstable female urethra. American Journal of Obstetrics and Gynecology 144: 93–97

Van der Merwe J, Kemerling R, Arendsen E, Mulder D, Hooijkaas H 1993 Sjögren's syndrome in patients with interstitial cystitis. Journal of Rheumatology 20: 962–966

Versi E, Cardozo L D 1985 Urethral instability in normal postmenopausal women. Proceedings of the 15th Annual International Continence Society, London, pp 115–116

Vessey M P, Metcalf M A, McPherson K, Yeates D 1987 Urinary tract infection in relation to diaphragm use and obesity. International Journal of Epidemiology 16: 1–4

Webb R J, Ramsden P D, Neal D E 1991 Ambulatory monitoring and electronic measurement of urinary leakage in the diagnosis of detrusor instability and incontinence. British Journal of Urology 68: 148–15

SECTION 3
CHAPTER

28

Bladder hypersensitivity

SARAH M CREIGHTON AND JOY DIXON

DEFINITION

The term hypersensitive bladder or sensory urgency is used to describe women with frequency and urgency not found to be due to organic disease such as detrusor instability or interstitial cystitis. The International Continence Society (1992) explains that urge incontinence has two causes; overactive detrusor function or hypersensitivity (sensory urgency). The definition is otherwise rather vague as no further guidelines on the clinical or urodynamic criteria required to make this diagnosis are given. Not only is the definition of sensory urgency vague, its aetiology is even less well understood. Thus treatment is often empirical and haphazard. Sensory urgency is generally accepted as urgency, frequency, nocturia and urge incontinence in the absence of detrusor instability. There is no other ICS definition but a urine culture must be sterile. Filling cystometry usually indicates a reduced volume at first desire to void and bladder capacity may be reduced. Some clinicians state that a cystoscopy must also be performed to exclude other causes such as interstitial cystitis, tumour or calculi.

PREVALENCE

There have been few formal studies looking at the prevalence of sensory urgency because the diagnosis is not clear-cut and most urodynamic units include these patients in their detrusor instability figures. Peattie et al (1988) estimated the incidence of sensory urgency in 558 women attending a teaching hospital urogynaecology clinic as 6% compared to 31% for detrusor instability.

AETIOLOGY

The aetiology of sensory urgency is unknown. Various theories have been proposed of a central nervous system problem as well as local bladder or urethral abnormalities. It has also been suggested that sensory urgency is an early form of detrusor instability and may just be earlier in the spectrum of disease.

Psychological factors

Sensory urgency may have an underlying psychological abnormality. Macaulay et al (1991) reported on the psychological aspects of 211 women attending a urodynamic unit. They found women with sensory urgency had a low feeling of self-esteem and were more anxious than women with genuine stress incontinence who showed features only seen in those with any long-standing complaint.

Creighton et al (1991) proposed that women with sensory urgency may have an abnormal perception of their own bladder size. This could in some way be similar to the abnormal perception of body size by women with anorexia. They studied 15 women with sensory urgency and compared them with 15 normal controls. Patients with symptoms of urgency and frequency and stable filling cystometry had their bladders slowly filled with a recorded volume of fluid. They were asked to estimate their bladder fullness using a visual analogue scale from 0 to 10, with 0 representing an empty bladder and 10 representing as full as possible. For all bladder volumes women with sensory urgency markedly overestimated their bladder fullness when compared to the normal controls (Fig 28.1). This may explain symptoms as they complained of a desire to void at a lower filled volume. They also studied a group of women with detrusor instability in a similar manner and found them to have very similar results to the sensory urgency group, i.e. a significant overestimation of bladder fullness when compared to normal controls. This of course may lend credence to the view that these conditions are of similar aetiology and indeed may be different facets of the same disease.

The success of psychological methods of treatment such as hypnosis, acupuncture and biofeedback may also confirm the role of psychological factors.

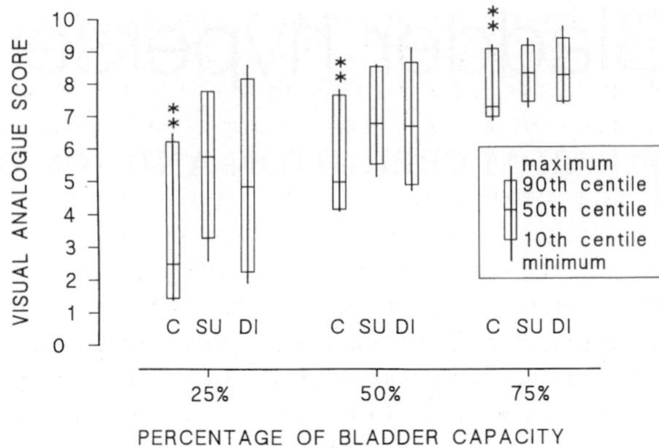

Fig. 28.1 Box and whisker plots of the visual analogue scores at 25, 50 and 75% of capacity for women with sensory urgency (SU), detrusor instability (DI) and normal controls (C). The normal controls had significantly lower perceptions of bladder fullness at each point: no differences being observed between the other two groups. (**p < 0.01).

Histological factors

Attempts have been made to define a histological difference in the detrusor muscle of women with sensory urgency. Frazer et al (1990) looked at the presence of mast cells in the detrusor muscle on biopsy in 27 women with idiopathic sensory urgency compared with 10 asymptomatic controls. They found a subgroup of eight women (30%) had a significant increase in the number of detrusor mast cells. This subgroup had no clinical or urodynamic features to distinguish them from the other sensory urgency patients. The increase in mast cells was not present in any of the controls. As detrusor mastocytosis is a feature of interstitial cystitis, they suggested that sensory urgency may be a forerunner of interstitial cystitis and thus should prompt extra vigilance in these women. This study only looked at small numbers of women and long-term follow-up of these patients is necessary.

Neurological factors

The sensory innervation of the bladder and urethra is an essential part of the bladder storage and voiding reflexes. There is a dual afferent innervation of the bladder with sympathetic afferents running to the thoracolumbar spinal cord and parasympathetic afferents projecting to the sacral segments. The location of the pelvic nerve afferents to sacral roots S2–4 have been confirmed by lesioning studies for relief of pain (White & Sweet 1955). In the normal bladder it is likely that there is a homogenous group of afferents which respond in a graded fashion to increase in intravesical pressure. These visceral afferents may encode information according to intensity rather than specificity theory. This would explain the variable sensation threshold (McMahon et al 1995). In studies of chemically induced inflammation of the bladder normally silent unmyelinated afferents are shown to be activated.

Nerve Growth Factor (NGF) is a member of a small group of secretory proteins known as neurotrophins. There is increasing evidence that NGF may regulate pain sensation in humans (Anand 1995). Increased concentrations of NGF have been found in patients with sensory urgency compared with a control group of patients with stress incontinence (Lowe et al 1997).

Capsaicin, a substance that can be extracted from red peppers, is known to be acutely irritant to cutaneous and other sensory endings when administered acutely, mainly because it releases substance P from nerve endings. It has selective actions on unmyelinated C fibres and A delta fibres. Most capsaicin-sensitive fibres are polymodal nociceptors which respond to a range of sensory stimuli. Although local application of capsaicin is initially algesic, repeated application leads to desensitization and results in long-lasting sensory deficits. It has been shown to give significant improvement in pain scores in such conditions as post-herpetic neuralgia (Bernstein et al 1989). In humans intravesical administration of capsaicin transiently reduces bladder sensation and irritative voiding symptoms. Malmgren et al (1990) showed an almost complete disappearance of substance P in the rat bladder 10 days after treatment with capsaicin. This implies that substance P or related peptides play a role in the regulation of the micturition threshold and the perception of pain from the bladder (Maggi et al 1989).

Bladder and urethral hypersensitivity

It has also been proposed that there may be an increased sensitivity of the bladder or urethra in these patients. Sensory threshold studies are performed using electrical stimuli applied via an electrode. Attempts have been made to study bladder sensitivity but equipment is complex and the appropriate stimuli not well worked out. Frazer & Haylen (1989) tested trigonal sensitivity but found no differences between women with sensory urgency or detrusor instability and normal controls. Although their study was relatively large, the number of control patients was small and they concluded that sensitivity values did not correlate with either first desire to void or cystometric bladder capacity.

Urethral hypersensitivity may be a more likely factor, as the most potent facilitative receptors for the micturition reflex are situated in the posterior urethra (Mahoney et al 1977). Several studies have looked at urethral sensitivity and results are conflicting.

The most appropriate method for testing sensory threshold is a 'method of limits' technique. This involves exposing the patient to a stimulus of changing intensity and asking the patient to indicate the onset of symptoms. Method of limits testing has been widely used in evaluating peripheral neuropathy and is the method of choice as it is both quick and accurate. Electrical stimuli have been used to estimate sensory thresholds for many years (Tursky & Watson 1964) but initially fell out of use due to technical difficulties. Recent introduction of improved stimulators has led to a resurgence of interest in this type of investigation. Electrical stimulation has been shown to be of use in screening for peripheral neuropathy, and values for thresholds obtained correlate with estimates of severity of neuropathy (Rendell et al 1989).

Kieswetter (1977) was first to try to investigate this possibility. He used bipolar ring electrodes mounted on a urethral catheter and found a lower urethral sensory threshold and thus increased urethral sensitivity in women with symptoms of urgency and frequency. Powell & Feneley (1980) used a similar technique to measure the sensitivity of the proximal urethra in clinically and urodynamically normal and abnormal patients. In those with a stable detrusor muscle, a positive correlation was found between the urethral sensory threshold and both first desire to void and bladder capacity. An increased urethral sensitivity was found in women with reduced bladder capacity but otherwise normal cystometry who complained of frequency and nocturia.

Both of the above studies used ring electrodes mounted on Foley urethral catheters. These produce relatively large electrical fields, for example that used by Powell & Feneley (1980) produces a field which penetrates the urethral tissue for a depth of 6 mm and a length of 17 mm. It was proposed that the areas of altered sensitivity may be confined to smaller sections of the urethra and thus more accurate measurements are needed.

To overcome this problem Creighton et al (1993) designed a catheter using the principle of urethral electrical conductance (UEC) already described in Chapter 12. The electrical current, if applied through the 1 mm gold-plated brass electrodes used for UEC measurements, only produces a field which penetrates tissue to a depth of 2 mm along a length of 3 mm. The principle of UEC can also be used to locate the electrodes at the bladder neck. The specially designed catheter contained three pairs of electrodes placed 1 cm apart, thus three known areas of the urethra can be studied (Fig. 28.2). A switch box was incorporated into the design to allow the catheter to be accurately located in the urethra and then a stimulatory current applied. This study compared urethral sensory threshold at three urethral sites between a group of women with sensory urgency and a group of normal controls. The results were surprising in that the women with sensory urgency had a significantly higher sensory threshold than the controls, rather than the expected lower result. The results were reproducible and occurred at all three points of testing. The significance of this is unknown and contradicts earlier work. However, peripheral neuropathies of varying significance can selectively involve small diameter myelinated and unmyelinated fibres. These small fibre neuropathies can present with a loss of sensory modalities conveyed by these fibres while large fibre dependent functions remain normal. This study may suggest that a peripheral neuropathy may be an aetiological factor in the development of sensory urgency. This remains to be investigated further.

PRESENTATION

Women with sensory urgency present with similar symptoms to those of detrusor instability and may be indistinguishable from this on clinical assessment. They complain of frequency and urgency and nocturia. They may also complain of urge incontinence. Vaginal examination rarely adds to information.

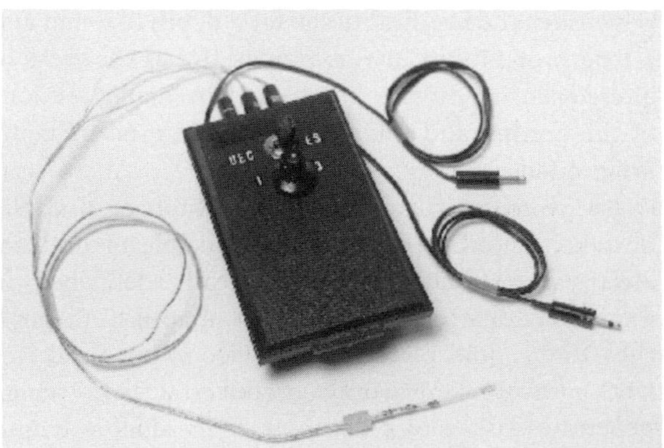

Fig. 28.2 The specially designed modified bladder neck electrical conductance catheter. The catheter contains three pairs of gold-plated brass electrodes. It is connected via a switch box to the UEC meter and a neurostimulator.

INVESTIGATION

Basic tests

Urinary frequency and nocturia can be confirmed with a urinary diary which eliminates excessive or inappropriate drinking as a cause for symptoms and can also be used as a basis for treatment such as bladder re-training. An idea of the true functional capacity can also be obtained. A mid-stream urine culture is imperative to exclude infection, and urine should also be sent for cytological examination, particularly if the symptoms are of sudden onset in an elderly woman.

Cystometry

Twin channel subtracted filling cystometry is necessary to exclude detrusor instability. In women with sensory urgency the bladder remains stable during cystometry despite provocation. Jarvis et al (1982) defined these women as having a reduced first desire to void of less than 75 ml and also a reduced bladder capacity of less than 400 ml, although not all clinicians adhere to these figures. This is essential and an absence of detrusor overactivity in the presence of the above symptoms leads to a diagnosis of sensory urgency. More recently, however, it has been shown that ambulatory cystometry may increase the detection of detrusor instability (Griffiths et al 1987). It may be that cases currently diagnosed as sensory urgency may really be covert detrusor instability which is missed on routine urodynamics. This may become clear as ambulatory testing becomes more widespread.

Bladder neck electrical conductance

If the above investigations are negative, urethral electrical conductance has been used to obtain more information (Ch. 12). An increase in bladder neck electrical conductance (BNEC) was noted to be associated with an increase in the symptoms of urgency (Holmes et al 1985). Peattie et al (1988) used the principle of bladder neck electrical conductance to locate the electrical conductance catheter at the bladder neck. The patients lay supine with 250 ml saline in the bladder while a continuous conductance reading was printed. The maximum deflection at rest (MDR) was measured and it was shown that the symptomatic women had a significantly increased MDR when compared to controls. The increase in bladder neck conductance occurs at bladder neck opening and is related to symptoms of urgency. This investigation is useful as it gives a positive finding in the presence of sensory urgency rather than using a diagnosis of exclusion as is made on cystometry.

Cystoscopy

In many units, a cystoscopy is also an integral part of investigation of sensory urgency. Interstitial cystitis can present with similar symptoms although usually there is bladder pain in addition. Features at cystoscopy have already been described in Chapter 13. Women with sensory urgency have a normal bladder capacity under general anaesthetic although this may be reduced on cystometry and on inspection of their urinary diary. A cystoscopy will also exclude tumour and calculi as a cause. In women who develop suspected sensory urgency after bladder neck surgery, a cystoscopy is imperative to ensure a stitch was not placed through the bladder.

TREATMENT

As the aetiology of sensory urgency is unknown, treatment is empirical and success rates unpredictable. As the clinical picture is so similar to detrusor instability, both conditions are treated similarly. The most common treatment is probably bladder retraining but other treatments include behavioural methods and drugs. Treatment outcomes are difficult to determine and there are few studies of long-term follow-up. The placebo response is high and thus objective studies have to be large, prospective and placebo-controlled. Aitchison et al (1989) found that at a 5-years follow-up, the natural history of sensory urgency is one of spontaneous resolution which must obviously be taken into account when assessing treatment.

Bladder re-training

Bladder re-training has been referred to in Chapter 27 as a useful treatment for urinary frequency and urgency, both due to detrusor instability and sensory urgency. The patient's urinary diary can be used to determine the starting point of training and the patient is asked to prolong the time between voiding. This may be done as an in-patient or out-patient. Success rates are higher in those women treated as in-patients although current medical resources are making this a financially impractical option. Cure rates for detrusor instability are high at over 90% (Jarvis 1982). Most units do not give separate figures for sensory urgency as opposed to detrusor instability although Holmes et al (1983) found the treatment to be more successful in those women without detrusor instability.

Biofeedback

Biofeedback entails demonstrating an autonomic function to the patient using visual or auditory means. The patient is then aware of that function and can learn to exert control over it. Biofeedback has been used with success in the treatment of detrusor instability (Cardozo et al 1978). This was done by using an amplifier which gave auditory evidence of increases in detrusor pressure. More recently Peattie et al (1988) have applied BNEC using this principle. The bladder neck opening associated with urgency can be shown to the patient on either a written printout or a meter dial. The patient can then attempt to exert control over this. A maximum of eight half-hour sessions were performed but most patients could control their bladder neck opening after three sessions. The mechanism of control is unknown but may be due to pelvic floor contraction. There was a significant improvement in both the BNEC variation and also the patients' symptoms. The disadvantages of treatment is that it requires an intensive course of one-to-one therapy with a specially trained nurse and doctor and is therefore expensive and time-consuming.

Dietary measures

Some patients do notice an improvement in symptoms with simple measures such as caffeine restriction. Patients should be warned that citrus fruit drinks and alcoholic drinks also exacerbate the irritative voiding symptoms. A dietary diary can be useful in eliciting these factors.

Behavioural therapies

Other methods such as psychotherapy, acupuncture and hypnosis have all been suggested for both detrusor instability and sensory urgency. In most studies numbers are small and placebo controls inappropriate. These may help individual patients but most are not available on the National Health Service. Treatment is expensive as again most require long periods of individual therapy on a one-to-one basis with a trained therapist.

Drug therapy

Drug therapy is the mainstay of treatment in detrusor instability. As the symptoms of sensory urgency are so similar, the same treatments are used. Most drugs such as anticholinergics act by reducing detrusor overactivity. As detrusor overactivity has been excluded in women with sensory urgency, it is hardly surprising that these drugs are usually ineffective. They appear to be effective in some women although these could perhaps represent women who have detrusor instability which has been missed. Unfortunately, as the numbers of women with sensory urgency is small, most drug studies do not look at them separately and the true success rates of treatment are unknown. If the underlying problem is psychological in nature, the placebo effect would be expected to be high. Further placebo-controlled, prospective trials are needed to elucidate this.

Neuromodulation

Electrical stimulation of the sacral nerve roots has been shown to modulate neural reflex behaviour of the lower urinary tract (Thon et al 1991). This concept of neuromodulation in the treatment of patients with conditions refractory to standard treatments has been assessed using percutaneous insertion of electrodes through the sacral foramina for a short period of time prior to insertion of a permanent implantable prosthesis. Thon et al (1991) described limited success in the treatment of patients with sensory urgency using this technique although success rates were higher in the detrusor instability group of patients in their study. At present this technique is not widely available on the NHS as the cost is prohibitive.

CONCLUSION

Sensory urgency is a poorly defined and poorly understood condition. Aetiological factors appear to include an underlying psychological abnormality. It is important to exclude detrusor instability and other bladder pathology before making the diagnosis. Treatment options are inadequately evaluated and there is no ideal method available. Much more work is needed to determine aetiology before any improvement can be made in treatment.

REFERENCES

Aitchison M, Carter R, Paterson P, Ferie B 1989 Is the treatment of urgency incontinence a placebo response? Results of a five year follow-up. British Journal of Urology 64(5): 478–480

Anand P 1995 Nerve Growth Factor regulates nociception in human health and disease. British Journal of Anaesthesia 75: 201–208

Bernstein J E, Korman N J, Bickers D R, Dahl M V, Millikan L E 1989 Topical capsaicin treatment of post herpetic neuralgia. Journal of the American Academy of Dermatology 21: 265–270

Cardozo L D, Abrams P H, Stanton S L, Feneley R C L 1978 Idiopathic detrusor instability treated by biofeedback. British Journal of Urology 50: 521–523

Creighton S M, Pearce J M, Robson I, Wang K, Stanton S L 1991 Sensory urgency: how full is your bladder? British Journal Obstetrics and Gynaecology 98(12): 1287–1289

Creighton S M, Plevnik S, Stanton S L 1993 Urethral sensitivity in the aetiology of sensory urgency. British Journal of Urology 73: 190–195

Frazer M I, Haylen B T 1989 Trigonal sensitivity testing in women. Journal of Urology 141(2); 356–358

Frazer M I, Haylen B T, Sisson M 1990 Do women with idiopathic sensory urgency have early interstitial cystitis. British Journal of Urology 66: 274–278

Griffiths C J, Assi M J, Style R A, Neal D E 1987 Ambulatory monitoring of bladder and detrusor pressure. British Journal of Urology 6: 161–162

Holmes D M, Stone A R, Bary P R, Richards C J, Stephenson T P 1983 Bladder training – 3 years on. British Journal of Urology 55: 660–664

Holmes D M, Plevnik S, Stanton S L 1985 Bladder neck electric conductance test in the investigation of sensory urgency and detrusor instability. Proceedings of the International Continence Society. London, 96–100

International Continence Society 1992 The standardisation of terminology of lower urinary tract function. Scandinavian Journal Urology and Nephrology suppl. 114.

Jarvis G J 1982 The management of urinary incontinence due to primary vesical sensory urgency by bladder drill. British Journal of Urology 54: 374–376

Kieswetter H 1977 Mucosal sensory thresholds of the urinary bladder and urethra measured electrically. Urologia Internationalis 32: 437–448

Lowe E M, Anand P, Fowler C J, Osborne J L 1997 Increased nerve growth factor in the urinary bladder of women with idiopathic season urgency and interstitial cystitis. British Journal of Urology 79(4): 572–7

Macaulay A J, Stern R S, Stanton S L 1991 Psychological aspects of 211 patients attending a urodynamic unit. Journal of Psychosomatic Research 35(1): 1–10

Maggi C A, Barbanti G, Santicioli P (1989) Cystometric evidence that capsaicin sensitive nerves modulate the afferent branch of micturition reflex in humans. Journal of Urology 142: 150–154.

Mahoney D T, Laferte R O, Blais D J 1977 Integral storage and voiding reflexes. Neurophysiologic concept of continence and micturition. Urology IX, 95–106

Malmgren A, Ekblad E, Sundler F, Andersson K E, Andersson P O 1990 Muscarinic supersensitivity in the rat urinary bladder after capsaicin pretreatment. Acta Physiologica Scandinavica 138(3): 377–387

McMahon S B, Dmitrieva N, Koltzenburg M (1995) Visceral pain. British Journal of Anaesthesia 75: 132–144

Peattie A B, Plevnik S. Stanton S L, 1988 The use of bladder neck electric conductance in the investigation and management of sensory urge incontinence in the female. Journal of the Royal Society of Medicine 81: 442

Powell P H, Feneley R C L 1980 The role of urethral sensation in clinical urology. British Journal of Urology 52: 539–541

Rendell M S, Katims J J, Richter R, Rowlands F 1989 A comparison of nerve conduction velocities and current perception thresholds as correlates of clinical severity of diabetic sensory neuropathy. Journal of Neurology, Neurosurgery and Psychiatry 52: 502–511

Thon W F, Baskin L S, Jonas U, Tanagho E A, Schmidt R A 1991 Neuromodulation of voiding dysfunction and pelvic pain. World Journal of Urology: 9: 138–141

Tursky B, Watson P D 1964 Controlled physical and subjective intensities of electric shock. Psychophysiology 1: 151–162

White J C, Sweet W H 1955 Pain. Its mechanisms and neurosurgical control. Thomas, Springfield, Illinois

SECTION 3
CHAPTER

29

Urinary tract infection

JOHN A THORNHILL AND JOHN M FITZPATRICK

INTRODUCTION

The adult woman is more susceptible to urinary tract infection than her male counterpart. Almost 4% of adolescent girls have bacteriuria on population screening and this increases roughly by 1 to 2% for every decade of age. Urinary infections may be repetitive at occasional or frequent intervals and this is especially so in elderly women or during pregnancy.

Infection of the female urinary tract can create a dilemma for the practising clinician. The diagnosis may be straightforward but subsequent decisions may be difficult; for example, the amount of investigation, the intensity and length of treatment, and whether to institute prophylaxis during follow-up. In addition to these difficult decisions there is the fear of missing some underlying pathology or ongoing destructive process that could ultimately lead to renal failure.

Fortunately, we can now successfully manage the vast majority of urinary tract infections (Iravani 1991). This is regardless of their severity and frequency and it is largely because our knowledge of the pathogenesis of female urinary infections has improved. We now know that the vulnerability to recurrent infections is due to carriage of abnormally high bacterial counts on the vaginal and urethral mucosa. These bacteria ascend and multiply in the bladder to cause infection. The bacteria on the perineum are spread from the rectum and they remain viable in large numbers in susceptible individuals because of special epithelial receptors. This disease model has implications for diagnosis and management: it underlines the limitations of interpreting bacterial counts in so-called mid-stream urine specimens because of the risk of contamination from the perineum. Antibiotics that affect the faecal flora by inducing bacterial resistance will make future treatment of urinary infections more difficult because it is these resistant organisms which become established on the perineum and thence predominate in any further urinary infection. This also explains how low-dose antibiotic prophylaxis with drugs which do not adversely affect the faecal reservoir are so effective in preventing recurrent urinary infection. The causative organisms in the urine, originating from the rectum, remain sensitive to the antibiotic which is excreted in the urine. We now have better diagnostic methods to identify underlying urological abnormalities that may cause bacterial persistence despite treatment. We are better equipped with newer antibiotics which have improved pharmacokinetics and a more specific spectrum of antimicrobial activity.

PATHOGENESIS

The establishment of an ascending urinary tract infection follows a sequence of events that is governed by host defence mechanisms and bacterial virulence factors (Bergman 1991). As already mentioned, studies have shown that urinary infection in the female is preceded by colonization of the vaginal and urethral mucosa. Stamey's meticulous investigations of the vaginal bacterial flora indicate that the incidence, duration and density of colonization by enterobacteria is greater among women who are susceptible to urinary infections (Stamey & Kaufman 1975). The reason for this phenomenon is that gram negative bacteria adhere more avidly *in vitro* to the squamous vaginal epithelium in susceptible women (Fowler & Stamey 1977). This adherence is due to a combination of bacterial virulence and impaired local immunity of the epithelial cell layer. Specific adhesions on the surface of *E. coli* have been identified and studies show that *in vitro* adherence can be divided into two types, dependent on the sensitivity to mannose. Sensitivity is due to mannose binding sites and is associated with micro-organisms that are heavily fimbriated. Mannose negative activity, that is *in vitro* adherence unaffected by the addition of D-mannose, is associated with non-fimbriated bacteria. Another group of mannose resistant bacteria with fimbriae have also been discovered. The different strains of *E. coli* can now by typed in terms of virulence by using these *in vitro* methods.

The association of bacterial adherence with the severity of clinical infection has been studied (Svanborg-Eden et al 1978). They and others (Orskov & Orskov 1983) correlated the susceptibility to recurrent infections with the adhesive properties of the bacteria in the urethra and vaginal vault and confirmed that adherence is associated with bacterial fimbriae. Other factors also play a role in the adherence of bacteria to vaginal cells. Adherence is greater in the early phase of the menstrual cycle and oestrogens have been implicated (Reid et al 1983). Colonization and bacteriuria are more common in postmenopausal women although it has not been possible to correlate this phenomenon with the alteration of oestrogen levels (Brocklehurst et al 1977). Parsons & Schmidt (1982) have shown the influence of vaginal pH on vaginal colonization in the postmenopausal group. Other studies demonstrate adherence of bacteria not only to vaginal squamous epithelium but also to buccal mucosa and this relationship suggests that receptors are present on squamous cells throughout the body. The concept of specific receptor sites in susceptible individuals has been investigated by Schaeffer who suggests that this is a specific genotypic trait (Schaeffer et al 1982). The antigen A3 has been identified in some patients, so HLA A3 may be a risk factor for recurrent urinary infections (Schaeffer 1989). Blood group antigen has also been implicated (Schaeffer et al 1993). The next phase in a developing infection is the passage of organisms into the bladder, and the ascent of bacteria along the female urethra is facilitated by its short anatomical length. This contrasts with the adult male in whom bacteriuria is rarely encountered even though preputal colonization is common, especially in uncircumcised males; the length of the urethra is therefore of significance. In paraplegic individuals, urethral organisms are the cause of bacteriuria but only in males using intermittent self-catheterization. Sexual intercourse can also cause the appearance of bacteria in a previously sterile bladder urine and epidemiological studies support the clinical impression that intercourse initiates bacteriuria. *E. coli* bacteriuria is also linked with the use of spermicidal foam and diaphragm contraceptive methods (Hooton et al 1991). However, the importance of sexual activity in the ascent of bacteria along the urethra is limited to those women who already have high colony counts on the vaginal mucosa (Elster et al 1981). Another predisposing factor for the spread of bacteria to the bladder relates to the histology of bladder outlet. The vagina, urethra and bladder trigone share the same embryological origin from the urogenital sinus. The squamous epithelium of the urethra, with its inherent susceptibility to bacterial adherence, therefore extends upwards and includes the bladder trigone.

There is no doubt that urine provides a good culture medium for bacteria but inoculation of organisms into the bladder rarely develops into florid infection. This confirms how the bladder itself can resist infection. There is little evidence to support an intrinsic bactericidal effect but there are other mechanisms which prevent infection (Cobbs & Kaye 1967). Vesical emptying and urine flow are particularly important in maintaining sterilization of the urinary tract. The bladder can also inhibit bacterial adherence to urothelial cells and this reduced adherence augments the effectiveness of the urine washout factor. The bladder may exert part of its antiadherence effect by secretion of antibodies. Secretory IgA has been implicated because of Uehling's studies which correlated decreased adherence with rising bladder antibody levels (Uehling et al 1982). The other major protective factor against adherence is the bladder's surface glycosaminoglycan layer. Early studies have shown how destruction of this secreted surface polysaccharide layer enables a marked increase in bacterial adherence (Parsons et al 1977). Further work has shown that if the glycosaminoglycan layer is removed, exogenous compounds such as heparin or pentosanpolysulfate are capable of immediately restoring antiadherence capability (Hanno 1978). The nature of this antiadherence mechanism is probably due to the hydrophillic properties of the polysaccharide layer (Parsons 1986). These surface compounds attract a layer of water to themselves and interpose this between the bladder and the urine. This water layer protects against bacterial adherence and also against toxic substances in the urine.

While the bladder has efficient physiological protective mechanisms against the development of infection, the dominant factor that prevents ascending urethral infection is the antireflux design of the vesicoureteric junction. This one-way valve allows the efflux of normally sterile ureteric urine but not the reflux of bladder urine with its higher propensity for bacterial contamination. This protective barrier may sometimes be ineffective, as occurs in cases with vesicoureteric reflux. This condition may be congenital in origin or can be secondary to a high-pressure or obstructed bladder. An infected bladder in association with reflux inevitably results in inoculation and spread of bacteria to the ureteric urine. Bacteria may also cross the normal vesicoureteric junction, although localization studies on the specific sites of infection confirm how rarely this event occurs, even in women who suffer recurrent bacteriuria (Neal 1989).

Bacterial motility becomes a significant factor in the event that bacteria enter the lower ureter. While the normal flow of urine down the ureter tends to wash out organisms, bacteria can ascend against the flow of a moving column of urine. This is due to the physics of laminar flow but animal studies also show that bacteria in the ureter can inhibit normal peristalsis (Roberts 1975). This reduction in peristalsis causes ureteric dilatation and the ureter may consequently act as a reservoir associated with intrarenal reflux of urine. In the presence of infection this form of intrarenal or high-grade reflux leads to severe inflammation and renal scarring. This sequence is more prevalent in infants and children because of the sensitivity of their renal papillae but it can persist into adulthood and may not present until that time. Also, while this damaging type of infection due to congenital vesicoureteric incompetence does not occur as a primary event in the adult female, a similar situation can arise in the presence of a combined ureteric obstruction and infection. Infections in infancy may predispose to problems in adulthood and animal studies show that experimental *E. coli* infection of the upper tract in young animals can prevent maturation of the vesicoureteric junction and the usual consequent disappearance of congenital reflux. This may explain why vesicoureteric reflux in children without infection generally disappears by the age of 4 while only 80% of cases with infection show resolution of their reflux (Baker et al 1966).

The primary response within the kidney is well documented and following intrarenal reflux, fimbriated *E. coli* attach to glycolipid receptors on the surface of the renal tubular epithelium (Roberts 1986). Bacterial multiplication loads the tubules and complement activation causes aggregation of platelets and white cells with subsequent prostaglandin release. Superoxide radicals produced within phagocytes are also liberated into the tubules, causing cell membrane disruption and tissue death.

The renal damage associated with bacterial infection may be rapid and extensive although this process can be prevented by early antibiotic treatment (Janson & Roberts 1978). Knowledge of the pathogenesis of urinary infection is important in interpreting the different clinical presentations with infection. It also helps in understanding the principles of current therapy and gives an insight into possible future treatment approaches.

CAUSATIVE ORGANISMS

Many bacterial species have been isolated from patients with urinary infection but the commonest organism responsible for adult female infection is *Escherichia coli* (Hooton & Stamm 1991). This is followed in frequency by *Proteus mirabilis* and other aerobes including *Klebsiella, Pseudomonas* and *Serratia*. The gram positive organisms include *Streptococcus faecalis* and coagulase negative *Staphylococci*. Non-coliform infections are more common in the chronic or complicated situation (Sobel & Kaye 1990). Anaerobic infections are rare, although fastidious organisms such as *Lactobacilli, Corynebacteria* and *Streptococcus milleri* have been isolated when appropriate culture methods are used. The full significance of anaerobic bacteria is not fully understood, although they have been implicated in the large group of cases with clinical infection but sterile urine routine aerobic culture methods. The role of *Chlamydia trachomatis* (which can be detected using immunohistochemical techniques to detect chlamydial antigens in bladder tissue) is also debated in this latter group (Shurbaji et al 1990).

CLINICAL FEATURES

Urinary infection can be divided into either upper or lower tract infection, depending on the principal site of involvement. The two groups are not mutually exclusive but they are usually clinically discernible. The distinction is important because the intensity of management differs between them. Many descriptive terms are used to cover the array of clinical presentation including pyelonephritis, pyelitis, cystitis and urethritis. Many of these terms were conceived before there was a proper understanding of the nature of urinary infection but they are still commonly used and therefore merit description.

Acute pyelonephritis

Historically, the term acute pyelonephritis was used by pathologists to describe the histological features associated with infection. Over the years, it has been adopted into clinical use and is now most commonly applied in the context of acute bacterial pyelonephritis. This is rather unfortunate because we now know that the histological features of pyelonephritis can be caused by a number of diseases other than acute infection. This condition is characterized by loin pain (which may be bilateral), rigors and pyrexia. Symptoms can be severe and there may be exquisite renal angle tenderness. The diagnosis is confirmed by the presence of pyuria and bacteriuria. There may also be symptoms of frequency, dysuria and urgency but the upper tract features are predominant. Intravenous urography is usually grossly normal but there may be suitable diagnostic clues such as renal enlargement, striations, impaired contrast excretion and non-obstructive dilatation of the collecting system and ureter (Kass et al 1976). Acute pyelonephritis does not generally carry a high morbidity but in elderly women or in those with renal impairment the course of the disease can be rapid and lead to gram negative septicaemia and/or acute renal failure.

Chronic pyelonephritis

In contrast to acute pyelonephritis which has recognizable clinical features, chronic pyelonephritis has no specific clinical diagnostic criteria. Similarly, while in adults there are generally no residual pathological sequelae after acute pyelonephritis, except for occasional focal scarring, in the chronic condition there are areas of chronic inflammation, scarring and atrophy. The condition may be detected incidentally for instance during pregnancy or the patient may present with an apparent 'simple' urinary infection. Alternatively, the condition may lead to renal failure in severe cases and the clinical features reflect this complication in such ways as high blood pressure, uraemia or simply generalized malaise. In the absence of clinical signs the diagnosis is usually made on intravenous urography. One or both kidneys appear shrunken on X-ray, with clubbing of the affected calyces and parenchymal thinning. If unilateral, then the opposite kidney may be hypertrophied or in bilateral cases there may be islands of preserved renal tissue that enlarge and appear as pseudotumours on X-ray. Approximately 1 in 4 patients in renal dialysis programmes have suffered chronic pyelonephritis and in one series 4% had suffered pyelonephritis during pregnancy (Schechter et al 1971). These figures underline the sinister potential of this condition but when viewed prospectively in adults diagnosed with unilateral disease the prognosis is 100% recovery and even in those with bilateral disease the 5-year survival is 95% (Gower 1976). It is mainly paediatricians who are exposed to cases with the most malignant disease course although, as discussed later, pregnant women are also at risk.

Pyonephrosis

Pyonephrosis is a complication of pyelonephritis in patients in whom there is obstruction of the renal tract. This is most commonly due to a calculus but it may be secondary to non-calculous hydronephrosis such as occurs with congenital pelviureteric junction obstruction. The resultant hydronephrosis becomes filled with pus, the patient develops a swinging pyrexia and may become gravely ill. The enlarged kidney may be palpable and very tender.

A nephrostomy drain can be inserted under X-ray or ultrasound control and this confirms the presence of pus. It is used for antegrade X-ray studies to determine the site and cause of obstruction and is left *in situ* to allow drainage of the obstructed system (Lang 1990). In the absence of an underlying calculous obstruction, the diagnosis of tuberculosis may be considered.

Cystitis

Cystitis simply means inflammation of the bladder but this pathological term is most commonly used to imply an acute infection of the bladder. In fact, the pathological findings vary widely depending on the cause, which may not be infective in origin. Cystitis is typically associated with symptoms of frequency, urgency and dysuria; there may also be suprapubic discomfort, and haematuria is commonly seen. The condition may be acute, recurrent or chronic and it can cause a variable level of morbidity. It is customary in the clinical setting to divide patients by their symptoms into those with infection of the bladder alone and those with associated upper tract involvement. This was based on the view that those infections with extension to the upper tracts were more difficult to eradicate and would be more susceptible to renal damage. However, localization studies have shown the inaccuracy of the clinical distinction between upper and lower tract infections. Also, the response to treatment is the same in uncomplicated cases.

The symptoms of frequency and dysuria suggest an infection of the lower urinary tract but it is important to remember that diagnostic confirmation requires the presence of significant bacteriuria. Several studies have identified a significant proportion of women with recurring frequency and dysuria that appear to have a sterile urine even on correctly timed and repeated cultures (Dans & Klaus 1976). The term 'urethral syndrome' is applied to this group with frequency and dysuria in the absence of significant bacteriuria. Unfortunately, in clinical practice patients are too often labelled with this condition without adequate urine testing. Accurate diagnosis demands careful and frequent urine cultures at the onset of symptoms and some would argue that specimens be taken by suprapubic aspiration. Many papers on the 'urethral syndrome' or 'frequency and dysuria syndrome' have failed to meet these criteria (Shortcliffe & Stamey 1986a). Another problem is that a proportion of these patients with non-infected urine have interstitial cystitis but this diagnosis is easily overlooked. In this latter condition there is panmural inflammation of the bladder and a variable level of resultant fibrosis. The aetiology remains obscure but there is marked leucocyte infiltration and mast cells in particular have been implicated as mediators of these pathological changes. The cardinal symptom is suprapubic pain relieved by micturition and this should always alert the clinician to the possibility of the diagnosis.

INVESTIGATIONS – URINE EXAMINATION

Bacteriuria

The only valid method of confirming urinary infection is by demonstrating 'significant' bacteriuria and by traditionally defined limits:

- Less than 10^3 bacteria/ml is probable contamination
- 10^3–10^5 bacteria/ml may be significant and requires a repeat assay
- Greater than 10^5 bacteria/ml probably represents an infection.

Overzealous application of these levels can however cause errors both in overdiagnosis and underdetection. For instance, in the general population, as many as 3–6% of asymptomatic sexually active women have bacteriuria and this level rises to 10% in the elderly. These findings prompted workers to suggest that such women, regardless of symptoms, should be treated. The aim was to prevent the situation of patients presenting with renal complications from infection by searching out and treating all women in the community that had bacteriuria. The hypothesis was false and it took several years before Asscher and others confirmed that this large subpopulation of females with asymptomatic bacteriuria do not represent a group at risk of developing serious renal disease, nor do they require treatment (Asscher et al 1969).

The problem of overdiagnosis of urinary infection arises from the method of urine sampling and it underlines the limitation of a strict 10^5/ml cut-off point. Women often carry large numbers of pathogenic bacteria on their perineum which can contaminate an otherwise sterile mid-stream urine sample. A single urine specimen showing more than 10^5 bacteria/ml has a 20% chance of being due to contamination alone.

The other problem with the 10^5/ml limit is one of underdetection and as many as 20–40% of women with symptomatic infections have less than 10^5 bacteria per ml. These lower than expected bacterial counts result from a combination of factors including the slow doubling time of bacteria in urine (45 minutes), frequent micturition (maybe every 39 minutes) due to irritation, and a high fluid intake. The problem of underdiagnosis is highlighted by Stamm who advises treating any symptomatic patient who has a bacterial count as low as 100 per ml (Stamm et al 1982).

Obtaining urine by the standard mid-stream method has therefore an intrinsic error when applying traditional colony count guidelines. Alternative techniques include suprapubic puncture, cystoscopy sampling or urethral catheterization. Even a low count obtained via suprapubic aspiration should be considered significant (Johnson 1991). However, these methods are invasive and are unwarranted in the majority of uncomplicated cases.

White cell count

The detection of pyuria supports a diagnosis of urinary infection, and especially so if the bacterial colony count is significant, but pyuria is only a sign of inflammation and it may not be bacterial in origin. Moreover, white cell contamination can occur in the absence of infection and lower counts than expected can be seen in cases with recurring infections. One of the principal roles of white cell counting is in diagnosing urinary infection in the acutely ill patient before cultures become available. It may also be of help in women with low colony counts, but who are strongly suspected of having significant infection. Lastly, the detection of white cell casts may lead one to suspect the presence of renal disease, and sterile pyuria may be the first clue in diagnosing tuberculosis.

Haematuria

Haematuria is commonly seen in women with urinary tract infection but this is variable and its detection is not reliable in making the diagnosis of infection. Haematuria is particularly important for another reason, and that is its association with urological tumours. It must always be considered significant until this diagnosis has been excluded by an adequate clinical, radiological and cystoscopic work-up. There is a further problem posed by a proportion of women who have recurrent episodes of haematuria associated with repetitive urinary infections. This can persist over a long period of time and it will then be necessary to repeat radiological investigations and cystoscopy with biopsies, even though initial tumour work-up some time previously had been normal. It is also important to emphasize that the radiological and cystoscopic findings may be quite unremarkable with carcinoma *in situ* of the bladder. This condition can only be confirmed by histology and one must therefore maintain a high index of suspicion and always proceed to bladder biopsies if there is any possibility of this diagnosis.

The presence of proteinuria is irrelevant to making a diagnosis of urinary infection although it may be an indication of a concomitant renal or extrarenal medical disorder. Its frequent detection irrespective of the presence or absence of disease is at least partially due to errors in interpreting the results of labstick urine tests.

SPECIALIZED INVESTIGATIONS

Specialized investigations are not necessary in the majority of simple urinary infections. Nor would it be feasible to investigate such large numbers of patients, the bulk of whom are treated at primary health care level. In addition, it is now recognized that progressive renal damage does not result from urinary tract infections in adults where the urinary tract is anatomically and physiologically normal. However, questions must be answered in any patient with urinary infection:

- Is there a possibility of renal damage?
- Can this be prevented by the detection and management of an underlying pathological cause such as calculus, reflux or obstruction?
- Could there be a concomitant tumour with secondary or incidental infection?

The problem therefore lies not in the choice of investigations but in the selection of patients for investigation from the large sub-population with bacteriuria.

The task is to divide cases into complicated and uncomplicated urinary tract infections and to do this one uses clinical predictors to identify the high-risk cases. The frequency of infection is important and isolated urinary infection, which is notoriously common in healthy adult females, can be presumed innocent. A proportion of women suffer recurrent infections over a period of time and they require investigation even though there is a low detection rate of underlying pathology. The severity of infection is also important and the clinical presentation may vary from an unpleasant symptomatic episode to the opposite end of the spectrum, with life-threatening septicaemia and severe debilitation. Prompt investigation in the latter group is clearly warranted to detect any remedial obstructive lesion.

Investigation is obviously indicated in patients with features suggestive of underlying renal tract disease or in those with a positive past history. Included in this list would be stone disease, polycystic kidneys or ureteric reflux as a child. In contrast to women with normal kidneys who generally do not suffer renal damage from infection, in this latter group the renal pathology and infection create an ongoing destructive cycle with loss of renal function. The classic example is where a small and innocent calculus which is metabolic in origin becomes infected and then grows rapidly because of infection to cause renal destruction.

There are also those cases who suffer urinary infection in the presence of concomitant generalized disease. Example are diabetes, analgesic abuse and neurological problems such as multiple sclerosis or spinal injury. These cases may initially have normal renal investigations but the combination of infection with their medical problem can lead to accelerated renal decompensation.

Another indication for further investigation is the identification of certain infecting organisms in the urine. The commonest example is *Proteus mirabilis*, a urea-splitting organism which is associated with the formation of struvite (Staghorn) renal calculi. *Proteus* has the unique feature of forming biofilms and subsequent encrustation, especially if there is a foreign body, e.g. a catheter, present (Reid et al 1992). Another organism which should not be overlooked is *Mycobacterium tuberculosis* and patients with sterile pyuria should have consecutive early morning urine samples examined with Ziehl Nielsen staining and special TB cultures as part of their work-up. As previously mentioned, the presence of haematuria either clinically or on microscopy is an absolute indication for further investigations, including cystoscopy. This rule applies even when a urinary infection is proven and is presumably the sole cause of the haematuria. Infection can occur concomitantly with a tumour anywhere in the renal tract and it is frequently seen in conjunction with bladder tumours which become necrotic and secondarily infected.

Renal ultrasound

Ultrasound has become increasingly popular as technology has improved and in many centres it has replaced the intravenous urogram as the primary investigation for the renal tract (Aslaksan et al 1990). It has the advantage of speed and it is totally non-invasive. There is no danger of allergy or radiation and it can be freely used in women of childbearing age. It has surpassed the IVU in assessing bladder tumours and is a sensitive measure of residual urine after micturition. Many contemporary gynaecologists and urologists are trained in ultrasound imaging and interpretation. Coupled with the low installation and maintenance costs, this means that ultrasound can now be adopted into office practice by clinicians who are confident to perform the procedure on their own. The principal drawback of ultrasound is its inability to visualize the mid-portion of the ureter. This is the site of many obstructive lesions and stones, but even in this instance any secondary hydronephrosis is detected which leads the clinician to more specific investigations.

Intravenous urogram (IVU)

Before ultrasonography was developed, the intravenous urogram used to be the cornerstone of investigation for the renal tract. The IVU is a reasonable determinant of the site and severity of ureteric obstructive lesions but its application in urinary tract infection has been disappointing, with at least 75% of investigations being normal. Its radiation risk also makes it unsuitable for routine use in sexually active women.

Micturating cystogram (MCU)

This investigation is used to detect and assess the severity of vesicoureteric reflux. This is one of the conditions which predispose to upper tract urinary infections that may require surgical intervention. The principal role for MCU is in children but, as discussed later, it is indicated in a proportion of women who suffer recurrent infection.

Modern teaching on reflux nephropathy tells us that it is ascending infection with reflux and not refluxing urine *per se* that causes renal damage (Rolleston et al 1975). Also, the most significant renal damage occurs in infancy or possibly even *in utero* and subsequent scarring and deterioration during childhood is principally a consequence of this initial major ascending infection (Smellie & Normand 1985). The aim in adults is therefore to prevent any further renal damage due to infection. This is primarily achieved by controlling lower tract bacteriuria with antibiotic prophylaxis which secondarily prevents the development of ascending infection (Smellie et al 1981; Smellie 1991). This theory and its application are attractive to many physicians because it shifts the emphasis from the control of reflux to the control of infection and it appears to remove the eventuality of surgery. It is imperative, however, that the management of reflux be kept in perspective and all cases with uncontrolled ascending infection secondary to reflux must be identified. The margin for further renal deterioration may be small and one must opt for surgical correction of reflux early if conservative measures fail to control the infection/destruction process.

The indications for an MCU in women are clear. It is required in women with clinically recurring upper tract infections. It is also indicated in women with clinical lower tract infections in whom one detects radiological evidence of upper tract damage. It should also be considered in women of childbearing age with uncontrolled lower tract infections. Although the upper tracts may be radiologically normal in this latter group, they would be at particular risk of pyelonephritis during pregnancy and this is compounded by the presence of reflux.

Computerized tomography (CT)

There is no doubt that CT offers the best anatomical detail of the urinary tract (Benson et al 1986), but it is not necessary in the vast majority of infections. Because of its ready availability it has almost become a first line investigation in some specialist centres in the United States but this approach cannot be justified elsewhere in terms of expense and time scale. It is more logical and practical to limit CT to the small minority of cases with complicated urinary infection and in whom both ultrasound and IVU are equivocal. In such cases there is a definite role for CT with its multidimensional imaging and its accuracy in assessing tissue density as well as size.

Cystoscopy

As with radiological investigations, cystoscopy is not used to diagnose urinary tract infection *per se*; rather it is used to detect an underlying cause, an associated complication, or most importantly to rule out urothelial carcinoma. It is primarily used to detect mucosal malignancy and, as already emphasized, it is always indicated if there is haematuria. In such cases the presence of a urinary infection does not preclude the existence of a concomitant bladder tumour. The role for cystoscopy in the remainder of cases is less clear. This group includes those with recurrent urinary infections but normal radiology and no haematuria. Cystoscopy generally has little to add to radiological procedures but the advent of small bore flexible fibreoptic instruments has made the procedure so quick, safe and acceptable to patients that it is easily performed in the out-patient department.

Radionuclide scanning

A very small proportion of cases with urinary infection will need radionuclide scanning and these are always complicated infections. Gallium scanning was previously used to detect infection, and especially a renal or perinephric abscess (Patel et al 1980), but this has been superseded by ultrasound and CT scanning. The nucleotide DMSA (dimercaptosuccinate 9 mm TC) is retained in the renal tubules and scanning therefore provides an anatomical and physiological map of renal tissue as well as a clear picture of the divided renal function. This knowledge about the precise distribution of non-functioning and healthy areas within a kidney is particularly useful if surgery, especially partial nephrectomy, is contemplated. DTPA (diethylenetriaminepenta-acetic acid) is currently the standard radionuclide used if there is a question of concomitant obstruction. Two important measurements can be made with the DTPA renogram: calculation of glomerular filtration rate and assessment of the contribution of each kidney to total renal function. The DTPA scan is a sensitive monitor of renal function where deterioration is suspected. The radionuclide scans with DTPA and DMSA therefore give information about the presence of obstruction and the amount of functioning renal tissue. They are appropriate baseline studies in patients with calculi or chronic pyelonephritis and are partially helpful if surgery is contemplated.

MANAGEMENT

There are four aspects to the management of urinary tract infections. General and supportive measures are used to eradicate infection and relieve symptoms. Antimicrobial therapy involves the correct choice, dosage and duration of appropriate antibiotic. An underlying cause for infection such as obstruction or calculus is sought. Lastly, the patient is observed for the development of complications such as septicaemia, pyonephrosis or the persistence of infection.

General and supportive measures

The intensity of supportive management depends on the severity of infection, which can range from a mild symptomatic episode to full-blown septicaemia. In all cases, except those in renal failure, fluid intake is increased to a minimum of 2 litres per day to encourage diuresis. In combination with regular bladder emptying, this simple measure can eradicate a significant proportion of cases with uncomplicated lower urinary tract infection. In a more severe attack, oral hydration may need to be supplemented by intravenous fluids. This is especially so if vomiting becomes a prominent feature, as can occur in pregnancy. In the most severe presentation of septicaemic shock there is an urgent need for volume expansion and intensive monitoring. Vasoactive drugs and assisted ventilation may be required. Current research is focused towards counteracting the effects of endotoxaemia by using antibodies against the cytokines which are implicated in this process (Roberts & Kaack 1993). Early identification of a potentially serious infection is also highly desirable (Leibovico et al 1992) and helps treatment.

Antimicrobial therapy

Antibiotics are the mainstay of treatment of urinary infection. Standard treatment eradicates up to 90% of first infections or re-infections in the normal host. A sterile urine can be achieved within hours of commencement of antibiotic when an appropriate agent is used. This predictable and remarkable outcome is due to the fact that most of the commonly available antimicrobials cover the necessary spectrum of bacteria. Sensitivity is therefore rarely an issue, even when an antibiotic has to be prescribed before the results of urine culture. The choice of antibiotic is based on a number of factors including site of infection, age of patient, complicating host factors and history of the infection (Faro 1992). Choice of antibiotic is also influenced by its pharmacokinetics, especially two factors: the level of absorption from the gastrointestinal tract and the percentage of drug excreted in the urine. Drugs which are poorly absorbed from the bowel alter the indigenous gut flora and initiate the development of resistant strains. Subsequent urinary re-infection with these resistant strains, as occurs in susceptible women, may then be more difficult to eradicate, although re-infection within 1 month of therapy is not common in practice (Harrison et al 1974; Kraft & Stamey 1977). Shortcliffe & Stamey (1986b) emphasize the importance of achieving a sterile urine during treatment and this end result is governed by urinary rather than serum antibiotic concentration. Fortunately, most of the oral antibiotics with gram negative activity are concentrated in the urine, so that the activity of many antimicrobials is substantially greater than suggested by *in vitro* testing.

The duration of antibiotic therapy has been widely debated and in practice treatment beyond 7 days is generally unwarranted. The results of further abbreviated treatment lasting 3 days or even a single-dose schedule are also comparable to more prolonged dosage (Savand-Feston et al 1982; Harbond & Gruneberg 1981; Leibovico & Wysenbeek 1991). This perhaps unexpected success rate with a single-dose schedule is because a loading dose of antimicrobial with a prolonged serum half-life such as trimethoprim will maintain inhibitory urine levels for as long as 3 days. The advantages of single-dose therapy include cost savings and improved patient compliance. In addition, postcoital antibiotic prophylaxis using a single dose of trimethoprim-sulfamethaxazole is highly effective for recurrent UTI following intercourse (Stapleton et al 1990). It must also be noted that the incidence of drug-related side-effects such as rashes, gastrointestinal upset and vaginitis are also significantly less than with conventional treatment regimens. The drawback with single-dose treatment is that a proportion of patients, especially those with severe infection, will not respond (Osterberg et al 1990). In some instances, there may be occult upper tract infection (Norrby 1990). Many of the reports advocating reduced dosage schedules exclude those patients with severe or complicated infection (Childs 1992). Despite many studies on this subject, the question of optional dosage schedule remains unanswered for the present (Fowler 1986).

At primary health care level it may be reasonable to use a single-dose schedule but for hospital referral cases it is prudent to adhere to a standard regimen lasting 7 days. This latter patient group includes those with complicated infections, many of whom have had previously unsuccessful treatment. In this latter group the fluoroquinolones may be highly effective, with low expected morbidity (Carson 1993).

URINARY TRACT INFECTION IN PREGNANCY

The incidence of overt urinary tract infections increases in pregnancy (see also Ch. 40), and 1–4% of pregnant women develop clinical acutepyelonephritis (Harris 1979). This is not because pregnant women are more susceptible to acquiring bacteriuria. In fact, the incidence of asymptomatic bacteriuria at first antenatal visit is the same as the general female population (2–6% for this age group). Rather, the anatomical and physiological changes associated with pregnancy alter the normal course of bacteriuria. They facilitate the development of infection, its spread to the upper tracts, and increase the risk of re-infection during the pregnancy. The only postulated change in bacteria has been linked to the predominance of *E. coli* fimbriae in pregnant patients – a known virulence factor and now apparently related to gestational age (Nowicki et al 1993).

The kidneys, ureters, bladder and urethra all undergo changes in pregnancy (Waltzer 1981). The kidneys expand in size due to increased renal vascular and interstitial volume. The glomerular filtration rate increases by 30–50% during the first trimester but renal tubular reabsorption does not rise correspondingly. Therefore, many substances including protein, glucose, urea and creatinine are excreted in larger than normal amounts. The normal reference values for serum urea and creatinine fall because of increased excretion and this is relevant because what might normally be considered as mild elevations in serum values may be indicative of significant renal impairment. Urinary protein excretion can rise to almost 300 mg in 24 hours before being considered pathological. These and other chemical alterations make the urine a better culture medium for bacteria. Urinary antibiotic clearance is increased, thus causing higher urinary concentrations but only in the short term because serum half-life is reduced.

Decreased peristalsis and progressive dilatation of the upper tracts occurs (Lindheimer & Katz 1970). There is resultant urinary stasis and ureteropelvic volume rises almost tenfold to 50 ml. These effects are primarily induced by progesterone secretion but they are exacerbated by pressure of the gravid uterus in the pelvis. The changes are usually obvious on the right side which may be explained by fetal lie. By 6 weeks postpartum these changes have usually reverted to normal.

The bladder is displaced and compressed by the enlarging uterus and urinary incontinence is not uncommon and is due to a combination of pelvic floor denervation and probably increasing intra-abdominal pressure.

The course of bacteriuria

Estimates vary but approximately 30% of women who have detectable bacteriuria in pregnancy will, if untreated, later develop an episode of clinical acute pyelonephritis (Kincaid-Smith & Bullen 1965). This complication is commonest in the third trimester when stasis is maximal. Before the introduction of antibiotics, premature delivery and perinatal mortality were associated with pyelonephritis in pregnancy but this condition is now treatable and there is no conclusive evidence that women with successfully treated acute pyelonephritis suffer an increased level of obstetric complications (McGrady et al 1985; Gilstrap et al 1981). Acute pyelonephritis in pregnancy is also largely preventable and initial treatment of asymptomatic bacteriuria can reduce the subsequent rate of upper tract infection to 3% or lower (Sweet 1977).

The 'normal' spontaneous clearance rates of asymptomatic bacteriuria are reduced in pregnancy and over 65% of women will remain infected throughout pregnancy if left untreated. Even when treated, about 25% will develop re-infection (Leverno et al 1981), but despite the risk of pyelonephritis and recurrent infections, the detection of bacteriuria does not imply any long-term maternal morbidity provided the renal tract and renal function were normal before conception. Recurrent infection and acute pyelonephritis can be expected in future pregnancies and almost 40% of women have bacteriuria over 15 years after delivery (Zinner & Kass 1971). End-stage renal disease rarely results from infections that are consequent on simple bacteriuria in pregnancy. In postmortem series, only 13 cases with end-stage renal disease were detected in over 8000 autopsies (Freedman 1967). The situation where bacteriuria is detected in women with known renal disease is very different to those with normal renal tracts, as there is a marked increase in the obstetric complication rate and a significant risk of further renal insufficiency. This leads to end-stage disease in almost 50% of cases within 18 months (Davison & Lindheimer 1978). The complication rate in those with less severe renal impairment is not as clear but these women benefit by full work-up and counselling before planning pregnancy. The problem in practice is that we often do not know whether women with detectable bacteriuria at first antenatal visit have concomitant renal disease. In the absence of a positive past history it is difficult to identify this small but important sub-group because serum biochemistry is frequently normal and radiological investigations are not appropriate.

Management

Based on our knowledge of the natural history of bacteriuria in pregnancy, all pregnant women with bacteriuria, whether symptomatic or not, should be treated to prevent subsequent development of pyelonephritis and to help to protect against renal damage should there be a pre-existing renal abnormality. The diagnosis of infection in pregnancy relies almost totally on urine testing. The symptoms of frequency, urgency and dysuria are so common in pregnancy that bacteriological proof is essential. Even in those with classic symptoms and associated pyrexia or loin pain, 50% of subsequent urine cultures will be negative.

For ethical and legal reasons, few antibiotics have been fully evaluated during pregnancy. The choice of antibiotic is important in pregnant women because of the risk of potential maternal or fetal side-effects. In practice, pregnant women have received a wide variety of medications and from this experience we can develop certain recommendations (Kreiger 1986; Doering & Stewart 1978). Tetracyclines are contraindicated throughout pregnancy because of the risk of maternal liver damage and effect on fetal bone and dental development. Erythromycin is not used because of potential liver toxic effects. Chloramphenicol is rarely used because of potential marrow toxicity but it is still available in some underdeveloped regions and it can cause fetal or neonatal death due to high tissue concentration in the fetus. Nitrofurantoin is generally safe except in cases with glucose-6-phosphate dehydrogenase deficiency, when haemolysis can occur. Trimethoprim is a folate antagonist and is therefore not recommended in early pregnancy because of potential teratogenic effects. Sulphonamides are not suitable because they may predispose to neonatal jaundice by competing for bilirubin binding sites.

Excluding these drugs leaves essentially only the penicillins and the cephalosporins. These two drugs have their usual risk of allergy but otherwise appear safe throughout pregnancy. Oral penicillin may be particularly suitable because of its high urinary concentration and low cost. In severe infections an aminoglycoside may be indicated. Its side-effects in pregnancy are no different from usual, therefore monitoring of serum levels is necessary. Antimicrobial therapy is usually continued for 7 days and a sterile urine must be documented by repeat culture. There are few trials as to whether a shorter course of treatment would suffice (Doering & Stewart 1978). If bacteriuria persists then a repeat course is prescribed but ultrasound is recommended to detect any stone or obstruction. In the small minority of cases of pyelonephritis who do not respond to parenteral treatment, it may be necessary to resort to plain X-ray and even intravenous urography. Surgery may be indicated in a small proportion of cases. All cases who have had infection require close scrutiny throughout pregnancy. If bacteriuria recurs, even though it may be asymptomatic, then low-dose antibiotic prophylaxis is indicated.

RECURRENT URINARY INFECTION

A seemingly infinite number of women are referred to a variety of hospital specialists because of recurrent urinary infection and this reflects the high frequency of bacteriuria in adult females. This group is important because of the potential for renal damage in the small proportion who have underlying renal tract pathology. Appropriate and effective treatment therefore demands a clear definition of the problem. Cases must be divided into the aforementioned 'complicated' group and the remaining vast majority who have recurrent urinary infections but with normal renal tracts and little potential for future renal decompensation. As a prerequisite, one must distinguish between relapsing urinary infection and recurrence of an infection.

In the relapsing situation, the focus of infection lies within the renal tract. Antibiotic treatment fails to eradicate infection and this may be for a number of reasons including inadequate tissue or urine concentration or underlying pathology such as stone, stricture or diverticulum. The original organisms remain identifiable in the urine and a full course of appropriate antimicrobial treatment should be restarted. If cultures remain infected then investigation is warranted to detect any surgically remedial cause. If pathology is present but is irreversible then it is reasonable to commence long-term suppressive antibiotic therapy to relieve symptoms and in an attempt to prevent further renal decompensation.

The pathogenesis of recurrent urinary tract infections has already been described. The source of infection is outside the renal tract and susceptibility is due to colonization of the vagina and urethra from the faecal reservoir. Abnormal biological factors render these women with recurrent infections susceptible to the colonization phenomenon.

Treatment

The principles of treatment of recurrent urinary infection differ little from the treatment of an isolated acute episode. Treatment combining general measures and antimicrobial therapy is always indicated in 'complicated' cases such as pregnancy, hypertension, renal disease, ascending infection or infections with *Proteus*. In uncomplicated cases the need for antimicrobial therapy is governed by the severity of symptoms. If attacks are frequently repetitive then antimicrobial prophylaxis is indicated.

It is important in all patients with recurrent urinary infections to explain their problem and create an atmosphere of self-help. There is frequently a functional overlay and there may be worries about developing renal failure and requiring dialysis. There may also be worries about personal hygiene or sexually transmitted diseases. Patients must be encouraged to increase fluid intake and practise regular voiding during the day and before bedtime. Double voiding should be practised if there is any suspicion of inadequate emptying. Micturition after intercourse is recommended if cystitis follows coitus, and vaginal lubricants may be of benefit. Personal hygiene is recommended but many authors condemn the use of bubble baths and vaginal sprays (Cattell 1985).

Antibiotic prophylaxis

Antimicrobials are given in the usual 5-day course to control acute infections but the key to preventing recurrent urinary infection is low-dose prophylaxis using a correctly chosen antibiotic. Prophylactic treatment is only justifiable when the frequency of proven infection exceeds two or more attacks every 6 months. Following a standard antibiotic course, the patient takes a daily single dose for 6 to 12 months. Nighttime dosage should ensure better compliance. Breakthrough infections are rare but can be treated by a conventional course of a different antibiotic and prophylaxis is subsequently restarted. Treatment can be stopped after a year but may need to be reinstated and some may need treatment for life.

Antimicrobial prophylaxis is effective in reducing the frequency of infections and the success of antimicrobial prophylaxis is dependent on the dosage and pharmacokinetics of the antibiotic agent. The aim is to achieve sufficient urinary antibiotic concentration to eradicate bacteria that are inoculated into the urine. At the same time, one wishes to maintain the normal faecal and vaginal flora and thus prevent the development of resistant strains (Lincoln et al 1970). Several antibiotics fulfil these criteria, including trimethoprim alone, trimethoprim and sulfamethoxazole, nitrofurantoin, nalidixic acid and cephalexin (Harding et al 1982). Side-effects are not seen, even after long-term therapy (Pearson et al 1979). Ronald & Harding (1981) concluded that published cumulative experience using trimethoprim 400 mg and sulfamethoxazole 200 mg exceeded 200 patient years and that infections were reduced tenfold to fewer than 0.2 infections per patient year. Unfortunately, while reducing the frequency of attacks, low-dose prophylaxis does not alter the natural history (or tendency) towards infection (Stamm et al 1991).

FUTURE APPROACHES

Our present level of success in treating acute urinary infections and in controlling re-infections by antibiotic prophylaxis is based on our current understanding of the pathogenesis of urinary infection. This knowledge has opened new avenues for research which concentrate on overcoming patient susceptibility and bacterial virulence. Five new approaches to treatment are under current investigation and these are based on bladder mucin layer replacement, competitive exclusion of introital colonizing bacteria, blockage of epithelial receptor sites, inactivation of bacterial haemolysins and, lastly, selective immunization. Much work has concentrated on diminishing bacterial virulence but work in spinal injuries patients, who are particularly susceptible to infections, suggests that focusing on host resistance factors may be more fruitful (Benton et al 1992).

Bladder mucin layer replacement

There is growing appreciation of the importance of the glycosaminoglycan (GAG) mucin layer in protecting the bladder against infection. How the mucin layer is synthesized and how it interferes with bacterial adherence is not fully understood but when adherence is established there is a subsequent sloughing of the mucin layer (Orskov et al 1980). This process facilitates further bacterial adherence and multiplication and the denuded epithelium is open to tissue invasion. The process by which bacteria can disrupt or digest the mucin layer remains undefined (Parsons et al 1984). Clinical estimates suggest that susceptible females may actually excrete reduced amounts of uromucoid (Sobel & Kaye 1985).

GAG replacing agents may therefore conceivably be useful in protecting against the development of infection. The intravesical instillation of synthetic glycosaminoglycans restores antiadherence capability in animals (Parsons 1982). There is also evidence that carbenoxolone can stimulate mucin production and bacterial clearance (Mooreville et al 1983). Further studies are needed to confirm the clinical efficiency of this approach.

Competitive exclusion

The concept whereby pathogenic bacteria colonizing the vagina and perineum might be displaced or replaced by non-pathogenic organisms has been termed 'competitive exclusion'. *Lactobacillus* strains have been identified in the normal flora of the cervix and *in vitro* studies have shown that adherence of *Lactobacillus* can block subsequent adherence of *E. coli* to uroepithelial cells (Chan et al 1984). *In vitro* placement of agar beads containing *Lactobacillus* into the bladder of rats prevents *E. coli* colonization but as yet similar human studies have not been performed (Reid et al 1985). These results are promising and theoretically at least support the concept of competitive exclusion causing a reduced susceptibility to infection. As more becomes known about bacterial adhesions and receptor sites on epithelial cells, attention has been given to preventing infections by the use of adherence blocking agents. Mannose and other disaccharides cause *in vitro* inhibition of *E. coli* adherence to epithelial cells but this experience has not been repeated in animal experiments (Kallenuis et al 1981; Aronson et al 1979). The inoculation of bacteria with 'blocking' disaccharide into the monkey bladder has paradoxically led to higher levels of bacteriuria in the long term (Roberts et al 1984). The practical application of receptor blockers therefore requires further careful evaluation.

Inactivation of bacterial haemolysins

It is well established that *E. coli* has the ability to lyse red cells *in vitro* and it is postulated that bacterial haemolysins play an active role in the development of infection by directly injuring the bladder mucosa (Welsh et al 1981). The genes responsible for haemolysin production are known to be closely linked in the *E. coli* chromosome and recombinant DNA technology can produce either a virulent non-haemolytic *E. coli* or colonies with haemolytic capability (Felmlee et al 1985). To date, no treatments have been developed that use this model but possible ways of preventing haemolytic activity might include either antibody production against haemolysin or an intravesical chemical inhibitor. Another possibility would be competitive exclusion with *E. coli* depleted of the haemolysin gene by recombinant technology.

Selective immunization

It is well recognized that an immune response follows urinary infection and this is reflected in increased urinary IgA levels (Uehling & Steihm 1971). The protective importance of this immune response is not fully established but it does support the concept of immunization against recurrent infections. The initial attempts at immunization in animals were based on systemic active immunization using attenuated *E. coli* or fimbriae but there was no protection against ascending urinary tract infections (Montgomerie et al 1972). Later studies on passive immunization using hybridoma antibodies against bacterial adhesions were more promising but they have not been repeated in humans because of the potential risks with systemic immunization (Silverblatt & Cohen 1979).

Because of the reservations about the safety and efficacy of systemic immunization, the emphasis has shifted towards the concept of local immunization. Experiments in the rat and dog show that intravesical immunization can be shown to decrease bacterial adherence and there is protection against ascending infection (Kaijser et al 1978; Uehling et al 1968). The problem with these experiments is that the catheter used to instill the antigen into the bladder is itself a cause of urinary infections. As a result, other workers have attempted vaginal immunization in monkeys using formalin killed *E. coli* (Uehling 1986). This immunogen evokes a definite local immune response and it appears that the rise in surface levels of anti-*E. coli* antibody are associated with faster clearance of urinary infections. This model is promising but the optional immunogen needs to be identified and local adjuvents to stimulate the immune response are needed. Further investigations are required but the concept of a regular vaginal instillation that prevents recurrent infections is simple and attractive.

The basic hypothesis behind these new approaches to the treatment of urinary infection is that infection is initiated by bacterial adherence to epithelial receptors at the introitus and lower urinary tract. The aim is that somehow a treatment can be developed which prevents or interferes with this adherence mechanism. This is a major shift in thinking from the traditional concept that bacteria appear almost by chance in the urinary tract and that antibiotics are therefore the logical and only solution.

Any change in emphasis should not detract from the unquestionable success of modern antibiotics in treating infections, but there is a new era of urological research which may discover an adjuvant to antibiotics. Hopefully a new agent can augment antibiotic activity in combating infection and also ablate the susceptibility to recurring urinary infections which is so common in women.

REFERENCES

Aronson M, Medilia O, Schori L et al 1979 Prevention of colonization of the urinary tract of mice with Escherichia coli by blocking of bacterial adherence with methyl l-D-manopyranoside. Journal of Infectious Diseases 139: 329–332

Aslaksan A, Boerheim A, Hunskaar S, Gothlin J H 1990 Intravenous urography versus ultrasonography in evaluation of women with recurrent urinary tract infection. Scandinavian Journal of Primary Health Care 8: 85–89

Asscher A W, Sussman M, Waters W E et al 1969 The clinical significance of asymptomatic bacteriuria in the non-pregnant woman. Journal of Infectious Diseases 120: 17–26

Baker R, Maxted W, Maylath J, Shuman I 1966 Relation of age, sex and infection to reflux: data indicating high spontaneous cure rate in paediatric patients. Journal of Urology 95: 27–32

Benson M, Lipuma J P, Resnich M I 1986 The role of imaging studies in urinary tract infection. Urologic Clinics of North America 13(4): 605–625

Benton J, Chawla J, Parry S, Stickler D 1992 Virulence factors in Escherichia coli from urinary tract infections in patients with spinal injuries. Journal of Hospital Infection 22: 117–27

Bergman A 1991 Urinary tract infections in women. Current Opinion in Obstetrics and Gynaecology 3(4): 541–544

Brocklehurst J C, Bee P, Jores D 1977 Bacteriuria in geriatric hospital patients. Its correlation and management. Age and Ageing. 6: 240–245

Carson C C 1993 Antimicrobial agents in urinary tract infections in patients with spinal cord injury. Urologic Clinics of North America 10(3): 443–452

Cattell W R 1985 Principles of management of urinary tract infections. In: Whitfield H N, Hendry W F (eds) Textbook of Genito Urinary Surgery. Churchill Livingstone, London, pp 479–513

Chan R C Y, Bruce A W, Reid G 1984 Adherence of cervical, vaginal and distal urethral normal microbial flora to human uroepithelial cells and the inhibition of adherence of gram negative uropathogens by competitive exclusion. Journal of Urology 131: 596–601

Childs S 1992 Current diagnosis and treatment of urinary tract infections. Urology 40(4): 295–299

Cobbs C G, Kaye D 1967 Antibacterial mechanism in the urinary bladder. Yale Journal of Biology and Medicine 40: 93–108

Dans P E, Klaus B 1976 Dysuria in women. Johns Hopkins Medical Journal 138: 13–18

Davison J M, Lindheimer M D 1978 Renal disease in pregnant women. Clinics in Obstetrics and Gynaecology 21: 411–427

Doering P, Stewart R 1978 The extent and character of drug consumption during pregnancy. Journal of the American Medical Association 239: 843–846

Elster A B, Lach P A, Roghmann K J 1981 Relationship between frequency of sexual intercourse and urinary tract infections in young women. Southern Medical Journal 74: 704–708

Faro S 1992 New considerations in treatment of urinary tract infections in adults. Urology 39: 1–11

Felmlee T, Pellett S, Welsh R A 1985 Nucleolide sequence of an Escherichia coli chromosomal hemolysin. Journal of Bacteriology 163: 94–105

Fowler J E 1986 Urinary tract infections in women. Urologic Clinics of North America 13(4): 673–683

Fowler J E, Stamey T A 1977 Studies of introital colonization in women with recurrent urinary infections; VII. The role of bacterial adherence. Journal of Urology 117: 472–476

Freedman L R 1967 Chronic pyelonephritis at autopsy. Annals of Internal Medicine 66: 697–710

Gilstrap L C, Leveno K J, cunningham F G et al 1981 Renal infection and pregnancy outcome. American Journal of Obstetrics and Gynecology 141: 709–716

Gower P E 1976 A prospective study of patients with radiologic pyelonephritis, papillary necrosis and obstructive atrophy. Quarterly Journal of Medicine 45: 315–419

Hanno P M 1978 The protective effect of heparin in experimental bladder infection. Journal of Surgical Research 25: 324–329

Harbond R B, Gruneberg R N 1981 Treatment of urinary infection with a single dose of amoxycillin, cotrimoxazole or trimethoprim. British Medical Journal 303: 409–415

Harding G K M, Ronald A R, Nicolle L E et al 1982 Long term antimicrobial prophylaxis for recurrent urinary tract infection in women. Review of Infectious Diseases 4: 438–443

Harris R E 1979 The significance of eradication of bacteriuria during pregnancy. Obstetrics and Gynecology 53: 71–73

Harrison W O, Holmes K K, Beldin M E, Wiesner P J, Turck M 1974 A prospective evaluation of recurrent urinary tract infection in women. Clinical Research 22: 125a (abstract)

Hooton T M, Stamm W E 1991 Management of acute uncomplicated urinary tract infection in adults. Medical Clinics of North America 75: 339–357

Hooton T M, Hilber S, Johnson C, Roberts P L, Stamm W E 1991 Escherichia coli bacteriuria and contraceptive method. Journal of the American Medical Association 265: 64–69

Iravani A 1991 Advances in the understanding and treatment of urinary tract infections in young women. Urology 37: 503–511

Janson K L, Roberts J A 1978 Experimental pyelonephritis: V. Functional characteristics of pyelonephritis. Investigative Urology 15: 397–400

Johnson C C 1991 Definitions, classification and clinical presentation of urinary tract infection. Medical Clinics of North America 75: 241–252

Kaijser B, Larsson P, Ollinj S 1978 Protection against ascending Escherichia coli pyelonephritis in rats and significance of local immunity. Infection and Immunity 20: 78–81

Kallenuis G, Mollbyr R, Hultberg H et al 1981 Structure of carbohydrate part of receptor on human uroepithelial cells for pyelonephritogenic Escherichia coli. The Lancet 2: 604–606

Kass E H, Silver T M, Kinnak J W et al 1976 The urographic findings in acute pyelonephritis: non obstructive hydronephrosis. Journal of Urology 116: 544–546

Kincaid-Smith P, Bullen M 1965 Bacteriuria in pregnancy. The Lancet 1: 395–399

Kraft J K, Stamey T A 1977 The natural history of symptomatic recurrent bacteriuria in women. Medicine 56: 55–60

Kreiger J N 1986 Complications and treatment of urinary tract infections in pregnancy. Urologic Clinics of North America 13(4): 685–693

Kunin C M, Sacha E, Paquim A J 1962 Urinary tract infections in children. Prevalence of bacteriuria and associated urological findings. New England Journal of Medicine 26: 1287–1289

Lang E K 1990 Renal, perirenal and pararenal abscess: percutaneous drainage. Radiology 174: 109–113

Leibovico L, Wysenbeek A J Single dose antibiotic treatment for symptomatic urinary tract infections in women: a meta-analysis of randomised trials. Quarterly Journal of Medicine 78: 43–57

Leibovico L, Greenshtain S, Cohen O, Weysenbeek A J 1992 Toward improved empiric management of moderate to severe urinary tract infections. Archives of Internal Medicine 152: 2481–2486

Leverno K J, Harris R E, Gilstrap L C 1981 Bladder versus renal bacteriuria during pregnancy: recurrence after treatment. American Journal of Obstetrics and Gynaecology 139: 403–406

Lincoln K, Lidin Janson G, Wimberg J 1970 Resistant urinary infections resulting from changes in the resistance pattern of faecal flora induced by antibiotics and hospital environment. British Medical Journal 3: 305–307

Lindheimer M D, Katz A J 1970 The kidney in pregnancy. New England Journal of Medicine 283: 1095–1097

McGrady G A, Daling J R, Peterson D R 1985 Maternal urinary tract infection and adverse fetal outcomes. American Journal of Epidemiology 121: 377–381

Montgomerie J Z, Kalmanson G M, Hubert E G et al 1972 Pyelonephritis: XIV. Effect of immunization on experimental Escherichia coli pyelonephritis. Infection and Immunity 6: 330–334

Mooreville M, Fritz R W, Mulholland S G 1983 Enhancement of the bladder defence mechanism by an exogenous agent. Journal of Urology 130: 607–609

Neal D E 1989 Localization of urinary tract infections. American Urologic Association Update. VIII (4): 26–29

Norrby S R 1990 Short term treatment of uncomplicated urinary tract infection in women. Review of Infectious Diseases 12: 458–467

Nowicki B, Martens M, Hart A, Moulds J, Nowicki S 1993 Gestational age dependent distribution of Escherichia coli fimbriae in pregnant patients with pyelonephritis. Journal of Urology 149 (4): 405A, 770–Abstract

Orskov I, Orskov F 1983 Serology of Escherichia coli fimbriae. Progress in Allergy 33: 80–105

Orskov I, Ferenz A, Orkov F 1980 Tamm-Horsfall protein or uromucoid in the normal urinary slime that traps type 1 fimbriated Escherichia coli. The Lancet 1: 887

Osterberg E, Abert H, Hallander H O, Kellner A, Lundin A 1990 Efficacy of single dose versus seven day trimethoprim treatment of cystitis in women: a randomized double-blind study. Journal of Infectious Diseases 161: 942–947

Parsons C L 1982 Prevention of urinary tract infection by the exogenous glycosaminoglycan sodium pentasanpolysulfate. Journal of Urology 127: 167–169

Parsons C L 1986 Pathogenesis of urinary tract infections. Urologic Clinics of North America 13 (4): 563–568

Parsons C, Schmidt J 1982 Control of recurrent lower urinary tract infection in the post menopausal woman. Journal of Urology 128: 1224–1226

Parsons C L, Grunspan C, Moore S W, Mulholland S G 1977 Role of surface mucin in primary antibacterial defence of bladder. Urology 9: 48–52

Parsons C L, Stauffer C, Mulholland S G et al 1984 Effect of ammonium on bacterial adherence to bladder transitional epithelium. Journal of Urology 132: 365–366

Patel R, Tanaka T, Mishkin R et al 1980 Gallium-67 scan aid to diagnosis and treatment of renal and perinephric infections. Urology 16: 225–228

Pearson N J, McSherry A M, Towner K J et al 1979 Emergence of trimethoprim-resistant enterobacteria in patients receiving long-term co-trimoxazole for the control of intractable urinary tract infection. The Lancet 1: 1205–1209

Reid G, Brooks J J L, Bacon D F 1983 In vitro attachment of Escherichia coli to human uroepithelial cells: variation in receptivity during the menstrual cycle and pregnancy. Journal of Infectious Diseases 148: 412–421

Reid G, Chan R C Y, Bruce E W et al 1985 Prevention of urinary tract infection in rats with an indigenous Lactobacillus case strain. Infection and Immunity 49: 320–324

Reid G, Denstedt J D, Karg Y S, Lam D, Nause C 1992 Microbial adhesion and biofem formation on ureteral stents in vitro and in vivo. Journal of Urology 148: 1592–1594

Roberts J A 1975 Experimental pyelonephritis in the monkey: III. Pathophysiology of ureteral malfunction induced by bacteria. Investigative Urology 13: 117–120

Roberts J A 1986 Pyelonephritis, cortical abscess and perinephric abscess. Urologic Clinics of North America 14 (4): 637–645

Roberts J A, Kaack B 1993 Events leading to septic death. Journal of Urology 149 (4): 404a, 767–abstract

Roberts J A, Kaach B, Kellenuis G et al 1984 Receptors for pyelonephritogenic Escherichia coli in primates. Journal of Urology 131: 163–168

Rolleston G L, Shannon F T, Utley W L 1975 Follow-up of vesico-ureteric reflux in the newborn. Kidney International 8: 59–64

Ronald A R, Harding G K M 1981 Urinary infection prophylaxis in women. Annals of Internal Medicine 94: 268–270

Savand-Feston M, Kenton B W, Rellon L B 1982 Single dose amoxycillin therapy with follow-up urine culture. American Journal of Medicine 73: 808–813

Schaeffer A J 1989 The role of bacterial adherence in urinary tract infection. American Urologic Association update. VIII (3): 18–23

Schaeffer A J, Jones J M, Duncan J L et al 1982 Adhesion of uropathogenic Escherichia coli to epithelial cells from women with recurrent urinary tract infection. Infection 10: 186–191

Schaeffer A J, Navas E L, Venegas M F et al 1993 Variation of blood group antigen expression on epithelial cells and mucus from women with and without history of urinary tract infections. Journal of Urology 149(4): 407A, 778–abstract

Schechter H, Leonard C B, Scribner B H 1971 Chronic pyelonephritis as a cause of renal failure in dialysis candidates. Analysis of 173 patients. Journal of the American Medical Association 216: 514–517

Shortcliffe L M D, Stamey T A 1986a Urinary infections in adult women. In: Walsh P C, Gittes R F, Perlmutter A D, Stamey T A (eds) Campbell's Urology, 5th edn, W B Saunders, Philadelphia, 1: 797–828

Shortcliffe L M D, Stamey T A 1986b Infections of the urinary tract: introduction and general principles. In: Walsh P C, Gittes R G, Perlmutter A D, Stamey T A (eds) Campbell's Urology, 5th Edn, W B Saunders, Philadelphia, 738–796

Shurbaji M S, Dumler J S, Gage W R, Petis G L, Gupta P K, Kuhaja F P 1990 Immunohistochemical detection of chlamydial antigens in association with cystitis. American Journal of Clinical Pathology 93: 363–366

Silverblatt F J, Cohen L S 1979 Antipili antibody affords protection against ascending pyelonephritis. Journal of Clinical Investigation 64: 333–336

Smellie J M 1991 Reflections of 30 years of treating children with urinary tract infections. Journal of Urology 146: 665–668

Smellie J M, Normand I C S 1985 Urinary infections in children 1985. Postgraduate Medical Journal 61: 895–905

Smellie J M, Normand I C S, Katz G 1981 Children with urinary infections: a comparison of those with and those without vesico-ureteric reflux. Kidney International 20: 717–722

Sobel J D, Kaye D 1985 Reduced uromucoid excretion in the elderly. Journal of Infectious Diseases 152: 653

Sobel J D, Kaye D 1990 Urinary tract infections. In: Mandell G L, Douglas R G, Bennett J E (eds) Principles and Practice of Infectious Diseases, 3rd edn, Churchill Livingstone, New York, 582–611

Stamey T A, Kaufman M F 1975 Studies of introital colonization in women with recurrent urinary infections: 11 A comparison of growth in normal vaginal fluid of common versus uncommon serogroups of escherichia coli. Journal of Urology 114: 264–267

Stamm W E, Courts G W, Running K R et al 1982 Diagnosis of coliform infection in acutely dysuric women. New England Journal of Medicine 307–463

Stamm W E, McKevitt M, Roberts P L, White N J 1991 Natural history of recurrent urinary tract infections in women. Review of Infectious Diseases 13: 77–84

Stapleton A, Latham R H, Johnson C, Stamm W E 1990 Postcoital antimicrobial prophylaxis for recurrent urinary tract infection: a randomized double blind placebo controlled trial. Journal of the American Medical Association 264: 703–706

Svanborg-Eden C, Eriksson B, Hanson L A et al 1978 Adhesion to normal human uroepithelial cells of Escherichia coli from children with various forms of urinary tract infections. Journal of Paediatrics 93: 398–403

Sweet R L 1977 Bacteriuria and pyelonephritis during pregnancy. Seminars in Perinatology 1: 25–40

Tolkoff-Rubin N E, Weber D, Fang L S T et al 1982 Single dose therapy with trimethoprim-sulfamethoxazole for urinary tract infection in women. Review of Infectious Diseases 4: 444–448

Uehling D T 1986 Future approaches to the management of urinary tract infection. Urologic Clinics of North America 13 (4): 749–750

Uehling D T, Steihm E R 1971 Elevated urinary secretory IgA in children with urinary tract infection. Paediatrics 47: 40–46

Uehling D T, Barnhart D D, Seastone C V 1968 Antibody production in urinary bladder infection. Investigative Urology 6: 211–222

Uehling D T, Jensen J, Balishe E 1982 Vaginal immunization against urinary tract infection. Journal of Urology 128: 1382–1384

Waltzer W C 1981 The urinary tract in pregnancy. Journal of Urology 125: 271–276

Welsh R A, Dellinger E P, Minshew B et al 1981 Haemolysin contributes to virulence of extraintestinal E. coli infections. Nature 294: 665–667

Zinner S H, Kass E H 1971 Long term 10–14 years follow-up of bacteriuria of pregnancy. New England Journal of Medicine 285: 820–824

Urethral lesions

CHARLOTTA PERSSON–JÜNEMANN AND HANSJÖRG MELCHIOR

TRAUMA

Trauma to the female urethra is uncommon, as the urethra is protected by the symphysis pubis and not as firmly anchored as the male urethra. The maximum incidence is in childhood, but iatrogenic injury to the female urethra is not uncommon and may follow surgical intervention or result from laceration during childbirth.

Aetiology

Only isolated case reports of injury to the female urethra in pelvic fractures have been reported, and the prepubertal female appears to be more prone to this injury than the adult (Webster 1984). In a series of 381 patients with traumatic rupture of the urethra, only seven were female, each of whom had an incomplete tear. Most of these resulted from traffic accidents. Separation or diastasis of the symphysis pubis following pelvic fracture leads to rupture of the posterior pubourethral ligament with loss of support for the bladder neck, laceration or transection of the urethra (Stanton et al 1981). Straddle injuries and the insertion of foreign bodies are also more common in children.

Surgical injury to the urethra may result from anterior vaginal wall repair, incontinence operations (especially sling-procedures; Cholhan & Stevenson 1996) or resection of a urethral diverticulum. Obstetrical injuries resulting from lacerations during forceps delivery as well as obstructed childbirth, with prolonged compression of the anterior vaginal wall against the symphysis pubis, result in ischaemia and necrosis, most prevalent in developing countries with poor obstetrical facilities.

Evaluation and treatment

Pelvic fracture with tearing or transection of the urethra, in most cases includes trauma to the vagina.

Symptoms may include profuse vaginal bleeding or gross haematuria. The diagnosis is confirmed by a speculum examination, retrograde urethrography or voiding cystourethrography, in most cases demonstrating the extravasation. Urethral catheterization should not be attempted, to avoid further damage to an incomplete transection of the urethra. Urethral trauma should be suspected in straddle injuries, penetrating injuries resulting from impalement trauma or gunshot wounds accompanied by profuse vaginal bleeding, gross haematuria or urinary incontinence.

Surgical trauma to the urethra will usually be identified at time of surgery. If undetected, a urethrovaginal fistula may result, and depending on the level of the lesion in relation to the sphincter mechanism, urinary incontinence. In addition to the above-mentioned investigation, X-ray using a double-balloon catheter and urethral instillation of dye during speculum examination is helpful.

Obstetrical injuries often present as postpartum incontinence when necrosis results in a urethrovaginal or more commonly, vesicovaginal fistula.

Management of urethral injuries is dictated by the extent of the lesion, time of diagnosis and the subsequent effect of the injury on urinary continence. Simple urethral contusions do not require surgical intervention, but temporary urinary diversion by suprapubic catheter is recommended.

Incomplete distal urethral tears are managed by vaginal debridement and suture repair in two layers over a stenting catheter. The transurethral catheter is removed at the end of the operation, and a suprapubic catheter is inserted for 7–10 days.

In *complete distal urethral tears*, primary repair over a stenting catheter can be attempted, but a circumferential end-to-end urethral reanastomosis may prove difficult. The alternative anastomosis of the torn proximal end of the urethra to the vaginal wall creating a neomeatus in a hypospadiac position, may result in urinary incontinence and voiding disorders.

Complete transsection of the proximal urethra or avulsion of the urethra from the bladder neck demands careful reconstruction. Most of these cases are associated with fracture of the pelvic bone in multitraumatized patients. Once the vital functions of the patient are stabilized, urethral reconstruction should be undertaken and may require a combined abdominovaginal approach. In many cases a primary retropubic approach can be indicated. From a suprapubic midline incision, the abdominal organs are explored and any pelvic haematoma evacuated. Following cystotomy, a 20 french transurethral catheter is inserted under visual and digital control. Debridement of the bladder neck and urethra is often difficult and unnecessary. Anastomosis of the bladder-neck and urethra is performed using six everting through-and-through, 0-dexon sutures. The transurethral catheter is removed and a suprapubic catheter inserted before the bladder is closed. If the anterior vaginal wall is disrupted, it is separately closed in two layers, making an attempt to avoid overlapping suture-lines, and in some cases using an omental pedicle-flap around the reconstructed area (Webster 1984). The retropubic and pelvic space are drained by suction. The suprapubic catheter is left in place until the patient is mobilized according to orthopaedic requirements.

URETHRAL PROLAPSE

Urethral prolapse denotes the complete circular eversion of the urethral mucosa through the external urethral meatus. This disorder is rare and involves premenarchal and postmenopausal females. About 90% of the affected infants are black, whereas in the menopausal group, only 15% are black (Owens & Morse 1968).

Aetiology

Fascial defects, poor bladder support, increased width or malformation of the urethra, and weakness of submucosal and elastic layers, have not been proven to be aetiologically relevant (Hepburn 1920; Richardson et al 1982; Zeigerman & Kimbrough 1948; Livermore 1921). Trauma, prolonged use of indwelling catheters, oestrogen deficiency, poor nutrition and medical conditions associated with sudden increase of intra-abdominal pressure, have been identified as predisposing factors (Turner 1973).

Presentation and treatment

There is a clear difference in symptoms between children and adults. Girls occasionally complain of itching or burning at the end of micturition. Generally parents notice blood stains on the underwear. The mild symptoms may result in delay of the correct diagnosis. Trauma or conditions with increased abdominal pressure are found in 35% of patients. In the menopausal group, pain is a significant factor associated with urinary retention, frequency, dysuria, urgency or incontinence. Bleeding is only found in 50% of the patients.

Physical examination reveals a sensitive bluish-purple mass which completely surrounds the urethral meatus and which may fill the entire vulva. Diagnosis is made on inspection, especially by identification of the urethral orifice. Urethral prolapse is the only tumour-like lesion in which the meatus is located in the centre of the mass. Biopsy is rarely necessary. Differential diagnosis in children includes prolapsed bladder or ureterocele, ectopic ureteral orifice and sarcoma. In adults, caruncle, carcinoma, periurethral abscess, polyps and condylomata must be excluded.

Treatment differs according to the different clinical presentations in child and adult patients. *Conservative treatment* consists of antibiotics and sitz-baths for children (Redmar 1982) and oestrogen cream for the older patients. Acute urinary symptoms and persistent pain will require *surgical management*.

Simple excision or high frequency electrocautery of the redundant mucosa with suturing of the corresponding wound margins are recommended (Moffett & Banks 1951; Abrams & Lewis 1954). A similar simple technique with 'four quadrant circumcision' and single sutures placed on either side, was described by Turner (1973). Fulguration and cryocautery were also applied (Friedrich 1977; Richardson et al 1982). Devine and Kessel (1980) favoured the attachment of the bladder-neck to the symphysis, believing that the urethral prolapse is a protrusion of all layers of the urethra. This procedure allows retraction of the prolapse and has the theoretical advantage of preserving the normal urethral length. Compared to alternative techniques, this approach seems difficult and time-consuming. Equally unadvisable is to tie a ligature around the protruding tissue over an indwelling catheter (Owens & Morse 1968).

ENDOMETRIOSIS

Endometriosis is the presence of endometrial tissue outside the uterus. It is found in approximately 15% of women between the ages of 25 and 45 years. It involves the urinary tract in 1.2% of the cases, the urethra is affected in only 2% of urinary tract involvement. Sole invasion of the urethra is extremely rare.

Aetiology

Several theories (embryonal, metaplastic and migratory) exist to explain the phenomenon. The most likely is the migratory theory, which includes traumatic dissemination and continuous invasion or metastasis by blood or lymphatic vessels (Arap et al 1984; Shook & Nyberg 1988).

Presentation and treatment

Times of presentation relate to menstrual activity. Clinical features depend on localization of the lesion. Endometriosis of the lower urinary tract often presents with the clinical triad of frequency, dysuria and haematuria. When the urethra is involved, dyspareunia is an additional symptom. Sometimes vague complaints of discomfort in the vesicovaginal region may be the only symptom, and the same applies with microscopic haematuria.

Diagnosis of urethral endometriosis is achieved with urethroscopy, preferably before or during menstruation. The typical appearence includes small bluish, protruding cysts. Diagnosis must be confirmed by biopsy, to exclude varices, angioma, papilloma and local inflammation or carcinoma.

Optimal treatment is to remove all endometriotic tissue as well as hormonal ovarian suppression or oophorectomy. Therapy, however, should be adjusted to the extent of the process, symptomatology and the individual biological situation. In cases of minor disturbance, hormonal treatment alone may be sufficient. Side-effects include nausea, breast tension, acne, weight gain and masculinization.

URETHRAL DIVERTICULUM

The incidence varies and is estimated between 0.6 and 1.7% of women with urological symptoms, although reports show an incidence as high as 5% in asymptomatic women and a sixfold higher incidence in black patients (Andersen 1967; Davis & Robinson 1970; Ganabathi et al 1994). Most diverticula are situated in the middle or distal third of the urethra; this distribution correlates with the topography of the female paraurethral ducts and glands.

Aetiology

The aetiology is often difficult to establish, including congenital lesions as well as acquired disease. The predominant hypothesis is that they are acquired as a result of infection, inflammation and/or obstruction of periurethral glands. Theories postulating trauma after urethral instrumentation or traumatic vaginal delivery, as well as meatal stenosis to be aetiologic factors have generally been rejected. The congenital theory assumes a secondary dilatation of preformed systems, finding support in anatomical findings describing a very high incidence of paraurethral ducts located particularly in the distal and dorsal region of the female urethra, prone to forming small cavities which could produce a diverticula (Huffman 1948).

Presentation

Urethral diverticula are most often found in the third to fifth decade. Usually there is a long history of characteristic symptoms including dyspareunia, dysuria, recurrent cystitis, postmicturition dribbling and urethral discharge. Less typical but suggestive of a diverticulum is significant urethral pain with normal urinalysis (Woodhouse et al 1980).

The female urethra is easily accessible to digital examination and therefore most diverticula can be diagnosed by transvaginal palpation. In its typical form, there is a tender cystic or resistent swelling felt suburethrally through the anterior vaginal wall. Often urine or purulent material can be expressed. Even blood may appear if the diverticulum contains a stone (1.5–10%) or tumour (Rajan et al 1993; Paik & Lee 1997; Oliva & Young 1996). Stasis and chronic infection increase the risk of stone formation (Leach & Bavendam 1987).

Evaluation and treatment

Diagnosis is made on the history and physical examination often supported by radiological studies and urethroscopy. Radiological studies alone are often insufficient, although an elevation of the bladder base can be suggestive of a proximal urethral diverticulum (Dretler et al 1972). Using a voiding cystourethrogram, performed in the standing position, it is possible to identify diverticula, showing the location, extent and configuration (Leach & Bavendam 1987). Retrograde positive pressure urethrography (double-balloon catheter) is better in distending and filling the assumed diverticulum (Davis & Cian 1956) (Fig. 30.1). Transvaginal sonography is superior in defining the localization and extent (Mouritsen & Bernstein 1996). Even careful cystourethroscopy can prove very difficult in finding the communicating area between the urethra and diverticulum in cases where the opening is very narrow.

The differential diagnosis includes a paraurethral cyst, abscess and the opening of an ectopic ureter.

If the patient is asymptomatic and there is no palpable induration indicating stone or tumour, no treatment is neccessary. If surgery is indicated, the preoperative evaluation of bladder function is indispensable for further management. In women with urinary stress incontinence, poor urethral support or a large proximal diverticulum, a simultaneous trans-

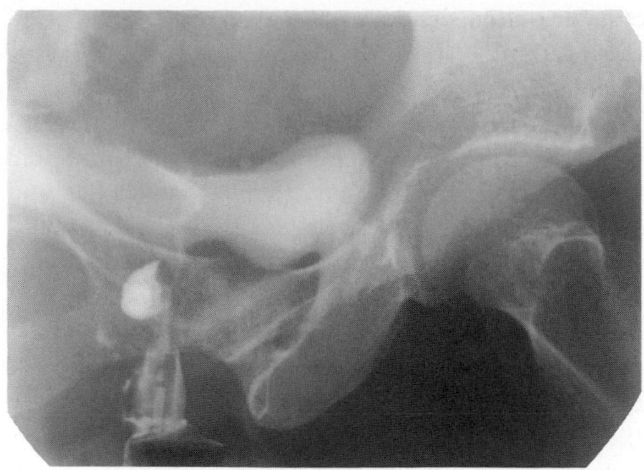

Fig. 30.1 Urethral diverticulum (retrograde urethrography).

vaginal bladder neck suspension should be combined with the diverticulectomy (Bass & Leach 1991; Ganabathi et al 1994; Raz 1994). Ideally, the diverticular sac should be separated completely and the urethral defect closed. Small diverticula and especially the lower ones can be removed transvaginally. Complications are rare, even if the incision leads from the external meatus through the bottom of the urethra into the orifice of the diverticulum, provided the diverticulum is in the distal urethra (Spence & Duckett 1970).

The complete removal of an infected large diverticulum attached to the bladder wall and trigone may be difficult. In such situations, the dissection of the diverticular neck by the vaginal route is recommended. This is followed by the removal of the urothelial layer of the sacculation and occlusion of the remaining cavity using fibrin sealant. In the vaginal approach, a curved longitudinal incision is advisable. This avoids overlapping of the urethral and vaginal sutures, in an attempt to avoid fistulae. In high-risk patients and cases with multilocular cysts, endoscopic incision of the diverticular orifice is simple and less traumatic (Frankenschmidt & Baumüller 1983; Vergunst et al 1996).

PARAURETHRAL CYSTS

Aetiology

A paraurethral cyst has the same aetiology as a urethral diverticulum but has no connection to the urethra. According to various embryological remnants, congenital cysts can be differentiated from müllerian, mesonephric or urothelial tissue (Das 1981). Acquired cysts are often the result of inflammation, occlusion of the urethral glands or secondary to delivery or trauma.

Presentation and treatment

Most often the cysts are asymptomatic and discovered upon routine gynaecological examination (Fig. 30.2). Otherwise, uncharacteristic symptoms of dysuria, dyspareunia and an abnormal voiding stream can be found in combination with a palpable vaginal mass.

Radiological studies are uninformative, needle aspiration and contrast injection may distinguish between an ectopic ureterocele or a paraurethral diverticulum.

In infants, paraurethral cysts seem to resolve spontaneously. In adults, spontaneous rupture is rare and may occur secondary to suppuration. Marsupialization can be successful in uninfected cysts, however in presence of infection or abscess formation, total excision of the cyst including the wall is usually neccessary (Fig. 30.3).

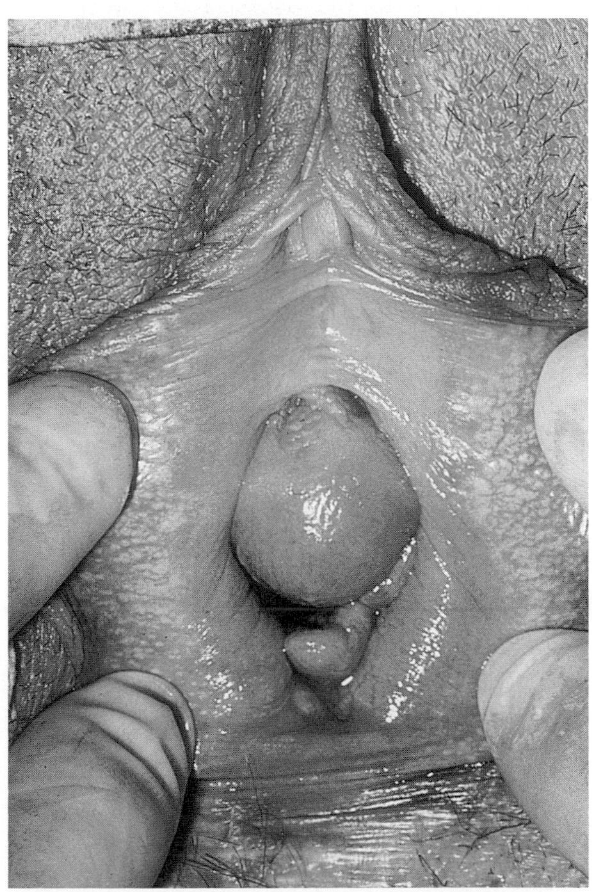

Fig. 30.2 Midline paraurethral cyst on vaginal examination.

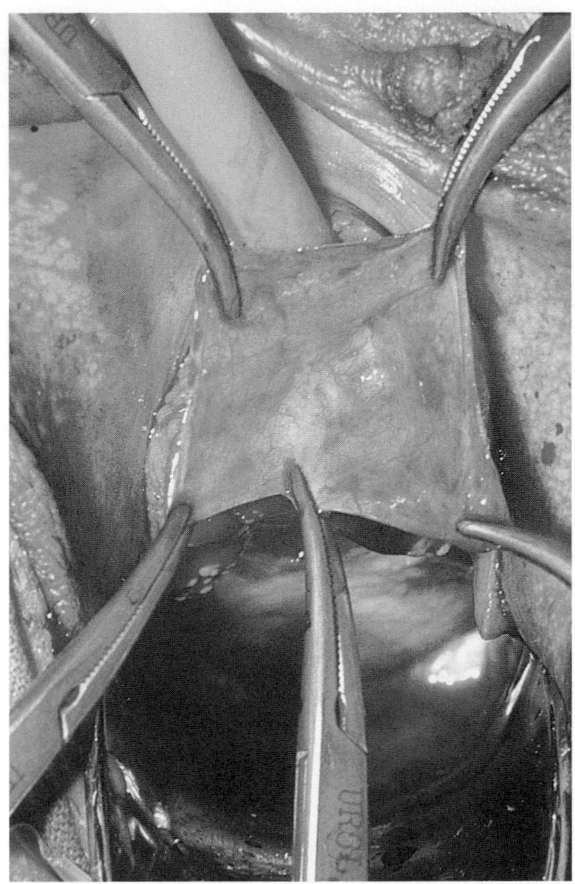

Fig. 30.3 Paraurethral cyst opened intraoperatively.

URETHRAL CARUNCLE

The urethral caruncle is the most common benign tumour of the female urethra and is most frequently found after the menopause. Symptoms may be nonspecific and include dysuria, dyspareunia, frequency, haematuria as well as a sensation of pressure in the perineum. Most often the caruncle is found on inspection, often in patients with transurethral catheters.

Presentation and treatment

Diagnosis is made on clinical and histological examination. A characteristic finding is a reddish, tender, polypoid excrescence protruding from the inferior position of the urethral meatus (Fig. 30.4). It is important to differentiate from carcinoma or urethral prolapse. Three histological types have been described: (1) The papillomatous caruncle, covered by transitional and squamous epithelium. Occasionally, nests of epithelial cells appear in crypts and may be

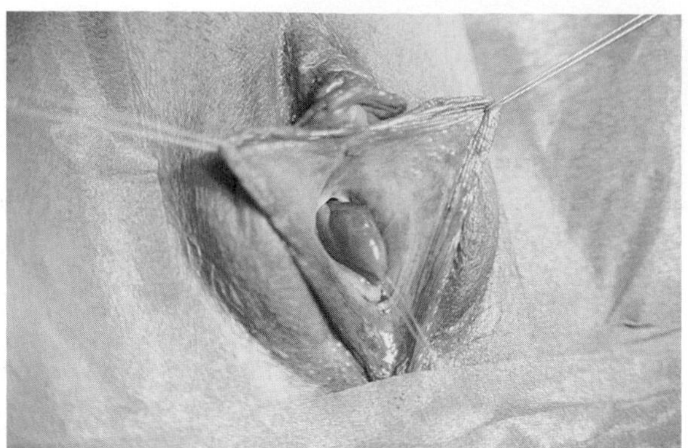

Fig. 30.4 Clinical presentation of a urethral caruncle.

confused with carcinoma. (2) The angiomatous lesion is more vascular, but otherwise similar. (3) The granulomatous type is composed entirely of granulation tissue without any epithelial hyperplasia.

Treatment is unneccessary if the lesion is unsuspicious or asymptomatic. Otherwise it should be completely excised followed by evertion of the normal mucosa or light cauterization and histological examination.

URETHRAL STENOSIS

In 1963, Lyon and Smith described a ring of fibrous tissue in the distal part of the female urethra, just inside the meatus which they termed 'distal urethral stenosis'. Later this stricture was suggested to be the cause of obscure persistent or recurrent urinary infections in women (Lyon & Tanagho 1965). Since then the existence, incidence, identification and functional effects of this disorder have been disputed (Graham et al 1967; Immergut & Wahmann 1968; Scholtmeijer & Griffiths 1985). There is some evidence suggesting that enlargement of the distal urethra has a beneficial effect on urinary infection and enuresis in girls (Halverstadt & Leadbetter 1968; Hendry et al 1973; Immergut & Gilbert 1973; Moormann et al 1974). It seems as if a normal funnel-shaped urethra allows a laminar urine flow, whereas a distal stricture leads to turbulent flow with resulting reflux of bacteria into the bladder, but further work is required to confirm this.

Presentation, evaluation and treatment

The clinical history should include characteristic symptoms of bladder obstruction. In girls, enuresis, frequency and dysuria are the predominant symptoms, generally associated with recurrent urinary infections or asymptomatic bacteriuria, and sometimes daytime wetting. Physical examination may reveal local inflammation of the urethral orifice and vulva or a ring of polyploid structures. Sometimes the meatal orifice is displaced in ventral direction, caused by a high insertion of the labia minora.

The most important diagnostic tool is the urethral calibration with bougie à boule, under general anaes-

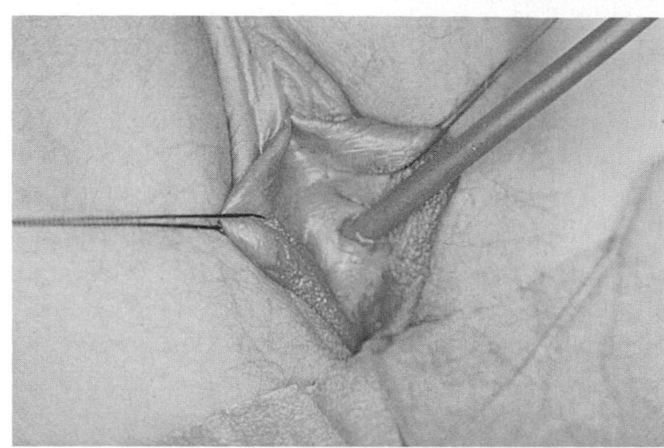

Fig. 30.5 Urethral calibration by bougie à boule.

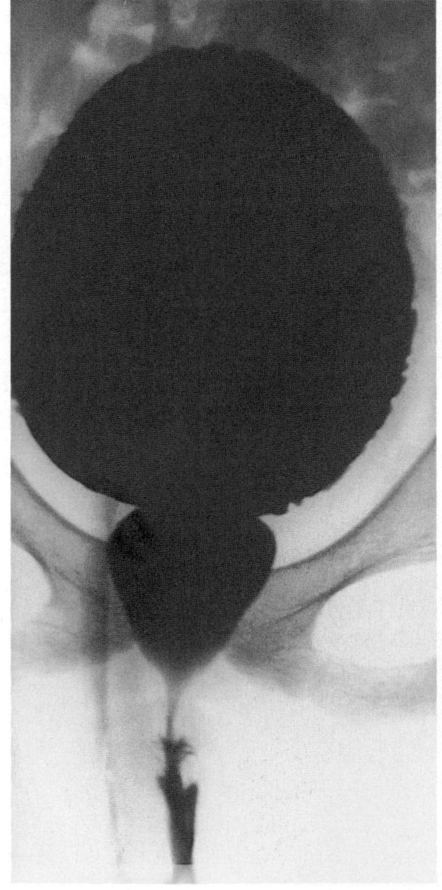

Fig. 30.6 Voiding cystourethrogram in a case of urethral stenosis.

thesia (Fig. 30.5). A sudden change in the urethral calibre seems important. A so-called 'spinning top' urethra in voiding cystourethrography can be suggestive, although functional disturbances such as bladder–sphincter dyscoordination reveal the same radiographic morphology (Fig. 30.6). The same applies to a high voiding pressure shown on cystometry. Residual urine and a thick bladder wall is common in both entities.

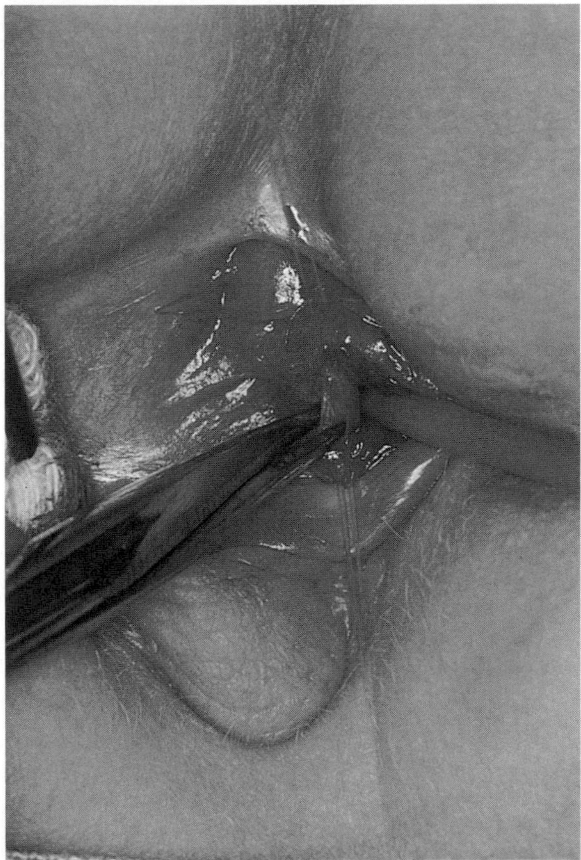

Fig. 30.7 Lateral meatotomy.

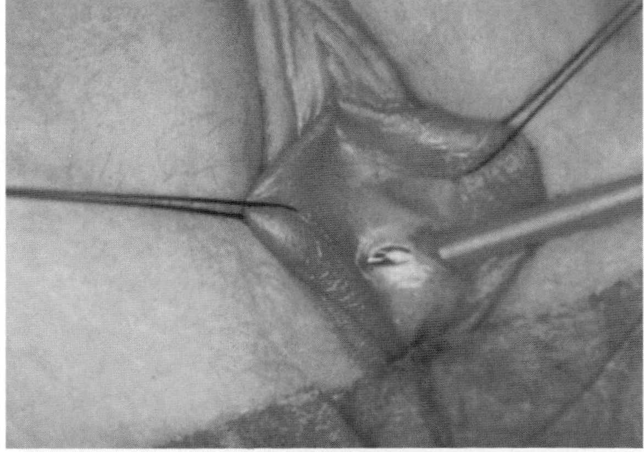

Fig. 30.8 Fibrous ring between the wound margins in a case of distal urethral stenosis.

Treatment in unequivocal cases of urethral stenosis can consist of dilatation of the tight urethral zone. Disadvantages include possible fissures of the mucosa which could lead to scars and new strictures. More common is the Otis urethrotomy, performing a longitudinal cut through the entire urethra. The use of this procedure demands caution or should be avoided, as cases of resulting incontinence have been described (Allen 1986; Kessler & Constantinou 1986). Preferable is a submucosal meatotomy (Moormann et al 1974) – a deep longitudinal incision is made at the meatus followed by the complete cutting of the fibrous ring, which can be seen between the wound margins (Figs 30.7 and 30.8). The incision is closed in a transverse, everting fashion using 6–0 catgut.

INFLAMMATION

Acute urethritis frequently occurs with gonorrheal infection in women; urethritis alone is uncommon. In most cases findings suggest a combined urethrocystitis. Microorganisms most often ascend into the lower urinary tract: from the rectum across the moist peritoneum and from the vagina to the external urethral orifice; in correlation fecal bacteria are predominant. Urethral malformations such as diverticulum or stenosis are predisposing factors. Non-bacterial urethrocystitis is a syndrome with the same symptoms and signs of infection, and the spectrum of causes includes chemically initiated inflammation (soaps, bathing lotion and deodorants), interstitial cystitis and senile urethritis.

Presentation and treatment

The symptoms include urgency, frequency and dysuria. Pyuria and haematuria may occur in severe infections or in some cases of allergic-toxic reactions. Clinical examination may show a tender urethra on palpation; ultrasonography of the urinary tract, including transvaginal sonography, should rule out any congenital or achieved morphological changes. Urinalysis may show significant count of bacteria; specific bacteriological samples and smears are important to rule out specific infections (e.g. chlamydia). Underlying urethral malformations can be visualized during micturition cystourethrography, urethrocystoscopy and meatal calibration. The functional evaluation however should be performed after adequate therapy of the acute inflammation.

Treatment of bacterial urethrocystitis corresponds to that of other urinary tract infections, namely antibiotics in accordance with the urine culture. Malformations of the urethra (urethral diverticulum, meatal stenosis) require surgery. The clinical symptoms of urgency, frequency and dysuria can be treated successfully using anticholinergic or antispasmotic drugs. In non-bacterial, allergic urethrocystitis, the responsible substances must be avoided.

CARCINOMA

Urethral cancer is the only genitourinary neoplasm which is more prevalent in women, the ratio being 4:1. It is rather rare; in 1986 Hopkins and Grabstald reported 1200 cases (Hopkins & Grabstaldt 1986). The maximum incidence is reported in the fifth and sixth decades, and white females are most often affected (85%).

Histopathology

The histological type depends on the cells of origin. The distal two thirds of the urethra is lined by a stratified squamous epithelium, and the proximal third by transitional epithelium. The periurethral Skenes glands and ducts (usually concentrated in the perimeatal region) are lined by pseudostratified and stratified epithelium. The lymphatics of the distal urethra drain into the inguinal lymph nodes while those of the proximal urethra drain into the pelvic chains (Hand 1970). Approximately 50% of the tumours arise from the distal urethra or vulvo-urethral junction. As a result, squamous-cell carcinoma predominates (68%), with adenocarcinoma and transitional-cell carcinoma being less common. Undifferentiated carcinoma, malignant melanoma, mixed tumours, clear cell carcinoma, and cloacogenic carcinoma account for the remaining lesions (Ziegerman & Gordon 1970; Grabstald 1973; Narayan & Konety 1992; Amin & Young 1997).

Chronic urethral irritation may predispose to development of urethral carcinoma, although no direct relationship has been documented. Urethral caruncles, fibrous polyps and condylomata can occur in association with urethral carcinoma in 2–11% of women. Carcinoma arising within a urethral diverticulum is extremely rare and has a different histological distribution (Seballos & Rich 1995). Leukoplakia of the urethra is considered a premalignant lesion.

Presentation and evaluation

Urethral bleeding or spotting is the most common symptom; gross haematuria is rare (Bracken et al 1976). Urinary frequency, dysuria, urinary obstruction and perineal pain are other non-specific complaints. Most of the tumours are discovered as an incidental finding during routine clinical examination, presenting as a palpable urethral mass or induration. Tumours arising from the distal urethra may protrude from the meatus (Fig. 30.9). Since an early carcinoma may be mistaken for a caruncle, any collar-like ring of induration or persistent ulceration or erosion of the urethra must be considered suspicious and should be biopsied (Marshall et al 1960). In more advanced disease, urethral carcinoma may be difficult to distinguish from a primary vaginal neoplasm. Examination of the groin and lower limbs is necessary to evaluate regional lymph nodes and for evidence of a lymphatic or venous stasis.

As well as visual inspection, urethrocystoscopy should if possible be performed. Retrograde urethrography or voiding cystourethrograms may demonstrate a filling defect (Fig. 30.10), alteration or fistula of the urethra. Computerized axial tomography is recommended for assessment of the pelvic and inguinal lymph node status.

Whilst tumours which arise at the meatus or per-

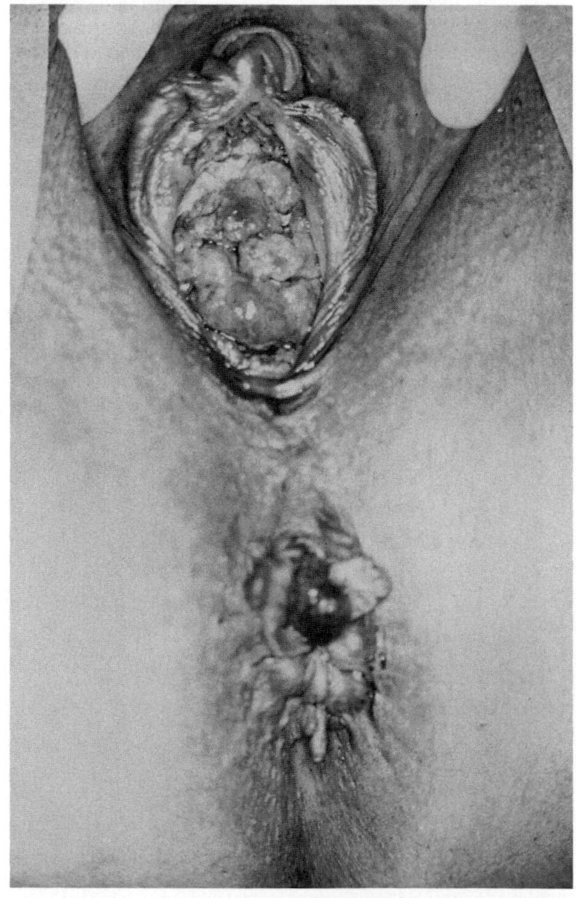

Fig. 30.9 Distal urethral carcinoma protruding through the meatus.

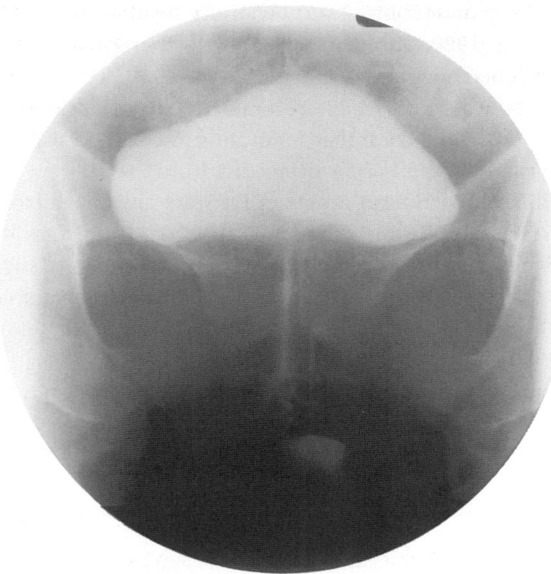

Fig. 30.10 Urethral obstruction by a squamous epithelial carcinoma (retrograde urethrography).

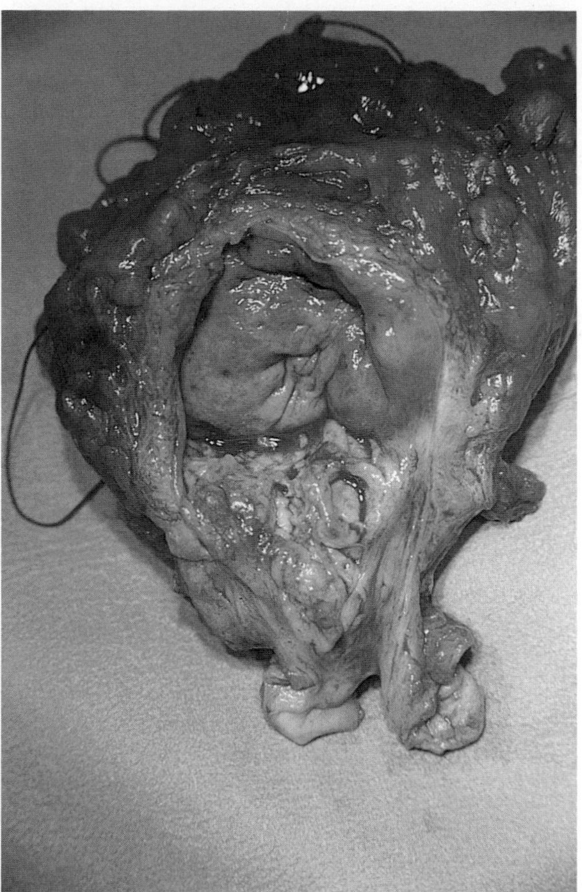

Fig. 30.11 Urethral cancer in a cystourethrectomy specimen.

imeatal region can be biopsied directly, proximal urethral tumours have to be biopsied transurethrally. The bladder and bladder neck must be carefully evaluated (Fig. 30.11). Primary bladder cancer with urethral extension or visa versa must be documented.

Incorporation of the TNM staging system for female urethral carcinoma is desirable; for practical reasons, the Chau and Green (1965) clinical classification is still in use (Table 30.1).

Tumour stage and location are more important in determining survival than the histopathological character (Sullivan & Grabstald 1978). An anterior carcinoma has generally a better prognosis than a posterior or entire urethral neoplasm; size, depth of invasion and lymph node status have significant prognostic importance (Bracken et al 1976).

Treatment

Superficial tumours of the distal urethra have been successfully treated by transurethral resection or local excision. Neoplasia infiltrating the urethral muscularis or periurethral tissue (stage 1 and 2) may be managed by partial urethrectomy. Partial or subtotal urethrectomy must not result in stress or total incontinence (Grigsby & Corn 1992). The 5-year survival rate for patients with a distal tumour treated by surgery is excellent (Narayan & Konety 1992). The results of megavoltage irradiation and interstitial brachytherapy using radium radon, gold or iridium for distal tumours are comparable to those of surgery (Delclos 1982; Prempree et al 1984; Micaili et al 1997). In particular, Iridium 192 using the after-loading technique has improved radiation distribution and has decreased morbidity.

Table 30.1 TNM Staging for female urethral carcinoma.

Stage 1	Tumour in the distal urethra
Stage 2	Tumour in the whole urethra infiltrating the periurethral tissue, excluding the vulva or bladder neck
Stage 3a	Tumour infiltrating the urethra and vulva
Stage 3b	Tumour infiltrating the vagina
Stage 3c	Tumour infiltrating the bladder neck
Stage 4a	Tumour infiltrating the parametrium or paracolpus
Stage 4b	Lymph node and/or distal metastasis

From Chau & Green (1965).

Neoplasia arising from the posterior urethra or involving the entire urethra are always of a higher stage and more than 50% have lymph node involvement (Johnson 1982). The treatment of choice of the posterior or entire tumours has been the anterior exenteration and urinary diversion, although the accumulated 5-year survival only ranges from 10 to 17%. Even the results of orthovoltage external beam and radium intracavitary radiation were discouraging; local failure approached 100% and severe complications were common. The results of an integrated approach using external beam radiation (20–50 Gy) followed by anterior exenteration and urinary diversion or brachytherapy to the interstitial tumour have not been impressive (Sailer et al 1988). The morbidity of these procedures is such that they require careful case selection (Hopkins et al 1983).

The inguinal lymph nodes are involved in a high percentage of distal third tumours, and the pelvic lymph nodes are involved in a high percentage of neoplasia arising from the posterior or involving the entire urethra. Because prophylactic lymphadenectomy has not been proven to be better than therapeutic node dissection, it has generally been discouraged (Levine 1980; Johnson 1982). Only therapeutic lymphadenectomy is recommended.

Several studies have recommended chemotherapy (M-VAC, or combined mitomycin-C and 5-fluorouracil) for palliation or as an adjunct to surgery or radiation, although long-term results are unavailable (Scher et al 1988; Tran et al 1995). The results of chemotherapy for other epithelioid carcinomas suggest that these tumours may be potentially responsive as well.

REFERENCES

Abrams M, Lewis M K 1954 Prolapse of the urethra in young girls. Journal of Urology 72: 222–225

Allen T D 1986 Internal urethrotomy in female subjects. Journal of Urology 136: 1280–1281

Amin M B, Young R H 1997 Primary carcinomas of the urethra. Seminars of Diagnostic Pathology 14 (2): 147–160

Andersen M J F 1967 The incidence of diverticula in the female urethra. Journal of Urology 98: 96–98

Arap N W, Lopes R N, Cury M, Montelatto N I D, Arap S 1984 Vesical endometriosis. Urology 24: 271–274

Bass J S, Leach G E 1991 Surgical treatment of concomitant urethral diverticulum and stress incontinence. Urologic Clinics of North America 18: 365–373

Bracker R B, Johnson D E, Miller L S, Ayala A G, Gomez J J, Rutledge F 1976 Primary carcinoma of the female urethra. Journal of Urology 116: 188–192

Chau P M, Grenn A E 1965 Radiotherapeutic management of malignant tumors of the vagina. Progress in Clinical Cancer 1: 728–750

Cholhan H J, Stevenson K R 1996 Sling transection of urethra: a rare complication. International Urogynecological Journal of Pelvic Floor Dysfunction 7 (6): 331–334

Das S P 1981 Paraurethral cysts in women. Journal of Urology 126: 41–43

Davis B L, Robinson D G 1970 Diverticula of the female urethra: assay of 120 cases. Journal of Urology 104: 850–853

Davis H, Cian L 1956 Positive pressure urethrography: A new diagnostic method. Journal of Urology 75: 753–757

Delclos L 1982 Carcinoma of the female. In: Johnson D E, Boileau M A (eds) Genitourinary Tumors. Fundamental principles and surgical techniques. Grune & Stratton, New York, pp 275–286

Devine P C, Kessel H C 1980 Surgical correction of urethral prolapse. Journal of Urology 123: 856–857

Dretler S P, Vermillion C D, McCullough D L 1972 The roentgenographic diagnosis of female urethral diverticula. Journal of Urology 107: 72–74

Frankenschmidt A, Baumüller A 1983 Weibliches Urethraldivertikel-Sichturethrotomie ausreichend? Aktuelle Urologie 14: 247–249

Friedrich E G 1977 Cryosurgery for urethral prolapse. Obstetrics and Gynecology 50: 359–361

Ganabathi K, Leach G E, Zimmern P E et al 1994 Experience with the management of urethral diverticulum in 63 women. Journal of Urology 152: 1445–1452

Grabstald H 1973 Tumors of the urethra in men and women. Cancer 32: 1236–1255

Graham J B, King L R, Kropp K A, Uehling D T 1967 The significance of distal urethral narrowing in young girls. Journal of Urology 97: 1045–1049

Grigsby P W, Corn B W 1992 Localized urethral tumours in women: Indications for conservative versus exenterative therapies. Journal of Urology 147: 1516–1520

Halverstadt D B, Leadbetter G W 1968 Internal urethrotomy and recurrent urinary infection in female children. 1. Results in the management of infections. Journal of Urology 100: 297–302

Hand J R 1970 Surgery of the penis and urethra. In: Campbell M F, Harrison J H (eds) Urology, vol 3. Saunders, Philadelphia, pp 2541–2647

Hendry W F, Stanton S L, Williams D I 1973 Recurrent urinary infection in girls; effect of urethral dilatation. British Journal of Urology 45: 72–83

Hepburn T N 1920 Prolapse of the female urethra. Surgery, Gynecology and Obstetrics 31: 83

Hopkins S C, Grabstald H 1986 Benign and malignant tumors of the male and female urethra. In: Walsh P C, Gittes R E, Perlmutter A D, Stamey T A (eds) Campbell's Urology, Vol 2, Saunders, Philadelphia, pp 1441–1448

Hopkins S C, Vider M, Nag S K, Tai D L, Soloway M S 1983 Carcinoma of the female urethra. Reassessment of modes of therapy. Journal of Urology 129: 958–961

Huffman J W 1948 The detailed anatomy of the paraurethral ducts in the adult human female. American Journal of Obstetrics and Gynecology 55: 86–101

Immergut M A, Gilbert E C 1973 Internal urethrotomy in recurrent urinary infections in girls. Journal of Urology 109: 126–127

Immergut M A, Wahman G E 1968 The urethral calibre of female children with recurrent urinary tract infections. Journal of Urology 99: 189–190

Johnson D E 1982 Cancer of the female urethra: Overview. In: Johnson D E, Boileau M A (eds) pp 267–274. Genitourinary Tumors. Fundamental principles and surgical techniques. Grune & Stratton, New York

Kessler R, Constantinou C E 1986 Internal urethrotomy in girls and its impact on the urethral intrinsic and extrinsic continence mechanisms. Journal of Urology 136: 1248–1253

Leach G F, Bavendam T G 1987 Female urethral diverticula. Urology 30: 407–415

Levine R L 1980 Urethral cancer. Cancer 45 (Suppl): 1965–1972
Livermore G R 1921 The treatment of prolapse of the urethra. Surgery, Gynecology and Obstetrics 32: 557
Lyon R P, Smith D R 1963 Distal urethral stenosis. Journal of Urology 89: 414–421
Lyon R P, Tanagho E A 1965 Distal urethral stenosis in little girls. Journal of Urology 93: 379–387
Marshall F C, Uson A C, Melicow M M 1960 Neoplasms and caruncles of the female urethra. Surgery, Gynecology and Obstetrics 110: 723–733
Micaili B, Dzeda M F, Miyamoto C T, Brady L W 1997 Brachytherapy for cancer of the female urethra. Seminars on Surgical Oncology 13(3): 208–214
Moffett J D, Banks R Jr 1951 Prolapse of the urethra in young girls. Journal of the American Medical Association 146: 1288–1289
Moormann J G, Kastert A B, Brausch K 1974 Diagnose und operative Therapie der distalen Stenose der weiblichen Harnröhre. Der Urologe A 13: 213–216
Mouritsen L, Bernstein I 1996 Vaginal ultrasonography: a diagnostic tool for urethral diverticulum. Acta Obstetrica et Gynecologica Scandinavica 75: 188–190
Narayan P, Konety B 1992 Surgical treatment of female urethral carcinoma. Urologic Clinics of North America 19: 373–382
Oliva Ti, Young R H 1996 Clear cell adenocarcinoma of the urethra: a clinicopathologic analysis of 19 cases. Modern Pathology 9 (5): 513–520
Owens S B, Morse W H 1968 Prolapse of the female urethra in children. Journal of Urology 100: 171–174
Paik S S, Lee J D 1997 Nephrogenic adenoma arising in an urethral diverticulum. British Journal of Urology 80 (1): 150
Prempree T, Amornmarn R, Patanaphan V 1984 Radiation therapy in primary carcinoma of the female urethra. II. An update on results. Cancer 54: 729–733
Rajan N, Tucci P, Mallouh C et al 1993 Carcinoma in female urethral diverticulum: case reports and review of management. Journal of Urology 150: 1911–1914
Raz S 1994 Fistulas, diverticula and incontinence. Journal of Urology 152: 1458–1459
Redmar J F 1982 Conservative management of urethral prolapse in female children. Urology 19: 505–506
Richardson D A, Haji S N, Herbst A L 1982 Medical treatment of urethral prolapse in children. Obstetrics and Gynecology 59: 69–74
Sailer S L, Shipley W U, Wang C C 1988 Carcinoma of the female urethra: A review of results with radiation therapy. Journal of Urology 140: 1–5.
Scher H I, Herr H W, Yagoda A et al 1988 Neoadjuvant M-VAC for extravesical urinary tract tumours. Journal of Urology 139: 475–477
Scholtmeijer R J, Griffiths D J 1985 Die distale Harnröhrenstenose bei Mädchen: Realität oder Traum? Aktuelle Urologie 16: 162–164
Seballos R M, Rich R R 1995 Clear cell adenocarcinoma arising from a urethral diverticulum. Journal of Urology 153(6): 1914–1915
Shook T E, Nyberg L M 1988 Endometriosis of the urinary tract. Urology 31: 1–6
Spence H M, Duckett J W Jr 1970 Diverticulum of the female urethra: clinical aspects and presentation of a simple operative technique for cure. Journal of Urology 104: 432–437
Stanton S L, Cardozo L, Riddle P 1981 Urological complications of traumatic diastasis of the symphysis pubis. British Journal of Urology 53: 453–454
Sullivan J, Grabstald H 1978 Management of carcinoma of the urethra. In: Skinner D G, De Kerion J B (eds) Genitourinary cancer. Saunders, Philadelphia, pp 419–429
Tran L N, Krieg R M, Szabo R J 1995 Combination chemotherapy and radiotherapy for a locally advanced squamous cell carcinoma of the urethra: a case report. Journal of Urology 153(2): 422–423
Turner R W 1973 Urethral prolapse in female children. Urology 2: 530–533
Vergunst H, Blom J H, De Spiegeleer A H, Miranda S I 1996 Management of female urethral diverticula by transurethral incision. British Journal of Urology 77(5): 745–746
Webster G D 1984 Urethral Trauma. In: Paulsen D F (ed.) Genitourinary surgery, Vol. 1 2, Churchill Livingstone, New York, pp 448–481
Woodhouse C R J, Flynn J T, Molland E A, Blandy J P 1980 Urethral diverticulum in females. British Journal of Urology 52: 305–310
Zeigerman J H, Gordon S F 1970 Cancer of the female urethra. A curable disease. Obstetrics and Gynecology 36: 785–789
Zeigerman J H, Kimbrough R A 1948 Circular prolapse of the urethra. American Journal of Obstetrics and Gynecology 56: 950–954

Pelvic organ prolapse

RICHARD C BUMP AND GEOFFREY W CUNDIFF

DEFINITION

Prolapse (from the late Latin *prolapsus*, a slipping forth) refers to the falling or slipping out of place of a part or viscus. In this chapter we use the term female pelvic organ prolapse to refer to the downward displacement of the pelvic organs towards or through the vaginal opening. The organs involved can include the urethra, urinary bladder, small and large bowel, omentum, and rectum, in addition to the vagina, cervix, uterus, and adnexa. Therefore, we prefer the term pelvic organ prolapse (POP) to genital or vaginal prolapse. POP occurring through other openings or defects – such as the urethral meatus (urethral prolapse), the anal canal (rectal prolapse and enterocele), or the levator plate (posterior rectocele) – will not be considered in this chapter.

Virtually all parous women and many active nulliparous women can be demonstrated to have less than perfect pelvic support on careful examination, although most have no symptoms related to this and fewer than 10–15% will require treatment in their lifetime (Hurt 1990a; Olsen et al 1997). Conversely, many women with vague symptoms often attributed to prolapse, such as pelvic or lower abdominal pain, pressure, or heaviness, have no or minor deficits of pelvic support. Our ability to distinguish clinically significant POP from normal variations in support is frustrated by an absence of longitudinal studies that identify symptoms consistently associated with prolapse and a dearth of controlled interventional trials that establish cure rates for these symptoms.

Until such studies are available, we arbitrarily define POP as a defect in normal pelvic support with the objective demonstration of descent of the pelvic organs towards or through the vaginal opening in a woman with bothersome urinary, bowel, sexual, or local pelvic symptoms that reasonably can be attributed to the descent.

AETIOLOGY

Structures essential to the maintenance of normal female pelvic organ support include the bony pelvis, the pelvic diaphragm, the urogenital diaphragm and perineal body, and the endopelvic fascia (Hurt 1990; DeLancey 1993; Wall 1993; Norton 1993; Richardson 1995). The bony pelvis is a hollow ring which surrounds the abdominopelvic organs and which articulates with the spinal column above and the femurs below. It provides the surfaces of attachment for the muscles and ligaments which contribute to the floor of the pelvis and to which the endopelvic fascia attaches. Rarely, significant abnormalities in the bony pelvis, such as occurs in patients with bladder exstrophy, contribute to frequent and early advanced prolapse (Mariona & Evans 1982; Blakeley & Mills 1981).

The muscles of the pelvic diaphragm form the dynamic floor of the pelvis. They normally contract tonically and reflexly to support the pelvic contents and maintain urinary and faecal continence. They relax to allow urination, defecation, parturition, and coitus. The pelvic diaphragm consists of the levator ani (puborectalis, pubococcygeus, and iliococcygeus portions) and coccygeus muscles. Arising from the pubic bone, arcus tendineus levator ani, and ischial spine, these paired muscles run posteriorly and medially to insert onto the perineal body, anal sphincter, anococcygeal raphe, and coccyx (Fig. 31.1A). Anterior to the perineal body, the levators separate to form the genital hiatus which is normally positioned far anterior near the pubic bone due to contraction of the

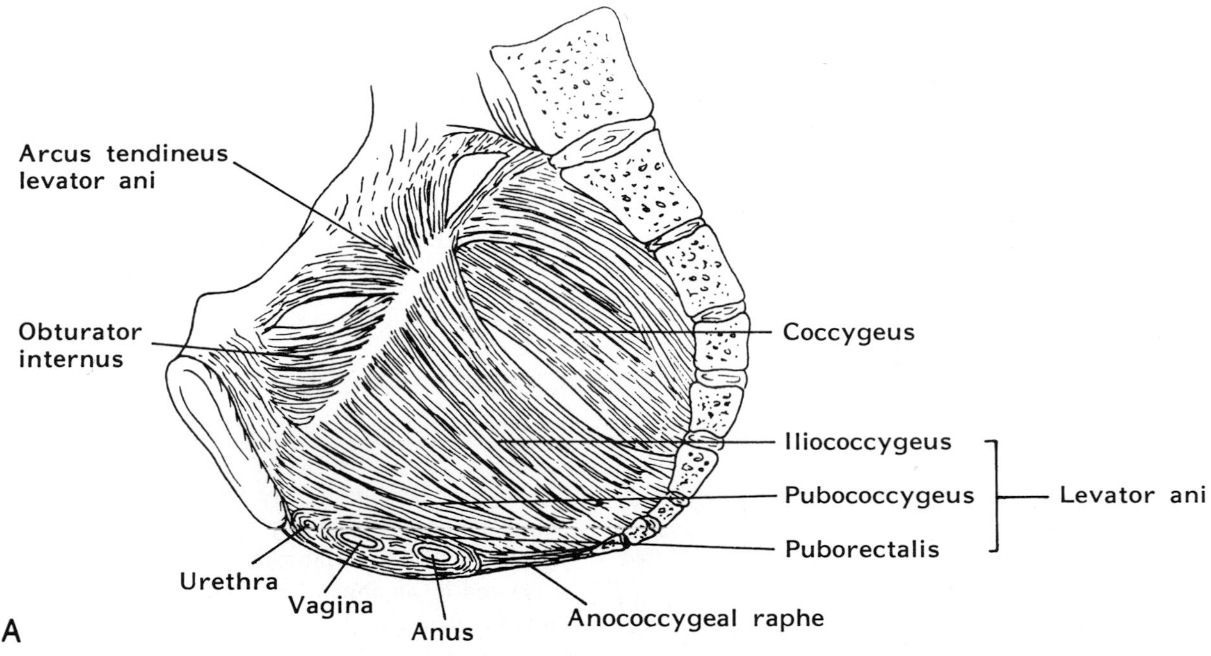

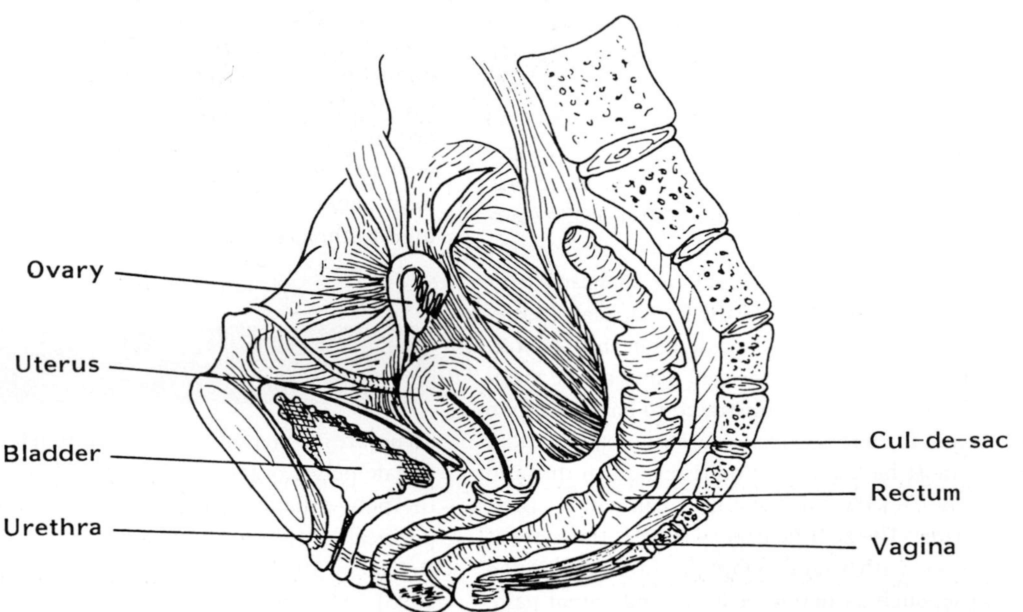

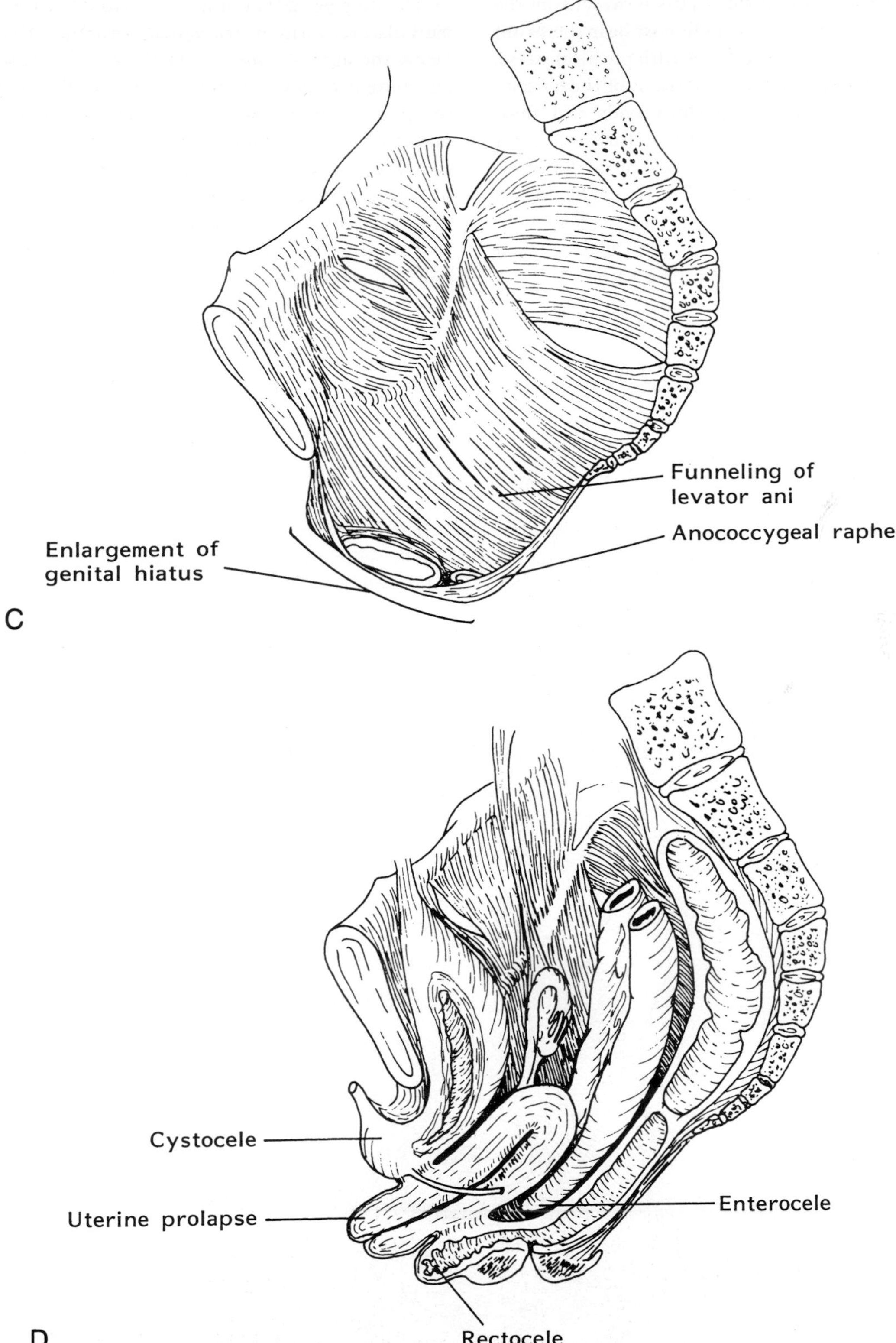

Fig. 31.1 **(A)** The pelvic diaphragm, consisting of the levator ani and coccygeus muscles. **(B)** The rectum, upper vagina, uterus and bladder lie on the pelvic diaphragm and are compressed against it in a flap-valve fashion during increases in abdominal pressure. **(C)** Damage to the pelvic diaphragm changes the orientation of the levator plate from horizontal to vertical, resulting in a widening of the genital hiatus in a posterior-inferior direction, making the hiatus the most dependent portion of the pelvis. **(D)** The increased load on the endopelvic fascia exceeds its limits, leading to breakage, detachment, and/or attenuation. The end result is prolapse of the pelvic organs through the genital hiatus. From Hurt (1990), pp 414–415, with permission.

levators. In this position the hiatus is away from the lowest point in the pelvis which must bear the brunt of abdominal pressure at rest and with physical stress. Posterior to the genital hiatus, portions of the muscles converge and attach to the perineal body and anus; posterior to the anus they fuse to form the levator plate, a shallow horizontal basin that normally forms the lowest part of the pelvic cavity. Upon the levator plate lie the nearly horizontally oriented rectum, upper vagina, uterus, and bladder, all of which are compressed against the contracting levator plate in a flap-valve fashion during increases in abdominal pressure (Fig. 31.1B) (Hurt 1990; DeLancey 1993; Wall 1993). Anatomic, neuropathic, and myopathic damage to the pelvic diaphragm changes the orientation of the levator plate from horizontal to vertical, resulting in a widening of the genital hiatus in a posterior-inferior direction, making the hiatus the most dependent portion of the pelvis (Fig. 31.1C) (Berglas & Rubin 1953). Once this occurs the endopelvic fascia, which until now needed only to stabilize the pelvic organs in position above the horizontal levator plate, is required to resist much more abdominal pressure. Ultimately this increased load surpasses the fascia's limits, leading to its breakage, detachment, and/or attenuation. The end result is prolapse of the pelvic organs through the genital hiatus (Fig. 31.1D). (Hurt 1990; DeLancey 1993; Norton 1993).

The urogenital diaphragm and superficial perineal musculature form a triangular structure that lies below the anterior segment of the pelvic diaphragm, attaching to the symphysis, the ischiopubic rami, and the perineal body. Based on their small bulk, it is unlikely that the diaphragm and superficial muscles contribute much to the support of the pelvic organs or to the active constriction of the genital hiatus (DeLancey 1993). The perineal body is a fibromuscular structure between the vagina and rectum which represents the confluence of the superficial perineal muscles, the external anal sphincter, the levator ani, and the posterior endopelvic fascia (Hurt 1990; Richardson 1995). The physical integrity and stability of the perineal body and the structures which contribute to it are essential to normal pelvic support. Excessive mobility and descent of the perineal body can both result from and contribute to progressive damage to the muscles of the pelvic floor.

The endopelvic fascia, a fibromuscular sheet continuous with the uterus, cervix, and vaginal wall, is composed of collagen, elastin and smooth muscle, and contains blood vessels and nerves. It envelops the vagina, cervix, and lower uterus and attaches and suspends these organs to the pelvic walls, aligning them about 30° above horizontal over the pelvic diaphragm (Fig. 31.2). It is useful conceptually to divide the endopelvic fascia into three levels, as

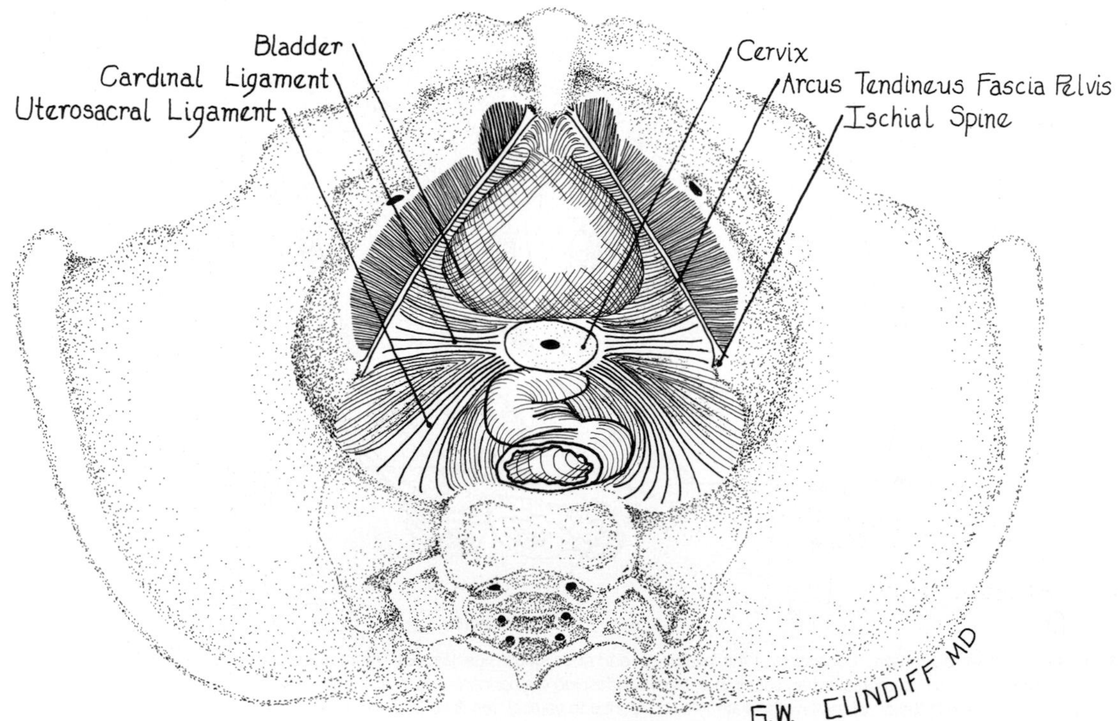

Fig. 31.2 The endopelvic fascia envelops the vagina, cervix, and lower uterus and attaches and suspends these organs to the pelvic walls, aligning them nearly horizontally over the pelvic diaphragm.

described by DeLancey (1992). Level I, the parametrium, is identified clinically as the uterosacral and cardinal ligament complex that attaches and suspends the uterus, cervix, and upper vagina to the pelvic side wall and the sacrum. Level II, the paracolpium, attaches the anterior and posterior vaginal walls to the lateral pelvic wall and is continuous with the endopelvic fascia of levels I and III. Anteriorly, this fibromuscular layer of the vaginal wall attaches to the arcus tendineus fascia pelvis overlying the obturator internus and levator ani muscles. The posterior wall fascia attaches to the superior fascia of the levator ani muscles laterally. At its inferior margins (level III), the endopelvic fascia of the vaginal walls fuses with surrounding structures. Anteriorly this fusion is with the urethra, the urogenital diaphragm, and the pubis, laterally it is with the levator ani fascia, and posteriorly it is with the perineal body. Discrete defects in the continuity of the endopelvic fascia or its peripheral attachments (Fig. 31.3), and rarely extreme attenuation of the fascia, can result in a variety of anatomic defects (Table 31.1). In summary, intact, continuous, and normally attached endopelvic fascia anteriorly, superiorly, and posteriorly prevents herniation of adjacent organs into the vagina; a healthy pelvic diaphragm prevents herniation of the vagina and adjacent viscera through the genital hiatus.

POP is the product of progressive failure of these pelvic support structures and mechanisms resulting from a series of predisposing, inciting, promoting, and decompensating factors (Table 31.2). The evidence is overwhelming that vaginal childbirth is the prerequisite inciting factor for the majority of prolapse. Delivery is capable of causing significant damage to the physical integrity of the endopelvic fascia and its attachments and injury to pelvic nerves and muscles. However, it is also clear that vaginal delivery does not result in clinically significant prolapse in the vast majority of women and that we cannot differentiate individual deliveries destined to result in prolapse from those that will not. The effect of birth trauma is quite variable and can contribute to prolapse of variable severity and sequence. In some instances, damage may be focal and very discrete, resulting in an isolated defect and minimal symptoms. For example, detachment of the anterior endopelvic fascia from the arcus tendineus fascia pelvis can result in a detachment cystocele that may be asymptomatic if good levator ani and pelvic diaphragm function is preserved. In another situa-

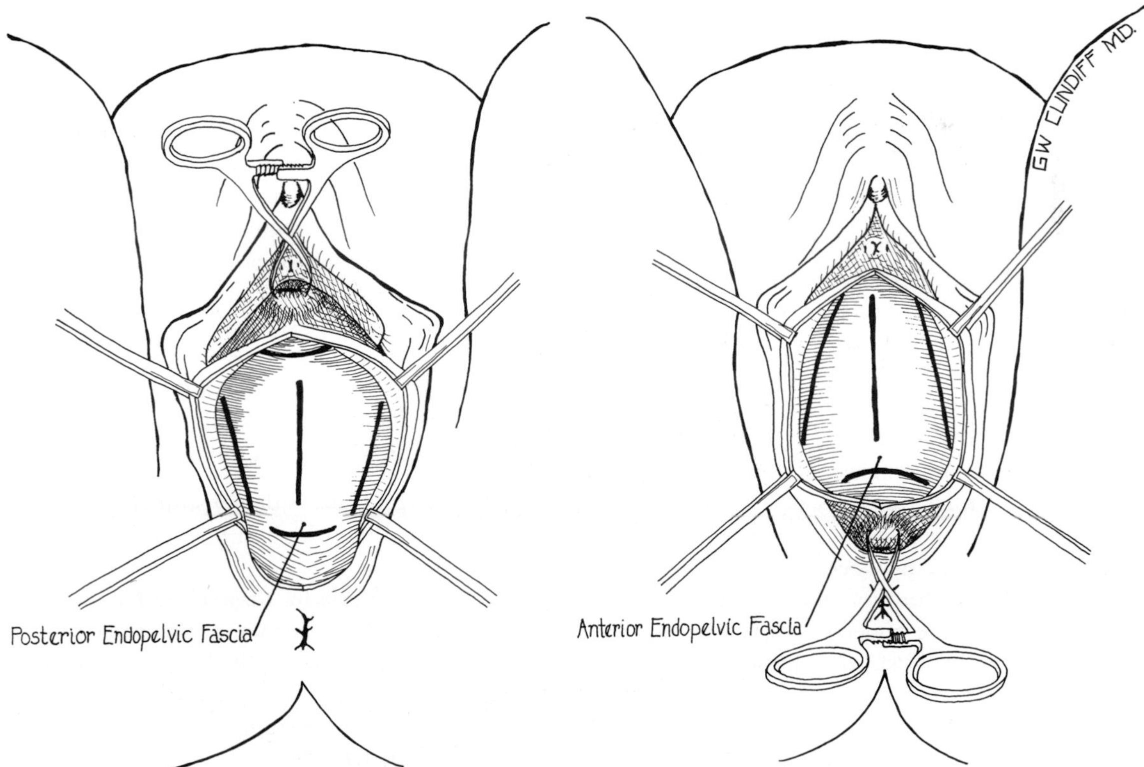

Fig. 31.3 Discrete defects can occur in the endopelvic fascia centrally as well as inferiorly, superiorly, or laterally at its peripheral attachments. Sites of discrete defects in the posterior endopelvic fascia (left) and the anterior endopelvic fascia (right) are depicted.

Table 31.1 Sequelae of some discrete fascial breaks or detachments.

Level	Structure	Sequelae
I	Uterosacral-cardinal complex	Uterovaginal prolapse
I-II junction	Anterior fascia	Superior cystocele, enterocele
	Posterior fascia	Perineal descent, enterocele
II lateral	Anterior fascia	Detachment cystocele (paravaginal defect)
II central	Anterior fascia	Central cystocele
II	Posterior fascia	High rectocele
III	Posterior fascia	Low detachment rectocele

Table 31.2 Factors contributing to pelvic organ prolapse.

Factors
Predisposing (congenital) factors
Skeletal
Neurological
Muscular
Connective tissue
Racial
Gender
Inciting (acquired) factors
Vaginal delivery
Surgery
Neurological
Promoting factors
Obesity
Smoking
Lung disease
Constipation
Recreational stresses
Occupational stresses
Surgery
Decompensating factors
Ageing
Menopause and hormonal deprivation
Neuropathy (progressive or acquired)
Myopathy (progressive or acquired)
Debilitation
Medications

tion, separation of the posterior fascia from the perineal body resulting in a distal rectocele can contribute to progressive prolapse if a feeling of incomplete defecation leads to excessive straining. Straining can effect sequential perineal descent, stretch injury to nerves, neuropathic muscle dysfunction, failure of the levator plate, detachment of the endopelvic fascia, and prolapse of the anterior and apical segments. Other examples of critical forks in the path to prolapse include, but are not limited to, the following: permanent, severe, delivery-induced pelvic neuropathy; failure to attach the uterosacral-cardinal complex to the upper vagina, close the cul-de-sac, and/or re-establish the continuity of the anterior and posterior endopelvic fascia at hysterectomy; spinal cord transection; isolated urethropexy for incontinence in a woman with multiple unrecognized support defects; uterosacral lysis for chronic pain (Davis 1996); or severe chronic cough induced by the initiation of an angiotensin-converting enzyme inhibitor for the treatment of hypertension.

Clearly, there are many scenarios which can lead to prolapse; in an individual patient a single factor in Table 31.2 may be so overwhelming that it alone will cause severe POP. More often, multiple sequential insults over a lifetime are responsible. The end result is damage to the integrity of the nerves, muscles, and fascia of the pelvis. The existing prolapse literature deals predominantly with the management of the end-stage disease. Future projects should attempt to identify and control or modulate the factors contributing to it.

CLASSIFICATION

One of the major deterrents to the scientific study of POP has been the lack of an accepted, objective, and validated system for describing the spectrum of pelvic support in individual patients and in study populations. In recognition of this problem, the International Continence Society (ICS) established an international, multidisciplinary terminology standardization committee for prolapse in 1993. The committee devised a site-specific quantitative description of support that locates six defined points around the vagina (two anterior, two posterior and two apical) with respect to their relationship to the hymen. Once measurements are obtained, subjects are assigned to one of five ordinal stages as follows:

Stage 0 – no prolapse is demonstrated, i.e. all points are at their highest possible level above the hymen

Stage I – the criteria for Stage 0 are not met but the most distal portion of the prolapse is more than 1 cm above the level of the hymen

Stage II – the most distal portion of the prolapse is 1 cm or less proximal to or distal to the plane of the hymen

Stage III – the most distal portion of the prolapse is more than 1 cm below the plane of the hymen but protrudes no further than 2 cm less than the total vaginal length in cm

Stage IV – essentially complete eversion of the total length of the lower genital tract is demonstrated.

In addition, the system calls for three other measurements: the anterior–posterior length of the genital hiatus and the perineal body and the total vaginal length. Prior to its acceptance, reproducibility studies in six centres in the United States and Europe were completed, documenting the inter- and intra-rater reliability and clinical utility of the system in 240 women (Athanasiou et al 1995; Schüssler & Peschers 1995; Montella & Cater 1995; Kobak et al 1995; Hall et al 1996) The standardization document was formally adopted by the ICS in 1995 and by the American Urogynecologic Society and the Society of Gynecologic Surgeons in 1996. It was published in 1996 (Bump et al 1996b) and is reproduced in its entirety in Appendix III.[1]

The ICS POP Quantitation and Staging system reliably describes the topographic position of six vaginal sites and gives information regarding perineal descent and the change in axis of the levator plate based on increases in genital hiatus and perineal body measurements. As such it is a useful tool to enhance communication among clinicians and researchers, to objectively follow changes in an individual patient over time, and to assess the success and durability of various surgical and non-surgical treatments. However, it does not identify the specific defect(s) in the pelvic support structures and mechanisms responsible for the topographic changes and cannot determine the surgical steps necessary for successful repair. Multiple ancillary procedures, including supplementary physical examination techniques, endoscopy, imaging procedures, photography, pelvic neuromuscle testing, and intraoperative identification of discrete fascial defects, play important roles in the formulation of a surgical strategy. These are considered in the standardization document and several are included in other chapters of this book.

The preoperative examination should (a) identify all defects in the endopelvic fascia that must be corrected to reduce the bulging or descent of organs through the vaginal wall and (b) consider the likelihood that the pelvic floor will act as an effective back-stop for the flap-valve support mechanism to prevent protrusion of the organs through the genital hiatus at the conclusion of the repair. To achieve the first aim, specific attention should be paid to the attachment of the anterior endopelvic fascia to the arcus tendineus fascia pelvis (Baden & Walker 1992), to the continuity of the anterior and posterior fascia at the vaginal apex, to the integrity of the superior vaginal attachments of the uterosacral-cardinal complex, to the continuity of the posterior fascia with the perineal body (Richardson 1993, 1995), to attachment of the posterior fascia to the levator fascia, and to discrete defects in the anterior and posterior fascia. The second aim is much more difficult to achieve accurately. A purely anatomic repair, usually performed vaginally, that re-attaches the vaginal apex to origins of the uterosacral-cardinal complex, corrects lateral and midline fascial defects, and reconnects the posterior fascia to the perineal body, will significantly narrow the genital hiatus and perineal body and restore the horizontal axis of the pelvic diaphragm. If the muscles of the diaphragm are healthy, restoration of axis and reloading will result in improved function and rehabilitation. Conversely, if the pelvic diaphragm is severely compromised on a neuropathic or myopathic basis, it will fail when re-aligned and reloaded, placing the anatomically repaired endopelvic fascia under excessive stress, leading to its failure and recurrent POP. In this instance, anatomic repair of fascial defects must be combined with a suspensory procedure using synthetic or heterologous materials, usually performed abdominally, to compensate for the critical dysfunction of the pelvic floor (Cundiff et al 1999). Efforts are currently being directed at evaluating the ability of imaging procedures (e.g. dynamic pelvic fluoroscopy, ultrasound, or MRI), neurophysiologic testing (e.g. computerized action potential analysis), functional testing of pelvic floor muscles, and physical examination measurements (e.g. assessment of perineal descent) to predict postoperative pelvic diaphragm function. Ultimately, the reliability of an evaluation scheme and surgical strategy for POP must be assessed in well-designed outcome studies that use standard, validated outcome measures involving multiple domains (e.g. anatomy, function, quality of life, cost effectiveness). The ICS POP quantitation and staging system seems to function well in the anatomic domain.

PRESENTATION

There is no agreement as to the symptoms caused by POP, which symptoms result exclusively from defects in pelvic support, and which symptoms reliably resolve following successful treatment of POP. Table 31.3 lists urinary, bowel, sexual, and other local symptoms considered in the ICS POP document. There is a need to develop, standardize, and psychometrically

Table 31.3 Symptoms associated with pelvic organ prolapse. From Bump et al (1996), with permission.

Symptoms
Urinary symptoms
Stress incontinence
Frequency (diurnal and nocturnal)
Urgency
Urge incontinence
Hesitancy
Weak or prolonged urinary stream
Feeling of incomplete emptying
Manual reduction to start or complete bladder emptying
Positional changes to start or complete voiding
Bowel symptoms
Difficulty with defecation
Incontinence of flatus, liquid stool, or solid stool
Faecal staining
Urgency of defecation
Discomfort with defecation
Digital manipulation of vagina, perineum or anus to complete defecation
Feeling of incomplete evacuation
Rectal protrusion during or after defecation
Sexual symptoms
Inability to have sexual activity
Inability to have vaginal coitus
Infrequent coitus
Dyspareunia
Lack of satisfaction or orgasm
Incontinence experienced during sexual activity
Other local symptoms
Vaginal pressure or heaviness
Vaginal or perineal pain
Sensation or awareness of tissue protrusion from the vagina
Low back pain
Abdominal pressure or pain
Observation or palpation of a mass

validate condition-specific quality of life instruments and scales for POP. Such instruments can be used both to determine the presence and severity of various symptoms and to assess the impact of POP on activities of daily living. Symptom severity and impact can be compared to the anatomic defect before and after treatment.

Some symptoms are clearly attributable to POP. Seeing and feeling massive external protrusion of tissues many centimetres beyond the hymen is an obvious example. Other symptoms are more ambiguous; will chronic constipation improve with prolapse reduction or did a lifetime of excessive straining cause the prolapse and pose a risk for its recurrence? Many patients present with a paucity of symptoms and are concerned only because they felt an internal 'bulge' while wiping after micturition or have been told that they 'have a cystocele' after a routine examination. In these situations, a careful recording of the POP quantitation exam measurements, words of explanation and reassurance, and a plan for longitudinal follow-up is usually the most prudent management strategy. In the end, it is the provider's responsibility to document the severity of the prolapse and to try to correlate the physical findings with the patient's symptoms and concerns. After this, frank and honest discussions with the patient should form the basis for her informed and involved consent in a plan of management or observation.

INVESTIGATIONS

The roles of the physical examination, imaging studies, neurophysiologic studies, and pelvic muscle testing were discussed in the earlier section on classification and are considered in other chapters. In this section, we will briefly consider two other evaluation modalities: urodynamics and upper urinary tract evaluations.

Urodynamic studies in women with POP have been recommended to evaluate for 'potential stress incontinence', to evaluate other overt urinary incontinence, and to evaluate emptying phase dysfunction. Women with advanced (Stage III or IV) POP involving the anterior segment rarely have genuine stress incontinence (GSI). In our experience with 184 consecutive women with such prolapse, none had GSI. It has been shown that severe POP, when accentuated by stress, will descend and obstruct the urethra, preventing GSI despite significant bladder neck hypermobility. Reduction of the prolapse with a barrier (a pessary or speculum) prevents the stress-activated urethral obstruction and reveals so-called occult or potential stress incontinence in 36–80% of women with advanced prolapse (Richardson et al 1983; Bump et al 1988; Bergman et al 1988; Rosenzweig et al 1992). It has been suggested that such tests should be used to identify patients at risk for GSI or intrinsic urethral sphincteric deficiency (ISD) so that they can receive a formal suspending urethropexy or a sling procedure, respectively, to prevent the development of GSI after prolapse reduction surgery. However, it has been shown retrospectively that only 10% of continent women undergoing vaginal prolapse surgery actually develop GSI, indicating that barrier testing drastically overestimates the risk of potential GSI (Beck et al 1991). A prospective, randomized trial from our units confirmed the lack of predictive value of barrier testing for both GSI and ISD (Bump et al 1996a). While barrier testing predicted potential stress incontinence in 10 of 15 subjects (67%) who underwent vaginal prolapse surgery without a suspending urethropexy, GSI was observed in only one subject (7%) at 6 months. Furthermore, we predicted that 7 of 29 women (24%) would have developed ISD whereas only one (3%) did. The fact that severe prolapse may mask potential GSI should be appreciated by every reconstructive pelvic surgeon. It should also be appreciated that a major aim of reconstructive surgery is for the patient to leave the operating room with durable and preferential support to the bladder neck. However, we should abandon the notion that preoperative barrier testing tells us which specific procedure should be performed to prevent GSI. Despite this conclusion, we continue to perform preoperative urodynamics on patients with Stage III and IV POP to evaluate their emptying function and their detrusor activity and compliance, as well as their sphincteric function. We do counsel patients with severe deterioration in sphincteric function that they have an increased risk for developing GSI and that they may need salvage therapy in the form of periurethral injections or a sling as a secondary procedure. Other patients are quoted an 8–10% risk of developing GSI and told that this is comparable to the failure rate of a Burch procedure performed for the treatment of GSI.

Patients with advanced prolapse have lower urinary flow rates and higher post-void residual volumes than other women. Nonetheless, most women with Stage III or IV POP empty quite efficiently. In a consecutive series of 184 such women, the mean and maximum flow rates averaged 13.6 and 20.0 ml/s and the mean post-void residual volume was 92 ml. Only 30% of this group had residuals over 100 ml (Coates et al 1997). We advise women with low flow rates and high post-void residuals that they may suffer persistent emptying phase dysfunction after prolapse surgery and that the potential need for prolonged intermittent self-catheterization is significant.

When a woman with Stage III or IV POP has urinary incontinence, it is likely that the basis for the incontinence is detrusor overactivity. An unstable detrusor or a poorly compliant detrusor in the face of partial physical urethral obstruction places such a patient at increased risk for vesicoureteral reflux, upper tract dilation, and renal damage. The urodyanamic evaluation of an incontinent prolapse patient should include an evaluation for detrusor instability, a determination of bladder compliance, and if either instability or decreased compliance is noted, a determination of the detrusor leak point pressure. Patients with a detrusor leak point ≥ 40 cm H_2O are at significant risk for upper tract damage (McGuire et al 1981). We recommend upper tract assessments (intravenous urogram or ultrasound) and serum creatinine determinations on all patients with stage III or IV POP who have poorly suppressed detrusor instability, detrusor instability with high post-void residual urine volumes, detrusor instability with recurrent infections, decreased bladder compliance (< 40 ml/cm H_2O), and detrusor leak point pressures ≥ 40 cm H_2O.

PREVENTION

There are several clinical interventions which may impact the future development of POP. As parturition appears to be a prominent inciting event, it deserves special attention. Obstetrical parameters associated with damage to the pelvic floor include nulliparity, macrosomia, and forceps delivery (Sultan et al 1993). It is obvious that the vaginal and perineal dilation necessary for descent and delivery of the fetal head is likely to be associated with trauma to the fascial supports. Vaginal delivery may also initiate damage to the pelvic floor musculature, either by direct injury to the muscles, damage to their innervation, or both (Toglia & DeLancey 1994). As compression or stretch injury caused by the fetal head in the birth canal appears to be a mechanism for nerve damage, a prolonged second stage and traumatic obstetrical interventions associated with it should be minimized when possible. The debate over the utility of episiotomy has waged for decades. There is evidence that episiotomy contributes to physical disruption of the internal and external anal sphincter (Sultan et al 1994). Conversely, episiotomy has been associated with a decreased incidence of cystocele and rectocele development, a protective effect that may be enhanced by the antepartum performance of pelvic muscle exercises (Taskin et al 1996). It is possible that a properly timed episiotomy and strong pelvic muscles can minimize distension and descent of the pelvic floor and concurrent nerve damage, although further studies are needed to confirm this hypothesis.

Although the preponderance of literature on pelvic floor exercises is in the treatment of GSI, Kegel's original work demonstrated a benefit in restoring the function of the pelvic muscles after parturition (Kegel 1948, 1949). Pelvic floor rehabilitation probably should be appreciated as playing a greater role in preventing POP. Minimizing other promoting factors (Table 31.2), such as chronically increased abdominal pressure, constipation, and oestrogen deficiency, cannot be overemphasized in efforts to prevent POP. Preventing POP after hysterectomy is another opportunity for the gynaecologist to intervene. Emphasis should be placed on obliteration of the cul-de-sac, providing superior support for the vagina, and re-establishing continuity of the superior endopelvic fascia at every abdominal and vaginal hysterectomy (Given 1992; Cruikshank 1987).

NON-SURGICAL TREATMENT

Although pelvic muscle exercises may be beneficial as primary therapy for early stages of POP and as adjunctive therapy for advanced stages, there are minimal data at this point to identify the best prospective candidates. Pessaries have traditionally been the mainstay of non-surgical therapy. Pessaries have been used to treat uterine malposition, dysmenorrhoea, menstrual irregularities, and incompetent cervix as well as POP (Browne 1962; Colmer 1953; Oster & Javert 1966). They are available in a variety of shapes and sizes that may allow tailoring of the pessary to a specific support defect and individual anatomy. Factors that jeopardize pessary effectiveness include a weak pelvic diaphragm, large genital hiatus, prior hysterectomy, and complete procidentia. Unfortunately, the same factors that contribute to severe stages of POP often can compromise the patient's ability to maintain the position of a pessary. While pessaries are effective in many women, they are not without potential complications, including vaginal wall ulceration due to an embedded pessary (Muram et al 1990), fistula formation (Goldstien et al 1990), and bowel herniation (Ott et al 1993). Complications can be minimized by choosing a pessary that does not exert excessive pressure on the vaginal epithelium and by emphasizing proper pessary care, including regular surveillance and cleaning and the use of oestrogen replacement therapy. Sulak et al (1993) described the following three types of patients that benefit from pessary use: the patient unfit for surgery, one awaiting surgery, and one who declines surgery. While pessaries were effective in managing such women, there was still a discontinuation rate of 20%.

SURGERY

There are numerous surgical techniques to correct POP from both the abdominal and vaginal approach. Too often, the choice of procedure and route of approach has been based on the surgeon's biases rather than on anatomic principles. Improved understanding of normal and abnormal pelvic anatomy and function now permit a more rational selection of procedure and route based on what is best for the individual patient.

Several considerations which impact the choice of procedure include the precise defects responsible for the POP, the aetiology of the defects, whether the inciting and promoting events are continuing processes, and the patients' desires and expectations. For the frail patient whose health status precludes prolonged extensive surgery, an obliterative procedure such as vaginectomy and colpocleisis affords symptom relief with minimal morbidity due to shorter operative time. Such a procedure is contraindicated, however, for any woman with a desire to maintain vaginal function. For a woman with discrete endopelvic fascia defects, an anatomic vaginal repair that corrects the defects of the indigenous tissues may be effective. Such repairs can be accomplished from the vaginal approach and are generally less stressful than procedures performed through an abdominal incision. As noted earlier, there are circumstances that may compromise the longevity of these repairs. Surgeries that utilize native tissues depend on normal muscular support and function and might be expected to fail in the presence of neuromuscular compromise of the pelvic diaphragm. Extreme attenuation of native tissues may also compromise the success of these repairs. Finally, women with recurrent POP, active lifestyles, or chronic ongoing aetiologies for POP may require a repair with more strength than is offered by anatomic repairs. Under these circumstances a compensatory repair that provides additional support mechanisms is indicated.

The primary advantage of obliterative procedures is the brevity of operating time which decreases acute perioperative morbidity. The vaginal approach and short operating time make regional or local anaesthesia with sedation an alternative to general anaesthesia for many chronically ill patients (Miklos et al 1995). While a short operating time is a goal of obliterative techniques, obtaining optimal results still demands attention to critical support defects. It is important to provide preferential support to the urethrovesical junction, and to adequately reduce the enterocele component of the prolapse during colpocleisis, if stress incontinence and recurrent prolapse are to be avoided. Since obliterative procedures preclude subsequent evaluation of the cervix and uterine cavity, vaginal hysterectomy should be performed prior to colpocleisis. Generally hysterectomy, enterocele repair, bladder neck support, vaginectomy, and colpocleisis can be completed in 90 minutes or less with limited blood loss. This is preferred over more delimited procedures such as a LeFort partial colpocleisis, in all but the most fragile patients.

In planning a reconstructive procedure designed

to maintain vaginal function, it is essential to address defects of support at all levels during both anatomic and compensatory procedures. While most women require multiple steps for successful repair, for the sake of organization we will address the vaginal apex, the anterior compartment, and the posterior compartment separately.

There are two important adjunct steps to ensuring durable apical support regardless of the anchoring site for the vaginal vault suspension. The first is establishing the continuity of the anterior and posterior vaginal fascia at the vaginal apex. Failure to approximate these fascial planes will result in a vault enterocele behind the thin vaginal epithelium lacking its myofascial layer. The second adjunct step is the closure of the cul-de-sac. Elimination of this potential space helps ensure the orientation of the vagina directly over the pelvic diaphragm.

There are many techniques for suspending the vaginal apex. For the patient with a functional pelvic diaphragm and good endopelvic fascia, a vaginal approach using native tissues is appropriate. An extensive culdoplasty that plicates the uterosacral ligaments and closes the cul-de-sac along with bilateral suspension of the vaginal vault from the origins of the uterosacral ligaments near the sacrum is one such approach (McCall 1957). Another option is to suspend the vault bilaterally to the fascia of the iliococcygeus muscle, just anterior to ischial spine (Shull et al 1993). Finally, unilateral or bilateral fixation of the apex to the sacrospinous ligament/coccygeus muscle complex is a widely advocated and utilized option (Richter & Albrich 1981; Nichols 1982; Myazakin 1987). Figure 31.4 illustrates each of these sites of attachment in relation to the normal anatomic position of the vagina. The lateral and posterior deflection of the vagina with the typical unilateral sacrospinous ligament fixation is clearly not anatomic and exposes the anterior superior vaginal wall to increased force during increases in abdominal pressure. While the iliococcygeus suspension maintains the normal alignment of the vaginal cylinder, the ischial spines are considerably inferior to the normal position of the vaginal apex. The origins of the uterosacral ligaments, if sufficiently strong on both sides, allow better vaginal depth with normal alignment. When attenuation of the ligaments mandates plication at the level of the suspension, the resulting midline suspension is not anatomic.

The woman with attenuated fascia, a compromised

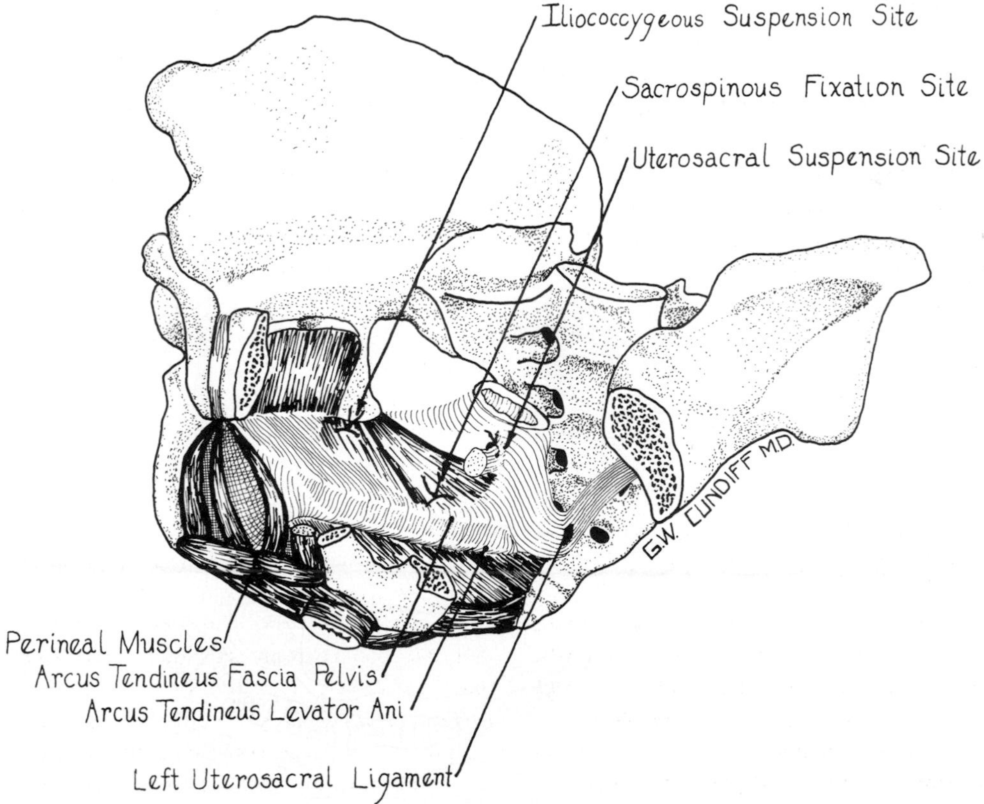

Fig. 31.4 Sites of attachment for suspension of the vaginal apex using the sacrospinous ligament/coccygeus muscle complex, the ileococcygeus muscle fascia, and the origins of the uterosacral ligaments. These sites of fixation are visualized through a window in a normally aligned vagina; oblique view with left public ramus removed.

pelvic floor, or severe ongoing physical stress is better served by a technique of vault suspension that provides compensatory support. Our preferred compensatory repair is the abdominal sacral colpopexy with interposition of a synthetic suspensory bridge between the prolapsed vagina and the anterior sacrum. This procedure maintains the normal axis of the vagina and is preferred to ventral fixation procedures. There is significant reported experience with this procedure which helps to define the important technical aspects. While early series attached the suspensory mesh to the sacrum at the S3–4 level, this site has been associated with an increased risk for significant haemorrhage and the sacral promontory to upper third of the sacrum appears to be a safer fixation area (Sutton et al 1981). Most failures occur due to avulsion of the mesh from the vagina (Addison et al 1989). This can be minimized by using a broad fixation of separate meshes to the anterior and posterior vaginal walls, being certain to include the entire wall (epithelium and fibromuscular layer) (Addison et al 1996). Any defect in the fibromuscular layer should be repaired before the mesh is attached. Reports of enterocele formation behind the posterior mesh emphasize the importance of a concurrent Halban's culdoplasty with permanent suture incorporating the posterior mesh into the anterior segment of the culdoplasty.

Defects in the anterior segment can occur laterally, superiorly, and in the midline (Fig. 31.3). Superior defects are addressed with closure of the cuff, establishing continuity of the anterior and posterior fascia. The original description of the repair of lateral defects, the paravaginal repair, utilized the vaginal approach (White 1912) but more recently the abdominal retropubic approach has been more popular (Richardson et al 1976). When performed vaginally, the epithelium is incised and dissected from the underlying endopelvic fascia beneath the descending pubic rami to the lateral pelvic wall. Abdominally, the retropubic space is dissected to expose several important landmarks including the arcus tendineus fascia pelvis running between the posterior aspect of the pubis and the ischial spine and the more superior and lateral obturator neurovascular bundle. Once landmarks are identified, the endopelvic fascia and lateral vaginal sulcus are sutured to the arcus with interrupted stitches using permanent suture. Central anterior defects can also be repaired from either a vaginal or abdominal approach. Vaginally, the epithe-

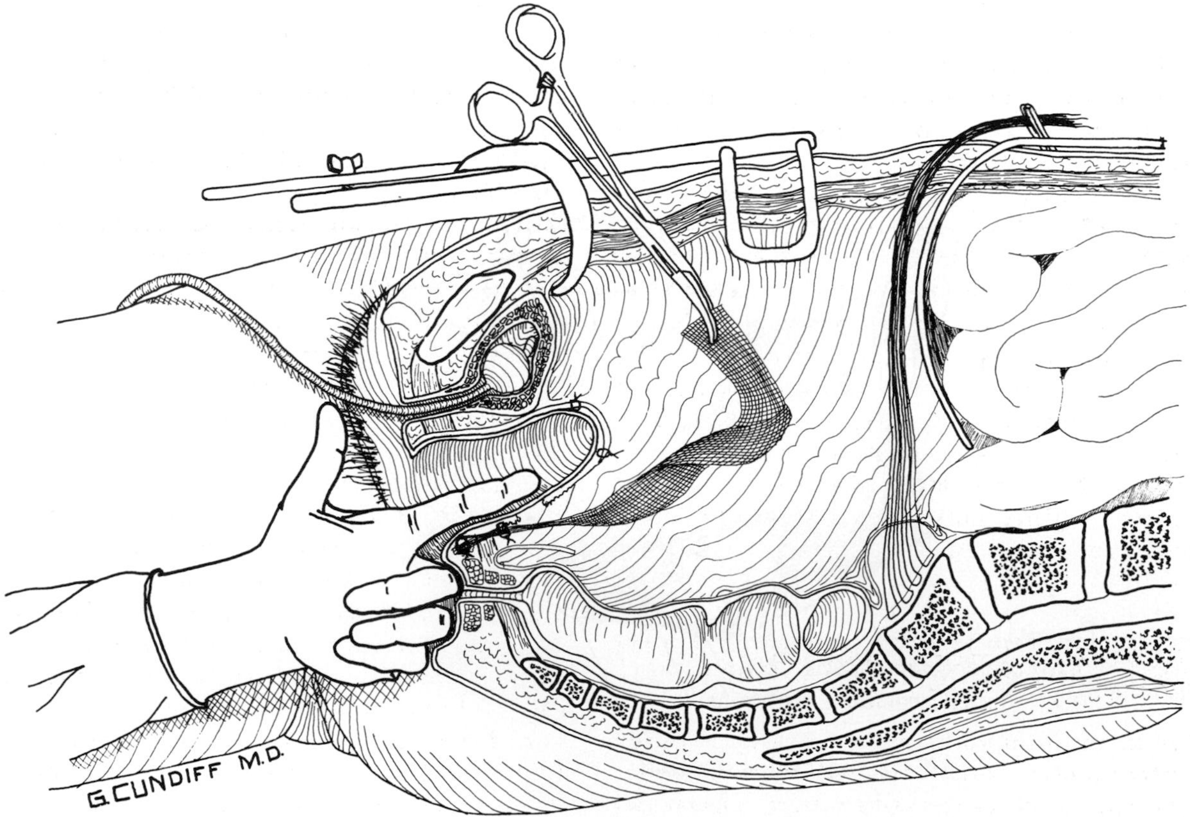

Fig. 31.5 Sagittal section illustrating dissection of the rectovaginal space and attachment of mesh to the perineal body which is elevated by the surgeon's hand.

lium is incised and dissected from the underlying endopelvic fascia until the defect is demonstrated. Access to the defect from the abdominal approach is achieved by opening the vesicouterine peritoneal reflection and mobilizing the bladder after clamping and ligating the bladder pillars (Macer 1978). For the occasional patient whose endopelvic fascia is too attenuated to repair, a piece of synthetic mesh or heterologous fascia can be used to substitute for the fascia (Nichols & Randall 1989). Following correction of all fascial defects, preferential support for the urethrovesical junction can be achieved either with vaginal plication of the endopelvic fascia (Hurt 1990b) or by a retropubic urethropexy.

Repair of posterior segment prolapse from a vaginal approach is similar to the technique described for the anterior wall (Richardson 1993). The epithelium is incised and dissected from the underlying endopelvic fascia out to its lateral attachments to the levator ani fascia. Identification of discrete fascial tears is facilitated by displacing the anterior rectal wall with a finger in the rectum and by avoiding the injection of haemostatic agents which distort and obscure the tissue planes. Careful attention to the attachment of the posterior endopelvic fascia to the perineal body is essential to prevent recurrent rectocele and to help correct perineal descent. We perform perineal reconstruction prior to fascial reattachment if the superficial perineal muscles are separated but avoid non-anatomic perineorrhaphy that artificially enlarges the perineum and superficially constricts the genital hiatus.

The abdominal sacral colpoperineopexy is an abdominal approach to the correction of posterior segment prolapse associated with severe perineal descent and vault prolapse (Cundiff et al 1997). Prior to attaching the posterior suspensory mesh, the rectovaginal septum is opened from above, permitting the mesh to be attached to the most superior aspect of the endopelvic fascia that remains contiguous with the perineal body (Fig. 31.5). For the patient with attenuated posterior fascia, the mesh is attached directly to the perineal body to provide compensatory support.

SURGICAL RESULTS AND COMPLICATIONS

Besides the usual complications associated with any surgery, prolapse surgery can result in new or continued dysfunction of the urinary tract, vagina, and bowel. The most disheartening complication, however, is recurrent POP. While some failures are inevitable, one must always question if a failure resulted from an incorrectly performed procedure or the choice of an inappropriate procedure.

The only prospective randomized study comparing vaginal and abdominal approaches for POP surgery was by Benson et al (1996). This study compared outcomes for all vaginal segments and noted a significantly higher rate of re-operation for recurrent prolapse with vaginal compared to abdominal surgery, 33% versus 16%. While the authors hypothesized that some of this difference was due to neuropathy caused by the vaginal dissection, some of the difference might also be explained by the use of the sacrospinous ligament suspension and needle urethropexies in the vaginal group. The majority of vaginal failures involved the anterior segment, and sacrospinous fixation has been shown to predispose to recurrent anterior wall prolapse (Paraiso et al 1996; Shull et al 1992; Morley & DeLancey 1988; Holley et al 1995) particularly when combined with needle bladder neck suspensions (Bump et al 1996a). Other complications described following sacrospinous fixation include vaginal shortening, sexual dysfunction, pain, and haemorrhage. The latter complications are related to the close proximity of pudendal nerves and vessels laterally and gluteal vessels and sacral nerve roots superiorly.

Although the technique of uterosacral suspension was described four decades ago, there is relatively little data regarding its efficacy. McCall (1957) reported no recurrent enteroceles during a 3-year follow-up and Given (1985) reported a 5% failure rate with an average follow-up of 7 years. Elkins et al (1995) compared high uterosacral suspension to sacrospinous ligament fixation and found a greater vaginal depth with the former (10.2 versus 8.3 cm). They cautioned about the proximity of the uterosacral ligaments to the ureters, averaging about 1.4 cm at the level of the cervix in cadaveric dissections.

In distinction to the sacrospinous and uterosacral ligaments, the iliococcygeus fascia does not have critical structures such as the pudendal nerve or ureter immediately adjacent to it. Meeks et al (1994) reported a 4% recurrence rate for anterior segment prolapse in 110 women following iliococcygeus suspension. This is better than the 19% failure rate in a study of 42 women reported by Shull et al (1993), although 10 women had minimal anterior defects and only 5% had failure of apical support.

Abdominal sacral colpopexy has a consistent cure rate of over 90% (Timmons et al 1992; Snyder & Krantz 1991; Creighton & Stanton 1991; Baker et al 1990). It is not without complications, including the risk of rare life-threatening intraoperative haemorrhage and a 3.3% incidence of vaginal mesh erosion (Timmons & Addison 1997). Erosions can usually be managed with vaginal excision of all or part of the mesh followed by partial colpocleisis. Our early experience with abdominal sacral colpoperineopexy demonstrates correction of severe recurrent prolapse to Stage 0 in 12 of 19 patients (63%), to Stage I in 4 (21%), and to Stage II in the remaining 3 (16%). Only 1 (5%) had a recurrent rectocele and two thirds of patients had resolution of chronic bowel symptoms (Cundiff et al 1998).

Discrete defect rectocele repairs have been shown to correct rectoceles in 82% of cases while achieving significant improvements in symptoms of constipation, tenesmus, and splinting of the vagina or perineum during defecation (Cundiff et al 1998). While there are considerable data regarding the efficacy of the abdominal paravaginal defect repair for GSI, its efficacy for anterior POP is not as well documented. Richardson (1976) reported a cure rate of 95% while Shull & Baden (1989) also reported a 5% recurrence rate for cystocele but noted a 6% incidence of vault prolapse and a 5% incidence of enterocele. Macer compared the vaginal and abdominal routes for midline anterior defect repairs, citing cure rates of 78% and 92% respectively, with a 4% incidence of bladder-flap haematomas using the abdominal approach (1978). Julian reported a 66% cure rate for standard vaginal anterior colporrhaphy for recurrent anterior prolapse compared to a 100% cure rate when Marlex mesh was used to substitute for the endopelvic fascia (1996). There was, however, a 25% incidence of mesh-related complications.

[1] A video tape demonstrating the method for completing and recording the POP quantitation examination is available at a nominal charge through the American Urogynecologic Society.

REFERENCES

Addison W A, Cundiff G W, Bump R C 1996 Sacral colpopexy is the preferred treatment for vaginal vault prolapse. Journal of Gynecologic Techniques 2: 69–74

Addison W A, Timmons M C, Wall L L, Livengood C H 1989 Failed abdominal sacral colpopexy: observations and recommendations. Obstetrics and Gynecology 74: 480–482

Athanasiou S, Hill S, Gleeson C, Anders K, Cardozo L 1995 Validation of the ICS proposed pelvic organ prolapse descriptive system. Neurourology and Urodynamics 14: 414–415

Baden W, Walker T. Surgical repair of vaginal defects. J B Lippincott, Philadelphia, pp 51–62

Baker K R, Beresford J M, Campbell C 1990 Colposacropexy with Prolene mesh. Surgery, Gynecology and Obstetrics 171: 51–54

Beck R P, McCormick S, Nordstrom L 1991 A 25-year experience with 519 anterior colporrhaphy procedures. Obstetrics and Gynecology 78: 1011–1018

Benson J T, Lucente V, McClellan E 1996 Vaginal versus abdominal reconstructive surgery for the treatment of pelvic support defects: a prospective randomized study with long-term outcome evaluation. American Journal of Obstetrics and Gynecology 175: 1418–1422

Berglas B, Rubin I C 1953 Study of the supportive structures of the uterus by levator myography. Surgery, Gynecology and Obstetrics 97: 677–692

Bergman A, Koonings P P, Ballard C A. Predicting postoperative urinary incontinence development in women undergoing operation for genitourinary prolapse. American Journal of Obstetrics and Gynecology 158: 1171–1175

Blakeley C R, Mills W G 1981 The obstetric and gynaecological complications of bladder exstrophy and epispadias. British Journal of Obsetetrics and Gynaecology 88: 167–173

Browne A D H 1962 Advances in obstetrics and gynecology. Practitioner 189: 428

Bump R C, Fantl J A, Hurt W G 1988 The mechanism of urinary continence in women with severe uterovaginal prolapse: results of barrier studies. Obstetrics and Gynecology 72: 291–295

Bump R C, Hurt W G, Theofrastous J P et al and the Continence Program for Women Research Group 1996a Randomized prospective comparison of needle colposuspension versus endopelvic fascia plication for potential stress incontinence prophylaxis in women undergoing vaginal reconstruction for stage III or IV pelvic organ prolapse. American Journal of Obstetrics and Gynecology 175: 326–335

Bump R C, Mattiasson A, Bø K et al 1996b The standardisation of terminology of female pelvic organ prolapse and pelvic floor dysfunction. American Journal of Obstetrics and Gynecology 175: 10–17

Coates K W, Harris R L, Cundiff G W, Bump R C 1997 Uroflowmetry in women with urinary incontinence and pelvic organ prolapse. British Journal of Urology 80: 217

Colmer W M 1953 Use of the pessary. American Journal of Obstetrics and Gynecology 65: 170

Creighton S M, Stanton S L 1991 The surgical management of vaginal vault prolapse. British Journal of Obstetrics and Gynecology 98: 1150–1154

Cruikshank S H 1987 Preventing posthysterectomy vaginal vault prolapse and enterocele during vaginal hysterectomy. American Journal of Obstetrics and Gynecology 156: 1433–1440

Cundiff G W, Harris R L, Coates K W, Low V B M, Bump R C, Addison W A 1997 Abdominal sacral colpoperineopexy: a new approach for correction of posterior compartment defects and perineal descent associated with vaginal vault prolapse. American Journal of Obstetrics and Gynecology 177: 1345–55

Cundiff G W, Weidner A C, Visco A G, Addison W A, Bump R C 1998 An anatomic and functional assessment of the discrete defect rectocele repair. American Journal of Obstetrics and Gynecology 179: 1451–7

Davis G D 1996 Uterine prolapse after laparoscopic uterosacral transection in nulliparous airborne trainees. Journal of Reproductive Medicine 41: 279–282

DeLancey J O L 1992. Anatomic aspects of vaginal eversion after hysterectomy. American Journal of Obstetrics and Gynecology 166: 1717–1728

DeLancey, J O L 1993 Anatomy and biomechanics of genital prolapse. Clinical Obstetrics and Gynecology 36: 897–909

Elkins T E, Hopper J B, Goodfellow K, Gasser R, Nolan T E, Schexnayder M C 1995 Initial report of anatomic and clinical comparison of the sacrospinous ligament fixation to the high McCall culdeplasty for vaginal cuff fixation at hysterectomy for uterine prolapse. Journal of Pelvic Surgery 1: 12–17

Given F T 1985 'Posterior culdeplasty': revisited. American Journal of Obstetrics and Gynecology 153: 135–139

Given F T 1992 Is posthysterectomy vaginal vault prolapse preventable? Journal of Gynecology Surgery 8: 201–209

Goldstien I, Wise G J, Tancer M L 1990 A vesicovaginal fistula and intravesical foreign body: a rare case of neglected pessary. American Journal of Obstetrics and Gynecology 163: 589–591

Hall A F, Theofrastous J P, Cundiff G C et al 1996 Inter- and intra-observer reliability of the proposed International Continence Society, Society of Gynecologic Surgeons, and American Urogynecologic Society pelvic organ prolapse classification system. American Journal of Obstetrics and Gynecology 175: 1467–71

Holley R L, Varner R E, Gleason B P, Apffel L A, Scott S 1995 recurrent pelvic support defects after sacrospinous ligament fixation for vaginal vault prolapse. Journal of the American College of Surgeons 180: 444–448

Hurt W G 1990a Pelvic organ prolapse. In. Shingleton H M, Hurt W G, (eds) Postreproductive Gynecology. Churchill Livingstone, New York, pp 413–440

Hurt W G 1990b Stress urinary incontinence In: Shingleton H M, Hurt W G (eds) Postreproductive Gynecology. Churchill Livingstone, New York, pp. 445–447

Julian T M 1996 The efficacy of Marlex mesh in the repair of severe, recurrent vaginal prolapse of the anterior midvaginal wall. American Journal of Obstetrics and Gynecology 175: 1472–1475

Kegel A H 1948 Progressive resistance exercise in the functional restoration of the perineal muscles. American Journal of Obstetrics and Gynecology 56: 238–248

Kegel A H 1949 The physiologic treatment of poor tone function of the genital muscles and of urinary incontinence. West Journal of Surgery, Obstetrics and Gynaecology 57: 527–535

Kobak W H, Rosenberg K, Walters M D 1995 Interobserver variation in the assessment of pelvic organ prolapse using the draft International Continence Society and Baden grading systems. International Urogynecology Journal 6: 304

McCall M L 1957 Posterior culdoplasty: surgical correction of enterocele during vaginal hysterectomy: a preliminary report. Obstetrics and Gynecology 10: 595–602

Macer G A 1978 Transabdominal repair of cystocele, a 20 year experience, compared with the traditional vaginal approach. American Journal of Obstetrics and Gynecology 131: 203–207

McGuire E J, Woodside J R, Borden T A, Weiss R M 1981 Prognostic value of urodynamic testing in myelodysplastic patients. Journal of Urology 126: 205–209

Mariona F G, Evans T N 1982 Pregnancy following repair of anal and vaginal atresia and bladder exstrophy. Obstetrics and Gynecology 59: 653–654

Meeks G R, Washburne J F, McGehee R P, Wiser W L 1994 Repair of vaginal vault prolapse by suspension of the vagina to iliococcygeus (prespinous) fascia. American Journal of Obstetrics and Gynecology 171: 1444–1454

Miklos J R, Sze E H M, Karram M M 1995 Vaginal correction of pelvic organ relaxation using local anesthesia. Obstetrics and Gynecology 86: 922–924

Montella J M, Cater J R 1995 Comparison of measurements obtained in supine and sitting position in the evaluation of pelvic organ prolapse. International Urogynecology Journal 6: 304

Morley G W, DeLancey J O L 1988 Sacrospinous ligament fixation for eversion of the vagina. American Journal of Obstetrics and Gynecology 158: 872–881

Muram D, Summitt R L, Feldment N 1990 Vaginal dilators for intermittent pelvic support: a case report. Journal of Reproductive Medicine 35: 303–304

Myazaki F S 1987 Miya hook ligature carrier for sacrospinous ligament suspension. Obstetrics and Gynecology 70: 286–288

Nichols D H 1982 Sacrospinous fixation for massive eversion of the vagina. American Journal of Obstetrics and Gynecology 142: 901–904

Nichols D H, Randall C L 1989 Vaginal Surgery, 3rd edn. Williams and Wilkins, Baltimore, p. 267

Norton P A 1993 Pelvic floor disorders: the role of fascia and ligaments. Clinical Obstetrics and Gynecology 36: 926–938

Olsen A L, Smith V J, Bergstrom J O, Colling J C, Clark A L. 1997 Epidemiology of surgically managed pelvic organ prolapse and urinary incontinence. Obstetrics and Gynaecology 89: 501–5

Oster S, Javert C T 1966. Treatment of the incompetent cervix with the Hodge pessary. Obstetrics and Gynecology 28: 206

Ott R, Richter H, Behr J, Scheele J 1993. Small bowel prolapse and incarceration caused by a vaginal ring pessary. British Journal of Surgery 80: 1157

Paraiso M F R, Ballard L A, Walters M D, Lee J C, Mitchinson A R 1996 Pelvic support defects and visceral and sexual function in women treated with sacrospinous ligament suspension and pelvic reconstruction. American Journal of Obstetrics and Gynecology 175: 1423–1431

Richardson A C 1993 The rectovaginal septum revisited: its relationship to rectocele and its importance in rectocele repair. Clinics in Obstetrics and Gynecology 36: 976–983

Richardson A C 1995 The anatomic defects in rectocele and enterocele. Journal of Pelvic Surgery 1: 214–221

Richardson A C, Lyon J B, Williams N L 1976 A new look at pelvic relaxation. American Journal of Obstetrics and Gynecology 568: 568–573

Richardson D A, Bent A E, Ostergard D R 1983 The effect of uterovaginal prolapse on urethrovesical pressure dynamics. American Journal of Obstetrics and Gynecology 146: 901–905

Richter K, Albrich W 1981 Long-term results following fixation of the vagina on the sacrospinal ligament by the vaginal route (vaginaefixatio sacrospinalis vaginalis). American Journal of Obstetrics and Gynecology 141: 811–816

Rosenzweig B A, Pushkin S, Blumenfeld D, Bhatia N N 1992 Prevalence of abnormal urodynamic test results in continent women with severe genitourinary prolapse. Obstetrics and Gynecology 79: 539–542

Schüssler B, Peschers U 1995 Standardisation of terminology of female genital prolapse according to the new ICS criteria: inter-examiner reproducibility. Neurourology and Urodynamics 14: 437–438

Shull B L, Baden W F 1989 A six year experience with paravaginal defect repair for stress urinary incontinence. American Journal of Obstetrics and Gynecology 160: 1432–1440

Shull B L, Capen C V, Riggs M W, Kuehl T J 1992 Preoperative and postoperative analysis of site-specific pelvic support defects in 81 women treated with sacrospinous ligament suspension and pelvic reconstruction. American Journal of Obstetrics and Gynecology 166: 1764–1771

Shull B L, Capen C V, Riggs M W, Kuehl T J 1993 Bilateral attachment of the vaginal cuff to iliococcygeus fascia: an effective method of cuff suspension. American Journal of Obstetrics and Gynecology 168: 19: 669–677

Snyder T E, Krantz K E 1991 Abdominal-retroperitoneal sacral colpopexy for the correction of vaginal prolapse. Obstetrics and Gynecology 77: 944–948

Sulak P J, Kuehl T J, Shull B L 1993 Vaginal pessaries and their use in pelvic relaxation. Journal of Reproductive Medicine 38: 919–923

Sultan A H, Kamm M A, Hudson C N, Thomas J M, Bartram C I 1993 Anal-sphincter disruption during vaginal delivery. New England Journal of Medicine 329: 1905–1911

Sultan A H, Kamm M A, Hudson C N, Bartram C I 1994 Third degree obstetrics anal sphincter tears: risk factors and outcome of primary repair. British Medical Journal 308: 887–891

Sutton G P, Addison W A, Livengood C H, Hammond C B 1981 Life-threatening hemorrhage complicating sacral colpopexy. American Journal of Obstetrics and Gynecology 140: 836–837

Taskin O, Wheeler J M, Yalcinoglu A I, Coksenim S 1996 The effects of episiotomy and Kegel exercises on postpartum pelvic relaxation: a prospective controlled study. Journal of Gynecology and Surgery 12: 123–27

Timmons M C, Addison W A 1997 Mesh erosion after abdominal sacral colpopexy. Journal of Pelvic Surgery 3: 75–80

Timmons M C, Addison W A, Addison S B, Cavenar M G 1992 Abdominal sacral colpopexy in 163 women with posthysterectomy vaginal vault prolapse and enterocele. Journal of Reproductive Medicine 37: 323–327

Toglia M R, DeLancey J O L 1994 Anal incontinence and the obstetrician-gynecologist. Obstetrics and Gynecology 84: 731–740

Wall L L 1993 The muscles of the pelvic floor. Clinical Obstetrics and Gynecology 36: 910–925

White G R 1912 An anatomic operation for cure of cystocele. American Journal of Obstetrics and Diseases of Women and Children 65: 286–290

Urogenital tract dysfunction and the menopause

CON J KELLEHER AND EBOO VERSI

INTRODUCTION

The lower urinary and genital tracts are embryologically and anatomically closely related. Both are sensitive to the effects of female sex steroids, and oestrogen receptors have been demonstrated in the vagina, urethra, bladder and pelvic floor (Blakeman et al 1996; Iosif et al 1981; Batra & Fosil 1983; Batra & Iosif 1987). Symptomatic, cytological and physiological changes in the urogenital tract occur during the menstrual cycle, in pregnancy and following the menopause (Van Geelen et al 1981; Tapp & Cardozo 1986; McCallin et al 1950; Solomon et al 1958; Versi 1994).

After the menopause the gradual atrophy of oestrogen-sensitive tissues results in a number of different urogenital complaints. These include an increased incidence of urinary symptoms of frequency, nocturia, urgency and incontinence, as well as the development of recurrent urinary tract infections. Dysuria may also be a symptom of oestrogen deficiency. Symptoms of vulvovaginal atrophy and vaginal dryness such as pruritis, burning and dyspareunia are also common amongst elderly postmenopausal women.

Epidemiological studies have attempted to relate the occurrence of urogenital symptoms to the menopause and subsequent oestrogen deficiency. Although an association undoubtedly exists, the urogenital tract is also affected by ageing processes and therefore aetiological factors other than oestrogen deficiency may be important. A cause and effect relationship is thus difficult to prove from available epidemiological data.

The aim of this chapter is to review the effects of oestrogens on the urogenital tract. Our knowledge is derived largely from epidemiological studies, and a number of clinical trials evaluating oestrogen replacement therapy for postmenopausal women.

OESTROGEN DEFICIENCY AND UROGENITAL SYMPTOMS

As a result of improvements in health and lifestyle expectancy women now spend a third of their lives in the oestrogen-deficient postmenopausal state. The prevalence of conditions occurring more frequently after the menopause is therefore likely to increase, with a similar expansion in health care expenditure. For this reason, ageing in the postmenopausal period has attracted increasing clinical and research interest, in an attempt to maintain the quality of life of elderly women.

In any discussion of menopausally related symptoms, it is important to appreciate that symptoms may be caused by absolute deficiency of sex steroids (e.g. osteoporosis-related symptoms) or may result from fluctuating levels of sex steroids during declining ovarian activity as in the climacteric (e.g. symptoms of vasomotor instability). It has been generally supposed that urogenital symptoms are due to the former but some of the symptoms may be due to the latter.

The symptoms of urogenital atrophy occur later after the menopause than vasomotor symptoms, and in contrast to the latter, do not disappear. Perhaps the most frequently reported symptoms are those of vaginal atrophy, namely dryness, burning, itching, and dyspareunia. In addition, discharge or postmenopausal bleeding may be troublesome secondary to vaginitis, irritation, or trauma of the vaginal or introital epithelium (Semmens & Wagner 1982).

Postmenopausal oestrogen deficiency also affects the lower urinary tract. Elderly women with lower urinary tract dysfunction often present with a combination of symptoms. The common complaints are stress incontinence, urgency, urge incontinence, frequency, possibly dysuria and recurrent urinary tract infection. An accurate diagnosis of the cause of urinary symptoms is made by careful assessment, including urodynamic studies.

UROGENITAL ATROPHY: PHYSIOLOGY

Oestrogen deficiency results in atrophy of all steroid hormone-sensitive urogenital tissues. Cytology is the most frequently used method of objective assessment. This is based on the classification of desquamated cells collected by vaginal and urethral smears, or from the urinary sediment. Cells are classified as parabasal, intermediate or superficial, depending on their degree of differentiation, and several different quota such as the KPI (karyopyknotic index), MV (maturation value), and MI (maturation index) can be calculated to express the degree of atrophy as a numeric value (Hammond 1977).

Vaginal cytology is based on the subjective judgement of a cytologist and this may explain the inconsistency between cytological and clinical findings (James et al 1984; Benjamin & Deutsch 1980). In order to standardize the evaluation of cytologic assessment, morphometric analysis of the characteristics of cell nuclei has been developed as well as immunohistochemical studies of the Ki-67 antigen, found in normal proliferating cells (McCormick et al 1993).

Maturation of postmenopausal atrophic vaginal epithelium can be induced by oestrogen replacement therapy. This is measured cytologically by a disappearance of parabasal cells and a significant increase in superficial cells on vaginal smear tests. In addition, an increased thickness and number of cell layers in the vaginal epithelium can be seen on vaginal biopsies, as well as the presence of Ki-67 antigen binding sites (Nilsson et al 1995). Oestrogen therapy has also been shown to increase vaginal blood flow (Semmens et al 1985), reduce vaginal dryness and lower vaginal pH (Nilsson et al 1995).

During the fertile years, the pH of the vagina is usually in the range 3.5–5.0. In postmenopausal women without oestrogen treatment, the vaginal pH is considerably higher, 5.5–6.8 (Semmens et al 1985). The low pH in premenopausal women is maintained by lactobacilli. Under the influence of oestrogen, glycogen is produced by exfoliating cells. This acts as a substrate for lactobacilli which convert glucose into lactic acid. In the oestrogen-deficient state, the vaginal epithelium becomes thinner and less glycogen is produced. Lactobacilli disappear and vaginal pH rises. This change is important with respect to vaginal and lower urinary tract colonization and infection by pathogenic organisms.

OSTROGEN DEFICIENCY AND URINARY INCONTINENCE: PHYSIOLOGY

The prevalence of urinary incontinence increases with age (Table 32.1), although there may be many reasons aside from the menopause why this should be

Table 32.1 Prevalence of incontinence amongst women residing independently in the community.

STUDY	PREVALENCE
Milne et al (1972)	
65 +-year-olds	34%
Thomas et al (1980)	
25–64-year-olds	18%
65+-year-olds	23%
Yarnell et al (1981) (women only)	
25–64-year-olds	46%
65+-year-olds	49%
Vetter et al (1981)	14%
Medical, Epidemiologic and Social Aspects of Aging study (Diokno et al 1986) (65+-year-olds)	30%
Iosif & Bekassy (1984) (61+-year-olds)	29%
Market Opinion Research International (MORI) survey (Brocklehurst 1990)	14%

so. Bladder and urethral function become less efficient with age (Rud et al 1980), and Malone Lee (1989) has shown that elderly women have a reduced urinary flow rate, an increased urinary residual, higher end-filling cystometric pressures (and maximum filling pressure), reduced bladder capacity and lower maximum voiding pressures. Additionally, whereas younger women excrete the bulk of their daily fluid intake before bedtime, many factors, including congestive cardiac failure and drugs, reverse this pattern in the elderly, nocturia becoming more common with advancing age. The major causes of urinary incontinence amongst women of all ages are listed in Table 32.2, and those affecting mainly older women are listed in Table 32.3. As is evident, aetiological factors in the elderly are usually not confined to the lower urinary tract (Resnick 1984).

Continence is maintained by a complex interaction of factors including the condition of the urethral epithelium, smooth muscle, urethral wall elasticity and vascularity, periurethral smooth muscle and urethral striated muscle and supporting structures. Urethral closure pressure and functional urethral length can be measured with a microtip transducer catheter (urethral pressure profilometry), and both decrease with age (Rud et al 1980; Edwards & Malvera 1974; Asmussen & Ulmsten 1976; Rud 1980a; Susset & Plante 1980).

Changes in urinary cytology are similar to the atrophic changes seen on vaginal cytologic assessment after the menopause (McCallin et al 1950), and both improve following oestrogen therapy (Solomon et al 1958). In addition, a decrease in periurethral striated muscle volume and urethral vascularity can be seen after the menopause (Versi & Cardozo 1988; Carlile et al 1988).

Table 32.2 The causes of urinary incontinence.

Genuine stress incontinence (GSI)[a]
Detrusor and/or urethral instability (DI)[a] (detrusor hyperreflexia)
Overflow incontinence
Fistulae (vesicovaginal, ureterovaginal, urethrovaginal)
Congenital
Urethral diverticulae
Temporary (eg. urinary tract infection, faecal impaction, drugs)
Functional (e.g. immobility, psychological)

[a]GSI and DI can coexist (mixed incontinence)

Table 32.3 Additional causes of transient incontinence in the elderly: *DIAPPERS*. Adapted from Resnick (1984); the misspelling is intentional.

D:	Dementia, delirium/confusional state
I:	Infection – urinary (symptomatic)
A:	Atrophic urethritis (oestrogen deficiency)
P:	Pharmaceuticals (e.g. hypnotics)
P:	Psychological, especially depression
E:	Excessive urine output (e.g. diuretics, renal, metabolic)
R:	Restricted mobility (e.g. change of environment)
S:	Stool impaction, heart failure

The bladder neck and urethra contain α-adrenoreceptors, the stimulation of which produces smooth muscle contraction and an increase in urethral closure pressure (Schreiter et al 1976). Oestrogen therapy modifies the response of the urethra and bladder to α-adrenergic stimulation (Callahan & Creed 1985), producing an increased sensitivity of the urethral smooth muscle. This is due, at least in part, to an increase in the number of postjunctional α_2-adrenoreceptors (Llarsson et al 1984).

Oestrogen therapy may improve urinary incontinence by a number of different mechanisms (Versi 1990). Firstly, the cytologic changes of the urethral mucosa may lead to an improved mucosal seal effect or 'hermetic closure'. The coaptation of the urethra is thought to be largely due to the softness of the urethral squamous epithelium (Zinner et al 1980, 1983) and the latter is under the influence of oestrogens (Everett 1941). In the neonate, squamous epithelium only covers the lumen of the distral urethra, but during the reproductive years this extends to line the entire urethra and trigone (Packham 1971). In addition, intrinsic urethral function may augment oestrogen action by increased periurethral vascularity (Raz et al 1972; Rud 1980b; Asmussen & Miller 1983; Versi & Cardozo 1985; Batra et al 1985), and improved urethral smooth muscle contractility (Callahan & Creed 1985).

It is interesting, in view of the successful pilot study of the effect of GTN on detrusor instability (James & Iacouvou 1993), that oestrogen therapy in sheep has recently been shown to increase the activity of nitric oxide synthase in sheep detrusor muscle (Robinson et al 1996). Although considerably larger studies are required to determine the effects of nitric oxide donors on human detrusor muscle function, this is an extremely important area for future research which may help to explain the mechanisms of postmenopausal urogenital dysfunction and the mechanism of action of oestrogen replacement therapy.

Although each of these factors may be important, it is also clear that urethral function depends on factors both intrinsic to and extrinsic to the urethra. These include the supporting ligaments (e.g. pubourethral ligament), the suburethral fascia and levator ani muscles, especially the pubococcygeus muscles. Thus integrity of the connective tissue is paramount, as it is integral to the above structures as well as being responsible for attaching myofibrils to each other and the muscles to their insertions.

Connective tissue is a very important component of the intrinsic female urethra, and collagen is its most abundant structural protein (Phillips & Davies 1981). To date, 14 different types of collagen have been identified and abnormal ratios of the type mix may result in structural weakness leading to hernias, vascular aneurysms and the Ehlers-Danlos syndrome (Norton et al 1991). Norton et al have shown that this may result in genital prolapse but its role in the genesis of stress urinary incontinence is, as yet, unclear.

Collagen is produced by fibroblasts which contain oestrogen receptors (Stumpf et al 1974). Brincat et al (1983, 1985) have shown that skin collagen declines after the menopause but that this decline can be reversed by oestrogen replacement therapy (Savvas et al 1993). Interestingly, Versi et al (1988) have shown that urethral closure pressure and functional urethral length correlate with skin collagen content, and therefore connective tissue factors may be fundamentally important to urethral function and continence. Recent studies indicate that oestrogen therapy stimulates collagen synthesis and turnover in postmenopausal urogenital tissues, but that initially degradation of aged tissues appears to exceed *de novo* collagen synthesis (Jackson et al 1996a), and therefore a long treatment interval may be required to produce a significant effect. This finding may explain the disappointing results of clinical trials on the effects of oestrogen replacement therapy on urinary incontinence (see below).

EPIDEMIOLOGY OF UROGENITAL ATROPHY AND URINARY INCONTINENCE

Symptoms of urogenital atrophy are extremely common amongst postmenopausal women although few receive appropriate treatment with oestrogen replacement therapy. Smith et al (1993) estimated that in Sweden, 40%–50% of 60–75-year-old women have symptoms of urogenital atrophy, but that only 10% receive oestrogen replacement. Iosif & Bekassy (1984) similarly found that 38% of postmenopausal women suffer from vaginal dryness and dyspareunia.

Epidemiological studies have attempted to document the prevalence of postmenopausal urinary incontinence. However, the true magnitude of this distressing condition is probably underestimated, due to the reluctance of women to admit to urinary symptoms (Table 32.4).

Although urinary incontinence is common in the postmenopausal years, prevalence data do not clearly indicate the role of oestrogen deficiency. In their large postal survey of almost 10 000 British women, Thomas et al (1980) showed that the prevalence of incontinence increased with age but not specifically at the time of the menopause. In contrast, Iosif and Bekassy (1984) found that 70% of incontinent elderly Swedish women related the onset of their symptoms to their last menstrual period. Jolleys (1988) reported that the prevalence of stress incontinence reached a peak at the age of 50 years and declined thereafter (Fig. 32.1). Kondo et al (1990) studied 1105 Japanese women and also found that the incidence of stress incontinence decreased after the age of 55 years, but showed that the incidence of urge incontinence increased with age (Fig. 32.2).

The only study to date analysing both urinary symptoms and urodynamic findings amongst climacteric women was performed at the Dulwich menopause clinic in London (Versi et al 1995). Two hundred and eighty-five women referred for various climacteric problems, but not complaining primarily of lower urinary tract symptoms, completed a detailed urinary symptom questionnaire and underwent urodynamic investigations comprising pad testing, uroflowmetry, videourodynamics and urethral pressure profilometry. Symptoms of stress inconti-

Table 32.4 Possible symptoms of urogenital atrophy.

Genital	Vaginal dryness, vaginal 'burning', pruritis, dyspareunia, prolapse.
Urinary	Urgency, frequency, dysuria, urinary tract infections, incontinence, voiding difficulties.

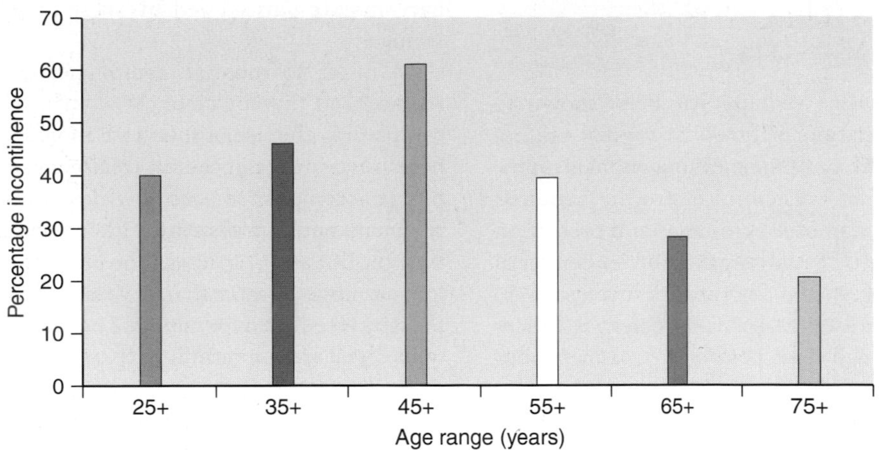

Fig. 32.1 The prevalence of stress incontinence in 833 British women. Note that it peaks in the 'climacteric' decade and declines therafter. Adapted from Jolleys (1988), with permission.

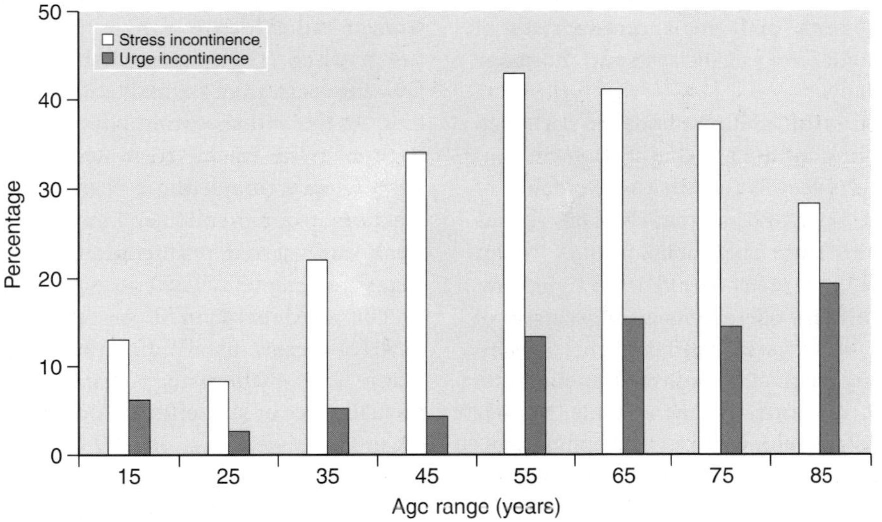

Fig. 32.2 The prevalence of stress and urge incontinence in 1105 Japanese women. Note that the pattern of stress incontinence peaks and then declines whereas that of urge incontinence increases after the age of 55 years. Adapted from Kondo et al (1990), with permission.

nence were reported in 53% of women and of urge incontinence in 26%. The symptoms of frequency (29%), nocturia (27%) and urgency (51%) were also common. Pain on micturition (11%) was less common, as were symptoms of voiding difficulties (about 15%). The urethral syndrome was rare (2%). Only 59% of these women had normal urodynamic investigations, common abnormalities being genuine stress incontinence (29%) with detrusor instability (10%) and voiding dysfunction (7%) being less common. Despite the common finding of urinary symptoms and urodynamic abnormalities, no correlation was seen with the timing of the menopause, except for the symptoms of frequency and nocturia, which appeared to increase 2 years after the menopause.

There is little evidence that stress incontinence is a result of the menopause, whereas urge incontinence and other irritative bladder symptoms may be. Although urinary symptoms are common in climacteric and postmenopausal women, and the lower urinary tract is known to be oestrogen sensitive, a causal relationship with the menopause is difficult to demonstrate. Unfortunately, epidemiological data are difficult to collect and incontinence in the elderly may be attributable to many other known factors. The menopause is a point in time and yet ovarian activity begins to decline before and continues to do so after the cessation of menses. Thus, any epidemiological study using the time of the menopause as a finite cut-off is likely to have flawed results.

OESTROGEN THERAPY FOR ATROPHIC VAGINITIS

Oestrogen replacement therapy has been shown to promote the maturation of atrophic vaginal epithelium and relieve the symptoms of urogenital atrophy. The high doses of systemic oestrogen required for the relief of vasomotor symptoms and protection against osteoporosis cause significant endometrial proliferation. Progestogen therapy is necessary to eliminate the increased risk of endometrial cancer with unopposed high-dose oestrogen treatment, but the regular uterine bleeding which usually occurs with this cyclical treatment may be difficult for many postmenopausal women to accept. Although continuous combined oestrogen/progestogen therapy can overcome this problem, elderly postmenopausal women may wish to avoid the systemic effects of oestrogen replacement, and the uncertain risks of breast cancer with long-term systemic hormone replacement therapy.

The major routes of administration of oestrogen therapy are shown in Table 32.5. One of the main benefits of non-oral delivery is that by the avoidance of first-pass hepatic metabolism the risk of venous thromboembolism may be minimized. Recent research has in fact demonstrated a significant increase in thromboembolic events amongst users of hormone replacement therapy, although not specifically related to any particular route of administration (Editorial, 1996). Additionally, more stable 24-hour oestradiol profiles are achieved and more physiological hormone profiles, maintaining the normal 2:1 oestradiol:oestrone ratio which is found in premenopausal women (Smith & Studd 1992). The inconvenience and skin irritation associated with oestrogen patches, and the small (3%) risk of tachyphylaxis (supraphysiological oestrogen levels) associated with implants are outweighed by these benefits for many women.

In order to increase compliance with oestrogen replacement therapy amongst women with urogenital complaints, the use of low-dose topical oestrogen has been advocated. Successful treatment of genital atrophy is accomplished with low-dose topical oestrogen regimens without systemic side-effects and endometrial proliferation. It does, however, appear that prolonged usage (greater than 1 year) of low-dose topical therapy is required for maximal benefit and that symptoms recur on discontinuing treatment (Iosif 1992).

Iosif (1992) reported a series of 48 women receiving treatment with 0.5 mg oestriol suppositories for 1–10 years. Vabra endometrial curettage showed the majority to have an inactive atrophic endometrium, with only 7 (15%) having a weakly proliferative endometrium after prolonged treatment. None of the women had evidence of hyperplasia or atypia. Mettler & Olsen (1991) assessed the effect of long-term low-dose oestradiol vaginal tablets (25 μg 17 β oestradiol) on the endometrium. Fifty-one women received once- or twice-weekly treatment for up to two years. All 9 women completing 2 years of treatment had an inactive atrophic endometrium, and only 3 cases of weak endometrial proliferation were found after 1 year's treatment.

The administration of oestrogen in vaginal pessaries or creams, by avoiding the enterohepatic circulation and by exerting mainly local effects, is virtually free of side-effects. A dose of 0.5 mg oestriol given twice weekly is usually effective treatment of atrophic vaginitis.

In order to overcome the messiness and inconvenience of these routes of administration, topical replacement therapy can be administered by the use of a sustained release silicone intravaginal ring. Smith et al (1993) evaluated a 55 mm diameter silicone vaginal ring releasing 5–10 μg oestradiol/24 h for a minimum of 90 days. Its efficacy, safety and acceptability were assessed in 222 postmenopausal women with symptoms and signs of vaginal atrophy. Maturation of the vaginal epithelium, measured cytologically, significantly improved during treatment, as well as symptoms of vaginal dryness, pruritus vulvae, dyspareunia and urinary urgency. Cure or improvement of atrophic vaginitis was recorded in more than 90% of subjects and the majority of the women found this form of treatment acceptable even during sexual intercourse (Smith et al 1993). As yet no placebo-controlled trial has been reported and this is eagerly awaited.

It is interesting to note that a recent study comparing the long-term effects (2–5 years) of systemic

Table 32.5 Routes of administration of oestrogen replacement therapy.

ROUTE	Proprietary name	Composition
Oral	e.g. Premarin	Conjugated equine oestrogen
	Progynova	Oestradiol valerate
	Ovestin	Oestriol
Transdermal	e.g. Estraderm	Oestradiol patches
Subcutaneous		Oestradiol implants
Transcutaneous	e.g. Oestragel	Oestradiol gel
Local/topical		
Vaginal cream	e.g. Premarin	Conjugated equine oestrogen
	Ovestin	Oestriol
Vaginal tablets	e.g. Vagifem	Oestradiol
Pessaries	e.g. Orthogynest	Oestriol
Vaginal ring	e.g. Estring	Oestradiol

transdermal oestrogen therapy and topical low-dose therapy (Estring) showed a significant improvement in cystometric parameters with Estring but not with systemic transdermal oestrogen (Voigt et al 1996). This, again, could be explained by the long-term beneficial effects of an intravaginal ring *per se* independent of oestrogen effects, as systemic oestrogen therapy has certainly been shown to induce maturation of urogenital tissues in a similar fashion to topical low-dose therapy. This again underscores the value of placebo-controlled trials.

An alternative therapy which has been shown to have a significant effect on the vagina (karyopyknotic index and maturation value), and to improve the symptoms of genital atrophy is tibolone (Livial, Organon) (Rymer et al 1994). This synthetic compound has oestrogenic, progestogenic and androgenic effects, and its oestrogenic potency is about 2% that of ethinyl-oestradiol. This mixed hormonal profile results in insignificant endometrial stimulation for the majority of users (Genazzani et al 1991; Trevoux et al 1983), eliminating the need for women to have a progestogen-induced withdrawal bleed.

Ultimately, the decision to use cyclical oestrogen/progestogen, continuous combined oestrogen/ progestogen, topical low-dose oestrogen, or tibolone, will depend on the wishes of the patient, and her need for the systemic or topical benefits of oestrogen replacement.

OESTROGEN THERAPY AND URINARY INCONTINENCE

A measure of the importance of oestrogen deficiency in the aetiology of urinary incontinence can be gauged by the improvement in symptoms, cytology and urodynamic assessment following oestrogen replacement therapy.

Unfortunately, those studies which have been performed vary in many important respects, namely the type, route, dose, mode and duration of administration of oestrogen, as well as the assessment of treatment efficacy.

A recent meta-analysis of 166 articles on this subject published in English from 1969–1992 included only six controlled and 17 uncontrolled trials of oestrogen therapy for the treatment of female urinary incontinence (Fantl et al 1994). Meta-analysis found an overall significant subjective improvement in incontinence symptoms following oestrogen therapy, but no evidence of objective improvement. As with all meta-analyses, caution has to be exercised when interpreting these results as they may be subject to publication bias as positive results are more likely to pass editorial scrutiny.

Oestrogens in undiagnosed incontinence

Early studies of the effect of oestrogens on the lower urinary tract predated urodynamic studies and were largely subjective and uncontrolled. The first report was in 1941 from Salmon et al who treated 16 women with dysuria, frequency, urgency and incontinence for 4 weeks using intramuscular oestrogen therapy. Symptomatic improvement was seen in 12 women. When treatment was discontinued, symptoms recurred and were again relieved by repeat intramuscular oestrogen therapy.

Thirty years later, Musiani (1972) gave 110 stress incontinent women quinestradol (which is no longer available), and reported a cure rate of 33% and an improvement rate of 39%. Schleyer-Saunders (1976) used oestradiol implants to treat 100 postmenopausal women with undiagnosed urinary incontinence and found that 70% were significantly improved, reducing the need for surgery.

Oestrogen therapy for urge incontinence

There have been few controlled studies reported in the literature despite the presence of a large placebo response in the treatment of urge incontinence. Samsioe et al (1985) entered 34 women aged 75 years into a double blind, placebo-controlled crossover study of oral oestriol 3 mg daily for 3 months. Despite the lack of objective assessment they found that urge incontinence and mixed incontinence were improved by oestriol, although in women with stress incontinence there was no difference between oestriol and placebo.

Cardozo et al (1993) reported the results of a double blind placebo-controlled randomized multi-centre study of oral oestriol 3 mg per day in the treatment of 64 postmenopausal women with 'the urge syndrome'. Women who entered the trial underwent urodynamic assessment and were divided into those with sensory urgency and those with detrusor instability. Treatment was for 3 months, after which patients were fully assessed both subjectively and objectively and side-effects were recorded. Patient compliance was confirmed by a significant improvement in the maturation index of vaginal wall smears with oestriol compared to placebo. Although oestriol produced both a subjective (particularly urgency and nocturia) and objective improvement in urinary function, it was not significantly better than placebo.

Iosif (1992) has shown that urogenital atrophy, a late manifestation of oestrogen deficiency, is only completely relieved after a year of treatment with 0.5 mg oestriol suppositories, and that symptoms recur with discontinuation of treatment. It is likely that Cardozo et al (1993) used too low a dose, the wrong route of administration or an inappropriate oestrogen, and it is unclear whether low-dose topical therapy, which improves genital atrophy without significant endometrial stimulation, is sufficient to treat urinary symptoms. Indeed, it is possible that oestrogen is actually no better than placebo for the management of postmenopausal women with this condition; although Fantl et al (1988) have suggested that oestrogen supplementation raises the sensory threshold of the bladder, reducing the symptom of nocturia.

In view of these disappointing results using oestriol in the management of postmenopausal urinary urgency, the efficacy of sustained release 17β-oestradiol vaginal tablets has been assessed (Vagifem, Novo Nordisk) (C Benness, MD thesis, personal communication, 1995). These are well absorbed from the vagina and have been shown to induce maturation of the vaginal epithelium within 14 days (Nilsson & Heimer 1992). One hundred and ten postmenopausal women suffering from urgency were randomized to receive either 25 μg 17β-oestradiol or matching placebo each day for 6 months. All underwent urodynamic investigations and were divided into three groups:

1 Detrusor instability
2 Sensory urgency
3 Normal urodynamics.

At the end of the treatment period the only significant difference between active and placebo therapy was the improvement in the symptom of urgency amongst women with a diagnosis of sensory urgency, which responded better to oestradiol than placebo. It is possible that localized atrophy causes or aggravates sensory urgency, and therefore topical oestrogen therapy is useful for its management.

Eriksen and Rasmussen (1992) showed, in a 12-week double blind randomized placebo-controlled trial, that treatment with 25 μg 17 β-oestradiol tablets significantly improved lower urinary tract symptoms of frequency, urgency, urge and stress incontinence compared to placebo. Unfortunately, they did not select women on the basis of their urinary symptoms and the study lacked the benefit of objective urodynamic assessment.

Oestrogen therapy for stress incontinence

The main variable which has been used to assess the efficacy of oestrogen therapy in the management of women with stress incontinence is urethral pressure profilometry. Caine & Raz (1973) showed that 26 of 40 (65%) women with stress incontinence had increased maximum urethral pressures and symptomatic improvement whilst taking conjugated oral oestrogen. Rud (1980) treated 24 stress incontinent women with high doses of oral oestradiol and oestriol in combination. He found a significant increase in transmission of intra-abdominal pressure to the urethra as well as an increase in maximum urethral pressure. Seventy per cent of women were symptomatically improved; however, high doses of oestrogen were employed over a short period of time and other studies have not all reported the same changes in urethral pressure profilometry.

Walter et al (1978) randomly allocated 29 incontinent, postmenopausal women with stable bladders to either oestradiol and oestriol or placebo (4 months cyclical treatment). They found a significant improvement in urgency and urge incontinence—7 out of 15 (47%) with oestrogen therapy—but no improvement in stress incontinence. They were unable to demonstrate a change in urethral pressure profile parameters. Similarly, Wilson et al (1987) entered 36 women with urodynamically proven genuine stress incontinence into a double blind, placebo-controlled study of cyclical oral oestrone for 3 months and showed no difference in the subjective response, urethral pressure profile parameters or quantity of urine loss.

A recent randomized placebo-controlled trial evaluated the effect of 6 months' treatment with oral oestradiol valerate (2 mg) on postmenopausal stress incontinence (Jackson et al 1996b). A significant subjective improvement in urinary symptoms was reported by both the active and placebo treatment groups, although no significant objective improvements were seen after either treatment.

The only study to date which has shown a significant objective improvement in genuine stress incontinence using oestrogen therapy was reported by Walter et al (1990). In a randomized placebo-controlled study using oestriol 4 mg daily, they showed that 9 out of 12 (75%) women preferred oestriol to placebo and that there was a significant objective decrease in urine loss with oestriol compared to placebo. However, the numbers in this study were small and it is the only study in the literature to report this effect!

Combination therapies

Oestrogen replacement therapy appears to be helpful for the symptoms of urgency and urge incontinence but not for stress incontinence, although there have been promising reports of combination therapy using an oestrogen and an α-adrenergic agonist. Beisland et al (1984) treated 24 menopausal women with genuine stress incontinence using phenylpropanolamine (50 mg twice daily orally) and oestriol (1 mg per day vaginally) separately and in combination. They found that the combination cured 8 women and improved a further 9, and was more effective than either drug alone. Hilton et al (1990) reported the results of a double blind, placebo-controlled study using oestrogen (oral or vaginal) alone or with phenylpropanolamine, in 60 postmenopausal women with urodynamically proven genuine stress incontinence. They found that the symptoms of frequency and nocturia improved more with combined treatment than with oestrogen alone, and that stress incontinence improved subjectively in all groups but objectively only in the combined group. It is likely that the effect of phenylpropanolamine on urethral α-adrenergic receptors is potentiated by the concomitant use of oestrogen replacement therapy in postmenopausal women. This form of treatment has not found widespread acceptance and is rarely employed, as other modalities of conservative treatment for stress incontinence are successful and associated with fewer side-effects.

OESTROGENS IN THE TREATMENT OF RECURRENT URINARY TRACT INFECTION

Oestrogen therapy has been shown to reverse urogenital atrophy and reduce the incidence of postmenopausal urinary tract infections.

Brandberg et al (1985) treated 41 elderly women with recurrent urinary tract infections with oral oestriol and showed that their vaginal flora was restored to the premenopausal type, and that they required fewer antibiotics. In an uncontrolled study, Privette et al (1988) evaluated 12 women who experienced frequent urinary tract infections. They were all found to have atrophic vaginitis and had suffered a mean of four infections per patient per year. Treatment consisted of a combination of short-term douche and antibiotic for 1 week, together with long-term oestrogen therapy. Follow-up was for 2–8 years and during that time there were only four infections in the entire group.

Kjaergaard et al (1990) studied 23 postmenopausal women with recurrent urinary tract infections. The women were treated with vaginal oestradiol or placebo for 5 months, following which there was improvement in vaginal cytology in the oestradiol group only, but no difference in the number of urinary tract infections or patient satisfaction between the two groups. Kirkengen et al (1992) randomized 40 elderly women with recurrent urinary tract infections to receive either oral oestriol 3 mg daily for 4 weeks, followed by 1 mg daily for 8 weeks or matching placebo. There was no difference between oestriol and placebo after the first treatment period but following the second treatment period, oestriol was significantly more effective than placebo at reducing the incidence of urinary tract infections.

More recently, in the largest study of its type to date, Raz & Stamm (1993) randomized 93 postmenopausal women with recurrent urinary tract infections to receive either intravaginal oestriol cream or placebo, and showed a significant reduction in the incidence of urinary tract infections with active treatment. Even oestriol, a weak oestrogen with minimal systemic effects, is effective in the prevention of recurrent urinary tract infections in women, suggesting that this is an important therapeutic role for oestrogen replacement therapy in postmenopausal women.

EFFECTS OF PROGESTERONE AND PROGESTOGENS ON THE URINARY TRACT

Cyclical progestogens are often used in conjunction with oestrogen replacement therapy in postmenopausal women to prevent endometrial hyperplasia and atypia attributable to unopposed oestrogen therapy. It is important, therefore, to consider briefly the effects of progesterone and progestogens on bladder and urethral function.

The effect of progesterone on the lower urinary tract has been most extensively studied during pregnancy, when a physiologically elevated serum progesterone level affects the ureters, bladder and urethra. During pregnancy, physiological hydroureter is attributed to both the smooth muscle relaxant effects of progesterone (Van Wagenen & Jenkins 1939) and obstruction by the gravid uterus. Langworth & Brack (1939) noted that during the course of experiments on vesical activity of healthy cats they had to exclude pregnant animals from the study as their bladder capacities were significantly increased. Similar studies were performed on pregnant rabbits, and again it was found that there was an almost 50% increase in the bladder capacity of these pregnant animals.

Youssef (1956) performed supine cystometrograms on 10 women throughout pregnancy, and noted an increase in bladder capacity and compliance. These changes have also been demonstrated following the administration of exogenous progesterone and during the luteal phase of the normal menstrual cycle (Gritsch & Brandsfetter 1954).

There are few studies of the effects of pregnancy or exogenous progestogen administration on the urethra. It is known that over 35% of pregnant women complain of stress incontinence at some time during their pregnancy and it has been suggested that this is related to progesterone levels (Stanton et al 1980). Van Geelen et al (1982) evaluated 43 pregnant women with urethral pressure profilometry, and also measured serum 17-hydroxyprogesterone levels. They found no change in the maximum urethral closure pressure, despite increasing levels of 17-hydroxyprogesterone and concluded that progesterone does not significantly alter the tone of the urethra. It is more likely that the increased prevalence of stress incontinence during pregnancy is due to transient detrusor instability (Cutner et al 1992).

Rud (1980) studied the effect of progesterone on the urethra of continent and incontinent women and found no change in maximal urethral closure pressure, but did find a decrease in urethral pressure transmission during the cough profile. Benness et al (1991) evaluated 14 postmenopausal women on continuous oestrogen and cyclical progestogen, and in 10 patients noted increased incontinence by pad testing during the progestational phase of the cycle. Eight of their patients had genuine stress incontinence, and in 7 of these, urethral sphincter incompetence was worse on progesterone. Raz et al (1973) have shown, however, that in continent women there is no change in the urethral pressure profile and no incontinence following the addition of the progestogen component to hormone replacement therapy. Progesterone may therefore inhibit the urethral closure mechanism by decreasing both the pressure transmission ratio and periurethral blood flow, and this is most profound in women with compromised urethral function who are already incontinent.

Burton et al (1992) questioned 217 women with premature ovarian failure on continuous oestrogen and cyclical progesterone therapy. He found an increase in the symptom of urgency during the progesterone phase of their cycle but no change in the incidence of urge incontinence or stress incontinence. These findings are in conflict with the expected action of progesterone on the lower urinary tract, but this was a questionnaire study with no objective measurements, and the women included were not complaining of lower urinary tract symptoms.

The clinical value of progesterone in patients with urinary complaints awaits evaluation. It may play a beneficial role in hormone replacement therapy in women with detrusor instability through its proposed β-adrenergic and anticholinergic properties. It may however, offset the beneficial effects of oestrogen in postmenopausal women with genuine stress incontinence (Benness et al 1991; Milne et al 1972), although in continent postmenopausal women this effect would appear to be minimal.

CONCLUSION

Urogenital atrophy is a common consequence of oestrogen deficiency and a cause of significant quality of life impairment for postmenopausal women. Atrophic vaginitis can be successfully treated with both systemic or topical low-dose oestrogen replacement, although long-term therapy is required to maintain symptomatic relief and cytologic maturation. The resolution of atrophic changes is also important for the restoration of normal vaginal bacterial flora and the prevention of vaginitis and recurrent urinary tract infections.

Systemic oestrogen replacement may alleviate the urinary symptoms of urgency, urge incontinence, frequency and nocturia, but not stress incontinence. To date, however, there have been few appropriate placebo-controlled studies using both subjective and objective outcome measures. Further confusion arises from the heterogeneity of different trials and consequently the best treatment in terms of dose, type of oestrogen and route of administration is unknown.

At present it is unclear whether low-dose oestrogen therapy has sufficient effect on the lower urinary tract to treat urinary incontinence. In addition, there is no conclusive evidence that oestrogen alone cures stress incontinence although, in combination with an α-adrenergic agonist, there may be a place for oestrogen therapy in the conservative management of genuine stress incontinence.

It is likely that urinary incontinence is the end result of a combination of many different factors; one of which is oestrogen deficiency. In this context, oestrogen replacement may be more important as an adjunct to other forms of treatment, rather than as a single modality of treatment in its own right.

Oestrogen supplementation undoubtedly offers many advantages to postmenopausal women and therefore makes them better able to cope with other disabilities; however, topical low-dose oestrogen is devoid of many of the benefits of systemic therapy.

REFERENCES

Asmussen M, Ulmsten U 1976 A new technique for measurement of urethral pressure profile. Acta Obstetrica et Gynecologica Scandinavica 55: 167–173

Asmussen M, Miller A 1983 Clinical Gynaecological Urology. Blackwell Scientific Publications, Oxford, p. 21

Batra S C, Fosil C S 1983 Female urethra, a target for estrogen action. Journal of Urology 129: 418–420

Batra S C Iosif L S 1987 Progesterone receptors in the female lower urinary tract. Journal of Urology 138: 1301–1304

Batra S, Bjellin L, Iosif S et al 1985 Effects of oestrogen and progesterone on the blood flow in the lower urinary tract of the rabbit. Acta Physiologica Scandinavica 123: 191–194

Beisland H O, Fossberg E, Moer A, Sander S 1984 Urethral sphincteric insufficiency in postmenopausal females: treatment with phenylpropanolamine and estriol separately and in combination. Urology International 39: 211–216

Benjamin F, Deutsch S 1980 Immunoreactive plasma estrogens and vaginal hormone cytology in postmenopausal women. International Journal of Gynecology and Obstetrics 17: 546–550

Benness C, Gangar K, Cardozo L D, Cutner A, Whitehead M 1991 Do progestogens exacerbate incontinence in women on HRT? Neurourology and Urodynamics 10: 316–318

Blakeman P J, Hilton P, Bulmer J N 1996 Mapping oestrogen and progesterone receptors throughout the female lower urinary tract. Neurourology and Urodynamics 15(4): 324–325

Brandberg A, Mellstrom D, Samsioe G 1985 Peroral estriol treatment of older women with urogenital infections. Lakartidningen 82: 3399–3401

Brincat M, Moniz C F, Studd J W W, Darby A J, Magos A, Cooper B 1983 Sex hormones and skin collagen content in postmenopausal women. British Medical Journal 287: 1337–1338

Brincat M, Moniz C F, Studd J W W 1985 Long term effects of the menopause and sex hormones on skin thickness. British Journal of Obstetrics and Gynaecology 92: 256–259

Brocklehurst J C 1993 Urinary incontinence in the community – analysis of a MORI poll. British Medical Journal 306: 832–834

Burton G, Cardozo L D, Abdalla H, Kirkland A, Studd J W 1992 The hormonal effects on the lower urinary tracts in 282 women with premature ovarian failure. Neurourology and Urodynamics 10: 318–319

Caine M, Raz S 1973 The role of female hormones in stress incontinence. Proceedings of the 16th Congress of the International Society of Urology, Amsterdam

Callahan S M, Creed K E 1985 The effect of estrogens on spontaneous activities and responses to phenylephrine of the mammalian urethra. Journal of Physiology 358: 35–46

Cardozo L D, Rekers H, Tapp A et al 1993 Oestriol in the treatment of postmenopausal urgency – a multicentre study. Maturitas 18: 47–53

Carlile A, Davies I, Rigby A, Brocklehurst J C 1988 Age changes in the female urethra, a morphometric study. Journal of Urology 139: 532–535

Cutner A, Cardozo L D, Benness C J 1992 Assessment of urinary symptoms in the second half of pregnancy. International Urogynaecology Journal 3: 30–32

Diokno A C, Brook B M, Brown M B 1986 Prevalence of urinary incontinence and other urological symptoms in the non institutionalised elderly. Journal of Urology 136: 1022

Editorial, The Lancet 1996 348, 9033: 977, 981

Edwards L, Malvern J 1974 The urethral pressure profile, theoretical considerations and clinical applications. British Journal of Urology 46: 325–334

Eriksen P S, Rasmussen H 1992 Low-dose 17 beta estradiol vaginal tablets in the treatment of atrophic vaginitis: a double-blind placebo controlled study. European Journal of Obstetrics and Gynaecology and Reproductive Biology 44: 137–144

Everett H S 1941 Urology in the female. American Journal of Surgery 52: 521–530

Fantl J A, Wyman J F, Anderson R L, Matt D W, Bump R C 1988 Postmenopausal urinary incontinence: comparison between non-estrogen supplement and estrogen-supplemented women. Obstetrics and Gynecology 71: 823–826

Fantl J A, Cardozo L D, Ekberg J, McClish D K, Heimer G 1994 Estrogen therapy in the management of urinary incontinence in postmenopausal women. A meta-analysis. Obstetrics and Gynaecology 83: 12–18

Genazzani A R, Benedek-Jaszman L J, Hart D M, Andolsek L, Kikovic P M, Tax L 1991 ORG OD 14 and the endometrium. Maturitas 13: 243–251

Gritsch E, Brandsfetter F 1954 Phasen Sphinktero-Zystometrie. Zentralblatt für Gunakologie 39: 1746–1750

Hammond D 1977 Cytological assessment of climacteric patients. Clinical Obstetrics and Gynecology 4: 49–70

Hilton P, Tweddel A L, Mayne C 1990 Oral and intravaginal estrogens alone and in combination with alpha adrenergic stimulation in genuine stress incontinence. International Urogynaecology Journal 12: 80–86

Iosif C S 1992 Effects of protracted administration of estriol on the lower genitourinary tract in postmenopausal women. Archives of Gynaecology and Obstetrics 251: 115–120

Iosif C S, Bekassy Z 1984 Prevalence of genito-urinary symptoms in the later menopause. Acta Obstetrica et Gynaecologica Scandinavica 63: 257–260

Iosif S, Batra S, Ek A, Astedt B 1981 Oestrogen receptors in the human female lower urinary tract. American Journal of Obstetrics and Gynecology 141: 817–820

Jackson S, Avery N, Shepherd A, Abrams P, Bailey A 1996a The effect of oestradiol on vaginal collagen in postmenopausal women with stress urinary incontinence. Neurourology and Urodynamics 15(4): 327–328

Jackson S, Shepherd A, Abrams P 1996b The effect of oestradiol on objective urinary leakage in postmenopausal stress incontinence: a double blind placebo controlled trial. Neurourology and Urodynamics 15(4): 322–323

James M J, Iacouvou J W 1993 The use of GTN patches in detrusor instability. A pilot study. Neurourology and Urodynamics 12(4): 399–400

James C, Breeson A, Kovacs G G et al 1984 The symptomatology of the climacteric in relation to hormonal and cytological factors. British Journal of Obstetrics and Gynaecology 91: 56–62

Jolleys J V 1988 Reported prevalence of urinary incontinence in women in general practice. British Medical Journal 296: 1300–1302

Kirkengen A L, Andersen P, Gjersoe E, Johannessen G A, Johnsen N, Bodd E 1992 Oestriol in the prophylactic treatment of recurrent urinary tract injections in post menopausal women. Scandinavian Journal of Prime Health Care 10: 139–142

Kjaergaard B, Walter S, Knudsen A, Johansen B, Barlebo H 1990 Treatment with low-dose vaginal estradiol in postmenopausal women. A double-blind controlled trial. Ugeskrift For Laegar 152: 658–659

Kondo A, Kato K, Saito M, Otani T 1990 Prevalence of hand washing urinary incontinence in females in comparison with stress and urge incontinence. Neurourology and Urodynamics 9: 330–331

Langworth O R, Brack C B 1939 The effect of pregnancy and the corpus luteum on vesical function. American Journal of Obstetrics and Gynecology 37: 121–125

Llarsson B, Anderson K E, Batra S, Mattiasson A, Sjögren C 1984 Effects of estradiol on norepinephrine induced contraction, alpha adrenoreceptor number and norepinephrine content in the female rabbit urethra. Journal of Pharmacology and Experimental Therapeutics 229: 557–562

McCallin P E, Stewart Taylor E, Whitehead R W 1950 A study of the changes in cytology of the urinary sediment during the menstrual cycle and pregnancy. American Journal of Obstetrics and Gynecology 60: 64–74

McCormick D, Chong H, Hobbs C, Datta C, Hall P A 1993 Detection of the Ki-67 antigen in fixed and wax embedded sections with the monoclonal antibody MIB1. Histopathology 22: 355–360

Malone Lee J 1989 Urodynamic measurement and urinary incontinence in the elderly. In: Brocklehurst J C (ed) Managing and measuring incontinence. Proceedings of Geriatric Workshop on Incontinence July 1988. Geriatric Medicine

Mettler L, Olsen P G 1991 Long term treatment of atrophic vaginitis with low dose oestradiol vaginal tablets. Maturitas 14: 23–31

Milne J S, Williamson J, Maule M M 1972 Urinary symptoms in older people. Modern Geriatrics 2: 198

Musiani U 1972 A partially successful attempt at medical treatment of urinary stress incontinence in women. Urology International 27: 405–410

Nilsson K, Heimer G 1992 Low dose oestradiol in the treatment of urogenital oestrogen deficiency – a pharmacokinetic and pharmacodynaamic study. Maturitas 15: 121–127

Nilsson K, Risberg B, Heimer G 1995 The vaginal epithelium in the postmenopause – cytology, histology and pH as methods of assessment. Maturitas 21: 51–56

Norton P, Friedman D, Boyd C et al 1991 Reduced type I: type III collagen ratios in men with recurrent inguinal hernias. Surgical Forum 42: 369

Norton P, Boyd C, Deak S 1992 Collagen synthesis in women with genital prolapse or stress urinary incontinence. Neurourology and Urodynamics 11: 300–301

Packham D A 1971 The epithelial lining of the female trigone and urethra. British Journal of Urology 43: 201–205

Phillips J I, Davies I 1981 A comparative morphometric analysis of the component tissues of the urethra in young and old female C57BL/ICRFAt mice. Investigations in Urology 18: 422–425

Privette M, Cade R, Peterson J, Mars D 1988 Prevention of recurrent urinary tract infections in postmenopausal women. Nephron 50: 24–27

Raz R, Stamm W E 1993 A controlled trial of intravaginal oestriol in post menopausal women with recurrent urinary tract infections. New England Journal of Medicine, 329(11): 753–756

Raz S, Caine M, Zeigler M 1972 The vascular component in the production of intraurethral pressure. Journal of Urology 108: 93–98

Raz S, Ziegler M, Laine M 1973 The effect of progesterone on the adrenergic receptors of the urethra. British Journal of Urology 45: 131–135

Resnick N M 1984 Urinary incontinence in the elderly. Medical Grand Rounds 3: 281

Resnick N M 1994 Urinary incontinence in the older woman. In: Kursh E D, McGuire E J (eds) Female Urology. Lippincott, Philadelphia, pp. 475–494

Robinson D, Massmann G A, Figueroa J P 1996 Characterisation of nitric oxide synthase (NOS) in overiectomised sheep bladder and the effects of estrogen. Neurourology and Urodynamics 15(4): 321–322

Rud T 1980a Urethral pressure profile in continent women from childhood to old age. Acta Obstetricia et Gynecologica Scandinavica 59: 331–335

Rud T 1980b The effects of oestrogens and gestagens on the urethral pressure profile in urinary continent and stress incontinent women. Acta Obstetricia et Gynecologica Scandinavica 59: 265–270

Rud T, Anderson K E, Asmussen M, Hunting A, Ulmsten U 1980. Factors maintaining the urethral pressure in women. Investigations in Urology 17: 343–347.

Rymer J, Chapman M G, Fogelman I, Wilson P O G 1994 A study of the effect of tibolone on the vagina in postmenopausal women. Maturitas 18: 127–133

Salmon U L, Walter R I, Gast S H 1941 The use of estrogens in the treatment of dysuria and incontinence in postmenopausal women. American Journal of Obstetrics and Gynecology 42: 845–847

Samsioe G, Jansson I, Mellstrom D, Svandborg A 1985 Occurrence, nature and treatment of urinary incontinence in a 70 year old female population. Maturitas 7: 335–342

Savvas M, Bishop J, Laurent G et al 1993 Type III collagen content in the skin of postmenopausal women receiving oestradiol and testosterone implants. British Journal of Obstetrics and Gynaecology 100: 154–156

Schleyer-Saunders E 1976 Hormone implants for urinary disorders in postmenopausal women. Journal of the American Geriatric Society 24: 337–339

Schreiter F, Fuchs P, Stockamp K 1976 Estrogen sensitivity of alpha receptors in the urethra musculature. Urologia Internationalis 31: 13–19

Semmens J P, Wagner G, 1982 Estrogen deprivation and vaginal function in postmenopausal women. Journal of the American Medical Association 248: 445–448

Semmens J, Tsai C, Curtis Semmens E, Loadholt C 1985 Effect of estrogens on vaginal physiology during menopause. Obstetrics and Gynecology 66: 15–18

Smith R N J, Studd J W W 1992 Hormone replacement therapy: a review. Journal of Drug Development 4: 235–244

Smith P, Heimer G, Lindskog M, Ulmsten U 1993 Oestradiol-releasing vaginal ring for treatment of post menopausal urogenital atrophy. Maturitas 16: 145–154

Solomon C, Panagotopoulous P, Oppenheim A 1958 Urinary cytology studies as an aid to diagnosis. American Journal of Obstetrics and Gynecology 76: 57–62

Stanton S L, Kerr-Wilson R, Harris G V 1980 The incidence of urological symptoms in normal pregnancy. British Journal of Obstetrics Gynaecology 87: 897–900

Stumpf W E, Sar M, Joshi S G 1974 Estrogen target cells in the skin. Experimentia 30: 196–198

Susset J, Plante P 1980 Studies of female urethral pressure profile. Part II. Urethral pressure profile in female incontinence. Journal of Urology 123: 70–74

Tapp A J S, Cardozo L D 1986 The postmenopausal bladder. British Journal of Hospital Medicine 35: 20–23

Thomas T M, Plymat K R, Blannin J 1980 Prevalence of urinary incontinence. British Medical Journal 281: 1243

Trevoux R, Dieulangard P, Blum A 1983 Efficacy and safety of

ORG OD 14 in the treatment of climacteric complaints. Maturitas 89–96

Van Geelen J M, Doesburg W H, Thomas C M G, Martin C B 1981 Urodynamic studies in the normal menstrual cycle: The relationship between hormonal changes in the menstrual cycle and urethral pressure profiles. American Journal of Obstetrics and Gynecology 141(4): 384–392

Van Geelen J M, Lemmens W A J G, Eskes T K A B, Martin L B Jr 1982 The urethral pressure profile in pregnancy and delivery in healthy nulliparous women. American Journal of Obstetrics and Gynecology 144: 636–649

Van Wagenen G, Jenkins R H 1939 An experimental examination of factors causing ureteral dilatation of pregnancy. Journal of Urology 42: 1010–1020

Versi E 1990 Incontinence in the climacteric. Clinical Obstetrics and Gynecology 33: 392–398

Versi E 1994 The bladder in menopause: lower urinary tract dysfunction during the climacteric. Current Problems in Obstetrics, Gynecology and Fertility 6: 193–232

Versi E, Cardozo L D 1985 Urethral vascular pulsations. Proceedings of the International Continence Society 15: 503–504

Versi E, Cardozo, L D 1988. Estrogens and lower urinary tract function. In: Studd JWW, Whitehead MI (eds) The Menopause. Blackwell Scientific Publications, pp 76–84

Versi E, Cardozo L, Brincat M, Cooper D, Montgomery J, Studd J W W 1988 Correlation of urethral physiology and skin collagen in postmenopausal women. British Journal of Obstetrics and Gynaecology 95: 147–152

Versi E, Cardozo L, Studd J, Brincat M, Cooper D 1995 Urinary disorders and the menopause. Menopause 2: 89–95

Vetter N J, Jones D A, Victor C R 1981 Urinary incontinence in the elderly at home. Lancet 2: 1275

Voigt R, Benninghoff B, Halaska M et al 1996 Influence of estraderm and Estring on urodynamic parameters in postmenopausal incontinent women. Neurourology and Urodynamics 15(4): 326–327

Walter S, Wolf H, Barlebo H, Jansen H 1978 Urinary incontinence in postmenopausal women treated with oestrogens: a double-blind clinical trial. Urologia Internationalis 33: 135–143

Walter S, Kjaergaard B, Lose G et al 1990 Stress urinary incontinence in postmenopausal women treated with oral estrogen (estriol) and alpha adrenoceptor–stimulating agent (phenylpropanolamine): a randomised double blind placebo controlled study. International Urogynecology Journal 12: 74–79

Wilson P D, Faragher B, Butler B, Bullock D, Robinson E L, Brown A D G 1987 Treatment with oral piperazine oestrone sulphate for genuine stress incontinence in post menopausal women. British Journal of Obstetrics and Gynaecology 94: 568–574

Yarnell J W G, St Leger A S 1981 The prevalence and severity of urinary incontinence in women. Journal of Epidemiology in Community Health 35: 71

Youssef A F 1956 Cystometric studies in gynaecology and obstetrics. Obstetrics and Gynecology 8: 181–188

Zinner N N, Sterling A M, Ritter R C 1980 The role of urethral softness in urinary incontinence. Urology 16: 115–117

Zinner N N, Sterling A M, Ritter R C 1983 Evaluation of inner urethral softness. Urology 22: 446–448

The elderly

JAMES MALONE-LEE

EPIDEMIOLOGY

In the United Kingdom the prevalence of urinary incontinence increases from 2% in men and 9% in women aged 15–64 to 7% of men and 12% of women aged 65 and over (Thomas et al 1980; Brocklehurst 1993). The increased prevalence of incontinence in late life reflects functional deterioration and coincidental disability, the two working additively (Ding et al 1996). There is some evidence that incontinence in an elderly person is an indicator of increased mortality rates although this probably reflects the fact that incontinence is more likely in the presence of greater morbidity (Diokno et al 1990).

In recent years it has often been stated that the future will see a marked explosion in the numbers of elderly in the population. This is, in fact, an exaggeration. The number of pensioners will rise by only 3% during the decade 1995 to 2005. During the 1920s and 1930s the birth rates were comparatively small and this has been reflected in the fall in the numbers of young elderly over the last 20 years. The coincident increase in the very elderly reflected the increased birth rates at the beginning of this century. Thus, the proportion of the population aged 75 and over in 1995 was 7.0%, this will be 7.4% in 2005 and 7.7% in 2015. Because of the baby boom after the Second World War, the decade 2000–2010 will see a rise in the number of people aged 45–59 by 13%. This is the age range of maximum earning power. During the next decade fewer elderly will find themselves living alone and more will have children. These data would suggest that the resources available for support of the very old will be greater than previously. Rising divorce rates and the greater participation in the workforce of women, who previously have provided a great deal of informal care, may influence the sociological scene. (Raleigh 1997).

The elderly are more prone to diseases that may influence the evolution of urinary incontinence. Cognitive impairment, graded as moderate or severe, is found in 2% in those aged 65–74, 7% in those aged 75–84 and 22% in those aged 85 and older. The absolute risk of cerebrovascular disease is related to age, as well as hypertension, with 50% of strokes occurring over the age of 75. Mobility problems are illustrated by the fact that one fifth of people aged 65 to 69 fall once or more during a year and this doubles by the age of 80. Diabetes is much more common in late life, with 50% of people aged over 70 demonstrating glucose intolerance. The immune defects associated with ageing are reflected in the fact that the prevalence of bacteriuria in women is about 20% between the ages of 65 and 75, increasing to between 20 and 50% over the age of 80.

Until recently, the elderly tended to be excluded from therapeutic trials because of a concern that they would prove unduly susceptible to adverse effects. We now have the benefit of data from interventional studies that deliberately recruited elderly people. A most striking observation is that often it has been found that the risk–benefit ratios greatly favour treatment being offered to the elderly (Goldberg & Chavin 1997). The increased sensitivity to drug therapy found in the elderly means that they are as susceptible to therapeutic effects as they are to side-effects. If the latter can be avoided by judicious dosing, there is a real chance of benefit. There are good reasons, therefore, to consider quite carefully the urogynaecology of the elderly.

CLINICAL SCIENCE

It is only possible to ascertain the effects of ageing itself by following a large cohort of people over many years. The Framingham and the Whitehall studies are examples of such experiments. However, an individual's response to ageing will be modified by many influences, examples being genotype, smoking or alcohol consumption. The number of putative factors which may influence the ageing process is vast. Unless you can control these extraneous influences you cannot ascribe observations to ageing alone. It is probable that we may never be able to describe the true process of normal ageing in humans, only ageing in particular genetic, environmental and historical circumstances.

Laboratory animal experiments do permit the study of the ageing of a species, because it is possible to keep genetically identical animals in constant, very well controlled environments. Indeed, some experiments on aged mice have provided some data on the associated changes in bladder function. However, it is now evident that species differences greatly limit the extrapolation of animal data to the human circumstance.

Many studies draw on cross-sectional samples of elderly people. It has to be understood that the observations made by such methods inform us only on what we should expect to find amongst other women who also fit the constraints of the sample. The data say nothing about the effects of ageing itself, or the experiences of women with other characteristics. Observations on nursing home residents of a certain age tell us little about women of similar age living independently. For this reason, age studies should report on the social and demographic characteristics of the samples in some detail.

There is a potential danger, however, in the misuse of detailed descriptive data. It is not difficult to collect a large data set of patient characteristics – computers help the process. The easy availability of sophisticated statistical software packages provide the opportunity to run the data through various multiple regression procedures which throw up factor associations supported by amazing '*p*' values ($p < 0.000001$!). This approach ignores the high probability of spurious correlations in large multivariate data sets and mistakenly uses the '*p*' value as a measure of association. There are many claimed associations between age and lower urinary tract dysfunction, which originate from this type of error.

As a general rule, clinical scientific discoveries can only be achieved by comparative experiments. Many age-related studies have not used comparative sampling of younger populations; such studies cannot be justifiably used to describe age-related phenomena.

There is a problem with the didactic use of ordinal classifications of pathophysiological phenomena; for example, a bladder is described as 'unstable or stable, obstructed or unobstructed', the term 'mixed incontinence' is used to describe the coincidence of two categories. Speciation apart, biological change, adaptive or destructive, invariably spans a continuum formed from the subtle interaction of many parts. It seems, therefore, very unwise to attempt to force the pathophysiology of the ageing lower urinary tract into arbitrary categories.

In a laboratory experiment it is usually possible to control the majority of factors which might influence the outcome. In clinical trials this is not the case so we circumvent a difficulty by using randomized sampling. This is certainly imperfect, but the best method that we have. Good practice entails the use of a very small number of outcome variables, which are used to test the effect of an intervention. There is an expectation that the samples will change over the period of observation, this often being for the better. This is not a placebo effect but results from the influence of a variety of factors, which, it is hoped, are represented evenly between the groups through randomization. We are not interested in this 'effect of history' but the differential effect of the intervention. Calculating the difference in the change in the test variable between groups assesses this.

Figures 33.1 and 33.2 illustrate the importance of a

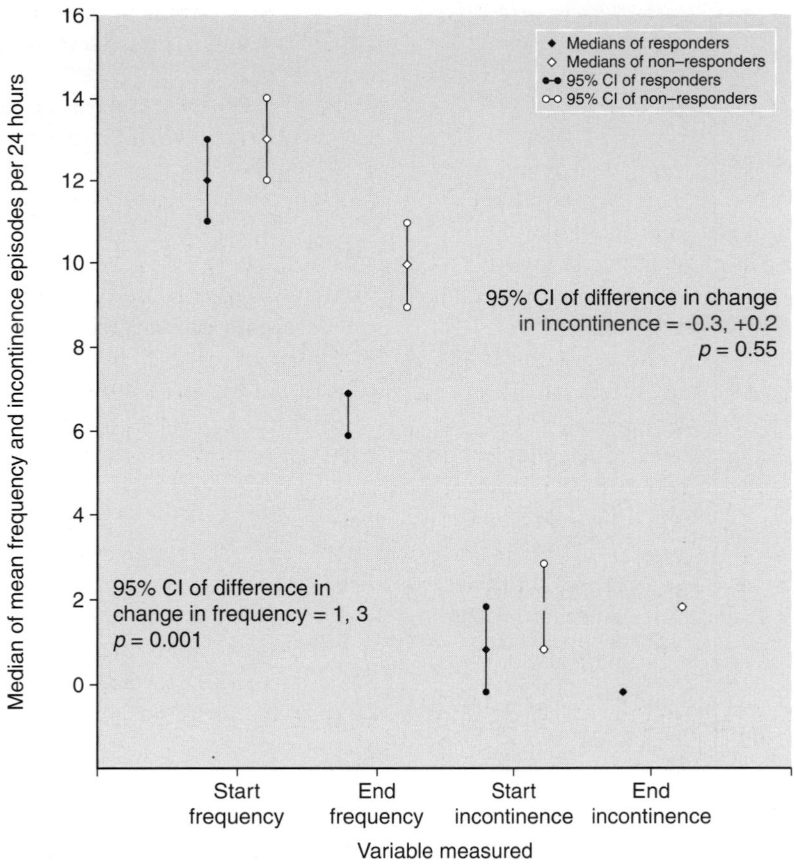

Fig. 33.1 Medians and 95% confidence intervals of daily urinary frequencies and incontinence episodes at the start and finish of treatment. 222 women aged less than 65 with detrusor instability, comparing responders with non-responders.

'between-group' analysis, whilst also demonstrating an important point in age-related clinical outcome studies. The data were taken from a pilot study, assessing outcome measure responses conducted on 300 women with detrusor instability (78 aged 65 and over). We followed these women over a 6–8 week period whilst they were being treated for detrusor instability with oxybutynin and bladder retraining. During this time they kept frequency/incontinence charts. At the end of the period they were divided into two groups: those who responded and those who did not. Analysis examined between-group difference in the change in daily frequencies and incontinence episodes, with an age-based subanalysis. Looking at the graphs the within-group differences are very striking, but these are not what we should analyse. It is the between-group analysis of the difference in change which is important and the 95% confidence intervals (CI) for these are quoted on the figures. It can be seen that, in the elderly, significant response differences were found in analysis of frequency and incontinence episodes, the former being more sensitive. Amongst younger adults only frequency showed significant differences in change. This is not a chance observation. Exactly the same patterns of outcome, in relation to age-group, were found in the multicentre, phase three studies of tolterodine. Younger people, being more mobile, can protect against incontinence, in the presence of detrusor instability, by raising frequency. The elderly are less able to do this and therefore differ in their reaction to disease and its treatment.

I have been involved in three clinical interventional studies of the treatment of detrusor instability in the elderly. In none of these studies have we ever detected a placebo response in the primary outcome variables. However, it is widely believed that detrusor instability is associated with a placebo response in the region of 30%. Why should this be? In all three studies the primary outcome measure was frequency and incontinence episodes recorded on diary charts. Between-group analysis demonstrated evidence of efficacy for an intervention in two of these trials. In all three studies there was no within-group change detected in those taking placebo (Wiseman et al 1991; Szonyi et al 1995), (Tolterodine in the elderly, data on file, Pharmacia & Upjohn, 1997).

During the studies, 'subjective' assessments of

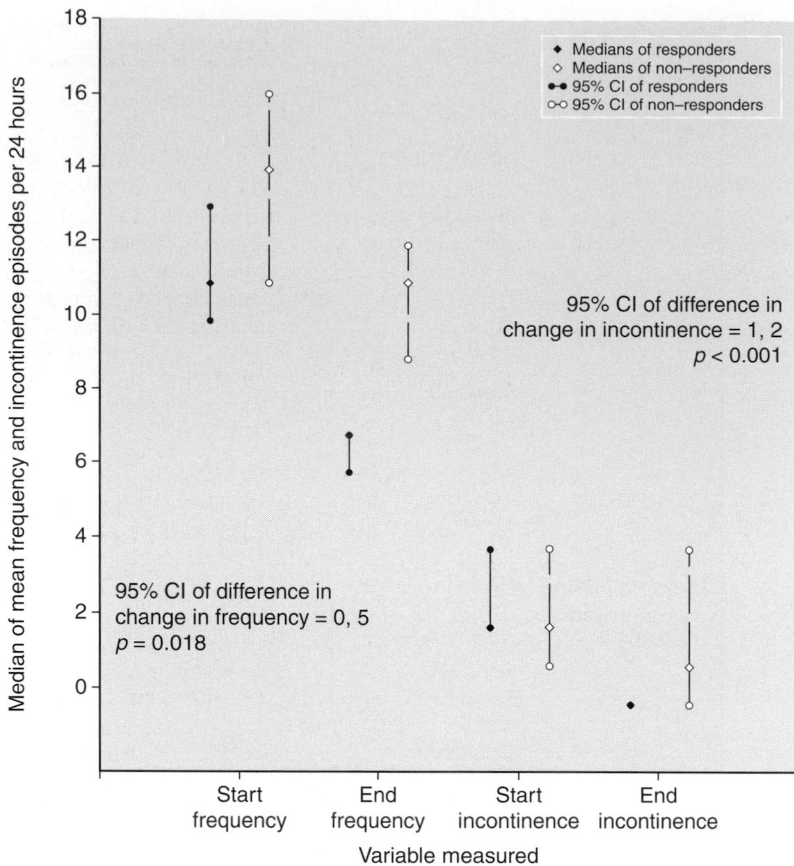

Fig. 33.2 Medians and 95% confidence intervals of daily urinary frequencies and incontinence episodes at the start and finish of treatment. 78 women aged 65 and over with detrusor instability, comparing responders with non-responders.

responses were collected onto ranked ordinal scales, the patients being asked to grade their responses at the end of the study. Within-group analysis of the subjective scales suggested a placebo response, but there were problems with the veracity of the analysis: (a) the sample sizes were too small for the scales used so that the data had to be forced into dichotomies; (b) such scales had never been validated as reliable outcome measures in clinical trials (frequency/volume charts) had; (c) the scales relied on recall over several weeks by people with variable short-term memory; (d) uncompared within-group changes are no evidence of a response. This is not an esoteric academic point; the drugs emmepronium, flavoxate, propantheline and flunnarazine have all been promoted using data derived from similar within-group analyses in the face of negative, comparative data. In clinical practice the use of these drugs is indeed very disappointing. Unvalidated, subjective scales, which rely on memory and recall over several weeks continue to be widely used to measure treatment outcomes.

THE URODYNAMICS OF OLD AGE

There are a number of age-related features of the pathophysiology of the lower urinary tract in women which have clinical significance. The descriptions of these differences will be prefaced by a brief description of the more advanced methods of urodynamics that were used to explore the age differences.

The filling phase

During the filling phase of a urodynamic study in a normal person, we expect to see a pressure rise reflecting the hydrostatic pressure head generated by the volume infused into the bladder. At 500 ml this is approximately 8 cm H_2O. In women with lower urinary tract symptoms, aged 75 and over, unstable contractions will be observed in 75–85%. Provided that the sphincter remains closed, these contractions will not involve any shortening of the detrusor fibres and will therefore be isometric. The filling pressures convey little about the isometric strength of the detrusor, but we can deduce that the active urethral sphincter can achieve at least the maximum filling pressure recorded.

Analysis of isometric strength requires calculation of the tension (T) generated in the wall of the bladder in order to achieve a pressure. According to Laplace's law the pressure generated by a tension in the wall of a curved vessel will vary inversely with respect to the radius.

$$P = \frac{2T}{R} \tag{1}$$

$$T = \frac{PR}{2} \tag{2}$$

Where T is the tension generated at a point on the bladder wall during a contraction, and R is the radius of the bladder, calculated from the known volume (V), treating the bladder as a sphere:

$$R = \left(\frac{3V}{4\pi}\right)^{\frac{1}{3}} \tag{3}$$

The detrusor pressure P_{det} results from the total force (F) generated by the tensions acting on the circumference of the bladder ($2\pi R$). The force of a detrusor contraction can therefore be calculated by multiplying equation 2 by $2\pi R$ as follows:

$$F = P_{det}\,\pi\left(\frac{3V}{4\pi}\right)^{\frac{2}{3}} \tag{4}$$

Figure 33.3 shows a plot of detrusor pressure against volume whilst an unstable bladder is being filled at a rate of 1 ml/s. The dotted curve is a plot of the calculated force (Equation 4). This figure has three important clinical implications.

1 The detrusor pressure is not a measure of detrusor strength.
2 The detrusor pressure is not a measure of the degree of unstable activity.
3 It is much harder to generate a contraction, for a given pressure, at higher capacities.

A force calculation has been used to examine differences in isometric strength between age groups (Malone-Lee & Wahedna 1993). Intuitively we might have expected less strength in late life. In fact, we found no differences in the maximum and total unstable forces generated by young and old with instability. There is a limitation to these data since

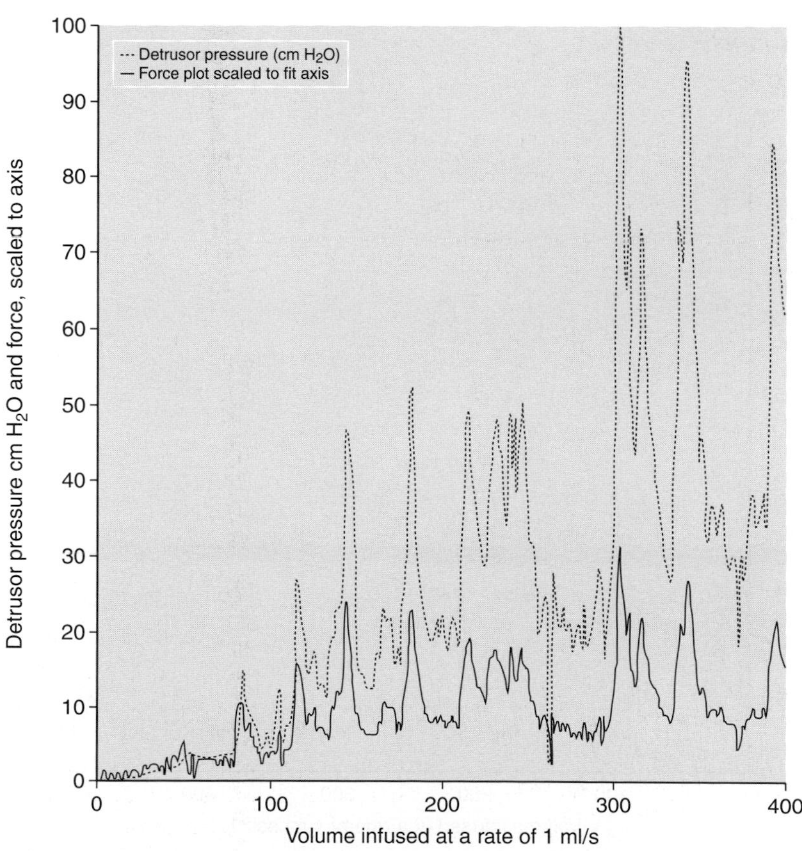

Fig. 33.3 Filling detrusor pressure against volume infused with force plot superimposed for comparison.

we did not know whether these contractions ever reach a true maximum.

Figure 33.3 does not tell us the whole story about detrusor instability. Figures 33.4A and 33.4B illustrate filling studies from two women with different patterns of detrusor instability. In Fig. 33.4A the pattern is of variable peaks of inconsistent amplitude with the contractions relaxing back completely. In Fig. 33.4B the pattern is of a motor summation with contractions building up, one upon another, with no relaxation between contractions. A method for describing the contraction patterns of unstable bladders numerically, using a data reduction technique, has permitted an exploration of the character differences in detrusor instability between age groups (Malone-Lee & Orugon 1993). Older women tend to demonstrate patterns of instability more akin to those illustrated in Fig. 33.4B and which are also more often seen in women with neurological disease (Gray et al 1997). Because of the similarities with detrusor hyperreflexia, it is tempting to suspect that, in late life, detrusor instability is associated with age-related neurological degeneration. This has yet to be explored. The bladder capacity associated with Fig. 33.4B was about 200 ml. Bladder capacities are lower amongst elderly women.

The idiopathic instability of younger women is more commonly of the type shown in Fig. 33.4A. There is a temptation to consider the instability of Fig. 33.4B to be more severe than that of Fig. 33.4A, but the bladder capacity recorded in B is much lower, so that underlying force will be less than at face value. The amplitude of the pressure waves will be ultimately limited by the strength of the sphincter (Fig. 33.4B). Low-pressure instability may simply reflect the limits of sphincter function. In instability, lower bladder capacities, more tenacious detrusor activity (Malone-Lee & Orugon 1993) and older age do not appear to be associated with a poorer therapeutic prognosis (Malone-Lee 1992). In fact, there do not appear to be any urodynamic variables indicative of a poorer prognosis for the treatment of detrusor instability (Wagg et al 1996). It is not appropriate therefore to talk of severity of detrusor instability.

Amongst women there are some interesting age-related changes involving bladder sensation. It has been found that the appreciation of bladder filling is reduced in association with age (Collas & Malone-Lee

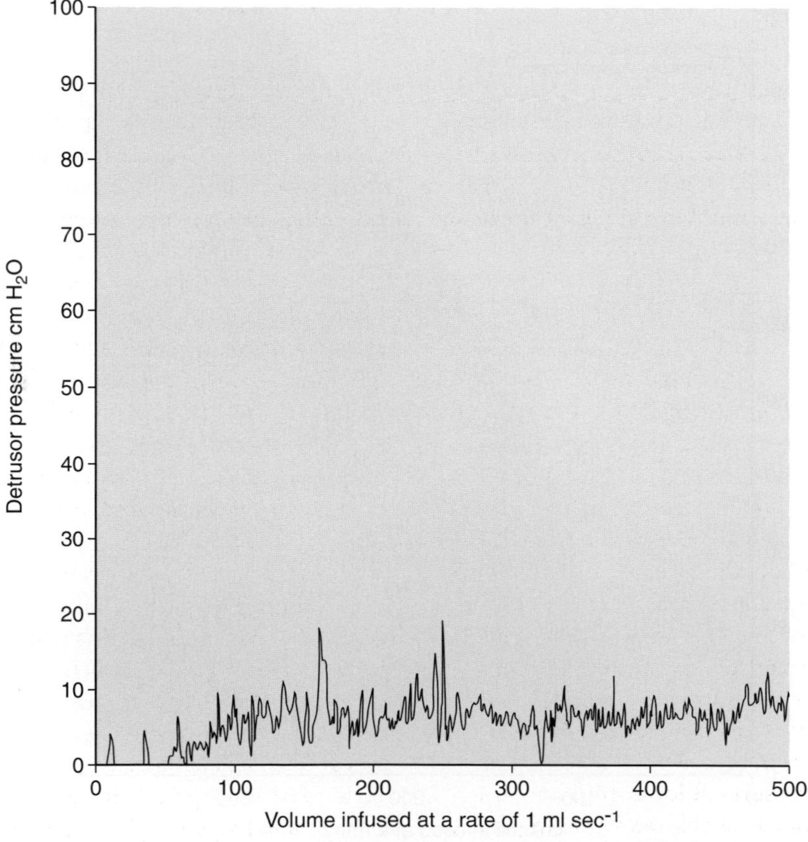

Fig. 33.4 (**A**) Filling detrusor pressure against volume infused. The recording is taken from a woman aged 45 with idiopathic instability

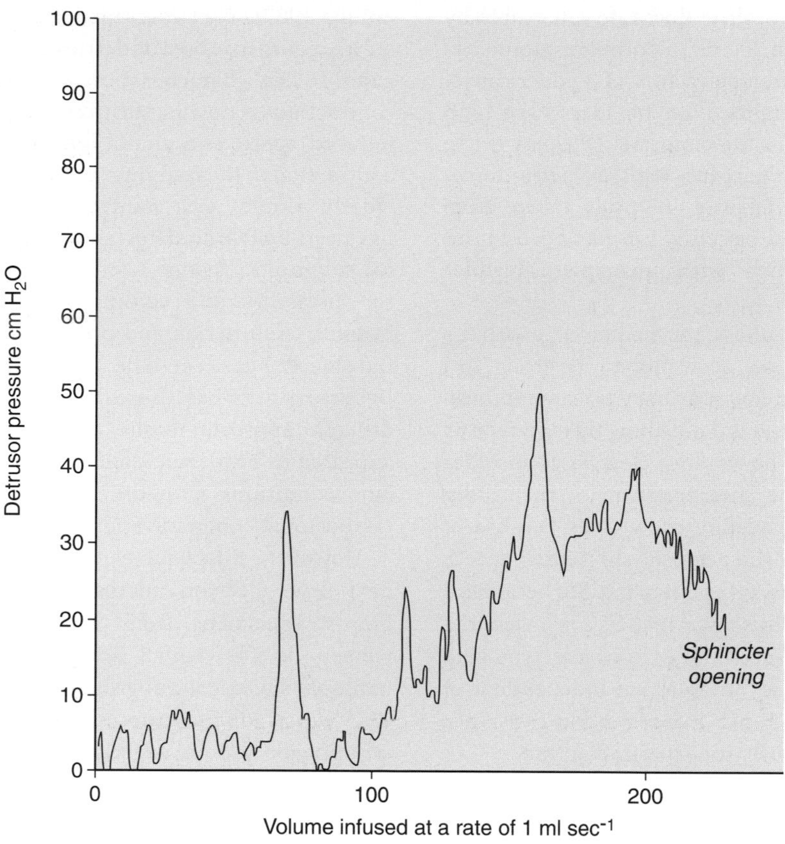

Fig. 33.4 (**B**) Filling detrusor pressure against volume infused. The recording is taken from a 70-year-old woman.

1996). Studies of bladder sensation, combined with tests of cortical perfusion and cognition, have shown that reduced bladder sensation in the elderly is associated with impaired cognition and reduced perfusion of specific parts of the cortex (Griffiths et al 1994a, 1994b).

The voiding phase

Whilst the isometric strength of the detrusor does not appear to be reduced in old age, isotonic voiding function is very different. The elderly void less successfully in late life and voiding is associated with higher residual urine volumes and a higher proportion of patients with incomplete bladder emptying (Resnick & Yalla 1987; Griffiths et al 1992; Malone-Lee & Wahedna 1993). The reasons for this are probably quite complicated and the study of the problem is the subject of some controversy at this time. During voiding, the detrusor must generate a pressure that will overcome the threshold of the relaxing sphincter. Laplace shows that it will be easier for the detrusor to generate threshold pressures at lower bladder capacities. Once the sphincter opens, and voiding commences, the detrusor needs to shorten and the faster the speed of shortening, the greater the voiding flow rate. Contractions involving muscle shortening are called isotonic. A purely isometric contraction involves force but no shortening, a purely isotonic contraction would involve shortening and no force. In nature we never see pure isotonic contractions; there is always an isometric component – reflected, in the case of the bladder, by the voiding detrusor pressures. The voiding pressure/flow plot of a cystometrogram offers an opportunity to assess the isotonic function of the detrusor under study by calculating the maximum shortening speed.

Derek Griffiths (1980) developed the method during the early days of urodynamics. He adapted the classic Hill equation, which describes the force/velocity relationship of striated muscle, to the bladder. It would be inappropriate to relate the mathematics of derivation in this chapter; it has been described thoroughly elsewhere. In practice, an equation called the 'bladder output relation' (BOR), is fitted to data collected from a filling/voiding cystometrogram which achieved a good estimate of the isometric detrusor potential, and a well recorded voiding pressure/flow plot. The variable of interest is called Q^*_{std} and it is an estimate of 25% of the maximum theoretical voiding flow rate achievable by a bladder voiding from 200 ml in entirely isotonic circumstances. It varies independently of bladder capacity and urethral resistance. Fast bladders have high Q^*_{std} and slow bladders the converse. Q^*_{std} has yet to be validated by comparison with *in vitro* force/velocity studies of detrusor biopsies taken from properly characterized patients, but has been found to be lower in women with incomplete bladder emptying.

Figure 33.5 shows a plot of the median Q^*_{std} with the 95% confidence intervals, according to age group, in a sample of women with lower urinary tract symptoms. A similar analysis of men did not show this age-related reduction, although the voiding flow rates in older men were lower. The interpretation is that older women have reduced voiding flow rates because of age-related slowing of the detrusor shortening speed, whereas in men the flow rates fall in late life because of the prostate. It has been shown that Q^*_{std} is lower, and urethral opening pressures higher in women who void incompletely. But these variables are independent of each other, so isotonic function and outflow resistance both contribute variously to urinary retention.

The combination of detrusor instability and incomplete bladder emptying in the elderly raises the controversy of 'detrusor hyperactivity and impaired contractility' (DHIC) (Resnick & Yalla 1987). This was described by Resnick and Yalla, when reporting on 32 elderly residents of a nursing home in 1987 (Resnick & Yalla 1987). They identified a specific physiological entity, being a subset of detrusor hyperreflexia in the elderly. The characteristics were unstable detrusor contractions, postmicturition residual urine, and reduced speed and amplitude of isometric detrusor contractions. In studying a much larger sample of elderly people, with younger comparators, my group has been unable to detect such a distinct physiological subgroup (Malone-Lee & Wahedna 1993). Detrusor instability and voiding problems, arising from isotonic dysfunction and urethral resistance, exist in the elderly but seem to be independent of each other. Derek Griffiths has also examined this issue, using a different approach to ours, and concluded that DHIC appeared to be a coincidental occurrence of two common conditions with different aetiologies (Griffiths DJ, personal communication, 1996).

However, Elbadawi et al (1993) have published data from electron microscopy studies of bladder biopsy specimens from elderly men (n=11) and women (n=24), which are in support of distinct pathophysiological subgroups of detrusor function. They reported four structural patterns, matching four urodynamic groups exactly, with no overlap. Additionally, two subsets, 'normal contractility' (n=11) and 'impaired contractility' (n=24) matched histological subsets exactly. These findings, despite attempts, have not been corroborated (Gosling JA, personal communication, 1996). Carey et al (1996) have reported finding some of the defining histological

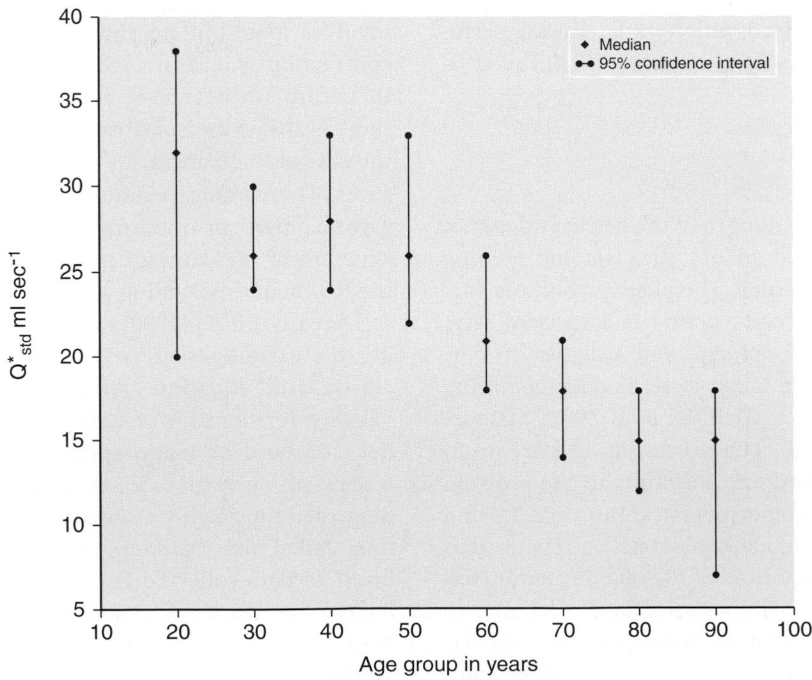

Fig. 33.5 Median Q^*_{std} and 95% CI by age group.

characteristics described by Elbadawi et al (1993) evenly distributed between normal women (n=15) and women with detrusor instability (n=22). Elbadawi et al (1997) have now published further corroborating evidence of their ultrastructural/urodynamic correlations, by drawing on data from 30 of their original subjects, with additional material from 14 new subjects. However, Carey et al (1997) have published data from a specific study on the elderly which again failed to support the findings of Elbadawi and colleagues. The difficulty with these controversies is that the studies depend on strict categorization to describe the pathological processes. This does not fit comfortably with what we know of biological systems.

There are changes in urethral function associated with ageing in women. Figure 33.6 demonstrates a plot of the voiding detrusor pressure against flow rate recorded from a urodynamic study. The pressure/flow plot is extremely important in urodynamic analysis and its properties have been well reviewed elsewhere (Griffiths 1980; Schafer 1992). It has been shown that the two pressure intercepts shown, $P_{det.close}$ and $P_{det.open}$ are invariably elevated in the presence of detrusor instability and reduced in the presence of genuine stress incontinence. Where both conditions exist, the values take the middle ground. Highest values are seen in neurological diseases such as multiple sclerosis (Fig. 33.7). It has been shown that greater age in women is associated with lower values of both $P_{det.close}$ and $P_{det.open}$, even in the presence of detrusor instability (Fig. 33.8) (Wagg et al 1996). So ageing, in women, is associated with a loss of urethral competence. The elevation of these pressures in association with detrusor instability results, fortuitously, in a compensatory mechanism which may protect against some incontinence arising from unstable bladder contractions. Elderly women are less able to benefit from this facility (Fig. 33.8). This coincidence of pathology illustrates an important principle in interpreting the disease process in elderly women. Unstable bladder contractions will be met by the resistance of the sphincter and relative degrees of sphincter failure may lead to incontinence, even though frank stress incontinence has not be demonstrated, nor described.

INFECTION

Old age is associated with a loss in immune competence and this is certainly reflected in the urinary tract. Mismanagement of urinary infection in the elderly can do a very great deal of damage (Gray & Malone-Lee 1995).

Asymptomatic bacteriuria is far more common in the elderly. About 20% of women and 3% of men aged 65–70 have bacteriuria and this rises to between 20 and 50% in women and about 20% of men aged over 80 (Gray & Malone-Lee 1995).

Greater morbidity has been associated with bacteriuria in the elderly (Gray & Malone-Lee 1995) but this may only be a reflection of susceptibility since there are no data that indicate that treating asymptomatic bacteriuria influences the general health state (Hooton & Stam 1991). There are no data available

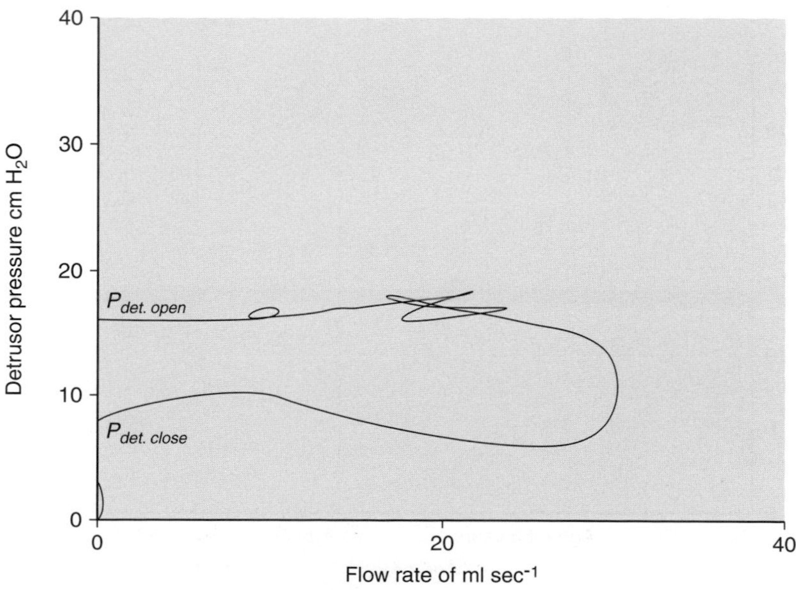

Fig. 33.6 Voiding detrusor pressure against flow rate.

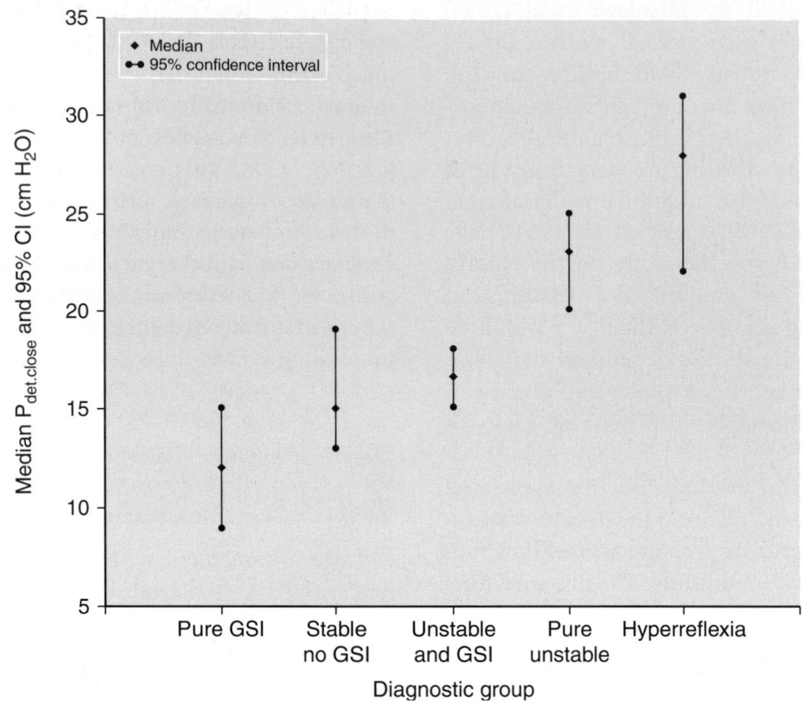

Fig. 33.7 Median $P_{det.close}$ and 95% CI by diagnostic group. Women with various combinations of instability and stress incontinence and women with hyperreflexia.

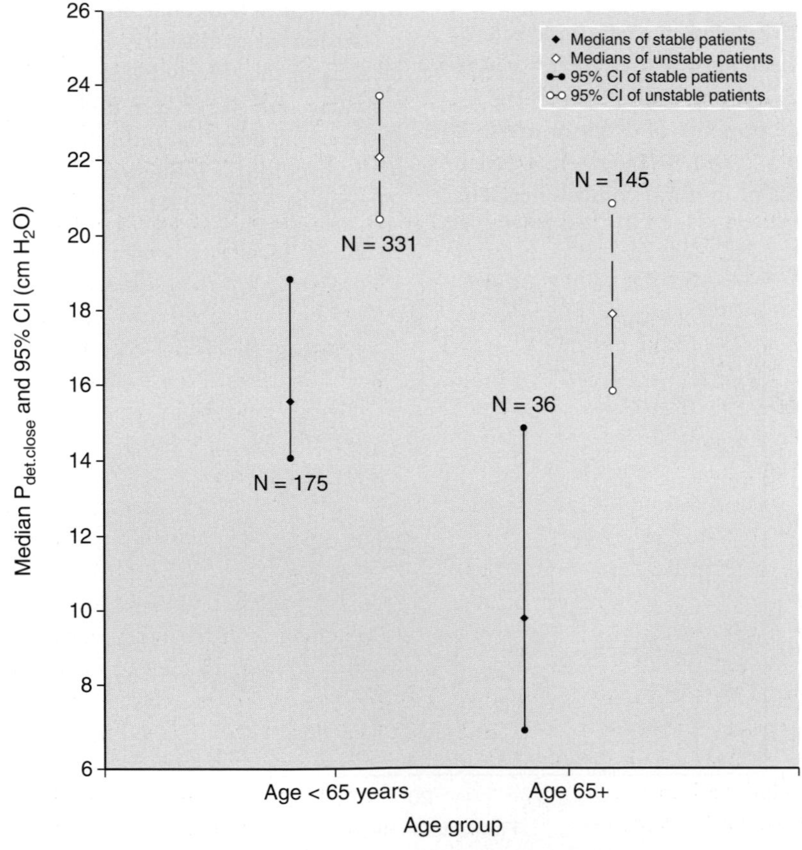

Fig. 33.8 Medians and 95% confidence intervals of $P_{det.close}$ for women with stable and unstable bladders, analysed by age group.

which support the treatment of non-acute dysuric bacteriuria in the incontinent elderly. It has been found that the detection of 'asymptomatic' bacteriuria in the elderly at the time of urodynamic assessment did not seem to be related to the course of events after investigation (Harari et al 1994). The injudicious treatment of asymptomatic bacteriuria in the elderly should be avoided because they are far more susceptible to the adverse effects of antibiotics, particularly *Clostridium difficile* infection of the colon.

In order to treat a urinary infection we need to choose a drug that is well absorbed from the gastrointestinal tract and therefore does not accumulate in the colon, that is excreted in the urine rapidly, not associated with high resistance rates and is inexpensive. Nitrofurantoin (Furadantin) fits this bill. Some patients experience nausea with nitrofurantoin and in these circumstances the macrocrystals (Macrodantin) prove useful. Trimethoprim (Monotrim) is a useful urinary antibiotic provided there is not a great deal of local resistance. Amoxycillin (Amoxil) continues to be recommended for urinary infections and is effective but particularly associated with the development of vaginal thrush infections. These occur in 25% of women prescribed amoxycillin. Nalidixic acid (Negram) is also a useful urinary antibiotic that is worth considering as a non-toxic first line treatment. The newer quinolones such as ciprofloxacin (Ciproxin) should really be used as second-line therapies for resistant infections (Hooton & Stamm 1991; Gray & Malone-Lee 1995).

The dose and duration should be designed to limit the period of treatment. A single dose may be effective but is unreliable and it is recommended that 3-day courses be used for managing uncomplicated acute cystitis. When urinary tract infection is complicated by hospitalization, instrumentation of the urinary tract, pregnancy, diabetes, immunosuppression, failure of previous therapy, more than three infections in the previous year, or symptoms lasting over 7 days, then a 7-day course should be used.

Elderly people are more likely than younger adults to require long-term catheterization because of urinary retention. Bacterial colonization of the long-term urethral catheters is universal. Suprapubic catheters have a lower prevalence of bacteriuria in some groups and also have advantages for comfort, convenience and ease of nursing. Catheter-associated bacteriuria is an important source of bacteraemia in hospitalized patients. However, treatment of asymptomatic bacteriuria in patients with long-term catheters is not indicated and treatment should be reserved for symptomatic patients only.

TREATING DETRUSOR INSTABILITY

The use of drugs in the elderly requires special consideration. Decreased renal clearance is primarily responsible for the increased sensitivity, but reduced organ reserve, loss of carrier proteins and the increased fat:water ratio also contribute. Whilst these factors give rise to more toxic effects it is becoming evident that there is also an increased propensity for gaining benefit from drugs. This dichotomy makes physiological sense, since both poles arise from enhanced sensitivity to medication. Previous experience has emphasized the importance of clinical efficacy and safety studies in treating the elderly (Editorial 1991; Thomas et al 1995). Three drugs can be given with efficacy and safety for the elderly with detrusor instability.

Imipramine is the oldest of the three (Castleden et al 1981, 1986). It is probably not as effective as oxybutynin but there are a number of references in the literature which report anecdotal observations of synergism in combination with oxybutynin, both drugs being administered in low dose, when treating particularly resistant patients (Karram & Bhatia 1989; Wall 1990).

Oxybutynin hydrochloride (Ditropan, Cystrin) seems to be the first choice drug of most centres in the treatment of the unstable bladder (Malone-Lee 1995). It is a tertiary amine with powerful anticholinergic, local anaesthetic and papaverine-like properties. It is very well absorbed from the gastrointestinal tract reaching maximum plasma concentration 30 minutes after ingestion. It is excreted by the kidneys and has a plasma half-life of about 3 hours (Hughes et al 1992). This is very slightly increased in the elderly. The side-effects involve a dry mouth, constipation, reflux oesophagitis (the usual reason for withdrawal of this medication), dry skin, visual accommodation problems and minor ankle swelling. There are no records of age-specific toxicity. Recent work has supported lower doses than those recommended in the data sheets for all age groups. We start all patients on 2.5 mg b.d. and titrate the dose in response to efficacy and side-effects (Malone-Lee et al 1992). We have recently completed a multicentre study of a new controlled release form of oxybutynin, being administered as a single dose of 10 mg daily. We found equal equivalence to oxybutynin 5 mg b.d., with 40% fewer side-effects (Birns & Malone-Lee 1997).

When we accomplished a placebo-controlled trial of oxybutynin in the elderly (Szonyi et al 1995) we noted an unexpected outcome. Both groups were using bladder retraining and kept diary charts throughout the course of the study. The separation between placebo and active groups started to evolve after 5 weeks and we did not know whether the plateau had been achieved at 6 weeks when the study terminated. The data coming from the four 12-week studies of tolterodine in adults has demonstrated a similar phenomenon with a plateau at about 8 weeks (Data on file, 1997, Pharmacia & Upjohn). It is therefore probably best to wait for 8 weeks between dose alterations as the dynamics of these drugs seem to be slower than the kinetics would suggest.

Tolterodine is a new, potent muscarinic receptor antagonist which exhibits a favourable selectivity for the bladder over salivary glands *in vivo*, in the anaesthetized cat (Nilvebrant et al 1997). As such it has significant potential for treating the overactive bladder. We have now completed a multinational, randomized, double blind, parallel group, comparative trial of tolterodine 1 mg b.d., 2 mg b.d. and placebo in patients of either sex, aged 65 or over, with urgency; urinary frequency of eight or more micturitions per 24 hours. The treatment period was 4 weeks (Data on file, 1997, Pharmacia & Upjohn).

There was a statistically significant difference in the reduction in episodes of incontinence and in the increase in volume voided/micturition in those taking tolterodine 2 mg b.d. compared to placebo. The commonest side-effect reported was a dry mouth that was found to be significantly dose-related. The withdrawal rate was low, although a higher incidence was found in the active treatment groups (placebo 2%, tolterodine 1 mg b.d. 7%, 2 mg b.d. 10%). The treatment groups did not demonstrate more numerous serious adverse events. In particular, no ECG differences were found between groups, especially no clinically significant alteration in the QTc interval. The latter was of particular relevance because of the previous toxicity of terodiline in the elderly (Nilvebrant et al 1997).

When treating detrusor instability in the elderly we always combine the antimuscarinic agent with an outpatient bladder retraining regimen because the oxybutynin study used bladder retraining in the treatment group. The more recent tolterodine data report active treatment without bladder retraining. The influence on bladder retraining of tolterodine will be tested shortly in a trial in the UK. Contrary to some recommendations, we do not use bladder retraining on its own because, as with placebo, we have never recorded a change in patients on placebo with bladder retraining (Wiseman et al 1991; Szonyi et al 1995)

INCONTINENCE AIDS

It is important to understand that where incontinence proves irreversible, it can be managed very well and safely by means of diapers. The government continues to fund clinical programmes designed to test the efficacy of the new products so that there are now readily available performance data which can guide the clinical staff in making choices on what best to use. As a rule of thumb, if the environment smells of urine, then the management strategy must be wrong.

REFERENCES

Birns J, Malone-Lee J G 1997 Controlled-release oxybutynin maintains efficacy with a 43% reduction in side effects compared with conventional oxybutynin treatment. Neurourology and Urodynamics 16(5): 429–430

Brocklehurst J C 1993 Urinary incontinence in the community – analysis of a MORI poll. British Medical Journal 306: 832–834

Carey M, Sapountzis K, Friedhuber A, Scurry J, Dwyer P 1996 Electron microscopy study of detrusor muscle cell junctions in women with detrusor instability and controls. Neurourology and Urodynamics 15(4): 431–432

Carey M, de Jong S, Moran P, Friedhuber A, Dwyer P, and Scurry J 1997 The unstable bladder: Is there an ultrastructural basis? Neurourology and Urodynamics 16(5): 423–425

Castleden C M, George C F, Renwick A G, Asher M J 1981 Imipramine a possible alternative to current therapy for urinary incontinence in the elderly. Journal of Urology 125: 318–320

Castleden C M, Duffin H M, Gulati R S 1986 Double-blind study of imipramine and placebo for incontinence due to bladder instability. Age and Ageing 15(5): 299–303

Collas D M, Malone-Lee J G 1996 Age associated changes in detrusor sensory function in patients with lower urinary tract symptoms. International Urogynecological Journal 7: 24–29

Ding Y Y, Lieu P K, Choo P W J, Tjia T T L 1996 Urinary incontinence after ischaemic stroke – Predictive factors for it prevalence. Neurourology and Urodynamics 15(4): 262–264

Diokno A C, Brock B M, Herzog A R, Bromberg J 1990 Medical correlates of urinary incontinence in the elderly. Journal of Urology 36(2): 129–138

Editorial 1991 Terodiline and torsades de pointes. British Medical Journal 303(6801): 519–520

Elbadawi A, Yalla S V, Resnick N M 1993 Structural basis of geriatric voiding dysfunction, I. Methods of a prospective ultrastructural/urodynamic study and an overview of the findings. Journal of Urology 150: 1650–1656

Elbadawi A, Hailmariam S, Yalla S V, and Resnick N M 1997 Structural basis of geriatric voiding dysfunction. VII. Prospective ultrastructural/urodynamic evaluation of its natural evolution. Journal of Urology 157: 1814–1822

Goldberg T H, Chavin S I 1997 Preventive medicine and screening in older adults. Journal of the American Geriatric Society 45(3): 344–354

Gray R P, Malone-Lee J 1995 Review: urinary tract infection in elderly people – time to review management? Age and Ageing 24(4): 341–345

Gray R, Wagg A and Malone-Lee J G 1997 Differences in detrusor contractile function in women with neuropathic and idiopathic detrusor instability. British Journal of Urology 80: 222–226

Griffiths D J 1980 Urodynamics: The mechanics and hydrodynamics of the lower urinary tract. Adam Hilger, Bristol

Griffiths D J, McCracken P N, Harrison G M, Gormley E A, Moore K, Hooper R, McEwan A J B, Triscott J 1994a Cerebral aetiology of urinary urge incontinence in elderly people. Age and Ageing 23: 246–250

Griffiths D J, McCracken P N, Harrison G M, Moore K N 1994b Urinary incontinence in the elderly: the brain factor. Scandinavian Journal of Urology and Nephrology 157: 83–88

Griffiths D J, McCracken P N, Harrison G M, Gormley E A 1992 Characteristics of urinary incontinence in elderly patients by 24-hour monitoring and urodynamic testing. Age and Ageing 21: 194–201

Harari D, Malone-Lee J G, Ridgway G L 1994 An age related investigation of urinary tract symptoms and infection following urodynamic studies. Age and Ageing 23: 62–64

Hooton T M, Stamm W E 1991 Management of acute uncomplicated urinary tract infection in adults. Medical Clinics of North America 75: 339–357

Hughes K M, Lang J C T, Lazare R, Gordon D, Stanton S L, Malone-Lee J, Geraint M 1992 The measurement of oxybutynin and its N-desethyl metabolite in plasma and its application to pharmacokinetic studies in young volunteers and elderly and frail elderly volunteers. Xenobiotica

Karram M M, Bhatia N N 1989 Management of coexistent stress and urge urinary incontinence. Obstetrics and Gynecology 73(1): 4–7.

Malone-Lee J G 1992 Incontinence. Reviews in Clinical Gerontology 2: 45–61

Malone-Lee J G, Wahedna I 1993 Characterisation of detrusor contractile function in relation to old-age. British Journal of Urology 72: 873–880

Malone-Lee J G, Orugon O 1993 A data reduction technique for describing and quantifying detrusor instability. International Urogynecological Journal 4: 204–211

Malone-Lee J G, Lubel D, Szonyi G 1992 Low dose oxybutynin for the unstable bladder. British Medical Journal 304: 1053

Malone-Lee J G 1995 The clinical efficacy of oxybutynin. Reviews in Contemporary Pharmacotherapy 5: 195–202

Nilvebrant L, Hallen B, Larsson G 1997 Tolterodine: a new bladder selective muscarinic receptor antagonist: Preclinical pharmacological and clinical data. Life Sciences 60: 1129–1136

Raleigh V S 1997 The demographic timebomb. British Medical Journal 315: 442–443

Resnick N M, Yalla S V 1987 Detrusor hyperactivity with impaired contractile function. An unrecognised but common cause of incontinence in elderly patients. Journal of the American Medical Association 257: 3076–3081

Schafer W 1992 Principles and clinical application of advanced urodynamic analysis of voiding function. Urologic Clinics of North America 17: 553–566

Szonyi G, Collas D M, Ding Y Y, Malone-Lee J G 1995 Oxybutynin with bladder retraining for detrusor instability in elderly people: a randomized controlled trial. Age and Ageing 24(4): 287–291

Thomas T M, Flymat K R, Blannin J, Meade T W 1980 The prevalence of urinary incontinence. British Medical Journal 281: 1243–1245

Thomas S H, Higham P D, Hartigan-Go K, Kamali F, Wood P, Campbell R W, Ford G A 1995 Concentration dependent cardiotoxicity of terodiline in patients treated for urinary incontinence. British Heart Journal 74(1): 53–56

Wall L L 1990 The management of detrusor instability. [Review]. Clinical Obstetrics and Gynecology 33(2): 367–377

Wagg A, Lieu P K, Ding Y Y, Malone Lee J G 1996 Age-related changes in female urethral function in association with detrusor instability. Journal of Urology 156: 1984–1988

Wagg A S, Bayliss M, Arnold K G, Malone-Lee J G 1996 Urodynamic prognosticators in detrusor instability. Neurourology and Urodynamics 15(4): 279–280

SECTION 3
CHAPTER

34

Urogynaecology in the developing world

JOHN KELLY

INTRODUCTION

The urological problems peculiar to developing countries are influenced by conditions of climate (many tropical), lack of resources, and poor communication (roads etc). There are various conditions which may affect urinary function or cause urinary tract pathology. Each of these will be considered in turn in this chapter.

OBSTRUCTED LABOUR

Incidence

The incidence of obstructed labour will vary depending on whether a hospital, or an area, or a country provides figures. It may be difficult or impossible to obtain national or regional figures because of the number of patients who never seek help, and those who die at home may not be included in statistics. The rates of abnormal delivery and ruptured uterus provide some indication of the incidence of obstructed labour. A 57-bed rural hospital in Ethiopia serving a population of 1.2 million reported an abnormal delivery rate of 52% and a ruptured uterus rate of 7% (Attat Hospital Reports 1993, 1994, 1995). Figures of 49.5% and 0.5% respectively were reported from a 193-bed hospital in south-east Tanzania (Nyangao Hospital Reports 1991, 1992). Ruptured uterus in a Nigerian teaching hospital was 0.4% (Faleimu et al 1990) compared with an incidence of 1 in 4366 in a Dublin teaching hospital (Gardeil et al 1994).

Predisposing causes

1 Small pelvis, due to chronic malnutrition and sometimes early age of first pregnancy. The multiparous patient whose obstructed labour is due to a transverse or oblique lie or a larger baby cannot understand why, having had previous babies normally, she cannot repeat a similar process.
2 Local customs – the patient may not seek help; she may only be allowed to seek the assistance of orthodox medicine after local remedies have failed and by this time she has been in labour for several days.
3 No help is readily available to diagnose and treat obstructed labour.
4 There is poor communication in some countries because of lack of roads and difficult terrain. Transporting the patient to a clinic or hospital for effective treatment may be a problem because of distance and/or costs. In Ethiopia, 75% of the population is, on average, 2.5 days' walk from an all-weather road.
5 Unbooked emergencies, rare in developed countries, account for over 80% of hospital maternal deaths in sub-Saharan Africa (Evans 1995). The two commonest complications in these unbooked patients were disproportion and ruptured uterus. Prevention of these problems includes improved education and better access to appropriate antepartum and intrapartum care.

Effect on urinary tract

The resultant damage to the urinary tract may be

1 A fistula from pressure necrosis
2 Injury to the bladder or ureters from extension of the uterine rupture, or during surgery under the difficult conditions of a ruptured uterus in the presence of sepsis and a severely shocked patient
3 Urinary tract infection.

SYMPHYSIOTOMY

The subcutaneous procedure of Zarate (1955) consists of division of the anterior ligament of the pubic symphysis and part of the inferior ligament, leaving the superior ligament intact. A firm polythene catheter is inserted into the bladder via the urethra; the urethra is pushed to one side while dividing the symphysis. The operator and the assistants who support the legs should be skilled in the technique. The assistants do not allow more than 90° abduction of the legs when the symphysis is divided and adduct the legs when the presenting part is crowned. A generous episiotomy is performed and the presenting part is displaced towards the rectum. The Ventouse is used in preference to forceps, which might damage the unsupported urethra.

If strict adherence to indications for the procedure are respected, then complications or sequelae are uncommon (Bergstrom et al 1994). The disproportion should be such that it cannot be overcome by better uterine action (augmentation) and not so gross that pelvic enlargement will be of no avail.

The presentation is usually cephalic but the procedure is also useful in the after coming head of a breech when the head is obstructed because of disproportion, or for shoulder dystocia. In a series of 1500 symphysiotomies in the years 1958–1988, in a voluntary agency hospital in rural Nigeria, there were only 3 traumatic injuries to the urethra. During this time many trainees were instructed in, and performed the procedure (Twomey D 1990, personal communication). If the patient presents late, then pressure necrosis may have already commenced.

FISTULAE

Vesicovaginal fistulae

Causes

The majority of vesicovaginal and/or rectovaginal fistulae in the developing world are obstetric in origin due to ischaemic necrosis from unrelieved obstructed labour. Operative delivery for obstetric complications may play a part; any pelvic surgery may result in damage to the bladder, urethra or ureters.

Malignancy such as cancer of the cervix or treatment of the malignancy may be associated with a fistula. Many patients still present with advanced carcinoma of the cervix and a vesicovaginal fistula.

Local practices to cure dyspareunia – an incision at the introitus may extend up the anterior vaginal wall causing a urethrovaginal and/or vesicovaginal fistula.

Lymphogranuloma venereum can cause a vesicovaginal fistula often in association with a rectovaginal fistula and destruction of the urethra.

The typical history of a fistula due to pressure necrosis (Fig. 34.1) is that of prolonged (i.e. days), and often unattended labour, resulting in a stillbirth and subsequent incontinence of urine, and perhaps also

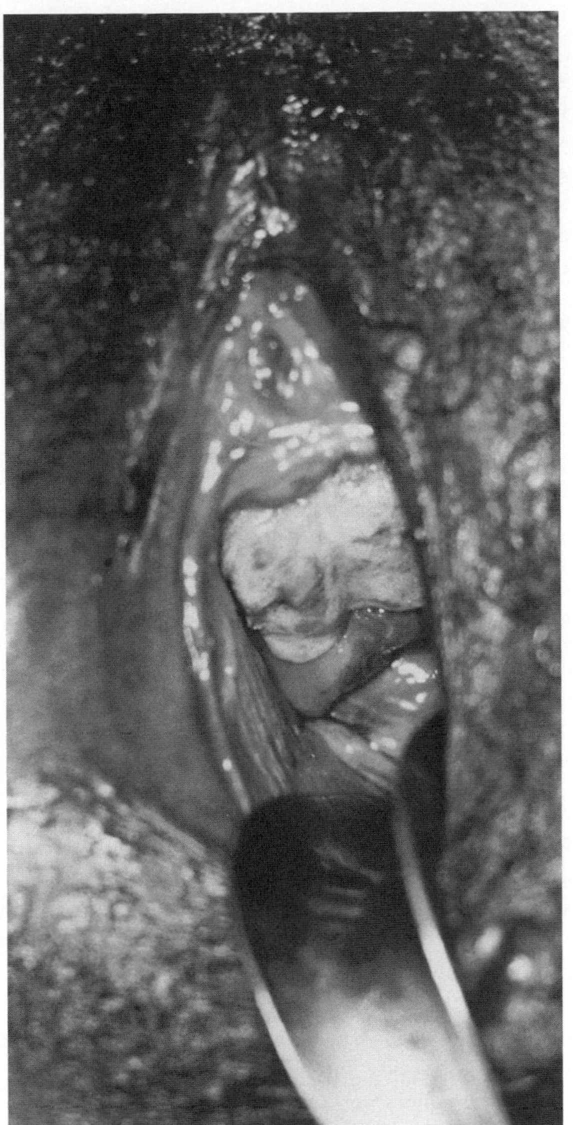

Fig. 34.1 Necrotic slough on anterior vaginal wall from a patient who had been in obstructed labour for several days. When the slough comes away there will be a vesicovaginal fistula.

of faeces. Such women, because of their offensiveness become outcasts of their family, friends and society. Many resort to begging to stay alive.

Incidence

Vesicovaginal fistulae are common in sub-Saharan Africa, stretching from Nigeria in the west to Ethiopia and Somalia in the east, and in northern Asia (Hamlin & Nicholson 1966; Kelly 1995). Approximately 1200 and 450 new cases a year are currently being treated in Addis Ababa, Ethiopia and Anua, Nigeria respectively (Hamlin C 1999, Ward A 1996, personal communications). The communiqué following the International workshop on Vesicovaginal Fistulae (March 1998, Nigeria) stated that 'vesicovaginal fistulae was a disease condition which afflicts about 2 million women in Africa and Asia, with Nigeria accounting for 200 000', and that it will take between 30 and 40 years to clear the existing backlog without attending to new cases in Nigeria. Regrettably there are many patients who suffer from a vesicovaginal fistula and have no ready access to efficient treatment. When a satisfactory therapeutic service becomes available, the number of patients seeking treatment increases progressively, as word gets around.

Classification

Vesicovaginal fistulae may be classified by anatomical site into high, mid or low. They may also be described as simple (good tissues and good access), or complicated (poor access, much loss of tissue, or poor tissue, much scarring, total destruction of the urethra, ureteric orifices opening close to, at the edge of, or even outside the margin of the fistula, and the presence of a rectovaginal fistula or a ureterovaginal fistula).

A high fistula may be vesicocervical or vesicouterine. Figure 34.2 shows a large vesicovaginal fistula with the bladder sound through the urethra.

Figure 34.3 shows a vesicovaginal fistula at the urethrovesical junction.

Figure 34.4 shows a large vesicovaginal fistula with the ureters close to the edge of the fistula. Both ureters have been catheterized.

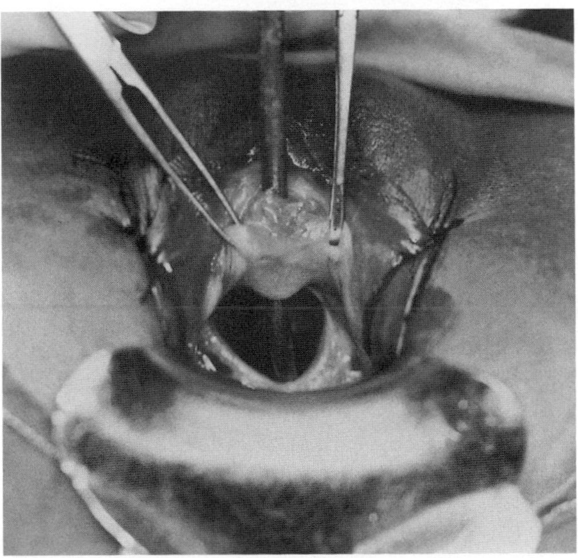

Fig. 34.2 Large vesicovaginal fistula. A sound has been passed per urethram.

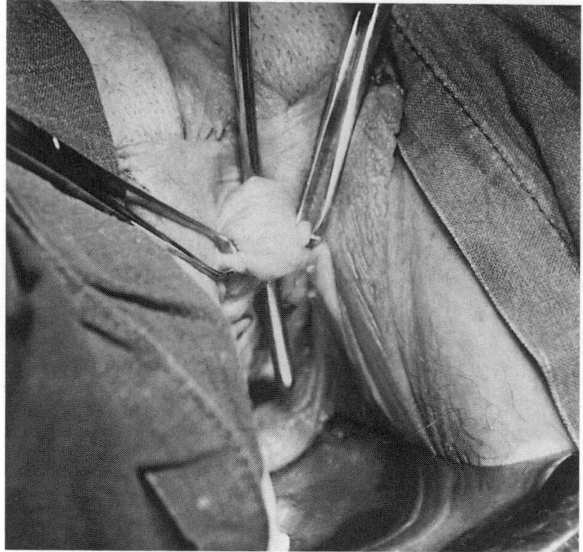

Fig. 34.3 Vesicovaginal fistula involving urethrovesical junction.

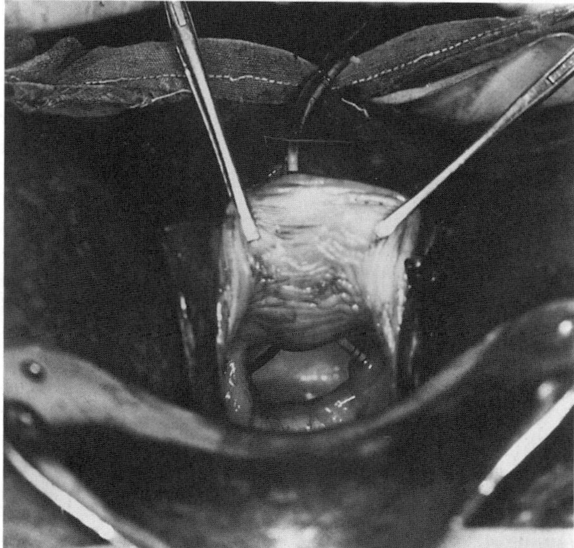

Fig. 34.4 Large vesicovaginal fistula with ureters at edge of fistula. Both ureters have been catheterized.

Preoperative assessment and diagnosis

Many fistulae can be demonstrated on palpation or with the patient in the exaggerated left lateral position, by inspection – a Sims' speculum and a simple anterior vaginal wall retractor are useful aids. Methylene blue or indigo carmine stained water or saline, as a 'dye test', may help reveal the opening of a small fistula. Cystoscopy may be of value in assessing the relationship of the fistula to the ureteric orifices; it may be impracticable where there is a large hole. Facilities for full intravenous urography may not be readily available in a developing country and may be too costly. At the preoperative assessment, which in a few patients may require anaesthesia, the plan of treatment will be decided. An abdominal or vaginal approach will be chosen according to the practice of the operator and the site of the fistula. A low vesicovaginal fistula and a urethrovaginal fistula should be approached vaginally. Urologists will usually prefer an abdominal approach and gynaecologists a vaginal approach. As most gynaecologists are used to the lithotomy position, this will often be preferred – shoulder pads and a steep Trendelenburg tilt are often useful. Some prefer the knee–chest position, especially for a fistula close to, and tucked under the urethral meatus. Any bladder calculi should be removed and reparative surgery deferred for at least a month. During this time, such a patient may benefit from bladder irrigation and treatment for any infection.

Biopsy, histology and appropriate therapy are necessary before attempt at repair in patients with a fistula associated with malignancy, lymphogranuloma venereum or schistosomiasis.

Timing of repair from the original injury (or previous attempt at repair)

A waiting period of 2–3 months is probably ideal. During this time the tissues become healthier, less friable and infection can be eradicated. Explanation should be given to the patient as to why the waiting period is an essential part of her treatment. During this time, she is given general measures to improve her health and specific treatment for any infection. A 'waiting hostel' is valuable for those who are weak, who have travelled long distances or require facilities for vulval toilet, not available at home. The patient with limb contractures resulting from prolonged immobilization will also benefit from physiotherapy. For radiation-induced fistulae the waiting interval is longer – at least a year. Blandy et al (1991) and Wang & Hadley (1990) have advocated early non-delayed repair of the simple small fistula. This may save the patient some weeks of waiting; however, some of these small fistulae will heal spontaneously, usually with the aid of catheter drainage (Kelly 1992a). As most vesicovaginal fistulae in the developing world are complicated, it is a wise precaution to wait 3 months.

Treatment

Anaesthesia for the repair operation in developing countries will usually be spinal, because of the shortage of trained anaesthetists. Where the operation lasts for more than 2 hours, then the spinal (heavy bupivacaine 2–3 ml) may require to be supplemented with some form of general anaesthesia or ketamine.

The vaginal approach

The basic points in the operative technique are:

1 Adequate exposure, which may only be achieved in some patients by performing an episiotomy and dividing fibrotic bands of dense scar tissue which may hide the fistula (Figs 34.5, 6 and 7).
2 Mobilization. Infiltration of a 1 in 250 000 solution of phenylephrine or adrenalin in saline helps to open up tissue planes and also acts as a vasoconstrictor. The fistula is circumcised using a small (number 15) blade and the vaginal skin is then dissected off the bladder with its fascia intact. The fibrous edge of the fistula is also excised, and any further scar tissue is divided to enable the fistula to be repaired in two layers without tension.
3 The fistula is closed with two layers of interrupted inverting sutures of 2/0 vicryl (or similar). A fish-hook type of needle (Symonds round-bodied size 9) is sometimes useful. Where the fistula is fixed to the pubic bone, an

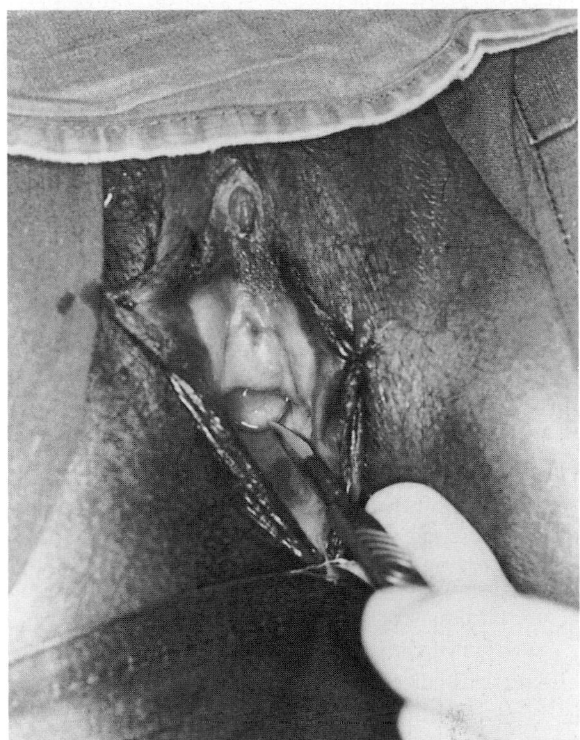

Fig. 34.6 Fibrotic band being divided at 4 o'clock to provide access for fistula repair.

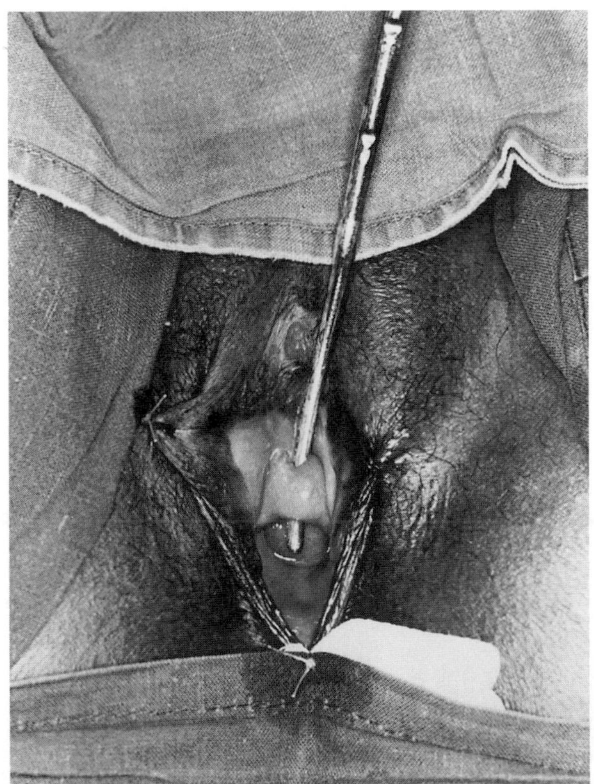

Fig. 34.5 Scar tissue posteriorly, severely limits access to vesicovaginal fistula which has destroyed most of bladder and part of urethra.

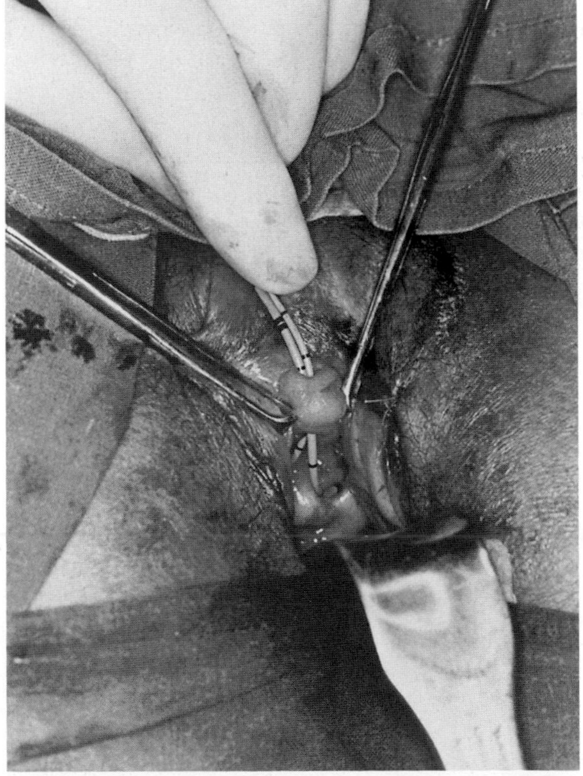

Fig. 34.7 Following division of fibrotic tissue, access is provided. The cervix is seen and the ureters which are close to the edge of the fistula have been catheterized.

aneurysm needle may be necessary to penetrate the periosteum.

4 A dye test is then performed to demonstrate that the fistula has been closed and also that another fistula has not been 'missed'.

5 The vaginal skin is closed with interrupted everting sutures: either absorbable 0, or 1 vicryl, or non-absorbable (nylon). Sometimes it is necessary to bring in skin flaps where there has been much loss of tissue.

6 The vagina is packed for 48 hours. Continuous bladder drainage for 14 days (usually a Foley catheter) is advised. Any drag or pull on the catheter is avoided by appropriate strapping. Nothing should enter the vagina for 3 months.

Additional points in the technique are used as appropriate; these may include the following:

1 The ureteric orifices should be sought. The ureter(s) may open anywhere on the edge of the fistula, even anteriorly, and occasionally outside the fistula directly on to the vagina (Fig. 34.8). Where the ureter is outside the margin of the fistula it should be mobilized and re-implanted into the bladder – the bladder on the side of the affected ureter will be mobilized accordingly. If both ureters are outside the margin of the fistula, then, as in the rare case of the double ureteric fistula approached by the abdominal route, the bladder has to be mobilized on both sides. Occasionally, re-implantation cannot be performed because of the wide separation of the ureter from the bladder, usually with dense scar tissue. The ureter might then be catheterized and the bladder repaired in an attempt to re-implant the ureter into the bladder by an abdominal approach then, or at a later date.

2 Where the urethra is absent, a new urethra has to be constructed.

3 A support graft is beneficial for complicated fistulae:

a) A Martius (1939) pedicle graft of fibro-fatty tissue (Figs 34.9 and 34.10) is brought down to cover and reinforce the repaired fistula and/or urethra, care being taken that the tunnel under the labia does not constrict the pedicle. Anchoring sutures secure the graft.

b) The Gracilis muscle pedicle graft (Figs 34.11 and 34.12) (Hamlin & Nicholson 1969) is very occasionally used where a new urethra has to be fashioned. The muscle is brought from the thigh to the introitus through a tunnel deep to the skin and superficial fascia of the upper thigh and labia, care being taken to preserve the neurovascular bundle (Fig. 34.12) which enters

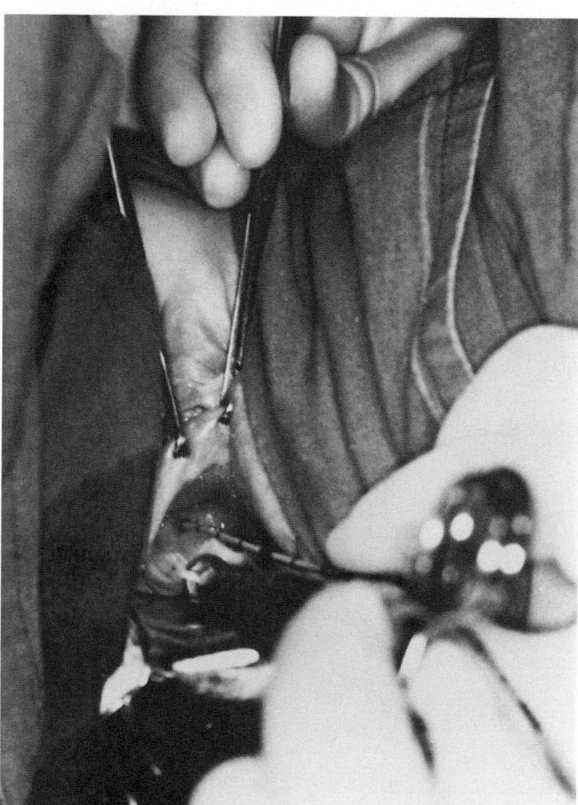

Fig. 34.8 Right ureter on edge of vesicovaginal fistula being catheterized.

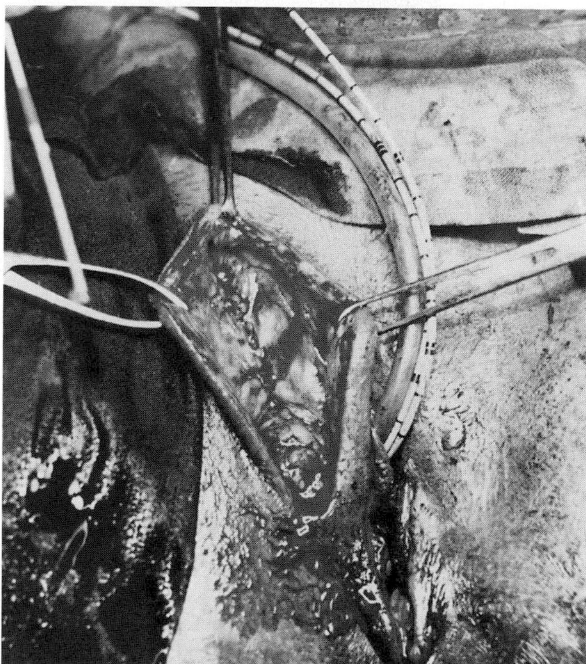

Fig. 34.9 Skin incised to display area from which right Martius pedicle graft will be dissected. Urine is seen draining from the ureteric catheters.

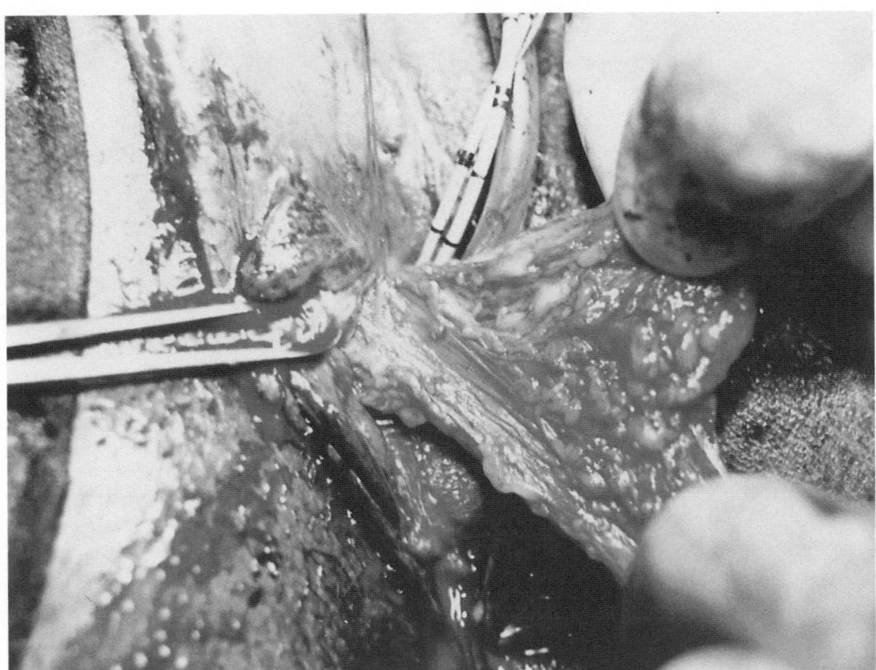

Fig. 34.10 Martius pedicle graft from right labium is displayed before it is anchored under the repaired fistula. A Foley catheter and ureteric catheters are seen.

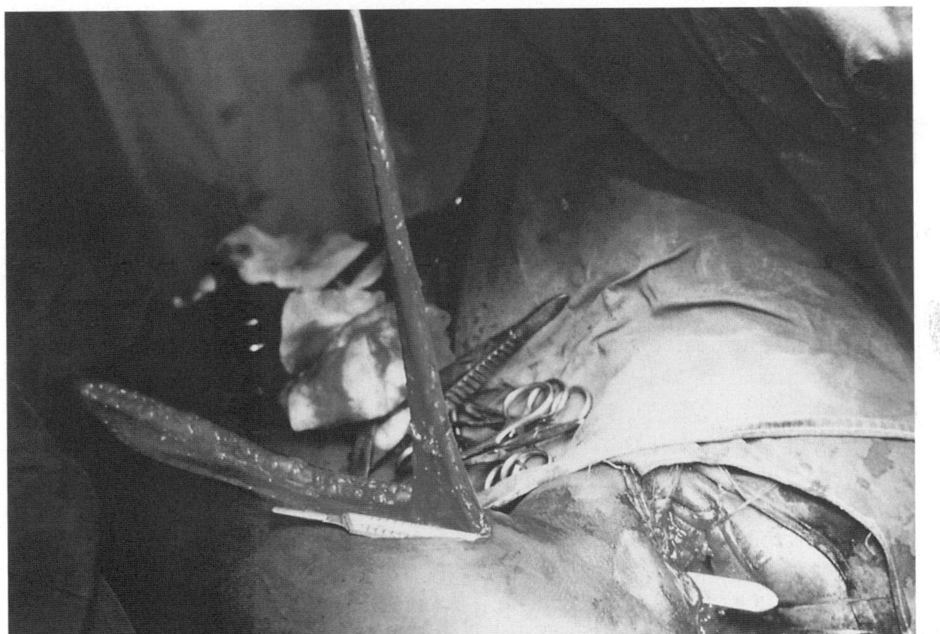

Fig. 34.11 Gracilis muscle graft from right thigh. Scalpel handle indicates the tunnel for the pedicle graft from thigh to support the repaired fistula.

the muscle on its lateral border, about 10 cm from the origin of the gracilis muscle. Five anchor sutures are used to secure the graft over the repair – the most important anchor is the one securing the muscle to the anterior aspect of the cervix, or to the remains of the uterus.

The abdominal approach

A transperitoneal approach is used. The bladder is bisected and the bladder and vagina widely mobilized. The ureters are catheterized to prevent inadvertent injury. The fistula track is excised, as is any

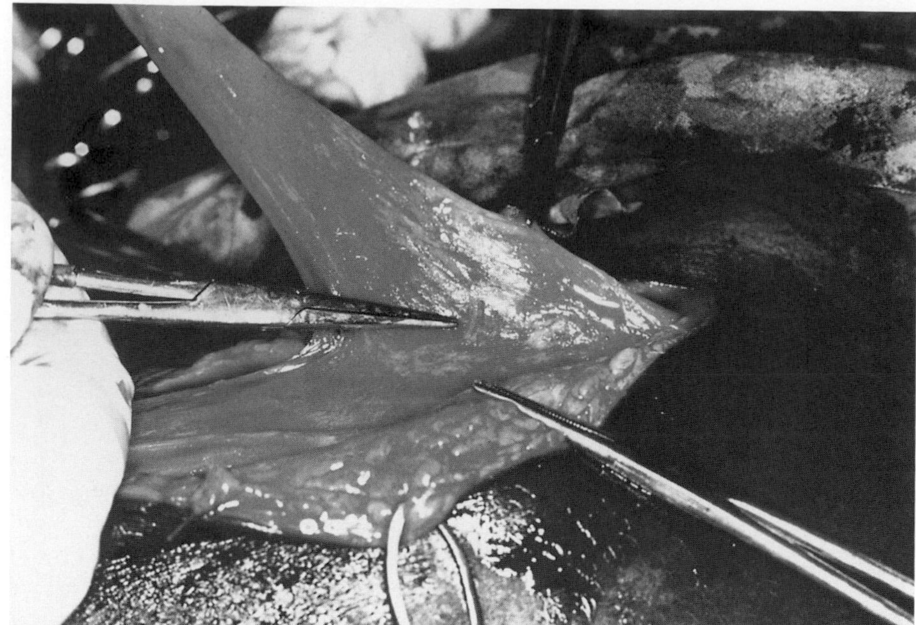

Fig. 34.12 Gracilis muscle pedicle graft. The neurovascular bundle, indicated by artery forceps, must be preserved.

unhealthy or scar tissue. The vaginal defect is closed in layers. A pedicled omental graft may then be introduced to reinforce the closure. The bladder is then closed in two layers, with 2/0 vicryl. In addition to the usual catheter drainage for 14 days, a suprapubic tubular drain is also useful for several days.

Other possible forms of therapy

Colpocleisis (rare) The vaginal epithelium surrounding the fistula is denuded. The anterior and posterior walls of the denuded upper part of the vagina are approximated to effect a partial colpocleisis.

Urinary diversion procedures (uncommon) These would be considered where the bladder had been completely destroyed. The ideal treatment would be implantation of the ureters into an isolated loop of ileum. However, in a developing society because an abdominal stoma is not acceptable, ureterosigmoidostomy is usually performed, provided there is an intact rectum and anal sphincter.

Rectovaginal fistula Where there is a rectovaginal fistula in addition to a vesicovaginal fistula, it can be repaired at the same operation as the vesicovaginal fistula is repaired. Temporary colostomy may be indicated where the rectovaginal fistula is high and difficult.

Social rehabilitation

Following curative surgery, the patient is provided with new clothes and sufficient funding for her journey home, where she will be reintegrated as a rightful member of her society.

The importance of seeking care during any subsequent pregnancy and delivery is emphasized to the patient. The majority of patients who become pregnant following a vesicovaginal fistula repair will be delivered by a caesarean section. Vaginal delivery may be possible where certain criteria are met (Kelly 1979):

1. The fistula was caused by a non-recurring factor such as malpresentation rather than grossly contracted pelvis.
2. The labour is conducted under skilled supervision in hospital with facilities for caesarean section.
3. A labial pedicled fat graft has been utilized in the repair – this is believed to protect the repair during labour.

The cured fistula patient is the source of referral to the Fistula Hospital for one third of patients (Kelly & Kwast 1993a); she is also an educator and primary health care provider in her own locality.

Ureterovaginal fistulae

These are less common than vesicovaginal fistulae. They may follow surgery, often when dealing with a ruptured uterus or uncontrolled bleeding at caesarean section; malignancy and/or radiotherapy may be causative.

The diagnosis is made by excluding a VVF on clinical examination and bladder dye test (beware that occasionally there may be both a vesicovaginal fistula and a uterovaginal fistula in the same patient). Cystoscopy will reveal the absence of efflux of urine from the injured side and the presence of efflux from the intact ureter. This can be aided by giving plenty of fluids, the use of a diuretic and perhaps intravenous methylene blue or indigo carmine. Further information can be obtained by attempting to pass a catheter up the affected side or injecting radio-opaque dye using a bulb catheter. Intravenous urography (where there is scarcity of resources for IVU, priority should be given to patients with ureteric fistulae) will show the state of renal function and any dilatation of the ureter consequent on obstruction.

Most ureterovaginal fistulae will present at about 2 to 6 weeks after injury and repair can be attempted from then onwards. The approach is primarily abdominal, either retroperitoneal or transperitoneal. (Ureteric re-implantation may be performed using a vaginal approach when the ureter has been found outside the edge of the fistula during a repair of a vesicovaginal fistula as previous described.)

Spontaneous healing can occasionally occur, especially when there has been incomplete division of the ureter and it has been possible to pass a catheter or a double-J stent up the ureter.

The site of the fistula is identified and the ureter is mobilized while maintaining its blood supply. The bladder is also mobilized towards the injured ureter so that the repair will not be under tension. If the site of injury is close to the bladder, the plan would be to reimplant the ureter into the base of the bladder. If the injury is higher, then a psoas hitch or a Boari flap procedure (or both) would be chosen and the ureter would be re-implanted into the posterolateral wall of the bladder.

The bladder is opened on its anterior aspect by a transverse incision nearer to the side of the injured ureter. A curved incision is used when a flap is planned. The intact ureter is catheterized, to prevent inadvertent injury. The ureter on the affected side is drawn into the bladder, which may be extended by the flap or mobilization, and then through a submucosal tunnel of 2–3 cm. The new ureteric orifice is freshened, spatulated and then sutured to the mucosa of the bladder with 3/0 or 4/0 vicryl. The implanted ureter is splintered with a 6 F infant feeding tube or a ureteric catheter. This splint or catheter is brought out through the cystostomy alongside a suprapubic catheter. The bladder is closed with two layers of 3/0 vicryl and drained with a urethral catheter (and for a few days also by the suprapubic catheter). The omentum can be used to wrap around the suture line to provide additional vascularity and protection. The area of repair is drained with a tubular drain.

URETHRAL DESTRUCTION

Causes

1 Pressure necrosis from obstructed labour may destroy the proximal or the entire urethra – there is usually also a vesicovaginal fistula.
2 Lymphogranuloma venereum may destroy the urethra – the process more commonly starts at the distal urethra (Fig 34.13).
3 Occasionally, local attempts to relieve introital stenosis, or surgical procedures in this area such

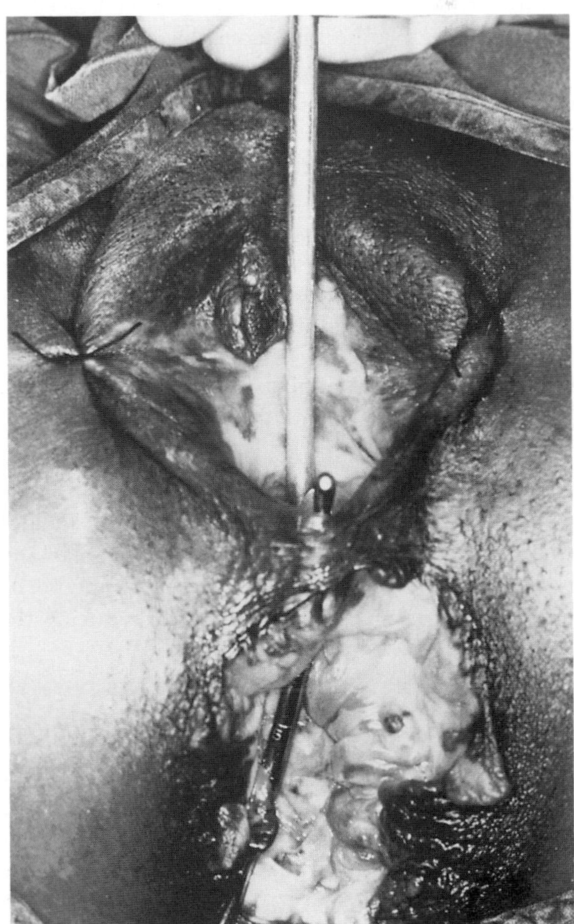

Fig. 34.13 Lymphogranuloma venereum. Absent urethra. Bladder sound goes straight into vesicovaginal fistula. Uterine sound demonstrates rectovaginal fistula.

as repair of a urethral diverticulum, may damage or destroy the urethra.

Management

This depends on the cause and the symptoms. Oxytetracycline therapy must be given to patients with lymphogranuloma venereum (see later) before considering them for surgery. A patient may still be continent if only the distal urethra is destroyed, when surgical intervention will not be indicated.

Surgical formation of a new urethra

Two vertical incisions 2.5 cm apart are made along the anterior wall of the skin of the vestibule, extending up to the bladder fistula usually at the site of the original internal urethral meatus. The vertical incisions then encircle the bladder fistula so that the result is a U-shaped incision. The edges are undermined to allow the new urethral tube to be created by approximating the skin edges without tension, using inverting interrupted sutures of 3/0 vicryl. The edges are brought together underneath a 12 F silicone catheter inserted into the bladder. The sutures at the bladder neck should be reinforced with a second layer of sutures to draw together the folds of the bladder muscle over this junction and to lessen the risk of stress incontinence. A second layer using paraurethral fibromuscular tissue from each side, again with interrupted sutures, is sutured in the midline over the new urethra. Tension is avoided by undermining and mobilizing the paraurethral fibromuscular tissue on both sides.

A support graft is highly recommended when creating a new urethra. This may be in the form of a Martius graft or by using the gracilis muscle (see above).

The skin closure, vaginal pack and bladder drainage are as for vesicovaginal fistulae. As following repair of vesicovaginal fistulae, physiotherapy in the form of perineal exercises is helpful in reducing the incidence of stress incontinence.

Results

The results of repair of vesicovaginal fistulae (including urethrovesico fistulae and creation of a new urethra), will be influenced by a variety of factors such as the severity of the lesion, the number of previous attempts at repair, the health of the patient, the available facilities and the experience and expertise of the whole team caring for the patient. The prospects for successful repair decline with each operation (Lawson 1978). In an evaluation of failed repairs at the Addis Ababa Fistula Hospital (Kelly & Kwast 1993b) failed repair was associated with a history of ruptured uterus, a history of previous unsuccessful attempts at repair, and more patients whose general condition was poor, whose fistula was complicated and required complicated operative procedures. The majority of the failures were cured by a further operation and at least 3% of these complicated fistulae closed spontaneously. It was possible that a further 6% may have closed as the patients did not re-attend. Eighty-eight per cent of patients were cured at the first attempt at repair at the Addis Ababa Fistula Hospital. Stress incontinence, unfortunately, was still a problem in 6% of patients even though the fistula was closed.

The author's personal series is now 1293 (267 also had a rectovaginal fistula repaired at the same operation) with results of:

Cured (at first attempt at repair)	84.5%
Stress incontinence	9.4%
Failed	6.1%

HIV INFECTION

AIDS in sub-Saharan Africa and parts of Asia is now a major problem with significant morbidity and mortality. Genitourinary manifestations may be the initial presentation of the disease. The clinical course of cervical carcinoma, pelvic inflammatory disease, peritonitis (sometimes associated with TB), syphilis, ulcerative lesions, condylomata and candidiasis may be altered or refractory to usual treatment (Korn & Landers 1995; Kwan & Lowe 1995; Maiman et al 1997).

Increasing degrees of immunosuppression cause failure of healing and in urogynaecology, fistula repairs are liable to be unsuccessful. Spontaneous rectovaginal fistulae in infants (Borgstein & Broadhead 1994; Hyde & Sarbah 1994) and in sexually active women (Verkuyl 1994) have been associated with HIV infection. Verkuyl (1995) suggested that HIV damage to the nervous system causes retention of urine. The only convincing intervention in reducing the incidence of HIV infection in Africa was that of improved control of sexually transmitted diseases (Grosskurth et al 1995). No association was found between condom use and HIV infection, either before or after adjustment for confounders (Quigley et al 1997).

GRANULOMA INGUINALE

This is caused by the bacterium, *Donovania granulomatis*, which is found inside large mononuclear cells in the affected tissue. It usually presents as a nodular thickening and elevation of the vulval skin, which breaks down to form an irregular ulcer affecting the clitoris, then the labia, the vagina and the flexures of the thighs. Strictures of the urethra may result or even septic cystitis. Characteristic Donovan bodies may be demonstrated on biopsy. Treatment is with streptomycin or tetracycline; ceftriaxone has proved useful in resistant cases (Marianos et al 1994). Genital ulcer disease, of any aetiology, is a recognized co-factor for HIV transmission (O'Farrell 1995).

LYMPHOGRANULOMA VENEREUM (LGV)

This is more common with a higher infectivity than granuloma inguinale and is caused by a virus of the *psittacosis-trachoma* or *Chlamydia* group. The primary sore is a small herpetiform ulcer in the posterior wall of the vagina; the anorectal lymph glands become involved and further spread produces involvement of the vulva and rectum – the genitoanorectal syndrome. The vulval and vaginal ulcers are painless but they can progress to destructive lesions with fenestration. The urethra, and less commonly the bladder, may be infiltrated followed by stricture and fistula formation. As the disease progresses, proctitis occurs followed by stricture of the rectum and rectovaginal fistula formation (Fig. 34.13), and in some cases complete destruction of the urethra. A diagnosis is made on the clinical picture and on histology. The treatment is by oxytetracycline in doses of 15–36 g over 15 to 30 days. Dilatation and graduated bougies may be useful. Attempts at any fistula repair should not be instituted until full medical treatment has been tried. Unfortunately, some of these patients require a colostomy or a urinary diversion (ureterocolic implantation is not advisable as LGV patients usually have a degree of rectal incontinence or a rectovaginal fistula which is difficult to cure). Rectal involvement in LGV is more common in women. Rectal stricture resembles and is known to predispose to rectal cancer (Chopda et al 1994).

SCHISTOSOMIASIS

Schistosomiasis is a group of diseases caused by trematodes of the genus *Schistosoma*. The intermediate host is the freshwater snail. Of the four known species, *S. haematobium* more commonly produces lesions in the female bladder and genital tract. It tends to live in the pelvic veins and deposits its ova in the bladder wall or urethra, and less commonly in the genital tract and rectum. The resulting disability from the infection in children is so mild, that many only seek medical help when dysuria and burning on micturition become severe. Haematuria may be accepted as a 'normal' event in children's lives in endemic areas.

The papillomatous or ulcerative lesions of the vulva, vagina and perhaps the cervix, like the more severe bladder features (polypoid lesions plus bladder calcification) appear in women in early reproductive life. Although vesicovaginal fistulae are uncommonly due to schistosomiasis of the bladder or vagina, when obstetric fistulae occur, in areas where schistosomiasis is hyperendemic, anti-schistosome treatment should be considered before surgery. Successful repair would be jeopardized in the presence of schistosoma bladder fibrosis. The diagnosis is confirmed by the identification of the ova in the urine. Where infection is light, a 24-hour specimen, or specimen after exercise may give positive results, provided that the last drops of urine expressed during micturition have not been missed. The treatment is by oral praziquantel, 40 mg/kg as a single oral dose. Treatment with anti-schistosome drugs should be avoided during pregnancy because of possible risks to the fetus.

The higher prevalence of the condition in males is due to greater opportunities for occupational exposure; in Muslim societies, women's exposure to infected water is restricted (Michelson 1993).

Although less common in the female, schistosomiasis is associated with bladder cancer (Lemmer & Fripp 1994).

FEMALE GENITAL MUTILATION (FGM) OR CIRCUMCISION (FIG. 34.14)

Three main types are practised:

1 Clitoridectomy or Sunna – the aim is removal of the prepuce, but usually involves removing the clitoris.

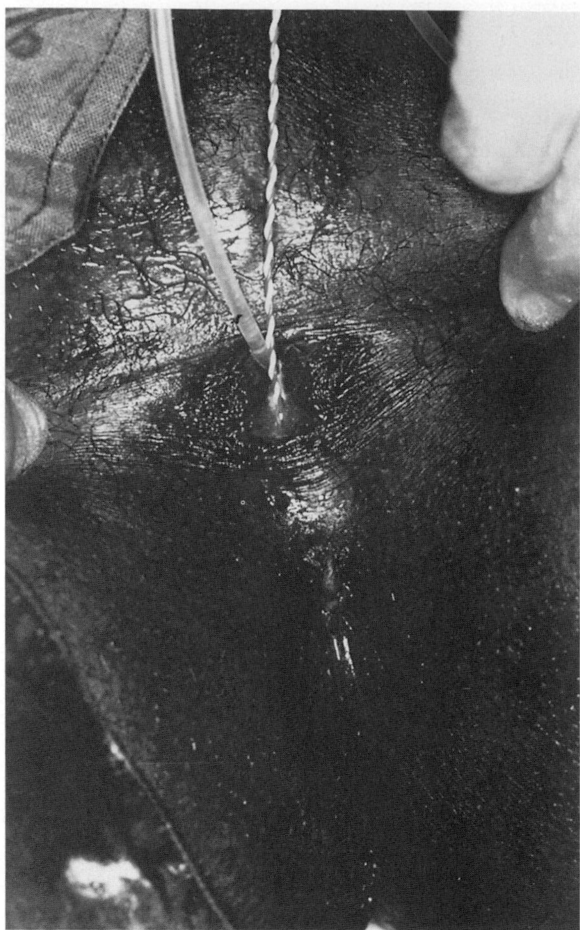

Fig. 34.14 Circumcision. This patient is being monitored in labour by a presenting part electrode and intrauterine pressure catheter. An 'anterior episiotomy' is necessary to aid vaginal delivery.

2 Excision – this involves type (1) plus removal of the clitoris plus part or all of both labia minora.
3 Infibulation – this involves type (2) plus removal of the inner surface of the labia majora; the cut edges of the two sides are made to fuse by various means – 'adhesive substances', use of thorns or string, or suturing. Infibulation or the pharaonic type was made illegal in the Sudan in the 1940s.

Space does not allow full discussion on the reasons given for FGM. Unfortunately, the victims of the practice (women) are also its strongest proponents. They can scarcely afford not to be. A poor uncircumcised woman may be stigmatized and not sought in marriage and has no prospect of support.

The urogynaecological implications or complications (all are more serious following the more serious type of FGM) are described below.

Immediate effects

These could involve acute urinary retention due to pain, damage to the urethra, or labial adhesions, resulting in urinary tract infections. These could also be caused by the use of unsterilized equipment, and the application of 'local' dressings, such as cow dung, etc.

Late effects

These may involve the following: chronic or recurrent urinary tract infection; dysuria consequent on scarring of the urethral meatus; calculus from urinary stasis plus infection. Another complication may be dyspareunia – sometimes when the husband is unable to effect penetration, he will try to enlarge the introitus with a knife which may damage the urethra or even the bladder. Problems arising at delivery include obstructed labour, with its consequences such as perinatal mortality and morbidity or even ruptured uterus or fistulae, either vesicovaginal or rectovaginal.

Management

Prevention involves recommending the abolition of FGM. This demands the education of men and women, all grades of health workers, and governments. The local community must acknowledge FGM as a dangerous and detrimental procedure and its members must be involved in any FGM eradication campaign. This will take time even among women themselves, because although 25% admitted to some complications due to circumcision, most requested recircumcision following delivery (Editorial 1983). Refashioning or re-infibulation of the original FGM in order 'to restore virginity' either in preparation for remarriage or to meet Allah resulted in severe haemorrhage in three patients, two of whom died (Khaled & Vause 1996). Treatment includes that for retention of urine, urinary tract infection and the prevention and treatment of calculi and strictures. Defibulation may be necessary in childhood for retention of urine and after marriage to allow consummation, or at delivery for outlet obstruction. Practitioners unaccustomed to dealing with delay in the second stage of labour because of circumcision, may find it strange to perform an 'anterior episiotomy' or even to perform in some patients decircumcision plus a perineotomy (McCaffrey et al 1995). The treatment of fistulae has already been discussed.

THE FUTURE

Our aim should be to promote health and fullness of life for all in the coming century. An integrated approach to preventative and curative health care for the individual and the community is required (Kelly 1992b). The local population should be actively involved in the formulation of health care activities, so that such care conforms with local needs, priorities, and resources. Everyone must have access to clean water, adequate food and housing, efficient sanitation and basic education. Training of the various health care workers at the appropriate level should be developed.

The introduction of trained traditional birth attendants (TTBAs) and ensuring their regular in-service training has resulted in a halving of the maternal mortality rate in a rural area of Nigeria (Brennan 1989; Ogar et al 1996). An encouraging side-effect, reflecting the acceptability of such training in the community was a tenfold increase in the uptake of childhood immunization programmes. Such interventions to reduce maternal mortality (obstructed labour was the main cause) will reduce the problems associated with ruptured uterus and obstetric fistulae (Fekadu et al 1997; Kelly et al 1998).

Adequate provision of health care workers and midwives may not be enough to prevent the tragic consequences of obstructed labour in countries with poor communications or transport. The construction of suitable roads in areas of difficult terrain may take some time, but will be necessary to enable patients in rural areas to be brought to centres where the necessary facilities exist for intravenous infusion or transfusion and appropriate operative delivery. In the meantime, the use of maternity waiting homes (Attat 1991, 1992, 1993, 1994; Poovan et al 1990) where 'at risk' women can reside during the latter months of pregnancy in close proximity to expert help, will reduce the number of women suffering from problems associated with obstructed labour.

Education is a key in the eradication of problems consequent on FGM, producing healthier mothers and babies, the prevention of exploitation of women, and the prevention and treatment of sexually transmitted diseases. Curing and preventing re-infection in schistosomiasis requires urine and stool surveys, chemotherapy, selective mollusciciding and modification of snail habitats.

Trainee health workers coming from the developing world to the West should receive the training in our society that best meets the needs of the developing country. Training in expensive high technology may be quite inappropriate. Experienced personnel from a developed society can provide valuable assistance, largely on a voluntary basis, in the developing countries. They may give a period of 2 years, or shorter periods in a locum capacity while the regular incumbents take well-earned leave. Those of us who have had the privilege of working in a developing society soon realize that we receive far more than we give.

The need for curative services will continue for a long time. Small units based on the models of the Addis Ababa Fistula Hospital and that of Dr Ann Ward in south-east Nigeria are probably the ideal for dealing with large numbers of patients suffering from vesicovaginal fistulae. Such units provide open access for patients, give an efficient service, train doctors and other health care workers and participate in audit and appropriate research (Kelly 1994). Part of the dedicated care required for treating fistulae can be provided by former patients who have been trained to perform duties normally carried out in a developed society by doctors and nurses (Kelly 1994). The main training of health care personnel in a developing country should be located in that country. The author has been involved in such training each year since 1969 in Ethiopia, and since 1985 in workshops, training local surgeons in fistula repair in parts of Africa where fistulae are prevalent – Ghana, Kenya, Somalia, Tanzania, Uganda and Zambia. Hopefully, as medical services and training evolve in such countries, fewer trainees will require to go abroad (Harrison et al 1995).

Internationally, attempts should be made to change policies which involve crippling debts and structured adjustment programmes. Imposing or increasing user fees for basic health care is one reason why maternal mortality and morbidity is not falling in the poorer countries of Africa – a caesarean section costs the equivalent of 9 months' average wage in Nigeria (Harrison 1996).

REFERENCES

Attat Hospital, Ethiopia, Annual Reports 1991–1995

Bergstrom S, Lublin H, Molin A 1994 Value of symphysiotomy and obstructed labour management and follow up of 31 cases. Gynaecologic and Obstetric Investigation 38: 31–35

Blandy J P, Badenoch D F, Fowler C G, Jenkins B J, Thomas N W M 1991 Early repair of iatrogenic injury to the ureter or bladder after gynecological surgery. Journal of Urology 146: 761–765

Borgstein E S, Broadhead R L 1994 Acquired rectovaginal fistula. Archives of Diseases in Childhood 71: 165–166

Brennan M 1989 Training traditional birth attendants. Post Graduate Doctor Africa 11: 16–18

Chopda N M, Desai D C, Sawant P D, Nanivadekar S A, Dave U R, Satarkar R P 1994 Rectal lymphogranuloma venereum in association with rectal adenocarcinoma. Indian Journal of Gastroenterology 13: 103–104

Evans J 1995 Sapping maternal health. Lancet 346: 1046

Faleimu B L, Ogunniyi S O, Makinde O O 1990 Rupture of gravid uterus in lfe-lfe, Nigeria. Tropical Doctor 20: 188–189

Fekadu S, Kelly J, Lancashire R, Poovan P, Redito A 1997 Ruptured uterus in Ethiopia. Lancet 349: 622

Gardeil F, Daly S, Turner M J 1994 Uterine rupture in pregnancy reviewed. European Journal of Obstetrics and Reproductive Biology 56: 107–110

Grosskurth H, Mosha F, Todd J 1995 Impact of improved treatment of sexually transmitted diseases on HIV infection in rural Tanzania: randomised controlled trial. Lancet 346: 530–536

Hamlin R J, Nicholson E C 1966 Experiences in the treatment of 600 vaginal fistulas and in the management of 80 labors which are followed by repair of these injuries. Ethiopian Medical Journal 4: 189–192

Hamlin R J, Nicholson E C 1969 Reconstruction of urethra totally destroyed in labour. British Medical Journal 4: 147–150

Harrison K A 1996 Poverty, deprivation and maternal health. In: Yearbook of the Royal College of Obstetricians and Gynaecologists. RCOG, London, pp. 33–44

Harrison N W, Eshleman J L, Ngugi P M 1995 Ethical issues in the developing world. British Journal of Urology 76, suppl 2: 93–96

Hyde G A, Sarbah S 1994 Acquired rectovaginal fistula in human immunodeficiency virus-positive children. Pediatrics 94: 940–941

Kelly J 1979 Vesico-vaginal fistulae. British Journal of Urology 51: 208–210

Kelly J 1992a Vesico-vaginal and recto-vaginal fistulae. Journal of the Royal Society of Medicine 85: 257–258

Kelly J 1992b Audit of health services in Gurage. Journal of Tropical Pediatrics 38: 206–207

Kelly J 1994 The Addis Ababa Fistula Hospital for poor women with childbirth injuries. In: Studd J (ed) Yearbook of the Royal College of Obstetricians and Gynaecologists. RCOG, London, pp. 2–6

Kelly J 1995 Obstetric fistulae. Contemporary Review Obstetrics Gynaecology 7: 156–159

Kelly J, Kwast B E 1993a Epidemiologic study of vesico-vaginal fistulae in Ethiopia. International Urogynecology Journal 4: 278–281

Kelly J, Kwast B E 1993b Obstetric vesico-vaginal fistulas: evaluation of failed repairs. International Urogynecology Journal 4: 271–273

Kelly J, Fekadu S, Lancashire R J, Poovan P, Redito A 1998 A follow-up of repair of ruptured uterus in Ethiopia. Journal of Obstetrics and Gynaecology 18(1): 50–52

Khaled K, Vause S 1996 Genital mutilation: a continued abuse. British Journal of Obstetrics and Gynaecology 103: 86–87

Korn A P, Landers D V 1995 Gynecologic disease in women infected with human immunodeficiency virus type I. Journal of Acquired Immune Deficiency Syndrome and Human Retrovirology 9 (4): 361–370

Kwan D T, Lowe F C 1995 Genitourinary manifestations of the acquired immunodeficiency syndrome. Urology 45: 13–27

Editorial: Female circumcision 1983 Lancet 1: 569

Lawson J 1978 The management of genito-urinary fistulae. Clinics in Obstetrics and Gynaecology 5: 209–236

Lemmer L B, Fripp P J 1994 Schistosomiasis and malignancy. South African Medical Journal 84: 211–215

McCaffrey M, Jankowska A, Gordon H 1995 Management of female genital mutilation: the Northwick Park Hospital experience. British Journal of Obstetrics and Gynaecology 102: 787–790

Maiman M, Fruchterrg R G, Clark M et al 1997 Cervical cancer as an AIDS-deficiency illness. Obstetrics and Gynecology 89: 76–80

Marianos A, Gilles M, Chuah J 1994 Ceftriaxone in the treatment of chronic donovanosis in central Australia. Genitourinary Medicine 70: 84–89

Martius H 1939 Vesico-genital and urethro-genital fistulas. In: Martius H, Newman Dorland W A (eds) Gynecologic Operations and their Topographic-anatomic Fundamentals. Debour, Chicago, pp. 353–399

Michelson E H 1993 Adam's rib awry? Women and schistosomiasis. Social Science and Medicine 37: 493 501

Nyangao Hospital, Tanzania, Annual Reports 1991, 1992

O'Farrell N 1995 Global eradication of donovanosis: an opportunity for limiting the spread of HIV-I infection. Genitourinary Medicine 71: 27–31

Ogar A M A, Umoh E S, Brennan M 1996. The effect of training traditional birth attendants on maternal mortality in area of Akwa Ibom State, Nigeria. Postgraduate Doctor Africa 18: 86–90

Poovan P, Kifle F, Kwast B E 1990 A maternity waiting home reduces obstetric catastrophes. World Health Forum 11: 440–445

Quigley M, Munguti K, Grosskurth H 1997 Sexual behaviour patterns and other risk factors for HIV infection in rural Tanzania: a case-control study. AIDS II: 237–248

Verkuyl D A A 1994 Repair of a recto-vaginal fistula with traction in a HIV positive patient. British Journal of Obstetrics and Gynaecology 101: 1088–1089

Verkuyl D A A 1995 Practising obstetrics and gynaecology in areas with a high prevalence of HIV infection. Lancet 346: 239–296

Wang Y, Hadley H R 1990 Non-delayed transvaginal repair of high lying vesico-vaginal fistula. Journal of Urology 144: 34–36

Zarate E 1955 Subcutaneous partial symphysiotomy. English edition, TICA, Buenos Aires

SECTION 3
CHAPTER

35 Psychological aspects of micturition disorders

ANDREW J MACAULAY

INTRODUCTION

The psychiatrist treats a number of serious psychiatric illnesses in which biological factors are particularly important (such as schizophrenia) and others in which the psychological and social dimensions are equally, or more, important. Thus, by training and clinical experience, the psychiatrist is attuned to considering the biological, psychological and social factors in each patient. The term 'psychosomatic medicine' is applied to physical disorders in which the psychological and social factors are perceived to play an important causal role.

Stress and life events

'Stress' is a term that can usefully be applied to a subjective feeling of dysphoria that is experienced by everyone from time to time when emotions become overwhelming.

The stress can be acute, such as a bereavement reaction, or it may be the suppressed frustration or hostility experienced with a chronic, unresolved marital problem. Thus, it has much to do with an inability to control personal circumstances, whether at work or in relationships.

'Life events' have been found to pre-date serious physical and psychological disease. As a result of a combination of diverse biological, social and personality factors, life events may precipitate schizophrenia in one patient and a myocardial infarction in another.

Patients with genuine stress incontinence may have psychological problems as a consequence, or independently, of their physical disorder. However, research suggests that the incidence is no greater than in other physical disorders (Macaulay et al 1987). It is, therefore, appropriate that most of this chapter is concerned with detrusor instability and sensory urgency.

Psychotherapy

Whilst the prescription of medication can appear reasonable and understandable, by contrast, psychotherapy can seem extremely mysterious, fanciful and on the fringes of conventional medical practice. However, in reality, most forms of psychotherapy fall into one of four types:

- Supportive psychotherapy
- Behavioural psychotherapy
- Cognitive psychotherapy
- Dynamic psychotherapy

Supportive psychotherapy

All clinicians practise supportive psychotherapy and it works by encouraging and supporting patients to use the coping skills they have. It does not attempt to bring about a fundamental change in personality or coping style, but can help the individual over a difficult patch (such as examination nerves, divorce, bereavement or serious physical illness).

Behavioural psychotherapy

The essence of behavioural psychotherapy is exposure to the feared object or situation. This can be a graded, stepwise, programme or by 'flooding' in which the individual stays in the feared situation until the panic has subsided. Behavioural psychotherapeutic techniques have been used in the treatment of phobias, marital and sexual problems.

Cognitive psychotherapy

Cognitive therapy attempts to help the patient recognize what may be 'false assumptions' and deal more appropriately and effectively with the situation. For example, a patient may experience a crippling social phobia and feel unable to walk into a room full of strangers. The therapist would seek to help the patient understand their thoughts about this situation and to recognize the 'false assumptions' such as, 'nobody will like me or want to talk to me', 'I am boring', or 'I wouldn't know where to start'.

Dynamic psychotherapy

Dynamic psychotherapy endeavours to uncover and resolve intrapsychic and relationship difficulties, and, as a consequence, result in change. For example, some individuals feel they have difficulty in making and sustaining relationships and it may be that this difficulty stems from their early childhood experiences. Within dynamic psychotherapy the patient is allowed to re-experience a range of emotions and thoughts and feelings which have their origin in earlier relationships, often with parental and sibling figures. The therapist allows a transference to develop. In this relationship, the patient treats the doctor as if he or she is the other person in the earlier relationship. By learning from the experience of the therapeutic relationship and through interpretation, the patient comes to a better understanding of the difficulties, why this may have arisen and how they might be able to change in the future.

Psychotherapy can be undertaken on a group basis and, indeed, there are some advantages. This is particularly so when there are difficulties in relationships.

LITERATURE REVIEW

Psychological factors and bladder function

There has been little published research on the relationship between the psyche and this particular area of the soma. Mosso & Pellicani (1882) found that strong emotion or the sound of running water led to detrusor contraction. Menninger (1941) suggested that, from a psychological standpoint, urination had many conscious and unconscious meanings, such as erotic and aggressive components. Thc importance of intrapsychic mechanisms was tested in an experimental setting by Straub et al (1949) who interviewed female patients during cystometry. When confronted with 'significant' psychodynamic sexual or aggressive issues, patients produced characteristic detrusor contractions.

This earlier work concentrated on the possible relationship between intrapsychic stress and bladder function. An alternative approach is to measure aspects of personality and neurotic symptomatology.

Jeffcoate & Francis (1966) gained a clinical impression that patients with urgency incontinence were anxious and introspective. Two studies (Rees & Farhoumand 1977; Stone & Judd 1978) have shown a relationship between detrusor instability and hysterical personality traits. This is not a consistent finding: Freeman et al (1985) did not find increased hysterical personality traits in their study of detrusor instability (DI). In a small study, Crisp & Sutherst (1984) found that those with DI and sensory urgency (SU) were significantly more anxious and neurotic. In a clinic survey on 211 patients, Macaulay et al (1987) found that approximately one quarter of the sample considered that their symptoms made life not worth living. This group of patients, regardless of diagnosis, were as anxious, depressed and phobic as psychiatric in-patients.

Although not life-threatening, chronic urinary symptoms may become incorporated into the patient's lifestyle and personality and are a source of significant morbidity. Patients with detrusor instability or sensory urgency are abnormally anxious, suggesting that anxiety is an important correlate of urgency, frequency, nocturia and urge incontinence. The patients also have a depressed mood, as might be expected in any patient with a longstanding, distressing condition.

Frewen (1972, 1976, 1978, 1980 and 1982) maintained that DI is a psychosomatic condition. His evidence rested, firstly, in the ability to elicit a history of emotional trauma antedating the onset of the symptom. Secondly, the efficacy of psychological treatment was thought to support a significant psychogenic component in the genesis of DI and SU. The fact that patients with emotional or social problems had a poor response to his treatment provided him with further support for his views on aetiology. However, factors that may be therapeutic need not imply any causality. (Headaches are not caused by a paracetamol deficiency!)

Morrison at al (1991) found that 47.9% of patients suffering from bladder dysfunction reached 'caseness' on the general health questionnaire – demonstrating significant psychiatric morbidity; 11.6% of their sample had a 'major depressive illness'. Pierson et al (1985) studied 23 patients with DI who were compared with 23 matched patients with GSI. Patients with DI had significantly higher scores on the Holmes & Rahe (1967) life stress measure, as well as being more depressed.

The literature is consistent on the association of urodynamic problems and psychiatric disorder, especially for patients with DI and SU. In fact, there is only one study that fails to support this (Lagro-Janssen et al 1992), although the number of patients were small and the trend was in line with other research. Thus, there have been positive findings suggesting that emotional factors are important in the causation and maintenance of urinary symptoms. Two themes emerge: firstly, there are personality traits related to DI and SU; secondly, there is a suggestion that such patients use characteristic intrapsychic mechanisms.

Treatment

Over the years a number of empirical treatments have been advocated and this review will consider the psychological methods.

Bladder training

Jeffcoate & Francis (1966) are credited as being the first to describe bladder training as a treatment for urge incontinence, quoting a symptomatic cure rate of 55%.

In 1978 Frewen referred to the additional use of supportive therapy, anxiolytic and anticholinergic drugs, and reported an objective cure rate of 82.5% at 3 months. The results were not broken down on an in-patient versus out-patient basis, so it is difficult to justify the author's conclusion that out-patient treatment is rarely helpful. Of the seven failures, five had chronically ill husbands. Frewen considered that their intractable social problems made it impossible for them to be amenable to any form of treatment.

Jarvis & Millar (1980) reported broadly similar findings in their controlled trial of in-patient bladder training for 60 patients, concluding that bladder training was the treatment of choice for detrusor instability. In 1982 Jarvis reported a study in which 20 of 33 patients became continent. Elder & Stephenson (1980) treated 21 patients with Frewen's regime and also concluded that the majority were cured or improved.

None of the above studies control for any possible non-specific influence of nursing or other paramedical staff, such as informal advice giving or counselling. The purpose of admission to hospital, or the use of additional techniques such as anxiolytic medication, was rarely defined. However, such criticism cannot be applied to Pengelly & Booth (1980). In their out-patient treatment study, patients with DI were provided with a micturition chart and measuring jug. In addition, the therapist explained the possibility of an emotional aetiology. These two aspects, the documentation of symptoms and explanation of the rationale of the treatment, form the basis of bladder training as understood today. Nineteen out of 25 patients were cured or improved symptomatically and 11 out of 25 cured or improved on cystometry. These results probably represent the most realistic cure rate for DI patients treated with out-patient bladder training.

Frewen (1982 and 1984) presented the results of out-patient bladder training, and quotes a cure rate of 86%. In his view, detrusor instability was caused by the patient's abnormal urinary symptom, and suggests that patients with SU go on to develop DI if the symptoms persist. Holmes et al (1983) reviewed 56 patients 1–5 years after in-patient bladder training. There was an overall 3-year response rate of 50%. Those with SU responded well to bladder training: 94% improved and of these only 6% relapsed. For those with idiopathic DI, the response rate was 90%

and the relapse rate 44%. There was a 55% response rate in patients with congenital or arteriosclerotic DI but all relapsed. Holmes concluded that patients with objectively stable bladders and the urge syndrome responded well to bladder training. These results highlight important differences between DI and SU. Three years is a good follow-up period. It would be interesting to know if at times of emotional stress and personal crisis their symptoms would return. Long-term follow-up is always difficult to undertake for very real practical reasons.

Hypnosis

Hypnotherapy has been used with success by Freeman & Baxby (1982). In this trial, 50 patients with detrusor instability underwent 12 sessions of hypnosis. The treatment consisted of induction of the hypnotic state, relaxation, ego strengthening and suggestions regarding symptom removal. Patients were instructed to practise daily at home using a prerecorded tape. At the end of the trial 29 patients were symptom-free, 14 improved and 7 were unchanged. This study also showed that hypnosis improved bladder function: 3 months after the end of the treatment 44 patients underwent cystometry and the objective measures obtained correlated positively with the reported symptomatic improvements. In addition to the hypnotic techniques described, the author (Freeman, 1985, personal communication) was aware that the patients also used the sessions to discuss personal stresses and worries.

Biofeedback

Cardozo et al (1978a) recruited patients who had failed to respond to other therapy. These were given an auditory signal which altered in tone in response to changes in bladder pressure as recorded by a bladder pressure catheter. Patients were asked to keep the tone low by whatever means possible. Using objective and subjective methods of assessment, 81% of the patients improved. These were good results but the procedure was time-consuming of staff and equipment.

Using the Hostility and Direction of Hostility Questionnaire (HDHQ) (Caine et al 1967), Cardozo et al (1978b) investigated the mental state of some of the patients who had taken part in the biofeedback trial. Those who improved or were cured scored a mean of 4.56, whereas those who were unchanged scored a mean of 11.8 (normal 0.5). Such patients might, perhaps, benefit from first attempting to correct the psychological mechanisms that led to abnormally high scores, before trying other behavioural treatments.

Psychotherapy

Hafner et al (1977) reported a study of patients with frequency, urgency and urge incontinence. They were divided into two groups on the basis of their neuroticism score on the Eysenck Personality Inventory (EPI) and Middlesex Hospital Questionnaire. All patients were treated with four to six sessions of autogenic training (a type of relaxation treatment), with the exception of the last four patients who received psychotherapy. Patients in the most neurotic group reported either a great or moderate improvement in urinary symptoms whilst the majority in the least neurotic group showed slight or no benefit. The authors suggested that this latter group of patients were denying or disclaiming their symptoms, citing as evidence the patients' biographical and medical histories. The authors did not record their measures of improvement, so it is difficult to draw any firm conclusions from this study.

Macaulay et al (1987) reported a randomized treatment trial on 50 patients with DI or SU. The psychotherapy group significantly improved on measures of urgency, incontinence and nocturia, though not on frequency. Bladder training was an effective treatment for frequency though there was little improvement in urgency or nocturia. Patients became less anxious and depressed. There was modest improvement in frequency of micturition for patients in the propantheline group. Thus, bladder training and psychotherapy were effective for different types of urinary symptoms.

Quality of life

It has come to light from prevalence studies that chronic urinary symptoms have a significant and often hidden effect on patients' lives. The mechanism is via interference with social relationships and restrictions imposed by incontinence and urinary frequency. Norton (1982) looked at the quality of life in operational terms such as ability to undertake domestic chores, social life, work relationships within the family and general well-being. Also included was a fear of odour and embarrassment as a cause of activity restriction. Patients are often embarrassed and unlikely to spontaneously volunteer how their urinary symptoms are affecting their lives. Wyman et al (1987) used an incontinence impact questionnaire and reported that a fifth of their sample had their social interactions moderately or severely interfered with by their symptoms. Norton et al (1988) found that over 60% avoided going away from home because of their symptoms. Sutherst (1979) reported that 48% of their sample reported sexual difficulties.

The data of Ouslander & Abelson (1990) suggests that the amount of leakage rather than the frequency of urine loss may have a greater negative psychosocial effect. However, Norton (1982) found that the degree of incontinence did not correlate with the degree of social disability. Wyman et al (1987) considered that the common association of urgency and frequency may be as significant as the incontinence itself. In general, being incontinent did not prevent most women from carrying out their normal activities and social relationships. However, there was a small group of women who did report moderate to severe psychosocial impact. Subjects with detrusor instability (DI) with or without sphincter incompetence appeared to perceive greater impairment than individuals with incompetence alone.

Wyman et al (1990) observed that 'there is no common method to measure psycho-social impact of urinary incontinence' and emphasize the need for the development of standardized research instruments. Research already presented shows that chronic urinary symptoms can have a dramatic and disabling long-term effect on the quality of life. It is also clear that it is important to appreciate that 'the experience of incontinence is unique to each individual and this should be considered in determining the most appropriate management strategy' (Wyman et al 1990).

Recently, several groups have attempted to produce appropriate quality of life scales, and these show promise for the future (for example, Jackson et al 1995; Kelleher et al 1995).

Summary

Patients with chronic urinary symptoms have characteristic personality traits, such as increased neuroticism scores, though not all studies agree on the type of profile.

Trials of psychological treatments seem promising, with the overall conclusion that patients with SU or idiopathic DI respond well. Regardless of the treatment offered, patients with gross psychological disturbances respond poorly.

PSYCHOLOGICAL ASPECTS OF CLINICAL MANAGEMENT

The 'psychological aspects' should naturally be an integral part of the investigation and treatment of patients with micturition disorders. Treatment will already have begun by taking a history and demonstrating a willingness to understand the problem. The history-taking will, of course, include questions of a psychological nature and it is often useful to have a few stock 'opening lines', such as 'I expect these difficulties have affected things at home'. Adolescent children are often a cause of anxiety and worry to their mothers. Marital disharmony is another area of current stress worthy of sensitive enquiry. A past history of early deprivation and childhood unhappiness, such as divorced alcoholic parents and sexual abuse can be important. It is surprising how often a termination of pregnancy is 'forgotten' and, when the matter is raised, it transpires that the patient's difficulties stem from such a time. Excessive alcohol intake may well account for some of the symptoms or, alternatively, it may be that the alcohol is being used as an anxiolytic.

Patients with genuine stress incontinence are likely to be offered physical treatments, should the severity of their symptoms warrant it. If this is the case, then they will need psychological support and encouragement. If the diagnosis is one of detrusor instability or sensory urgency, then it is likely that psychological approaches will be a mainstay of any treatment offered.

If the main complaint is frequency and the symptom appears to be habit disorder without any significant secondary gain operating, bladder training is likely to be successful. If it is urgency with, or without, incontinence, or nocturia, or if the interview suggests anxieties, distress or conflicts, then the therapeutic thrust should be more towards 'talking about the things that are worrying you'.

I believe that a combination of out-patient bladder training and psychotherapy appropriate to the patient's needs represents the best approach for patients with detrusor instability or sensory urgency.

Thus it can be seen that there are four aspects to treatment:

- Education and explanation about symptoms
- Bladder training
- A chance to talk about anxieties and worries (psychotherapy)
- Medication.

Education and explanation

Many patients value, and are reassured by, an explanation for their symptoms, whether it is in biological terms (a basic explanation of anatomy) or in psychological terms, perhaps even using an example (such as the common association of urgency and frequency prior to examinations).

Bladder training

Bladder training has a chapter devoted to it. However, it is right to emphasize that it is most likely to be effective when it is a part of an overall treatment strategy.

Psychotherapy

The history may well have highlighted some serious emotional difficulties. The treatment package needs to offer an opportunity for psychotherapy. It is surprising how effective this can be, even if this only amounts to two or three sessions of perhaps half an hour's duration. Counselling and effective listening skills can be taught.

Medication

Given the realities of clinical life, the question of psychotropic medication usually arises. Antidepressants are useful for patients who, in addition to urinary symptoms, present with 'biological' symptoms of depression, such as early morning wakening, diurnal variation of mood and suicidal feelings. Some of the original tricyclic antidepressants have quite troublesome side-effects. Monoaminoxidase inhibitors are not used as first line antidepressants. It is useful to be acquainted with one or two antidepressants, for example, one which is sedative (e.g. trazodone 150 mg at night) and one that has no effect on arousal (e.g. lofepramine 70 mg b.d. or sertraline 50 mg daily). Unfortunately, all take time to lift mood, usually two to three weeks, although the sedative effect starts with the first tablet. The dosage should be built up gradually over a couple of weeks. Most patients stay on a maintenance dose for several months. Occasionally their physical symptoms dominate the patient's thoughts. Small doses of medication, such as sulpiride (200 mg b.d.) or trifluoperazine (2 mg b.d.), can help.

It is perfectly reasonable and proper that physicians and surgeons prescribe psychotropic medication and this is to be commended. Patients will find it easier to accept medication from the doctor they have seen for their urinary problems, rather than to be referred off to see the 'shrink' or 'the doctor who sees lunatics'.

Anxiolytics may help in the short-term, but are probably best avoided in patients who have difficulty in acknowledging emotional distress or conflict; it is just such patients who become 'addicted' to medication as a way of avoiding dealing with life's difficulties. For initial night insomnia a short-acting drug is usually recommended, whilst longer-acting drugs are used for the complaint of anxiety. However, drugs do not cure marital disharmony and abolishing the symptoms may deter patients from confronting and dealing with their difficulties.

Role of the psychiatrist

Rather than referring the occasional patient, it might prove more useful to involve the psychiatrist in discussion of difficult patients. Most urodynamic units have a continence nurse adviser who supervises bladder training already and may welcome the opportunity to discuss problem patients with a psychiatrist. Your hospital will have a psychology department and it is likely that they are able to offer skills in behavioural psychotherapy and might welcome an approach. Early discussion with the patient's general practitioner can offer novel therapeutic avenues as many have practice counsellors.

Summary

Psychological, social and biological factors are intimately enmeshed in the genesis and treatment of micturition disorders. This chapter has reviewed the literature concerning the aetiology and treatment. The suggested clinical management mirrors the research findings.

REFERENCES

Caine T M, Fould G A, Hope K 1967 Manual of the Hostility and Direction of Hostility Questionnaire. University of London Press, London

Cardozo L D, Stanton S L, Hafner J, Allen V 1978a Biofeedback in the treatment of detrusor instability. British Journal of Urology 50: 250–254

Cardozo L D, Abrams P D, Stanton S L, Feneley R C L 1978b Idiopathic bladder instability treated by biofeedback. British Journal of Urology 50: 521–523

Crisp A, Sutherst J 1984 Psychological factors in women with urinary incontinence. Proceedings of the International Continence Society/UDS 1: 174–176

Elder D D, Stephenson T P 1980 An assessment of the Frewen Regime in the treatment of detrusor dysfunction in females. British Journal of Urology 52: 467–471

Freeman R M, Baxby K 1982 Hypnotherapy for incontinence caused by the unstable detrusor. British Medical Journal 284: 1831–1834

Freeman R M, McPherson F M, Baxby K 1985 Psychological features of women with idiopathic detrusor instability. Urologia Internationalis 40: 257–259
Frewen W K 1972 Urgency incontinence. Review of 100 cases. Journal of Obstetrics and Gynaecology of the British Commonwealth 79: 77–79
Frewen W K 1976 Urgency incontinence. British Journal of Sexual Medicine 3: 21–24
Frewen W K 1978 An objective assessment of the unstable bladder of psychosomatic origin. British Journal of Urology 50: 246–249
Frewen W K 1980 The management of urgency and frequency of micturition. British Journal of Urology 52: 367–369
Frewen W K 1982 Bladder training in general practice. Practitioner 226: 1847–1849
Frewen W K 1984 The significance of the psychosomatic factor in urge incontinence. British Journal of Urology 56: 330
Hafner R J, Stanton S L, Guy J 1977 A psychiatric study of women with urgency and urgency incontinence. British Journal of Urology 40: 211–214
Holmes T H, Rahe R H 1967 The social readjustment rating scale. Journal of Psychosomatic Research 11: 213–218
Holmes D M, Stone A R, Bary P R, Richards C J, Stephenson T P 1983 Bladder training – 3 years on. British Journal of Urology 55: 660–664
Jackson S, Donovan J, Kent L, Abrams P 1995 The ICS-PBH study: preliminary findings concerning the reliability of the ICS-BPH questionnaire. Proceedings of the International Continence Society vol. 14: 536–537
Jarvis G J 1982 The management of urinary incontinence due to primary vesical sensory urgency by bladder drill. British Journal of Urology 54: 374–376
Jarvis G J, Millar D R 1980 Controlled trial of bladder drill for detrusor instability. British Medical Journal 281: 1322–1323
Jeffcoate T N A, Francis W J A 1966 Urgency incontinence in the female. American Journal of Obstetrics and Gynecology 94: 604–618
Kelleher V, Salvatore S, Cardozo L D, Yip A, Kelleher C J 1995 The importance of urinary symptoms and urodynamic parameters in quality of life assessment. Proceeding of the International Continence Society vol. 14, no.5, pp 540–542.
Lagro-Janssen A L, Debruyne F M, Van Weel C et al 1992 Psychological aspects of female urinary incontinence in general practice. British Journal of Urology 70: 499–502
Macaulay A J, Stanton S L, Stern R S, Holmes D M 1987 Micturition and the mind: psychological factors in the aetiology and treatment of urinary disorders in women. British Medical Journal 294: 540–543
Menninger K A 1941 Some observations on the psychological factors in urination and genito-urinary afflictions. Psychoanalytical Review 28: 117–129
Morrison M et al 1991 Psychiatric aspects of female incontinence. International Urogynecology Journal 2: 69–72
Mosso A, Pellicani P 1882 Sur les fonctions de la bessie. Archives Italiennes de Biologie 1: 97–128
Norton C 1982 The effects of urinary incontinence in women. International Rehabilitative Medicine 4(1): 9–14
Norton P A, MacDonald L D, Sedgwick P M, Stanton S L 1988 Distress and delay associated with urinary incontinence, frequency and urgency in women. British Medical Journal 297: 1187
Ouslander J G, Abelson S 1990 Perceptions of urinary incontinence among elderly outpatients. Gerontologist 30(3): 369–372
Pengelly A W, Booth C M, 1980 A prospective trial of bladder training as treatment for detrusor instability. British Journal of Urology 52: 463–466.
Pierson C A, Meyer C B, Ostergard D R 1985 Vesical instability, a stress related entity. Proceedings of the International Continence Society 1: 176–177
Rees D L P, Farhoumand N 1977 Psychiatric aspects of recurrent cystitis in women. British Journal of Urology 49: 651–658.
Stone C B, Judd G E 1978 Psychogenic aspects of urinary incontinence in women. Clinics in Obstetrics and Gynaecology 21(3): 807–815
Straub L R, Ripley H S, Wolf S 1949 Disturbances of bladder function associated with emotional states. Journal of the American Medical Association 141: 1139–1143
Sutherst J R 1979 Sexual dysfunction and urinary incontinence. British Journal of Obstentrics and Gynaecology 86: 387
Sutherst J R, Brown M, Shawer M 1981 Assessing the severity of urinary incontinence by weighing perineal pads. Lancet I: 1128–1130
Wyman J F, Harkins S W, Choi S C, Taylor J R, Fantl J A 1987 Psychosocial impact of urinary incontinence in women. Obstetrics and Gynecology 70: 378–381
Wyman J F, Harkins S W, Fantl J A 1990 Psychosocial impact of urinary incontinence in the community-dwelling population. Journal of the American Gynecology Society 38: 282–2

Nocturnal enuresis

JOHN HINDMARSH

INTRODUCTION

Gaining bladder control

Bladder control is one of the most difficult skills the child has to learn. The skill is usually attained by the age of 4 to 5 years and there are three components for this to be successful. Firstly, there must be a mature central nervous system able to interpret the afferent signals from the bladder and an efferent pathway to respond appropriately. Secondly, the bladder must be of sufficient capacity to be able to hold a night's output of urine and, thirdly there must be acquisition by the child of the circadian rhythm with respect to antidiuretic hormone (ADH).

Diurnal and bladder control

Bladder control during the daytime occurs in the second year of life when the child learns how to postpone micturition by inhibiting the detrusor motor cortex and by use of the striated muscle of the pelvic floor. The process is accelerated by the child's desire to remain dry, by parental encouragement and increase in bladder capacity. Once the child is reliably dry by day, night-time continence usually follows quickly.

Failure to gain bladder control

If this basic skill of bladder control has not been mastered by the age of 4 to 5, reliable bladder control becomes more difficult to achieve and parental understanding with professional support should be sought. This basic skill can easily be delayed by external stressful events, such as family breakup.

Patterns of enuresis and associated symptoms

Children with nocturnal incontinence beyond the age of 7 are termed enuretic, the condition affecting about 8% of all 7-year-olds. Persistence of nocturnal enuresis through childhood into adult life is more commonly associated with the diurnal symptoms of frequency, urgency and urge incontinence. Those adults who do eventually gain night control frequently become nocturic. These patients under stressful circumstances, either physical or mental, will have occasional episodes of nocturnal incontinence and also a tendency to diurnal urgency with urge incontinence due to persisting bladder instability which is never fully supressed in enuretics. Urogynaecologists need to be aware of this when investigating stress incontinent patients with a past history of enuresis with diurnal symptoms.

Enuresis – the symptom and the cause

Enuresis has become synonymous with bedwetting and is often regarded as a disease in its own right, rather than a symptom of many different causes, from maturational delay of the CNS through to neurological damage, psychiatric abnormalities and local bladder dysfunction. The symptom of enuresis requires qualification to differentiate those children or adults who have never gained bladder control from those who have gained bladder control and subsequently lost it. It is also important to differentiate between those who have nocturnal enuresis alone (monosymptomatic), and those who have associated diurnal symptoms.

Definition (Table 36.1)

Primary nocturnal enuresis is defined as a reflex act of micturition occurring at night in an individual who has failed to gain bladder control at the normal age in the absence of an organic pathology. A secondary or late onset enuretic is a child who has gained control at the normal age for at least a 6-month period and then become wet again. The use of the term 'nocturnal enuresis' for adults who wet the bed should be resisted as the incontinence will be as a result of a known organic pathology.

Table 36.1 Classification of enuresis.

Type	Duration
Primary with no diurnal symptoms (monosymptomatic)	Lifelong
Primary with diurnal symptoms	Lifelong
Recurrent enuresis	Enuresis persisted beyond 7 but control was gained but later lost
Late onset enuresis	Individual attained bladder control at normal age but later became enuretic

Normal development of bladder control

Under normal circumstances, the functional bladder capacity doubles between the age of 2.5 and 4 years at about 30 ml/year which is achieved in part by bladder growth and in part by cortical suppression of infantile reflexes. For voluntary control to occur, bladder sensation must be intact to carry the afferent impulses from the bladder mucosa, bladder muscle, pelvic sensory ganglia and pelvic floor to the cortex and for the brain to be mature enough to respond in an appropriate way by inhibiting detrusor motor activity until voiding is desired. Bladder inhibition is mainly achieved by contraction of the striated muscles of the distal sphincter complex. The maturational delay of neural pathways results in the child's inability to consciously or subconsciously suppress the voiding reflex. When the voiding reflex is activated the sensation of bladder contraction and the passage of urine may not produce a very powerful afferent bombardment, resulting in a failure of the appropriate inhibiting pathway to be activated, which results in failure of the bladder to enlarge.

FACTORS PREVENTING BLADDER CONTROL

Maturational delay

Maturational delay does not imply that the rate of myelination of the nerve fibres is slower than normal, but is a term used for slow learning of bladder control. EEG studies have demonstrated both failure of the central nervous system to respond to bladder fullness or contraction when asleep and failure of the central nervous system to inhibit the micturitional reflex.

Antidiuretic hormone (ADH)

Diurnal variation of ADH (arginine vasopressin) has been found to be absent in some primary enuretics, resulting in large volumes of urine being passed at night (nocturnal polyuria). In most children and young adults with primary enuresis, ADH can be found in the bloodstream at night, but essentially the diurnal rhythm is blunt. This results in the nocturnal output of urine being close to the daytime figure of 50 ml per hour instead of 20 ml per hour (Rittig et al 1995).

Genetic factors

Some factors adversely affecting the gaining of bladder control have been identified. Bakwin (1971) was the first to show that monozygotic twins are concordant for enuresis twice as frequently as dizygotic twins and suggested that the frequency in other members of the family is directly related to the closeness of the genetic relationship. The location of the gene has been found to be an autosomal dominant with 90% penetration.

Environmental factors

Other studies have demonstrated that environmental factors also influence the failing of gaining bladder control, such as overcrowding, the sharing of bedrooms and the children of semi-skilled and unskilled workers.

Maternal and birth factors

Other positive associations have been found between young mothers, low birth weight and second children. Children who were small for gestational age, who suffered asphyxia or showed neurological symptoms during the neonatal period, have a higher risk of developing both daytime and nighttime enuresis.

Neurological factors

In addition to this, enuretics have been found to have greater fine and gross motor clumsiness and perceptual dysfunction than controls, as well as slower growth rates than controls (Jarvelin 1989). Jarvelin suggests that there is a maturational delay alone accounting for nocturnal enuresis whereas there is genuine neurological damage to those who have enuresis and diurnal symptoms. Clinically there is a large overlap between the two groups (Lunsing et al 1991).

Emotional

Children who have gained bladder control and then some months or years later lose control frequently will be found to have an emotional cause for the wetting. This holds more strongly for girls than for boys. These patients represent only a small number of children with nocturnal enuresis.

Sleep

EEG studies

Deep sleep has been frequently quoted as a major associated cause of enuresis, but the evidence is not strong. Many children sleep deeply but do not wet the bed and EEG studies have confirmed that enuretic episodes are primarily related to the bladder filling and then emptying at a certain point but this point is not related to specific sleep stages. Further studies on sleep cystometry have demonstrated that enuresis occurs at the awake bladder capacity and is independent of the depth of sleep (Norgaard et al 1985).

Urodynamic studies

Some authorities have claimed that obstructive uropathy is an important component of enuresis; however it is difficult to interpret urodynamic data and cystoscope findings in young children and most authorities quote a figure of 1–3%.

Spontaneous remission (Fig. 36.1)

The recorded rate of spontaneous remission is approximately 16% per annum so that the by the age of 15 the incidence of nocturnal enuresis is approximately 1% of the population. Those individuals who reach adulthood and yet remain enuretic are the hardcore patients who have a high incidence of diurnal symptoms with severe cystometric bladder abnormality (small capacity unstable bladder). A third of all adult women with bladder instability have a previous history of nocturnal enuresis (Moore et al 1991).

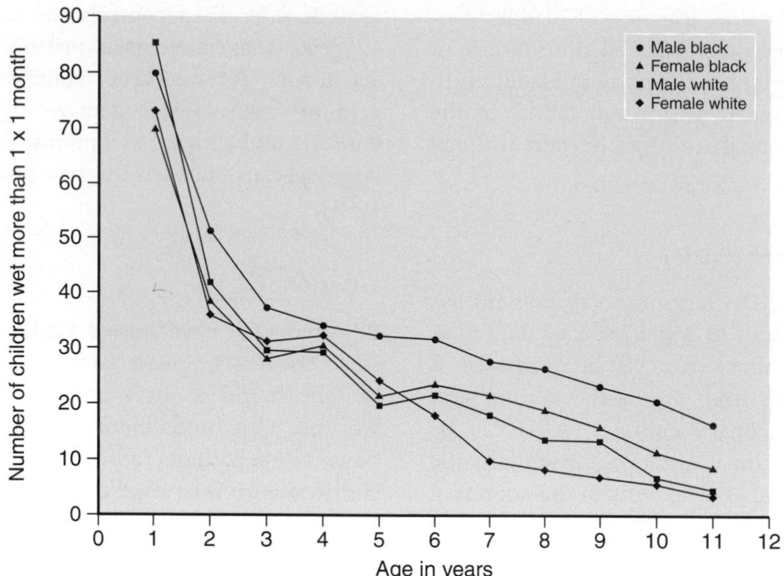

Fig. 36.1 The age of attaining bladder control. From Oppel et al (1968), with permission.

ACCESS TO PROFESSIONAL ADVICE

Parental and self-referral

Enuresis is an unusual condition in that it is the parent often distressed by the amount of washing that has to be done who seeks advice on behalf of the child. The primary care physician will refer the patient to a specific clinic dealing with enuresis for the patient and family to seek help and advice. If the enuresis persists to the age of 14, the child will often self-refer as she is anxious about wetting the bed when she goes away on camp or to stay with friends and relatives. Children who are still enuretic at the age of 16 become withdrawn and fearful of seeking advice because of the social stigma associated with bedwetting.

Advisory service

The Continence Advisory Service staffed by nurses experienced in dealing with enuretics is particularly valuable in dealing with these families and in particular in supporting the family during treatment. These nurses will have access to information on patient and parent support groups and guidelines on minimum standards of clinical practice.

Full history

Enuretic episodes

Whichever professional sees the patient first, it is important to record whether the enuresis is lifelong or of recent onset, how many nights per week or month the patient is wet, and the longest dry period, often only one or two weeks in total. Further information on the time of the night that the enuresis occurs, the number of nights per week and the particular day per week that the bed is wet and whether it is associated with menstruation, anxiety or bouts of heavy drinking should be noted. These will form the baseline from which the effects of any medical management can be gauged.

Daytime symptoms

Daytime symptoms should also be recorded, particularly those of frequency, urgency and urge incontinence which are present in a high percentage (70%) of adult enuretics although the incidence is less so in children. Enuretics restrict their fluid intake so that an apparent normal pattern of voiding will occur. It is important to ask about the effect of large fluid loads in these patients. Urgency may be induced by the sound of running water, anxiety or on reaching the front door, known as 'latch-key' incontinence. The presence of diurnal symptoms unfortunately has an adverse effect on the patient's chances of gaining reliable bladder control lifelong.

Associated symptoms

The stream of an enuretic patient is classically short and fast in the older patient with diurnal symptoms, and thus a history of hesitancy and poor stream should alert the clinician to an urethral disorder. Women patients with large, floppy bladders and nocturnal enuresis will often void by abdominal strain due to detrusor hypotonia.

Family history

A family history of enuresis can be found in 30% of children with primary enuresis. In addition, there is a high incidence of enuresis in those patients whose parents are of low social class and amongst second siblings of large families. Neurological abnormalities such as alteration in sensation or weakness of limbs in the older enuretic should be sought as it may be an early symptom of multiple sclerosis.

Factors causing enuresis

Factors that exacerbate and reduce the number of nights wet should be sought, as simply withholding or reducing these factors will help in the management. Tiredness, anxiety and premenstrual tension, when associated with excess fluid consumption, will increase the number of episodes of enuresis, whereas fluid restriction, staying away from home and relaxation are associated with less frequent episodes of wetting.

INVESTIGATIONS

Prepuberty

Children up to puberty with primary nocturnal enuresis do not require detailed investigation. However, a careful examination is mandatory to exclude evidence of spina bifida and a chronically distended bladder and examination of the external genitalia for meatal stenosis is necessary. A mid-stream urine test should always be performed; cystoscopy and IVU are unrewarding but X-rays of the lumbar spine and sacrum may reveal spina bifida occulta or an absent sacrum.

Postpuberty

Teenagers and young adults should be investigated fully after clinical examination as above; in addition the lower limbs and perianal area are examined for sensory loss and tone. The number of enuretics who have neurological damage to the bladder without stigmata of neurological disease is thought to be between 5 and 10%.

Post-childbirth

Local trauma following childbirth exacerbates the urgency experienced by women who have in the past been enuretic. Childbirth also predisposes to stress incontinence, resulting in a mixed picture of stress and urge incontinence.

Urine analysis

Mid-stream urine is sent for microscopy, culture and sensitivity and tested for specific gravity and glucose to exclude diabetes insipidus and mellitus. Enuretics with superimposed urinary tract infection have marked exacerbation of their urinary symptoms both by day and night.

Urodynamics

Urine flow rate

The enuretic urinary flow is very distinctive: it is of short duration, high peak flow and low volume. A small number have evidence of urethral narrowing characterized by a low peak flow and others with acontractile bladders void by abdominal strain. A postvoid bladder scan is performed to ensure that the bladder is empty; if not, this suggests an obstructed or neuropathic bladder.

Video urodynamics

Video urodynamics is the single most important investigation of bladder function which combines cystography with pressure studies, both during the filling and voiding phase of the micturition cycle. In teenagers and adults, the pressure lines are passed via the urethra rather than suprapubically as in the child. A high incidence of bladder instability has been identified using video cystometry in enuretic children and adults and, in those adults with diurnal symptoms, the incidence of bladder instability rises to about 80%. It is therefore important to enquire before submitting a patient to corrective surgery for stress incontinence if they had enuresis as children, as the instability is not reversible (Moore et al 1991).

Filling cystometry reveals the presence or absence of detrusor instability which is demonstrated as large phasic bladder contractions, capable of opening the bladder neck and producing an acute sense of urgency in the patient. The sensory pathways are tested by recording at the first sensation of fullness and at the point of urgency. The volume and the infused pressure at bladder capacity are important end points, as the bladder capacity in enuretics is lower than normal (350 ml) and the pressure higher (low compliance). Urgency due to detrusor contraction is associated with opening of the bladder neck and ballooning of the urethra due to voluntary contraction of the distal sphincter mechanism. During the voiding phase, the detrusor pressure may be normal but the flow rate high, but when the patient is commanded to interrupt the flow, the isometric pressure rise is very high. A small number of enuretics have urodynamic evidence of outflow obstruction but, if the urethral closure pressures are measured, the peak urethral pressure at the level of the distal sphincter mechanism will be very high when the patient is asked to inhibit detrusor contraction or to voluntarily grip the pelvic floor muscles. This is a result of repeated contraction of the distal sphincter mechanism when the bladder becomes unstable, to prevent urge leakage.

Electrophysiological studies of the urethra and anal sphincter mechanism by needle or ring electrodes confirm sensory deficiency of the posterior urethra and impairment of the bulbocavernosus reflexion some cases.

Cystoscopy under general anaesthetic

The urethra is calibrated and visualized to ensure that there is no meatal stenosis, bladder neck stenosis or urethral valves present to account for the enuresis. In the enuretic patient the proximal urethra and bladder neck are commonly inflamed in patients with urgency due to the high pressure being transmitted from the bladder to the urethra during unstable contractions. The bladder capacity under anaesthesia in children is normal but in adults it is low. After bladder filling the finding of submucosal punctate haemorrhages throughout the bladder is typical when the bladder is distended beyond its functional capacity. Mild to severe trabeculation of the bladder is a feature of enuretics with proven bladder instability, particularly in men whose bladder contracts against the closed distal sphincter mechanism to prevent leakage. Cystoscopy can be rewarding in certain enuretics as it seems to stimulate the afferent pathways or dilate the urethra, altering the sensation and urethral resistance to flow.

TREATMENT (Fig. 36.2)

Bladder training

The aim of bladder training is to enlarge the bladder capacity by subconsciously increasing the sensory awareness of bladder filling and to reduce the depth of sleep so that the bladder can accommodate a night's output of urine. It is important that the nurse practitioner in charge of management is enthusiastic and follows the progress actively, involving both parent and child and rewarding the child for good progress.

Star charts

By encouraging children to fill in star charts, denoting dry versus wet nights, and encouraging the child to hold on to urine for longer and longer periods of time during the day, the best results are obtained. In paediatric studies, the use of star charts and enuresis alarms proved successful, with the child remaining

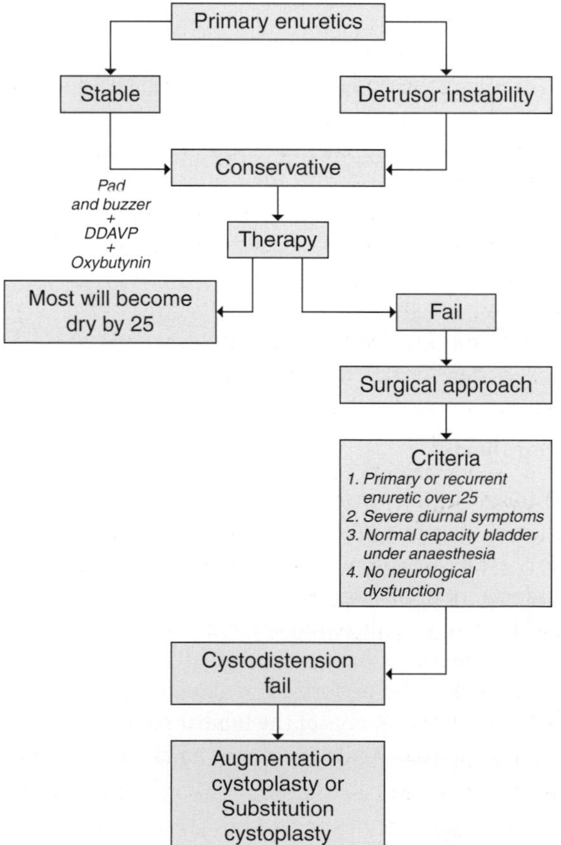

Fig. 36.2 Adult enuresis.

reliably dry in 40–50% of cases for up to a year (Devlin & O'Caithan 1990).

Modern alarms

Modern alarms that do not wake up the whole house are available in the form of vibration wrist bands. All alarms work on the principle that urine seeping onto a pad completes an electrical circuit triggering the alarm. It is thought that the effectiveness of this treatment is related to the increased central awareness of bladder and urethral afferents during sleep, with an appropriate increase in pelvic floor EMG and bladder inhibition. Evaluations of the different alarms have been undertaken and there has been little significant difference in their success rate. Parents preferred the Eastleigh Urilarm Delux which had fewer false alarms or breakdowns and is generally more durable than the alternatives. It must be emphasized that the results do depend heavily on the enthusiasm of the physician, the nurse practitioner and the parent. The follow-up visits by the nurse adviser are essential to correct any malfunction and particularly to support the parents. When a decision about which alarm to use has been made, each night when the child goes to bed the alarm is set, and when activated the child is awoken and the bed is changed. A record is kept of the number of wet nights versus dry nights and the apparatus is used for a minimum of 3 months. After several weeks of conditioning, the child is usually awake before micturition occurs; the majority of studies conducted to date have reported that 50% of children are dry at the end of 3–4 months with a relapse rate of only 20%.

Conditioning with the alarm is reported to have even better results where the individual is encouraged to increase fluid intake at night over time, so that the subconscious sensory awareness is overstimulated. This technique is known as over-learning, with reported results of 60% of children staying dry at one year. A small series of adults with enuresis have been treated by the alarms and noted a small beneficial effect. If the pad and bell is not successful after 3 months, it may be combined with desmopressin.

Desmopressin

The use of the antidiuretic hormone desmopressin (DDAVP) has been shown to be effective in children, both by nasal spray and in tablet form. Twenty-five per cent of children were reported reliably dry after cessation of DDAVP (Moffatt et al 1993). In adults, similarly controlled trials have demonstrated its efficacy in reducing the number of episodes of nocturnal incontinence. The reason for the effectiveness of this drug is due to an alteration in the diurnal rhythm of AVP production in the enuretic patient, the DDAVP supporting the nocturnal deficiency of AVP. The major indication for the use of this drug on its own in adults is to give them a reliably dry night when away from home, staying with friends or on holiday.

Pharmacology

There are no drugs capable of curing an 'enuretic child' at present; however, there are some capable of reducing the time it takes for spontaneous remission to occur. Imipramine has been widely used in the past and has been shown to be significantly better than placebo, although fears of cardiotoxic side-effects and the possibility of overdosing have resulted in pediatricians being resistant to prescribing it.

Anticholinergic drugs such as propantheline bromide and oxybutynin have been unsuccessful when tested against placebo in monosymptomatic enuresis but are of benefit in those with associated diurnal symptoms and in adults who have become nocturic.

Psychotherapy

This mode of therapy may be of value in late onset enuretics whose condition has a stronger association with emotional and behavioural disturbances than the primary enuretic. The effectiveness of psychotherapy is produced by improving the behaviour and emotions rather than on the episodes of incontinence. There is no evidence that psychotherapy has any place in the management of adult enuresis but it may be of value in patients who suddenly become incontinent at night without physical cause.

Surgical treatment

Surgery is contraindicated in patients who have noctural enuresis without diurnal symptoms, as spontaneous remission can be expected to occur in primary enuretics by the age of 25. The adult enuretic with associated diurnal symptoms resistant to medical treatment will have such severity of bladder dysfunction that the quality of their life is poor and they will frequently demand treatment. Patients should only be considered for surgery if they are over 20, have severe frequency, urgency and urge incontinence resistant to the currently available medical treatment and, thirdly, have urodynamically proven bladder instability. The aim of surgery is to reduce the detrusor motor activity (instability), reduce the bladder power and increase the functional bladder capacity, particularly at night. Women with severe diurnal symptoms with stable bladders do not respond so well to surgical techniques directed towards the bladder, probably because the primary cause is urethral instability.

Stretching the bladder and myotomy

Simple hydrostatic distension of the bladder up to pressures of 100 cm H_20 will improve the patient symptomatically, but only for a short time. This method works by stretching the bladder wall and weakening the bladder muscles. The use of a more prolonged distension using a balloon was popular in the 1980s, but the 2-year results demonstrated the majority of these patients' symptoms had returned.

There have been several methods described to reduce the power of the detrusor muscle directly by incision of the muscle by myotomy and/or by transecting the bladder above the ureterical orifices. A small percentage of patients do gain long-term benefit from these procedures; however, in the majority the symptoms return after 2 years.

Denervation procedures

A number of centres have reported their results on sacral neurectomy and to date the long-term results have proved disappointing, although more selective sacral neurectomies in the future may be more satisfactory.

Bladder enlarging procedures/diversion

If cystodistension and bladder myotomy/transection do not result in long-term improvement, either urinary diversion or augmentation can be undertaken. The 'clam cystoplasty' has been used extensively in such patients with overactive bladders with good effect. A patch of ileum is placed into the divided bladder over the vault which acts as a low pressure point, so that when the detrusor contracts the pressure remains low due to the patch. If this technique proves unsuccessful, a substitution cystoplasty, where the supratrigonal bladder muscle is removed, may be the only alternative available to urinary diversion.

CONCLUSION

Before a management policy can be adopted, the presence or absence of bladder instability and the integrity of the neural pathways are determined. Those patients with mild symptoms benefit from bladder drill, conditioning apparatus and pharmacotherapy. Patients unresponsive to these simple measures are frequently found to have severe symptoms and grossly unstable bladders. They may initially respond to cystodistension and bladder myotomy/transection but the only reliable longer term management of value is bladder augmentation by clam cystoplasty or substitution enterocystoplasty.

Women who were enuretic as children or young adults who then develop incontinence as adults after childbirth will not respond well to standard anti-incontinence procedures, as their instability will be exacerbated by the outlet resistance.

REFERENCES

Bakwin H 1971 Enuresis in twins. American Journal of Diseases of Children 121: 222–228

Devlin J B, O'Caithan C 1990 Predicting treatment outcomes in enuresis. American Journal of Diseases of Children 65: 1158–1161

Jarvelin M R 1989 Developmental history and neurological findings in enuretic children. Developmental Medicine and Child Neurology 31: 728–736

Lunsing R J, Hadders-Algra M, Touwen B C L, Huisjes H J 1991 Nocturnal enuresis and minor neurological dysfunction at 12 years: a follow up study. Developmental Medicine and Child Neurology 37: 439–445

Moffatt M E K, Harlos S, Kirshen A J, Burd L 1993 Desmopresin acetate and nocturnal enuresis: How much do we know? Paediatrics 92: 420–425

Moore H K, Richmond D H, Parys B T 1991 Sex distribution of adult idiopathic detrusor instability in relation to childhood bed wetting. British Journal of Urology 68: 479–482

Norgaard J P, Petersen E B, Djurhuus J C 1985 Diurnal antidiuretic hormone levels in enuretics. Journal of Urology 134: 1029–1031

Oppel W C, Harper P A, Rider R V 1968 The age of attaining bladder control. Paediatrics 42: 627–641

Rittig S, Mattiesen T B, Hunsballe J M, Pederson E B, Djurhuus J C 1995 Age related change in circadian control of urine output. Scandinavian Journal of Urology and Nephrology suppl. 173: 71–74

SECTION 3
CHAPTER

37

Sexual problems

FRAN READER

INTRODUCTION

Urological symptoms can be associated with sexual problems in three main ways:

1 They may be the direct cause of sexual difficulties where none previously existed.
2 They may be the apparent cause of a sexual problem: in this case the development of an organically based bladder problem may be conveniently used, consciously or unconsciously, to avoid further sexual contact when there is a pre-existing but unacknowledged sexual problem.
3 They may be the presenting symptom of underlying sexual conflict and the emotional stress that this can create.

Sexual problems, perhaps better defined as sexual presenting symptoms, can affect any phase of the sexual response cycle. There may be reduction in the frequency of sexual activity due to loss of desire or sexual avoidance. Alternatively, sexual arousal may be affected or women may present with anorgasmia. Other urological problems can lead to dyspareunia which may present as sexual avoidance. Sexual problems in the woman can affect the man's sexual responsiveness, resulting in such symptoms as loss of desire, premature ejaculation and partial or even complete erectile failure.

INCIDENCE

Sutherst (1979) evaluated 103 patients attending an incontinence clinic: 48 patients admitted that their urinary problems adversely affected their sexual life. In 36 patients, intercourse took place less frequently than before and in 12 patients it had ceased altogether.

Reasons given for this were dyspareunia, leakage of urine during intercourse, decreased libido, depression or simply embarrassment. More recently, Vierhout & Gianotten (1993) studied 245 women with urinary incontinence; of the 80% who were sexually active, 66 (34%) complained of incontinence during sexual activity with a strong negative effect on their sexual relationships.

In general, the incidence of such problems is likely to be underestimated. Many patients are too embarrassed to disclose problems of such an intimate nature. This supposition was supported by Hilton (1988), who assessed 400 consecutive women presenting to a gynaecological urology clinic. Only 2 of the 324 who were sexually active volunteered the specific complaint of incontinence during intercourse. On direct questioning, however, a further 77 (34%) admitted to this problem, which occurred on penetration in 53 women and during orgasm in 26. They all considered it to be a significant problem and welcomed the opportunity for discussion.

These studies highlight the need for inclusion of questions relating to the patient's sexuality in routine history taking. Information concerning the presence of a sexual problem and the more detailed information subsequently elicited may influence the direction of treatment for any given urological symptom.

HISTORY TAKING

Before considering more detailed aspects of history taking, it is important to acknowledge that sex can be a highly emotive subject for patients and doctors. Unfortunately, patients are highly sensitive to any signs of embarrassment or discomfort displayed by the doctor when sexual matters are raised. This can inhibit disclosure of a sexual problem or prevent its more detailed discussion. Initial denial of a problem should not always be accepted at face value. Observation of body language, tone of voice and slight hesitations in speech may provide valuable clues, in which case the line of questioning should be resumed later, perhaps in a different way and when greater rapport has been established.

If the patient acknowledges a sexual problem, direct referral to a trained sex therapist may be appropriate. Alternatively, if there is time, and the clinic doctor or nurse is comfortable with more detailed history taking and discussion, the following guidelines may help.

Guidelines for history taking

1. Ask open-ended questions to encourage open disclosure about the problem.
2. Avoid being judgemental about the patient's sexual behaviour, values or beliefs.
3. Use simple, non-technical language.
4. Elicit and accept the patient's feelings and thoughts associated with the problem.
5. Be sensitive to the patient's attitude to the problem, e.g. open-minded or inhibited.
6. Ensure you have time and privacy, and reassure about confidentiality.

The details of taking a sexual history have been covered by Hawton (1985), Woody (1992) and Webster (1997). Hawton recommended that history taking should lead to a formulation of the predisposing, precipitating and maintaining factors for the presenting sexual problems. Considering the history in sequence of childhood, adolescence, early adult and current experiences gives a framework for eliciting the necessary information.

Topics to cover in taking a sexual history

1. Childhood experiences should include exploration of the family, social and religious backgrounds especially relationships that formed attitudes towards sex, nudity, and open discussion about sexual matters.
2. Adolescent experiences should include feelings about the onset of menstruation and body changes and early experiences of sexual experimentation, whether these were pleasant or unpleasant and associated with guilt or anxiety.
3. Past relationships.
4. Current experiences
   - (a) Quality of the general relationship, previous levels of enjoyment of sexual activity with the current partner and the extent of disharmony caused by the sexual problem.
   - (b) The onset of the sexual problem, especially in relation to that of the urological symptoms.
   - (c) The patient's self-image and level of acceptance of her own sexuality.

UROLOGICAL SYMPTOMS AND SEXUAL PROBLEMS

Urological symptoms may cause sexual problems but careful history taking is required to exclude pre-existing sexual problems that have been exacerbated by the urological symptoms. In this case, the urinary symptoms are likely to increase the severity of the sexual problem and may well be used, consciously or unconsciously, as a convenient excuse for avoiding further sexual contact. Alternatively, the urological symptoms may present as a manifestation of the anxiety caused by a sexual problem. Sexual problems can undoubtedly create considerable emotional stress and the relationship between emotional stress and idiopathic detrusor instability has been well documented (Frewen 1978; Walters et al 1990; Vereeken 1989). When this is the only demonstrable abnormality of bladder dysfunction, the relationship between the two problems is more clear cut, but cause and effect may be more difficult to disentangle.

The main urological symptom likely to cause a sexual problem is incontinence during intercourse or on orgasm. Other symptoms such as urgency, frequency or dysuria may also be contributory. It is more likely that urological symptoms will be found to be the major cause rather than the effect of any sexual problems in the following circumstances:

1. Symptoms are caused by sphincter incompetence, neuropathic bladder disorders or non-neuropathic instability.
2. Medical or surgical intervention has proven unsuccessful.
3. The underlying lesion is untreatable (Walters et al 1990; Wheeler 1990).

Psychological findings

The psychological morbidity experienced by women with chronic urinary problems is considerable (Morrison et al 1991; Walters et al 1990; Wyman 1994). Morrison et al (1991) described a psychiatric survey of 169 female patients suffering from bladder dysfunction. Results showed that 47.9% had significant psychiatric morbidity, especially depression. Anxiety symptoms were more prevalent in those women with detrusor instability and sensory urgency. Studies have suggested that detrusor instability and sensory urgency are more frequently associated with psychological problems and sexual dysfunction than genuine stress incontinence (Vereeken 1989).

Incontinence during intercourse or orgasm

Little is known about the normal urodynamic responses which take place during penetration and orgasm, but Hilton (1988) found significant differences in urodynamic diagnoses within four groups of a total of 400 women studied. Not only were differences found between women who experienced incontinence in sexual situations and those who did not, or were sexually inactive, but also between those who experienced incontinence on penetration or during orgasm.

Of the 209 patients shown to have genuine stress incontinence, 48 experienced incontinence during intercourse, 37 (18%) on penetration and 11 (5%) on orgasm. Of the 57 women with detrusor instability, 11 had noted urinary leakage during intercourse, experienced by 2 (3%) only on penetration and by 9 (16%) during orgasm. These symptom distributions were significantly different from that seen in the 66 women in whom no urodynamic diagnosis was established, in whom only 5 had experienced leakage during intercourse, 3 on penetration and 2 on orgasm.

Khan and his colleagues (1988) used urodynamic investigations before and during masturbation, to study 3 women who complained of incontinence during orgasm. The studies showed incontinence to be due to either detrusor contraction or urethral relaxation, or a combination of both.

Although the problem may be found in patients with all urodynamic diagnoses, urinary incontinence during vaginal penetration is more likely with genuine stress incontinence, whereas those women with detrusor instability have a greater incidence of incontinence on orgasm.

Cystitis

The urge to pass urine during or immediately after intercourse is experienced by many women. Masters & Johnson (1966) associated this symptom with a rigid perineum and nulliparity, causing the posterior wall of the bladder to be irritated with repeated penile thrusting. Postcoital dysuria, commonly known as 'honeymoon cystitis' results, sometimes followed by a urinary tract infection. It is suggested that organisms are introduced into the bladder during intercourse and if they are not voided soon after, they multiply and cause infection (Dalton & Bergquist 1987).

Apart from 'honeymoon cystitis', many women experience acute urinary tract infections in association with sexual activity. Simple measures such as perineal hygiene and voiding after intercourse may solve the problem. Some women with recurrent cystitis after sex have a urethra that is closer to the vaginal opening than usual. If this anatomical variation is found then the female superior position may help avoid urethral trauma, as can a pillow under the woman's buttocks, to angle her pelvis upwards, if the male is in the superior position. For acute attacks, a high fluid intake combined with bicarbonate to alter the pH of the urine and a short course of antibiotics such as trimethoprim or nitrofurantoin are recommended. Trimethoprim 200 mg, taken prophylactically after sex may reduce episodes of cystitis.

Contraceptive diaphragm users were found in one study (Vessey et al 1987) to have a 2–3 times higher risk than among well-matched controls of referral to a hospital for urinary tract infections (see Ch. 29).

Postmenopausal atrophic vaginitis can also cause dysuria, urgency and urinary tract infection after coitus. The use of vaginal lubricants, such as Senselle or Replens, and topical or systemic oestrogen replacement therapy should be considered. Recurrent urinary tract infections associated with sexual activity can lead to sexual avoidance by the woman because of fear of pain and illness, and by the man because of the fear of damaging or contaminating his partner. In addition to taking the above physical measures, counselling may be required to help the couple adjust to this problem, especially where physical treatment has proven ineffective (Gibbons 1990; Webster 1993).

Enuresis

Enuresis is frequently associated with other personality disorders, notably difficulty in open expression of emotions. Since treatment for enuresis usually includes training in the control of body functions, this in itself can interfere detrimentally with sexual expression. The women is afraid to 'let go' and give up control in the way that is needed for the experience of full sexual arousal and orgasm. She may find her vulval area to be a source of embarrassment and disgust and therefore be reluctant to share her bed with a partner. In helping enuretic women with sexual problems, much patience is called for, since the concomitant personality difficulties can make treatment slow and at times discouraging. Vaginismus may be present, and specialist referral is usually necessary in such circumstances.

Prolapse

Prolapse may cause incontinence and make penetration difficult. It is important that the couple understand the nature of the anatomical changes that have occurred. Couple counselling may be appropriate pre- and postoperatively:

During surgery the use of vaginal trainers (dilators) can help to ensure vaginal capacity is adequate. The circumference of the partner's erect penis may be larger than the surgeon's two examining fingers, especially if the surgeon is female. Occasionally dyspareunia or loss of vaginal sensations occurs as a result of surgery, or as a result of the woman's psychological response to her altered body. General enquiry into the quality of the patient's sexual life is indicated at the postoperative follow-up. The daily use of vaginal trainers by the patient can be beneficial from 2 weeks postoperatively until her out-patient follow-up. This will help to maintain vaginal capacity and will help the woman to gain confidence that penetrative sex will be possible and pain-free. If penetrative sex has become mechanically difficult then non-penetrative forms of sexual expression, such as mutual masturbation or oral sex, can be explored as alternatives.

MANAGEMENT

It has been found that women who leak during penetration and have urodynamically proven genuine stress incontinence benefit from bladder neck surgery (Cardozo 1988; Vierhout & Gianotten 1993). A few women, however, develop this for the first time after surgery, even though the stress incontinence has been cured. Imipramine 50 mg taken during the evening has been found to help some, and women who have detrusor instability may respond to oxybutynin chloride 5 mg three times a day (Cardozo 1988). Benefit may also be gained from a bladder re-training programme or improving pelvic floor muscle tone with Kegel exercises or vaginal cones (Peattie et al 1988) (see also Chs 47 and 49). In addition to any physical measures implemented, full discussion of the patient's sexual difficulties should take place. Macaulay et al (1987) showed by a cost benefit analysis that in the management of detrusor instability psychotherapy and bladder training are less expensive than medical management, and recommended the increased availability of bladder training and psychotherapy. Vereeken's review (1989) highlighted the value of a multidisciplinary approach.

Where urological symptoms are not resolved by physical interventions, management consists largely with helping the couple to come to terms with their disability and learn how to maximize the quality of their sexual relationship.

The single most important measure that can be taken to deal with such a problem is to ensure that the patient and her partner talk openly and honestly with each other and share their feelings about the situation. It may be insufficient to tell the patient to go home and talk about it with her partner and therefore it is sometimes preferable to see the couple together and thus facilitate this communication. Often in the joint interview it becomes apparent that misunderstandings exist between the couple. For example, a woman incontinent during orgasm may think that her partner is far more disturbed by this than he actually is. Indeed, some men find this to be erotically stimulating but have previously been hesitant to acknowledge the fact.

Discussion of practical measures that can be taken to minimize the intrusion of the woman's symptoms into lovemaking is important, e.g. advising the woman to empty her bladder before starting sexual activity and to use a waterproof sheet on the bed. Such common-sense counselling need not be unduly time-consuming and may well be all that is necessary to bring about a substantial improvement in the quality of the patient's sexual life. However, some cases may need to be dealt with more fully by a trained sex therapist.

General principles of psychological treatment

Psychological factors that can underlie sexual problems are shown in Figure 37.1. Whatever the relationship of thc urological problem to the sexual problem, it will be found that lack of knowledge, acceptance of cultural myths and taboos and failure of effective communication between the couple (Stanley 1981a) can also play their part, either as a major cause of the problem or by acting to perpetuate it. Therefore, use of the broad therapeutic strategies of education, permission giving and teaching communication skills (Stanley 1981b), are helpful. In addition, once sexual failure has been experienced for whatever reason, the vicious circle of failure and fear of failure leading to further failure becomes established. Performance pressure and unrealistic concepts of sexual success feed into this vicious circle.

Education

Lack of knowledge about the basic anatomy and physiology of the sexual response (Masters & Johnson 1966) and misconceptions about the normality of certain sexual practices are widespread and therefore some degree of education is frequently beneficial. Many couples feel that they are unique and isolated in their difficulties, and this, together with lack of information of the anatomy and physiology of the physical response, gives rise to irrational and inhibiting fears and fantasies. Straightforward information using models or pictures can do much to reduce anxieties and facilitate communication. Using a hand-held mirror to help give the woman a guided tour of her external genitalia can be highly educational and also contains a strong element of permission giving (Stanley 1981b).

Permission giving

Whatever other reasons can be found for a couple experiencing a sexual problem, the cultural myths and taboos surrounding the topic of sex and its open discussion are frequently a contributing factor. Sensitively challenging myths and giving permission to change can be therapeutic. Although 'permission giving' may seem to be a somewhat abstract concept, it is occurring throughout the consultation spent discussing sexual matters, simply because the physician is listening and talking in a frank and open way, as

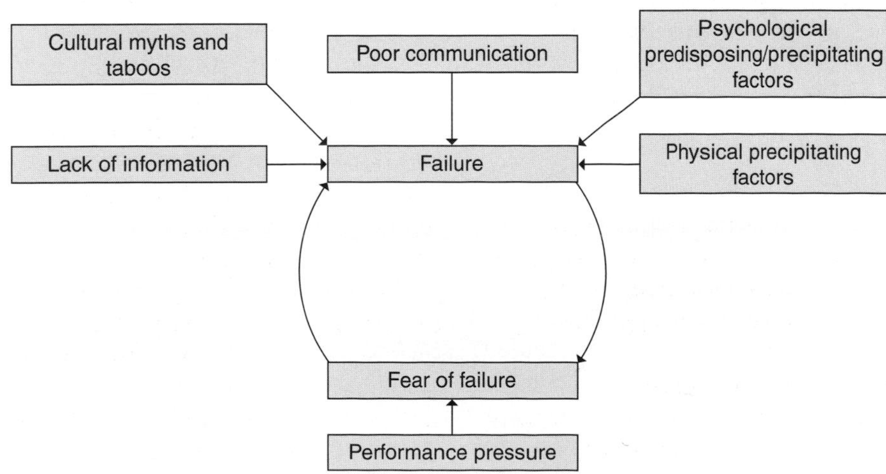

Fig. 37.1 Cycle of failure – fear of failure.

would occur during discussion of any other medical topic.

Teaching communication skills

Part of teaching communication skills is telling patients that, contrary to popular myth, they do need to let each other know what they like and dislike during lovemaking. A slightly more complex aspect of communication, which appears to be central to the development of intimacy, is the ability to share emotional feelings. It is particularly important to share the more negative ones in an honest and constructive way.

Important concepts for good communication

1 Understanding the difference between thoughts and feelings.
2 Recognition and acceptance of your own thoughts and feelings.
3 Active listening.
4 Recognition and acceptance of your partner's thoughts and feelings.
5 Accepting ownership of your feelings by using 'I feel' when expressing feelings.
6 Say what you mean and mean what you say.
7 When asserting 'no', separate the action you are saying 'no' to from the person.

Redefining success

One aspect of treatment involves helping couples define for themselves a broad and more realistic concept of 'normal' and 'successful' sex. A specific therapeutic measure that may help this process is the staircase concept (Fig. 37.2). A staircase of five steps is used as the basis for discussion. The ground and each rung of the staircase are defined in terms of the level of intensity of physical pleasure experienced, relating these to the sexual response cycle and the body changes occurring with increasing sexual arousal. The banister represents the phase of resolution after the sexual experience. By using the staircase as a framework for discussion, the couple can begin to review their ideas of what for them could constitute sexual 'success'.

Ideas to consider from the staircase concept

1 The pleasure they experience on any given step of the staircase can be valued in its own right and shared with their partner without necessarily progressing to higher steps every time.
2 It is possible to go up and down different steps on the staircase without having to dash to the top every time.
3 A mutually satisfying sexual experience need not demand that both partners progress up the staircase at the same pace, always arriving at the top together.
4 Orgasm is not necessarily essential for individual satisfaction.
5 Each individual is responsible for the level of the staircase they get to on each sexual experience. They can choose to get off the staircase and slide down the banister whenever they wish.

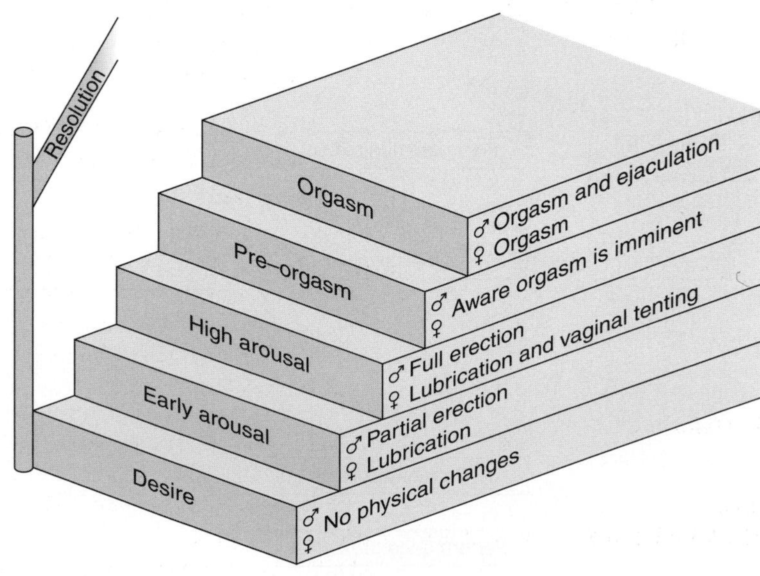

Fig. 37.2 Staircase concept.

6 What is important at the end of each sexual experience are the thoughts and emotions carried within each individual as they slide down the banister. Feelings of fulfilment and pleasure will reinforce the sexual activity as a positive experience and one that is worthwhile repeating.

Removing performance pressures

A common fantasy exists that to have good sex, an erect penis must penetrate a lubricated vagina and that it should result in mutual orgasm. It may seem that the staircase concept can go some way towards removing the pressure to 'perform'. In addition, a modification of the Masters & Johnson sensate focus programme can be used (Reader 1991). Sensate focus uses behavioural/cognitive strategies to remove performance pressure and open up communication about sexual likes and dislikes so that couples learn, from the insights gained, how to maximize the aspects that will enhance sexual pleasure and to avoid those that will sabotage sexual pleasure. Similar self-pleasuring exercises can be used to help women who attend for therapy on their own.

RESOURCES

Books for professionals

Human Sexuality and its Problems
Bancroft, Churchill Livingstone

An in-depth fully referenced text book and reference book for physical and psychological aspects of human sexuality.

Sex Therapy – A Practical Guide
Hawton, Oxford Medical Press

A concise guide for professionals which includes details of how to make an assessment to ensure that neither the physical nor the psychological aspects are overlooked.

Self-help books

The Relate Guide to Loving Relationships
Livintoff, Vermillion

An informative and easy-to-read book with suggested exercises to help couples work through their problems.

Living, Loving and Aging: Sexual and Personal Relationships in Later Life
Greengross and Greengross, Age Concern

A sensitively written and practical book dealing realistically with sexuality in later life, including all the possible physical problems that can affect sex, such as incontinence.

Medical suppliers

Owen Mumford Ltd – vaginal trainers
Brook Hill, Woodstock, Oxford, OX20 1TU
01993 812021

Colgate Medical – vaginal cones
Guildford Business Park, Middleton Road, Guildford, Surrey GU2 5LZ
01483 302222

Organizations

British Association for Sexual and Relationship Therapy (BASRT)
PO Box 13686, London SWZO 9ZH
020 8543 2707
Multidisciplinary organization of sex therapists trained through approved training schemes who work with couples and individuals with brief therapeutic approaches that integrate behavioural and cognitive with systemic and psychodynamic theories. Fully trained therapists are accredited by the organization and are also registered with the United Kingdom Council of Psychotherapists (UKCP).

RELATE
Herbert Gray College, Little Church Street, Rugby CV21 3AP
RELATE counsellors can extend their general couple training to specialize in psychosexual work. Their training is approved by BASRT.

Institute of Psychosexual Medicine
11 Chandos Street, London W1M 9DE
020 7580 0631
Doctors who have trained in psychosexual medicine through the Institute have attended seminar training that focuses on the doctor–patient relationship. The genital examination is used as an important window into the patient's perception of their sexuality and sexual problems.

SPOD – Association to aid sexual and personal relationships of people with a disability
286 Camden Road, London N7 0BJ
020 7607 8851/2
SPOD run a telephone helpline for patients and health professionals. They also have excellent leaflets.

REFERENCES

Cardozo L D 1988 Sex and the bladder. British Medical Journal 296: 579–588

Dalton J R, Bergquist E J 1987 Urinary tract infections. Crown Helm, London

Frewen W K 1978 An objective assessment of the unstable bladder of psychosomatic origin. British Journal of Urology 50: 246–249

Gibbons P 1990 Cystitis in the sexually active female. Nursing Times 86(2): 33–35

Hawton K 1985 Sex therapy: a practical guide. Oxford Medical Publications, Oxford

Hilton P 1988 Urinary incontinence during sexual intercourse: a common but rarely volunteered symptom. British Journal of Obstetrics and Gynaecology 50: 919–934

Khan Z, Bhola A, Starer P 1988 Urinary incontinence during orgasm. Urology 31(3): 279–282

Macaulay A J, Stern R S, Holmes D M, Stanton S L 1987 Micturition and the mind: Psychological factors in the aetiology and treatment of urinary symptoms in women. British Medical Journal 294: 540–543

Masters W J, Johnson V E 1966 Human Sexual Response. J & A Churchill, London

Morrison L M, Morrison M, Small D R et al 1991 Psychiatric aspects of female incontinence. The International Urogynaecology Journal 2: 69–72

Peattie A B, Plevnik S, Stanton S L 1988 Vaginal cones: a conservative method of treating genuine stress incontinence. British Journal of Obstetrics and Gynaecology 95: 1049–1053

Reader F 1991 Disorders of female sexuality. In: Studd J (ed) Progress in Obstetrics and Gynaecology. Churchill Livingstone, Edinburgh, pp. 303–317

Stanley E M G 1981a Non-organic causes of sexual problems. British Medical Journal 282: 1042–1048

Stanley E M G 1981b Principles of managing sexual problems. British Medical Journal 282: 1200–1202

Sutherst J R 1979 Sexual dysfunction and urinary incontinence. British Journal of Obstetrics and Gynaecology 86: 387–388

Vereeken R L 1989 Psychological and sexual aspects of different types of bladder dysfunction (Review). Psychotherapy and Psychosomatics 51 (3): 128–134

Vessey M P, Metcalfe M A, McPherson K, Yeats D 1987 Urinary tract infection in relation to diaphragm use and obesity. International Journal of Epidemiology 16: 1–4

Vierhout M E, Gianotten W L 1993 Unintended urine loss in women during sexual activities: An exploratory study. Nederlands Tijdschrift Voor Geneeskunde 137 (18): 913–916

Walters M D, Taylor S, Schoenfeld L S 1990 Psychosexual study of women with detrusor instability. Obstetrics and Gynaecology 75(1): 22–26

Webster D C 1993 Sex and interstitial cystitis: Explaining the pain and planning of self-care. Urologic Nursing 13(1): 4–11

Webster L 1997 Taking a sexual history. The Diplomate 4(4): 266–269

Wheeler V 1990 A new kind of loving? The effect of continence problems on sexuality. Professional Nurse 5(9): 492–496

Woody J D 1992 Treating sexual distress: integrative systems therapy. Sage Publications, Newbury Park

Wyman J F 1994 The psychiatric and emotional impact of pelvic floor dysfunction. Current Opinion in Obstetrics and Gynaecology 6 (4): 336–339

Lower intestinal tract disease

MICHAEL M HENRY AND ABDUL H SULTAN

Functional disorders of the anorectum are frequently the consequence of the same aetiopathological mechanisms as those giving rise to a disturbance of function within the genitourinary tract, and therefore a brief account can be justified in a text largely concerned with gynaecological disease. Patients frequently have symptoms referrable to both systems, suggesting that a combined approach to management should be offered whenever possible. In practice, as a consequence of ever-increasing degrees of specialization, this is rarely achieved.

PELVIC FLOOR AND ANORECTAL CONTINENCE (TABLE 38.1)

It is generally believed by proctologists that the pelvic floor plays a key role in the maintenance of anorectal continence in the normal state. If a pressure probe is inserted into the rectum and withdrawn caudally through the anal canal at centimetre intervals, a stepwise increase in pressure is recorded over an area approximately corresponding to the internal anal sphincter (IAS) (Fig. 38.1). Resting anal pressure has been shown to be largely a functional IAS contraction with a small contribution made by the external anal sphincter (EAS) (Bennett & Duthie 1964). If the subject is requested to contract the EAS maximally, the intra-anal pressure doubles. The role of the IAS and EAS in anorectal control continues to be disputed. Surgical division of the IAS rarely gives rise to any significant functional deficit. Internal sphincter loss in most patients usually leads to only a minor degree of incontinence, mostly restricted to loss of control of flatus and to liquid stool. On the other hand, some patients who develop severe faecal incontinence may

Table 38.1 Factors responsible for normal anorectal continence.

Anal sphincters
Pelvic floor
Sensory factors
Miscellaneous factors
Internal sphincter
Innervated hypogastric and sacral parasympathetic nerves
External sphincter
Innervated pudendal nerves
Anorectal angle (flap-valve)
Innervated from above by direct branches of the sacral plexus
Receptors in the pelvic floor
Rectosphincteric inhibitory reflex (sampling)
Valves of Houston
Anal cushions
Vectors acting in the cephalad direction

on physiological testing be found to have idiopathic IAS deficiency as the primary abnormality, with relative sparing of the EAS and pelvic floor muscles. Similarly, the true function of the EAS as a separate entity remains uncertain, since in most patients division of the muscle ring does not give rise to significant anorectal incontinence other than urgency and soiling in the presence of diarrhoea. However, some patients with neuropathic damage of EAS (see below), where the pelvic floor is relatively spared, may experience severe functional disturbance.

The puborectalis, because of its intimate relationship to the lower rectum and upper anal canal, is the most relevant of the levator muscles. In company with the remainder of the muscles which comprise the pelvic floor and the EAS, this muscle displays the unusual property (for skeletal muscle) of continuous resting electrical tone. This function is maintained without conscious effort and during sleep (Floyd & Walls 1953), and has been demonstrated to be the consequence of a spinal reflex (Parks et al 1962). Hence disruption of any limb of this reflex (e.g. in tabes dorsalis) will result in complete cessation of resting tone and anorectal incontinence.

Contraction of the puborectalis muscle in turn generates an angle between the lower rectum and upper anal canal – the anorectal angle (Fig. 38.2). There is again dispute concerning the true importance of this anatomical entity. Parks (1975) believed that the angle is of prime importance for the maintenance of normal control because it permits a flap-valve mechanism to operate. He believed that intra-abdominal pressure was conducted via the anterior rectal wall such that any increase (e.g. from coughing or sneezing) caused it to close over the top of the anal canal and effectively excluded the anus from the intrarectal contents. However, Bartolo (1986) failed to demonstrate by radiographic techniques any increase in the angle in a group of normal controls in whom intra-abdominal pressure was increased by performing the Valsalva manoeuvre. There is no question, however, that during a cough impulse there is a considerable recordable reflex increase in the pelvic floor muscle electrical activity (presumably to cause an increase in anorectal angulation), and on sigmoidoscopy the anterior rectal wall can be clearly seen moving downwards as it is forced on to the upper part of the anal canal.

The sensation of a full rectum, alerting the individual to the possibility of an impending need to defecate, is also an important element of normal continence. Sensory receptors have never been clearly identified within the wall or mucosa of the rectum itself, and sensation seems to be preserved in patients undergoing rectal excision and coloanal anastomosis (Lane & Parks 1977). These lines of evidence suggest that the requisite receptors probably reside within the pelvic floor muscles, which cradle and lie in intimate contact with the rectum. Evidence in favour is the demonstration of stretch receptors (Winkler 1958) and muscle spindles (Walls 1959) in these muscles.

An important contributing factor to sensation facilitating a locally mediated visceral reflex is

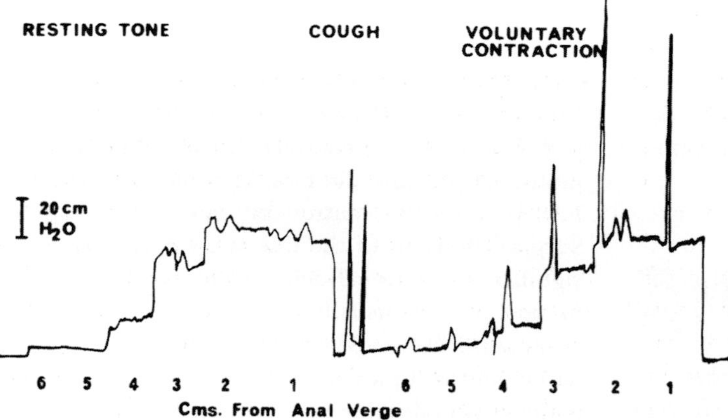

Fig. 38.1 A normal anal pressure profile. In the first section of the tracing the pressure probe has been inserted into the rectum and is withdrawn at centimetre intervals with the patient in the resting state and lying in the left lateral position. The internal sphincter is responsible for a zone of high pressure (maximum 60 cm H_2O) over the distal 4 cm. The pressure profile is repeated but on this occasion the patient is requested to contract the external anal sphincter. Intra-anal pressures are thereby increased during contraction by at least a factor of two.

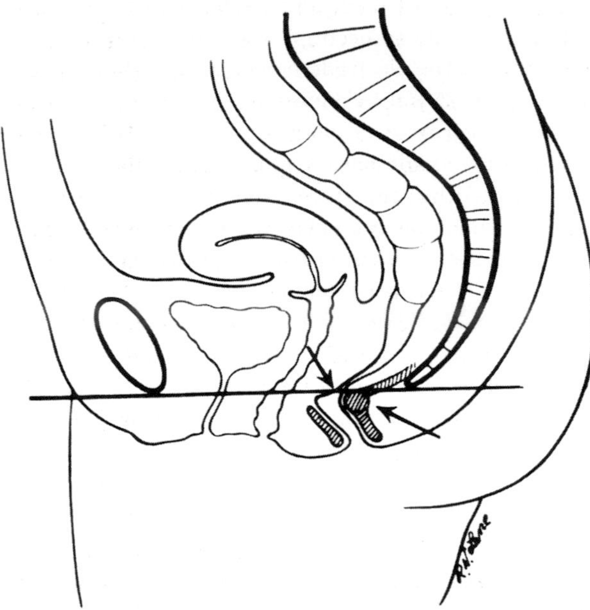

Fig. 38.2 The normal anorectal angle created by the forward pull of the puborectalis muscle (lower arrow). Abdominal pressure is conducted onto the anterior rectal wall (upper arrow) helping to prevent leakage of rectal contents when intra-abdominal pressure is raised (e.g. by coughing, lifting, etc).

referred to as the rectosphincteric inhibitory reflex. The reflex, first described by Gowers (1877) refers to inhibition of the internal anal sphincter as a consequence of rectal distension, e.g. by flatus or by faeces. The reflex can be shown to be independent of extrinsic neural sources and is abolished by rectal myotomy (Lubowski et al 1987), confirming that the reflexes are mediated via the intramural neural pathways. Under normal conditions the reflex acts to permit a small amount of rectal contents to enter the proximal anal canal in response to IAS relaxation. At the dentate line the contents make contact with the profuse sensory receptors which are concentrated at this level, and therefore permit discrimination between faeces and flatus. If faeces are perceived to be present, there is vigorous contraction of the EAS and the anal contents are propelled back to the rectum until the time is propitious for defecation to proceed. Sampling occurs at a regular and frequent basis during the daytime in all normal individuals.

There are certainly other factors that may play a part, and these have yet to be elucidated. For example, the role of haemorrhoids in providing cushions of tissue has never been properly explained, but minor degrees of incontinence are common after haemorrhoidectomy and this cannot be explained on the basis of damage to either of the sphincters.

DEFECATION

When the patient is ready to defecate complex physiological mechanisms are instituted which, like those responsible for continence, are incompletely understood. There is no dispute that, under normal circumstances, defecation is preceded by a reflex inhibition of electrical activity within the pelvic floor and EAS. This is turn facilitates defecation by causing increased obliquity of the anorectal angle. The passage of the faecal bolus is further assisted by reflex relaxation of the IAS in response to rectal distension. The actual vector forces responsible for evacuation probably arise from increased intra-abdominal pressure, rather than from peristaltic activity within the rectum itself. At the completion of the defecatory effort there is a rapid burst of electrical activity within the EAS and pelvic floor to restore the anorectal angle. At the same time, tone is regained within the IAS. Central mechanisms in the nervous control of defecation are ill understood. Urge incontinence is a feature of inflammatory conditions of the rectum and of spinal and cerebral disorders alike. Recent evidence has suggested that there is a fast-conducting direct pyramidal pathway to the sacral anterior horn cells supplying the pelvic floor and EAS; this suggests that the cortex plays an important role in the normal control of these muscles.

INVESTIGATION OF PELVIC FLOOR DISORDERS

Over recent years there has been a marked development in techniques designed to provide an objective assessment of pelvic floor function. This has been a direct consequence of an accelerating interest in the treatment of these conditions.

Manometry

This is the most endurable method, since it is simple, cheap and a relatively non-invasive means of assessing IAS and EAS function. Pressures can be recorded simply by using either water-filled balloons or a water-perfusion system. The latter is vulnerable because the intrusion of faecal contents may introduce artefact. More accurate measurement of complex systems are available, e.g. using transducers and radiotransmitters. However, these are generally only required in units where research commitments are predominant. Recording systems should then be connected via a suitable transducer to a device capable of producing a clear and preferably permanent tracing.

Manometry is currently the only practical method for assessing IAS function, and also the only means of testing the integrity of the rectosphincteric inhibitory reflex. Assessment of the EAS manometrically is less satisfactory, as it requires the patient's subjective ability to comprehend and cooperate during maximal voluntary contraction.

Electromyography

A more accurate approach to the assessment of EAS and pelvic floor function is gained by conventional, and more especially by single-fibre, electromyography (EMG). The former uses either surface electrodes or relatively broad-diameter needle electrodes, both of which record from a wide surface area, and is largely useful in identifying skeletal muscle. The identification of muscle and its anatomical position may be particularly relevant after muscle has been divided (e.g. following a third-degree perineal tear) providing the surgeon with precise anatomical detail of the position of the retracted EAS prior to its repair. In children, EMG exploration may be helpful in identifying the pelvic floor in rectal atresia prior to pull-through surgery.

To determine whether the skeletal muscle under investigation has undergone denervation (see below) the more sophisticated technique of single-fibre EMG must be used. With concentric needle electrodes individual muscle fibre action potentials cannot be recognized reliably within the motor unit action potential. Single muscle fibre action potentials can be recorded extracellularly by using an electrode whose recording surface consists of a central wire, which opens at the midshaft of the electrode in a small circular leading-off surface 25 μm in diameter (Fig. 38.3). In normal muscle, recordings of motor units are made in which one or two single muscle fibre action potentials are obtained within the uptake area of the electrode. In muscle which has been denervated and subsequently reinnervated, the number of components will be increased. An average of the positive components is taken from 20 different sites in the muscle and the figure is referred to as the fibre density for that muscle. The normal values obtained in the external anal sphincter are 1.3 in men, 1.5 in women (Jameson et al 1994a).

Nerve stimulation studies

Having established that denervation has occurred within the pelvic floor muscles it may be relevant to determine whether the anatomical site of the neurological damage is central (cauda equina) or peripheral (pudendal nerves).

The central component can be studied by means of transcutaneous lumbar spinal stimulation (Merton et al 1982). A single impulse of 800–1500 V decaying with a time constant of 50 ms is delivered through an electrode placed on the spinous process of L1 and repeated at L4. The evoked contraction associated with the pelvic floor response can be detected either by surface or by needle electrode. Pathology affecting the cauda equina will give rise to a more pronounced delay at L1 than at L4. If the neuronal damage results from peripheral disease, the delay at L1 and L4 will be increased to a similar degree (Snooks et al 1985a).

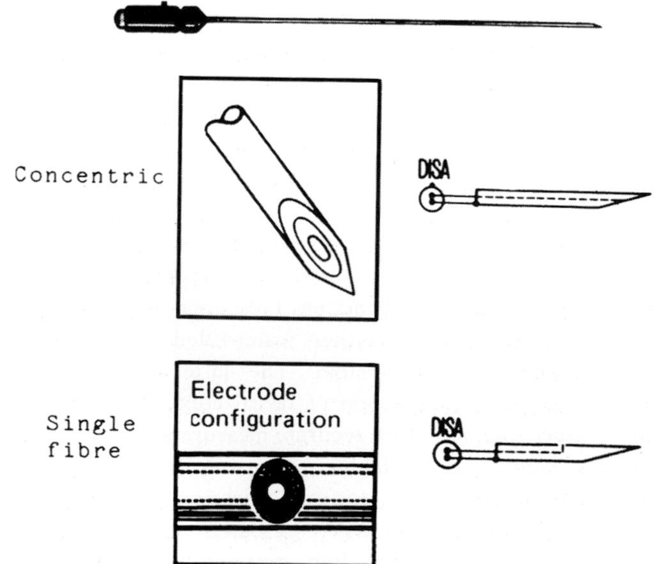

Fig. 38.3 Electrodes employed for electromyography. Upper electrode is of conventional concentric type with its recording surface at the tip. The lower electrode is of single-fibre type with its recording surface situated on the surface of its shank near the tip.

The peripheral component (i.e. the pudendal nerves) is tested by means of a disposable glove stimulating electrode, which comprises a glove consisting of two stimulating electrodes at the tip and two recording electrodes at the base. The glove is inserted into the rectum and, with the patient in the left lateral position, the tip is brought into contact with the pudendal nerve at the level of the ischial spine. The nerve is then stimulated electrically with a square-wave stimulus of 0.1 ms duration and 50 V amplitude, and the evoked response in the EAS is detected electrically by the surface recording electrodes situated at the base of the glove. The procedure is then repeated for the opposite side and the latency of the EAS muscle responses is measured on the paper printout of the EMG apparatus from the onset of the stimulus to the onset of the response. The normal value of the pudendal response is 1.9 ms and a latency of greater than 2.4 ms is considered abnormal.

It has recently been shown that pudendal motor latency can be measured vaginally with equal reproducibility as the transrectal route (Tetzschner et al 1997). Recording electrodes can also be mounted on to a Foley catheter and the urinary sphincter contraction response to direct stimulation of the pudendal nerve can be recorded. This is particularly relevant in the investigation of patients with stress incontinence of urine. In a recent study by Vernava et al (1993) it was found that the pudendal nerve terminal latency was much more accurate in determining evidence of denervation than the application of manometric techniques. However neurophysiologists maintain that a prolonged pudendal latency measurement is a poor measure of pudendal neuropathy as it only reflects conduction delay in the fast conducting fibres of the pudendal nerve. Even with destruction of 75% of the nerve fibres there is minimal prolongation of latency. A prolonged latency may reflect a neuropraxia (Sultan et al 1994c) and therefore not always equate to pudendal neuropathy; abnormal latency measurements should be interpreted with caution.

Sacral reflexes

Using the technique described by Bradley (1972), reflex anal contraction following stimulation of the bladder neck can be recorded, and these reflexes are found to be increased in neuropathic disorders affecting the pelvic floor as well as cauda equina disease. The bulbocavernosus reflex, the latent interval between stimulation of the bulbocavernosus muscle, the clitoris and the evoked response within the anal sphincter, has been investigated by Vernava et al (1993), and has been shown to be helpful in detecting motor neurone lesions.

Evoked potentials

Stimulation of the pudendal nerve, from either the anal sphincter or the bladder, can lead to potentials which, by computer averaging, can be distinguished by electrodes placed over the cerebral cortex. Recording of such evoked potentials could be delayed in the presence of spinal disorders, and this is therefore a method for detecting possible spinal disease. However, there is considerable variation in the latencies considered by different groups (Loening-Baucke & Reid 1990). In a study carried out at St Mark's Hospital of 13 patients and 16 healthy controls, reproducible evoked potentials could be recorded after anorectal stimulation only in a minority of subjects, and when recordable they showed a marked inter- and intrasubject variation (Speakman et al 1990).

Anal endosonography

Until the advent of anal ultrasound, structural defects of the internal sphincter could only be inferred indirectly by measuring the resting anal pressure and defects of the external anal sphincter by using the painful technique of needle EMG. The development of anal endosonography (Law & Bartram 1989) and subsequent scientific re-definition and validation of images (Sultan et al 1993a) has radically altered understanding of the pathogenesis of anal incontinence. Patients who had previously been believed to be suffering from pure neurogenic faecal incontinence were subsequently found to have anal sphincter defects identified by ultrasound. Consequently anal endosonography is now the gold standard investigation in the assessment of anal sphincter integrity.

In order to determine the incidence and relationship between nerve and muscle trauma during childbirth, Sultan et al (1993b) performed anal endosonography and neurophysiological tests in a prospective study of 202 women before and 150 women 6 weeks after delivery. Occult anal sphincter defects were identified in 35% of primiparous and 44% of multiparous women. Although only one third to a half of the women with sphincter defects were symptomatic, there was a strong correlation with defecatory symptoms. It is noteworthy that although pudendal nerve motor latency measurements were significantly prolonged at 6 weeks postpartum, this did not correlate with the development of defecatory symptoms and recovery appeared to take place in the majority by 6 months. Women having their first vaginal delivery were at greatest risk of sphincter damage and only 4% of multiparous women developed new sphincter damage. Forceps delivery was identified as the single independent factor associated with sphincter trauma (Fig. 38.4). Subsequent randomized studies have shown that vacuum extraction is less likely to inflict mechanical trauma to the anal sphincters (Sultan et al 1998). No new defects or symptoms were identified in women delivered by caesarean section although women who had a caesarean section following a long labour had prolonged pudendal nerve latencies. The high prevalence of defecatory symptoms and occult anal sphincter damage has also been demonstrated by another larger prospective study (Donnelly et al 1998a).

Recent studies have shown that despite primary repair of obstetric third/fourth degree tears, up to 50% of these women suffer anal incontinence. Furthermore, using anal endosonography it has been demonstrated that poor outcome is related to persistent sphincter defects in about 85% of women (Sultan et al 1994a, Poen et al 1998a). By contrast, secondary sphincter repair for the treatment of established fecal incontinence using the overlap technique of anterior sphincter repair is associated with a good outcome in 80% of patients (Engel et al 1994). Recently, Sultan et al (1999) demonstrated the feasibility of the overlap repair as a primary procedure ($n = 27$) for obstetric third and fourth degree tears (Fig. 38.5). They reported anal incontinence (flatus only) in 8% and persistent external sphincter defects in 15%. It now remains for a randomized study of end-to-end vs. overlap repair to be completed.

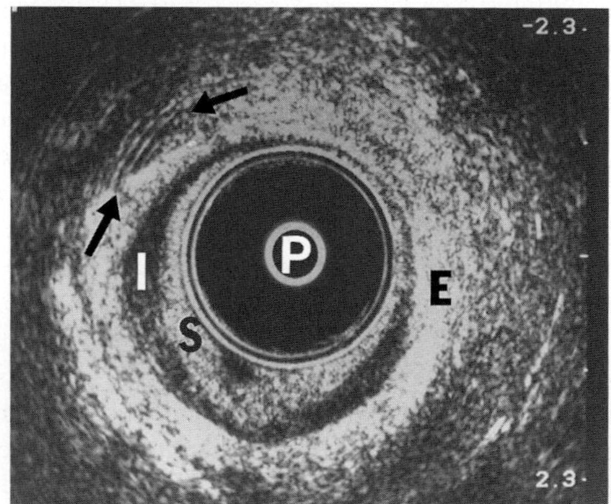

Fig. 38.4 Anal endosonographic image (B & K Medical, Gentofte, Denmark: 10 MHz probe) of a woman who became incontinent after a forceps delivery. P, probe in anal canal; S, submucosa; E, external anal sphincter; I, internal sphincter. The injury to the external sphincter (between arrows) was not recognized at delivery. The internal sphincter is also abnormally thin anteriorly indicative of injury. A haemorrhoid can be seen in the submucosal layer at the 6–7 o'clock position.

Imaging the undisturbed anal sphincter by transvaginal endosonography (Sultan et al 1994b) and transperineal ultrasound (Peschers et al 1997) is a more recent development. Transvaginal ultrasound can be complementary to anal endosonography particularly in the evaluation of perineal sepsis (Poen et al 1998b).

Evacuation proctography

This radiological technique, also known as a defecography, serves to demonstrate normal anatomy of the anorectum as well as disorders of rectal evacuation. The technique involves filling the rectum with a thick barium paste, seating the patient on a radiolucent commode and recording images during bowel evacuation. The vagina may be opacified with barium paste to improve anatomical orientation.

Evacuation proctography allows measurement of the anorectal angle and provides objective evidence of rectocele size and emptying. It also enables identification of enteroceles (herniation of small bowel into the rectovaginal space), rectal intussusception and mucosal prolapse, and may suggest the diagnosis of anismus otherwise known as spastic pelvic floor (Kelvin et al 1994). A rectocele of less than 2 cm in depth which rarely retains barium at the end of evacuation can be identified in 80% of asymptomatic women (Bartram et al 1988). Proctography may aid in differentiating between completely emptying rectoceles that may not cause defecatory symptoms from those that retain barium and are symptomatic. However neither the quantity of barium trapped nor the rate of evacuation bears a consistent relationship to defecatory symptoms (Halligan & Bartram 1995).

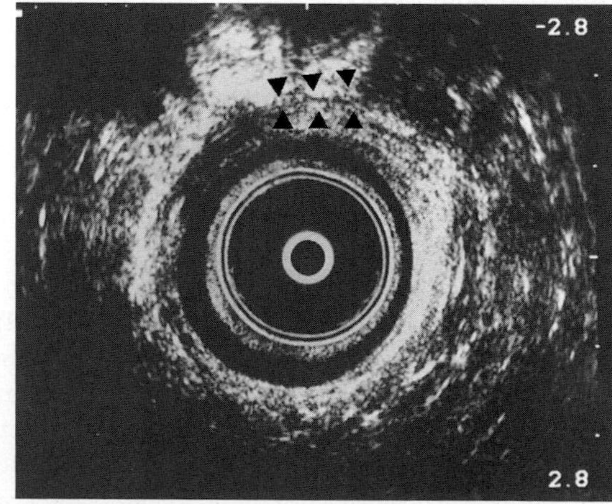

Fig. 38.5 Anal endosonographic image taken 6 weeks after a primary overlap anal sphincter repair immediately after an obstetric third degree tear. The arrows indicate the site where the ends of the external sphincter have been overlapped.

Proctography diagnoses other obstructive causes such as rectal intussusception, anismus and identifies coexistent enteroceles, 50% of which are missed on clinical assessment. However as barium paste is of a different consistency to the condensed faeces present in obstructed defecation, proctography may not be representative of *in vivo* pathophysiology. Furthermore, as the technique involves considerable radiation to the pelvis, it should be performed judiciously, particularly in women of childbearing age.

Scintigraphic defecography

This is a more accurate quantitative technique that measures the rate and degree of evacuation in addition to allowing measurement of the anorectal angle and assessment of pelvic floor descent. An artificial stool is made by adding water containing technetium-99m to oatmeal (Hutchinson et al 1993) or rehydrated potatoes. Radioactive markers are placed over the pubis, lumbosacral junction and coccyx and the artificial stool mixture is inserted into the rectum via a 50 ml syringe and lubricated tubing. The patient is then seated over a commode in front of a gamma camera and serial images are taken every 5 seconds. Although this technique involves a lower radiation dose than barium proctography, it lacks anatomical detail to define other pelvic floor structures and, like barium proctography, the correlation between symptoms and rectocele size is inconsistent.

Dynamic pelvic fluoroscopy

This technique, also known as four-contrast cystocolpodefecography, involves opacification of the bladder, vagina, small bowel and rectum (Brubaker & Heit 1993). Two hours before defecography, the patient ingests a barium sulfate solution. The bladder is filled with 200 ml of a water-soluble contrast via a catheter and thick barium paste is injected into the vagina. Barium paste is also instilled into the rectum via a caulking gun or a 50 ml nozzle-syringe until an urge to defecate occurs. Radio-opaque markers are placed on the perineum and anal verge. The patient is then seated upright on a radiolucent commode. Digital fluoroscopy minimizes radiation exposure. Images are then taken at rest, squeezing and straining and dynamic screening is performed during attempts to evacuate the bowel and bladder. As pelvic floor defects usually affect more than one compartment, pelvic fluoroscopy is useful both as a diagnostic tool and in the planning of appropriate surgery (Brubaker et al 1993). It is particularly useful in identifying coexisting enteroceles and sigmoidoceles (herniation of the sigmoid colon into the rectovaginal space). However, in some women widening of the rectovaginal space can be demonstrated during straining without contrast-filled small bowel. Simultaneous injection of contrast into the peritoneal cavity can differentiate between a peritoneocele and an enterocele (Bremmer et al 1995).

Magnetic resonance imaging (MRI)

In contrast to pelvic fluoroscopy, MRI can demonstrate uterovaginal prolapse and ballooning of the pelvic floor, thereby providing a more global picture of the pelvic floor and visceral relationships (Steiner et al 1998). However, pelvic fluoroscopy is more physiological as it is performed in the upright position and involves evacuation rather than straining. Recent advances with MRI in the upright position (Fielding et al 1996) and dynamic MR combined with colpocystoproctography (Lienemann et al 1997) are promising imaging techniques that will prove particularly useful in complex and recurrent prolapse.

PATHOPHYSIOLOGY OF FUNCTIONAL ANORECTAL DISEASE

Porter (1962), employing conventional EMG techniques, made the observation that many patients with rectal prolapse and faecal incontinence could be shown to have abnormal electrical activity of the pelvic floor. The explanation for these changes was clarified by histochemical studies of pelvic floor muscle biopsies in which features consistent with denervation were demonstrated by Parks et al (1977). That these muscles have been denervated in patients with rectal prolapse and anal incontinence was later confirmed by electrophysiological studies (Neil & Swash 1980). Application of nerve stimulation studies showed that the site of neuronal damage was peripheral, i.e. pudendal, in most patients (Snooks et al 1985a). Denervation has since also been demonstrated to have been an important feature in patients with constipation (Snooks et al 1985b), solitary rectal ulcer syndrome (Snooks et al 1985c), urinary incontinence (Snooks & Swash 1984) and the descending perineum syndrome (Henry et al 1982).

The source of denervation is almost certainly multifactorial and is still a subject for speculation. There seems to be no doubt that many patients develop pelvic floor failure as a consequence of traumatic childbirth (Snooks et al 1984). The innervation of the pelvic floor may be damaged by vaginal delivery, but it appears to be less damaged by caesarean section.

Damage is most prominent in multiparae, and correlates most strongly with a prolonged second stage of labour and with forceps delivery.

Pudendal nerve injury may also be the consequence of a peripheral neuropathy occurring in diabetes mellitus (Rogers et al 1988), or in direct injury from surgery or road traffic accident. Lower motor neurone lesions may result from disease affecting the cauda equina, but these are generally considered to be rare.

DISORDERS OF THE PELVIC FLOOR

Faecal incontinence

The consequences for the individual affected by anorectal incontinence are often serious, since such patients may perceive themselves to be in a state of social and professional isolation. At St Mark's Hospital, London, of those patients who presented for treatment the disorder appears to be most common in middle age and is eight times more common in women than in men.

Minor faecal incontinence is defined as the inadvertent passage of flatus or soiling in the presence of diarrhoea. This state is usually associated with poor internal anal sphincter function, which in turn is often the consequence of previous anal surgery (anal stretch, haemorrhoidectomy), or may accompany minor anal rectal disorders such as condylomata or second-degree haemorrhoids. Sometimes the condition may occur spontaneously, and this is associated with pharmacological disorders of the internal anal sphincter (Speakman et al 1993). Partial denervation of the pelvic floor and EAS may similarly give rise to lesser degrees of incontinence in which the deficit is only present when challenged by the presence of liquid stool.

These patients are not usually greatly restricted by this handicap, and their management is largely conservative. Anorectal pathology should be looked for on clinical examination and treated accordingly. Where impaction occurs normal function can frequently be readily restored by the use of aperients and rectal washouts. If the IAS alone is deficient, surgery is unlikely to benefit the patient and management usually consists of a combination of codeine phosphate (to constipate) and an irritant suppository to induce complete rectal evacuation.

Major faecal incontinence is defined as the inadvertent passage of formed stool on at least a twice-weekly basis. As discussed above, the majority of patients will be of middle age with a history of obstetric trauma which precedes the onset of incontinence by a period varying from several days to several decades. Sultan et al (1993b) found in a study of 202 consecutive women that 35% of primiparous women developed an anal sphincter defect demonstrated by ultrasonography during vaginal delivery (see above). None of the 23 women who underwent caesarean section developed a sphincter defect following delivery. Vaginal delivery resulted in significant prolongation of the pudendal nerve latency bilaterally in primiparous women (Sultan et al 1994c). In multiparous women (n = 32) six admitted to anal incontinence dating back to previous deliveries, and similarly the pudendal nerve latencies were significantly increased bilaterally following vaginal delivery. There was greater damage recorded on the left side rather than on the right, and the pudendal nerve latency was not altered in those women who were delivered by elective caesarean section. When the obstetric variables were analysed in detail it was found that both a heavy fetus and a long second stage of labour strongly correlated with the significant prolongation of pudendal latency. After the sixth decade the muscle denervates as a normal physiological response to ageing, and this contributes further to the loss of anal function and helps to explain why some patients fail to develop problems until later life. Previous trauma responsible for division of the anal sphincter ring (e.g. fracture of the bony pelvis, third degree perineal tear, anal fistula surgery or sexual assault) may be relevant, and if there is a history of incontinence associated with a history of perineal pain and/or disseminated neurological symptoms, a neurological cause should be considered.

Examination of patients with anorectal incontinence is customarily conducted with the patient in the left lateral position, having first examined the abdomen. On inspection, soiling of the perianal skin with faecal matter may be apparent and when the patient is requested to strain there may be perineal descent associated with genital and/or rectal prolapse. The anal canal itself may gape (if there is IAS deficiency), and on digital examination of the anus both resting tone (IAS and squeeze tone EAS) may be deficient. The anal reflex will be absent to clinical testing and there may be diminished sensation in the perianal skin.

Before embarking on treatment these patients should be investigated by anorectal physiology tests and, if a neurological or sensory cause is suspected, lumbar myelography should be included. All patients with rectal symptoms should undergo sigmoidoscopy and, where relevant, a barium enema to exclude malignancy. If there are urological symptoms urodynamics, including videocystourethrography, should be considered.

Treatment

By virtue of the degree of their disability these patients require energetic, and often surgical, treatment. Where there is complete rectal prolapse rectopexy is indicated. The majority of patients with prolapse regain near-normal anorectal continence if the prolapse is successfully controlled. In a small subgroup who remain incontinent, pelvic floor surgery can be considered as a secondary procedure.

Anal sphincter repair

Anal sphincter repair can be responsible for near-total recovery of function in 80% of patients, provided that there is no coincidental denervation of the muscle (Lauerberg et al 1988). Engel and colleagues (1994), however, found no evidence to suggest that a prolonged preoperative pudendal latency was necessarily related to a poor outcome for anal sphincter repair in a series of 55 patients from St Mark's Hospital, London. In this series, improvement in function was more closely related to the success in obtaining an anatomically intact external anal sphincter ring as judged by anal ultrasound examination.

Before surgery patients should be investigated physiologically to determine whether there is denervation, and also by anal ultrasound to locate the anatomical positions of the retracted ends of the EAS. The operation is usually performed with the patient in the lithotomy position, and some surgeons prefer to carry out a defunctioning colostomy to permit the repair to heal in a relatively uncontaminated environment. The fibrous scar filling the space between the retracted muscle is excised and the mucosa approximated with an absorbable suture. The muscle is then repaired by an overlapping technique using non-absorbable suture material (Fig. 38.6). The wound is left open to heal by secondary intention.

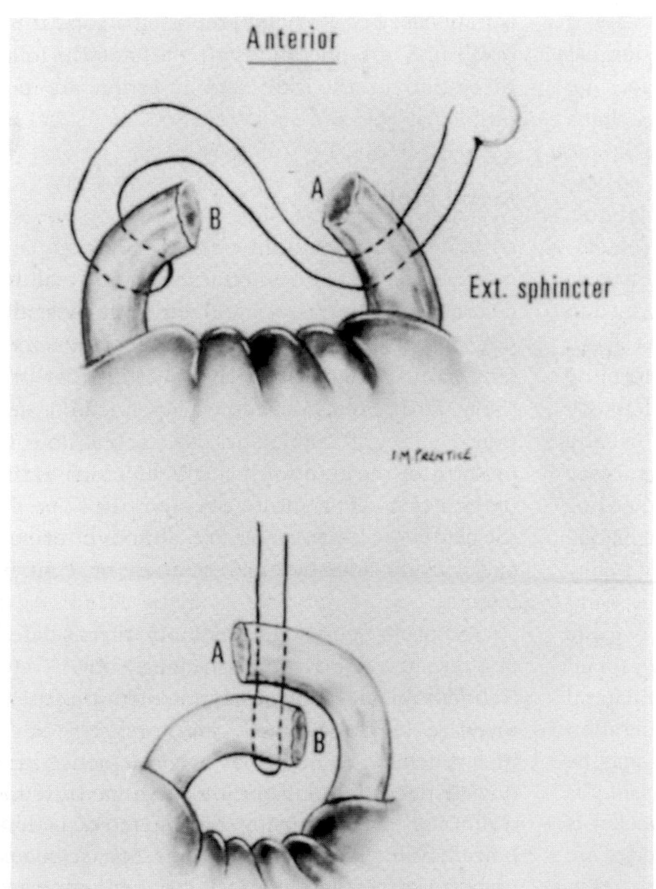

Fig. 38.6 External anal sphincter repair. The muscle ends are overlapped and sutured with a non-absorbable material.

Postanal repair

In the presence of established denervation of the pelvic floor, the preferred procedure in the UK is the operation devised by the late Sir Alan Parks (1975). The procedure can restore continence in about 80% of patients initially, but falls to about 60% after 3 years (Jameson et al 1994b). Parks originally believed that the anorectal angle could be restored, but there is little evidence to support this. It seems more likely that improved function is the consequence of increasing the length of the anal canal and of improving the mechanical advantage of the muscle fibres (Womack et al 1988).

A V-shaped incision is created just behind the anus and the space between the IAS and EAS dissected until Waldeyer's fascia is reached. The fascia has to be divided to obtain access to the pelvis. The levator muscles and EAS are then plicated sequentially using non-absorbable suture material. The skin is partially closed leaving a portion of the wound to heal by secondary intention (Henry & Porter 1988).

Neuromuscular stimulated gracilis transplant

In the USA attempts have been made to treat anal incontinence by transposing the tendon of the gracilis muscle around the anal canal to create a neosphincter (Pickerell et al 1954). The operation has severe limitations because the gracilis muscle does not possess tonic activity. This led to the discovery that a chronic constant stimulation of skeletal muscle can convert a fast twitch fatiguable muscle to a slow twitch muscle capable of contraction without fatigue. The first stimulated graciloplasty in which stimulating electrodes were inserted into the gracilis muscle with the tendon encircling the anus was performed in Maastricht in 1986 by Baeten et al (1995). At about the same time Williams et al (1991) were performing similar operations in London. Dynamic graciloplasty is now an accepted surgical procedure usually reserved for patients in whom conventional surgery has failed. The procedure may be done in either one or two stages. The first stage involves making a medial incision in the thigh and a second incision just below the knee. The tendon is detached at its insertion and delivered into the thigh wound. An incision is made on each side of the anus and the tendon is wrapped around the anus and secured to the contralateral ischial tuberosity. The second stage of the operation involves implantation of the stimulator which may be performed at a later date. A transverse incision is made in the anterior abdominal wall and a pocket is created for the stimulator. Stimulating electrodes are then placed adjacent to the gracilis nerve branches at the top of the thigh and then tunnelled through the stimulator. The stimulator is activated after 4–6 weeks to allow healing to take place. In order to allow defecation to occur the muscle needs to relax and therefore the stimulator must be switched off. Following dynamic graciloplasty, restoration of continence to both liquid and solid stool has been reported in up to 78% of patients (Baeten et al 1995; Geerdes et al 1996). The main complications appear to relate to technical problems with the muscle wrap and stimulator. Other problems include infection and difficulty in defecation, particularly in those who have had a long history of bowel evacuation problems. Perianal sepsis is a contraindication and therefore this procedure cannot be used in patients suffering from Crohn's disease. Although no unwanted effects have been demonstrated with an active stimulator during pregnancy, it is recommended that the stimulator be turned off (Vaisey et al 1998a).

Artificial bowel sphincter

The artificial bowel sphincter was introduced in 1996 (Wong et al 1996) following the introduction of the artificial urinary sphincter in 1972. Although long-term results are still awaited, early results are encouraging. Vaisey et al (1998b) reported a good functional result in 5 of 6 operations after 10 months follow-up. Ulceration of the skin and infection are potential problems.

Rectal prolapse

Although this condition is observed at any age, it is most common at the extremes of life. In children the disorder may be associated with mucoviscidosis; if not, it is usually a transient phenomenon requiring minimal treatment. There is no doubt that in adults the majority are associated with pelvic floor denervation (Neill et al 1981). The weak pelvic floor favours prolapse of the anterior rectal wall, which in turn initiates a rectorectal intussusception. In some patients the aetiology remains obscure, although malnutrition and chronic constipation seem to be contributing factors.

The prolapse may develop only during defecation, or alternatively may be permanently down, requiring frequent manual replacement. Sometimes patients are unaware of the prolapse and present with faecal incontinence, occurring as a consequence of pelvic floor denervation and the IAS damage caused by the trauma of the prolapsing four layers of oedematous bowel wall. Rarely, the prolapsing segment may undergo strangulation and subsequent rupture.

Treatment

Most patients require surgical treatment, since persistent prolapse causes cumulative damage to the anal sphincters and the condition itself causes great distress. The preferred procedure in the UK is rectopexy, an operation whereby the rectum is tethered to the sacrum by an inert implant (e.g. Mersilene). The operation can be performed traditionally by an open procedure or, more recently, by laparoscopic methods. For those patients at high anaesthetic risk, the procedure described by Delorme (1900) can be attempted. This is a perineal operation in which the redundant mucosa is excised and the underlying muscle plicated.

Descending perineum syndrome, perineal pain syndrome and solitary rectal ulcer syndrome

These uncommon conditions are discussed under a single heading because they are closely allied to each other and may be different manifestations of the same entity. The plane of the perineum normally lies above that of the bony outlet of the pelvis, both in the resting state and during straining. In patients with the descending perineum syndrome, however, the perineum balloons down well below the bony pelvis, particularly during straining (Henry et al 1982). The pelvic muscles are usually denervated and it is far from clear whether this is a primary or secondary event. In other words, it is possible that the pudendal nerves are stretched by elongation caused by the pelvic floor descent. Many patients with this syndrome develop anal incontinence. In the early stages there is prolapse of the anterior rectal wall mucosa into the anal canal. This has the effect of obstructing the passage of the faecal bolus during defecation, and forces the patient to strain excessively to achieve voiding. At the completion of the defecatory effort the redundant mucosa may remain in the anal canal, where it is perceived as retained faecal matter. The patient continues to strain fruitlessly in an effort to void what is in essence part of their own rectal wall.

Because the pudendal nerve is a mixed motor/sensory nerve perineal, descent may cause a constant perineal aching pain, which is provoked by prolonged standing and relieved by lying flat.

Perineal descent is also associated with a condition in which there is a shallow, usually solitary, discrete ulcer in the midrectum—solitary rectal ulcer syndrome. The ulcer is usually sited anteriorly or anterolaterally at a level 4–10 cm from the anal verge. These patients similarly strain excessively at defecation, and it is believed that the ulcer is traumatic in origin. The ulcer may be painful and give rise to substantial rectal bleeding.

Treatment

The treatment of these disorders is frequently unsatisfactory. In the early stages the anterior rectal mucosal prolapse may be treated by injection or by surgical excision, combined with advice on improvement in bowel function and, in particular, to avoid straining. Where solitary rectal ulcer syndrome develops in combination with radiological evidence of internal prolapse, rectopexy may prove beneficial (Halligan et al 1995).

Irritable bowel syndrome

Irritable bowel syndrome (IBS) is the second commonest functional gastrointestinal disorder in both primary and secondary care with a male to female ratio of 1:3. It affects about 20% of adults in the western world and is probably the commonest clinical problem seen by gastroenterologists (Harvey et al 1983).

The diagnosis of irritable bowel syndrome (IBS) is only made after other pathology has been excluded. The condition represents a spectrum of symptoms, any combination of which can present. There is no objective test by which the condition may be diagnosed and there is no recognizable underlying aetiopathology. There appears to be strong evidence to support the concept that there is a disorder of intestinal motility, but whether this is primary or secondary remains unresolved (Rogers et al 1989). Episodes of pain correlate closely with periods of elevated intraluminal pressure in the colon and small bowel.

In 1978, Manning et al described a list of symptoms likely to be present with IBS. Talley et al (1990) validated the diagnostic value of these symptoms and reported a high sensitivity but a suboptimal specificity. An international working party has now published a more specific and defined symptom criteria (Thompson et al 1989) for the diagnosis for IBS (Table 38.2).

The site of the abdominal pain can vary from patient to patient and within individual patients. There is usually a clear relationship between symptoms and periods of stress/anxiety. Alternation in bowel habit is almost always present; usually there are periods of constipation alternating with periods of diarrhoea.

However, IBS is also associated with extraintestinal symptoms suggestive of vasomotor instability,

Table 38.2 The 'Rome' diagnostic criteria for irritable bowel syndrome.

Continuous or recurrent symptoms for at least 3 months of:
- Abdominal pain relieved by defecation or associated with a change in frequency or consistency of stool
- Defacatory disturbance on at least a quarter of the time:
  - Frequency of bowel actions (>3/day or <3/week)
  - Consistency of stool (hard/loose/watery)
  - Passage of stool (straining/urgency/tenesmus)
  - Mucus passage
  - Abdominal distension

mood or behavioural abnormalities, fatigue, dyspareunia, bronchial hyperactivity and urinary symptoms and a history of sexual abuse. Approximately half the patients with IBS who seek medical assistance have psychological symptoms of depression and/or anxiety. Monga et al (1997) studied 16 premenopausal women with IBS and 16 controls. Although they found no relationship between oesophageal and bladder sensory thresholds they demonstrated that symptoms of urinary urgency, frequency and urodynamically proven detrusor instability occurred significantly more frequently in the IBS group (37.5% vs. 6.2%). This finding suggested that IBS is part of a generalized disorder of smooth muscle giving rise to an irritable bladder. Donnelly et al (1998b) studied 208 pregnant women prospectively before and after first childbirth and found an existing diagnosis of IBS in 11%. At 6 weeks postpartum women with IBS had a higher incidence of defecatory urgency (64% vs. 10%) and flatus incontinence (35% vs. 13%). Women with IBS also had an increased anal mucosal electrosensitivity of the upper anal canal before and after delivery but were not at an increased risk of sustaining mechanical sphincter disruption.

Treatment

As IBS is a chronic, relapsing, functional bowel disorder of unknown aetiology, no consistently successful treatment exists. The first line of management after a detailed history and examination to exclude an organic cause would be reassurance, education, dietary modification and behavioural therapy. Identification of food trigger factors (lactose, fructose, sorbitol and caffeine) may be identified by keeping a symptom and food diary for 2–4 weeks. However, management of IBS ultimately implies end-organ control of the most debilitating symptom. If diarrhoea is the main symptom then drugs such as loperamide, diphenoxylate and cholestyramine can be used. If constipation is the main symptom then advice on increasing dietary fibre should be given and osmotic laxatives, stool softeners or enemas could be used as a last resort. Abdominal bloating can be treated with anticholinergic agents of mebeverine. Central treatment with antidepressants appear not to work in non-depressed patients (Farthing 1995). Clinicians treating IBS need to be aware of drug side-effects namely, the tricyclic antidepressant imipramine slows intestinal transit whereas the serotonin reuptake inhibitor, paroxetine acclerates motility in the small intestine. Inadvertent success with central treatment can therefore be easily confused and equated with an affective disorder.

Constipation

A patient is defined as suffering from constipation if she complains of either infrequent defecation (less than two bowel actions per week) or difficult defecation (straining and difficulty in evacuating the rectum). Under normal conditions the first priority must be the exclusion of any obstructing lesions, such as carcinoma, hence sigmoidoscopy and barium enema should be regarded as mandatory in most patients. A classification of the important causes is given in Table 38.3.

Where no obvious cause can be identified the standard approach is to investigate colonic transit and pelvic floor function in an attempt to distinguish between patients with slow-transit constipation and those with pelvic floor dysfunction (anismus). It is not always possible to differentiate between the two

Table 38.3 Classification of constipation in adults.

No structural abnormality of anus, rectum or colon and no associated physical disorder
Faulty diet
Pregnancy
Old age
Idiopathic slow-transit constipation
Irritable bowel syndrome
Structural disease of anus, rectum or colon
Anal pain/stenosis
Colonic stricture
Aganglionosis
Megarectum/megacolon
Secondary to abnormality outside colon
Endocrine/metabolic
Hypothyroidism
Hypercalcaemia
Porphyria
Neurological
Sacral outflow/spinal cord disorders
Cerebral disorders
Systemic sclerosis and other connective tissue disorders
Psychological
Drug side-effects

conditions, since some patients will be found to have a combination of both.

Slow-transit constipation

This can be defined by the simple radiological technique described by Hinton and colleagues (1969). A capsule containing 20 radio-opaque solid markers is ingested and on the fifth day a plain abdominal X-ray is performed. Under normal circumstances 80% of the markers should have been voided; if more than 20% remain, the patient can be assumed to have delayed colonic transit.

This condition is prevalent in women at the time of the menarche and can be associated with severe degrees of constipation, with bowel function proving refractory to laxatives. The colon is of normal diameter, in distinction to primary megacolon, the latter being a functional disorder which occurs in men and women in equal numbers.

Pelvic floor dysfunction

Recently it has been clearly established that some patients have normal transit but are quite unable to empty a full rectum. This occurs in some patients because of increased electrical activity within the pelvic floor musculature during attempted defecation. The aetiology of this paradoxical contraction in the pelvic floor cannot be explained. In some patients it may be a behavioural abnormality which is the consequence of an abnormal pattern of defecation instituted from early childhood. In others the disorder is due to spasticity of the muscle secondary to upper motor neurone lesions; this is frequently observed in patients with multiple sclerosis, for example (Gill et al 1994).

Patients with denervation of the pelvic floor may similarly experience difficulty with defecation, which is aggravated by the presence of a rectocele. Patients with this disorder frequently need to insert a digit either into the anal canal or into the vagina to assist emptying of a full rectum. The diagnosis of pelvic floor dysfunction is usually made by evacuation proctography (Mahieu et al 1984). A barium paste is introduced into the rectum and cineradiography is performed while the patient attempts defecation. The films are studied for paradoxical puborectalis contraction and intrarectal intussusception. In the latter case obstructed defecation is the consequence of a prolapsing rectum, which may not necessarily be overt and hence cannot be diagnosed by any method other than by defecography.

Treatment of constipation

Under normal circumstances dietary adjustments and/or simple laxatives are adequate means of restoring normal bowel function where there is no underlying obstructive cause. In the severe forms of slow-transit constipation surgery may be indicated. It is now generally accepted that partial resection (e.g. sigmoid colectomy) leads to an early recurrence of symptoms. The treatment of choice is total colectomy and ileorectal anastomosis. This operation restores bowel function at the expense of causing diarrhoea. The abdominal pain these patients describe preoperatively often persists postoperatively, suggesting that the disorder is part of a generalized motility disorder affecting the whole length of the gut.

Patients with pelvic floor dysfunction pose a particular problem in management. Wherever possible, conservative measures to induce liquid stool (by laxatives) and to encourage rectal emptying by the use of irritant suppositories (e.g. glycerine) should be employed. Surgical excision of anterior prolapsing mucosa and repair of rectocoele has been reported as sucessfully controlling symptoms in up to 50% of patients (Janssen & Van Dijke 1994). Biofeedback techniques to encourage the patient to relax the pelvic floor during attempted defecation are time-consuming but have proved helpful in some cases (Turnbull & Ritvo 1992).

REFERENCES

Bartolo D C C 1986 Flap-valve theory of anorectal continence. British Journal of Surgery 73: 1012–1014

Bartram C I, Turnbull G K, Lennard-Jones J E 1988 Evacuation proctography: An investigation of rectal expulsion in 20 subjects without defecatory disturbance. Gastrointestinal Radiology 13: 72–80

Baeten C G, Geerdes B P, Adang E M M et al 1995 Anal dynamic graciloplasty in the treatment of intractible fecal incontinence. New England Journal of Medicine 332: 1600–1605

Bennett R C, Duthie H L 1964 The functional importance of the internal sphincter. British Journal of Surgery 51: 355–357

Bradley W E 1972 Urethral electromyelography. Journal of Urology 119: 563–564

Bremmer S, Ahlback S, Uden R, Mellgran A 1995 Simultaneous defecography and peritoneography in defecation disorders. Diseases of the Colon and Rectum 38: 969–973

Brubaker L, Heit M H 1993 Radiology of the pelvic floor. Clinical Obstetrics and Gynecology 36(4): 952–49

Brubaker L, Retzy S, Smith C, Saclarides T 1993 Pelvic floor evaluation with dynamic fluoroscopy. Obstetrics and Gynecology 82: 863–8

Delorme R 1900 Sur le traitement des prolapses du rectum totaux pour l'excision de la muquese rectable au rectocolique. Bulletin des Members de la Société Chirurgical de Paris 26: 498–499

Donnelly V S, Fynes M, Campbell D, Johnson H, O'Connell R, O'Herlihy C 1998a Obstetric events leading to anal sphincter damage. Obstetrics and Gynecology 92: 955–61

Donnelly V S, O'Herlihy C, Campbell D M, O'Connell P R 1998b Postpartum fecal incontinence is more common in women with irritable bowel syndrome. Diseases of the Colon and Rectum 41: 586–9

Engel A F, Kamm M A, Sultan A H, Bartram C I, Nicholls R J 1994 Anterior anal sphincter repair in patients with obstetric trauma, British Journal of Surgery 81: 1231–4

Farthing M J G 1995 Irritable bowel, irritable body, or irritable brain. British Medical Journal 310: 171–5

Fielding J R, Versi E, Mulkern R V, Lerner M H, Griffiths D J, Jolesz F A. 1996 MR imaging of the female pelvic floor in the supine and upright positions. Journal of Magnetic Resonance Imaging 6: 961–3

Floyd W F, Walls E W 1953 Electromyography of the sphincter ani externus in man. Journal of Physiology 122: 599–609

Geerdes B P, Heineman E, Konsten J, Soeters P B, Baeten C G 1996 Dynamic graciloplasty. Complications and management. Diseases of the Colon and Rectum 39: 912–917

Gill K P, Chia Y W, Henry M M, Shorvon P J 1994 Defecography in multiple sclerosis patients with severe constipation. Radiology 191: 553–556

Gowers W R 1877 The automatic action of the sphincter ani. Proceedings of the Royal Society of London 26: 498–499

Halligan S, Bartram C I 1995 Is barium trapping in rectoceles significant? Diseases of the Colon and Rectum 38: 764–768

Halligan S, Nicholls R J, Bartram C I 1995 Proctographic changes after rectopexy for solitary rectal ulcer syndrome and preoperative predictive factors for a successful outcome. British Journal of Surgery 82: 314–317

Harvey R F, Salih S Y, Read A E 1983 Organic and functional disorders in 200 gastroenterology outpatients. Lancet 1983: I: 632–4

Henry M M, Porter N H 1988 A colour atlas of faecal incontinence and rectal prolapse. Wolfe Publications, London.

Henry M M, Parks A G, Swash M 1982 The pelvic floor muscle in the descending perineum syndrome. British Journal of Surgery 62: 470–472

Hinton J M, Lennard Jones J E, Young A C 1969 A new method for studying gut transit times using radio-opaque markers. Gut 10: 842–847

Hutchinson R, Mostafa A B, Grant E A et al 1993 Scintigraphic defecography: quantitive and dynamic assessment of anorectal function. Diseases of the Colon and Rectum 36: 1132–1138

Jameson J S, Chia Y W, Kamm M A, Speakman C T M, Chye Y H, Henry M M 1994a Effect of age, sex and parity on anorectal function. British Journal of Surgery 81: 1689–1692

Jameson J S, Speakman C T, Darzi A, Chia Y W, Henry M M 1994b. Audit of postanal repair in the treatment of faecal incontinence. Diseases of the Colon and Rectum 37: 369–372.

Janssen L W M, Van Dijke C F 1994 Selection criteria for anterior rectal wall repair in symptomatic rectocoele and anterior rectal wall prolapse. Diseases of the Colon and Rectum 37: 1100–1107

Kelvin F M, Maglinte D D T, Benson J T 1994 Evacuation proctography (defecography): An aid to the investigation of pelvic floor disorders. Obstetrics and Gynecology 83: 307–314

Lane R H S, Parks A G 1977 Function of the anal sphincters following colo-anal anastomosis. British Journal of Surgery 64: 596–599

Lauerberg S, Swash M, Henry M M 1988 Delayed external sphincter repair for obstetric tear. British Journal of Surgery 75: 786–788

Law P J, Bartram C I 1989 Anal endosonography – technique and normal anatomy. Gastrointestinal Radiology 14: 349–353

Lienemann A, Anthuber C, Baron A, Kohz P, Reiser M 1997 Dynamic M R colpocytorectography assessing pelvic-floor descent. European Radiology 1997; 7(8): 1309–1317

Loening-Baucke V, Read N W 1990 Cortical evoked potential recorded after electrical endorectal stimulation in human volunteers. Gastroenterology 98: A371

Lubowski D Z, Nicholls R J, Swash M, Jordan M J 1987 Neural control of internal anal sphincter function. British Journal of Surgery 74: 668–670

Mahieu P, Pringot J, Bodart O 1984 Defecography: 1. Description of a new procedure and results in normal patients. Gastrointestinal Radiology 9: 253–261

Manning A P, Thompson W G, Heaton K W, Morris A F 1978 Towards positive diagnosis of the irritable bowel syndrome. British Medical Journal ii: 653–654

Merton P A, Hill D K, Morton H B, Marsden C D 1982 Scope of a technique for electrical stimulation of human brain, spinal cord and muscle. Lancet ii: 597–600

Monga A K, Marrero J M, Stanton S L, Lemieux M C, Maxwell J D 1997 Is there an irritable bladder in the irritable bowel syndrome. British Journal of Obstetrics and Gynaecology 104: 1409–12

Neill M E, Swash M 1980 Increased motor unit fibre density in the external sphincter in anorectal incontinence: a single fibre EMG study. Journal of Neurology, Neurosurgery and Psychiatry 43: 343–347

Neill M E, Parks A G, Swash M 1981 Physiological studies of the anal sphincter musculature in faecal incontinence and rectal prolapse. British Journal of Surgery 68: 531–536

Parks A G 1975 Anorectal incontinence. Proceedings of the Royal Society of Medicine 68: 681–690.

Parks A G, Porter N H, Melzack J 1962 Experimental study of the reflex mechanicm controlling the muscles of the pelvic floor. Diseases of the Colon and Rectum 5: 407–414

Parks A G, Swash M, Urich H 1977 Sphincter denervation in anorectal incontinence and rectal prolapse. Gut 18: 656–665

Peschers U M, DeLancey J O L, Schaer G N, Schuessler B 1997 Exoanal ultrasound of the anal sphincter: normal anatomy and sphincter defects. British Journal of Obstetrics and Gynaecology 104: 999–1003

Pickerell K, Masters F, Georgiade N, Horton C 1954 Rectal sphincter reconstruction using gracilis muscle transplant. Plastic and Reconstructive Surgery. 13: 46–55

Poen A C, Felt-Bersma R J F, Strijers R L M, Dekkers G A, Cuesta M A, Meuwissen S G M 1988a Third-degree obstetric perineal tear: long-term clinical and functional results after primary repair. British Journal of Surgery 85: 1433–38

Poen A C, Felt-Bersma R J F, Cuesta M A, Meuwissen S G M 1988b Vaginal endoscopy of the anal sphincter complex is important in the assessment of faecal incontinence and perianal sepsis. British Journal of Surgery 85: 359–63

Porter N H 1962 Physiological study of the pelvic floor in rectal prolapse. Annals of the Royal College of Surgeons of England 31: 379–404

Rogers J, Levy D M, Henry M M, Misiewicz J J 1988 Pelvic floor neuropathy: a comparative study of diabetes mellitus and idiopathic faecal incontinence. Gut 29: 756–761

Rogers J, Henry M M, Misiewicz J J 1989 Increased segmental activity and intraluminal pressures in the sigmoid colon of patients with irritable bowel syndrome. Gut 30: 634–641

Snooks S J, Swash M 1984 Abnormalities of the innervation of the urethral striated sphincter muscle in incontinence. British Journal of Urology 56: 401–405

Snooks S J, Swash M, Henry M M, Setchell M E 1984 Injury to innervation of pelvic floor sphincter musculature in childbirth. Lancet ii: 546–550

Snooks S J, Swash M, Henry M M 1985a Abnormalities in central and peripheral nerve conduction in patients with anorectal incontinence. Journal of the Royal Society of Medicine 78: 294–300

Snooks S J, Barnes P R H, Swash M, Henry M M 1985b Damage to the innervation of the pelvic floor musculature in chronic constipation. Gastroenterology 89: 977–981

Snooks S J, Nicholls R J, Henry M M, Swash M 1985c Electrophysiological and manometric assessment of the pelvic floor in solitary rectal ulcer syndrome. British Journal of Surgery 72: 131–133

Speakman C T M, Kamm M A, Swash M 1990 Cerebral evoked potentials – are they of value in anorectal disease? Gut 31: A1173

Speakman C T M, Hoyle C H V, Kamm M A, Henry M M, Nicholls R J, Burnstock G 1993 Neuropeptides in the internal anal sphincter in neurogenic faecal incontinence. International Journal of Colorectal Disease 8: 201–205

Steiner R A, Healy J C 1998 Patterns of prolapse in women with symptoms of pelvic floor weakness: magnetic resonance imaging and laparoscopic treatment. Current Opinion in Obstetrics and Gynecology 10: 295–301

Sultan A H, Nicholls R J, Kamm M A, Hudson C N, Beynon J, Bartram C I 1993a Anal endosonography and correlation with in vitro and in vivo anatomy. British Journal of Surgery 80: 508–511

Sultan A H, Kamm M A, Hudson C N, Thomas J M, Bartram C I 1993b Anal sphincter disruption during vaginal delivery. New England Journal of Medicine 329: 1902–11

Sultan A H, Kamm M A, Hudson C N, Bartram C I 1994a Third degree obstetric anal sphincter tears: risk factors and outcome of primary repair. British Medical Journal 308: 887–891

Sultan A H, Loder P B, Bartram C I, Kamm M A, Hudson C N 1994b Vaginal endosonography: a new technique to image the undisturbed anal sphincter. Diseases of the Colon and Rectum 37: 1296–99

Sultan A H, Kamm M A, Hudson C N 1994c Pudendal nerve damage during labour: prospective study before and after childbirth. British Journal of Obstetrics and Gynaecology 101: 22–28

Sultan A H, Johanson R B, Carter J E 1998 Occult anal sphincter trauma following randomized forceps and vacuum delivery. International Journal of Gynecology and Obstetrics 61: 113–119

Sultan A H, Monga A K, Kumar D, Stanton S L 1999 Primary repair of obstetric anal sphincter rupture using the overlap technique. British Journal of Obstetrics and Gynaecology 106: 318–323

Talley N J, Phillips S F, Melton L J, Zinsmeister A R 1990 Diagnostic value of the Manning criteria in irritable bowel syndrome. Gut 31: 77–81

Tetzschner T, Sorensen M, Lose G, Christiansen J 1997 Vaginal pudendal nerve stimulation: a new technique for assessment of pudendal nerve latency. Acta Obstetrica et Gynecologica Scandinavica 76: 294–299

Thompson W G, Dotevall G, Drossman D A, Heaton K W, Kruis W 1989 Irritable bowel syndrome; guidelines for the diagnosis. Gastroenterology International 2: 92–95

Vaisey C J, Kamm M A, Nicholls R J 1998a Recent advances in the surgical treatment of faecal incontinence. British Journal of Surgery 85: 596–603

Vaisey C J, Kamm M A, Gold D M, Bartram C I, Halligan S, Nicholls R J 1998b Clinical, physiological, and radiological study of a new purpose-designed artificial bowel sphincter. Lancet 352: 105–9

Vernava A M, Longo, W E, Danel R N 1993 Pudendal neuropathy and the importance of EMG evaluation of fecal incontinence. Diseases of the Colon and Rectum 36: 23–27

Walls E W 1959 Recent observations of the anatomy of the anal canal. Proceedings of the Royal Society of Medicine 52(suppl): 85–87

Williams N S, Patel J, George B D, Itallan R I, Watkins E S 1991 Development of an electrically stimulated neoanal sphincter: Lancet 338: 1166–1169

Winkler G 1958 Remarques sur la morphologie et l'innervation du muscle releveur de l'anus. Archives d'Anatomie et Histologie et Embryologie, Strasbourg 41: 77–95

Womack N R, Morrison J F B, Williams N S 1988 Prospective study of the effects of postanal repair in neurogenic faecal incontinence. British Journal of Surgery 75: 48–52

Wong W D, Jensen L L, Bartolo D C C, Rothernberger D A 1996 Artificial anal sphincter. Diseases of the Colon and Rectum 39: 1345–51

SECTION 3
CHAPTER
39

Clinical neuropathology of the urethra

BJØRN KLEVMARK AND SIGURD KULSENG-HANSSEN

BACKGROUND AND DEFINITION

During micturition the bladder neck and the proximal urethra are funnel-shaped, and the size and form of the urethra remain fairly unchanged until the bladder is empty.

The urethra is innervated by all three types of nerve: sympathetic, parasympathetic and somatic, with an unknown proportion of each (see Ch. 1). Against this background the previously used concept 'neuropathic urethra' has turned out to be impossible to define and use. The concept 'neurogenic bladder' has survived for almost 100 years, because in the bladder the parasympathetic innervation is dominant. Thus, the various types of neurogenic bladder have consistent, well-known clinical–urodynamic symptoms and signs.

The term 'neuropathic urethra' was introduced by Abel et al (1974) and used to some degree for the next 10–15 years (Gibbon 1977; Madersbacher 1977; Sham Sunder et al 1978; McGuire 1984). However, the 'neuropathic urethra' was always part of a larger clinical condition of the neurogenic bladder, which resulted in unclear definition of the concept of the 'neuropathic urethra'.

In this chapter we use the term 'neuropathology'. We define clinical neuropathological conditions of the urethra as conditions where neurogenic dysfunction is supposed to be the main aetiological factor, and where the bladder is neurogenically normal. Accordingly, we will deal with the following three conditions:

- Detrusor–bladder neck dyssynergia
- Detrusor–sphincter dyssynergia (the functional or psychosomatic type)
- Unstable urethra.

DETRUSOR–BLADDER NECK DYSSYNERGIA

This is well known in men who have a circular sphincter muscle in the bladder neck, which contracts during ejaculation and provides antegrade ejaculation (Andersen et al 1976; Fryjordet 1979). However, detrusor–bladder neck dyssynergia has been described in women as a rare condition (Diokno et al 1984; Klevmark 1985). Even if a woman has no genital sphincter, she has circular smooth muscle fibres and ample adrenergic innervation at the bladder neck (Ek et al 1977a,b; Gosling et al 1977; Alm

1978; Klück 1980; Thind 1995). Diokno et al (1984) demonstrated histologically marked circular muscle hypertrophy in one of their operated cases. The genital sphincter in men has an adrenergic innervation (α-adrenoceptors) and α-adrenoceptor blocking agents have a clinical therapeutic effect. This effect is not observed in women.

The patients usually have a long history of bothersome desire to void, low flow-rate (Fig. 39.1), residual urine and recurrent cystitis. Abdominal straining will not improve the bladder emptying. No obstruction is seen during endoscopy and the urethra has a normal calibre. The bladder wall may be trabeculated with signs of infection.

A pressure-flow-EMG study will show a high detrusor pressure, low flow-rate and a silent EMG. When there is no increased resistance at the pelvic floor level, it must be located at the bladder neck and is shown by voiding cystourethrography (VCU) (Fig. 39.2).

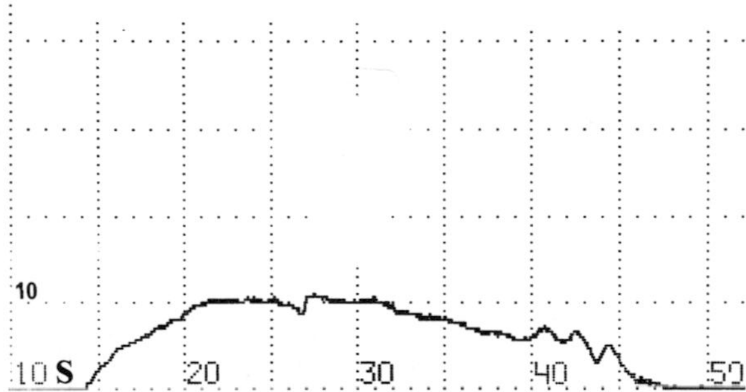

Fig. 39.1 Detrusor–bladder neck dyssynergia. Female, 27 years. Spontaneous uroflowmetry. Voided 246 ml, residual urine 50 ml. Maximum flow-rate 11.2 ml/s, average 7.5 ml/s. Flow curve consistent with outlet resistance.

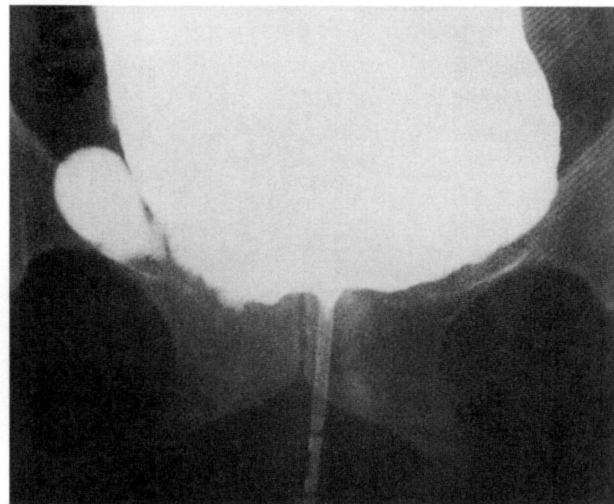

Fig. 39.2 Detrusor–bladder neck dyssynergia. Voiding cystourethrography. Female 33 years. Micturition against narrow bladder neck. Bladder diverticulum and uneven bladder wall indicating trabeculation. Maximum flow-rate 1.8 ml/s, detrusor pressure 200 cm H_2O, residual urine 250 ml. From Diokno et al (1984) with permission.

The condition can only be cured by surgical intervention. Urethral dilatation or transurethral incision of the bladder neck is insufficient. It is necessary to make a suprapubic approach to perform a Y-V plasty of the bladder neck. In most cases there is a firm ring at the bladder neck which can be felt when it is cut through. When the ring has been cut, the urethra is palpated as soft and distensible. It is necessary to cut approximately 1 cm down through the anterior wall of the urethra to obtain a satisfactory interposition of normal bladder wall tissue at the level of the bladder neck. VCU will now show a funnel-shaped bladder neck, the flow-rate has become normal and there is no residual urine (Fig. 39.3).

The patient in Figure 39.1 had a preoperative pressure-flow-EMG study showing detrusor pressure of 95 cm H_2O, maximum flow-rate 14 ml/s, a silent

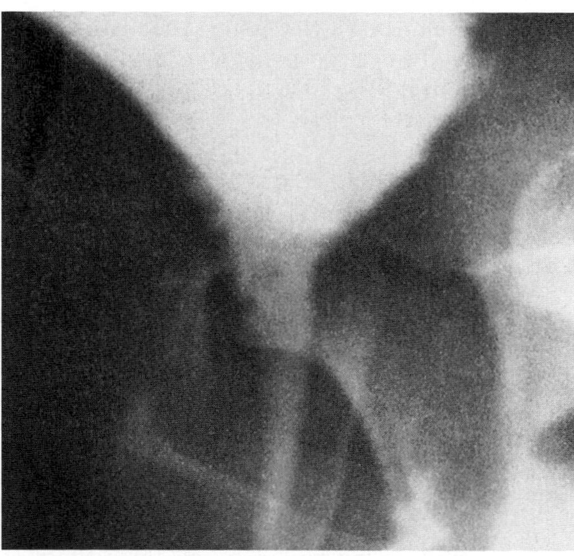

Fig. 39.3 Detrusor–bladder neck dyssynergia. Same patient as in Figure 39.2. After open Y-V plasty the bladder neck has become funnel-shaped and bladder emptying normal. From Diokno et al (1984) with permission.

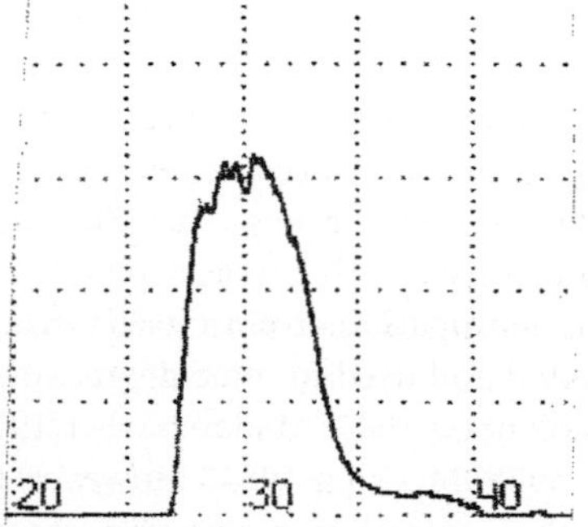

Fig. 39.4 Detrusor–bladder neck dyssynergia. Same patient as in Figure 39.1, 16 months after open Y-V plasty of the bladder neck. Spontaneous uroflowmetry. Voided 182 ml, no residual urine. Maximum flow-rate 32.3 ml/s, average 13.0.

EMG and 50 ml residual urine. Two months postoperatively, the corresponding numbers were 55 cm H_2O, 29 ml/s and no residual urine. The maximum flow-rate 16 months after the operation was 32.3 ml/s (Fig. 39.4).

If there are contraindications for surgery, intermittent self-catheterization can be tried. However, the patients are often young or middle-aged and catheterization will be unsatisfactory in the long run. Postoperative incontinence has not occurred (Diokno et al 1984; Klevmark, personal communication, 1998), which indicates that the bladder neck is not an essential part of the normal continence mechanism.

Is detrusor–bladder neck dyssynergia in women a clinical neuropathological condition? The aetiology is unknown. It could be that sympathetic nervous overactivity initiates the process which then ends in morphological changes.

DETRUSOR–SPHINCTER DYSSYNERGIA (FUNCTIONAL)

Detrusor–sphincter dyssynergia is defined by the International Continence Society Committee on Standardization of Terminology (Abrams et al 1988) as follows:

> Detrusor–sphincter dyssynergia describes a detrusor contraction concurrent with an involuntary contraction of the urethral and/or periurethral striated muscle. In the adult, detrusor–sphincter dyssynergia is a feature of neurological voiding disorders. In the absence of neurological features the validity of this diagnosis should be questioned ... Overactivity of the urethral sphincter may occur during voiding in the absence of neurological disease and is termed dysfunctional voiding.

Detrusor–sphincter dyssynergia without signs of neurological disorder is present in young adults, mostly women. This has been termed the functional or psychosomatic type of detrusor–sphincter dyssynergia by many clinicians. According to our definition, we shall only deal with neuropathological conditions of the urethra where the bladder is neurogenically normal. Detrusor–sphincter dyssynergia in cases of neurological disorders (usually myelopathia) is always combined with neurogenic disturbance of the bladder, usually detrusor hyperreflexia. Dysfunctional voiding, as proposed by the ICS, is a non-specific term.

In the functional detrusor–sphincter dyssynergia the urethral and periurethral striated muscles contract before the detrusor contraction is fulfilled, and there are variable volumes of residual urine. The condition is usually found in girls and very young women, and is probably a behavioural disturbance related to various intrinsic and extrinsic factors in childhood and during puberty (in the family and/or at school).

The diagnosis is based on the case history, with recurrent cystitis as the main symptom, and repeated

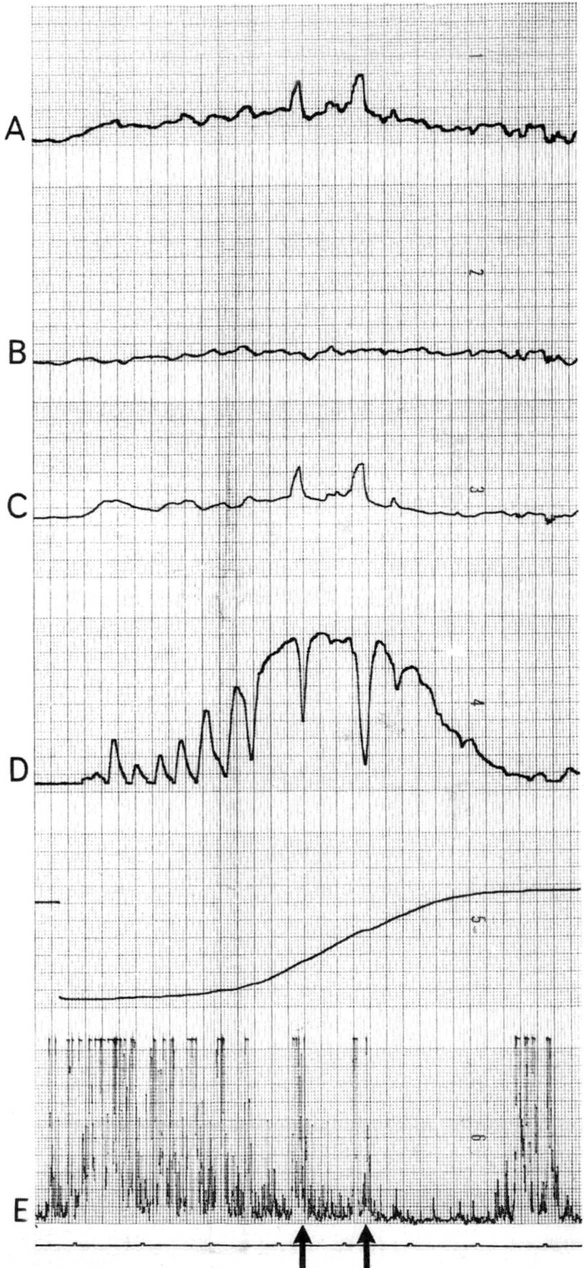

Fig. 39.5 Detrusor–sphincter dyssynergia, Female, 19 years. Pressure-flow-EMG study. (**A**) Bladder pressure. (**B**) Rectal pressure. (**C**) Detrusor pressure. (**D**) Flow-rate. (**E**) EMG from urethral striated muscle. At maximum flow-rate the flow is first reduced and then interrupted due to contractions of urethral striated muscle (arrows). Detrusor responds simultaneously to the obstruction with marked pressure rise.

uroflowmetry studies with measurement of residual urine. To verify the diagnosis it is necessary to do a pressure-flow-EMG study. There are two situations. The first is demonstrated in Figure 39.5 and the other is in Figures 39.6 and 39.7.

Figure 39.5 is from a 19-year-old woman with recurrent cystitis. At maximum flow-rate there are two marked changes of the flow curve which correspond with two sharp moderate increases of detrusor pressure (as in a stop-test). The EMG shows urethral striated muscle contractions corresponding with the reduction in flow-rate and increase in detrusor pressure. This patient had a normal maximum flow-rate of 21 ml/s.

Figures 39.6 and 39.7 are from a 20-year-old woman with recurrent cystitis from the age of 15. Spontaneous flowmetry shows 'superflow' of 46 ml/s (Fig. 39.6). Normal women, and the patient described above with two short interruptions of flow, will not develop a flow-rate of more than 25–30 ml/s. That is because micturition is usually performed by a pronounced initial fall in urethral pressure, which only requires the supplement of a relatively small detrusor contraction to provide optimal flow-rate.

Pronounced 'superflow' may occur when a very strong detrusor overcomes a large urethral resistance, or a paretic bladder is emptied by abdominal straining. This can only be evaluated by a pressure-flow-EMG study as shown in Figure 39.7. Other measurements of residual urine in this patient showed variation between 8 ml and 100 ml. In a case like this the detrusor may be able to develop very high pressure, but is not always able to continue the contraction until the bladder is emptied completely. The same high pressure-high flow voiding is well known in some men with prostatic obstruction complaining of urgency and frequency.

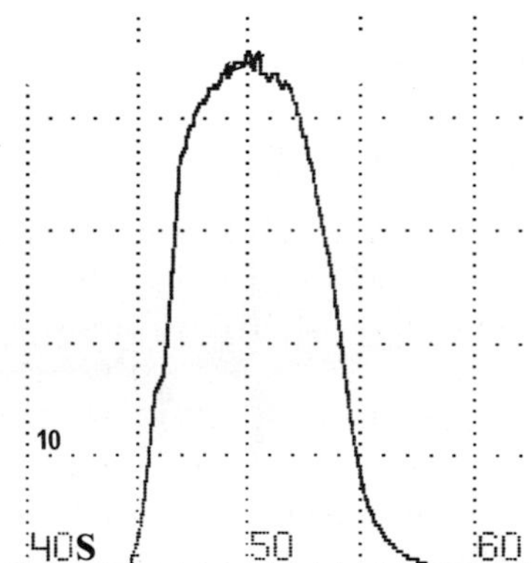

Fig. 39.6 Detrusor–sphincter dyssynergia. Female 20 years. Spontaneous uroflowmetry. Voided 317 ml, 8 ml residual urine. Maximum flow-rate 46 ml/s, average 26.4.

Treatment of functional detrusor–sphincter dyssynergia is by relaxation training, preferably using biofeedback. Neuromodulation (electrical stimulation of sacral roots) should be tried for impaired sphincter relaxation (Everaert et al 1997). Intermittent self-catheterization once or twice a day to get rid of residual urine may be necessary in cases of recurrent infection. A correct combination of intermittent catheterization and antibiotics will usually be successful. It should be stressed that all cases of 'superflow' in women need a pressure-flow-EMG study.

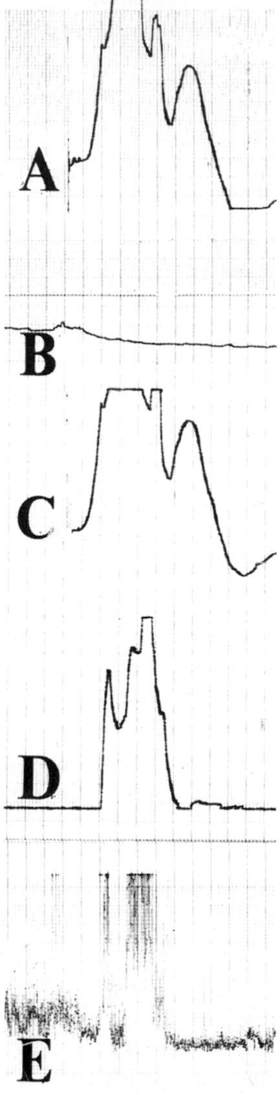

Fig. 39.7 Detrusor–sphincter dyssynergia. Same patient as in Figure 39.6. Pressure-flow-EMG study. (**A**) Bladder pressure. (**B**) Rectal pressure. (**C**) Detrusor pressure. (**D**) Flow-rate. (**E**) EMG from urethral striated muscle. Voided volume 380 ml. Maximum flow-rate 45 ml/s, 100 ml residual urine. Detrusor pressure 138 cm H_2O. No increase in rectal pressure. This patient compensates for the marked urethral striated muscle contraction with an extraordinarily high detrusor pressure, which results in very high maximum flow (superflow), but the detrusor is not able to continue the contraction long enough to empty the bladder completely.

UNSTABLE URETHRA

Urethral pressure variations were first described by Karlson (1953). It has been shown that urethral pressure variation is a physiological phenomenon which is present in variable degree in women with neurourological symptoms as well as in normal women (Kulseng-Hanssen 1983; Versi & Cardozo 1986; Hilton 1988; Sørensen 1992). Previous attempts to define urethral pressure variations as a pathological phenomenon on a quantitative basis were arbitrary and are no longer of any interest. The pressure level from which the variations take place may be of pathological significance. During ambulatory recording, incontinence is most often due to a large urethral pressure fall and a relatively small detrusor contraction (Fig. 39.8). Kulseng-Hanssen et al (1987a, b) found that the variation of the urethral pressure was due to variable activity of the urethral smooth and striated muscles.

In several reports sudden urethral relaxation has been described as the only cause of urinary incontinence (Bradley et al 1973; Torrens & Collins 1975; McGuire 1978, 1984; Woodside & Borden 1983). 'Unstable urethra' was defined by the ICS (Bates et al 1981) as 'a condition where a patient is leaking urine due to sudden urethral pressure fall without concomitant detrusor contraction'. Abrams (1997) prefers to call the condition 'inappropriate urethral relaxation'. 'Unstable urethra' may be a case of detrusor instability where the urethral pressure fall in itself is large enough to give leakage, and is therefore not followed by a detrusor contraction.

Previously, urge incontinent women were studied with simultaneous urethrocystometry (SUCM). However, in many cases it was not possible to demonstrate the leakage the patients said they felt during daily activity. To improve the diagnosis an ambulant method was introduced – ambulatory urethro-cysto-recto-metry (AUCRM) (Kulseng-Hanssen & Klevmark 1988). In the first study comprising 26 women the leakage mechanism was demonstrated with AUCRM in 21 patients, while only in 13 patients with SUCM. A case of unstable urethra is shown in Figure 39.9.

Unstable urethra is a rare condition. Kulseng-Hanssen & Klevmark (1996) found 3% of unstable urethra among 110 patients with urethral pressure variations. Thind (1995) found in pharmacological studies of healthy women that striated muscle is far more functionally important in the urethral wall than smooth muscle. Probably, for some functional reason, unstable urethra is caused by a sudden reduction in somatic and/or sympathetic nerve activity. Because the condition is rare, therapeutical experience is difficult to obtain. Pharmacological agents, such as α-adrenoceptor agonists, may be tried.

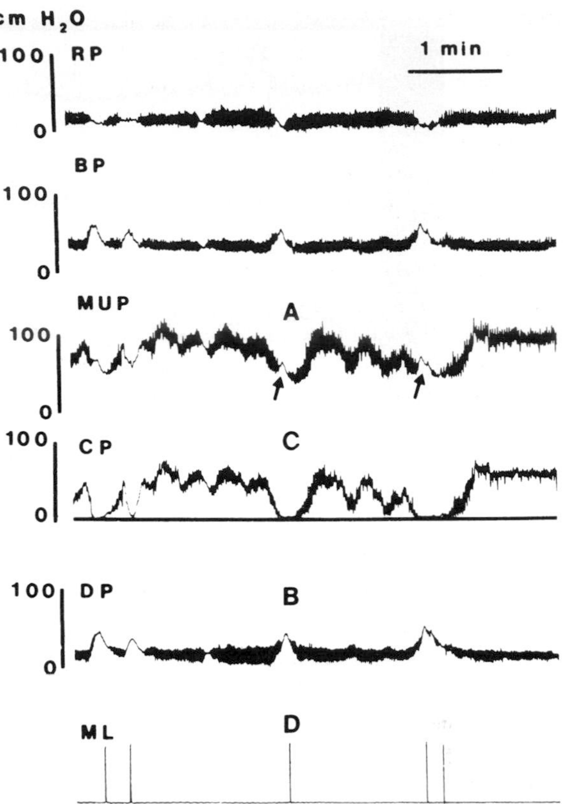

Fig. 39.8 Detrusor instability. Ambulatory urethro-cysto-rectometry (AUCRM). RP: Rectal pressure; BP: Bladder pressure; MUP: Maximum urethral pressure; CP: Closure pressure; DP: Detrusor pressure and ML: Leakage detector. The patient is leaking due to a maximum urethral pressure fall of 56 cm H_2O (A) and a detrusor contraction of 23 cm H_2O (B). Closure pressure becomes 0 cm H_2O (C) and leakage is verified by the leakage detector (D). The arrows point to urethral pressure waves occurring concomitantly with the detrusor pressure rise. From Kulseng-Hanssen & Klevmark (1988), with permission.

CONCLUSION

The three different clinical neuropathological conditions described in this chapter have three features in common. Neurogenic dysfunction is supposed to be the main aetiological factor while the bladder is neurogenically normal. Diagnosis depends upon the most elaborate urodynamic studies, namely pressure-flow-EMG (for the dyssynergias) and ambulatory monitoring of urethral, bladder and abdominal pressure (for the unstable urethra). In addition, the level of an urethral obstruction can be visualized by voiding cystourethrography.

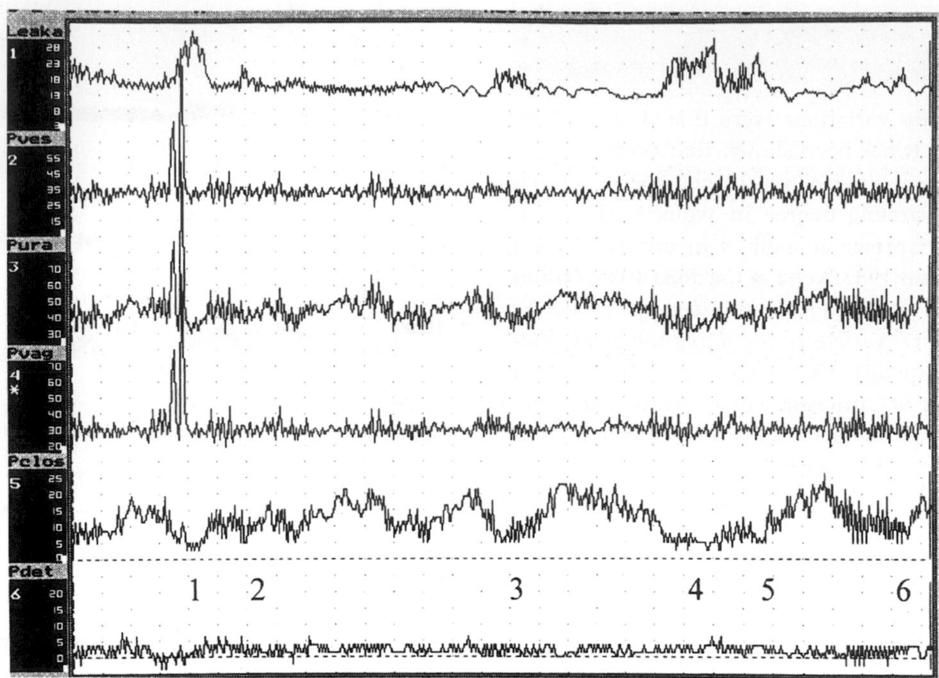

Fig. 39.9 Unstable urethra. Ambulatory urethro-cysto-rectometry (AUCRM). The first leakage is caused by a cough. A urethral pressure decrease with leakage during and some seconds after the cough is seen. The detrusor pressure is stable. The urethral and closure pressures decrease and leakage is seen another five times. This figure shows a four times compressed recording (5 min). Due to calibration procedures, the true zero closure pressure is +12 cm H_2O. From Kulseng-Hanssen & Klevmark (1996), with permission.

REFERENCES

Abel B J, Jameson R M, Gibbon N O K, Krisnan K R 1974 The neuropathic urethra. Lancet 2: 1229–1230

Abrams P 1997 Urodynamics, 2nd edn. Springer, London

Abrams P, Blaivas J G, Stanton S L, Andersen J T (chairman) 1988 The standardisation of terminology of lower urinary tract function. International Continence Society Committee on Standardization of Terminology. Scandinavian Journal of Urology and Nephrology Supp 114

Alm P 1978 Cholinergic innervation of the human urethra and urinary bladder. Acta Pharmacology and Toxicology 43: 56–62

Andersen J T, Jacobsen O, Gammelgaard P A, Hald T 1976 Dysfunction of the bladder neck: a urodynamic study. Urology International 31: 78–86

Bates P, Bradley W E, Glen E et al 1981 Fourth report on the standardisation of terminology of lower urinary tract function. Terminology related to neuromuscular dysfunction of lower urinary tract. British Journal of Urology 52: 333–335

Bradley W E, Logothesis J L, Timm G W 1973 Cystometric and sphincter abnormalities in multiple sclerosis. Neurology 23: 1131–1139

Diokno A C, Hollander J B, Bennett C J 1984 Bladder neck obstruction in women: a real entity. The Journal of Urology 132: 294–298

Ek A, Alm P, Andersson K-E, Persson C G A 1977a Adrenoceptor and cholinoceptor mediated responses of the isolated human urethra. Scandinavian Journal of Urology and Nephrology 12: 97–104

Ek A, Alm P, Andersson K-E, Persson C G A 1977b Adrenergic and cholinergic nerves of the human urethra and urinary bladder. A histochemical study. Acta Physiologica Scandinavica 99: 345–352

Everaert K, Plancke F, Lefevere F, Oosterlinck W 1997 The urodynamic evaluation of neuromodulation in patients with voiding dysfunction. British Journal of Urology 79: 702–707

Fryjordet A 1979 Dyskinesia of the bladder neck. Journal of the Norwegian Medical Association 99: 1180–1181 (In Norwegian. Summary in English)

Gibbon N O K 1977 The neuropathic urethra. Royal College of Surgeons, Edinburgh 22: 118–126

Gosling J A, Dixon J A, Lendon R G 1977 The autonomic innervation of the human male and female bladder neck and proximal urethra. Journal of Urology 118: 302–305

Hilton P 1988 Unstable urethral pressure: Toward a more relevant definition. Neurourology and Urodynamics 6: 411–418

Karlson S 1953 Experimental studies on the functioning of the female urinary bladder and urethra. Acta Obstetrica et Gynecologica Scandinavica 32: 285–307

Klevmark B 1985 Functional bladder neck obstruction in women. Scientific proceedings, Norwegian Surgical Society p. 23 (in Norwegian)

Klück P 1980 The autonomic innervation of the human urinary bladder, bladder neck and urethra. Anatomical Records 198: 439–447

Kulseng-Hanssen S 1983 Prevalence and pattern of unstable urethral pressure in one hundred seventy-four gynecologic patients referred for urodynamic investigation. American Journal of Obstetrics and Gynecology 146/8: 895–900

Kulseng-Hanssen S, Klevmark B 1996 Ambulatory urodynamic

monitoring of women. Scandinavian Journal of Urology and Nephrology 30 (Suppl. 179): 27–37

Kulseng-Hanssen S, Klevmark B 1988 Ambulatory urethro-cysto-rectometry: A new technique. Neurourology and Urodynamics 7: 119–130

Kulseng-Hanssen S, Stranden A 1987b Urethral pressure variations in women with neurourological symptoms: III. Relationship to urethral wall venous plexus. Neurourology and Urodynamics 6: 87–93

Kulseng-Hanssen S, Stien R, Fønstelien E 1987a Urethral pressure variations in women with neurourological symptoms: I. Relationship to urethral and pelvic floor striated muscle. Neurourology and Urodynamics 6: 71–78

McGuire E J 1978 Reflex urethral instability. British Journal of Urology 50: 200–304

McGuire E J 1984 The neuropathic urethra. In: Mundy T, Stephenson T, Wein A J (eds) Urodynamics. Churchill Livingstone, Edinburgh, pp 287–295

Madersbacher H 1977 The neuropathic urethra: urethrogram and pathophysiological aspects. European Journal of Urology 3: 321–332

Sham Sunder G, Parsons K F, Gibbon O K 1978 Outflow obstruction in neuropathic bladder dysfunction: the neuropathic urethra. British Journal of Urology 57: 422–426

Sørensen S 1992 Urethral pressure variations in healthy and incontinent women. Neurourology and Urodynamics 11: 549–591

Thind P 1995 The significance of smooth and striated muscles in sphincter function of the urethra in healthy women (thesis). Neurourology and Urodynamics 14: 6

Torrens M, Collins C D 1975 The urodynamic assessment of adult enuresis. British Journal of Urology 47: 433–440

Versi E, Cardozo L 1986 Urethral instability: Diagnosis based on variations of the maximum urethral pressure in normal climacteric women. Neurourology and Urodynamics 5: 535–541

Woodside J R, Borden T A 1983 Central nervous system lesion causing urethral instability and urinary incontinence. Journal of Urology 130: 136–137

SECTION 4

Urinary tract in pregnancy

Upper urinary tract in pregnancy

JOHN M DAVISON

During normal pregnancy the changes in the urinary tract are so extensive that non-pregnant norms are inappropriate for the management of antenatal patients. Awareness of this is essential if early signs of renal dysfunction are to be detected and/or if proper advice is to be given to women with renal problems who seek guidance on the advisability of conceiving or continuing a pregnancy already in progress.

URINARY TRACT CHANGES IN NORMAL PREGNANCY

Glomerular filtration (GFR) and renal plasma flow are 50–70% higher than non-pregnancy values (Sturgiss et al 1994). GFR, as 24-hour creatinine clearance, increases immediately in early pregnancy and serum levels of creatinine and urea, which average 73 µmol/l and 4.3 mmol/l, respectively, in non-pregnant women, decrease to mean values of 51 µmol/l, and 3.3 mmol/l in pregnancy. Values of creatinine of 75 µmol/l and urea of 4.5 mmol/l, which are acceptable in non-pregnant women, are suspect in pregnancy. Caution is necessary when serially assessing renal function on the basis of serum creatinine levels alone (especially in the presence of renal disease) because even when up to 50% of renal function has been lost, serum creatinine can still be less than 130 mmol/l.

The gestational increase in GFR is entirely due to renal vasodilation without glomerular blood pressure being significantly elevated or any long-term damaging effects on the maternal kidney (Baylis 1994). Both total protein and albumin excretion are significantly increased after 20 weeks' gestation, with means (and upper limits) of 200 mg (260 mg) and 15 mg (30 mg) respectively near term (Baylis & Davison 1998).

The kidneys enlarge because both vascular volume and interstitial space increase, with a 70% increase overall in renal volume by the third trimester (Sturgiss et al 1994). Although the calyces, renal pelves and ureters dilate markedly. There is no effect on the frequency and symmetry of ureteral jets. (Asrat et al

1998). The anatomical changes are invariably more prominent on the right side and evident in 90% of women by the third trimester. The important clinical implications are:

- Mistakenly diagnosing obstructive uropathy
- Stasis of urine within the ureters may contribute to the tendency in pregnant women with asymptomatic bacteriuria to develop frank pyelonephritis
- Errors in tests based on timed urine collections
- Postpartum X-ray assessment of the renal tract should be delayed until at least 4 months postpartum to allow changes to resolve.

URINARY TRACT INFECTIONS

Diagnosis is difficult because normal pregnant symptoms include urinary frequency, dysuria, nocturia and urgency; it must be based on laboratory evidence. A standard definition of infection is a colony count greater than 100 000 bacteria per ml of urine, although counts as low as 20 000 may represent active infection in pregnancy (Cunningham & Lucas 1994). Urinary white cell count tends to increase in pregnancy such that moderate pyuria may be normal. *Escherichia coli* is the predominant infecting organism (75–90% of cases); *Klebsiella, Proteus* and *Enterobacter* account for most of the remainder.

For urinary tract infections, see also Chapter 29.

Asymptomatic bacteriuria

In pregnancy, 5% of women will have a covert urinary infection, 30% of whom will develop a symptomatic infection if untreated (McGladdery et al 1992). Urinary infection confers an increased risk of pregnancy complications, including premature labour, fetal growth retardation and pre-eclampsia. Most obstetricians advocate routine screening at antenatal booking, with additional screening (monthly) in women with a past history of urinary infections and/or renal disorders, a policy that would predict 70% of those destined to have symptomatic infections. Treatment should be governed by organism sensitivity and continued for at least 7–10 days for initial infections and 21 days for recurrences. Regardless of the antimicrobial used or duration of treatment, 30% of women will relapse. Some authorities advocate prophylactic therapy following re-infections (Stein & Funfstuck 1999).

There is no evidence that asymptomatic infections cause permanent renal damage in adults with normal urinary tracts. Radiological abnormalities of the urinary tract are present in 20% of pregnant women with asymptomatic bacteriuria, although the association in some is incidental.

Acute pyelonephritis

Ureteric dilatation may increase susceptibility to pyelonephritis in pregnancy; despite routine screening it still complicates 1% of pregnancies (3% in unscreened populations). High fever (often fluctuating), vomiting, rigors and severe loin pain are common findings, but may be absent in the early stages. Diagnosis should be supported by urine microscopy and culture. Severe infections can have serious sequelae, including septic shock, adult respiratory distress syndrome and perinephritic abscess formation (Cunningham & Lucas 1994; Shieve et al 1994).

In pregnancy, the differential diagnosis is similar to that in non-pregnant subjects but, in addition, loin pain may be due to an acute hydroureter/ hydronephrosis (see later) or it may be referred from the lumbosacral vertebra or sacroiliac joints (due to increased lumbar lordosis and softening of pelvic ligaments). Abdominal pain may also be due to abruptio placentae, degenerating fibroids, chorioamnionitis or acute appendicitis, the latter presenting atypically in late pregnancy when the uterus is maximally enlarged (Twickler et al 1994).

Treatment should be aggressive and undertaken in hospital. Fluid and electrolye balance should be monitored and intravenous fluids given to correct hypovolaemia. Fetal tachycardia is common, making fetal heart monitoring difficult to interpret. There is a risk of premature labour, although prevention by treatment with β-sympathomimetics may exacerbate endotoxin-induced cardiovascular effects and increase the risk of respiratory complications. A penicillin or cephalosporin should be administered intravenously pending confirmation of organism sensitivity and oral therapy continued for 2 weeks. Failure to respond to treatment may indicate an underlying pelvi-ureteric or ureteric obstruction or the presence of calculi and warrants further investigation.

If Gram-negative sepsis is suspected, blood cultures should be taken and an aminoglycoside (gentamycin or tobramycin) added to the regimen, although the newer penicillins appear to be equally effective with reduced risk to the fetus. Blood levels of an aminoglycoside should be monitored, since its clearance is altered in pregnancy.

HYDROURETER/HYDRONEPHROSIS

Ureteropelvic dilatation is common in pregnancy and may cause loin pain. Urine microscopy demonstrates few or no red cells, repeat urine cultures are negative and the diagnosis is confirmed by ultrasound. Positioning the patient in the knee–chest position may relieve discomfort and promote spontaneous drainage. Rarely is ureteric catheterization (stenting) or nephrostomy necessary to preserve renal function, unless there is a solitary kidney (Davison 1998).

UROLITHIASIS (RENAL TRACT CALCULI)

Interestingly, whilst the factors associated with renal stone formation are known to increase in pregnancy, namely, urinary stasis, ascending infections and excretion of stone forming salts (e.g. calcium, urate and cystine), the incidence of renal calculi is low (1 in 2000 pregnancies; Maikranz et al 1994). Furthermore, pregnancy does not appear to increase symptomatic calculi in known 'stone formers'. Enhanced excretion of inhibitors of calcium stone formation such as magnesium, citrate and nephrocalcin as well as increased alkalinity of the urine afford some protection.

The presentation of renal calculi is similar to that in non-pregnant subjects. Most ureteric colic occurs in the second or third trimester when ureteric dilatation is greatest and perhaps previously asymptomatic stones pass into the ureter, only to become stuck at the pelvic brim. The mainstay of diagnosis of calculi is ultrasound. Asymmetry of ureteral jets, manifesting as absence of flow or sluggish continuous flow from the affected side, implies ureteral calculi (Asrat et al 1998). Interpretation of findings and visualization of the ureter can be difficult but may be enhanced with colour flow Doppler scanning. Radiological examination is undesirable because of potential effects on the fetus, although limited exposure may be warranted. Renal function should be assessed and infection excluded but any in-depth analysis of urine and serum biochemistry to determine the cause of stone formation should be delayed until well after delivery, when non-pregnant 'norms' can be applied.

Conservative management is usually successful or delivery can be effected before undertaking surgical or minimally invasive intervention. Any definitive surgery should be delayed until at least 4 months post-delivery. The safety of lithotripsy has not been validated in pregnancy. Drugs used to treat 'stone formers' (thiazides, xanthine oxidase inhibitors, D-penicillamine) are best avoided.

CHRONIC RENAL DISEASE

In general, fertility and the ability to sustain an uncomplicated pregnancy are linked to the degree of functional impairment and the presence, or not, of hypertension rather than to the renal pathology *per se* (Davison & Baylis 1998). This is best considered, albeit arbitrarily, by assignment of women to one of three categories (1) *preserved or only mildly impaired renal function* (serum creatinine ≤ 125 μmol/l) and no hypertension, (2) *moderate renal insufficiency* [serum creatinine 133–275 μmol/l (some use 221 μmol/l as the upper limit)] and (3) *severe renal insufficiency* (serum creatinine ≥ 275 μmol/l).

Women in the first category usually have successful obstetric outcomes and pregnancy does not appear to affect adversely the underlying disease; perinatal mortality in this group is now less than 3% and irreversible renal functional loss in the mother is negligible. This generalization, however, may not hold true for certain kidney diseases: for instance, patients with scleroderma and periarteritis nodosa, disorders often associated with hypertension, do poorly, and pregnancy is best discouraged. Women with lupus nephritis do not do well as patients with primary glomerulopathies, especially if the disease has flared within 6 months of conception. Although there is still controversy about whether or not pregnancy adversely affects the natural history of IgA nephritis, focal glomerular sclerosis, membranoproliferative nephritis, and reflux nephropathy, the current view is that there is little supporting evidence for an ill-effect (Lindheimer & Katz 1994).

Overall across the three categories, the more the dysfunction (with or without hypertension), the worse are outcomes in terms of obstetric success and

Table 40.1 Categories of renal disease and outcome for pregnancy.

Prospects	Category		
	Mild	Moderate	Severe
Pregnancy complications (%)	26	47	86
Successful obstetric outcome (%)	96(85)	90(69)	75(71)
Long-term sequelae (%)	<3 (9)	25(71)	53(92)

Estimates are based on 2477 women/3602 pregnancies (1973–1997) and do not include collagen diseases. Numbers in parentheses refer to prospects when complication(s) develop before 28 weeks' gestation (Davison & Baylis 1998 and unpublished data).

maternal prognosis (Table 40.1) (Jungers et al 1995, Abe 1997, 1996, Holley et al 1996, Jones & Hayslett 1996). The following issues are important, in addition to the routine antenatal care provision and specific considerations for particular diseases (Table 40.2).

Blood pressure

During pregnancy most of the specific risks of hypertension appear to be related to superimposed pre-eclampsia (Lindheimer 1996). The true incidence of superimposed pre-eclampsia in women with pre-existing renal disease is difficult to establish because diagnosis cannot be made with certainty on clinical grounds alone; hypertension and proteinuria may be manifestations of the underlying renal disease (Sibai 1996). What is known, however, is that hypertension is a major factor in fetal prognosis, with the relative risk of fetal loss being ten times greater when hypertension is present pre-pregnancy or in early pregnancy then when blood pressure in spontaneously normal or well controlled (Jungers et al 1997). Indeed, whilst treatment of mild hypertension (diastolic blood pressure below 95 mmHg in the second trimester or less than 100 mmHg in the third) is not necessary during normal pregnancy, many would treat women with underlying renal disease more aggressively, believing that this improves obstetric outcome and preserves kidney function (Baksis 1996).

Renal function

If renal function deteriorates significantly, then reversible causes, such as urinary infection, subtle dehydration and/or electrolyte imbalance (occasionally precipitated by inadvertent diuretic therapy) should be sought (Lindheimer & Katz 1994). Near term, as in normal pregnancy, a decrease in function of 15–20%, which affects serum creatinine minimally, is permissible. Failure to detect a reversible cause of a significant decrement is a reason to deliver. When proteinuria occurs and persists, but blood pressure is normal and renal function preserved, pregnancy can be allowed to continue.

Antenatal surveillance and timing of delivery

Serial fetal monitoring is essential since renal disease can be associated with intrauterine growth retardation. When complications do arise, the correct moment for intervention must be judged in relation to fetal status. (The same applies to dialysis and transplant patients.) Current technology should minimize the incidence of intrauterine fetal death as well as neona-

Table 40.2 Specific renal diseases and pregnancy.

Renal disease	Effects and outcomes
Chronic glomerulonephritis	Usually no adverse effect in the absence of hypertension. One view is that glomerulonephritis is adversely affected by the coagulation changes of pregnancy. Urinary tract infections may occur more frequently
IgA nephropathy	Risks of uncontrolled and/or sudden escalating hypertension and worsening of renal function
Pyelonephritis	Bacteriuria in pregnancy can lead to exacerbation. Multiple organ system derangements may ensue including adult RDS
Reflux nephropathy	Risks of sudden escalating hypertension and worsening of renal function
Urolithiasis	Infections can be more frequent, but ureteral dilatation and stasis do not seem to affect natural history. Limited data on lithotripsy, thus best avoided
Polycystic disease	Functional impairment and hypertension usually minimal in childbearing years
Diabetic nephropathy	Usually no adverse effect on the renal lesion, but there is increased frequency of infection, oedema and/or pre-eclampsia
Systemic lupus erythematosus (SLE)	Controversial; prognosis most favourable if disease in remission >6 months prior to conception. Steroid dosage should be increased postpartum
Perarteritis nodosa	Fetal prognosis is dismal and maternal death often occurs
Scleroderma	If onset during pregnancy then can be rapid overall deterioration. Reactivation of quiescent scleroderma may occur postpartum
Previous urinary tract surgery	Might be associated with other malformations of the urogenital tract. Urinary tract infection common during pregnancy. Renal function may undergo reversible decrease. No significant obstructive problem but caesarean section often needed for abnormal presentation and/or to avoid disruption of the continence mechanism if artificial sphincter present. If caesarean section needed in patient with clam cystoplasty then classical approach may be advisable.
After nephrectomy, solitary kidney and pelvic kidney	Might be associated with other malformations of urogenital tract. Pregnancy well tolerated. Dystocia rarely occurs with pelvic kidney
Wegener's granulomatosis	Limited information. Proteinuria (± hypertension) is common. Immunosuppressives are safe but cytotoxic drugs are best avoided
Renal artery stenosis	May present as chronic hypertension or as recurrent isolated pre-eclampsia. If diagnosed then transluminal angioplasty can be undertaken in pregnancy if appropriate

tal morbidity and mortality. Preterm delivery may be needed if there is evidence of impending fetal death, if renal function deteriorates substantially, if uncontrollable hypertension supervenes or if eclampsia occurs.

Long-term outlook

With moderate or severe insufficiency, pregnancy-related loss of renal function occurs in up to 50% of women, of whom at least 10% progress rapidly post-delivery to endstage failure, most of them having had severe hypertension and heavy proteinuria pre-pregnancy (Jones & Hayslett 1996; Jungers et al 1997). Furthermore, there can be little doubt that a serum creatinine >250–300 μmol/l pre-pregnancy (corresponding to a creatinine clearance of ≤25 ml/min) implies a serious risk of both accelerated deterioration of maternal kidney function and unsuccessful fetal outcome (Jungers & Chauvean 1997).

Why does pregnancy exacerbate renal disease? It might be related to an increase in intraglomerular pressure as a mechanism to augment GFR and or be due to superimposition of platelet and fibrin deposition onto the already damaged kidney, along with microvascular coagulation and endothelial dysfunction as part of the pre-eclamptic process.

ACUTE OBSTETRIC RENAL FAILURE

Complications of pregnancy used to be a common cause of acute renal failure (ARF) but are now rare in western countries. Improved obstetric management, particularly of pre-eclampsia and acute haemorrhage, as well as liberalization of abortion laws, preventing the need for illegal procedures which may lead to sepsis, have dramatically reduced the incidence of ARF. Most cases are now related to pre-eclampsia and its complications, although any cause of ARF may arise in pregnancy (Pertuiset & Grünfeld 1994).

Acute tubular necrosis is usually the underlying lesion but a higher proportion are due to renal cortical necrosis than in non-pregnant subjects. Nevertheless, when ARF is associated with pregnancy-specific conditions such as pre-eclampsia and the Haemolysis, Elevated Liver enzymes and Low Platelets (HELLP) syndrome, spontaneous recovery can be surprisingly rapid following delivery.

Invariably pregnancy has advanced far enough for the fetus to be viable and coordination with the neonatal team allows optimal timing of delivery. In the obstetric setting, however, the current pregnancy may represent the best chance of perinatal success so, with the exclusion of pre-eclampsia, many would advocate early and frequent dialysis to prolong the pregnancy.

Pre-eclampsia

In this common condition, characterized by generalized vasoconstriction and often associated with minor renal dysfunction, ARF is rare unless there are other complications such as HELLP syndrome or abruptio placentae (Lindheimer 1996).

Uterine sepsis and pyelonephritis

Serious postpartum and post-abortion sepsis is now rare. Improved supportive therapy and evacuation of retained products of conception usually prevents serious sequelae. Clostridial infection can rapidly supervene, resulting in ARF, haemolysis, coagulopathy and hypocalcaemia, although death is usually due to overwhelming sepsis rather than renal failure. Surgical removal of the uterus is often recommended but some prefer conservative management, stating that complications make surgery too risky.

Acute primary pyelonephritis is rarely associated with renal dysfunction or ARF in non-pregnant women. In pregnancy, however, decrements in creatinine clearance are common and the risk of ARF appears to be greater, perhaps due to increased sensitivity of renal vasculature to bacterial endotoxins.

Acute fatty liver of pregnancy (AFLP)

This condition occurs in late pregnancy or early puerperium and is associated with severe hepatic dysfunction and coagulopathy. Renal dysfunction may be mild, although ARF is not uncommon. Despite its rarity, awareness of AFLP is essential as its initial presentation may be subtle (nausea, vomiting, mild jaundice) or complicated by other conditions such as pulmonary embolus (PE) in which case there may be rapid progress to severe maternal and fetal compromise. Mortality rates for both mother and baby have been quoted at greater than 70%, although nowadays earlier recognition and intervention has reduced mortality rates to less than 20%. Other causes of hepatic dysfunction must be excluded and delivery effected immediately, followed by maximal supportive care.

Idiopathic postpartum renal failure

Idiopathic postpartum renal failure is rare but is a recognized cause of ARF in the first few weeks following delivery. Its aetiology is obscure but there are histological similarities with haemolytic uraemic syndrome and malignant nephrosclerosis. The outcome is poor; few women make a complete recovery.

LONG-TERM DIALYSIS

Despite reduced libido and significant infertility, women on haemodialysis and peritoneal dialysis can conceive and must therefore use contraception if they wish to avoid pregnancy. Pregnancy is not common, with an incidence of 1–2% being quoted (Okundaye et al 1998), its true frequency is unknown because at least 30% of pregnancies end in early spontaneous abortion, there is a 10–15% therapeutic abortion rate and until recently the literature was skewed towards reporting success (Hou & Firanek 1998). Pregnancy is three times less common in peritoneal dialysis patients than in haemodialysis patients.

There has been a move away from thinking that pregnancy is a disastrous accident, with evidence accruing from specialist centres that pregnancy should be another goal of rehabilitation (Romaõ et al 1998). This is not to say, however, that these women will have non-hectic pregnancies: they are prone to volume overload, severe exacerbations of their hypertension and/or superimposed pre-eclampsia as well as polyhydramnios. They also have high fetal wastage at all stages in pregnancy. Even when therapeutic terminations are excluded, the live birth outcome at very best is 40–50% (Bagon et al 1998; Toma et al 1999).

Women frequently present for care in advanced pregnancy because pregnancy was not suspected. Irregular menstruation is common in dialysis patients and missed periods are usually ignored. Ultrasound is needed to confirm and date the pregnancy. It could be argued that peritoneal dialysis is the method of choice in pregnancy because, theoretically, it should maintain a more stable environment for the fetus in terms of fluid and electrolyte homeostasis and cardiovascular stability (Redrow et al 1988). Whatever the route, the dialysis strategy involves a 50% increase to more than 20 hours/week (Hou & Firanek 1998). There are several aims:

- To maintain serum urea < 20 mmol/l; some would argue < 15 mmol/l, as intrauterine death is more likely if levels are much in excess of 20 mmol/l. Success has occasionally been achieved despite levels of 25 mmol/l for many weeks.
- To avoid hypotension during dialysis, which could be damaging to the fetus. In late pregnancy the uterus and the supine posture may aggravate this by decreasing venous return.
- To maintain strict control of blood pressure.
- To avoid rapid fluctuations in intravascular volume, by limiting interdialysis weight gain to about 1 kg until late pregnancy.
- To scrutinize carefully for preterm labour, as dialysis and uterine contractions are associated.
- To monitor calcium levels closely to avoid hypercalcaemia.

Dialysis patients are usually anaemic which is invariably aggravated further in pregnancy. Blood transfusion may be needed, especially before delivery. Caution is necessary because transfusion may exacerbate hypertension and impair the ability to control circulatory overload even with extra dialysis. Treatment of anaemia with low dose synthetic erythropoietin (rHuEpo) has been used in pregnancy without ill-effect (McGregor et al 1991) and, indeed, requirements may double or triple. An interesting clinical point is that the need to increase rHuEpo dose in an otherwise stable patient may be a clue that she is pregnant (Maruyama & Arakawa 1997).

RENAL TRANSPLANTATION

Following a kidney transplant, renal, endocrine and sexual functions return rapidly (Davison 1995). About 1 in 50 women of childbearing age with a functioning transplant become pregnant. Of these, 35% do not go beyond the first trimester because of spontaneous or therapeutic abortion, but 95% of pregnancies that do continue end successfully (Table 40.3).

A woman should be counselled from the onset of her renal failure when the potential for optimal rehabilitation is discussed (Davison 1994). Couples who want a child should be encouraged to discuss all the implications, including the harsh realities of maternal survival prospects (London et al 1995). In most patients, a wait of 18 months to 2 years post-transplant is advised, by which time she will have recovered from the surgery, graft function will have stabilized and immunosuppression will be at mainte-

Table 40.3 Pregnancy implications for renal transplant recipients.

Problems in pregnancy	Successful obstetric outcome	Long-term problems
49%	95%(70%)	12%(25%)

Estimates based on 3690 women in 4680 pregnancies which attained at least 28 weeks gestation (1961–1966). Figures in brackets refer to implications when complication(s) developed prior to 28 weeks' gestation (Davison & Baylis 1998, and unpublished data).

nance levels. Also, if function is well maintained at 2 years, there is a high probability of allograft survival at 5 years. Table 40.4 lists a suitable set of guidelines, with emphasis on the fact that the criteria are relative.

In most pregnancies renal function is augmented. Towards term there may be transient deterioration (with or without proteinuria) and in 15% of women there is a slight but permanent functional loss afterwards. Despite an overall complication rate of 46%, the chances of success are 95%, reduced to 75% if complications (usually hypertension, renal deterioration and/or rejection) occur before 28 weeks. There is a 30% chance of developing hypertension, pre-eclampsia or both. Preterm delivery occurs in 40–60% and intrauterine growth retardation in at least 20–40% of pregnancies (Toma et al 1999). Despite its pelvic location, the graft rarely produces dystocia and is not injured during vaginal delivery. Caesarean section should be reserved for obstetric reasons only.

Neonatal complications include respiratory distress syndrome, leukopenia, thrombocytopenia, adrenocortical insufficiency and infection. More information is needed about the intrauterine effects and neonatal aftermath of immunosuppression which, at maintenance levels, is apparently harmless.

More information is needed about the intrauterine effects and neonatal aftermath of immunosuppression which, at maintenance levels, appears to be harmless (Ghandour et al 1998). Many of the data relate to azathioprine (Imuran®) and steroids, with problems being minimal. There are now more reports on pregnancies in women taking cyclosporin (Sandimmune®) and although numerous adverse effects are attributed to this drug in the non-pregnant, the overall pregnancy success rates are compatible with routine immunosuppression. Of importance is that blood cyclosporin levels may decrease at the beginning of the second trimester, necessitating an increased dosage, with return to pre-pregnancy dosage following delivery to avoid the dangers of toxicity. A new cyclosporin preparation (Neoral®) apparently has improved bioavailability, enabling easier maintenance

Table 40.4 Guidelines for pre-pregnancy counselling for renal transplant patients.

- Good general health for about 2 years after transplantation
- Stature compatible with good obstetric outcome
- No or minimal proteinuria
- No hypertension. Due to high incidence of hypertension in women on cyclosporin well controlled hypertension is perhaps more appropriate
- No evidence of graft rejection
- No pelvi-calcyeal distension apparent on a recent intravenous urogram or ultrasonography
- Stable renal function with plasma creatinine of 180 μmol/l (2 mg/dl) and preferably <125 μmol/l (4.4 mg/dl)
- Drug therapy reduced to maintenance levels: prednisone, 15 mg/day or less, and azathioprine, 2 mg/kg/day or less

of blood drug concentration in the therapeutic range.

Data are not yet available for tacrolimus (FK506/Progref®), mycophenolate (MMF/Cell Cept®), antithymocytic globulin (ATG/Atgam®) and orthoclone (OKT3®) but good outcomes in liver recipients have been reported (Jain et al 1997). As little is known about the excretion or biological significance of immunosuppressive agents in breast milk (which does of course confer many benefits), breastfeeding is usually discouraged.

There are data to indicate that pregnancy does not compromise long-term renal prognosis (First et al 1995; Sturgiss & Davison 1995) and that repeated pregnancies do not adversely affect graft function, provided renal function is well preserved prior to pregnancy (Ehrich et al 1996). Another long-term consideration is that these patients, like others on immunosuppression, have a malignancy rate many times greater than normal (Opelz 1996) and genital tract malignancies are no exception.

Transplantation medicine is changing rapidly nowadays (Knoll & Bell 1999) and the only logical way of studying all types of outcome with post-transplant pregnancies will involve the establishment of a UK National Registry (Davison & Redman 1997), akin to that operational in the US since 1991, which has accrued information from almost 800 pregnancies (Armenti et al 1995, 1998; Gaughan et al 1996).

REFERENCES

Abe S 1996 Pregnancy in glomerulonephritic patients with decreased renal function. Hypertension in Pregnancy 15: 305–312

Armenti V T, Stefanosky E V, Cater J R, McGory C H, Radomski J S, Mortiz M J 1995 Pregnancy in transplant recipients. Journal of Transplant Coordination 5: 130–136

Armenti V T, Moritz M J, Davison J M 1998 Medical management of the pregnant transplant recipient. Advances in Renal Repair Therapy 5: 14–23

Asrat T, Roossin M C, Miller E I 1998 Ultrasonographic detection of ureteral jets in normal pregnancy. American Journal of Obstetrics and Gynecology 178: 1194–1198

Bagon J A, Vernaeve H, De Muylder X, Lafountaine J J, Martens J, Van Roost G 1998 Pregnancy and dialysis. American Journal of Kidney Diseases 31: 756–765

Baksis G L 1996 Is the level of arterial pressure reduction important for preservation of renal function. Nephrology Dialysis and Transplantation 11: 2383–2397

Baylis C 1994 Glomerular filtration and volume regulation in gravid animal models. In: Lindheimer M D, Davison J M (eds) Bailliere's Clinical Obstetrics and Gynaecology Vol 8 (2) Bailliere Tindall, London, pp 235–264

Baylis C, Davison J M 1998 The normal renal physiological changes which occur during pregnancy. In: Davison A M, Cameron J S, Grünfeld J-P, Kerr D N S, Ritz E (eds) Oxford Textbook of Clinical Nephrology, 2nd edn. Oxford University Press, Oxford pp 2297–2315

Cunningham F G, Lucas M J 1994 Urinary tract infections complicating pregnancy. In: Lindheimer M D, Davison J M (eds) Bailliere's Clinical Obstetrics and Gynaecology Vol 8(2) Bailliere Tindall, London, pp 353–373

Davison J M 1994 Pregnancy in renal allograft recipients: problems, prognosis and practicalities. Bailliere's Clinical Obstetrics and Gynaecology 8: 501–525.

Davison J M 1995 Towards longterm graft survival in renal transplantation: pregnancy. Nephrology Dialysis and Transplantation 10 (Suppl 1): 85–89

Davison J M, Redman C W G 1997 Pregnancy post-transplant: the establishment of a UK registry. British Journal of Obstetrics and Gynaecology 104, 1106–1107

Davison J M 1998 Renal complications which can occur in pregnancy. In: Davison A M, Cameron J S, Grünfeld J-P, Kerr D N S, Ritz E (eds) Oxford Textbook of Clinical Nephrology, 2nd edn. Oxford University Press, Oxford pp 2317–2325

Davison J M, Baylis C 1998 Pregnancy in patients with underlying renal disease. In: Davison A M, Cameron J S, Grünfeld J-P, Kerr D N S, Ritz E (eds) Oxford Textbook of Clinical Nephrology (2E), Oxford University Press, Oxford, pp 2327–2348

Ehrich J H H, Loirat C, Davison J M, Rizzoni G, Wittkop B, Selwood N H, Mallick N P 1996 Repeated successful pregnancies after kidney transplantation in 102 women. Nephrology Dialysis and Transplantation 11: 1314–1317.

First M R, Combs C A, Weiskittel P, Miodovinik M 1995 Lack of effect of pregnancy on renal allograft survival or function. Transplantation 59: 472–477

Ghandour F Z, Krauss T C, Hricik D E 1998 Immunosuppressive drugs in pregnancy. Advances in Renal Repair Therapy 5: 31–37

Gaughan W J, Moritz M J, Radomski J S, Burke J F, Armenti V T 1996 National Transplantation Pregnancy Registry – Report on outcomes in cyclosporine-treated female kidney transplant recipients with an interval from transplant to pregnancy of greater than 5 years. American Journal of Kidney Diseases 28: 266–269

Holley J L, Bernardini J, Quadri K H M, Greenberg A, Laifer S A 1996 Pregnancy outcomes in a prospective matched control study of pregnancy and renal disease. Clinical Nephrology 45: 77–82

Hou S H 1996 Pregnancy in women treated with peritoneal dialysis: viewpoint. Peritoneal Dialysis International 16: 442–443

Hou S H, Firanek C 1998. Management of the pregnant dialysis patient. Advances in Renal Repair Therapy 5: 24–30

Jain A, Venkataramanan R, Fung J J et al 1997 Pregnancy after liver transplantation under tacrolimus. Transplantation 64: 559–565

Jones D C, Hayslett J P 1996 Outcome of pregnancy in women with moderate or severe renal insufficiency. New England Journal of Medicine 335: 226–232

Jungers P, Chauveau D 1997 Pregnancy in renal disease. Kidney International 52: 871–885

Jungers P, Houillier P, Forget D, Labrunie M, Skkiri H, Giatras I, Descamps-Latscha B 1995 Influence of pregnancy on the course of primary chronic glomerulonephritis. Lancet 346: 1122–24

Jungers P, Chauveau D, Choukronn G et al 1997 Pregnancy in women with impaired renal function. Clinical Nephrology 47: 281–288

Knoll G A, Bell R C 1999 Tacrolimus versus cyclosporin for immunosuppression in renal transplantation: meta-analysis of randomised trials. British Medical Journal 318: 1104–1107

Lindheimer M D 1996 Pre-eclampsia – eclampsia 1996: preventable? Have the disputes on its treatment been resolved? Current Opinion in Nephrology and Hypertension 5: 452–458

Lindheimer M D, Katz A I 1994 Gestation in women with kidney disease: prognosis and management. Bailliere's Clinical Obstetrics and Gynaecology 8: 387–404

London N, Farmery S M, Will E J, Davison A M, Lodge J P A 1995 Risk of neoplasia in renal transplant patients. Lancet 346: 403–406

McGladdery S L, Aparicio S, Verrier-Jones K 1992 Outcome of pregnancy in an Oxford/Cardiff cohort of women with previous bacteriuria. Quarterly Journal of Medicine 303: 533–539

McGregor E, Stewart G, Junor B J R, Rodger R S C 1991 Successful use of recombinant human erythropoietin in pregnancy. Nephrology Dialysis and Transplantation 6: 292–293

Maikranz P, Lindheimer M D, Coe F 1994 Nephrolithiasis in pregnancy. Bailliere's Clinical Obstetrics and Gynaecology 375–386

Maruyama H, Arakawa M 1997 Diagnostic clue to pregnancy in hemodialysis patients: progressive anemia resistant to erythropoietin. Journal of the American Society of Nephrology 8: A1130

Okundaye I B, Abrinko P, Hou S H 1998 Registry of pregnancy in dialysis patients. American Journal of Kidney Diseases 31: 766–773

Opelz G 1996 Are post-transplant lymphomas inevitable? Nephrology Dialysis and Transplantation 11: 1952–1955

Pertuiset N, Grunfeld J P 1994 Acute renal failure in pregnancy. Bailliere's Clinical Obstetrics and Gynaecology 8: 333–351

Sturgiss S N, Davison J M 1995 Effect of pregnancy on long-term function of renal allografts. American Journal of Kidney Diseases 26: 54–56

Redrow M, Chereum L, Elliott J et al 1988 Dialysis in the management of pregnant patients with renal insufficiency. Medicine 67: 199–208

Romão J E, Luders C, Kahhale S et al 1998 Pregnancy in women on chronic dialysis. Nephron 78: 416–422

Shieve L A, Handler A, Hershow R, Persky V Davis F 1994 Urinary tract infections during pregnancy: its association with maternal morbidity and perinatal outcome. Obstetrical and Gynecological Survey 49: 596–597

Sibai B H 1996 Treatment of hypertension in pregnant women. New England Journal of Medicine 335: 257–264

Stein G, Funfstuck R 1999 Asymptomatic bacteriuria – what to do. Nephrology, Dialysis and Transplantation 14: 1618–1621

Sturgiss S N, Dunlop W, Davison J M 1994 Renal haemodynamics and tubular function in human pregnancy. Bailliere's Clinical Obstetrics and Gynaecology 8: 209–234

Toma H, Tanabe K, Tokumoto T, Kobayashi C, Yagisawa T 1999 Pregnancy in women receiving dialysis or transplantation in Japan: a nationwide survey. Nephrology, Dialysis and Transplantation 14: 1511–1516

Twickler D M, Lucas M J, Bowe L et al 1994 Ultrasonic evaluation of central and end-organ hemodynamics in antepartum pyelonephritis. American Journal of Obstetrics and Gynecology 170: 814–818

Lower urinary tract in pregnancy

ALFRED CUTNER AND RICHARD KERR-WILSON

INTRODUCTION

Earlier reviews (Brown 1978, 1981; Marchant 1978; Waltzer 1981) have tended to concentrate on pathological effects of pregnancy. This chapter will review the physiological and pathophysiological changes that take place in the lower urinary tract during pregnancy.

ANTENATAL

Urinary symptoms and their aetiology

Frequency

One of the earliest symptoms of pregnancy is urinary frequency. This may be noticed even before the first missed period. There have been several published reports (Francis 1960a; Parboosingh & Doig 1973a, 1973b; Stanton et al 1980; Cutner et al 1992a, 1992b; Cutner 1993) on the prevalence of frequency and nocturia but different authors have used varying definitions and this may reflect the difference in findings.

The first large-scale study of bladder function in pregnancy was by Francis (1960a). She assessed 400 women and defined frequency as at least 7 daytime voids and 1 nighttime void. Fifty-nine point five percent experienced frequency of micturition in early pregnancy, 61% in mid-pregnancy and 81% in late pregnancy. She found the prevalence increased as pregnancy progressed. Parboosingh & Doig (1973a) defined nocturia as voiding at least three nights in a week. In their cross-sectional study, they found a prevalence of 58% in the first trimester, 57% in the second trimester and 66% in the third trimester. Most of their patients accepted nocturia as being a normal feature of pregnancy and less than 4% were actually distressed by it.

Stanton et al (1980) defined frequency as seven or more daytime voids and nocturia as two or more nighttime voids. Although frequency was more common in nulliparous than multiparous women, this difference was only significant at 38 weeks and 40 weeks of gestation (Fig. 41.1). Cutner et al (1992a) and

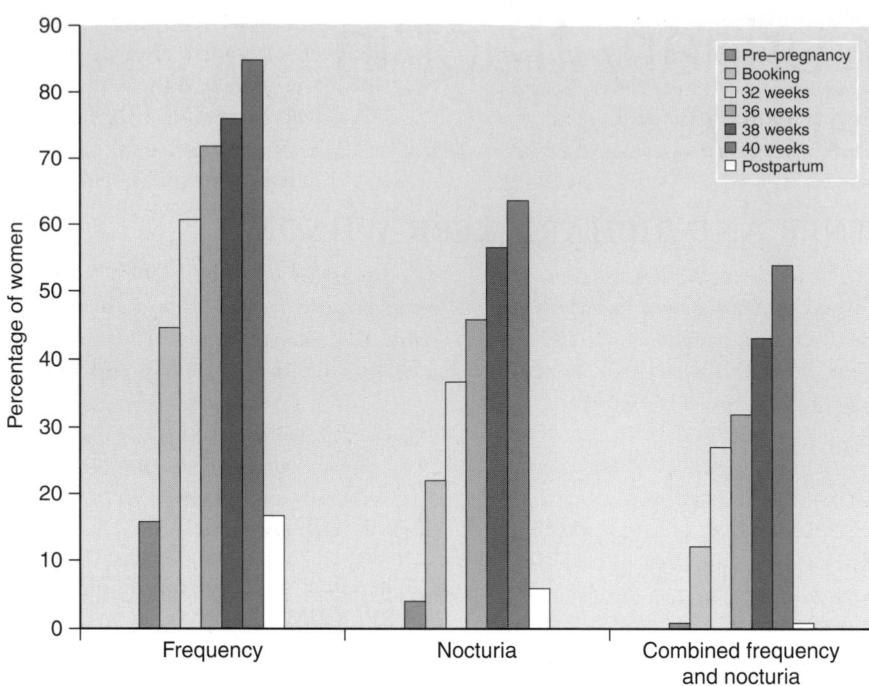

Fig. 41.1 Frequency and nocturia in pregnancy. From Stanton et al (1980), with permission.

Cutner (1993) found that 43% of women complained of diurnal frequency and 34% of nocturia in early pregnancy; 91% overall complained of an increased voiding pattern. In addition, Cutner (1993) looked at the effect of parity and race on voiding patterns in early pregnancy and found an increased prevalence of frequency in black, nulliparous women compared to white, nulliparous women and an increased prevalence of nocturia in black parous women compared to white parous women.

Both Stanton et al (1980) and Cutner (1993) found no relationship between engagement of the fetal head and frequency in the last 4 weeks of pregnancy. However, Cutner (1993) demonstrated that although increased voiding patterns tend to resolve, those women who suffer a worse increase in their number of voids during pregnancy are more likely to suffer from these symptoms postpartum. It has been demonstrated that increased voiding correlates with both increased fluid intake and increased urine output (Francis 1960a; Parboosingh & Doig 1973a; Cutner 1993) but whether increased urine output follows increased fluid intake or vice versa is unknown.

Parboosingh & Doig (1973a, 1973b) suggest that increased sodium excretion at night results in increased urine production, leading to nocturia. Nocturnal urine production decreases in the third trimester but decreased bladder capacity at this stage of pregnancy prevents improvement in nocturia. Francis (1960a) and Cutner (1993) have shown no correlation between the maximum volume of urine voided and diurnal frequency and nocturia. However, nighttime voiding at all stages of pregnancy is a function of the number of hours spent in bed (Cutner et al 1992a, 1992b; Cutner 1993). Cutner (1993) demonstrated a correlation between the maximum voided volumes and the first sensation and bladder capacity. In addition, urodynamic studies demonstrated that women with low compliance had a reduced first sensation and a reduced bladder capacity. If the number of voids is related to the first sensation and bladder capacity, which in turn is related to the presence of low compliance, one might expect that this effect would be more marked in the day than at night when the uterus would no longer have such a marked pressure effect on the bladder. Thus, whether or not pressure from an enlarged uterus results in frequency remains controversial (Shutter 1922; Hundley et al 1938; Malpas et al 1949; Francis 1960a; Langer et al 1990).

Stress incontinence

Stress incontinence is associated with increased parity but whether pregnancy itself or childbirth is the primary cause remains in doubt. There have been four prospective studies of the symptom of stress incontinence in pregnancy (Francis 1960b; Stanton et al 1980; Cutner 1993; Viktrup et al 1992).

Francis (1960b) found that 53% of nulliparous

women and 84% of multiparous women complained of the symptoms of stress incontinence antenatally and that it rarely occurred for the first time postpartum. This is in agreement with other studies (Stanton et al 1980; Cutner 1993; Viktrup et al 1992). The prevalence of stress incontinence is shown in Figure 41.2.

Beck & Hsu (1965) looked at 1000 women retrospectively who were attending their gynaecological out-patient clinic. Thirty-one per cent admitted to the symptom of stress incontinence and, of the 246 women whose stress incontinence was associated with the previous pregnancy, 82% said it first occurred antenatally.

Iosif (Iosif 1981; Iosif & Ingemarsson 1982) performed two retrospective studies and concluded that pregnancy was the cause of this symptom rather than delivery. They found no significant difference between women with stress incontinence and continent controls with respect to the duration of labour, mode of delivery or infant weight. In addition they found that the incidence of stress incontinence in the mothers of patients with stress incontinence was five times greater than in the control group.

Stoner et al (1994) reported that caesarean section protected against the development of stress incontinence and that having a mother who complained of stress incontinence was associated with an increased risk.

Wilson et al (1996), in a postal questionnaire study, found a significant reduction in the prevalence of incontinence for women after their first caesarean section; however there was little difference between elective caesarean section or emergency caesarean in the first or second stage. In addition, the prevalence of incontinence was similar between those women having three or more caesarean sections and those women delivered vaginally. These studies suggest that pregnancy and hereditary factors are more influential in causing permanent stress incontinence than childbirth itself. However, the symptom of stress incontinence is not synonymous with a diagnosis of genuine stress incontinence, i.e. urethral sphincter weakness. Cutner (1993) has demonstrated a significant correlation between the length of the first stage of labour and the degree of the symptom of stress incontinence postnatally.

The possibility of a predisposition has been substantiated by King & Freeman (1996) who performed perineal ultrasound scans in 128 primigravid women antenatally and again 10–14 weeks postnatally. They found a significant increase in bladder neck mobility antenatally in those women who subsequently experienced postpartum stress incontinence compared with the continent postpartum group.

Retention of urine

The classic cause of urinary retention in early pregnancy is incarceration of the retroverted uterus at

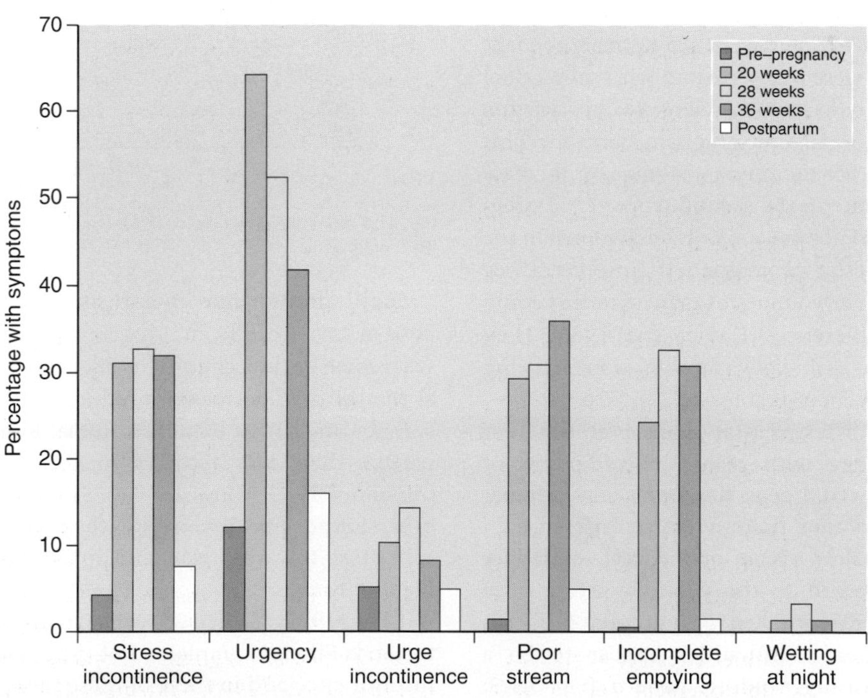

Fig. 41.2 Lower urinary tract symptoms in pregnancy. From Cutner (1993), with permission.

12–14 weeks gestation. This has been attributed to mechanical pressure on the bladder neck with elongation of the urethra. However, there is little difficulty in passing a catheter in these cases. Therefore it is unlikely that the retertion is caused by direct pressure of the uterus on the bladder neck or urethra. In addition, Francis (1960a) examined the radiographs of six women who had urethrocystography carried out at the time of retention. She demonstrated that there is no elongation of the urethra and no elevation of the urethrovesical junction in these patients. She suggested that retention is caused by the retroverted uterus interfering with the normal opening mechanism of the internal urethral meatus. Once retention has been present for some time, oedema of the bladder neck may make it difficult to pass a catheter as a secondary effect.

Prophylaxis includes resting in a prone or semi-prone position. Once retention has occurred, the bladder should be kept empty and if the uterus still remains retroverted in the pelvis, gentle vaginal or rectal manipulation should be tried. If this is unsuccessful it is suggested that pressure should be exerted on the fundus while traction is applied to the anterior lip of the cervix, with the patient in the knee–chest position (Myerscough 1982).

Urodynamics

There have been two studies on uroflowmetry in pregnancy. Fischer & Kittel (1990) measured the peak flow rate and volume voided at different stages of pregnancy in 290 women. There were 128 normal pregnancies and 103 who were being treated with salbutamol for premature labour. There were 46 postpartum women and 19 normal non-pregnant controls. This study concluded that there was a significant increase in the peak flow rate in the second trimester of pregnancy compared to normal controls and women in the first or third trimester of pregnancy. However, these women passed larger volumes of urine and this could account for the differences (Haylen et al 1989). They also found lower peak flow rates in women being treated with intravenous tocolytics.

Cutner (1993) assessed 400 women at different stages of pregnancy with regard to symptoms of voiding difficulties and peak flow rates and volumes voided. He found that there was no difference in the symptoms of slow stream or incomplete bladder emptying with regard to the peak flow rate once the volume voided was taken into account. Indeed, symptoms of voiding difficulties appear to be a function of increasing voiding pattern (Fig. 41.3; Table 41.1)

Table 41.1 Equations for the peak flow rate and average flow rate in pregnancy.

$$\text{Ln (peak flow rate)} = 0.140 + 0.587 \times \text{Ln (volume)}$$
[Root mean square error = 0.358]

$$\text{Square root (average flow rate)} = -1.140 + 0.957 \times \text{Ln (volume)}$$
[Root mean square error = 0.560]

From Cutner (1993), with permission.

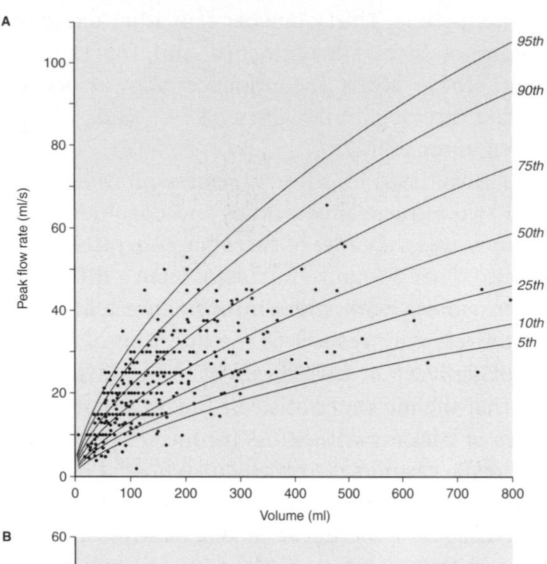

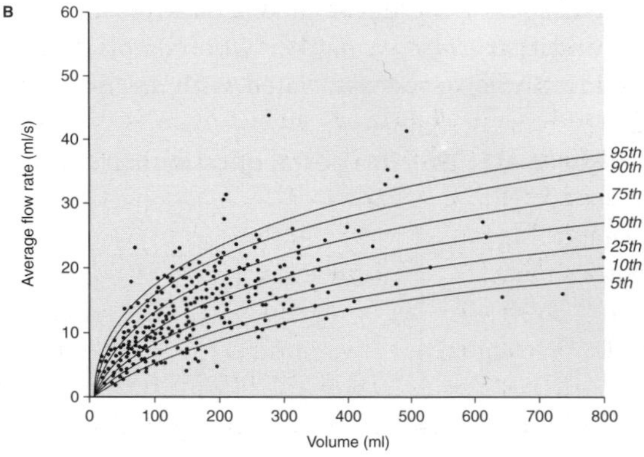

Fig. 41.3 Nomograms for the peak flow rate (**A**) and average flow rate (**B**) in pregnancy.

Early urodynamic investigations utilized simple cystometry. Results in pregnancy were conflicting, with some authors finding evidence of bladder atony at the third trimester with reduced intravesical pressure for any given bladder volume. By 6 weeks postpartum there was a return to normal bladder tone (Muellner 1939; Youssef 1956). Francis (1960b), however, found the reverse, with decreasing bladder capacities towards term and evidence of increased bladder tone.

Clow (1975) studied 25 women with subtracted cystometry. Fifteen complained of the symptom of stress incontinence and in three of these there was evidence of detrusor instability which improved postpartum.

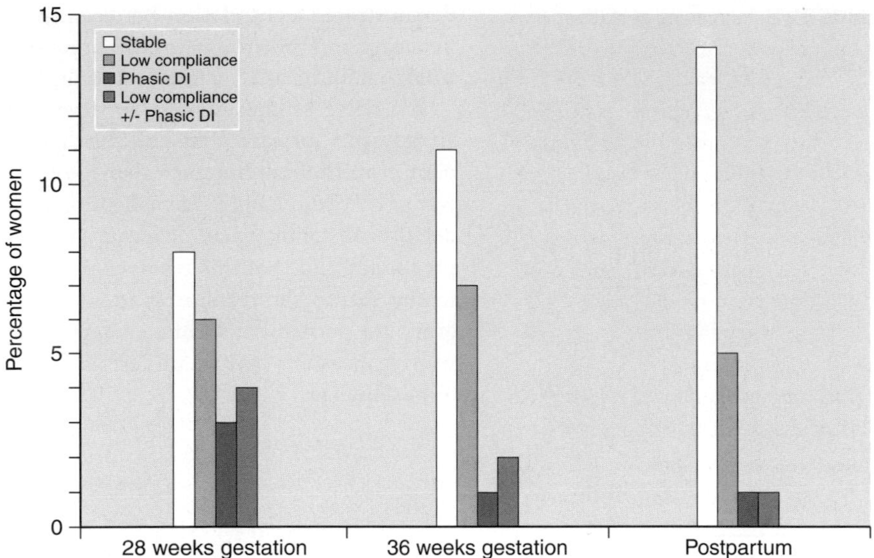

Fig. 41.4 Detrusor instability in pregnancy. From Cutner & Cardozo (1996), with permission.

Cutner (Cutner et al 1990; Cutner et al 1991; Cutner et al 1992b; Cutner 1993; Cutner & Cardozo 1996) found poor correlation between lower urinary tract symptoms and urodynamic investigations in pregnancy. There was evidence of increased detrusor instability in pregnancy which appeared to resolve postpartum (Fig. 41.4). In early pregnancy, women with low compliance had an earlier first sensation to void compared with women with a stable bladder, and they had a lower bladder capacity compared to those women with detrusor instability or a stable bladder. In addition, women with phasic detrusor instability had an increased prevalence of urethral instability in pregnancy. These findings would suggest that the two conditions (low compliance and phasic detrusor instability) may well have different aetiologies in pregnancy although in the non-pregnant state they may lead to similar symptomatology.

Iosif (Iosif et al 1980; Iosif & Ulmsten 1981) performed simultaneous urethrocystometry in pregnant women who complained of the symptom of stress incontinence and those who did not. They found differences in maximum urethral closure pressure and functional urethral length between the two groups (Fig. 41.5). This is in agreement with Cutner (1993) who also found that black women compared to white women had greater maximum urethral closure pressure, maximum urethral pressure, functional urethral length and anatomical urethral length in pregnancy compared to white women. In the asymptomatic women Iosif (Iosif et al 1980) found a rise in bladder pressure from the 12th to the 38th weeks of pregnancy which was compensated for by a corresponding increase in urethral closure pressure and ensured continence.

Van Geelen et al (1982) repeated similar work to Iosif in 43 pregnant women (see Fig. 41.5). Although they found increases in maximum urethral pressure and urethral length and bladder pressure, they failed to show increases in maximum urethral closure pressure or functional urethral length with increasing gestation. However, their data included 12 women who complained of the symptom of stress incontinence.

Postpartum, van Geelen et al (1982) found urethral length and pressure measurements decreased significantly after vaginal delivery, which was in contrast to 6 women who were delivered by caesarean section before or early in labour. In the latter group, the urethral length parameters were similar to those in nulliparous women and in early pregnancy, although the urethral pressures were still reduced. One woman was delivered by caesarean section late in the second stage after a failed attempt at vacuum extraction and in this case the postpartum changes were similar to those observed in the vaginal delivery group. The postpartum changes observed after vaginal delivery were not influenced by the duration of the second stage, the presence or absence of episiotomy; nor were they related to the weight of the infant.

Iosif et al (1981) compared two groups of patients with urinary incontinence during pregnancy or immediately after childbirth and carried out simultaneous urethrocystometry 7–14 days after delivery. The first group had only occasional urine leakage but the second reported more severe and prolonged stress incontinence. In the first group they found that urethral length

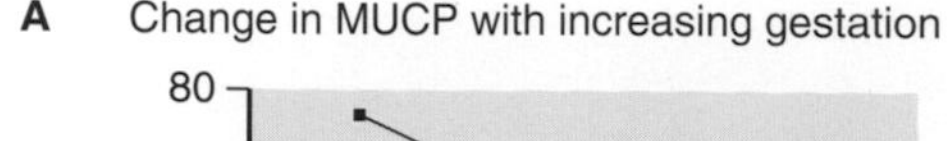

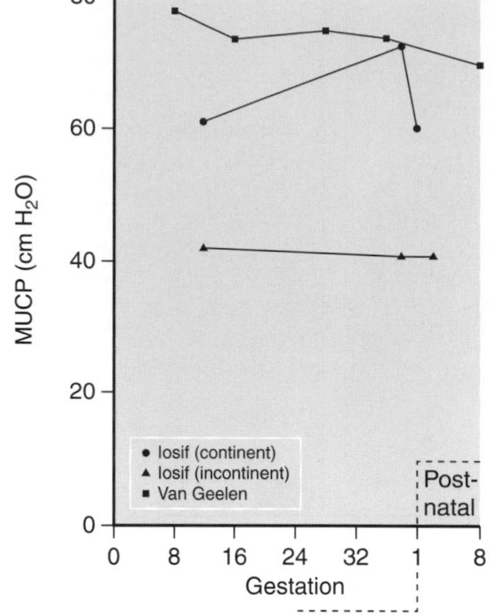

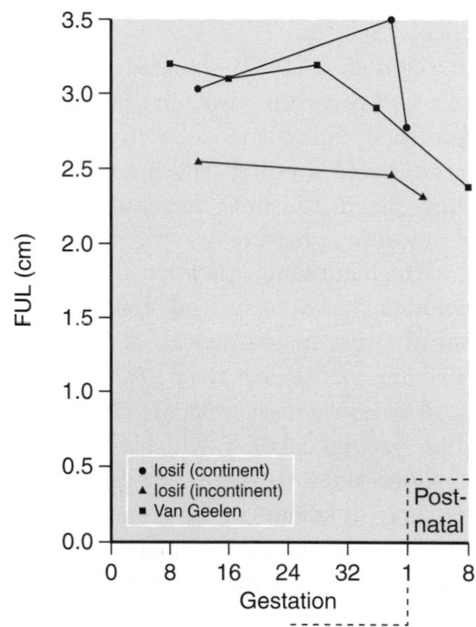

Fig. 41.5 Urethral pressure profile parameters in pregnancy. (**A**) Change in MUCP with increasing gestation. (**B**) Change in FUL with increasing gestation. MUCP: Maximum urethral closure pressure; FUL: Functional urethral length. From the studies by Iosif et al 1980; Iosif & Ulmsten 1981; van Geel et al 1982, with permisison.

and pressures were similar to continent females. The second group had negative cough pressure profiles, with shorter urethral lengths and lower resting pressures than the first group. They postulated that the incontinence in the first group may merely be the result of pressure on the bladder by the pregnant uterus combined with hormonal relaxation of the mechanism of urethral suspension. In the second group, however, they suggest that irreversible damage had occurred to the urethral suspension mechanism. Cutner (1993) has demonstrated a correlation between the length of the first stage and the drop in urethral pressure parameters from that found at 36 weeks gestation.

All these studies would support the hypothesis already put forward that childbirth leads to permanent urethral sphincter damage in susceptible women. Urodynamic investigations suggest that detrusor instability may be a cause of incontinence in pregnancy and that this resolves postpartum. Studies in the future should aim at identifying a high-risk group for permanent sphincter damage such that preventive measures may be undertaken to prevent long-term sequelae.

LABOUR

The effect of the bladder on labour

Although a full bladder was originally believed to slow the progress of labour (Kantor et al 1949; Toppozada et al 1967), more recent reports indicate that a full bladder does not affect the course of normal established labour (Read et al 1980; Kerr-Wilson et al 1983).

Kantor et al (1949) carried out radiographic and simple cystometric studies on patients during labour. They found that the distended bladder can obstruct descent early in labour until the presenting part is well below the ischial spines. However, once the presenting part is on or near the pelvic floor, the bladder usually causes no obstruction. Early in labour, a large portion of the bladder remains in the pelvis, but when the presenting part is deep in the pelvis, the bladder is mostly abdominal. In addition, they showed that the application of low forceps did not impinge on the bladder. They recommend that evacuation of the bladder is essential early in labour, but routine catheterization is unnecessary prior to spontaneous labour or low forceps delivery. This study is unique and can probably never be repeated in view of the potential radiation risks. Toppozada et al (1967) assessed the effect of catheterization on 'tocodynagraphic' activity in 42 patients in the first stage of labour. Each woman had at least 300 ml of urine in her bladder and, after catheterization, there was an overall increase in uterine activity. They concluded that their results confirmed the belief in the inhibitory effect of the full bladder.

Read et al (1980) suggested that emptying the urinary bladder has no effect on the course of labour. They studied 68 patients in the active phase of labour for 30 minutes before and after catheterization. They

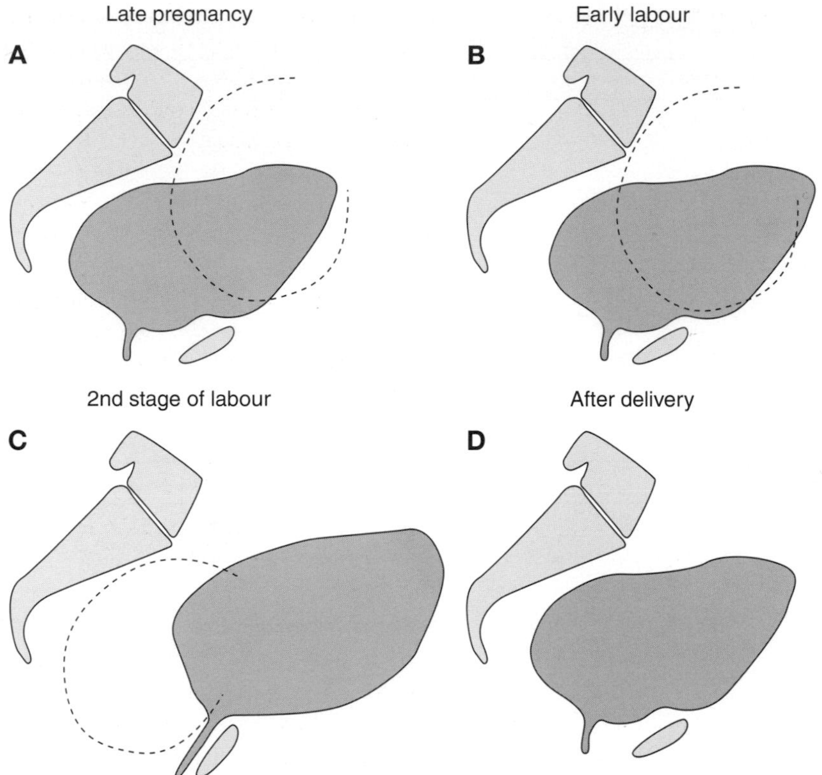

Fig. 41.6 Movements of the bladder in labour. (**A**) Late pregnancy. (**B**) Early labour. (**C**) Second stage of labour. (**D**) After delivery. Modified from Malpas et al (1949).

found no changes in uterine activity, cervical dilatation and descent of the fetal presenting part. However, less than half their patients had more than 300 ml of urine in their bladders at the time of catheterization.

In order to confirm this finding, Kerr-Wilson et al (1983) examined the effect of a full bladder containing at least 300 ml of urine during normal established labour in 20 patients. They were compared with 10 controls, who had 250 ml of urine or less when catheterized. All patients were in the active phase of labour and had uterine activity measured by means of an intrauterine pressure catheter. No patients had labour augmented nor epidural analgesia, and all ended in spontaneous vertex deliveries. Progress of labour was assessed by estimation of cervical dilatation and descent of the fetal head on vaginal examination before and after catheterization. Uterine activity was calculated in Montivideo units. Both before and after catheterization, the slope of the partogram in patients with full bladders was similar to the controls in both nulliparae and multiparae. Although there was a significant increase in uterine activity after catheterization in patients with full bladders, there was also an increase in the control group. They concluded that a full bladder does not affect the course of normal established labour, and it is therefore unnecessary to catheterize patients in the active phase in order to attempt to accelerate progress.

The effect of labour on the bladder

Malpas et al (1949) examined the effect of labour on the position of the bladder and urethra in 32 women radiologically during labour. They found that as labour advanced, the bladder neck became displaced forward but not upward, and the length of the urethra remained unchanged. The vesicourethral junction became funnel-shaped as a result of the bladder base being rolled up towards the lower abdomen. After delivery there was immediate return of the bladder base and urethra to normal (Fig. 41.6). They concluded that it was rotation of the bladder base from the horizontal to the vertical that stretched the fascial investment and led to stress incontinence. Indeed Landon et al (1990) demonstrated that fascial tensile strength is reduced in pregnancy and it may be that the support of the pregnant urethrovesical junction is particularly susceptible to stretching. These views are supported by other studies (Kantor et al 1949; Bennetts & Judd 1941; Funnel et al 1954; Seski & Duprey 1961).

Table 41.2 Postpartum urodynamic data in primiparae.

Data	48 hours	4 weeks	P
PFR (ml/s)	22.3 ± 2.7	23.5 ± 2.7	NS
Volume voided (ml)	363.0 ± 54.1	385.0 ± 43.2	NS
Residual (ml)	29.0 ± 9.5	24.5 ± 6.8	NS
FDV (ml)	277.0 ± 26.1	224.0 ± 29.4	.05
Capacity (ml)	392.5 ± 37.1	331.0 ± 33.6	.04
PR_1 (cm H_2O)	7.8 ± 3.1	5.1 ± 0.9	NS
PR_2 (cm H_2O)	3.8 ± 1.4	1.8 ± 0.8	NS

PFR: peak flow rate; FDV: first desire to void; PR_1: detrusor pressure rise on filling; PR_2: detrusor pressure rise on standing; NS: not significant.
Mean ± SEM
From Kerr-Wilson et al (1984), with permission from the American College of Obstetricians and Gynecologists.

Table 41.3 Urodynamic data in multiparae.

Data	48 hours	4 weeks	P
PFR (ml/s)	24.5 ± 3.4	20.5 ± 2.3	NS
Volume voided (ml)	358.0 ± 50.7	302.5 ± 35.5	NS
Residual (ml)	30.3 ± 10.1	18.0 ± 4.9	NS
FDV (ml)	227 ± 32.9	200.0 ± 19.3	NS
Capacity (ml)	430 ± 37.6	335 ± 27.5	.03
PR_1 (cm H_2O)	7.0 ± 1.7	9.8 ± 3.9	NS
PR_2 (cm H_2O)	6.0 ± 2.4	3.2 ± 0.8	NS

Abbreviations as in Table 41.1
*Mean ± SEM
From Kerr-Wilson et al (1984), with permission from the American College of Obstetricians and Gynecologists.

Bennetts & Judd (1941) suggested that labour resulted in a hypotonic bladder. They performed cystoscopy and intravesical pressure measurements using simple cystometry in 105 women from 36 to 60 hours after vaginal delivery. Residual urine was measured in 94 patients, of whom 34% had a volume greater than 250 ml and in 6% the volume was in excess of 500 ml. At cystometry, they found hypotonic bladders, with decreased bladder sensation and increased bladder capacity in over 80% of their patients. Forty-five per cent of their patients had no pain or desire to micturate with the bladder distended to one litre. These findings were independent of the type of delivery, degree of trauma or intrapartum analgesia.

Youssef (1956) in his series of only 10 patients had similar results with marked hypotonia and increased bladder capacity postpartum. He indicated that this may be an important factor in predisposing patients to postpartum retention and the formation of residual urine. Kerr-Wilson et al (1984) however, suggest that changes in the management of labour may have gone some way to prevent such dramatic effects on the bladder. They carried out urodynamic investigations in 10 primiparae and 10 multiparae at 48 hours and 4 weeks after vaginal delivery. Eight patients had epidural analgesia, 15 had an episiotomy, and 3 had an instrumental delivery. The mean duration of the first and second stages of labour was 8.5 hours and 32 minutes respectively. The patients were catheterized 4–6 hours after delivery if they were unable to void. The results are given in Tables 41.2 and 41.3. The mean urodynamic values were all within normal limits, although there were differences between the 48-hour and 4-week recordings. There was a positive correlation in primiparae between duration of labour and residual urine at 48 hours but no correlation with either episiotomy or fetal weight. The authors concluded that modern obstetric practice does not predispose to postpartum bladder hypotonia, which is chiefly caused by prolonged labour and the failure to catheterize early after delivery.

PUERPERIUM

Early

Although the modern management of labour may have decreased the incidence of postpartum retention, it is still the commonest time for retention to occur in relation to pregnancy and may lead to long-term sequaelae (Dolman 1992).

Possible predisposing factors for postpartum retention are trauma, analgesia and prolonged labour. Spasm of the external urethral sphincter caused by pain was thought to be the cause of retention following vaginal delivery by Francis (1960a). Crawford (1972) Grove (1973) and Krantz & Edwards (1974) believed that instrumental delivery was the primary cause of postpartum lower urinary tract dysfunction and that epidural analgesia did not have any influence but Weil et al (1983) concluded that patients who give birth vaginally with an epidural block may be at greater risk of developing asymptomatic urinary retention.

Tapp et al (1987) found that women who had epidural analgesia had a significantly larger residual of urine on day 2 and day 5 than those women who had other forms of analgesia. Weil et al (1983) also found that the second stage of labour was significantly longer in the group that had residual urine in excess of 100 ml. Although they found that epidural analgesia and a prolonged second stage appeared to contribute to the formation of residual urine, this was only temporary and all patients were voiding normally by 6 weeks.

The effect of epidural analgesia on bladder function following caesarean section has been assessed by Kerr-Wilson & McNally (1986). They concluded that epidural analgesia may predispose to urinary retention following caesarean section, and advocated the use of an indwelling catheter at the time of surgery in these patients.

Khullar & Cardozo (1993) demonstrated that the bladder takes up to 8 hours to regain its sensation after the last top-up of epidural and it is within this time that a diuresis may occur and, therefore, the woman is particularly susceptible to overdistension. This overdistension may result in permanent detrusor damage. Changes in epidural techniques, including drugs administered, whether top-ups are intermittent or continuous and the advent of mobile epidurals, means that the epidural type needs to be cited in studies reported (Russell & Reynolds 1993).

Postpartum retention is associated with long-term sequelae. Tapp et al (1987) reported 6 women who developed acute retention postpartum. Two patients had permanent voiding difficulties, 2 required self-catheterization 6 months postpartum and 2 had altered bladder sensation although they were voiding normally. Five of the 6 patients had epidural analgesia, and 4 had an instrumental delivery. Four of the patients had residual urine volumes in excess of one litre when catheterized. However, this small retrospective study does not preclude the possibility that these patients may have had an underlying neuropathy, rather than retention secondary to labour, which resulted in their voiding difficulties.

Care of the bladder following delivery requires particular vigilance. Attention should be paid to those patients at risk of developing retention, including those who have had a traumatic delivery, prolonged labour, epidural analgesia or caesarean section. Voiding alone is not adequate assessment of bladder function since it may be incomplete, leading to increasingly large residuals of urine. Input–output charts are generally inadequate following delivery as a diuresis may occur and women are encouraged to increase their fluid intake to promote breast-feeding. The minimum requirement is that women at risk should be on an output chart to ensure they are voiding at least 200 ml urine at more than 2-hourly intervals. Frequent small volumes of urine indicates incomplete voiding. If necessary, a disposable catheter can be passed to ensure the bladder is empty. If a woman is unable to void after delivery she should not be left more than 6–8 hours before a catheter is passed to avoid overdistension of the bladder. If a second catheterization is required then it is advisable to leave an indwelling catheter in position for 48 hours. If, after this, voiding is still unsatisfactory then a suprapubic catheter is recommended, together with investigations for possible underlying causes of retention. A suprapubic catheter will also allow the mother to leave hospital with her baby after being given instructions on how to manage the catheter, with arrangements having been made for its removal. However, some patients may prefer a urethral catheter for 2 weeks and then an in-out catheter to check for urinary residual.

Late

Although symptoms of stress incontinence usually appear first during pregnancy, it is probably the effect of vaginal delivery which causes this to become permanent. Schuessler et al (1988) noted no stress incontinence 6 months after caesarean section in a group of 58 patients, whereas 22 out of 366 women (6%) who delivered vaginally had persisting stress incontinence. Suggested reasons for this are either stretching or denervation of the pelvic floor musculature during vaginal delivery.

Allen et al (1990) studied 96 nulliparous women who delivered vaginally. They were examined at 36 weeks gestation, 2–5 days and 2 months after delivery. Perineometer readings were made on each occasion. They found an initial reduction in pelvic floor contraction immediately postpartum, with some recovery later. Electromyography revealed evidence of reinnervation of the pelvic floor which varied from mild in some cases to severe in those women who had marked incontinence. The only factor in labour which was associated with severe damage was a long, active second stage. However, evidence of denervation may well reflect a propensity to develop prolapse in later life rather than genuine stress incontinence. Smith et al (1989) have shown evidence of partial denervation of the pelvic floor using electromyography in women with both stress incontinence and genital tract prolapse and supported these findings with histochemical studies of the pubococcygeus muscle in symptomatic women (Gilpin et al 1989). Cutner (1993), looking 6 weeks postpartum, has found a correlation between a long first stage of labour and a drop in urethral pressure profile parameters from that found at 36 weeks gestation.

Schuessler et al (1988) suggested that epidural analgesia appears to prevent the development of stress incontinence and he proposes that relaxation of the pelvic floor during labour by this form of analgesia is the mechanism by which it works. However, these findings are challenged by Viktrup & Lose (1993).

It would thus appear that a long first stage of labour and a long, active second stage of labour increase the chances of the development of permanent stress incontinence following delivery. Again, it must be recognized that most of these studies have not performed urodynamic investigations and, therefore, stress incontinence as a symptom may not be synonymous with genuine stress incontinence as a diagnosis.

CONCLUSION

The relationship between the lower urinary tract, the pregnant uterus, labour and delivery are close but complex. Frequency of micturition appears to be a function of fluid intake or urine output but may also be related to low compliance. Nocturia appears to be related to urine production, the hours spent in bed and again possibly decreased bladder capacity. Although stress incontinence is a very common symptom it may be a symptom due to other causes such as detrusor instability or it may be a physiological event which will resolve postpartum. It may also indicate a susceptibility to the development of permanent genuine stress incontinence following a difficult delivery.

During labour a full bladder does not appear to effect the progress of labour once it is established. Immediately after delivery the bladder does appear to be hypotonic, particularly following prolonged labour with epidural analgesia. Vigilance is necessary to prevent the development of long-term voiding difficulties.

Vaginal delivery definitely does have a deleterious effect on the pelvic floor and urethral sphincter function but the exact factors and those women who are at risk have yet to be identified. It may be that future studies will identify these women and prophylactic caesarean section will be a possibility but until they can be correctly identified this would be a high price to pay.

REFERENCES

Allen R E, Hosker G L, Smith A R B, Warrell D W 1990 Pelvic floor damage and childbirth: a neurophysiological study. British Journal of Obstetrics and Gynaecology 97: 770–779

Beck R P, Hsu N 1965 Pregnancy, childbirth, and the menopause related to the development of stress incontinence. American Journal of Obstetrics and Gynecology 91: 820–823

Bennetts F A, Judd G E 1941 Studies of the post-partum bladder. American Journal of Obstetrics and Gynecology 40: 419–427

Brown A D G 1978 The effects of pregnancy on the lower urinary tract. Clinics in Obstetrics and Gynaecology 5: 151–168

Brown A D G 1981 Urinary tract problems. Hospital Update. 7: 529–536

Clow W M 1975 Effect of posture on bladder and urethral function in normal pregnancy. Urologia Internationalis 30: 9–15

Crawford J S 1972 Lumbar epidural block in labour: a clinical analysis. British Journal of Anaesthetics 44: 66–74

Cutner A 1993 The lower urinary tract in pregnancy. MD thesis, University of London

Cutner A, Cardozo L D 1996 The association between pregnancy and abnormal detrusor activity. Journal of Obstetrics and Gynaecology 16: 143–145

Cutner A, Cardozo L D, Benness C J, Carey A Cooper D 1990 Detrusor instability in early pregnancy. Neurourology and Urodynamics 9: 328–329

Cutner A, Cardozo L D, Benness C J 1991 Assessment of urinary symptoms in early pregnancy. British Journal of Obstetrics and Gynaecology 98: 1283–1286

Cutner A, Carey A, Cardozo L D 1992a Lower urinary tract symptoms in early pregnancy. Journal of Obstetrics and Gynaecology 12: 75–78

Cutner A, Cardozo L D, Benness C J 1992b Assessment of urinary symptoms in the second half of pregnancy. International Urogynecology Journal 3: 30–32

Dolman M 1992 Midwives' recording of urinary output. Nursing Standard. 6(27): 25–27

Fischer W, Kittel K 1990 Harnfluβmessungen in der Schwangerschaft und im Wochenbett (Urine flow studies in pregnancy and puerperium). Zentralblatt fur Gynakologie 112: 593–600

Francis W J A 1960a Disturbances of bladder function in relation to pregnancy. Journal of Obstetrics and Gynaecology of the British Empire 67: 353–366

Francis W J A 1960b The onset of stress incontinence. Journal of Obstetrics and Gynaecology of the British Empire 67: 899–903

Funnell J W, Klawans A H, Cottrell T L C 1954 The postpartum bladder. American Journal of Obstetrics and Gynaecology 67: 1249–1256

Gilpin S A, Gosling J A, Smith A R B, Warrell D W 1989 The pathogenesis of genitourinary prolapse and stress incontinence of urine. A histological and histochemical study. British Journal of Obstetrics and Gynaecology 96: 15–23

Grove L H 1973 Backache, headache, and bladder dysfunction after delivery. British Journal of Anaesthetics 45: 1147–1149

Haylen B T, Ashby D, Sutherst J R, Frazer M I, West C R 1989 Maximum and average flow rates in normal male and female populations – the Liverpool nomograms. British Journal of Urology 64: 30–38

Hundley Jr J M, Siegel I A, Hachtel F W, Dumler J C 1938 Some physiological and pathological observations on the urinary tract during pregnancy. Surgery, Gynecology and Obstetrics 66: 360–379

Iosif S 1981 Stress incontinence during pregnancy and in puerperium. International Journal of Gynecology and Obstetrics 19: 13–20

Iosif C S, Ingemarsson I 1982 Prevalence of stress incontinence among women delivered by elective cesarian section. International Journal of Gynaecology and Obstetrics 20: 87–89

Iosif S, Ulmsten U 1981 Comparative urodynamic studies of continent and stress incontinent women in pregnancy and in the puerperium. American Journal of Obstetrics and Gynecology 140: 645–650

Iosif S, Ingemarsson I, Ulmsten U 1980 Urodynamic studies in normal pregnancy and in puerperium. American Journal of Obstetrics and Gynecology 137: 696–700

Iosif S, Henriksson L, Ulmsten U 1981 Postpartum incontinence. Urologia Internationalis 36: 53–58

Kantor H I, Miller J E, Dunlap J C 1949 The urinary bladder during labor. American Journal of Obstetrics and Gynecology 48: 354–365

Kerr-Wilson, R H J, McNally S 1986 Bladder drainage for caesarean section under epidural analgesia. British Journal of Obstetrics and Gynaecology 93: 28–30

Kerr-Wilson R H J, Parham G P, Orr, J W 1983 The effect of a full bladder on labour. Obstetrics and Gynecology 62: 319–323

Kerr-Wilson R H J, Thompson S W, Orr J W, Davis R O, Cloud G A, 1984 Effect of labor on the postpartum bladder. Obstetrics and Gynecology 64: 115–118

Khullar V, Cardozo L D 1993 Bladder sensation after epidural analgesia. Neurourology and Urodynamics 12(4) 424–425

King J, Freeman R 1996 Can we predict antenatally those patients at risk of postpartum stress incontinence? Neurourology and Urodynamics 15(4): 130–131

Krantz M L, Edwards W L 1974 Anaesthesia and urinary retention in obstetrics. Journal of the Indian State Medical Association. 76: 329–330

Landon C R, Crofts C E, Smith A R B, Trowbridge E A 1990 Mechanical properties of fascia during pregnancy: a possible factor in the development of stress incontinence of urine. Contemporary Review of Obstetrics and Gynaecology 2: 40–46

Langer R, Golan A, Neuman M, Schneider D, Bukovsky I, Caspi E 1990 The effect of large uterine fibroids on urinary bladder function and symptoms. American Journal of Obstetrics Gynecology 163: 1139–1141

Malpas P, Jeffcoate T N A, Lister U M 1949 The displacement of the bladder and urethra during labour. Journal of Obstetrics and Gynaecology of the British Empire 56: 949–960

Marchant D J 1978 The urinary tract in pregnancy. Clinics in Obstetrics and Gynaecology 21: 817–914

Muellner S R 1939 Physiological bladder changes during pregnancy and the puerperium. J. Urol. 41: 691–695

Myerscough P R 1982 Munro Kerr's Operative Obstetrics, 10th edn. Bailliere Tindall, London

Parboosingh J, Doig A 1973a Studies of nocturia in normal pregnancy. Journal of Obstetrics and Gynaecology of the British Commonwealth 80: 888–895

Parboosingh J, Doig A 1973b Renal nyctohemeral excretory patterns of water and solutes in normal human pregnancy. American Journal of Obstetrics and Gynaecology 116: 609–615

Read J A, Miller F C, Yeh S-Y, Platt L D 1980 Urinary bladder distension: effect on labour and uterine activity. Obstetrics and Gynecology 56: 565–570

Russell R, Reynolds F 1993 Epidural analgesia: not just one technique. British Journal of Obstetrics and Gynaecology (letter) 100: 1155–1156

Schuessler B, Hesse U, Dimpfl T, Anthuber C 1988 Epidural anaesthesia and avoidance of postpartum stress urinary incontinence. Lancet 1: 762

Seski A G, Duprey W M 1961 Postpartum intravesical photography. Obstetrics and Gynecology 18: 548–556

Shutter H W 1922 Care of the bladder in pregnancy, labor and the puerperium. Journal of the American Medical Association 79: 449–453

Skoner M M, Thompson W D, Caron V A 1994 Factors associated with risk of stress urinary incontinence in women. Nursing Research 43(5): 301–306

Smith A R B, Hosker G L, Warrell D W 1989 The role of pudendal nerve damage in the aetiology of genuine stress incontinence in women. British Journal of Obstetrics and Gynaecology 96: 29–32

Stanton S L, Kerr-Wilson R, Harris G V 1980 The incidence of urological symptoms in normal pregnancy. British Journal of Obstetrics and Gynaecology 87: 897–900

Tapp A J S, Meir H, Cardozo L D 1987 The effect of epidural analgesia on post-partum voiding. Neurourology and Urodynamics 6: 235–237

Toppozada H K, Gaafar A A, El-Sahwi S 1967 The urinary bladder and uterine activity. American Journal of Obstetrics and Gynecology 144: 636–649

Van Geelen J M, Lemmens W A J G, Eskes T K A B, Martin, C B, 1982 The urethral pressure profile in pregnancy and after delivery in healthy nulliparous women. American Journal Obstetrics and Gynecology 144: 636–649

Viktrup L, Lose G 1993 Epidural anesthesia during labour and stress incontinence after delivery. Obstetrics and Gynecology 82 (6): 984–986

Viktrup L, Lose G, Roff M, Barfoed K 1992 The symptom of stress incontinence caused by pregnancy or delivery in primipara. Obstetrics and Gynecology 79(6): 945–949

Waltzer W C 1981 The urinary tract in pregnancy. Journal of Urology 125: 271–276

Weil A, Reyes H, Rottenberg, R D, Beguin F, Herrmann W L 1983 Effect of lumbar epidural analgesia on lower urinary tract function in the immediate postpartum period. British Journal of Obstetrics and Gynaecology 90: 428–432

Wilson P D, Herbison R M, Herbison G P 1996 Obstetric practice and the prevalence of urinary incontinence three months after delivery. British Journal of Obstetrics and Gynaecology 103(2): 154–161

Youssef A F 1956 Cystometric studies in gynecology and obstetrics. Obstetrics and Gynecology 8: 181–188

SECTION

5

Treatment

Applied pharmacology

ALAN J WEIN AND ASH K MONGA

INTRODUCTION

Many recent reviews are available which describe the physiology and pharmacology of the micturition cycle. There are two relatively discrete phases: a filling–storage phase of micturition and an emptying phase. Normal urine storage and continence require:

1. Accommodation of increasing volumes of urine at a low intravesical pressure and with appropriate sensory appreciation
2. A bladder outlet that is closed during rest and during increases in intra-abdominal pressure
3. Absence of inappropriate bladder contractions (detrusor instability or detrusor hyperreflexia).

Normal emptying requires:

1. A coordinated bladder contraction of significant magnitude and duration
2. Concomitant lowering of resistance at the level of the smooth muscle of the bladder neck and proximal urethra (smooth sphincter) and of the periurethral and intramural urethral striated musculature (striated sphincter)
3. Absence of anatomical obstruction.

All types of therapy for voiding dysfunction can, then, be most logically considered within a purely functional classification based on whether the primary problem seems to be one of bladder filling and urine storage or one of bladder emptying. Individual methods of therapy can also be subclarified as to whether they affect the bladder or the bladder outlet. The following outlines illustrate such a functional classification (Tables 42.1 and 42.2).

PRINCIPLES OF PHARMACOLOGICAL THERAPY

Most pharmacological agents produce their effects by combining with specialized functional components of cells, known as receptors. The drug–receptor interaction alters the function of the cell and initiates the

Table 42.1 Therapy to facilitate bladder emptying.

- Increasing intravesical pressure\bladder contractility
- External compression, Valsalva promotion or initiation of reflex contractions
  - Trigger zones or manoeuvres
  - Bladder training, tidal drainage
- Pharmacological therapy
  - Parasympathomimetic agents
  - Prostaglandins
  - Blockers of inhibition – α-adrenergic antagonists; Opioid antagonists
- Electrical stimulation
  - Directly to the bladder
  - To the spinal cord or nerve roots
- Reduction cystoplasty
- Decreasing outlet resistance
  - At a site of anatomical obstruction
    - α-adrenergic antagonists
    - Urethral stricture repair\dilattion
  - At the level of the smooth sphincter
    - Transurethral resection or incision of the bladder neck
    - Y-V plasty of the bladder neck
    - Pharmacological therapy
      - α-adrenergic antagonists
      - β-adrenergic agonists
  - At the level of the striated sphincter
    - External sphincterotomy
    - Urethral overdilatation
    - Pudendal nerve block or interruption
    - Pharmacological therapy
      - Skeletal muscle relaxants
      - Centrally acting relaxants
      - Dantrolene
      - Baclofen
      - α-adrenergic antagonists
    - Biofeedback, psychotherapy
- Circumventing problem
- Intermittent catheterization
- Continuous catheterization
- Urinary diversion

Table 42.2 Therapy to facilitate urine storage.

- Inhibiting bladder contractilty decreasing sensory input\increasing bladder capacity; timed bladder emptying
  - Pharmacological therapy
    - Anticholinergic agents
    - Musculotropic relaxants
    - Polysynaptic inhibitors
    - Calcium antagonists
    - β-adrenergic agonists
    - α-adrenergic antagonists
    - Prostaglandin inhibitors
    - Tricyclic antidepressants
    - Dimethyl sulfoxide
    - Bromocriptine
  - Biofeedback, bladder re-training
  - Bladder overdistention
  - Electrical stimulation (reflex inhibition)
  - Interruption of innervation
    - Central (subarachnoid block)
    - Peripheral (sacral rhizotomy, selective sacral rhizotomy)
    - Perivesical (peripheral bladder denervation)
  - Augmentation cystoplasty
- Increasing outlet resistance
  - Physiotherapy
    - Electrical stimulation of the pelvic floor
  - Pharmacological therapy
    - α-adrenergic agonists
    - Tricyclic antidepressants
    - β-adrenergic antagonists
    - Oestrogen
  - Vesicourethral suspension (SUI)
  - Bladder outlet reconstruction
  - Surgical mechanical compression
  - Non-surgical mechanical compression
- Circumventing problem
  - Antidiuretic hormone
  - External collecting device
  - Intermittent catheterization
  - Continuous catheterization
  - Urinary diversion

series of biochemical and physiological changes that characterize the effects produced by the agent. Most of the agents which alter the urodynamics of the lower urinary tract affect the synthesis, transport, storage or release of neurotransmitter, the combination of the neurotransmitter with postjunctional receptors, or the inactivation, degradation or re-uptake of neurotransmitter. Complex metabolic changes occur after receptor activation, and these mechanisms, which are 'metabolically distal' to membrane receptor sites are also potential sites of stimulation, inhibition or modulation.

One must be thoroughly familiar with the literature surrounding the use of a particular pharmacological agent and remember that:

1 Agents may act at more than one site and even at several sites within a neural pathway or muscle
2 They may have different effects *in vitro* and *in vivo* and at different concentrations
3 They may have different effects in different species
4 They may have different acute and long-term effects
5 They may have multiple effects at any of the levels of action, each within a different time frame
6 The sensitivity, number, and type of receptors within a particular tissue can be affected by its physiological state (denervation, distension, hypertrophy, inflammation, ischaemia) and by the drug itself.

Generally speaking, the simplest and least hazardous form of pharmacological therapy should be tried first. If single-agent therapy fails, a combination of therapeutic manoeuvres or pharmacological agents can sometimes be used to achieve a particular effect, especially if their mechanisms of action are different and if their side-effects are not synergistic. Finally, it should be noted by physician and patient alike that although great improvement often occurs with rational pharmacological therapy, a perfect result (restoration to normal status) with no side-effects is seldom, if ever, achieved.

FACILITATION OF BLADDER EMPTYING

Absolute or relative failure to empty results from decreased bladder contractility, increased outlet resistance, or both (Wein 1992). Absolute or relative failure of adequate bladder contractility may result from temporary or permanent alteration in any one of the neuromuscular mechanisms necessary for initiating and maintaining a normal detrusor contraction. Inhibition of the micturition reflex in a neurologically normal individual may occur via a reflex mechanism secondary to painful stimuli especially from the pelvic and perineal areas, or may be psychogenic. Non-neurogenic causes include impairment of bladder smooth muscle function, which may result from overdistension, severe infection or fibrosis. Drug therapy may also inhibit bladder contractility, either through neurological or myogenic mechanisms. Increased outlet resistance is generally secondary to anatomical obstruction, but may be secondary to a failure of coordination of the smooth or striated sphincter during bladder contraction. Treatment for failure to empty generally consists of attempts to increase intravesical pressure or facilitate the micturition reflex, to decrease outlet resistance, or both.

Increasing intravesical pressure

Parasympathomimetic agents

Since a large part of the final common pathway for physiological bladder contraction is stimulation of the muscarinic cholinergic receptor sites at the postganglionic parasympathetic neuromuscular junction (Wein 1992), agents which imitate the actions of acetylcholine (ACh) might be expected to be useful in the management of patients who cannot empty because of inadequate bladder contractility. ACh itself cannot be used for therapeutic purposes because of actions at central and ganglionic levels and because of its rapid hydrolysis by acetylcholinesterase and by non-specific cholinesterase (Taylor 1990). Many acetylcholine-like drugs exist. However, only bethanechol chloride (BC) exhibits a relatively selective action on the urinary bladder and gut with little or no action at therapeutic dosages on ganglia or on the cardiovascular system (Taylor 1990). It is cholinesterase-resistant and causes contraction *in vitro* of smooth muscle from all areas of the bladder (Raezer et al 1973; Wein 1992).

BC, or agents with a similar action, have long been recommended (Starr & Ferguson 1940) for the treatment of postoperative or postpartum urinary retention. For over 30 years it has been used in the treatment of atonic or hypotonic bladder (Lee 1949) and has been reported to be effective in achieving 'rehabilitation' of the chronically atonic or hypotonic detrusor (Sonda et al 1979). When so used, it is recommended that the drug be initially administered subcutaneously in a 5–10 mg dose (usually 7.5 mg) every 4–6 hours. The patient is asked to try to void 20–30 minutes after each dose. Bethanechol has also been used to stimulate reflex bladder contractions in patients with suprasacral spinal cord injury (Perkash 1975).

Although BC has been reported to increase gastrointestinal motility and has been used in the treatment of gastro-oesophageal reflux, only anecdotal success in specific patients with voiding dysfunction is reported. Short-term studies in which the drug was the only variable have generally failed to demonstrate significant efficacy in terms of flow and residual urine volume data (Barrett 1981). Farrell and colleagues (1990) conducted a double-blind randomized trial that looked at the effects of two catheter management protocols and the effect of BC on postoperative urinary retention following gynaecological incontinence surgery. They concluded that BC was not helpful at all in this setting. In adequate doses, BC is capable of increasing tension in bladder smooth muscle, as would be expected from *in vitro* studies, but its ability to stimulate a coordinated and sustained bladder contraction in patients with voiding dysfunction has been unimpressive (Barrett & Wein 1991).

It is difficult to find reproducible urodynamic data which support recommendations for the usage of BC in any specific category of patients. Most, if not all, 'long-term' reports in such patients are neither prospective nor double-blind and do not exclude the effects of other simultaneous regimens (such as treatment of urinary infection, bladder decompression or timed emptying.

Other methods of achieving a cholinergic effect are seldom used. Philip et al (1980) reported that a 4 mg oral dose of carbachol, a cholinergic agonist which also possesses some ganglionic-stimulation properties, had a much more favourable effect on urodynamic parameters in patients with cholinergic supersensitivity than a 50 mg oral dose of BC, with no apparent increase in side-effects. Voided volumes were reduced, detrusor pressures increased, and the length of contraction shortened. Hedlund & Andersson (1988) treated patients with benign prostatic hyperplasia with 2–4 mg three times a day of carbachol. There were no changes in urodynamic variables despite the occurrence of gastrointestinal side-effects. Taylor (1990) states that carbachol is 'no longer available' because of its nicotinic action. Anticholinesterase agents also have the net effect of producing or enhancing cholinergic stimulation. Philip & Thomas (1980) reported that parenteral but not oral distigmine improved voiding efficiency in patients with neurogenic bladder dysfunction with reflex detrusor activity.

No agreement exists about whether cholinergic stimulation produces an increase in urethral resistance (Wein et al 1980a,b). It appears that pharmacologically active doses do in fact increase urethral closure pressure, at least in patients with detrusor hyperreflexia (Sporer et al 1978). This would, of course, tend to inhibit bladder emptying. As to whether cholinergic agonists can be combined with agents to decrease outlet resistance to facilitate emptying and achieve an additive or synergistic effect, our own experience with such therapy, using even as much as 200 mg of oral BC daily, has been extremely disappointing. The potential side-effects of cholinomimetic drugs include flushing, nausea, vomiting, diarrhoea, gastrointestinal cramps, bronchospasm, headache, salivation, sweating, and difficulty with visual accommodation (Taylor 1990). Intramuscular and intravenous use can precipitate acute and severe side-effects, resulting in acute circulatory failure and cardiac arrest, and is therefore prohibited. Contraindications to the use of this general category of drug include bronchial asthma, peptic ulcer, bowel obstruction, enteritis, recent gastrointestinal surgery, cardiac arrhythmia, hyperthyroidism, and any type of bladder outlet obstruction.

One potential way of increasing bladder contractility is cholinergic enhancement. Such an action might be useful alone or in combination with a parasympathomimetic agent. Metoclopramide (Reglan) is a dopamine antagonist with cholinergic properties. It has a central antiemetic effect in the chemoreceptor trigger zone and peripherally increases the tone of the lower oesophageal sphincter, promoting gastric emptying. Its effects seem to be related to its ability to antagonize the inhibitory action of dopamine, to augment ACh release, and to sensitize the muscarinic receptors of gastrointestinal smooth muscle (Albibi & McCallum 1983). Some data in the dog suggest that this agent can increase detrusor contractility (Mitchell & Venable 1985) and there is one anecdotal case report of improved bladder function in a diabetic patient treated with this agent (originally) for gastroparesis (Nestler et al 1983). Cisapride is a substituted synthetic benzamide that enhances the release of ACh in Auerbach's plexus. In 15 patients with complete spinal cord injury treated with 10 mg of cisapride three times a day for 3 days, Carone and associates (1993) noted earlier and higher amplitude reflex contractions in those with hypoactive bladders and there was significant decrease in compliance. There was also increased activity and decreased compliance of the anorectal ampulla with no alteration in striated sphincter activity.

Prostaglandins

The reported use of prostaglandins (PG) to facilitate emptying is based on the hypothesis that these substances contribute to the maintenance of bladder tone and bladder contractile activity. PGE_2 and PGF_{2a} cause *in vitro* and *in vivo* bladder contractile response. PGE_2 seems to cause a net decrease in urethral smooth muscle tone; PGE_{2a} causes an increase. Bultitude and colleagues (1976) reported that instillation of 0.5 mg PGE_2 into the bladders of women with varying degrees of urinary retention resulted in acute emptying and an improvement of long-term emptying (several months) in two thirds of the patients studied ($n = 22$). In general, they reported a decrease in the volume at which voiding was initiated, an increase in bladder pressure, and a decrease in residual urine. Desmond and co-workers (1980) reported the results of intravesical use of 1.5 mg of this agent (diluted with 20 ml of 0.2% neomycin solution) in patients whose bladders exhibited no contractile activity or in whom bladder contractility was relatively impaired. Twenty of 36 patients showed a strongly positive response, and six showed a weakly positive immediate response. Fourteen patients were reported to show prolonged beneficial effects, all but one of whom had shown a strongly positive immediate response. The authors noted additionally that the effects of PGE_2 appeared to be additive or synergistic with cholinergic stimulation in some patients.

Vaidyanathan and colleagues (1981b) reported that intravesical instillation of 7.5 mg of PGF_{2a} produced reflex voiding in some patients with incomplete suprasacral spinal cord lesions. The favourable response to a single dose of drug, when present, lasted from 1.0 to 2.5 months. Tammela and associates (1987) reported that one intravesical administration of 10 mg of PGF_{2a} facilitated voiding in women who were in retention 3 days after surgery for stress urinary incontinence. The drug was administered in 50 ml of saline as a single dose and retained for 2 hours. However, in these 'successfully' treated patients, the average maximum flow rate was 10.6 ml/second with a mean residual urine volume of 107 ml; also, the authors state that 'bladder emptying deteriorated in most patients on the day after treatment'.

Jaschevatsky and colleagues (1985) reported that 16 mg of PGF_{2a} in 40 ml of saline given intravesically reduced the frequency of urinary retention in a group of women undergoing gynaecological surgery. Inexplicably, however, this only occurred in women undergoing vaginal hysterectomy with vaginal repair, not in those undergoing vaginal repair with urethral plication or vaginal repair alone. Koonings and colleagues (1990) reported that daily intravesical doses of PGF_{2a} and intravaginal PGE_2 reduced the number of days required for catheterization after stress incontinence surgery compared to a control group receiving intravesical saline. Other investigators, however, have reported conflicting (negative) results. Stanton et al (1979) and Delaere and co-workers (1981) reported no success using intravesical PGE_2 in doses similar to those reported earlier. Delaere and co-workers similarly reported no success using PGF_{2a} in a group of women with emptying difficulties of various causes, although it should be noted that they used lower doses than those reported earlier. Wagner and colleagues (1985) utilized PGE_2 in doses of 0.75–2.25 mg and reported no effect on urinary retention in a group of patients after anterior colporrhaphy. Schubler (1990) reported that both intravesical PGE_2 and sulprostone (a derivative) caused a strong sensation of urgency in normal women volunteers, resulting in reduced bladder capacity and instability. Both agents also decreased resting urethral closure pressure. PGE increased detrusor pressure at opening and during maximum flow. Sulprostone slightly decreased these latter two parameters. All effects had disappeared 24 hours after administration. Prostaglandins have a relatively short half-life, and it is difficult to understand how any effects after a single application can last up to several months. If such an effect does occur, it must be the result of a 'triggering effect' on some as yet unknown physiological or metabolic mechanism. Potential side-effects of prostaglandin usage include bronchospasm, chills, tachycardia, cardiac arrhythmia, convulsions, hypocalcaemia, vomiting, diarrhoea, pyrexia, hypertension and hypotension (Rall 1990).

Blockers of inhibition

De Groat and co-workers (Wein et al 1991a; de Groat & Booth 1984; de Groat 1993) have demonstrated in the cat a sympathetic reflex during bladder filling which, promotes urine storage partly by exerting an α-adrenergic inhibitory effect on pelvic parasympathetic ganglionic transmission. Some investigators have suggested that α-adrenergic blockage, in addition to decreasing outlet resistance, may in fact facilitate transmission through these ganglia and thereby enhance bladder contractility. On this basis, Raz & Smith (1976) first advocated a trial of an α-adrenergic blocking agent for the treatment of non-obstructive urinary retention. Tammela (1986) reported that phenoxybenzamine (POB) was more effective in preventing recurrent retention after initial catheterization in a group of postoperative patients than was either carbachol or placebo. Golman and colleagues (1988) reported on a prospective randomized study of 102 patients over age 60 undergoing hernia repair. Fifty-eight patients were given POB 10 mg the night before and 2 hours before surgery, and twice a day for 3 days afterwards. None of the treated patients developed postoperative retention, whereas 26 of the 44 controls developed postoperative retention. In 21 of 26 patients with urinary retention, the retention disappeared within 48 hours after POB administration (and bladder decompression). Although such an effect may be due solely to an α-adrenergic effect on the outlet (see next section, 'Decreasing outlet resistance'), it may be that α-adrenergic blockade can, under certain circumstances, facilitate the detrusor reflex, either through a direct effect on parasympathetic ganglia or an indirect one (a mechanism associated with a decrease in urethral resistance).

Opioid antagonists

Recent advances in neuropeptide physiology and pharmacology have provided new insights into lower urinary tract function and its potential pharmacological alteration. It has been hypothesized that endogenous opioids may exert a tonic inhibitory effect on the micturition reflex at various levels (Wein et al 1991a; Steers 1992), and agents such as narcotic antagonists therefore may offer possibilities for stimulating reflex bladder activity. Thor and associates (1983) were able to stimulate a micturition contraction with naloxone, an opiate antagonist, in unanaesthetized cats with chronic spinal disease. The effects, however, were transient, and tachyphylaxis developed. Vaidyanathan et al (1981a) reported that an intravenous injection of 0.4 mg of naloxone enhanced detrusor reflex activity in 5 of 7 patients with neuropathic bladder dysfunction caused by incomplete suprasacral spinal cord lesions. The maximum effect occurred within 1 to 2 minutes after intravenous injection and the effect was gone by 5 minutes. Murray & Feneley (1982) reported that in a group of patients with idiopathic detrusor instability, 0.4 mg of naloxone caused an increase in detrusor pressure at zero volume, and at first desire to void a decrease in the maximum cystometric capacity and a worsening of the degree of instability. Galeano and co-workers (1986) reported that naloxone, although it increased bladder contractility in the cat with chronic spinal disease, also aggravated striated sphincter dyssynergia and spasticity – a potential problem in the treatment of patients with emptying failure. Wheeler and colleagues (1987), however, noted no significant cystometric changes in a group of 15 patients with spinal cord injury following intravenous naloxone, and 11 of the 15 showed decreased perineal electromyographic (EMG) activity. Although this issue is intriguing, it is of little practical use at present.

Decreasing outlet resistance

Inhibition of the striated sphincter

Classic detrusor-striated sphincter dyssynergia is generally seen only in patients with overt neurological damage or disease between the brain stem and the sacral spinal cord. A disorder that is at least qualitatively similar can be seen in patients without an apparent structural or neurological defect and falls into one of the syndromes of incoordination. There is no class of pharmacological agent which selectively relaxes the striated musculature of the pelvic floor. Three different types of drug have been used to treat voiding dysfunction secondary to outlet obstruction at the level of the striated sphincter: the benzodiazepines, dantrolene, and baclofen. All are characterized generally as antispasticity drugs (Cedarbaum & Schleifer 1990). Baclofen and diazepam act predominantly within the central nervous system, whereas dantrolene acts directly on skeletal muscle. Glycine and gamma-aminobutyric acid (GABA) have been identified as the major inhibitory neurotransmitters in the spinal cord (Bloom 1990). Evidence favours glycine as the mediator of intraspinal postsynaptic inhibition and the most likely inhibitory transmitter in the reticular formation. GABA appears to mediate presynaptic inhibition in the spinal cord and the inhibitory action of local interneurones in the brain. The specific substrate for spinal cord inhibition consists of the synapses located on the terminals of the primary afferent fibres. GABA is the transmitter secreted by these synapses and activates specific receptors, resulting in a decrease in the amount of excitatory transmitter released by impulses from primary afferent fibres, consequently reducing the amplitude of the excitatory postsynaptic potentials. The inhibitory action of GABA in the brain occurs through an increase in chloride conductance with hyperpolarization of the membrane.

Benzodiazepines Benzodiazapines are extensively used for the treatment of anxiety and related disorders, (Shader & Greenblatt 1993) although pharmacologically they can also be classified as centrally acting muscle relaxants.

Side-effects include non-specific central nervous system depression, manifested as sedation, lethargy, drowsiness, slowing of thought processes, ataxia, and decreased ability to acquire or store information (Shader & Greenblatt 1993).

The benzodiazepines potentiate the action of GABA at both presynaptic and postsynaptic sites in the brain and spinal cord (Davidoff 1985; Lader 1987), and increase the affinity of the GABA receptor sites on central nervous system membranes, thus increasing the frequency with which the chloride channels open in response to a given amount of GABA. Presynaptic inhibition is augmented, and it is thought that this reduces the release of excitatory transmitters from afferent fibres.

There are few available references that provide valuable data on the use of any of the benzodiazepines for treatment of functional obstruction at the level of the striated sphincter. The few articles which specifically mention diazepam report that it is more effective than oral POB, intravesical PGE or oral BC in promoting spontaneous voiding after colposuspension surgery. We have not found the recommended oral doses of diazepam effective in controlling the classic type of detrusor-striated sphincter dyssynergia secondary to neurological disease. If the cause of incomplete emptying in a neurologicaly normal patient is obscure, and the patient has what appears urodynamically to be inadequate relaxation of the pelvic floor striated musculature (e.g. occult neuropathic bladder, the Hinman syndrome), a trial of such an agent may be worthwhile. The rationale for its use is relaxation of the pelvic floor striated musculature during bladder contraction, with associated removal of an inhibitory stimulus to reflex bladder activity. However, improvement under such circumstances may simply be due to the antianxiety effect of the drug or to the intensive explanation, encouragement, and modified biofeedback therapy that usually accompanies such treatment in these patients.

Baclofen Baclofen (Lioresal) depresses monosynaptic and polysynaptic excitation of motor neurones and interneurones in the spinal cord and was originally thought to function as a GABA agonist (Cedarbaum & Schleifer 1990; Davidoff 1985). Currently, it is thought that activation of the GABA receptors by Baclofen causes a decrease in the release of excitatory transmitters on to motor neurones by increasing potassium conductance or by inhibiting calcium influx. Baclofen's primary site of action is the spinal cord, but it is also reported to be active at more rostral sites in the central nervous system. Milanov (1991) states that, like a GABA agonist, baclofen suppresses excitatory neurotransmitter release but also has direct GABAergic activity. Its effect in reducing spasticity is caused primarily by normalizing interneurone activity and decreasing motor neurone activity (perhaps secondary to normalizing interneurone activity).

Baclofen has been found useful for the treatment of skeletal spasticity due to a variety of causes (especially multiple sclerosis and traumatic spinal cord lesions) (Cedarbaum & Schleifer 1990). With reference to voiding dysfunction, Hachen & Krucker (1977) found that a daily oral dose of 75 mg was ineffective in patients with striated sphincter dyssynergia and traumatic paraplegia, whereas a daily intravenous dose of 20 mg was highly effective. Florante and associates (1980) reported that 73% of their patients with voiding dysfunction secondary to acute and chronic spinal cord injury had lower striated sphincter responses and decreased residual urine volume following baclofen treatment, but only with an average daily oral dose of 120 mg. Potential side-effects of baclofen include drowsiness, insomnia, rash, pruritus, dizziness and weakness. It may impair the ability to walk or stand and is not recommended for the management of spasticity due to cerebral lesions or disease. Sudden withdrawal has been shown to provoke hallucinations, anxiety and tachycardia; hallucinations due to reductions in dosage during treatment have also been reported.

Drug delivery often frustrates adequate pharmacological treatment, and baclofen is a good example of this. Intrathecal infusion bypasses the blood–brain barrier. Cerebrospinal fluid (CSF) levels 10 times higher than those reached with oral administration are achieved with infusion amounts 100 times less than those taken orally (Penn et al 1989). Direct administration into the subarachnoid space by an implanted infusion pump has shown promising results not only for skeletal spasticity but for striated sphincter dyssynergia and bladder hyperactivity as well. Nanning and colleagues (1989) reported on such administration to 7 patients with intractable bladder spasticity. All patients experienced a general decrease in spasticity, and the amount of striated sphincter activity during bladder contraction decreased; 6 showed an increase in bladder capacity. Four previously incontinent patients were able to stay dry with clean intermittent catheterization (CIC). The action of baclofen on bladder hyperactivity is not unexpected, given its spinal cord mechanism of action, and this inhibition of bladder contractility when the drug is administered intrathecally may in fact prove to be its most important benefit. Loubser and colleagues (1991) studied 9 patients with spinal cord injury and refractory spasticity, using an external pump to test the initial response. Eight showed objective improvement in functional ability; 3 of 7 studied urodynamically showed an increase in bladder capacity. Kums & Delhaas (1991) reported on 9 men who were paraplegic or quadriplegic secondary to trauma or multiple sclerosis and also had intractable muscle spasticity; they were treated with intrathecal baclofen. After a successful test period during which the drug was administered through an external catheter, a drug delivery system was implanted and connected to a spinal catheter. Doses ranged from 74 to 840 mg/24 hours. Patients were studied before and 4 to 6 weeks after initiation of therapy. Mean residual urine volume fell from 224 to 110 ml (p = .01), mean urodynamic bladder capacity rose from 162 to 263 ml (p<.005), and pelvic floor spasm decreased at both baseline and maximum bladder capacity (p<.005 and .025, respectively). Three subjects became continent. Additionally, CIC was no longer complicated by adductor spasm. Development of tolerance to intrathecal baclofen with a consequent requirement for increasing doses may prove to be a problem with long-term chronic use, and studies are under way to investigate this.

Dantrolene Dantrolene (Dantrium) exerts its effects by direct peripheral action on skeletal muscle (Cedarbaum & Schleifer 1990; Davidoff 1985). It is thought to inhibit the excitation-induced release of calcium ions from the sarcoplasmic reticulum of striated muscle fibres, thereby inhibiting excitation–contraction coupling and diminishing the mechanical force of contraction. The blockade of calcium release is not complete, however, and contraction is not completely abolished. It reduces reflex more than voluntary contractions, probably because of a preferential action on fast-twitch rather than slow-twitch skeletal muscle fibres. It has been shown to have therapeutic benefits for chronic spasticity associated with central nervous system disorders. The drug improves voiding function in some patients with classic detrusor-striated sphincter dyssynergia and was initially reported to be very successful in doing so (Murdock et al 1976). In adults the recommended starting dose is 25 mg daily, gradually increasing by increments of 25 mg every 4–7 days to a maximum oral dose of 400 mg given in four divided doses. Hackler and colleagues (1980) reported improvement in voiding function in approximately half of their patients treated with dantrolene but found that such improvement required oral doses of 600 mg daily. Although no inhibitory effect on bladder smooth muscle seems to occur (Harris & Benson 1980), the generalized weakness that dantrolene can induce is often significant enough to compromise its therapeutic effects. Other potential side-effects include euphoria, dizziness, diarrhoea and hepatotoxicity.

Other agents Beta-adrenergic agonists, especially those with prominent β-2 characteristics, are able to produce relaxation of some skeletal muscles of the slow-twitch type (Olsson et al 1979; Holmberg & Waldeck 1980). This kind of action may account at least in part for the decrease in urethral profile parameters seen with terbutaline (see earlier section, Decreasing outlet resistance at the level of the smooth sphincter). This area of pharmacology and its clinical relevance is somewhat confusing at the moment because β-2 adrenergic drugs have been reported to potentiate periurethral striated muscle contraction, albeit in a different *in vitro* system (see later section, Increasing outlet resistance). Botulinum toxin (an inhibitor of acetylcholine release at the neuromuscular junction of striated muscle) has been injected directly into the striated sphincter to treat dyssynergia (Dykstra & Sidi 1990). Injection carried out weekly for 3 weeks can achieve a duration of effect averaging 2 months. The number of patients tested so far is small, and more information is needed about criteria for success and about side-effects.

Inhibition of the smooth sphincter

Alpha-adrenergic antagonists There is no question that the smooth muscle of the bladder and urethra of a variety of experimental animals and of man contains both α- and β-adrenergic receptors (Andersson 1993; Wein et al 1991b). The smooth muscle of the bladder base and proximal urethra contains predominantly α-adrenergic receptors. The bladder body contains both varieties of adrenergic receptors, the β variety being more common. The suggestion that α-adrenergic blockade could be useful in certain patients who cannot empty their bladder was actually first made by Kleeman in 1970. Krane & Olsson (1973a,b) were among the first to endorse the concept of a physiological internal sphincter which is partially controlled by tonic sympathetic stimulation of contractile α-adrenergic receptors in the smooth musculature of the bladder neck and proximal urethra. Further, they hypothesized that some obstructions which occur at this level during detrusor contraction result from an inadequate opening of the bladder neck or an inadequate decrease in resistance in the area of the proximal urethra.

Abel and colleagues (1974) pointed out that such a functional obstruction, which they, too, presumed to be mediated by the sympathetic nervous system, could be maximal at a urethral rather than bladder neck level, and coined the term 'neuropathic urethra'. Many others have subsequently confirmed the utility of α-blockade in the treatment of what is now usually referred to as smooth sphincter or bladder neck dyssynergia or dysfunction. Successful results, usually defined as an increase in flow rate, a decrease in residual urine, and an improvement in upper tract appearance (when that is pathological), can often be correlated with an objective decrease in urethral profile closure pressures. One would expect such success with α-adrenergic blockade in treating emptying failure to be least evident in patients with detrusor-striated sphincter dyssynergia, as reported by Hachen (1980). Much of the confusion relative to whether or not α blockers have a direct (as opposed to an indirect) inhibitory effect on the striated sphincter relate to the interpretation of observations about their effect on urethral pressure and periurethral striated muscle EMG activity in the region of the urogenital diaphragm. It is impossible to tell by pressure tracings alone whether a decrease in resistance in one area of the urethra is secondary to a decrease in smooth or in striated muscle activity.

Alpha-adrenergic blocking agents have also been used to treat both bladder and outlet abnormalities in patients with so-called autonomous bladders (Norlen 1982). These include those with myelodysplasia, sacral or infrasacral spinal cord neural injury, and voiding dysfunction following radical pelvic surgery. Parasympathetic decentralization has been reported to lead to a marked increase in adrenergic innervation of the bladder, resulting in conversion of the usual beta (relaxant) bladder response to sympathetic stimulation to an alpha (contractile) response (Sundin et al 1977). Although the alterations in innervation have been disputed, the alterations in receptor function have not. Koyangi (1979) demonstrated urethral supersensitivity to α-adrenergic stimulation in a group of patients with autonomous neurogenic bladders, implying that a change had occurred in adrenergic receptor function in the urethra following parasympathetic decentralization. Parsons & Turton (1980) observed the same phenomenon but ascribed the cause to adrenergic supersensitivity of the urethral smooth muscle caused by sympathetic decentralization. Nordling and colleagues (1981) described a similar phenomenon in women who had undergone radical hysterectomy and ascribed this change to damage to the sympathetic innervation. Decreased bladder compliance is often a clinical problem in such patients and this, along with a fixed urethral sphincter tone, results in the paradoxical occurrence of both storage and emptying failure. Norlen (1982) has summarized the supporting evidence for the success of α-adrenolytic treatment in these patients. Phenoxybenzamine is capable of increasing bladder compliance (increasing storage) and decreasing urethral resistance (facilitating emptying). Andersson and co-workers (1981) used prazosin (Minipress) in such patients and found that maximum urethral pressure during filling was decreased, whereas 'autonomous waves' were reduced. McGuire & Savastano (1985) reported that phenoxybenzamine decreased filling cystometric pressure in the decentralized primate bladder.

Alpha-adrenergic blockade can decrease bladder contractility in patients with voiding dysfunction by another mechanism. Jensen reported an increase in the 'α-adrenergic effect' in bladders characterized as 'uninhibited' (Jensen 1981a,b,c). Short- and long-term prazosin administration increased bladder capacity and decreased the amplitude of contractions. Thomas and colleagues (1984) found that intravenous phentolamine produced a significant reduction in maximum voiding detrusor pressure, voiding volumes, and peak flow rates in patients with suprasacral spinal cord injury with no reduction of outflow obstruction.

POB was the α-adrenergic agent originally used for the treatment of voiding dysfunction. It and phentolamine have blocking properties at both α-1 and α-2 receptor sites. The initial adult dosage of this agent is 10 mg\day, and the usual daily dose for voiding dysfunction is 10 to 20 mg. Daily doses larger than 10 mg are generally divided and given every 8–12 hours. After the drug has been discontinued, the effects of administration may persist for days because the drug irreversibly inactivates α-receptors, and the duration of effect depends on the rate of receptor resynthesis (Hoffman & Lefkowitz 1990b). Potential side-effects include orthostatic hypotension, reflex tachycardia, nasal congestion, diarrhoea, miosis, sedation, nausea and vomiting (secondary to local irritation).

Prazosin hydrochloride (Minipress) is a potent selective α-1 antagonist (Hoffman & Lefkowitz 1990b) and its clinical use to lower outlet resistance has already been mentioned. The duration of action is 4–6 hours; therapy is generally begun in daily divided doses of 2–3 mg. The dose may be gradually increased to a maximum of 20 mg daily, although it is seldom more than 9–10 mg daily used for voiding dysfunction. The potential side-effects of prazosin are a consequence of its α-1 blockade. Occasionally, there occurs a 'first-dose' phenomenon, a symptom complex of faintness, dizziness, palpitations and, infrequently, syncope, thought to be due to acute postural hypotension. The incidence of this phenomenon can be minimized by restricting the initial dose of the drug to 1 mg and administering this at bedtime.

Terazosin (Hytrin) and doxazosin (Cardura) are two of the latest in the series of highly selective postsynaptic α-1 blocking drugs. They are readily absorbed and have a high bioavailability and a long plasma half-life, enabling their activity to be maintained over 24 hours following a single dose (Taylor 1989; Lepor 1990). Because of the α-1 receptor content of the prostatic stroma and capsule, the use of these drugs has recently been promoted for the treatment of voiding dysfunction secondary to benign prostatic hyperplasia (BPH). Their side-effects are similar to those of prazosin (Wilde et al 1993b). Alfluzosin is a new agent that is reported to be a selective and competitive antagonist of α-1 mediated contraction of the prostate capsule, bladder base, and proximal urethral smooth muscle. It is said to be more specific for such receptors in the genitourinary tract than in the vasculature, raising the possibility that voiding may be facilitated by doses that have minimal vasodilatory effects, thus minimizing postural hypotension (Wilde et al 1993a). The drug requires three times daily dosing (7.5 to 10 mg total). Our own experience suggests that a trial of an agent with α-adrenergic blocking properties is certainly worthwhile because its effect or non-effect will become obvious in a matter of days, and the pharmacological side-effects are of course reversible. However, our results with such therapy for non-BPH-related voiding dysfunction have been less spectacular than those of some other investigators.

Other potential non-specific therapy Beta-adrenergic stimulation has been shown experimentally to decrease the urethral pressure profile and thus urethral resistance (Raz & Caine 1971). It seems doubtful that a β agonist will prove clinically useful in facilitating bladder emptying by decreasing outlet resistance. Progesterone has been suggested as a possible treatment for emptying abnormalities in women. In a study of normal women looking at the effects of oestrogen alone (E) versus oestrogen plus progesterone (E+P), maximum flow in the E only group increased from 26 to 38 ml/second. A sphincteric effect was hypothesized (Burton & Dobson 1993). Finally, nitric oxide (NO) has been suggested to be a mediator of non-adrenergic non-cholinergic (NANC) relaxation of the smooth muscle of the bladder outlet which occurs with bladder contraction (Andersson 1993). Whether this means that analogues or substances which release NO *in vivo* will prove useful in decreasing smooth muscle-related outlet resistance in humans remains to be seen. If so, one could envisage a role for NO synthetase inhibitors in stabilizing urethral pressure or increasing outlet resistance. NO is a ubiquitous molecule, however, and exerts inhibitor effects on the detrusor body *in vitro* (see later section, 'Decreasing bladder contractility'). Opposite functional effects on the bladder and outlet (on contractility and resistance) could well frustrate any clinical application.

FACILITATION OF URINE STORAGE

Excluding fistulae and mental incompetence, the pathophysiology of failure of the lower urinary tract to fill with or store urine adequately may be secondary to reasons related to the bladder, to the outlet, or both (Wein et al 1991a). Hyperactivity of the bladder during filling can be expressed as discrete involuntary contractions (IVC) or as reduced compliance with or without phasic contraction. Purely sensory urgency may also account for storage failure. A fixed decrease in outlet resistance may result from damage to innervation of the structural elements of the smooth or striated sphincter or from neurological disease or injury, surgical or other mechanical trauma, or ageing. Classic genuine stress incontinence in women seems primarily to be a sphincter dysfunction caused by a failure of the normal transmission of increases in intra-abdominal pressure to the area of the bladder neck and proximal urethra. The pathophysiology of genuine stress incontinence may also involve a decrease in the reflex striated sphincter contraction, which occurs with a number of manoeuvres which increase intra-abdominal pressure. Treatment of abnormalities related to the filling or storage phase of micturition is directed towards inhibiting bladder contractility, increasing bladdder capacity, or decreasing sensory input during filling, or towards increasing outlet resistance, either continuously or only during abdominal straining.

Decreasing bladder contractility

Anticholinergic agents

Because a large part of the neurohumoral stimulus for physiological bladder contraction is acetylcholine-induced stimulation to postganglionic parasympathetic muscarinic cholinergic receptor sites on bladder smooth muscle (Andersson 1993; Wein et al 1991b), atropine and atropine-like agents will depress true involuntary bladder contractions of any aetiology (Andersson 1988; Blaivas et al 1980; Jensen 1981a). In such conditions the volume at the first involuntary contraction will generally be increased, the amplitude of the contractions decreased, and the total bladder capacity increased, with a proportionate reduction in symptomatology. Interestingly, bladder compliance in normal individuals and in those with detrusor hyperreflexia in whom the initial slope of the filling curve on cystometry is normal prior to the involuntary contraction, does not seem to be significantly altered (Jensen 1981b). Outlet resistance, at least as reflected by urethral pressure measurements, does not seem to be clinically affected by anticholinergic therapy.

Although these agents generally produce significant clinical improvement in patients with involuntary bladder contractions and symptoms consequent to these, only partial inhibition generally results. In many animal models atropine only partially antagonizes the response of the whole bladder to pelvic nerve stimulation and of bladder strips to field stimulation, although it does completely inhibit the response of bladder smooth muscle to exogenous cholinergic stimulation. Of the theories proposed to explain this phenomenon, called 'atropine resistance', the most attractive and most commonly cited is the idea that a major portion of the neurotransmission involved in the final common pathway of bladder contraction is non-adrenergic and non-cholinergic, secondary to a release of a transmitter other than acetylcholine or norepinephrine (Andersson 1993; Wein et al 1991b). Although the existence of atropine resistance in human bladder muscle is by no means agreed on, this concept is the most common hypothesis invoked to explain clinical difficulty in abolishing IVC with anticholinergic agents alone, and it is also used to support the rationale of treatment of such types of bladder activity with agents that have different mechanisms of action.

Receptor subtyping is particularly relevant for drug development in general and for antimuscarinic compounds in particular. Subtyping can be based on functional assays, on radioligand-binding affinity, and on receptor cloning and expression. At least five different genetically established (by cloning) muscarinic subtypes exist (designated M_1 to M_5) (Bonner 1989). The nomenclature M_1 to M_3 describes the pharmacologically defined (using subtype selective agonists and antagonists) muscarinic subtypes (Andersson 1993; Poli et al 1992). Pirenzepine (a selective muscarinic blocker) was originally used to subdivide muscarinic receptors into M_1 and M_2 categories; using this subclassification, detrusor muscarinic receptors have been found to be the M_2 type (Andersson 1993; Levin et al 1988a, b). On further analysis of the M_2 receptor population, a small proportion of glandular M_2 receptors was found which could represent the pharmacologic type responsible for muscarinic agonist-induced contractions. This subtype is now called the M_3 receptor and, although a systematic subclassification of human detrusor M receptors remains to be made, indirect evidence suggests that human detrusor also contains this subtype (Andersson 1993; Poli et al 1992).

In treating patients, it appears that some become relatively refractory to anticholinergic drugs after a while. Such an effect could have many causes, but one pharmacological fact which could contribute to such a phenomenon is a change in receptor density in response to certain stimuli (up- or down-regulation). Experimentally, at least, Levin and colleagues (1988a) have shown that an increase in peripheral muscarinic receptor density occurs with chronic atropine administration (in the rat). On the other hand, certain pathological states may be associated with changes in receptor density, which may in turn affect the response to anticholinergic (and other) agents. Restorick & Mundy (1989) described a decrease in density of muscarinic cholinergic receptors and an increase in density of α-adrenergic receptors in bladder dome samples from humans with detrusor hyperreflexia; β-adrenergic receptor density remained unchanged. Lepor and associates (1989) described a similar decrease in cholinergic receptor density in bladder specimens from children and adults with voiding dysfunction due to myelomeningocele, spinal cord injury, or multiple sclerosis, all of whom had involuntary bladder contractions. Proposed mechanisms include down-regulation due to hyperactivity, smooth muscle hypertrophy and bladder wall fibrosis.

Specific drugs

Propantheline bromide (Pro-Banthine and others) is the classically described oral agent for producing an antimuscarinic effect in the lower urinary tract. The usual adult oral dose is 15 to 30 mg every 4 to 6 hours, although higher doses are often necessary. Propantheline is a quaternary ammonium compound, which is poorly absorbed after oral administration (Brown 1990). Oral administration in the fasting state, rather than with or after meals, is preferable from the standpoint of drug bioavailability (Gibaldi & Grundhofer 1975). Although there are obviously many other considerations in accounting for the effect of a given dose of drug on the lower urinary tract, there is no oral drug available whose direct *in vitro* antimuscarinic binding potential approximates that of atropine better than the long available and relatively inexpensive propantheline bromide (Levin et al 1982; Peterson et al 1990). There is a surprising lack of valuable data on the effectiveness of propantheline for the treatment of bladder hyperactivity. As Andersson points out (1988), anticholinergic drugs in general have been reported to have both great and poor efficacy for this indication. To show the range of variation, Zorzitto and colleagues (1986) concluded that propantheline bromide administered orally in doses of 30 mg four times a day to a group of institutionalized incontinent geriatric patients had marginal benefits which were outweighed by the side-effects. Blaivas and colleagues (1980) on the other hand, by increasing the dose of propantheline (up to 60 mg four times a day) until incontinence was eliminated or side-effects precluded further use, obtained a complete response in 25 to 26 patients with involuntary bladder contractions. Differences in bioavailability, selective drug delivery, receptor selectivity, receptor density, atropine resistance, pathophysiology, susceptibility to dose-limiting side-effects and mental status are all potential factors which could explain such disparate results. The Agency for Health Care Policy and Research (AHCPR) clinical practice guidelines (Weiner et al 1986) lists five randomized controlled trials for propantheline, in which 82% of the patients were women. Percentage cures (all figures refer to per cent minus per cent on placebo) are listed as 0–5, per cent reduction in urge incontinence as 0–53, per cent side-effects 0–50, and per cent dropouts 0–9.

Scopolamine is another belladonna alkaloid marketed as a soluble salt. It has prominent central depressive effects at low doses, probably due to its greater penetration (compared to atropine) through the blood–brain barrier. Transdermal scopolamine has been used for treating involuntary bladder contractions (Cornella et al 1990). The 'patch' provides continuous delivery of 0.5 mg daily to the circulation for 3 days. Cornella and associates, however, reported poor results with this form of drug in treating 10 patients with detrusor instability (Greenstein et al 1992). Only 2 patients showed a positive response, an additional one showed a slight improvement, and in 8 of 10 it had to be discontinued because of side-effects. Side-effects were related to the central nervous system (ataxia, dizziness) and included blurred vision and dry mouth.

Although methantheline (Banthine) has a higher ratio of ganglion-blocking to antimuscarinic activity than does propantheline, the latter drug seems to be at least as potent in each respect, clinical dose for dose. Methantheline does have similar effects on the lower urinary tract, and some clinicians still prefer it over other anticholinergic agents. Few real data are available regarding its efficacy.

A lack of selectivity is a major problem with all antimuscarinic compounds because they tend to affect parasympathetically innervated organs in the same order; generally larger doses are required to inhibit bladder activity than to affect salivary, bronchial, nasopharyngeal and sweat secretions. The potential side-effects of all antimuscarinic agents include inhibition of salivary secretion (dry mouth), blockade of the ciliary muscle of the lens to cholinergic stimulation (blurred vision for near objects), tachycardia, drowsiness, and inhibition of gut motility. Those agents which possess some ganglion-blocking activity may also cause orthostatic hypotension and impotence at high doses (generally required for nicotinic activity to become manifest). Antimuscarinic agents are generally contraindicated in patients with narrow angle glaucoma, and should be used with caution in patients with significant bladder outlet obstruction because complete urinary retention may be precipitated.

Musculotropic relaxants

These agents fall under the general heading of direct-acting smooth muscle depressants, whose 'antispasmodic' activity reportedly affects smooth muscle directly at a site that is metabolically distal to the cholinergic or other contractile receptor mechanism. Although all of the agents discussed in this section do relax smooth muscle *in vitro* by a papaverine-like (direct) action, all have been found to possess variable anticholinergic and local anaesthetic properties in addition. There is still some uncertainty about how much of their clinical efficacy is due only to their atropine-like effect. If, in fact, any of these agents do exert a clinically significant inhibitory effect that is independent of antimuscarinic action, a therapeutic rationale exists for combining them with a relatively pure anticholenergic agent.

Oxybutynin chloride (Ditropan) is a moderately potent anticholinergic agent which has strong independent musculotropic relaxant activity as well as local anaesthetic activity. Comparatively higher concentrations *in vitro* are necessary to produce direct spasmolytic effects, which may be due to calcium channel blockade (Kachur et al 1988; Thompson & Lauvetz 1976). The recommended oral adult dose is 5 mg three or four times a day, although in the elderly a dose of 2.5 mg twice daily is equally effective with reduced side-effects; side-effects are antimuscarinic and dose-related. Initial reports documented success in depressing detrusor hyperreflexia in patients with neurogenic bladder dysfunction (Thompson & Lauvetz 1976) and subsequent reports documented success in inhibiting other types of bladder hyperactivity as well (Andersson 1988). A randomized double-blind, placebo-controlled study comparing oxybutynin 5 mg three times a day with placebo in 30 patients with detrusor instability was carried out by Moisey and colleagues (1980). Seventeen of 23 patients who completed the study with oxybutynin had symptomatic improvement, and 9 showed evidence of urodynamic improvement, mainly an increase in maximum bladder capacity. Hehir & Fitzpatrick (1985) reported that 16 of 24 patients with neuropathic voiding dysfunction secondary to myelomeningocele were cured or improved (17% dry, 50% improved) with oxybutynin treatment. Average bladder capacity increased from 197 ml to 299 ml (with drug) versus 218 ml (with placebo). Maximum bladder filling pressure decreased from 47 to 37 cm H_2O (with placebo).

In a prospective randomized study of 34 patients with voiding dysfunction secondary to multiple sclerosis, Gajewski & Awad (1986) found that a dose of 5 mg three times a day of oral oxybutynin produced a good response more frequently than 15 mg of propantheline three times a day. They concluded that oxybutynin was more effective in the treatment of detrusor hyperreflexia secondary to multiple sclerosis. Holmes and associates (1989) compared the results of oxybutynin and propantheline in a small group of women with detrusor instability. The experimental design was a randomized crossover trial with a patient-regulated variable dose regimen. This kind of dose titration study allows the patient to increase the drug dose to whatever he or she perceives to be the optimum ratio between clinical improvement and side-effects – an interesting way of comparing two drugs while minimizing differences in oral absorption. Of the 23 women in the trial, 14 reported subjective improvement with oxybutynin, as opposed to 11 with propantheline. Both drugs significantly increased the maximum cystometric capacity and reduced the maximum detrusor pressure on filling. The only significant objective difference was a greater increase in the maximum cystometric capacity with oxybutynin. The mean total daily dose of oxybutynin tolerated was 15 mg (range, 7.5–30) and that of propantheline was 90 mg (range, 45–145). Thuroff and colleagues (1991) compared oxybutynin to propantheline and placebo in a group with symptoms of instability and either detrusor instability or hyperreflexia. Oxybutynin (5 mg three times a day) performed best, but propantheline was used at a relatively low dose – 15 mg three times a day. The rate of side-effects was higher for oxybutynin at just about the level of clinical and urodynamic improvement. The mean grade of improvement on a visual analogue scale was higher for oxybutynin (58.2%)

versus propantheline (44.7%) and placebo (43.4%). Urodynamic volume at the first involuntary bladder contraction increased more with oxybutynin (51 vs. 11.2 vs. 9.7 ml), as did the change in maximum cystometric capacity (80.1 vs. 48.9 vs. 22.5 ml). Residual urine volume also increased more (27.0 vs. 2.2 vs. 1.9 ml).

Zeegers and colleagues (1987) reported on a double-blind prospective crossover study comparing oxybutynin, flavoxate (see later in this section), emepronium, and placebo. There was a high dropout rate (19 of 60 patients) and the entry criteria were vague (frequency, urgency, urge incontinence). The results were scored as 5 (excellent overall effect) to 1 (no improvement) by both patient and physician, and the results were combined into a single number. The percentages of results in categories 3 to 5 for the agents used were oxybutynin 61%, placebo 41%, emperonium 34%, and flavoxate 31%. The results of the first treatment above gave corresponding percentages of 63%, 29%, 18% (probably reflecting eight dropouts due to side-effects), and 44%.

Ambulatory urodynamic monitoring and pad weighing were used to assess the effects of oxybutynin on detrusor hyperactivity by Van Doorn & Zwiers (1990). The 24-hour average frequency of involuntary bladder contractions decreased from 8.7 to 3.4, the maximum contraction amplitude decreased from 32 to 22 cm H_2O, and the duration of the average involuntary bladder contraction decreased from 90 to 60 seconds. However, daily micturition frequency did not change (11 to 10), nor the amount of urine lost – findings the authors try to minimize by pointing out that some patients had sphincteric incontinence as well and that a higher fluid intake during treatment may have occurred. The AHCPR guideline (Weiner et al 1986) lists six randomized controlled trials for oxybutynin; 90% of patients were women. The percentage of cures (all figures refer to percentage *minus* percentage on placebo) is listed as 28% and 44%, percentage of reduction in urge incontinence is 9% and 56%, and the percentages of side-effects and dropouts are 2% and 66% and 3% and 45% respectively.

There are some negative reports on the efficacy of oxybutynin. Zorzitto and colleagues (1989) came to conclusions similar to those resulting from their study of propantheline (see earlier) in a double-blind placebo-controlled trial conducted in 24 incontinent geriatric institutionalized patients; oxybutynin 5 mg twice a day was no more effective than placebo with scheduled toileting in treating incontinence in this type of population with detrusor hyperactivity. An incontinence profile was used to assess results. The only significant difference noted was an increase in residual urine volume (159 vs. 92 ml). Ouslander and colleagues (1988a,b) reported similar conclusions in a smaller study of geriatric patients, and they concluded simply that the drug is safe for use in the elderly at doses of 2.5–5 mg three times a day.

Topical application of oxybutynin and other agents to normal or intestinal bladders has been suggested and tried (Kato et al 1989). This conceptually attractive form of alternative drug administration, delivered either by periodic intravesical instillation of liquid or timed-released pellets, awaits further clinical trials and the development of preparations specifically formulated for this purpose. Madersbacher & Jilg (1991) reviewed such usage of oxybutynin and presented data on 13 patients with complete suprasacral cord lesions who were on CIC. One 5 mg tablet was dissolved in 30 ml of distilled water, and the solution was instilled intravesically. Of the 10 patients who were incontinent, 9 remained dry for 6 hours. For the group, the changes in bladder capacity and maximum detrusor pressure were statistically significant. Some data were given in a figure showing plasma oxybutynin levels in a group of patients in whom administration was intravesical or oral. The level following an oral dose rose to 7.3 mg/ml but was less than 2 mg/ml at 4 hours. Following intravesical administration, the level rose gradually to a peak of about 6.2 mg/ml at 3.5 hours, but at 6 hours it was still greater than 4 mg/ml, and at 9 hours it was still between 3 and 4 mg/ml. Did the intravesically applied drug act locally or systemically? Weese and colleagues (1993) reported on a similar dose of oxybutynin (5 mg in 30 ml of sterile water) to treat 42 patients with involuntary bladder contractions who had either failed oral anticholinergic therapy (11 patients) or had intolerable side-effects (31 patients). Twenty had hyperreflexia, 19 had instability, and 3 had bowel or bladder hyperactivity after augmentation. The drug was instilled two or three times a day for 10 minutes by catheter. Twenty-one per cent (9 patients) dropped out because they were unable to tolerate CIC or retain the solution properly, but there were no reported side-effects. Fifty-five per cent of patients (18 out of 33) who were able to follow the protocol reported at least a moderate subjective improvement in incontinence and urgency. Nine patients became totally continent and experienced complete resolution of their symptoms; 18 patients improved and experienced a decrease of 2.5 pads per day. There were no urodynamic data. Follow-up ranged from 5 to 35 months (mean, 18.4 months). The lack of side-effects prompted some speculation about the mechanism of drug action. One possibility suggested was simply a more prolonged rate of absorption. Another and more intriguing one was a decreased pass through the liver and therefore a decrease in metabolites, the hypothesis being that perhaps the metabolites and not the primary compound are responsible for the side-effects. Anyone who is prescribed oxybutynin will agree that 'dry mouth' is one of the most troublesome side-effects and one which causes many patients to discontinue therapy.

Kelleher and co-workers (1998) attempted to contact 348 women who had a diagnosis of detrusor instability 6 months after the diagnosis was made. Of these, 256 responded for follow up and the majority had received oxybutynin treatment. Only 18.2% continued with treatment because of the side-effects, particularly dry mouth. It has been proposed that side-effects may be reduced by trying a controlled release preparation or even a rectal preparation.

Collas and Malone-Lee (1997) reported the pharmacokinetic properties of rectal oxybutynin. The study was an open, cross over, new design comparing 5 mg oxybutynin given orally with 5 mg given rectally by suppository. Twenty volunteer students were used throughout the study. The plasma level was a more steady state. Side-effects were much lower than the oral route of administration. Delaere and Branje (1998) performed a pilot study with 15 patients with overactive detrusors. All had stopped oral oxybutynin because of marked side-effects. Of the 15 patients, three withdrew because of diarrhoea and stomach problems and four complained of problems with a minor dry mouth. Eleven continued their treatment because of benefit and minimal, or no, side-effects. Winkler and Sand (1998) in a retrospective study also showed a marked reduction in side-effects. This route of administration appears promising but larger trials are required to evaluate it thoroughly.

Relatively recently, new medications, or new formulations of old medications, have been introduced which specifically address the problem of improved tolerability of pure anticholinergic agents or agents purported to have a 'combined action' but whose clinical activity seems to reside in the anticholinergic component.

Tolterodine is a drug specifically developed for the treatment of patients with bladder overactivity. It is a potent, competitive, cholinergic receptor antagonist, non-selective for any particular cholinergic receptor type (Nilvebrant et al 1997a). Its major metabolite exhibits a similar pharmacological profile. Tolterodine has been reported to demonstrate bladder selectivity both in vitro and in the anaesthetised cat model (Nilvebrant et al 1997b). In these latter studies, the drug and its metabolite showed a more pronounced effect on acetylcholine induced bladder contraction than on electrically induced salivation. While the dose-response curves for bladder contraction inhibition were similar for tolterodine and oxybutynin, oxybutynin showed the opposite tissue selectivity profile. This selectivity is yet to be explained pharmacologically, but seems to exist in humans as well. Stahl and colleagues (1995) studied the effect of a single 6.4 mg dose of tolterodine on bladder and salivary function and found that the inhibitory effect on bladder function persisted up to 5 hours, but stimulated salivation was inhibited only around the time of peak serum levels. In clinical studies, tolterodine has been compared to placebo and to the prior gold standard of treatment, immediate release oxybutynin. Appell (1997) reported on a pooled analysis of a total of 1120 patients in whom tolterodine at doses of 1 or 2 mg twice daily was compared to oxybutynin 5 mg 3 times daily or placebo. Both active drugs significantly decreased incontinence episodes for 24 hours, decreased the number of micturitions for 24 hours, and increased the volume voided per micturition compared to placebo. There was no difference in effectiveness between the 2 mg dose of tolterodine and the 5 mg dose of oxybutynin, but tolerance was significantly improved with tolterodine when adverse events, dry mouth (both frequency and intensity), dose reductions, and patient withdrawals were considered.

Once daily formulations of oxybutynin have been developed, also with the purpose of increasing tolerability while maintaining efficacy. One formulation, oxybutynin XL, uses an ingenious osmotic drug delivery system to release the agent at a controlled rate over 24 hours. This formulation overcomes the marked peak-to-trough fluctuations in plasma levels of both the drug and its major metabolite, also metabolically active, that occur with immediate release oxybutynin (Gupta and Sathyan 1999). A trend towards a lower incidence of dry mouth with oxybutynin XL was attributed to reduced first pass metabolism and to maintenance of lower and less fluctuating plasma levels of drug. Clinical trials have concentrated on comparing oxybutynin XL with immediate release oxybutynin. Anderson et al (1999) reported on a 13-centre study, which showed globally that this extended release formulation had comparable efficacy to the immediate release formulation, but with improved tolerability. One can use this study, however, only to compare the two drugs, as only patients who had previously responded to treatment with oxybutynin were selected for participation. Whether this selection process included those who experienced favourable efficacy but poor tolerability was not stated. Weekly urge incontinence episodes were the primary outcome measure, and this decreased substantially in both groups, with no difference between the two. Dry mouth was reported in 68% of patients receiving the controlled release formulation, and 87% of those receiving immediate release. Corresponding numbers for moderate to severe dry mouth were 25% and 46% respectively. From this standpoint, the controlled release formulation seems better tolerated than the immediate release formulation. However, somnolence was reported in 38% of the controlled release group and 40% of the immediate release group, blurred vision in 28% and 17% respectively, constipation in 30% and 31% respectively, and dizziness in 28% and 38% respectively. Normal voiding frequency increased 54% in the controlled release group and 17% in the immediate release group. Another extended release form of oxybutynin was utilized by Birns and co-workers (1997), who reported comparable efficacy of a 10 mg preparation compared with 5 mg twice daily of immediate release oxybutynin. Efficacy was similar, but the extended release formulation was better tolerated, with patients reporting only approximately half the total number of adverse events compared with those treated with the immediate release preparation. Nilsson and co-workers (1997), however, failed to demonstrate improved tolerability for the controlled release formulation.

Trospium chloride is a non-selective anticholinergic drug with primarily peripheral (antimuscarinic) activity, but also, at least in vitro, some ganglionic (nicotinic) effects as well (Thuroff et al 1998). Stohrer and colleagues (1991) reported on a double blind placebo study with this agent in patients with detrusor hyperreflexia. With few side-effects, the drug was reported to increase maximum cystometric capacity, decrease maximal detrusor pressure, and increase compliance. Madersbacher and co-workers (1995) found the drug to be equally as effective as oxybutynin in patients with hyperreflexia due to spinal cord injury, but with fewer side-effects. There is little else available in the literature on the effects of trospium. One study did look at the influence of trospium versus oxybutynin on quantitative EEG parameters in healthy volunteers (Pietzko et al 1994). Quantitative evaluation shows statistically significant decreases in α and β-1 activity after oxybutynin, but not after trospium.

Propiverine is an agent reported to have a pharmacological profile similar to that of oxybutynin: anticholinergic direct myotrophic relaxant and local anaesthetic activity, with anticholinergic activity prominent in the clinical setting (Thuroff et al 1998). Most of the references which cite propiverine's effectiveness in the treatment of patients with detrusor overactivity are in abstract form or in the German literature (see Thuroff et al 1998; Andersson et al 1999). It has been suggested in these reports that the drug may have equal efficacy to oxybutynin, but fewer side-effects. Andersson and co-workers (1999) state that its place in therapy is difficult to evaluate and requires further comparative studies.

Darifenacin is a very selective M_3 receptor antagonist with possible selectivity for urinary bladder over salivary gland (Wallis & Napier 1999). In a small placebo controlled study published only in abstract form, a single 10 mg dose of darifenacin showed improvement in urodynamic parameters in patients with overactive bladder, though significant reductions in salivary flow were also apparent (Rosario et al 1996). Little other clinical data is available, and studies are ongoing to determine the efficacy/tolerability profile of this agent.

Concerning hyperactivity in augmented or intestinal neo-bladders, for which there is no separate section in this chapter, Andersson and colleagues (1992) recently reviewed this phenomenon and its pharmacological treatment. They noted few instances of positive results with agents given systemically. Locally applied agents were thought to offer more promise. A list of possibilities and their assessments was included. Pure anticholinergics have produced no good results, either locally or systemically. Oxybutynin has shown poor results with systemic therapy but some good results with local therapy. Alpha agonists have produced no effect; β agonists have shown no local effects and equivocal effects when administered subcutaneously, but the comment was made that such use will probably be limited by side-effects. Other possibilities mentioned for future use included opioid agonists (diphenoxylate – a component of Lomotil – and loperamide), calcium antagonists, potassium channel openers, and NO donors.

Dicyclomine hydrochloride (Bentyl) is also reported to exert a direct relaxant effect on smooth muscle, in addition to an antimuscarinic action (Downie et al 1977). An oral dose of 20 mg three times a day in adults has been reported to increase bladder capacity in patients with detrusor hyperreflexia (Fischer et al 1978). Beck and co-workers (1976) compared the use of 10 mg dicyclomine, 15 mg propantheline and placebo, three times a day, in patients with detrusor hyperactivity. The cure or improved rates, respectively, were 62%, 73% and 20%. Awad and associates (1977) reported that 20 mg of dicyclomine three times a day caused resolution or significant improvement in 24 of 27 patients with involuntary bladder contractions.

Flavoxate hydrochloride (Urispas) has a direct

inhibitory action on smooth muscle but very weak anticholinergic properties (Andersson 1988; Ruffman 1988). Overall favourable clinical effects have been noted in some series of patients with frequency, urgency, and incontinence, and in patients with urodynamically documented detrusor hyperreflexia (Jonas et al 1979; Delaere et al 1977). The recommended adult dosage is 100–200 mg three or four times a day. As with all agents in this group, a short clinical trial may be worthwhile. Reported side-effects are few.

Calcium antagonists

The role of calcium as a messenger in linking extracellular stimuli to the intracellular environment is well established, including its involvement in excitation–contraction coupling in striated, cardiac and smooth muscle (Wein et al 1991a; Andersson 1993). The dependence of contractile activity on changes in cytosolic calcium varies from tissue to tissue, as do the characteristics of the calcium channels involved, but interference with calcium inflow or intracellular release is a very potent potential mechanism for bladder smooth muscle relaxation.

Nifedipine has been shown to be an effective inhibitor of contraction induced by several mechanisms in human and guinea-pig bladder muscle (Andersson 1988; Forman et al 1978). It has also been shown to block completely the non-cholinergic portion of the contraction produced by electrical field stimulation in rabbit bladder (Husted et al 1980). Nifedipine more effectively inhibited contractions induced by potassium than by carbachol in rabbit bladder strips, whereas terodiline, an agent with both calcium antagonistic and anticholinergic properties, had the opposite effect. However, terodiline did cause complete inhibition of the response of rabbit bladder to electrical field stimulation. At low concentrations terodiline has mainly an antimuscarinic action, whereas at higher concentration a calcium antagonistic effect becomes evident. *In vitro* experiments appeared to show that these two effects were additive with regard to bladder contractility. Other experimental studies have confirmed the inhibitory effect of the calcium antagonists nifedipine, verapamil, and diltiazem on a variety of experimental models of the activity of spontaneous and induced bladder muscle strips and whole bladder preparations (Finkbeiner 1983; Malkowicz et al 1985). Andersson and colleagues (1986) showed that nifedipine effectively and with some selectivity inhibited the non-muscarinic portion of the contraction of rabbit detrusor strips. This was in contrast to verapamil, diltiazem, flunarizine and lidoflazine, which caused a marked depression of both the total and the non-muscarinic parts of the contraction, suggesting that differences exist between various calcium channel blockers with respect to their effects on at least electrically induced bladder muscle contraction. These results were used as support for the view that, even if 'atropine resistant' contractions in rabbit and human bladder had different causes, combined muscarinic receptor and calcium channel blockade might offer a more effective way of treating bladder hyperactivity than the single-mechanism therapies presently available.

A number of clinical studies on the inhibitory action of terodiline on bladder hyperactivity have shown clinical effectiveness. The AHCPR guidelines (Weiner et al 1986) list seven randomized controlled trials for terodiline; 94% of patients were women. The percentage of cures (all figures refer to percentage minus percentage on placebo) is listed as 18% and 33%; percentage of reduction in urge incontinence is 14% and 83%, and the percentages of side-effects and dropouts are 14% and 40% and 2% and 8%, respectively. Terodiline also exhibits an inhibitory effect on experimental hyperreflexia in the rabbit whole bladder model, suggesting a possible role for local administration as well (Levin et al 1993).

Terodiline is almost completely absorbed from the gastrointestinal tract and has a low serum clearance. The recommended dosage in adults is 25 mg twice a day, reduced to an initial dose of 12 mg twice a day in geriatric patients. The common side-effects seen with calcium antagonists (hypotension, facial flushing, headache, dizziness, abdominal discomfort, constipation, nausea, rash, weakness and palpitations) have not been reported in larger initial clinical studies with terodiline, side-effects consisting primarily of those consequent to its anticholinergic action. However, questions have been raised about the occurrence of a rare arrhythmia (torsade de pointes) in patients taking terodiline simultaneously with antidepressants or antiarrhythmic drugs (Veldhuis & Inman 1991; Connolly et al 1991). Stewart and colleagues (1992) reported a prolongation of QT and QTC intervals and a reduction in heart rate in elderly patients taking 12.5 mg of terodiline twice a day. These effects were apparent after 1 week but not after 1 day of therapy. These investigators also reported polymorphic ventricular tachycardia in 4 patients (3 over age 80) receiving the drug. They advised avoiding using the drug in patients with cardiac disease requiring cardioactive drugs or those with hypokalaemia, or in combination with other drugs which can prolong the QT interval, such as tricyclic antidepressants or antipsychotics. After other reports of apparent cardiac toxicity, the drug was voluntarily withdrawn by the manufacturer pending the results of further safety studies. The studies conducted for approval by the Food and Drug Administration (FDA) were likewise voluntarily halted by the manufacturer; there is current activity directed towards their reinstitution.

Other calcium antagonist drugs have not been widely used to treat voiding dysfunction. Palmer and colleagues (1981) reported a double-blind placebo trial with a single 20 mg daily dose of flunarizine in 14 women with detrusor instability and consequent symptoms. A statistically significant decrease in urgency was produced in the drug-treated group, but there was no change in the frequency of micturition. Although a trend towards improvement of cystometric parameters occurred, it was not statistically significant ($p>0.05$). Nifedipine is useful as prophylaxis against the development of autonomic hyperreflexia during endoscopic examination in patients with high spinal injury. A 10-mg dose given 30 minutes prior to the examination has been successful, and a sublingual dose of 10 mg has been effective in relieving an episode (Dykstra et al 1987).

Potassium channel openers

Potassium channel openers efficiently relax various types of smooth muscle by increasing potassium efflux, resulting in membrane hyperpolarization. Hyperpolarization reduces the opening probability of ion channels involved in membrane depolarization, and excitation is reduced. Vaidyanathan et al (1981b) summarized studies showing that, in isolated human and animal detrusor muscle, potassium channel openers reduce spontaneous contractions and contractions occurring in response to electrical stimulation, carbachol, and low (but not high) external potassium concentrations. There are some suggestions that bladder instability, at least that associated with intravesical obstruction and detrusor hypertrophy, may be secondary to supersensitivity to depolarizing stimuli. Theoretically, then, potassium channel openers might be an attractive alternative for the treatment of detrusor instability in such circumstances, without inhibiting the normal voluntary contractions necessary for bladder emptying (Malgren et al 1990). Pinacidil is a compound which, in a concentration-dependent fashion, inhibits not only spontaneous myogenic contractions but also contractile responses induced by electrical field stimulation and carbachol in isolated human detrusor (Fovaeus et al 1989) and in normal and hypertrophied rat detrusor. Unfortunately, a preliminary study of this agent in a double-blind crossover format produced no effects on symptoms in 9 patients with detrusor instability and bladder outlet obstruction (Hedlund et al 1990).

Nurse and associates (1991) reported on the use of cromakalim, another potassium channel opener, in 17 patients who had refractory detrusor instability or hyperreflexia or had stopped other drug therapy because of intolerable side-effects. Six of 16 (35%) patients who completed the study showed a decrease in frequency and an increase in voided volume. Long-term observation was not possible because the drug was withdrawn owing to reported adverse effects of high doses in animal toxicological studies. Potassium channel openers are not at present very specific for the bladder and are more potent in relaxing other tissues – hence their potential utility in the treatment of hypertension, asthma, and angina. If tissue-selective potassium activator drugs can be developed, they may prove very useful for the treatment of detrusor instability, irritable bowel and epilepsy (Longman & Hamilton 1992). Intravesical use has also been suggested (Levin et al 1992).

Side-effects of pinacidil include headache, peripheral oedema (in 25–50% of patients and dose-related), weight gain, palpitations, dizziness and rhinitis. Hypertrichosis and symptomatic T-wave changes have also been reported (30%). Fewer data are available on cromakalim, which can produce dose-related headache but rarely oedema (Vaidyanathan et al 1981b).

Prostaglandin inhibitors

Prostaglandins (PG) are ubiquitous compounds which have a potential role in the excitatory neurotransmission to the bladder, the development of bladder contractility or tension occurring during filling, the emptying contractile response of bladder smooth muscle to neurostimulation, and even the maintenance of urethral tone during the storage phase of micturition, as well as the release of this tone during the emptying phase. Downie & Karmazyn (1984) suggest a different type of contractile influence of PG on detrusor muscle. They found that mechanical irritation of the epithelium of rabbit bladder increased basal tension and spontaneous activity in response to electrical stimulation, and that these responses, related to the intensity of the irritative trauma, were mimicked by prostaglandins, increasing afferent input at a given degree of bladder filling and contributing to the triggering of involuntary bladder contractions at a small bladder volume (Andersson 1988). Thus, there are many mechanisms whereby PG synthesis inhibitors might decrease bladder contractility in response to various stimuli. However, objective evidence of this is scant.

Cardozo and colleagues (1980) reported a double-blind placebo study on the effects of 50 mg three times a day of flurbiprofen, a PG synthetase inhibitor, on 30 women with detrusor instability. They concluded that the drug did not abolish involuntary bladder contractions or abnormal bladder activity but did not delay the intravesical pressure rise to a greater degree of distension. Forty-three per cent of the patients experienced side-effects, primarily nausea, vomiting, headache, indigestion, gastric distress, constipation and rash. Cardozo & Stanton (1979) reported symptomatic improvement in patients with detrusor instability who were given indomethacin in doses of 50–200 mg daily, but this was a short-term study with no cystometric data, and the drug was compared only with bromocriptine. The incidence of side-effects was high (19 of 32 patients), although no patient had to stop treatment because of them. Numerous PG synthetase inhibitors exist, most of which belong in the category of non-steroidal anti-inflammatory drugs, and every clinician has a favourite. It should be remembered that these drugs can interfere with platelet function and contribute to excess bleeding in surgical patients; some may have adverse renal effects as well (Brooks & Day 1991).

Beta-adrenergic agonists

The presence of β-adrenergic receptors in human bladder muscle has prompted attempts to increase bladder capacity with β-adrenergic stimulation. Such stimulation can cause significant increases in the capacity of animal bladders, which contain a moderate density of β-adrenergic receptors. *In vitro* studies show a strong dose-related relaxant effect of β-2 agonists on the bladder body of rabbits but little effect on the bladder base or proximal urethra. Terbutaline, in oral doses of 5 mg three times a day, has been reported to have a 'good clinical effect' in some patients with urgency and urge incontinence, but no significant effect on the bladders of neurologically normal humans without voiding difficulty (Fatigati & Murphy 1984). Although these results are compatible with those seen in other organ systems (β-adrenergic stimulation causes no acute change in total lung capacity in normal humans but does favourably affect patients with bronchial asthma), there are few adequate studies of the effects of β-adrenergic stimulation in patients with detrusor hyperactivity.

Lindholm & Lose (1986) used 5 mg three times a day of terbutaline in 8 women with motor and 7 with sensory urge incontinence. After 3 months of treatment, 14 patients claimed to have experienced beneficial effects, and 12 became subjectively continent. In 6 of 8 cases, the detrusor became stable on cystometric examination. Interestingly, the volume at first desire to void increased in the patients with originally unstable bladders from a mean of 200 to 302 ml, but the maximum cystometric capacity did not change. Nine patients had transient side-effects, including palpitations, tachycardia, or hand tremor, and in three of these, side-effects continued but were acceptable to the patient. In one patient the drug was discontinued because of severe adverse symptoms.

Gruneberger (1984), in a double-blind study, reported that clenbuterol had produced a good therapeutic effect in 15 of 20 patients with motor urge incontinence. Unfavourable results of β-agonist usage for bladder hyperactivity were published by Castleden & Morgan (1980) and Naglo et al (1989).

Tricyclic antidepressants

Many clinicians have found that tricyclic antidepressants, particularly imipramine hydrochloride, are especially useful for facilitating urine storage, both by decreasing bladder contractility and by increasing outlet resistance (Barrett & Wein 1991). These agents have been the subject of a voluminous and highly sophisticated pharmacological investigation to determine the mechanisms of action responsible for their varied effects (Baldesarini 1990; Richelson 1990; Hollister 1986). Most data have been accumulated as a result of trying to explain the antidepressant properties of these agonists, and consequently involve primarily central nervous system tissue. The results, conclusions and speculations based on the data are extremely interesting, but it should be emphasized that it is essentially unknown whether they apply to or have relevance for the lower urinary tract. In varying degrees, all of these agents have three major pharmacological actions. They have central and peripheral anticholinergic effects at some (but not all) sites; they block the active transport system in the presynaptic nerve ending which is responsible for the re-uptake of the release amine neurotransmitters norepinephrine and serotonin; and they are sedatives, an action which occurs presumably on a central basis but is perhaps related to antihistaminic properties (at H_1 receptors, though they also antagonize H_2 receptors to some extent). There is also evidence that these agents desensitize at least some α-2 and some β adrenoreceptors. Paradoxically, they have also been shown to block some α and serotonin-1 receptors. Imipramine has a prominent systemic anticholinergic effect but only a weak antimuscarinic effect on bladder smooth muscle (Olubadewo 1980; Levin et al 1983). It does have a strong direct inhibitory effect on bladder smooth muscle, however, that is neither anticholinergic nor adrenergic (Benson et al 1977; Olubadewo 1980; Levin & Wein 1984). This may be due to a local anaesthetic-like action at the nerve terminals in the adjacent effector membrane, an effect that seems to occur also in cardiac muscle (Bigger et al 1977), or it may be due to an inhibition of the participation of calcium in the excitation–contraction coupling process (Olubadewo 1980; Malkowicz et al 1987).

Akah (1986) has provided supportive evidence in the rat bladder that desipramine, the active metabolite of imipramine, depresses the response to electrical field stimulation by interfering with calcium movement perhaps not only extracellular calcium movement but also internal translocation and binding. Direct evidence suggesting that the effect of imipramine on norepinephrine re-uptake occurs in lower urinary tract tissue as well as brain tissue has been provided by Foreman & McNulty (1993) in the rabbit. In addition, they describe a significantly greater but similar effect of tomoxetine in the bladder and urethra in this model. Tomoxetine inhibits norepinephrine re-uptake selectively, whereas imipramine has a non-selective effect. This fact suggests a potential new clinical approach to the use of more selective and potent re-uptake inhibitors for the treatment of incontinence. In attempting to correlate clinical effects with mechanisms of action, one might also postulate a β receptor-induced decrease in bladder body contractility if peripheral blockade of norepinephrine re-uptake does occur there, owing to the increased concentration of β receptors compared to α-adrenergic receptors in that area. An enhanced α-adrenergic effect in the smooth muscle of the bladder base and proximal urethra, where α receptors outnumber β receptors, is generally considered to be the mechanism whereby imipramine increases outlet resistance.

Clinically, imipramine (Tofranil and others) seems to be effective in decreasing bladder contractility and increasing outlet resistance (Raezer et al 1977; Cole & Fried 1972; Tulloch & Creed 1981; Castleden et al 1981). Castleden and colleagues (1981) began therapy in elderly patients with detrusor instability with a single 25 mg nighttime dose of imipramine, which was increased every third day by 25 mg until the patient either was continent or had side-effects, or a dose of 150 mg was reached. Six of 10 patients became continent and, in those who underwent repeated cystometry, bladder capacity increased by a mean of 105 ml and bladder pressure at capacity decreased by a mean of 18 cm H_2O. Maximum urethral pressure (MUP) increased by a mean of 30 cm H_2O. Although our subjective impression (Raezer et al 1977) was that the bladder effects became evident only after several days of treatment, some patients in the Castleden series became continent after only 3–5 days of therapy. Our usual adult dose for treatment of voiding dysfunction is 25 mg four times a day; less frequent administration is possible because of the drug's long half-life. Half that dose is given in elderly patients, in whom the drug half-life may be prolonged. In our experience, the effects of imipramine on the lower urinary tract are often additive to those of atropine-like agents; consequently a combination of imipramine and an antimuscarinic or an antispasmodic is sometimes especially useful for decreasing bladder contractility (Raezer et al 1977). If imipramine is used in conjunction with an atropine-like agent, it should be noted that the anticholinergic side-effects of the drugs may be additive. It has been known for many years that impramine is relatively effective for the treatment of nocturnal enuresis in children. Doses for this condition range from 10 to 50 mg daily. Whether the mechanisms of drug action in this situation are the same as those for decreasing bladder contractility, is unknown. Korczyn & Kish (1979) have presented evidence that the antienuretic effect results from a different mechanism than the peripheral anticholinergic effect and the drug's antidepressant effect. The antienuretic effect occurs soon after initial administration, whereas the antidepressant effects generally take 2–4 weeks to develop.

Doxepin (Sinequan) is another tricyclic antidepressant which has been found to be more potent, using *in vitro* rabbit bladder strips, than other tricyclic compounds with respect to antimuscarinic and musculotropic relaxant activity (Levin & Wein 1984). Lose and colleagues (1989), in a randomized double-blind crossover study of women with involuntary bladder contractions and either frequency, urgency, or urge incontinence, found that this agent caused a significant increase in control over nighttime frequency and incontinence episodes and a near-significant decrease in urine loss (by the pad weighing test) and in the cystometric parameters of first sensation and maximum bladder capacity. The dose of doxepin used was either a single 50 mg bedtime dose or this dose plus an additional 25 mg in the morning. The number of daytime incontinence episodes decreased in both doxepin and placebo groups, and the difference was not statistically significant. Doxepin treatment was preferred by 14 patients, whereas 2 preferred placebo. Three patients had no preference. Of the 14 patients who stated a preference for doxepin, 12 claimed that they became continent during treatment, and 2 claimed improvement. The 2 patients who preferred placebo claimed improvement. The AHCPR guidelines combine results for imipramine and doxepin, citing only three randomized controlled trials, with an unknown percentage of women patients. The percentage of cures (all figures refer to percentage minus the percentage on placebo) are listed as 31%, percentage of reduction in urge incontinence as 20–88%, and percentage of side-effects as 0–70%.

When used in the generally larger doses employed for antidepressant effects, the most frequent side-effects of the tricyclic antidepressants are those attributable to their systemic anticholinergic activity (Baldesarini 1990; Richelson 1990). Allergic phenomena, including rash, hepatic dysfunction, obstructive jaundice, and agranulocytosis may also occur, but are rare. Central nervous system side-effects may include weakness, fatigue, parkinsonian effect, fine tremors noted mostly in the upper extremities, a manic or schizophrenic picture and sedation, probably from an antihistaminic effect. Postural hypotension may also be seen, presumably due to selective blockade (a paradoxical effect) of α-1 adrenergic receptors in some vascular smooth muscle. Tricyclic antidepressants may also cause excess sweating of obscure origin and a delay in orgasm, or orgasmic impotence, whose cause is likewise unclear. They may also produce arrhythmias and can interact in deleterious ways with other drugs – thus caution must be observed in using these drugs in patients with cardiac disease (Baldesarini 1990). Whether cardiotoxicity will prove to be a legitimate concern in patients receiving smaller doses (smaller than those used for treatment of depression) for lower urinary tract dysfunction remains to be seen but is a matter of potential concern. Consultation with a patient's cardiologist is always helpful before such therapy is instituted in questionable situations. The use of imipramine is contraindicated in patients receiving monoamine oxidase inhibitors because severe central nervous system toxicity can be precipitated, including hyperpyrexia, seizures and coma. Some potential side-effects of antidepressants may be, especially in the elderly, weakness, fatigue and postural hypotension. If imipramine or any of the tricyclic antidepressants is to be prescribed for the treatment of voiding dysfunction, the patient should be thoroughly informed about the fact that this is not the usual indication for this drug and that potential side-effects exist. Reports of significant side-effects (severe abdominal distress, nausea, vomiting, headache, lethargy and irritability) following abrupt cessation of high doses of imipramine in children suggest that the drug should be discontinued gradually, especially in patients receiving high doses.

Dimethyl sulfoxide (DMSO)

DMSO is a relatively simple, naturally occurring organic compound that has been used as an industrial solvent for many years. It has multiple pharmacological actions (membrane penetrating, anti-inflammatory, local analgesic, bacteriostatic, diuretic, cholinesterase-inhibitory, collagen solvent, vasodilator) and has been used for the treatment of arthritis and other musculoskeletal disorders, generally in a 70% solution. The formulation for human intravesical use is a 50% solution. Sant (1987) has summarized the pharmacology and clinical usage of DMSO and has tabulated good to excellent results in 50–90% of collected series of patients treated with intravesical instillations for interstitial cystitis. However, DMSO has not been shown to be useful in the treatment of detrusor hyperreflexia or instability or in any patient with urgency or frequency but without interstitial cystitis. The subject of interstitial cystitis and its treatment is considered in Chapter 27.

Polysynaptic inhibitors

Baclofen has been discussed previously with agents that decrease outlet resistance secondary to striated sphincter dyssynergia. It is also capable of depressing detrusor hyperreflexia. A double-blind crossover study reported that it was very effective in decreasing both day and night urinary frequency and incontinence in patients with idiopathic instability (Taylor & Bates 1979). Cystometric changes were not recorded, however, and considerable improvement was also obtained in the placebo group. The intrathecal use of baclofen for treatment of detrusor hyperactivity is a potentially exciting area (see prior discussion), and further reports are awaited.

Other potential agents

Nitric oxide (NO) is hypothesized to be a mediator of the non-adrenergic non-cholinergic relaxation of the outlet smooth muscle which occurs with bladder contraction. Evidence exists that it is also involved in relaxation of bladder body smooth muscle (James et al 1993) and this provides interesting fodder for speculation: is relaxation impaired in some types of hyperactivity and can NO analogues or synthetase stimulators be developed as agents to inhibit detrusor contractility? Glyceryl trinitrate releases NO *in vivo* and achieves its cardiovascular effects by relaxing vascular smooth muscle. A pilot study of 10 patients with instability given transdermal NO showed significant decreases in episodes (per 24 hours) of frequency (9.7–6.7), nocturia (1.84–1.09), and incontinence (0.61–0.36) (James & Iacovou 1993). Although the ubiquity of NO might seem to lessen its potential use in treating bladder hyperactivity (unless more organ-specific substrates or receptors are found), randomized controlled trials should be done.

Soulard and colleagues (1992) have described the effects of JO-1870 on bladder activity in the rat. This non-anticholinergic probable opioid agonist increased bladder capacity and threshold pressure responsible for micturition in a dose-dependent fashion, raising the possibility of the use or development of opioid agonists with selectivity for receptors involved in the micturition reflex. Propiverine has been described by Haruno (1992) to inhibit spontaneous or agonist-induced bladder contractility in various preparations by either an anticholinergic or calcium channel blocking effect; it has relative selectivity (10–100 times) for bladder and ileum. No clinical trials have been reported.

Constantinou (1992a,b) described the effects of thiphenamil hydrochloride on the lower urinary tract of healthy women volunteers and those with detrusor incontinence. In a randomized controlled trial, based on diary records from 14 patients with instability, it was reported that voiding frequency per day decreased significantly (from 10.3 to 8.0 times), but placebo values were not given. Daily incontinence episodes decreased in 9 patients from 2.3 to 1.6 (not significant, placebo values not given) with pad dryness (rated on a 0–4 scale) improving from 1.6 to 1.2 (significant, but no placebo data given). Objective urodynamic results (in 16 patients) showed no flowmetry changes, no changes in bladder capacity, some increase in first sensation of fullness, and a significant decrease in detrusor voiding pressure (46.1–31.9 cm H_2O) over placebo. The data and interpretation in this article are confusing to me, especially because the study of healthy volunteers showed no urodynamic differences except an increase in maximum flow rate (from 16.9 to 27.7 ml/second), at a dose of 800 mg of drug. This drug was said to be a 'synthetic antispasmodic'. The most that can be said about the clinical use of thiphenamil is that, now that a question has been raised, it needs to be addressed by further 'cleaner' studies with internally consistent results.

Increasing bladder capacity by decreasing sensory (afferent) input

Decreasing afferent input peripherally is the ideal treatment for both sensory urgency and instability or hyperreflexia in a bladder with relatively normal elastic or viscoelastic properties in which the sensory afferents constitute the first limb in the abnormal micturition reflex. Capsaicin. (Maggi et al 1989; Maggi 1991, 1992) Capsaicin is an irritant and algogenic compound obtained from hot red peppers that has highly selective effects on a subset of mammalian sensory neurones, including polymodal receptors and warm thermoreceptors (Maggi et al 1989; Maggi 1991, 1992; Dray 1993). Capsaicin produces pain by selectively activating polymodal nociceptive neurones by membrane depolarization and opening a certain-selective ion channel, which can be blocked by ruthenium red. Repeated administration induces desensitization and inactivation of sensory neurones by several mechanisms. Systemic and topical capsaicin produces a reversible antinociceptive and anti-inflammatory action after an initially undesirable algesic effect. Local or topical application blocks C-fibre conduction and inactivates neuropeptide release from peripheral nerve endings, accounting for local antinociception by activating specific receptors on afferent nerve terminals in the spinal cord; spinal neurotransmission is subsequently blocked by a prolonged inactivation of sensory neurotransmitter release. With local administration (intravesical) the potential advantage of capsaicin is a lack of systemic side-effects. The actions are highly specific when the drug is applied locally – the compound affects primarily small-diameter nociceptive afferents, leaving the sensations of touch and pressure unchanged, although heat (not cold) perception may be reduced. Motor fibres are not affected (Craft & Porreca 1992). The effects are reversible, although it is not known whether initial levels of sensitivity are regained. Craft & Porreca list intravesical doses in the rat as 0.03–10.0 μM for 15–30 minutes and in humans a maximum of 1–2 mM.

Maggi (1992) reviewed the therapeutic potential of capsaicin-like molecules. Capsaicin-sensitive primary afferents (CSPA) innervate the human bladder, and intravesical instillation of capsaicin into human bladder produces a concentration dependent decrease in first desire to void, decreased bladder capacity and a warm burning sensation. Maggi used doses of 0.01, 1.0, and 10 μM, administered in ascending order at 10- to 15-minute intervals as constant infusions of 20 ml/minute until micturition occurred (Maggi et al 1989). Five capsaicin-treated patients with 'hypersensitive disorder' reported either a complete disappearance of symptoms (4 patients) or marked attenuation of symptoms (1 patient), beginning 2–3 days after administration and lasting 4–16 days. After that time, the symptoms gradually reappeared but were no worse. Fowler and colleagues (1992) found that considerably higher doses (up to 1–2 mM for 30 minutes) were necessary to produce an effect in humans. However, these investigators reported that bladder control improved within 2 days, and the improvement lasted for 3–6 months. Lower doses (0.1–100 μM) produced 'no long lasting benefit'. An efferent function of CSPA is the release of neurotransmitters from the peripheral endings of these sensory neurones, such as tachykinins and calcitonin gene-related peptide (CGRP) (Maggi 1992). These neurotransmitters can produce events collectively known as neurogenic inflammation, which can include: all or some smooth muscle contractions, increased plasma protein extravasation, vasodilation, mast cell degranulation, facilitation of transmitter release from nerve terminals, recruitment of inflammatory cells and so on. This is another reason why intravesical capsaicin could theoretically be useful in treating the pain and related problems of interstitial cystitis and certain types of bladder hyperactivity which originate in primary afferents.

The peripheral terminals of CSPA form a dense plexus just below the bladder urothelium, and fibres penetrating the urothelium come into contact with the lumen. This location, combined with the peculiar chemosensitivity of the CSPA, permits them to detect 'backflow' of chemicals across the urothelium, which is thought to occur during conditions leading to breakdown of the 'barrier function' of the urothelium (Maggi 1992). If the 'barrier' theory or 'leaky urothelium' theory (see Ch. 27) of the pathogenesis of the interstitial cystitis is true for some of many patients with this condition, the CSPA in such patients may be stimulated by urine constituents leaking back across the urothelium. Under these circumstances, a local release of neuropeptides may well contribute in producing neurogenic inflammation. If this is so, as Maggi suggests, a local treatment leading to desensitization of CSPA would be doubly advantageous. With capsaicin, however, excitation precedes desensitization, somewhat limiting the potential for therapy in humans. A preferable analogue would produce the latter action while reducing or eliminating the former one. Finally, Maggi discusses the possible long-term disadvantages of such therapy as related to the potential physiological roles, trophic or protective, of CSPA and their secretions in response to stimulation.

Increasing outlet resistance

Alpha-adrenergic agonists

The bladder neck and proximal urethra contain a preponderance of α-adrenergic receptor sites which, when stimulated, produce smooth muscle contraction (Wein et al 1991a,b; Andersson 1993). The static infusion urethral pressure profile is altered by such stimulation, producing an increase in maximum urethral pressure (MUP) and maximum urethral closure pressure (MUCP). Various orally administered pharmacological agents producing α-adrenergic stimulation are available. Generally, outlet resistance is increased to a variable degree by such an action. The potential side-effects of all these agents include blood pressure elevation, anxiety and insomnia due to stimulation of the central nervous system, headache, tremor, weakness, palpitations, cardiac arrhythmias and respiratory difficulties. All such agents should be used with caution in patients with hypertension, cardiovascular disease or hyperthyroidism (Dray 1993).

The use of ephedrine to treat SUI was mentioned as early as 1948 (Rashbaum & Mandelbaum 1948). This is a noncatecholamine sympathomimetic agent which enhances release of norepinephrine from sympathetic neurones and directly stimulates both α- and β-adrenergic receptors (Hoffman & Lefkowitz 1990a). The oral adult dosage is 25–50 mg four times a day. Some tachyphylaxis develops in response to its peripheral actions, probably as a result of depletion of norepinephrine stores.

Pseudoephedrine, a steriosomer of ephedrine, is used for similar indications and carries similar precautions. The adult dosage is 30–60 mg four times a day. Diokno & Taub (1975) reported a 'good to excellent' result in 27–38 patients with sphincteric incontinence treated with ephedrine sulfate. Beneficial effects were most often achieved in those with minimal to moderate wetting; little benefit was achieved in patients with severe stress incontinence. A dose of 75–100 mg of norephedrine chloride has been shown to increase MUP and MUCP in women with urinary stress incontinence (Ek et al 1978). At a bladder volume of 300 ml, MUP rose from 82 to 110 cm H_2O, and MUCP rose from 63 to 93 cm H_2O. The functional profile length did not change significantly. O'Brink & Bunne (1978), however, noted that 100 mg of norephedrine chloride given twice a day did not provide an alternative to surgical treatment. Lose & Lindholm (1997) treated 20 women with stress incontinence with norfenefrine, an α agonist, given as a slow-release tablet. Nineteen patients reported reduced urinary leakage; 10 reported no further stress incontinence. MUCP increased in 16 patients during treatment, the mean rise being 53–64 cm H_2O.

The group at Kolding Hospital in Denmark has published three other articles of note on the use of norfenefrine for sphincteric incontinence. The results are interesting. Forty-four patients with SUI were randomized to treatment with norfenefrine 15–30 mg three times a day versus placebo for 6 weeks (Sanchez-Ferrer et al 1989). Subjectively, 12 of 23 (52%) of the norfenefrine group reported improvement as opposed to 7 of 21 (33%) of the placebo group, a difference which was not significant. Continence was reported by 6 (26%) norfenefrine patients and 3 (14%) placebo patients (not significant). Judged by a stress test, 7 patients in each group became continent; 11 of 23 (48%) improved both subjectively and objectively in the norfenefrine group as opposed to 5 of 21 (24%) in the placebo group ($p = .09$). MUCP increased significantly, from 50 to 55 cm H_2O in the norfenefrine group, and from 55 to 65 cm H_2O in the placebo group. Although the patients were said to have 'genuine stress incontinence', 5 of 12 with 'urge incontinence' were reported cured with norfenefrine, and 4 of 7 with placebo.

Diernoes and associates (1989) reported on the results of a 1-hour pad test in 33 women with either SUI or combined stress incontinence and urgency treated with 30 mg three times a day of norfenefrine. Leakage of more than 10 g was required for entry into the study. Subjective improvement was reported by 10 patients (30%). Continence as shown by pad test was found in 6 patients (18%). Pad tests are graded on a scale of 1–4. At 12 weeks, 20 patients (61%) had improved by at least one grade (patient .05), but at 3 weeks the number was 13 (39%) (not significant).

In a study by Lose and colleagues (1988), 44 consecutive patients with genuine stress incontinence were treated with norfenefrine 15–30 mg three times daily in a 6-week, double-blind and parallel, placebo-controlled study. Subjectively, 52% were improved and 26% became continent during norfenefrine treatment. Objectively (stress test), 30% became continent and MUCP increased 10%, which was statistically significant. These results, however, were not statistically different from those of placebo treatment. Simultaneously, subjective and objective improvement was seen more often in patients given norfenefrine compared to placebo ($p<0.1$). In patients with the most severe incontinence according to urodynamic criteria, the effect of norfenefrine was statistically significantly better than placebo. A low incidence of side-effects was observed and no differences between norfenefrine and placebo were found. It is concluded that norfenefrine may be of value in the treatment of female stress incontinence.

Phenylpropanolamine hydrochloride (PPA) shares the pharmacological properties of ephedrine and is approximately equal in peripheral potency while causing less central stimulation (Hoffman & Lefkowitz 1990a). It is available in 25- to 50-mg tablets and 75-mg timed-release capsules and is a component of numerous proprietary mixtures marketed for the treatment of nasal and sinus congestion (usually in combination with an H_1 antihistamine) and as appetite suppressants. Using doses of 50 mg three times a day, Awad and associates (1978) found that 11 of 13 women and 6 of 7 men with stress incontinence were significantly improved after 4 weeks of therapy. MUCP increased from a mean of 47 to 72 cm H_2O in patients with an empty bladder and from 43 to 58 cm H_2O in patients with a full bladder. Using a capsule containing 50 mg of PPA, 8 mg of chlorpheniramine (an antihistamine), and 2 mg of isopropamide (an antimuscarinic), Stewart and colleagues (1976) found that, of 77 women with SUI, 18 were completely cured with one sustained-release capsule. Twenty-eight patients were 'much better', 6 were 'slightly better' and 25 were no better. In 11 men with post-prostatectomy stress incontinence, the numbers in the corresponding categories were 1, 2, 1 and 7. The formulation of Ornade has now been changed, and each capsule of drug contains 75 mg of PPA and 12 mg of chlorpheniramine. One study reported on a group of 24 women with SUI treated with PPA or placebo with a crossover after 2 weeks. Severity of SUI was graded 1 (slight) or 2 (moderate). Average MUCP overall increased significantly with PPA compared to placebo (48 to 55 vs. 48 to 49 cm H_2O). This was a significant difference in grade 2 but not in grade 1 patients. The average number of leakage episodes per 48 hours was reduced significantly overall for PPA patients but not in placebo patients (5 to 2 vs. 5 to 6). This was significant for grade 1 but not for grade 2 patients. Subjectively, 6–24 patients thought that both PPA and placebo were ineffective. Among the 18 patients (of 24) who reported a subjective preference, 14 preferred PPA and 4 placebo. Improvements were rated subjectively as good, moderately good and slight. Improvements obtained with PPA were significant compared with those for placebo for the entire population and for both groups separately. The AHCPR guidelines (Weiner et al 1986) reported 8 randomized controlled trials with PPA 50 mg twice a day for SUI in women. Percentage cures (all figures refer to per cent minus per cent on placebo) are listed as 0–14; reduction in incontinence as 19–60%, side-effects and dropouts as 5–33% and 0–4.3%, respectively.

Some authors have emphasized the potential complications of phenylpropanolamine. Baggioni et al (1987) emphasized the possibility of blood pressure elevation, especially in patients with autonomic impairment. Caution should still be exercised in individuals known to be significantly hypertensive and in elderly patients, in whom pharmacokinetic function may be altered.

Midodrine is a long-acting α-adrenergic agonist reported to be useful in the treatment of seminal emission and ejaculation disorders following retroperitoneal lymphadenectomy. Treatment with 5 mg twice a day for 4 weeks in 20 patients with stress incontinence produced a cure in 1 and improvement in 14 (Kieswetter et al 1983). MUCP rose by 8.3%, and the plaometric index of the continence area on profilometry increased by 9%. The actions of imipramine have already been discussed. On a theoretical basis, an increase in urethral resistance might be expected if indeed an enhanced α-adrenergic effect at this level resulted from an inhibition of norepinephrine re-uptake. However, as mentioned previously, imipramine also causes α-adrenergic blocking effects, at least in vascular smooth muscle. Many clinicians have noted improvement in patients treated with imipramine primarily for bladder hyperactivity but who had, in addition, some component of sphincteric incontinence. Gilja and colleagues (1984) reported a study of 30 women with stress incontinence who were treated with 75 mg of imipramine daily for 4 weeks. Twenty-one women subjectively reported continence. Mean MUCP for the group increased from 34.06 to 48.23 mmHg.

Although some clinicians have reported spectacular cure and improvement rates with α-adrenergic agonists and agonists which produce an α-adrenergic effect in the outlet of patients with sphincteric urinary incontinence, our own experience coincides with those who report that such treatment often produces satisfactory or some improvement in mild cases but rarely total dryness in patients with severe or even moderate stress incontinence. A clinical trial, when possible, is certainly worthwhile, however, especially in conjunction with pelvic floor physiotherapy or biofeedback.

Beta-adrenergic antagonists and agonists

Theoretically, β-adrenergic blocking agents might be expected to 'unmask' or potentiate an α-adrenergic effect, thereby increasing urethral resistance. Gleason and colleagues (1974) reported success in treating certain patients with SUI with propranolol, using oral doses of 10 mg four times a day. The beneficial effect became manifest only after 4–10 weeks of treatment. Cardiac effects occur rather promptly after administration of this drug, but hypotensive effects do not usually appear as rapidly, although it is difficult to explain such a long delay in onset of the therapeutic effect on incontinence on this basis. Kaisary (1984) also reported success with propranolol in the treatment of stress incontinence. Although such treatment has been suggested as an alternative to α agonists in patients with sphincteric incontinence and hypertension, few if any subsequent reports of such efficacy have appeared. Others have reported no significant changes in urethral profile pressures in normal women after β-adrenergic blockade (Donker & Van Der Sluis 1976). Although 10 mg four times a day is a relatively small dose of propranolol, it should be recalled that the major potential side-effects of the drug are related to this therapeutic β-blocking effect.

Beta-adrenergic stimulation is generally conceded to decrease urethral pressure but β-2 agonists have been reported to increase the contractility of fast-contracting striated muscle fibres (extensor digitorum longus) from guinea-pigs, and suppress that of slow-contracting fibres (soleus) (Fellenius et al 1980). Clenbuterol, a selective β-2 agonist, has been reported to potentiate, in a dose-dependent fashion, the field stimulation-induced contraction in isolated periurethral muscle preparation in the rabbit. The potentiation is greater that that produced by isoproterenol and is suppressed by propranolol (Kishimoto et al 1991). The authors reported an increase in urethral pressure with clinical use of clenbuterol and speculate on its promise in the treatment of sphincteric incontinence.

Oestrogens

Although oestrogens were recommended for the treatment of urinary incontinence in women as early as 1941 (Salmon et al 1941), there is still controversy over their use and benefit–risk ratio for this purpose. This subject is a good example of why it is sometimes difficult to obtain a consensus about the efficacy or non-efficacy of a particular category of drug for the treatment of incontinence. There is an impressive basic science literature on the effects of oestrogen on the lower urinary tract, but no strictly appropriate experimental model of either stress incontinence or detrusor hyperactivity or hypersensitivity. There are numerous clinical trials, some controlled and some not, some using oestrogen alone and some using oestrogen plus α agonists. There is little consistency in methodology, and the manner in which some authors have chosen to express their data and conclusions is confusing. In some cases, raw data seem to be ignored in favour of statistics but, as always, there is no lack of opinions.

Much attention has been paid to the innervation, physiology and pharmacology of the smooth muscle of the uterus. Oestrogens have been found to affect many related properties including excitability, neuronal influences on the muscle, receptor density and sensitivity, and transmitter metabolism, especially in adrenergic nerves. The urethra (and trigone) are embryologically related to the uterus, and significant work has also been done on the effects of oestrogenic hormones on the lower urinary tract. Hodgson et al (1978) reported that the sensitivity of the rabbit urethra to α-adrenergic stimulation was oestrogen-dependent; castration caused decreased sensitivity, and treatment with low levels of oestrogen reversed this. Levin and co-workers (1980, 1981) showed that parenteral oestrogen administration can change the autonomic receptor content and the innervation of the lower urinary tract of immature female rabbits. A marked increase in response to α-adrenergic, muscarinic, and purinergic stimulation occurred in the bladder body but not the base, and there was a significant increase in the number of α-adrenergic and muscarinic receptors in the bladder body but not the base.

Larsson and associates (1984) reported that oestrogen treatment of the isolated female rabbit urethra caused an increased sensitivity to norepinephrine. It was suggested that the mechanism was related to a more than twofold increase in the α-adrenergic receptor number. Callahan and Creed (1985) reported that pre-treatment with oestrogen of oophorectomized dogs and wallabies did increase sensitivity of urethral strips to α-adrenergic stimulation, but that this did not occur in the rabbit or guinea-pig. Bump and Friedman (1986) reported that sex hormone replacement with oestrogen, but not testosterone, enhanced the urethral sphincter mechanism in the castrated female baboon by effects that were unrelated to skeletal muscle. They added that these effects might not be related just to changes in the urethral wall. Batra and colleagues (1986) have shown that two doses of oestradiol and oestratriol increased blood perfusion into the urethra (as well as the vagina and uterus) of oophorectomized mature female rabbits. After menopause, urethral pressure parameters normally decrease somewhat (Rud 1980a) and although this change is generally conceded to be related in some way to decreased oestrogen levels, it is still largely a matter of speculation whether the actual changes occur in smooth muscle, blood circulation, supporting tissues, or the 'mucosal and seal mechanism.' Versi and associates (1988) describe a positive correlation between skin collagen content, which does decline with declining oestrogen status, and parameters of the urethral pressure profile, suggesting that the oestrogen effect on the urethra may be predicted, at least in part, by changes in the collagen component. Eika and colleagues (1990) reported that bladders from oopharectomized rats weighed less and had a higher collagen content and lower atropine resistance than controls, and that oestrogen substitution reversed these parameters.

Raz and co-workers (1973a) reported that progesterone enhanced the β-adrenergic response of the dog urethra and ureter. Progesterone receptors have been identified in the human urethra (Batra & Iosif 1987), but Rud reported that treatment with progestogens had no effect on urethral profile parameters (Rud 1980b). Raz et al (1973b) reported that oral medroxyprogesterone acetate 20 mg daily exacerbated stress incontinence in 60% of women so treated, with corresponding changes in urethral pressures.

Raz and associates (1973b) found that a daily dose of 2.5 mg of Premarin (conjugated oestrogens) improved stress incontinence and increased urethral pressure in 65% of postmenopausal patients, effects that the authors attributed to mucosal proliferation with a consequently improved 'mucosal seal effect' and to enhancement of the α-adrenergic contractile response of urethral smooth muscle to endogenous catecholamines. Schreiter and associates (1976) reported similar benefits after 10 days of treatment with daily divided doses of 6 mg of oestriol. They also presented evidence that the effects of oestrogen and of exogenous α-adrenergic stimulation were additive. In one of the first studies which presented some quantitative data on oestrogen, Rud (1980b) reported the effects of 4 mg doses of oestradiol and 8 mg daily doses of oestriol on 30 women with an average age of 61, 24 of whom had SUI. Small but statistically significant increases occurred in the MUP (59–63 cm H_2O), functional urethral length (25–28 mm), and actual urethral length (33–37 mm). No statistically significant change occurred in urethral closure pressure (37–39 cm H_2O). Eight of the 24 incontinent patients experienced subjective and objective improvement, 9 experienced subjective improvement only, and 7 experienced neither subjective nor objective improvement. There was no correlation between subjective or objective improvement and urodynamic parameters. However, of 18 patients in whom pressure transmission to the urethra was recorded during cough, 7 improved. All of these reported subjective improvement, and 5 were shown objectively to be dry. Rud pointed out that it is hard to believe that the small changes in urodynamic measurements which occurred, although statistically significant, were directly related to resumption of continence. It was noted that the increased pressure transmission ratio might be due to factors outside the urethra – either in the striated musculature of the pelvic floor or in the periurethral vasculature or supporting tissues. Rud also studied proflowmetry during the menstrual cycle and found no correlation between oestrogen levels and MUP. It may be, as suggested, that at physiological levels oestrogens have little influence on urodynamic measurements related to continence and that only pharmacological doses cause urodynamically significant changes. Pharmacological doses may also alter responses to other exogenous autonomic stimulation, particularly α-adrenergic stimulation, as laboratory experiments suggest.

Beisland and colleagues (1984) carried out a randomized, open, comparative crossover trial in 20 postmenopausal women with urethral sphincteric insufficiency. Both oral PPA (phenylpropanolamine hydrochloride), 50 mg twice a day, and oestriol vaginal suppositories, 1 mg daily, significantly increased the MUCP and the continence area on profilometry. PPA was clinically more effective than oestriol but not sufficiently so to obtain complete continence. However, with combined treatment, 8 patients became completely continent, 9 were considerably improved, and only one remained unchanged. Two patients dropped out of the study because of side-effects. Bhatia and colleagues (1989) used 2 g daily of conjugated oestrogen vaginal cream for 6 weeks in 11 postmenopausal women with SUI. Six were cured or improved significantly. Favourable response was correlated with increased closure pressure and increased pressure transmission. In an accompanying article, Karram and associates (1989) reported that oestrogen administration in 6 women with premature ovarian failure (but without lower urinary tract problems) did not produce any change in urethral pressure, functional length or cystometric parameters. However, a significant increase in the pressure transmission ratio to the proximal and mid-urethra (89–109% and 86–100%, respectively) was noted after oral oestrogen, although serum E-2 levels and cytological changes were similar in the two modes of administration. Negative effects from oestrogen alone on stress incontinence were reported by Walter and colleagues (1978), Hilton & Stanton (1983) and Samsioe et al (1985), but in each of these studies urge symptomatology was favourably affected. In a review article, Cardozo (1990) concluded that 'there is no conclusive evidence that oestrogen even improves, let alone cures, stress incontinence', although it 'apparently alleviates urgency, urge incontinence, frequency, nocturia and dysuria.'

Walter and colleagues (1990) completed a complicated but logical study of 28 postmenopausal women with SUI (out of 38 original subjects). After 4 weeks of a placebo run-in, patients were randomized to oral oestriol (E3) or PPA alone for 4 weeks, and then to combined therapy for 4 weeks. In the group which sequentially received placebo, PPA and PPA/E3, the percentages reporting cure or improvement, respectively, were 0 and 13%, 13 and 20%, and 21 and 14%. In the group receiving placebo, E3, and E3/PPA, the corresponding percentages were 0 and 0%, 14 and 29%, and 64 and 7%. Objective parameters showed the following: the number of leak episodes per 24 hours in patients treated with PPA first showed a 31% decrease (~ 3 to 2) compared to placebo (p<0.003). For those treated with E3 first, the change was not significant (~1.5 to 0.8). Combined treatment produced a mean decrease of 48% over placebo. There was a greater effect with E3/PPA than with PPA/E3. Pad weights (in grams in a 1-hour test) decreased significantly with PPA alone (~27 to 6 g), but there was no difference between PPA and PPA/E3. E3 alone significantly decreased pad weights (~47 to 15 g). Although E3/PPA was not significantly different, there was further numerical loss from ~15 to 3 g. The overall conclusions were that E3 and PPA are each effective in treating SUI in postmenopausal women and, based on subjective data, combined therapy is better than either drug alone. This conclusion was substantiated by a significant decrease in the number of leak episodes in the patients in whom E3 was given, as measured by pad-weighing tests.

Hilton and colleagues (1990) published the results of a double-blind study of 60 (originally) postmenopausal women with SUI who were treated for 4 weeks with oral and vaginal oestrogen alone and in combination with PPA. There were six groups in this study: vaginal oestrogen (VE) and PPA; VE and oral placebo (OP); oral oestrogen (OE) and PPA; OE and OP; vaginal placebo (VP) and PPA; VP and OP. Subjective symptoms and reported pads per day decreased in all groups; the greatest reduction occurred in those treated with VE, although the reduction in groups 1,2,4 and 6 were all significant. Objective pad weight after exercise testing showed a slight decrease in all groups except the double placebo one. Reduction was maximal in the VE/PPA group (22 to 8 g), but the pre-treatment values for pads per day and pad weight varied greatly (<0.5 to ~3.5 pads per day; <5 g to 22 g). There was no change in cystometric or urethral profilometric evaluation, either resting or under stress.

Jackson and co-workers (1997) produced a double blind, placebo-controlled randomized trial of unopposed oestradiol in 68 women with genuine stress incontinence. Using a standardized questionnaire before and afterwards, they showed no improvement of the symptom of stress incontinence or any other urinary symptom.

A unique new method for delivering vaginal

oestrogen involves a silicone ring with an oestradiol-loaded core containing 2 mg of 17-beta oestradiol. The device is inserted into the vagina, by the patient or the physician. A low, constant dose (5–10 g/24 hours) is delivered over a period of 90 days (Bachmann et al 1997). This mode of administration is not only more acceptable to certain women (Ayton et al 1996); it offers a more continuous delivery of oestrogen to the affected tissues (Johnston 1996).

Circumventing the problem

Antidiuretic hormone-like agents

The synthetic antidiuretic hormone (ADH) peptide analogue DDAVP (1-deaminino-8-D-arginine vasopressin) has been used for the symptomatic relief of refractory nocturnal enuresis in both children and adults. (Norgaard et al 1989). The drug can be administered conveniently by intranasal spray at bedtime (in a dose of 10–40 μg) and effectively suppresses urine production for 7–10 hours. Its clinical long-term safety has been established by continued use in patients with diabetes insipidus. Normal water deprivation tests in the Rew and Rundle article (1989) seem to indicate that long-term use does not cause depression of endogenous ADH secretion, at least in patients with nocturnal enuresis. Changes in diuresis during 2 months of treatment in an elderly group of 6 men and 12 women with increased nocturia and decreased ADH secretion have been reported. Nocturia decreased 20% (in volume) in men and 34% in women. However, the number of voids from 8 p.m. to 8 a.m. decreased from 4.5 to 4.3 in men and from 3.5 to 2.8 in women, but the drug was not given until 8 p.m. At present, this novel circumventive approach to the treatment of urinary frequency and incontinence has been largely restricted to those with nocturnal enuresis or diabetes insipidus. The fact that the drug seems to be much more effective than simple fluid restriction alone for the former condition is perhaps explained by relatively recent reports suggesting a decreased nocturnal secretion of ADH by such patients (Norgaard et al 1989). Recently, suggestions have been made that DDAVP might be useful in patients with refractory nocturnal frequency and incontinence who do not belong in the category of primary nocturnal enuresis. Kinn & Larsson (1990) reported that micturition frequency 'decreased significantly' in 13 patients with multiple sclerosis and urge incontinence who were treated with oral tablets of desmopressin and that less leakage occurred. The actual approximate average change in the number of voids during the 6 hours after drug intake was 3.2 to 2.5. A similar circumventive approach is to give a rapidly acting loop diuretic 4–6 hours before bedtime. This, of course, assumes that the nocturia is not due to obstructive uropathy. A randomized double-blind crossover study of this approach using bumetanide in a group of 14 general practice patients was reported by Pedersen & Johansen (1988). Control nocturia episodes per week averaged 17.5; with placebo, this decreased to 12(!), and with drug to 8. It remains to be seen whether any drug company pursues this avenue of treatment.

EFFECTS OF VARIOUS PHARMACOLOGICAL AGENTS ON URINE STORAGE AND EMPTYING

It is obvious from the foregoing discussion that any one of a number of agents prescribed for reasons unrelated to voiding dysfunction can affect autonomic nervous system and receptor function and can thereby influence urine storage, urine emptying, or both. Agents which decrease outlet resistance may predispose a patient to stress or sphincteric incontinence, or worsen an already existing condition. Agents which increase intravesical pressure by increasing bladder muscle contractility may decrease functional bladder capacity, since the threshold pressure at which the sensation of distension is perceived will be reached at a lower intravesical volume. Thus an increase in urinary frequency and perhaps a feeling of urgency may occur under these circumstances. Agents that inhibit bladder contractility may decrease the urinary flow rate and may cause relative or even complete urinary retention. If emptying is inhibited, an increase in residual urine may well occur, with an increase in urinary frequency because of a decreased functional capacity. Compounds which increase outlet resistance can cause the same end effects on voiding efficiency as those which decrease bladder contractility. It is obvious that adverse and unwanted pharmacological effects on lower urinary tract function do not occur in the great majority of patients treated with agents which have this potential. Such effects are usually most manifest in those patients whose pre-treatment voiding status already borders on being pathological.

REFERENCES

Abel B, Gibbon N, Jameson R 1974 The neuropathic urethra. Lancet 2: 1229

Akah P A 1986 Tricyclic antidepressant inhibition of the electrical evoked responses of the rat urinary bladder strip-effect of variation in extracellular Ca{+2+} concentration. Archives Internationales de Pharmacodynamie et de Therapie 284: 231

Albibi R, McCallum R W 1983 Metoclopramide: pharmacology and clinical application. Annals of Internal Medicine 98: 86

Anderson R U, Mobley D, Blank B, et al 1999 Once daily controlled versus immediate release oxybutynin chloride for urge incontinence. Journal of Urology 161: 1809–1812

Andersson K E, Ek A, Hedlund H 1981 Effects of prazosin in isolated human urethra and in patients with lower neuron lesions. Investigative Urology 19: 39

Andersson K E, Fovaeus M, Morgan E E 1986 Comparative effects of five different calcium channel blockers on the atropine-resistant contraction in electrically stimulated rabbit urinary bladder. Neurourology and Urodynamics 5: 579

Andersson K E 1988 Current concepts in the treatment of disorders of micturition. Drugs 35: 477

Andersson K E, Hedlund H, Mansson W 1992 Pharmacologic treatment of bladder hyperactivity after augmentation and substitution enterocystoplasty. Scandinavian Journal of Urology are Nephrology 142: 42–46.

Andersson K E 1993 Pharmacology of lower urinary tract smooth muscles and penile erectile tissues. Pharmacological Reviews 45: 253

Andersson K E, Appell R, Cardozo L, et al 1999 Pharmacological treatment of urinary incontinence. In: Abrams P, Khoury S, Wein A (eds) Incontinence Plymbridge Distributors, Plymouth 447–486

Appell R A 1997 Clinical efficacy and safety of tolterodine in the treatment of overactive bladder: a pooled analysis. Urology 50 (suppl GA): 90–96

Awad S A, Bryniak S, Downie J W, Bruce A W 1977 The treatment of the uninhibited bladder with dicyclomine. Journal of Urology 114: 161

Awad S A, Downie J, Kirulita J 1978 Alpha adrenergic agents in urinary disorders of the proximal urethra: I. Stress incontinence. British Journal of Urology 50: 332

Ayton R A, Darling G M, Murkies A I, et al 1996 A comparative study of safety and efficacy of continuous low dose estriadiol released from a vaginal ring compared with conjugated equine estrogen vaginal cream in the treatment of postmenopausal urogenital atrophy. British Journal of Obstetrics and Gynaecology 103: 351–358

Bachmann G, Notelovitz M, Nachtigall L, Birgerson L 1997 A comparative study of a low-dose estradiol vaginal ring and conjugated estrogen cream for postmenopausal urogenital atrophy. Elsevier Science Inc. 4: 109

Baggioni I, Onrot J, Stewart C K, Robertson D 1987 The potent pressor effect of phenylpropanolamine in patients with autonomic impairment. Journal of the American Medical Association 258: 236

Baldesarini R J 1990 Drugs and the treatment of psychiatric disorders. In: Gilman A G, Rall T W, Nies A S, Taylor P (eds) Goodman and Gilman's The Pharmacological Basis of Therapeutics, 8th edn, Pergamon Press, New York, pp 383–435

Barrett D M 1981 The effects of oral bethanechol chloride on voiding in female patients with excessive residual urine: a randomized double-blind study. Journal of Urology 126: 640

Barrett D M, Wein A J 1991 Voiding dysfunction: diagnosis, classification and management. In: Gillenwater J Y, Grayhack J T, Howards S T, Duckett J W (eds) Adult and Pediatric Urology, 2nd edn, Mosby-Year Book, St. Louis, pp 1001–1099

Batra S, Byellin L, Sjögren C 1986 Increases in blood flow of the female rabbit urethra following low dose estrogens. Journal of Urology 136: 1360

Batra S C, Iosif C S 1987 Progesterone receptors in the female lower urinary tract. Journal of Urology 138: 1301

Beck R P, Anausch T, King C 1976 Results in testing 210 patients with detrusor overactivity incontinence of urine. American Journal of Obstetrics and Gynecology 125: 593

Beisland H O, Fossberg E, Moer A E 1984 Urethral sphincter insuffciency in postmenopausal females: treatment with phenylpropanolamine and estriol separately and in combination. Urologia Internationalis 39: 211

Benson G S, Sarshik S A, Raezer D M, Wein A J 1977 Bladder muscle contractility: Comparative effects and mechanisms of action of atropine, propantheline, flavoxate and imipramine. Urology 9: 31

Bhatia N N, Bergman A, Karram M M 1989 Effects of estrogen on urethral function in women with urinary incontinence. American Journal of Obstetrics and Gynecology 160: 176

Bigger J, Giardino E, Perel J E 1977 Cardiac antiarrhythmic effect of imipramine hydrochloride. New England Journal of Medicine 296: 206

Birns J, Malone-Lee J G and the Oxybutynin CR Study Group 1997 Controlled release oxybutynin maintains efficacy with a 43% reduction in side effects compared with conventional oxybutynin treatment. Neurourology and Urodynamics 16: 429–430 (abstract)

Blaivas J, Labib K, Michalik S E 1980 Cystometric response to propantheline in detrusor hyperreflexia: therapeutic implications. Journal of Urology 124: 259

Bloom F E 1990 Neurohumoral transmission and the central nervous system. In: Gilman A G, Rall T W, Nies A S, Taylor P (eds) Goodman and Gilman's The Pharmacological Basis of Therapeutics, 8th edn, Pergamon Press, New York, pp 244–268

Bonner T I 1989 The molecular basis of muscarinic receptor diversity. Trends in Neurosciences 12: 148

Brooks P M, Day R O 1991 Non-steroidal anti-inflammatory drugs – differences and similarities. New England Journal of Medicine 324: 1716

Brown J H 1990 Atropine, scopolamine and related antimuscarinic drugs. In: Gilman A G, Rall T W, Nies A S, Taylor P. (eds) Goodman and Gilman's The Pharmacological Basis of Therapeutics, 8th edn. Pergamon Press, New York, pp 150–165

Bultitude M, Hills N, Shuttleworth K 1976 Clinical and experimental studies on the action of prostaglandins and their synthesis inhibitors on detrusor muscle in vitro and in vivo. British Journal of Urology 48: 631

Bump R C, Friedman C I 1986 Intraluminal urethral pressure measurements in the female baboon: effects of hormonal manipulation. Journal of Urology 136: 508

Burton G, Dobson C 1993 Progesterone increases flow rates. A new treatment for voiding abnormalities? Neurourology and Urodynamics 12: 398

Callahan S M, Creed K E 1985 The effects of oestrogens on spontaneous activity and responses to phenylephrine of the mammalian urethra. Journal of Physiology 358: 35–46

Cardozo L 1990 Role of estrogens in the treatment of female urinary incontinence. Journal of the American Geriatric Society 38: 326

Cardozo L, Stanton S L 1979 An objective comparison of the effects of parenterally administered drugs in patients suffering from detrusor instability. Journal of Urology 122: 58–59

Cardozo L D, Stanton S L, Robinson H, Hole D 1980 Evaluation of flurbiprofen in detrusor instability. British Medical Journal 280: 281–282

Carone R, Vercella D, Bertapelli P 1993 Effects of cisapride on anorectal and vesicourethral function in spinal cord injured patients. Paraplegia 31: 125

Castleden C M, George C F, Renwick A G, Asher M J 1981 Imipramine – a possible alternative to current therapy for urinary incontinence in elderly. Journal of Urology 125: 218

Castleden C M, Morgan B 1980 The effect of beta adrenoceptor agonists on urinary incontinence in the elderly. British Journal of Clinical Pharmacology 10: 619

Cedarbaum J M, Schleifer L S 1990 Drugs for Parkinson's disease spasticity, and acute muscle spasms. In: Gilman A G, Rall T W, Nies A S, Taylor P (eds) Goodman and Gilman's The Pharmacological Basis of Therapeutics, 8th edn. Pergamon Press, New York, pp 463–484

Cole A, Fried F 1972 Favorable experiences with imipramine in the treatment of neurogenic bladder. Journal of Urology 107: 44

Collas D, Malone-Lee J G 1997 The pharmacokinetic properties of rectal oxybutynin – a possible alternative to intravesical administration. Neurourology and Urodynamics 16: 3–4

Connolly M J, Astridge P S, White E G E 1991 Torsade de pointes ventricular tachycardia and terodilene. Lancet 338: 344

Constantinou C E 1992a Pharmacologic treatment of detrusor incontinence with thiphenamil HCL. Urologia Internationalis 48: 42

Constantinou C E 1992b Pharmacologic effect of thiphenamil HCL on lower urinary tract function of healthy asymptomatic volunteers. Urologia Internationalis 48: 293

Cornella J L, Bent A E, Ostergard D R, Horbach N S 1990 Prospective study utilizing transdermal scopolamine in detrusor instability. Urology 35: 96

Craft R M, Porreca F 1992 Treatment parameters of desensitization to capsaicin. Life Sciences 51: 1767

Davidoff R A 1985 Antispasticity drugs: mechanisms of action. Annals of Neurology 17: 107

de Groat W C 1993 Anatomy and physiology of the lower urinary tract. Urologic Clinics of North America 20: 383–401

de Groat W C, Booth A M 1984 Autonomic systems to the urinary bladder and sexual organs In: Dyck P J, Thomas P K, Lambert E H (eds) Peripheral Neuropathy. W B Saunders, Philadelphia pp 285–299

Delaere K J P, Michiels H G E, Debruyne F M J, Moonen W A 1977 Flavoxate hydrochloride in the treatment of detrusor instability. Urologia Internationalis 32: 377

Delaere K J P, Thomas C M G, Moonen W A, Debruyne F M J 1981 The value of intravesical prostaglandin F2a and E2 in women with abnormalities of bladder emptying. British Journal of Urology 53: 306

Delaere K P J, Branje J Ph A 1998 Rectal administration of oxybutynin in the treatment of detrusor instability: preliminary promising results of a pilot study. Neurourology and Urodynamics 17: 319–320

Desmond A, Bultitude M, Hills N, Shuttleworth K 1980 Clinical experience with intravesical prostaglandin E{–2}: a prospective study of 36 patients. British Journal of Urology 53: 357

Diernoes E, Rix P, Sorenson T, Alexander N 1989 Norfenefrine in the treatment of female urinary stress incontinence assessed by one hour pad weighing test. Urologia Internationalis 44: 28

Diokno A, Taub M 1975 Ephedrine in treatment of urinary incontinence. Urology 5: 624

Donker P, Van Der Sluis C 1976 Action of beta adrenergic blocking agents on the urethral pressure profile. Urologia Internationalis 31: 6

Downie J, Twiddy D, Awad S A 1977 Antimuscarinic and non-competitive antagonist properties of dicyclomine hydrochloride in isolated human and rabbit bladder muscle. Journal of Pharmacology and Experimental Therapeutics 201: 662

Downie J W, Karmazyn M 1984 Mechanical trauma to bladder epithelium liberates prostanoids which modulate neurotransmission in rabbit detrusor muscle. Journal of Pharmacology and Experimental Therapeutics 230: 445–449

Dray A 1993 Mechanism of action of capsaicin-like molecules on sensory neurons. Life Sciences 51: 1759

Dykstra D D, Sidi A A, Anderson L 1987 The effect of nifedipine on cystoscopy-induced autonomic hyperreflexia in patients with high spinal cord injuries. Journal of Urology 138: 1155

Dykstra D D, Sidi A A 1990 Treatment of detrusor-striated sphincter dyssynergia with botulinum A toxin. Archives of Physical Medicine and Rehabilitation 71: 24

Eika B, Salling L N, Christensen L L, Andersen A, Laurberg S, Danielsen C C 1990 Long-term observation of the detrusor smooth muscle in rats. Its relationship to ovariectomy and estrogen treatment. Urological Research 18: 439

Ek A, Andersson K E, Gullberg B, Ulmsten K 1978 The effects of long-term treatment with norephedrine on stress incontinence and urethral closure pressure profile. Scandinavian Journal of Urology and Neurology 12: 105

Farrell S A, Webster R D, Higgins L M, Steeves R A 1990 Duration of postoperative catheterization: a randomized double-blind trial comparing two catheter management protocols and the effect of bethanechol chloride. International Urogynecology Journal and Pelvic Floor Dysfunction 1: 132

Fatigati V, Murphy R A 1984 Actin and tropomyosin variants in smooth muscles. Dependence on tissue type. Journal of Biological Chemistry 259: 14383–14388

Fellenius E, Hedberg R, Holmberg E E 1980 Functional and metabolic effects of terbutaline and propranolol in fast and slow contracting skeletal muscle in vitro. Acta Physiologica Scandinavica 109: 89

Finkbeiner A E 1983 Effect of extracellular calcium and calcium-blocking agents on detrusor contractility: an in vitro study. Neurourology and Urodynamics 2: 245

Fischer C, Diokno A, Lapides J 1978 The anticholinergic effects of dicyclomine hydrochloiride in inhibited neurogenic bladder dysfunction. Journal of Urology 120: 328

Florante J, Leyson J, Martin B, Sporer A 1980 Baclofen in the treatment of detrusor sphincter dyssynergy in spinal cord injury patients. Journal of Urology 124: 82

Foreman M M, McNulty A M 1993 Alterations in K+-evoked release of H-3- norepinephrine and contractile responses in urethral and bladder tissues induced by norepinephrine reuptake inhibition. Life Sciences 53: 193

Forman A, Andersson K, Henriksson L, Rud T, Ulmsten U 1978 Effects of nifedipine on the smooth muscle of the human urinary tract {in vitro} and {in vivo}. Acta Pharmacologica et Toxicologica 43: 111–118

Fovaeus M, Andersson K E, Hedlund H 1989 The action of pinacidil in isolated human bladder. Journal of Urology 141: 637

Fowler C J, Jewkes D, McDonald W I E 1992 Intravesical capsaicin for neurogenic bladder dysfunction. Lancet 329: 1239

Gajewski J, Awad J A 1986 Oxybutynin versus propantheline in patients with multiple sclerosis and detrusor hyperreflexia. Journal of Urology 135: 966

Galeano C, Jubelin B, Biron L, Guenette L 1986 Effect of naloxone on detrusor-sphincter dyssynergia in chronic spinal injured cat. Neurourology and Urodynamics 5: 203

Gibaldi M, Grundhofer B 1975 Biopharmaceutic influences on the anticholinergic effects of propantheline. Clinical Pharmacology and Therapeutics 18: 457

Gilja I, Radej M, Kovacic M, Parazajder J 1984 Conservative treatment of female stress incontinence with imipramine. Journal of Urology 132: 909

Gleason D, Reilly R, Bottaccinin M, Pierce M J 1974 The urethral continence zone and its relation to stress incontinence. Journal of urology 112: 81

Golman G, Levian A, Mazor A 1988 Alpha-adrenergic blocker for posthernioplasty urinary retention. Archives of Surgery 123: 35–36

Greenstein A, Chen J, Matzkin H E 1992 Transdermal scoploamine in prevention of post open prostatectomy bladder contractions. Urology 39: 215

Gruneberger A 1984 Treatment of motor urge incontinence with clenbuterol and flavoxate hydrochloride. British Journal of Obstetrics and Gynaecology 91: 275

Gupta S K, Sathyan G 1999 Pharmacokinetics of an oral once-a-day controlled release oxybutynin formulation compared with immediate release oxybutynin. Journal of Clinical Pharmacology 39: 289–296

Hachen H 1980 Clinical and urodynamic assessment of alpha adrenolytic therapy in patients with neurogenic bladder function. Paraplegia 18: 229

Hachen H, Krucker V 1977 Clinical and laboratory assessment of the efficacy of baclofen on urethral sphincter spasticity in patients with traumatic paraplegia. European Urology 3: 327

Hackler R, Broecker B, Klein F, Brady S 1980 A clinical experience with dantrolene sodium for external urinary sphincter hypertonicity in spinal cord injured patients. Journal of Urology 124: 78

Harris J D, Benson G S 1980 Effect of dantrolene on canine bladder contractility. Urology 16: 229

Haruno A 1992 Inhibitory effects of propiverine hydrochloride on the agonist-induced or spontaneous contractions of various isolated muscle preparations. Drug Research 42: 815

Hedlund H, Mattiasson A, Andersson K E 1990 Lack of effect of pinacidil on detrusor instability in men with bladder outlet obstruction. Journal of Urology 143: 369A

Hedlung H, Andersson K E 1988 Effects of prazosin and carbochol in patients with benign prostatic obstruction. Scandinavian Journal of Urology and Nephology 22: 19

Hehir M, Fitzpatrick J M 1985 Oxybutynin and the prevention of urinary incontinence in spinal bifida. European Urology 11: 254

Hilton P, Tweddell A L, Mayne C 1990 Oral and intravaginal estrogens alone and in combination with alpha-adrenergic stimulation in genuine stress incontinence. International Urogynecology Journal and Pelvic Floor Dysfunction 1: 80

Hilton P, Stanton S L 1983 The use of intravaginal estrogen cream in genuine stress incontinence. British Journal of Obstetrics and Gynaecology 90: 940

Hodgson B J, Dumas S, Bolling D R, Heesch C M 1978 Effect of estrogen on sensitivity of rabbit bladder and urethra to phenylephrine. Investigative Urology 16: 67

Hoffman B B, Lefkowitz R J 1990a Catecholmines and sympathomimetic drugs. In: Gilman A G, Rall T W, Nies A S, Taylor P (eds) Goodman and Gilman's The Pharmacological Basis of Therapeutics, 8th edn. Pergamon Press, New York pp 187–220

Hoffman B B, Lefkowitz R J 1990b Adrenergic receptor agoinsts. In: Gilman A G, Rall T W, Nies A S, Taylor P (eds) Goodman and Gilman's The Pharmacological Basis of Therapeutics, 8th edn. Pergamon Press, New York pp 221–243

Hollister L E 1986 Current antidepressants. Annual Review of Pharmacology and Toxicology 26: 23

Holmberg E, Waldeck B. 1980 On the possible role of potassium ions on the action of terbutaline on skeletal muscle contractions. Acta Pharmacologica et Toxicologica 46: 141

Holmes D, Montz F, Stanton S L 1989 Oxybutynin v. propantheline in the management of detrusor instability: a patient regulated variable dose trial. British Journal of Obstetrics and Gynaecology 96: 607–612

Husted S, Andersson K E, Sommer L 1980 Anticholinergic and calcium antagonistic effects of terodilene in rabbit urinary bladder Acta Pharmacologica et Toxicologica 46: 20

Jackson S, Shepherd A, Abrams P 1997 Does oestrogen supplementation improve the symptoms of postmenopausal urinary stress incontinence? A double blind placebo controlled trial. Neurourology and Urodynamics 16: 350–351

James M J, Birmingham A T, Hill S J 1993 Partial mediation by nitric oxide of the relaxation of human isolated detrusor strips in response to electrical field stimulation. British Journal of Clinical Pharmacology 35: 366

James M J, Iacovou J W 1993 The case of GTN patches in detrusor instability: a pilot study. Neurourology and Urodynamics 12: 399

Jaschevatsky O E, Anderman S, Shalit A 1985 Prostaglandin F2a for prevention of urinary retention after vaginal hysterectomy. Obstetrics and Gynecology 66: 244

Jensen D, Jr 1981a Pharmacological studies of the uninhibited neurogenic bladder. Acta Neurologica Scandinavica 64: 145–174

Jensen D, Jr 1981b Altered adrenergic innervation in the uninhibited neurogenic bladder. Scandinavian Journal of Urology and Nephrology. 60: 61

Jensen D, Jr 1981c Uninhibited neurogenic bladder treated with prazosin. Scandinavian Journal of Urology and Nephrology 15: 229–233

Johnston A 1996 Estrogens-pharmacokinetics and pharmacodynamics with special reference to vaginal administration and the new estradiol formulation Esting. Acta Obstetrica et Gynecologica Scandinavica 165: 16–25

Jonas U, Petri E, Kissal J 1979 The effect of flavoxate on hyperactive detrusor muscle. European Urology 5: 106

Kachur J F, Peterson J S, Carter J P, Rzeszotarski W J, Hanson R C, Noronha-Blob L 1988 R and S enantiomers of oxybutynin: pharmacological effects in guinea pig bladder and intestine. Journal of Pharmacology and Experimental Therapeutics 247: 867–872

Kaisary A U 1984 Beta adrenoceptor blaockade in the treatment of female stress urinary incontinence. Annales d'Urologie 90: 351

Karram M M, Yeko T R, Sauer M V, Bhatia N N 1989 Urodynamic changes following hormonal replacement therapy in women with premature ovarian failure. Obstetrics and Gynecology 74: 208

Kato K, Kitada S, Chun A, Wein A J, Levin R M 1989 In vitro intravesical instillation of anticholinergic, antispasmodic and calcium blocking agents (rabbit whole bladder model). Journal of Urology 141: 1471–1475

Kelleher C J, Cardozo L D, Khullar V, Salvatore S 1998 A medium-term analysis of the subjective efficacy of treatment for

women with detrusor instability and low bladder compliance. British Journal of Obstetrics and Gynaecology 104: 988–993
Kieswetter H, Hennrich F, Englisch M 1983 Clinical and pharmacologic therapy of stress incontinence. Urologia Internationalis 38: 58
Kinn A C, Larsson P O 1990 Desmopressin: a new principle for symptomatic treatment of urgency and incontinence in patients with multiple sclerosis. Scandinavian Journal of Urology and Nephrology 24: 109
Kishimoto T, Morita T, Okamiyo Y 1991 Effect of clenbuterol on contractile response in periurethral striated muscle of rabbits. Tohoku Journal of Experimental Medicine 165: 243
Kleeman F J 1970 The physiology of the internal urinary sphincter. Journal of Urology 104: 549
Koonings P, Bergman A, Ballard C A 1990 Prostaglandins for enhancing detrusor function after surgery for stress incontinence in women. Journal of Reproductive Medicine 35: 1
Korczyn A D, Kish I 1979 The mechanism of imipramine in enuresis nocturna. Clinical and Experimental Pharmacology and Physiology 6: 31
Koyangi T 1979 Further observation on the denervation supersensitivity of the urethra in patients with chronic neurogenic bladders. Journal of Urology 122: 348
Krane R, Olsson C 1973a Phenoxybenzamine in neurogenic bladder dysfunction: I. Clinical considerations. Journal of Urology 110: 653
Krane R, Olsson C 1973b Phenoxybenzamine in neurogenic bladder dysfunction. II. Clinical considerations. Journal of Urology 110: 653
Kums J J M, Delhaas E M 1991 Intrathecal baclofen infusion in patients with spasticity and neurogenic bladder disease. World Journal of Urology 9: 99
Lader M 1987 Clinical pharmacology of benzodiazepines. Annual Review of Medicine 38: 19
Larsson B, Andersson K, Batra S, Mattiasson, A Sjögren C. 1984 Effects of estradiol on norepinephrine-induced contraction, alpha adrenoceptor number and norepinephrine content in Journal of Pharmacology and Experimental Therapeutics 229: 557
Lee L 1949 The clinical use of urecholine in dysfunctions of the bladder. Journal of Urology 62: 300
Lepor H, Gup D, Shapiro E, Baumann M 1989 Muscarinic cholinergic receptors in the normal and neurogenic human bladder. Journal of Urology 142: 869
Lepor H 1990 Role of long acting selective alpha-1 blockers in the treatment of benign prostatic hyperplasia. Urologic Clinics of North America 17: 651
Levin R M, Shofer F S, Wein A J 1980 Estrogen-induced alterations in the autonomic responses of the rabbit urinary bladder. Journal of Pharmacology and Experimental therapeutics 215: 614
Levin R M, Jacobowitz D, Wein A J 1981 Autonomic innervation of rabbit urinary bladder following estrogen administration. Urology 17: 449
Levin R M, Staskin D, Wein A J 1982 The muscarinic cholinergic binding kinetics of the human urinary bladder. Neurourology and Urodynamics 1: 221
Levin R M, Staskin D, Wein A J 1983 Analysis of the anticholinergic and musculotropic effects of desmethylimipramine on the rabbit urinary bladder. Urological Research 11: 259
Levin R M, Ruggieri M R, Lee W, Wein A J 1988a Effect of chronic atropine administration on the rat urinary bladder Journal of Urology 139: 1347
Levin R M, Ruggieri M R, Wein A J 1988b Identification of receptor subtypes in the rabbit and human urinary bladder by selective radio-ligand binding. Journal of Urology 139: 844
Levin R M, Hayes L, Zhao Y, Wein A J 1992 Effect of pinacidil on spontaneous and evoked contractile activity. Pharmacology 45: 1–8
Levin R M, Scheiner S, Zhao Y, Wein A J 1993 The effect of terodiline on hyperreflexia (in vitro) and the in vitro response of isolated strips of rabbit to field stimulation, bethanechol and KCI. Pharmacology 46: 346
Levin R M, Wein A J 1984 Comparative effects of five tricyclic compounds on the rabbit urinary bladder. Neurourology and Urodynamics 3: 127
Lindholm P, Lose G 1986 Terbutaline (Bricanyl) in the treatment of female urge incontinence. Urologia Internationalis 41: 158
Longman S D, Hamilton T C 1992 Potassium channel activator drugs – mechanism of action, pharmacological properties, and therapeutic potential. Medical Research Review 12: 73–148
Lose G, Rix P, Diernaes E, Alexander N 1988 Norfenefrine in the treatment of female stress incontinence. A double-blind controlled trial. Urologia Internationalis 43(1): 11–15.
Lose G, Jorgensen L, Thunedborg P 1989 Doxepin in the treatment of female detrusor overactivity: a randomized double-blind crossover study. Journal of Urology 142: 1024
Lose G, Lindholm D 1997 Clinical and urodynamic effects of nofenefrine in women with stress incontinence. Urologia Internationalis 39: 298
Loubser P G, Narayan R K, Sadin K J 1991 Continuous infusion of intrathecal baclofen: Long term effects on spasticity in spinal cord injury. Paraplegia 29: 48
Madersbacher H, Jilg G 1991 Control of detrusor hyperreflexia by the intravesical instillation of oxybutynin hydrochloride. Paraplegia 19: 84
Madersbacher H, Stohrer M, Richter R, et al 1995 Trospium chloride versus oxybutynin: a randomized double blind, multicentre trial in the treatment of detrusor hyperreflexia. British Journal of Urology 75: 452–446
Maggi C A, Barbanti G, Santicioli P et al 1989 Cystometric evidence that capsaicin-sensitive nerves modulate the afferent branch of micturition reflex in humans. Journal of Urology 142: 150–154
Maggi C A 1991 Capsaicin and primary afferent neurons: from basic science to human therapy? Journal of the Autonomic Nervous System 33: 1–14
Maggi C A 1992 Therapeutic potential of capsaicin-like molecules – studies in animals and humans. Life Sciences 51: 1777–1781
Malkowicz S B, Wein A J, Brendler K, Levin R M 1985 Effect of diltiazem on in vitro rabbit bladder function. Pharmacology 31: 24–33
Malkowicz S B, Wein A J, Ruggieri M R, Levin R M 1987 Comparison of calcium antagonist properties of antispasmodic agents. Journal of Urology 138: 667–670
Malgren A, Andersson K, Andersson P O, Fovaeus M, Sjögren C 1990 Effects of cromakalim (BRL 34915) and pinacidil on normal and hypertrophied rat detrusor in vitro. Journal of Urology 143: 828–834
McGuire E, Savastano J 1985 Effect of alpha adrenergic blockade and anticholinergic agents on the decentralized primate bladder. Neurourology and Urodynamics 4: 139
Milanov I G 1991 Mechanisms of baclofen action on spasticity. Acta Neurologica Scandinavica 85: 304
Mitchell W C, Venable D D 1985 Effects of metoclopramide on detrusor function. Journal of Urology 135: 791
Moisey C, Stephenson T, Brendler C 1980 The urodynamic and subjective results of treatment of detrusor instability with oxybutynin chloride. British Journal of Urology 52: 472

Murdock M, Sax D, Krane R 1976 Use of dantrolene sodium in external sphincter spasm. Urology 8: 133
Murray K H A, Feneley R C I 1982 Endorphins: a role in urinary tract function? The effect of opioid blockade on the detrusor and urethral sphincter mechanisms. British Journal of Urology 54: 638
Naglo A S, Nergardh A, Boreus L O 1989 Influence of atropine and isoprenoline on detrusor hyperactivity in children with neurogenic bladder. Scandinavian Journal of Urology and Nephrology 15: 97
Nanning J, Frost F, Penn R 1989 Effect of intrathecal baclofen on bladder and sphincter function. Journal of Urology 142: 101
Nestler J E, Stratton M A, Hakin C A 1983 Effect of metoclopramide on diabetic neurogenic bladder. Clinical Pharmacology 2, 83
Nilsson C G, Lukkari E, Haarala M, et al 1997 Comparison with a 10 mg controlled release oxybutynin tablet with a 5 mg oxybutynin tablet in urge incontinent patients. Neurourology and Urodynamics 16: 533–542
Nilvebrant L, Hallen B, Larsson B 1997a Tolterodine – a new bladder selective muscarinic receptor antagonist: preclinical pharmacological and clinical data. Life Sciences 60: 1129–1136
Nilvebrant L, Andersson K-E, Gillberg P-G, et al 1997b Tolterodine – a new bladder selective antimuscarinic agent. European Journal of Pharmacology 27: 195–207
Nordling J, Meyhoff H, Hald T 1981 Sympatholytic effect on striated urethral sphincter. A peripheral or central nervous system effect? Scandinavian Journal of Urology and Nephrology 15: 173
Norgaard J P, Rillig S, Djurhuus J C 1989 Nocturnal enuresis: an approach to treatment based on pathogenesis. Journal of Pediatrics 114: 705
Norlen L 1982 Influence of the sympathetic nervous system on the lower urinary tract and its clinical implications. Neurourology and Urodynamics 1: 129
Nurse D E, Restorick J M, Mundy A R 1991 The effect of cromakalim on the normal and hyper-reflexic human detrusor muscle. British Journal of Urology 68: 27–31
O'Brink A, Bunne G 1978 The effect of alpha adrenergic stimulation in stress incontinence. Urologia Internationalis 12: 205
Olsson A, Swanberg E, Scedinger I 1979 Effects of beta adrenoceptor agonists on airway smooth muscle and on slow contracting skeletal muscle: in vitro and in vivo results compared. Acta Pharmacologica et Toxicologica 44: 272
Olubadewo J 1980 The effect of imipramine on rat detrusor muscle contractility. Archives Internationales de Pharmacodynamie et de Therapie 145: 84
Ouslander J G, Blaustein J, Connor H 1988a Pharmacokinetics and clinical effects of oxybutynin in geriatric patients. Journal of Urology 140: 47
Ouslander J G, Blaustein J, Connor H 1988b Habit training and oxybutynin for incontinence in nursing home patients: a placebo-controlled trial. Journal of the American Geriatric Society 36: 40
Palmer J, Worth P, Exton-Smith A 1981 Flunarizine: a once daily therapy for urinary incontinence. Lancet 2: 279
Parsons K, Turton M 1980 Urethral supersensitivity and occult urethral neuropathy. British Journal of Urology 52: 131
Pederson E, Torring J, Kleman B 1980 Effect of the alpha-adrenergic blocking agent thymoxamine on the neurogenic bladder and urethra. Acta Neurologica Scandinavica 61: 107
Pederson P A, Johansen P B 1988 Prophylactic treatment of adult nocturia with bumetanide. British Journal of Urology 62: 145
Penn R D, Savoy S M Corcos D E 1989 Intrathecal baclofen for severe spinal spasticity. New England Journal of Medicine 320: 1517
Perkash I 1975 Intermittent catheterization and bladder rehabilitation in spinal cord injury patients. Journal of Urology 114: 230
Peterson J S, Patton A J Noronha-Blob L 1990 Mini-pig urinary bladder function: comparisons of {in vitro} anticholinergic responses and {in vivo} cystometry with drugs indicated for urinary incontinence. Journal of Autonomic Pharmacology 10: 65–73
Philip N, Thomas D, Clark S 1980 Drug effects on the voiding cystometrogram: a comparison of oral bethanechol and carbachol. British Journal of Urology 52: 484
Philip N H, Thomas D G 1980 The effect of distigmine bromide on voiding in male paraplegic patients with reflex micturition. British Journal of Urology 52: 492
Pietzko A, Dimpfel W, Schwantes U, Topfmeier P 1994 Influences of trospium chloride and oxybutynin on quantitative EEG in healthy volunteers. European Journal of Clinical Pharmacology 47: 337–343
Poli E, Monica B, Zappia L E 1992 Antimuscarinic activity of telemyepine on isolated human urinary bladder: no role for M-1 receptors. Genetic Pharmacology 23: 659
Raezer D M, Wein A J, Jacobowitz D M E 1973 Autonomic innervation of canine urinary bladder. Cholinergic and adrenergic contributions and interaction of sympathetic and parasympathetic systems in bladder function. Urology 2: 211
Raezer D M, Benson G S, Wein A J 1977 The functional approach to the management of the pediatric neuropathic bladder: a clinical study. Journal of Urology 117: 649
Rall T W 1990 Oxytocin prostaglandins, ergot alkaloids and other drugs: tocolytic agents. In: Gilman A G, Rall T W, Nies A S, Taylor P (eds) Goodman and Gilman's The Pharmacological Basis of Therapeutics, 8th edn. Pergamon Press, New York pp 933–953
Rashbaum M, Mandelbaum C C 1948 Non-operative treatment of urinary incontinence in women. American Journal of Obstetrics and Gynecology 56: 777
Raz S, Zeigler M, Caine M 1973a The effect of progesterone on the adrenergic receptors of the urethra. British Journal of Urology 45: 663–667
Raz S, Ziegler M, Caine M 1973b The role of female hormones in stress incontinence. In: Proceedings of 16th Congress Société Internationale d'Urologie, Paris, vol. 1 pp 397–402
Raz S, Caine M 1971 Adrenergic receptors in the female canine urethra. Investigative Urology 9: 319
Raz S, Smith R B 1976 External sphincter spasticity syndrome in female patients. Journal of Urology 115: 443
Restorick J M, Mundy A R 1989 The density of cholinergic and alpha and beta adrenergic receptors in the normal and hyper-reflexic human detrusor. British Journal of Urology 63: 32
Rew D A, Rundle J S H 1989 Assessment of the safety of regular DDAVP therapy on primary nocturnal enuresis. British Journal of Urology 63: 352
Richelson E 1990 Antidepressants and brain neurochemistry Mayo Clinic Proceedings 65: 1227
Rosario D J, Cutinha P R, Chapple C R, et al 1996 The effects of single dose darifenacin on cystometric parameters and salivary flow in patients with urge incontinence secondary to detrusor instability. European Urology 30 (suppl 2): 240 (abstract)
Rud T 1980a Urethral pressure profile in continent women from childhood to old age. Acta Obstetrica et Gynecologica Scandinavica 59: 331
Rud T 1980b The effects of estrogens and gestagens on the

urethral pressure profile of urinary continent and stress incontinent women. Acta Obstetrica et Gynecologica Scandinavica 59: 265

Ruffman R 1988 A review of flavoxate hydrochloride in the treatment of urge incontinence. Journal of International Medical Research 16: 317

Salmon U J, Walter R I, Geist S H 1941 The use of estrogens in the treatment of dysuria and incontinence in postmenopausal women. American Journal of Obstetrics and Gynecology 42: 845

Samsioe G, Jansson I, Mellström D, Svanborg A 1985 Occurrence, nature and treatment of urinary incontinence in a 70-year-old female population. Maturitas 7: 335

Sanchez-Ferrer C F, Roman R J, Harder D R 1989 Pressure-dependent contraction of rat juxtamedullary afferent arterioles. Circulation Research 64: 790–798

Sant G R 1987 Intravesical 50% dimethyl sulfoxide (Rimso-50) in treatment of interstitial cystitis. Urology 4 (suppl): 17

Schreiter F, Fuchs P, Stockamp K 1976 Estrogenic sensitivity of α-receptors in the urethra musculature. Urologia Internationalis 31: 13

Schubler B 1990 Comparison of the mode of action of PGE2 and sulprostone, a PGE2 derivative, on the lower urinary tract in healthy women. Urological Research 18: 349

Shader R I, Greenblatt, D J 1993 Use of benzodiazepines in anxiety disorders. New England Journal of Medicine 328: 1398

Sonda L, Gershon C, Diokno A 1979 Further observations on the cystometric and uroflowmetric effects of bethanechol chloride on the human bladder. Journal of Urology 122: 775

Soulard C, Pascaud X, Roman F J, Grouhel A, Junien J L 1992 Pharmacological evaluation of JO-1870-relation to the potential treatment of urinary bladder incontinence. Journal of Pharmacology and Experimental Therapeutic 260: 1152

Sporer A, Leyson J, Martin B 1978 Effects of bethanechol chloride on the external urethral sphincter in spinal cord injury patients. Journal of Urology 120: 62

Stahl M M, Ekstrom B, Sparf B, Mattiasson A, Andersson K E 1995 Urodynamic and other effects of tolterodine: a novel antimuscarinic drug for the treatment of detrusor overactivity. Neurourology and Urodynamics 14: 647–655

Stanton D L, Cardozo L D, Ken-Wilson R 1979 Treatment of delayed onset of spontaneous voiding after surgery for incontinence. Urology 13: 494

Starr I, Ferguson C K 1940 Beta methylcholine urethane. Its action in various normal and abnormal conditions, especially postoperative urinary retention. American Journal of the Medical Sciences 200: 372

Steers W D 1992 Physiology of the urinary bladder. In: Walsh P C, Retik A B, Stamey T A, Vaughan E D (eds) Campbell's Urology, 6th edn. WB Saunders, Philadelphia, pp 142–169

Stewart B, Borowsky L, Montague D 1976 Stress incontinence: conservative therapy with sympathomimetic drugs. Journal of Urology 115: 558

Stewart D A, Taylor J, Ghosh S, MacPhee G J A, Abdullah I, McLenachan J M, Stott D J 1992 Terodiline causes polymorphic ventricular tachycardia due to reduced heart rate and prolongation of QT interval. European Journal of Clinical Pharmacology 42: 577–580

Stohrer M, Bauer P, Giannetti B M, et al 1991 Effect of trospium chloride on urodynamic parameters in patients with detrusor hyperreflexia due to spinal cord injuries: a multicentre placebo controlled double-blind trial. Urologia Internationalis 47: 138–143

Sundin T, Dahlstom A, Norlen L, Svedmyr N 1977 The sympathetic innervation and adrenoreceptor function of the human lower urinary tract in the normal state and after parasympathetic denervation. Investigative Urology 14: 322

Tammela T L 1986 Prevention of prolonged voiding problems after unexpected postoperative urinary retention: comparison of phenoxybenzamine and carbachol. Journal of Urology 136: 1254

Tammela T L, Kontturi M, Lukkarinen O 1987 Intravesical prostaglandin F2 for promoting bladder emptying after surgery for female stress incontinence. British Journal of Urology 60: 43

Taylor M C, Bates C P 1979 A double-blind crossover trial of baclofen: a new treatment for the unstable bladder syndrome. British Journal of Urology 51: 505

Taylor P 1990 Cholinergic agonists. In: Gilman A G, Rall T W, Nies A S, Taylor P (eds) Goodman and Gilman's The Pharmacological Basis of Therapeutics, 8th edn. Pergamon Press, New York pp 122–130

Taylor S H 1989 Clinical pharmacotherapeutics of doxazosin. American Journal of Medicine 87 (suppl 2A): 25

Thomas D G, Philp N H, McDermott T E 1984 The use of urodynamic studies to assess the effect of pharmacological agents with particular references to alpha blockade. Paraplegia 22: 162

Thompson I, Lauvetz R 1976 Oxybutynin in bladder spasm, neurogenic bladder and enuresis. Urology 8: 452

Thor K B, Roppolo J R, de Groat W C 1983 Naloxone-induced micturition in unanesthesized paraplegic cats. Journal of Urology 129: 202

Thuroff J, Bunke B, Ebner A e 1991 Randomized double-blind multicenter trial on treatment of frequency, urgency and incontinence related to detrusor hyperactivity: oxybutynin vs. propanthelene vs. placebo. Journal of Urology 145: 813

Thuroff J, Chartier-Kasker E, Corcus J, et al 1998 Medical treatment and medical side-effects in urinary incontinence in the elderly. World Journal of Urology 16(suppl 1): 48–61

Tulloch A G S, Creed K E 1981 A comparison between propantheline and imipramine on bladder and salivary gland function. British Journal of Urology 125: 218

Vaidyanathan S, Rao M, Chary K S N 1981a Enhancement of detrusor reflex activity by naloxone in patients with chronic neurogenic bladder dysfunction. Journal of Urology 126: 500

Vaidyanathan S, Rao M, Mapa M 1981b Study of instillation of 15(S)-15-methyl prostaglandin F2a in patients with neurogenic bladder dysfunction. Journal of Urology 126: 81

Van Doorn E S C, Zweirs W 1990 Ambulant monitoring to assess the efficacy of oxybutynin chloride in patients with mixed incontinence. European Urology 18: 49

Veldhuis G, Inman J 1991 Terodilene and torsade de pointes (letter to the editor). British Medical Journal 303: 519

Versi E, Cardozo L, Buncat L E 1988 Correlation of urethral physiology and skin collagen in post menopausal women. British Journal of Urology and Gynaecology 95: 147

Wagner G, Husstein P, Enzelsberger H 1985 Is prostaglandin E2 really of therapeutic value for postoperative urinary retention? Results of a prospectively randomized double-blind study. American Journal of Obstetrics and Gynecology 151: 375

Wallis R M, Napier C M 1999 Muscarinic antagonists in development for disorders of smooth muscle function. Life Sciences 64: 395–401

Walter S, Wolf H, Barleto H, Jensen H K 1978 Urinary incontinence in post menopausal women treated with estrogens. Urologia Internationalis 33: 135

Walter S, Kjærgaard B, Lose G et al 1990 Stress urinary incontinence in postmenopausal women treated with oral estrogen (estriol) and an alpha-adrenoceptor-stimulating agent (phenylpropanolamine): a randomized double-blind placebo-controlled study. International Urogynecology Journal and Pelvic Floor Dysfunction 1: 74

Weese D L, Roskamp D A, Leach G E, Zimmern P E 1993 Intravesical oxybutynin chloride: experience with 42 patients. Urology 41: 527

Wein A J, Malloy T, Shofar F e 1980a The effects of bethanechol chloride on urodynamic parameters in normal women and in women with significant residual urine volumes. Journal of Urology 124: 397

Wein A J, Raezer D D, Malloy T 1980b Failure of the bethanechol supersensitivity test to predict improved voiding after subcutaneous bethanechol administration. Journal of Urology 123: 202

Wein A J, Levin R M, Barrett D M 1991a Voiding function: relevant anatomy, physiology, and pharmacology. In: Duckett J W, Howards S T, Grayhack J T, Gillenwater, J Y (eds) Adult and Pediatric Urology, 2nd edn. Mosby-Year Book, St. Louis pp 933–999

Wein A J, Van Arsdalen K N, Levin R M 1991b Pharmacologic therapy. In: Krane R J, Siroky M B (eds) Clinical-neuro-urology, Little Brown, Boston pp 523–558

Wein A J 1992 Neuromuscular dysfunction of the lower urinary tract. In: Walsh P C, Retik A B, Stamey T A, Vaughan E D J (eds) Campbell's Urology, 6th edn. WB Saunders, Philadelphia pp 573–642

Weiner L B, Baum N H, Suarez G M 1986 New method for management of detrusor instability: transdermal scopolamine. Urology 28: 208

Wheeler J S, Jr. Robinson C J, Culkin D J, Nemchausky B A 1987 Naloxone efficacy in bladder rehabilitation of spinal cord injury patients. Journal of Urology 137: 1202

Wilde M, Fitton A, McTavish D 1993a Alfuzosin – a review of its pharmacodynamic and pharmacokinetic properties and its therapeutic potential in BPH. Drugs 45: 410

Wilde M, Fitton A, Sorkin E 1993b Terazosin: a review of its pharmacodynamic and pharmacokinetic properties and therapeutic potential in BPH. Drugs and Aging 3: 258

Winkler H A, Sand P K 1998 Treatment of detrusor instability with oxybutynin rectal suppositories. International Journal of Urogynaecology and Pelvic Floor Dysfunction 9: 100–102

Zeegers A, Kiesswetter H, Kramer A, Jonas U 1987 Conservative therapy of frequency, urgency and urge incontinence: a double-blind clinical trial of flavoxate, oxybutynin emepronium and placebo. World Journal of Urology 5: 57

Zorzitto M L, Jewett M A, Fernie G R e 1986 Effectiveness of propantheline bromide in the treatment of geriatric patients with detrusor instability. Neurourology and Urodynamics 5: 133

Zorzitto M L, Holliday P J, Jewett M A 1989 Oxybutynin chloride for geriatric urinary dysfunction: a double-blind placebo controlled study. Age and Ageing 18: 195

43

Electrical therapy

STANISLAV PLEVNIK, DAVID B VODUŠEK, NICOLAS P BRYAN, STEPHEN C RADLEY AND CHRISTOPHER R CHAPPLE

Part One: Non-implanted

Part Two: Implants

Part One: Non-implanted

Stanislav Plevnik and David B Vodušek

INTRODUCTION

Non-implanted electrical stimulation is becoming accepted as a useful non-invasive mode of therapy for female urinary incontinence by an increasing number of clinicians who believe that the most conservative treatment approaches should be tried first. Such an approach has been supported by the US Department of Health and Human Services (1996).

Electrical stimulation (ES) has been introduced to treat lower urinary tract disturbances with the aim of providing a substitute for what is lacking in the functional integrity of the system. Early workers have drawn parallels to ES as used in physical medicine, where functional (electrical) prostheses have been developed to improve walking in paretic (hemiparetic) patients (preventing foot-drop). Since then some have been stuck with the term 'functional electrical stimulation' in the therapy of micturition disorders, although it needs to be realized that – strictly speaking – only those therapeutic strategies should be called 'functional' which substitute electrical stimuli for absent neural control.

Some therapeutic applications of ES in lower urinary tract disorders aim to improve function (particularly to achieve continence), but achieve this 'indirectly' (or rather through their short- or long-term carry-over effects). To call all the different ES strategies 'functional' would be confusing; instead we employ the term 'therapeutic electrostimulation'. Under this heading we include 'electric pessary' (Alexander & Rowan 1968), maximum perineal electrical stimulation (Moore & Schofield 1967), intravaginal electrical stimulation (Erlandson et al 1978), acute electrical stimulation (Godec & Cass 1978), maximal electrical stimulation (Janež et al 1981), electrical sphincter stimulation (Vereecken et al 1984), short-term electric stimulation (Plevnik et al 1986a) and maximal pelvic floor stimulation (Eriksen et al 1989). All these methods have a common denominator: they have been proposed or are used for treating lower urinary tract disorders, but they cannot really be applied as a 'real time substitute' for absent neural control. They are (or have been) used in a therapeutic fashion. Their immediate effects are thought to be understood, but their long-term (carry-over) effects are probably more relevant for therapeutic results. Thus these methods are in a sense closer to physiotherapy (or perhaps even pharmacological treatment) than to pacemakers.

This chapter attempts to review critically the non-implanted therapeutic ES methods and devices used for the treatment of lower urinary tract dysfunction.

PHYSIOLOGY OF ELECTRICAL STIMULATION

Basic principles

The excitable membrane of the nerve or muscle cell becomes depolarized in changing electrical fields. In principle both muscle and nerve, and both motor and sensory nerve fibres can be excited. It is often not possible to excite separately only one particular type of neural fibre, as they lie anatomically very close together. On the other hand, there are morphological and physiological differences between the excitable structures, which makes them differentially sensitive to various parameters of electrical stimulation. So, for instance, the threshold for depolarization is much lower for the motor nerve fibres than for the muscles. If a muscle is innervated it is, as a rule, activated through depolarization of its motor nerve, if both are exposed to a changing electrical field. Therefore 'pelvic floor stimulation' is something of a misnomer, if taken to mean direct stimulation of muscle.

Although few of the published methods of ES explicitly say so, it seems reasonable to propose that their effects are mediated through excitation of motor and sensory nerve fibres in the particular region where the electrodes are applied.

Depolarization of motor nerve fibres

Excitation of motor fibres leads to activation of the muscle which this nerve innervates. We can call this the direct effect. In depolarizing motor nerve fibres the depolarization travels not only distally to activate the muscle, but also proximally. The latter – the so-called antidromic activation – is not usually mentioned, and we do not know if it leads to any relevant effects in therapeutic ES. A single stimulus depolarizing the motor nerve will lead to a single muscle contraction (which can be easily recorded on stimulation of pudendal nerve – Vodušek et al 1983). If the stimulation is performed as a continuous delivery of stimuli at a certain rate, a so-called tetanic muscle contraction will be achieved, which is (mechanically) much stronger than the individual contraction. To achieve such a contraction frequencies from 20 to 50 Hz are usually applied. One has, however, to consider that muscle is fatiguable and that higher frequencies lead to fatigue much faster. Using an intermittent type of stimulation with trains of stimuli interrupted by pauses, the muscle fatigue can be limited to a certain extent (Rotembourg et al 1976). Motor units in muscles consist of different types of muscle fibres, and these are defined through the type of neurocontrol. Tonic fibres are innervated by motor neurones producing low frequency activation for longer periods of time, whereas phasic motor fibres are innervated by motor neurones producing fast rates of activation for short periods. Due to the reliance of muscle fibres' metabolism on rate of activation, muscle fibres can be changed by ES from one type to another. Therefore prolonged ES of a muscle causes not only hypertrophy of muscle fibres, but also a change in motor unit properties (Salmons & Vrbova 1969).

Depolarization of sensory nerve fibres

Depolarization of sensory fibres leads not only to various reflex responses, but really to widespread 'invasion' into the CNS, which also leads to perception of stimulation. The easily measurable effects of stimulation of sacral afferents are reflex contractions of pelvic floor muscles (the so-called sacral reflexes) (Vodušek 1996). On the other hand, a decrease in pelvic floor spasticity on ES has also been described (Schmidt & Tanagho 1991; Bosch & Groen 1995a). Stimulation of sacral afferents has also been shown to interfere with sensory input from visceral afferents (Jiang et al 1991). Therapeutically, the vesicoinhibitory influence of perineal ES seems to be of greatest relevance. De Groat & Ryall (1969) demonstrated inhibitory postsynaptic potentials and inhibition of discharges of parasympathetic neurones due to a spinal reflex with a somatic (pudendal) afferent limb. They also reported that stimulation of these somatic afferents may have both an excitatory and an inhibitory influence on the bladder, depending on whether intravesical pressure was low or high respectively. Stimulation of pudendal afferents was observed to induce bladder inhibition due to pudendal–hypogastric (Sundin & Carlsson 1972) as well as to pudendal–pelvic spinal reflexes (Sundin et al 1974). The latter is assumed to be of main importance for detrusor inhibition in humans. Intravaginal electrical stimulation activated the same reflex mechanisms in cats (Fall et al 1977a). Bladder contraction inhibition has been achieved optimally with frequencies between 5 and 10 Hz (Erlandson et al 1978; Lindström et al 1983). The belief that primary activation of perineal (sphincter) muscles is the triggering factor of (reciprocal) bladder inhibition seems to be widespread. However, it has been shown in animals that sphincter muscle contraction is not necessary to achieve detrusor inhibition by afferent stimuli (De Groat & Ryall 1969; Lindström et al 1983).

Strength of electrical stimulation

In humans, bladder inhibition occurs on ES of non-muscular pudendal afferents, i.e. the dorsal penile nerve (Vodušek et al 1986), even with a stimulus that is sub-threshold for the bulbocavernosus reflex response. Most of the authors who used vaginal, anal or perineal needle electrodes for vesicoinhibitory ES in their clinical studies used rather strong stimuli (Plevnik et al 1991). However, electrodes placed in close proximity to the pudendal nerve have led to bladder inhibition with substantially weaker stimuli (Vodusek et al 1986, 1988) (Fig. 43.1). High amplitudes may be necessary because of higher nerve–electrodes distances in the case of anal or vaginal stimulation.

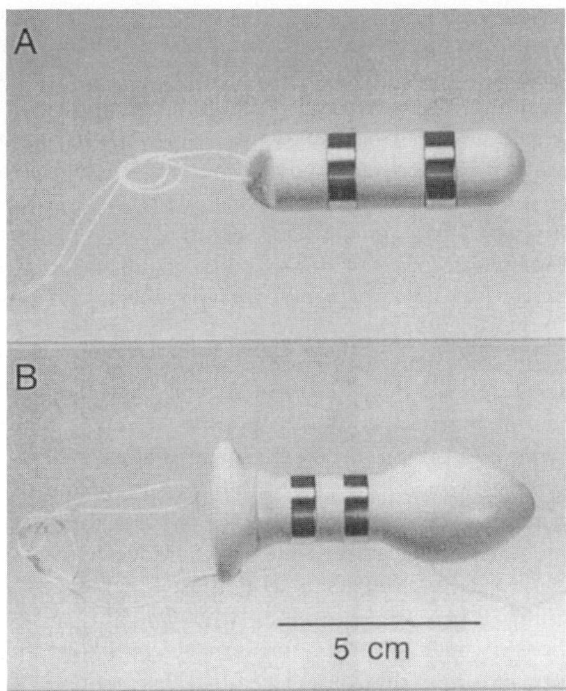

Fig. 43.1 Devices for long-term automatic vaginal (**A**) or anal (**B**) electrical stimulation. The plug contains electrodes, a pulse generator which generates a current-controlled biphasic, charge-balanced, intermittent stimulation pattern, and has an automatic ON/OFF switch (Medicon, Norway).

Carry-over effects of electrical stimulation

ES of motor and sensory sacral nerve fibres in the pudendal nerves may lead both to pelvic floor contraction, and inhibition of the active detrusor (Vodušek et al 1986, 1988). All these effects have been demonstrated during stimulation. But there are delayed or carry-over effects of such stimulation as well. Short-term carry-over detrusor inhibition has been demonstrated (Vodušek et al 1986), and might be due to the activation of the spinal opioid system (Dray & Metsch 1984). Long-term effects which are known from therapeutic application of strong, short electrostimulation (Plevnik et al 1991) are as yet not clarified. A change in the bladder receptor properties has been postulated (Janež et al 1981), but not confirmed (Jiang & Lindström 1996). Carry-over effects of prolonged muscle contraction include hypertrophy of muscle and change of motor unit types. It seems attractive to analyse ES therapeutic effectiveness in terms of control theory concepts: the electrically induced afferent input replaces the lost physiological neural control by (a) setting the threshold for micturition (b) adjusting the gain of bladder and/or sphincter contraction and (c) operating switches to regain lost coordination. As an illustration of such mechanisms we can refer to a study of a small group of women with poor tonic motor unit activity in sphincter muscles, and lack of voluntary contraction thereof: increases in tonic activity and a regaining of voluntary contraction were demonstrated after perineal ES (Vodušek & Kralj 1979). In another experimental study, intravesical ES induced a prolonged modulation of the micturition reflex without a change in tension sensitivity of bladder mechanoreceptors in the rat, thus requiring central changes as an explanation for the effect (Jiang & Lindström 1996).

Indeed, it is necessary to postulate rather neutral interferences of electrostimulation in integrated neural control, as quite opposite effects can be observed by ES in different patient groups. Whereas hyperreflexive bladders are inhibited (e.g. to improve storage; Godec et al 1976), hypo- or areflexive bladders can become activated (e.g. to improve emptying; Plevnik et al 1984). It is as if the disrupted neural control is rearranged by electrostimulation by 'hitting the switches', and thus turning the control mechanism as a rule towards a more functional status.

THERAPEUTIC ELECTRICAL STIMULATION IN CLINICAL PRACTICE

Although therapeutic effects in lower urinary tract dysfunction have been achieved by vaginal (De Soldenhoff & McDonnel 1969; Fall et al 1977b), anal (Hopkinson & Lightwood 1967), clitoral (Vodušek et al 1986) and even tibial nerve ES (McGuire et al 1983), the presently commercially available devices mostly use vaginal or anal electrodes. Such ES we shall call perineal (Fig. 43.2). Another type of non-implantable ES is the intravesical ES, which is used particularly to improve bladder function in patients with residual urine or retention (Katona & Eckstein 1974; Madersbacher et al 1987).

Electrical stimulation in incontinent patients

We propose that different methods of therapeutic perineal ES may be most practically distinguished by the different time course of treatment, and by the different strengths of the electrical pulses used. All proposed methods may therefore actually be classified as either long-term (weak) stimulation or short-term (strong) electrical stimulation. Long-term ES (also called 'chronic') is characterized by prolonged application of low-strength stimuli for many hours a day and/or night for a period of several months, which is prescribed as a home treatment programme. Short-term strong ES is characterized by pulses of strong intensities, which are applied for short periods of time (15–20 min), usually several times in consecutive days, for various periods, and either as in-patient or home treatment. Technical characteristics of long-term and short-term ES methods are described and discussed in detail later in this chapter.

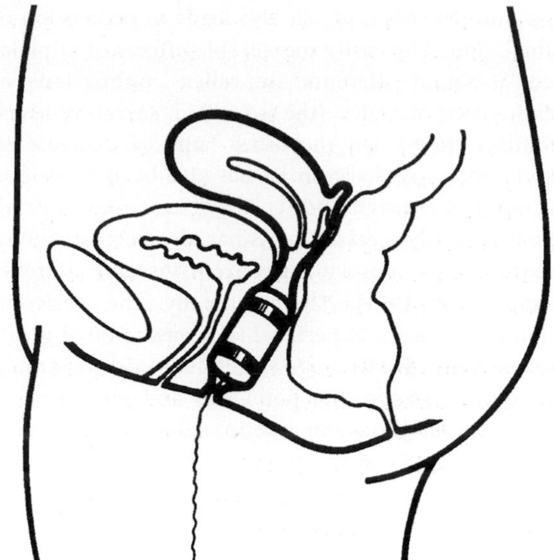

Fig. 43.2 Electrode placement during vaginal stimulation.

Long-term electrical stimulation

Long-term ES has been used to treat urinary incontinence due to urethral weakness and/or detrusor overactivity. Treatment with vaginal or anal plug electrodes was successful in 37% of stress incontinent, 42% of urge incontinent, and 75% of patients with mixed stress and urge incontinence (Doyle et al 1974). Plevnik et al (1977) have reported a success in 67% of patients with stress incontinence treated with vaginal plug or anal plug long-term ES. Fall et al (1977c) were using an inflatable vaginal electrode and reported success in 48% of stress and 100% of urge and mixed incontinence patients. Treatment with automatic anal ES (Fig. 43.1) (Eriksen et al 1987) has been reported as successful in 79% of stress, 78% of urge and 76% of mixed stress and urge incontinent patients, the follow-up being 9–36 months. No placebo-controlled studies using long-term ES are known to the authors.

Short-term strong electrical stimulation

Faradic stimulation or faradism can be ranked among short-term ES methods, although it is only of historic interest. Faradic stimulation has been performed in clinic with either one sacral and one suprapubic surface electrode or with one sacral and one vaginal or anal electrode. The stimulation was of an intermittent pattern. A 55% cure rate in a group of stress incontinent patients was reported by Moore & Schofield (1967). The mode of action of faradic stimulation is unclear; it could be stipulated that when using one sacral and one vaginal (or anal) electrode the acute effects of stimulation are at least partially due to the excitation of pudendal nerves.

Out-patient and home short-term strong electrical stimulation Following early reports on out-patient short-term application of strong ES (Godec et al 1975; Godec & Cass 1978; Janež et al 1979; Plevnik & Janež 1979) a more convenient and practical technique, i.e. short-term strong electrical stimulation for home treatment of incontinence, was developed and clinically tested (Plevnik et al 1986a). In non-controlled trials of strong short-term ES, Plevnik et al (1984) have reported success rates between 47 and 79% in patients with stress, urge, or mixed incontinence and enuresis using vaginal and anal electrodes, and Schiøtz (1994) has reported a 45% success rate in stress incontinent patients. Several other non-controlled trials with positive results were reported, but it is particularly important to mention some recent placebo-controlled trials of short-term strong ES delivered as home therapy. Sand et al (1995) have reported on a multicentre prospective randomized double-blind placebo-controlled trial of ES in treatment of stress incontinent patients. Success rates of 48% (subjective) and 62% (objective assessment), as opposed to 13 and 19% in the placebo-treated group were obtained, respectively. This difference was significant, but the drop-out rate in the ES treated group was somewhat larger (20%) than in the placebo-treated group (6%). A 'compliance monitor' was employed in the study.

Significant success in treatment with ES as opposed to placebo in patients with stress incontinence was also reported by Yamanishi et al (1996), using a treatment schedule of 2–3 daily treatments for 1 month. In the double-blind randomized controlled study of the efficiacy of 3 months' short-term ES in stress incontinent patients, Luber & Wolde-Tsadik (1997) reported no differences in subjectively and objectively assessed outcomes between ES and placebo-treated groups. Contrary to Sand et al (1995), Yamanishi et al (1996) and Luber & Wolde-Tsadik (1997), who used sham devices in their control groups, Bo et al (1999) offered continence guard to the control group in their multicentre single-blind randomized controlled study of 6 months' home ES in the treatment of stress incontinent patients, and reported 3 out of 25 patients (12%) as being subjectively cured in the ES group as compared to 1 out of 30 patients (3.3%) in the control group. Objectively, the differences between ES and control group were significant only in some secondary outcome measures. In urge incontinent patients Brubaker et al (1996) reported a 50% success rate in ES treated versus 13% in the placebo-treated group, the difference being significant. Tršinar & Kralj (1996) reported on a placebo-controlled study of strong short-term ES in children with unstable bladder and nocturnal enuresis and/or daytime incontinence. At 4.5 months after treatment 75% of stimulated children were cured or improved by 50% or more, in comparison with 14% of the placebo group, the difference being significant.

Using short-term strong ES as an out-patient procedure Abel et al (1996) reported a placebo-controlled trial in urge incontinent patients with a success rate of 91% versus 45% (subjective assessment) and 54% versus 27% (objective assessment), the difference being significant only for the subjective assessment. Their drop-out was 21% in the ES treated group.

Controlled studies have confirmed the beneficial effects of short-term strong ES in both stress and urge incontinent patients and in children with unstable bladders and incontinence. We have been using the short-term strong ES for over 20 years in Ljubljana with good therapeutic effects and without any serious side-effects. Our treatment programme consists of repeated (daily) application of 'strong' anal or vaginal continuous ES (maximum current up to 90 mA, maximum voltage 38 V, pulse duration 0.75 ms, frequency 20 Hz), lasting 20 minutes per session for 1 month. In a minority of refractory cases a treatment programme of several months has been used. The stimulation unit used consists of a battery-driven stimulator connected by cable to the stimulating anal or vaginal plug electrodes (Fig. 43.3). Treatment sessions are patient-controlled: after the plug is inserted the patient switches the stimulation on and is encouraged to continuously adjust the stimulation strength to just below the level of discomfort, i.e. to the level of the feeling of strong (but not painful) ES.

Interferential electrical stimulation **(interferential therapy)** is an out-patient short-term ES which is used for treatment of genuine stress incontinence. Traditionally, two pairs of surface electrodes have been used, one pair placed on both medial aspects of upper thighs, with the other placed on the lower abdomen. Alternating high frequency currents of slightly different frequencies are delivered from each pair of electrodes and it is postulated that they

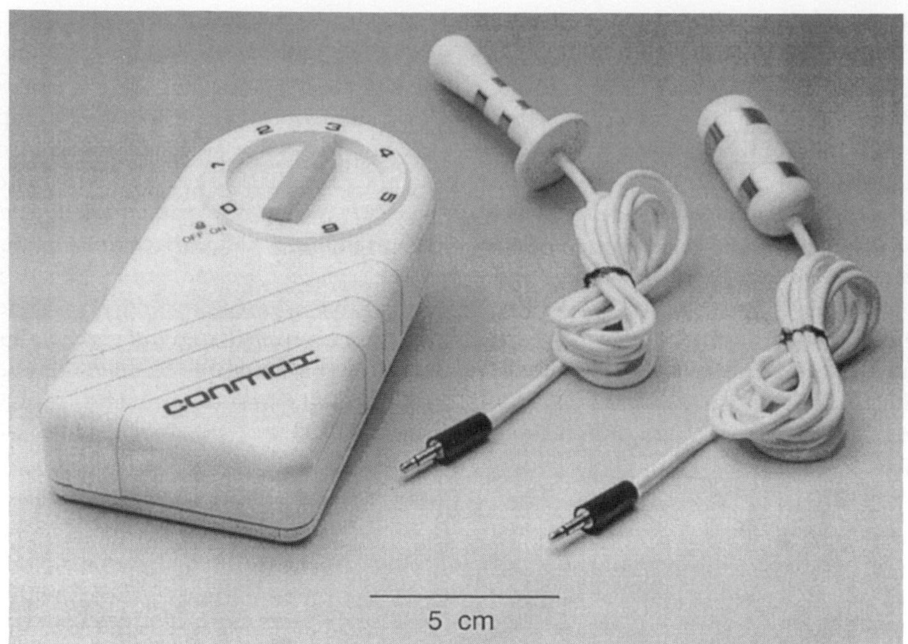

Fig. 43.3 Electrical stimulator for short-term strong electrical therapy with cylindrical vaginal or anal electrodes. Current-controlled biphasic, charge-balanced continuous or intermittent stimulation is automatically switched off after 20 minutes of use (Conmax®, Slovenia).

interact to produce low frequency electrical pulses which excite neuromuscular structures of the pelvic floor (Laycock et al 1994). The amplitude of the current is adjusted to the level which is comfortable to the patient and which produces a barely perceptible contraction of the pelvic floor. The patient is as a rule instructed to voluntarily contract pelvic floor during the duration of electrical pulses, similarly as in the case of faradic stimulation. Two to three 15–30-minute sessions are usually performed weekly for a period of 4–6 weeks. Cure rates from 60–90% have been reported (Olah et al 1990). A bipolar electrode arrangement with electronically produced amplitude-modulated current has been advocated as superior to the above described classic technique (Laycock & Green 1988).

Long-term vs. short-term electrical stimulation

A mean success rate of above 50% can be expected for various types of incontinent patients. No firm conclusions can be drawn from the results of non-comparative studies as to whether long-term or short-term ES is to be preferred. Short-term ES would seem to be more convenient and practical for patients since it does not require carrying the stimulator during the day or removal for voiding and/or defecation. The applied stimulation in long-term ES is so weak that it does not even reach sensory threshold in many patients. The beneficial effects achieved by such stimulation performed in the erect position could be at least partially attributed to pelvic floor exercises with vaginal cones (Plevnik 1985; Peattie et al 1988) which may be reflexly performed by the patients when they make an effort to hold, i.e. to prevent the electrode plug from sliding out of the vagina.

Predictability of the success of treatment

Perineal contraction visually observed during the trial stimulation has been suggested as a predictor of success of prolonged ES in stress (and urge) incontinent patients, but a considerable false negative (40%) and false positive prediction rate (25%) was found (Harrison & Paterson 1970). An increased urethral closure pressure during trial stimulation is a poor predictor of success of short-term ES in genuine stress incontinence (Plevnik et al 1986a). The cystometrically determined acute effect (i.e. present or absent detrusor inhibition) of a trial vaginal or anal ES correlated poorly with success rate of failure of short-term home ES (Plevnik et al 1986a). High success rates with prolonged ES in patients with incontinence due to an overactive detrusor were achieved in those patients whose perineal muscles were not completely denervated, and in whom a trial stimulation produced an increase in pressure as measured in the anal canal (Godec et al 1976). However, some patients showed improvement of incontinence after ES even though marked denervation has been shown in the perineal muscles on EMG (Plevnik et al 1986a). We can conclude that no valid procedure for identification of ES responsive patients has been found as yet.

Selection of patients for perineal ES

Clinical evaluation of all factors involved in generating the patient's symptoms is necessary. Underlying conditions, when present, should be treated accordingly. Theoretically, neuromuscular structures involved in lower urinary tract function must be at least partially preserved in order to achieve success with ES. In practice, the integrity of the sacral neuromuscular system can be evaluated both clinically and electrophysiologically and only patients without completely disrupted sacral reflex arcs could conceivably gain from ES. Most patients, however, will not have neurological lesions.

Patients' cooperation and ability to manipulate the device is essential for the success of therapy. Furthermore, the vaginal and the anal canal should provide satisfactory retention of electrodes during stimulation. Except for mucosal irritation and constipation (Plevnik et al 1986a) no other side-effects of perineal ES are known. It should be kept in mind that safety of stimulation during pregnancy and menstruation has not been established. Furthermore, in patients with heart pacemakers, ES should be avoided.

Non-implanted ES is non-invasive and (as a home treatment programme) cost-efficient, and should in our opinion be seriously considered in every incontinent patient, provided that the previously mentioned general criteria of selection are fulfilled. No particular diagnostic group has to be excluded.

We conclude that ES can be suggested prior to surgery for genuine stress incontinence. ES can be prescribed regardless of factors such as age, parity and previous surgery, which were shown to correlate inversely with success of surgical therapy (Harrison & Paterson 1970; Edwards & Malvern 1972; Doyle et al 1974).

In a comparative study of oxybutinin and short-term strong ES, Wise et al (1993) concluded that both oxybutinin and ES reduce the severity of urinary symptoms in women with detrusor instability and that ES is less effective but more acceptable. It has been our practice to offer ES prior to pharmacological treatment of detrusor overactivity because of similar experience with our patients.

Electrical stimulation in patients with urinary retention

Perineal electrical stimulation

Perineal anal or vaginal short-term strong ES in a group of 6 paraplegic patients with urinary retention resulted in cure or improvement in 5 patients (Plevnik et al 1984). ES induced bladder facilitation with inhibition of overactive periurethral sphincters, as shown urodynamically.

Intravesical (transurethral) electrical stimulation

Intravesical ES was started by Katona in the late 1950s in patients with neurogenic bladders with the aim of activating the detrusor (Katona & Eckstein 1974). The procedure consists of filling the bladder with saline to approximately one third capacity. Electric current is delivered via a monopolar electrode placed transurethrally (with the inactive electrode placed on a normally sensitive skin area). The technique involves several sessions lasting 1 to 2 hours daily for 1 to several months. The method was suggested particularly for incontinent myelodysplastic patients, in whom Madersbacher (1992) reported 30–40% improvement rates. The technique has often been applied together with a biofeedback procedure controlling intravesical volume. It has been demonstrated that excitation of bladder mechanoreceptor afferents of the A delta type is achieved by intravesical ES (Ebner et al 1992). A randomized placebo-controlled study has not shown efficacy beyond that of placebo (Boone et al 1992) but the study has been criticized on the grounds of poor patient selection. Recent uncontrolled studies have supported the efficacy of the technique using intravesical ES with current intensities of 10–20 mA (varying according to the patient's sensory threshold). Monophasic rectangular 1–6 ms long pulses were used at frequencies of 10–50 Hz in packages of 3–10 s, a rise time of 2–6 s, and pauses of 3–10 s. The stimulation time for a single stimulation session was 90 minutes (Del Popolo et al 1996). The treatment has also been called 'transurethral ES' (Primus et al 1996), and has been proposed for bladder rehabilitation after gynaecological surgery (Madersbacher et al 1995). Intravesical ES is very time consuming as an out-patient technique; it has, however, been suggested as a home treatment procedure in patients who are on clean intermittent catheterization (Risi et al 1996).

We conclude that intravesical ES has gained some acceptance as a means to improve or restore bladder function in patients with residual urine or retention. Reflecting the proposed mode of action, this particular ES procedure would seem logical for this purpose; but actually no comparison to the less invasive perineal ES in patients with retention has been reported.

TECHNICAL ASPECTS AND FURTHER DEVELOPMENT

Stimulators

Therapeutic stimulators generate either continuous or intermittent pattern of either mono- or biphasic pulses. The latter minimize electrode corrosion. In case of intermittent stimulation, times of 'stimulation off' and 'stimulation on' are usually in the range of a few seconds. Frequency and pulse duration are 10–50 Hz and 0.2–1 ms respectively. Stimulators consist of a battery operated external pulse generator connected to vaginal or anal electrodes by wire (Fig. 43.3). The pulse generator has a knob for adjustment of stimulation intensity. Maximum pulse intensity among available short-term strong electric stimulators is 120 mA (pulse duration 0.2 ms, maximum pulse charge 24 μC; MS 106, Medicon, Norway), while maximum and still safe pulse charge is 67.5 μC (pulse duration 0.75 ms, pulse intensity 90 mA; Conmax®, Slovenia).

Practicality of devices for prolonged ES has been improved by placing the complete system, together with the battery and electronic circuit, in the stimulating vaginal plug (Šuhel 1976) (Fig. 43.1A) and anal plug (Eriksen et al 1987) (Fig. 43.1B). These devices are automatically switched on when the electrodes come in contact with mucosa and produce gradual increase of the stimulation current at the insertion of the stimulator up to the pre-adjusted constant stimulation intensity from 0–25 mA (pulse duration 0.5 ms, maximum pulse charge 12.5 μC, frequency 25 Hz; PSV, Medicon, Norway).

The possibility of control of pulse intensity is important; it avoids discomfort during onset of stimulation and at the same time increases the patient's self-confidence, which is needed to overcome the fear of the electric current. After the electrodes are inserted, it allows for a gradual increase in stimulation intensity to the desired level, i.e. until the sensation of strong contraction is reached. It also allows for any decrease in intensity if discomfort or even pain occurs, due to e.g. displacement of stimulation electrodes.

Further developments

ES for therapy of urinary incontinence may not be optimal in terms of the stimulus parameters and its mode of application. The stimulus parameters of available therapeutic stimulators were determined rather empirically. Optimization of stimulation, however, requires knowledge of the mechanism of its long-term action. Recording the strength/duration curves for a constant current, rectangular charge-balanced electrical pulse, a duration of 0.2 ms has been found to be optimal, both for inducing sensations and muscle contraction in the perineal region at minimum pulse energy (Plevnik et al 1986b). The ascertained optimal pulse duration is much shorter than the commonly employed pulse durations. It provides the same excitation of somatic nerve fibres at two to three times less charge and energy pulse as a 1 ms long pulse.

Frequency in the train of stimuli applied to the patient was chosen empirically by most authors. Erlandson et al (1978) determined, on the basis of experimental data, that a frequency between 20 and 50 Hz was optimal for sphincter closure and 5 to 10 Hz for bladder inhibition. In practice, it seems that there is no difference using 5, 10 or 20 Hz for bladder inhibition in patients (Vereecken et al 1984), but frequencies below 10 Hz are poorly tolerated by patients. There is something to be said for simplicity of design to have a single stimulator for treatment of incontinence (i.e. with 20 Hz). Further clinical studies should justify the present vogue to have a range of frequency options. Similarly, the question of continuous versus intermittent stimulation has not been answered yet. Although there is not sufficient physiological evidence to support the preferential use of any of the two methods, many clinicians are using the intermittent pattern of ES, which is, however, more complicated in electronic design. Furthermore, intermittent ES may be suboptimal for detrusor inhibition (Fall & Madersbacher 1994).

Since the carry-over effects of therapeutic ES are not yet physiologically elucidated, the proper afferent input from ES cannot yet be properly ascertained. Most authors seem to feel that the strongest, yet safe (and bearable) stimulation is most likely to be efficient.

Electrodes

Different designs and sizes of electrodes have been tested for perineal ES, e.g. vaginal ring pessary (Alexander & Rowan 1968), cylindrical vaginal electrodes (De Soldenhoff & McDonnel 1969), expandable vaginal electrodes (Fall et al 1977c) and anal plug electrodes (Hopkinson & Lightwood 1967). Clip electrodes (as proposed for pudendal somatosensory evoked potentials; Vodušek 1990) stimulating the dorsal clitoral nerve, have been found to be quite effective. Electrodes are usually made of stainless steel and are incorporated into inconductive and inert material.

Perineal sites of stimulation have been chosen empirically for therapeutic electrical stimulation in incontinent patients. It has been demonstrated that stimulating the clitoral branch of the pudendal nerve is more important for the therapeutic effect than stimulating the pelvic floor branches (Lindström & Sudsuang 1989). Intravaginal stimulation is practical and comes close to pudendal nerves via surface electrodes. The anal approach will probably remain necessary for some groups of patients where the vaginal approach is not possible, e.g. for children.

The early investigators assumed that stronger ES would be more effective and used (in clinic) simultaneous multi-site stimulation, e.g. vaginal, anal and perineal needle stimulation (Kralj et al 1977) or anal and perineal needle stimulation (Godec & Cass 1978). Although using only a single stimulation site (anal or vaginal) has been justified in many clinical studies, some clinicians are still using more complicated simultaneous anal and vaginal stimulation (Abel et al 1996). The necessity to use such an ES regime has not been well demonstrated.

Temporary mode of application

The optimal time course of ES therapy (duration of ES sessions, number of ES sessions per day/week) has not been ascertained. It is not clear how long ES therapy should be administered before assessing treatment or abandoning therapy.

Out-patient versus home treatment

The common perception of clinicians that out-patient (i.e. clinician-controlled) ES is more effective than home therapy (i.e. self-administered) should also be verified. Comparative studies of out-patient therapy versus home therapy, with electronic controller of usage time of the home stimulator, should be encouraged.

Discomfort

At present, some discomfort is associated with therapeutic ES in most patient groups treated. This should in the future be minimized by optimization of electrical stimulation parameters, site of stimulation and electrode configuration. As discomfort is a very subjective experience and the sensation of ES varies during the period of application (becoming less and less – Plevnik et al 1986a), therapy with a variable (controllable) output stimulator is to be preferred. It is to be stressed that current-controlled (constant current) stimulators are to be preferred. Only these will provide an adequate and controllable depolarization of nerve fibres independently from tissue impedance, which has been shown to vary with intensity of stimulation (Vrtačnik et al 1985).

Safety

With any ES there are hazards of inadvertent excitation of the heart and local tissue damage at the site of stimulating electrodes. The Association for the Advancement of Medical Instrumentation (AAMI) proposed standards for transcutaneous electrical nerve stimulation (TENS) devices (Association for the Advancement of Medical Instrumentation 1980) based on the work of Zoll & Linenthal (1964) defining the maximum safe charge per pulse (75 μC). The AAMI also proposed the maximum safe average current output (10 mA). These standards should provide guidelines for perineal stimulation.

Regulated current (constant current) charge-balanced biphasic ES has been shown to minimize electrochemical processes at the metal–tissue interface, thus minimizing tissue injury and electrode corrosion (Mortimer 1981). According to the same author, the limitation for charge density of such stimulation in healthy muscle should be 0.4 $\mu C/mm^2$. He also established that healthy muscle tissue can tolerate monophasic stimulation, provided that current density does not exceed 10 mA/mm^2.

CONCLUSION

Although seemingly paradoxical, therapeutic ES seems to balance favourably the integrated reflex activity of bladder and urethra in a significant proportion of patients with quite diverse functional abnormalities.

It is expected that further clinical experience and controlled trials in well-defined patient groups with sphincter weakness and/or unstable or hyperreflexic detrusors will make perineal ES more widely accepted by doctors, and thus more widely available to patients with urinary incontinence. Controlled trials should further delineate the role of intravesical (transurethral) ES in patients with hypocontractile bladders. The fact that ES in the perineal region not only acutely compensates for the lack of insufficient detrusor inhibition in detrusor incontinence and/or insufficient urethral closure in sphincter incontinence, but that it also induces long-term (post-stimulation) beneficial effects which persist (for various time intervals) after termination of treatment, warrants further investigation with the final aim of improving patient selection. Results on the possible placebo and/or physiotherapy effects of long-term ES are still missing.

We feel that patient and doctor acceptance of therapeutic ES can be heightened by an appropriate physiologically oriented explanation (i.e. that the therapeutic programme supplements and improves the use of the available neuromuscular structures).

Also we feel that the patients should be encouraged to profit from the increased awareness of the pelvic floor muscles or bladder that the ES provides. This should facilitate any physiotherapy or biofeedback therapy, which might be added to ES in a logically combined and adjuvant treatment programme.

ACKNOWLEDGEMENT

The authors are grateful to Mr Miloš Kogej for his help in the preparation of this manuscript.

Part Two: Implants

Nicolas P Bryan, Stephen C Radley and Christopher R Chapple

INTRODUCTION

The use of electrical therapy, administered via implants, can be divided into two types: those that stimulate voiding when required and those that modulate the lower urinary tract by chronic stimulation. Stimulation of voiding has been confined to spinal cord injured patients. The strong stimulus required is too painful for patients with intact pain pathways, unless the additional ablative procedure of deafferentation is carried out. The main protagonists who developed sacral anterior root stimulation (SARS) were Brindley et al (1986), with the original intradural stimulator, and Tanagho and Schmidt (1988) who subsequently developed an extradural stimulator.

Chronic electrical stimulation has been employed for treating urinary incontinence since Caldwell (1963) successfully implanted electrodes into the pelvic floor musculature and used electrical stimulation to treat stress incontinence (Caldwell et al 1968). Certainly stress incontinence can be improved by external direct stimulation of the efferent nerve supply to the pelvic floor and urethral sphincter. This requires an intact nerve supply to these muscular structures, perhaps explaining the limited success of electrical nerve stimulation in treating this condition. This remains a treatment to be used in conjunction with pelvic floor training and surgical procedures, e.g. colposuspension.

The use of the early implanted electrodes was limited by equipment failure and sepsis. New techniques have been developed, in conjunction with technological advances, using electrical stimulation to treat a variety of lower urinary tract conditions; no single method has yet emerged as superior to all others. Significant technical advances have been achieved with miniaturization and better biocompatability.

There is no broad consensus over the optimal site or parameters of stimulation, though the 3rd sacral nerve root is generally favoured in chronic electrical stimulation. SARS uses a book of electrodes to stimulate all or a selected group of nerve roots.

There are two theories as to how electrical stimulation may modulate lower urinary tract function. The first is based on work using SARS in patients with a neuropathy due to suprasacral lesions of the spinal column. Tanagho espoused stimulation of the sacral nerve roots innervating the urethral sphincter postulating that this had a direct effect on the striated urinary sphincter and resulted in reflex inhibition of detrusor activity (Tanagho 1993). An alternative concept is based on the presence of the local spinal reflexes some of whose afferent peripheral nerves enter the sacral spinal cord via the sacral roots, which do not necessarily involve the urethra, but when stimulated can still inhibit detrusor activity. The exact pathway whereby electrical stimulation alters lower urinary tract function remains obscure but may become clearer with further advances in our understanding of neuroanatomy and neurophysiology.

It is important to understand the underlying anatomical and physiological principles of action of the different methods of implanted nerve stimulators.

ANATOMY AND PHYSIOLOGY

Somatic innervation

The sacral plexus provides a somatic innervation to the pelvic floor via the pudendal nerve. This nerve is derived from the 2nd to 4th anterior sacral nerve roots (S2–S4). The major contributions to this nerve are from S2 and S3. Efferent nerve fibres originate from the nucleus of Onufrowicz (Onuf's nucleus) in the anterior horn of S2 to S4 (Onufrowicz 1899, Blaivas 1982) while the afferent fibres enter the corresponding dorsal roots to terminate in several layers of the sacral dorsal horn, from whence ascending tracts originate. Some afferent fibres project to Onuf's nucleus (Blaivas 1985), forming a local reflex loop. Onuf's nucleus also receives nerves from descending spinal tracts originating mainly in the pons.

The pudendal nerve re-enters the pelvis via the lesser sciatic foramen and runs along the underside of the pelvic floor (Fig. 43.4), giving branches to the dorsal nerve of the penis/clitoris, levator ani, external anal sphincter, perineal muscles, rhabdosphincter of the external urethral sphincter (Tanagho et al 1969; Bradley 1978; de Araujo et al 1982) and receiving sensory branches (Jünemann et al 1988). The pudendal nerve is not the only somatic nerve supply; a number of direct unnamed branches arise from the sacral roots before the pudendal nerve is formed, running close to the pelvic plexus to innervate the levator ani, external anal sphincter and rhabdosphincter of the urethra (Matzel et al 1990; Zvara et al 1994).

The sacral nerve roots S2 and S3 also contribute to the sciatic nerves and cutaneous nerves of the perineum. S2 innervates some of the lateral hip rotators, biceps femoris, muscles of the calf and some intrinsic foot muscles while S3 usually only supplies intrinsic foot muscles (especially those producing plantar-flexion of the hallux) (Williams et al 1989).

Parasympathetic innervation

The parasympathetic supply to the lower urinary tract originates from the intermediolateral column of grey matter (IMLC) at the level of S2 to S4 (Sheehan 1941). Branches arise from the corresponding roots as they emerge from the sacral foramina, to form the pelvic nerves and pelvic plexus on the deep surface of the sacrum and levator ani (Mitchell 1953; Elbadawi 1982) and supply the detrusor muscle via ganglia which occur throughout the course of the efferent parasympathetic pathways, including within the detrusor muscle itself (Fig. 43.4). Parasympathetic afferents project to the IMLC, so providing feedback to the efferent parasympathetics, as well as synapsing with second order neurones that ascend to the higher centres (Morgan et al 1981).

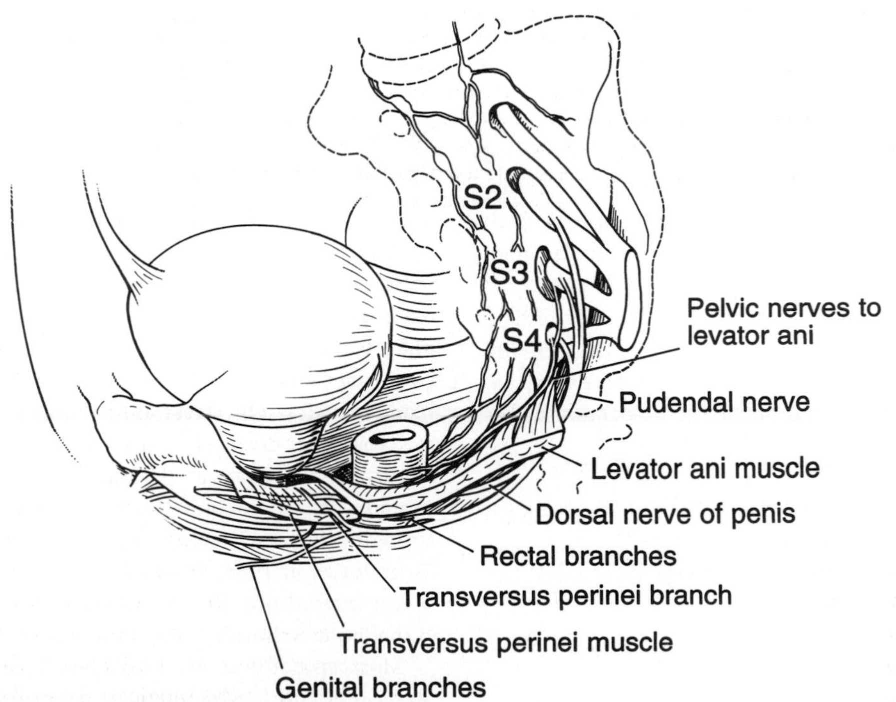

Fig. 43.4 Innervation of the lower urinary tract and pelvic floor.

Parasympathetic and somatic afferent nerves synapse in similar regions at the level of the sacral spinal cord (Tanagho et al 1982; McKenna & Nadelhaft 1985; Roppola et al 1985).

Sympathetic innervation

Sympathetic nerves also contribute to the plexuses within the pelvis; after having emerged from the T10 to L2 segments they pass through the sympathetic chain to the superior hypogastric plexus, then via hypogastric nerves to the inferior hypogastric plexus and combine with parasympathetic nerve fibres within the pelvis (Chai & Steers 1996). A few sympathetic fibres pass directly to organs or blood vessels. Many autonomic fibres synapse within the plexuses, from which postganglionic fibres continue, whilst others pass directly to ganglia in the detrusor wall itself. Sympathetic afferents may detect deep pain at the T10–L2 level (Habler et al 1990). Interconnections between the sympathetic and parasympathetic nervous system occur on every level and there are also short neurones within the ganglia (Elbadawi & Schenk 1968, 1971, deGroat & Saum 1976) all of which potentially act as modulators of impulses passing through the postganglionic nerves.

From the above description it is clear that extensive interconnections exist between somatic and autonomic nerves, both within the autonomic nervous system and between motor and sensory nerves. This arrangement permits extensive and complex reflex arcs involved in both urine storage and micturition which are also controlled by descending pathways from the higher centres of the central nervous system. These interconnections and reflex arcs continue to be investigated and ultimately may be understood to such a degree that the precise pathways may be identified and electrical stimulation applied with greater precision to modulate lower urinary tract function.

Currently a major limiting factor is the lack of data available in the human. The majority of the existing literature is based on animal studies, with extrapolation to the human, with all of the associated drawbacks and limitations.

ELECTRICAL STIMULATION OF NERVES

Stimulation of excitable tissues, such as nerves, depends on a number of factors:

1 The excitability of the nerve
2 Strength of the stimulus at the tissue
3 The form of electrical stimulus used.

Large, myelinated fibres are easiest to stimulate with an electrical pulse compared to small, unmyelinated fibres.

The strength of the electrical stimulus necessary at nerves is dictated by the level of current density at the nerve. Too high a current density will damage the nerve. The current density is determined by: the distance from the electrode to the nerve (inverse square law), the distance between the cathode and anode and the size of the electrode. Furthermore, the available energy is limited by battery life.

The most appropriate electrical stimulus is an alternating current. This will stimulate the nerve every time the polarity is altered and has the effect of giving the nerve a pulsed stimulus. The parameters that can be altered are the frequency, pulse width and pulse shape (most commonly a square wave). A pulse width of less than 30 μs cannot be compensated for by a higher current and a pulse width of greater than 500 μs cannot compensate for an inadequate current (Gleason 1991). These parameters therefore apply limits to the available pulse widths. As a general rule, shorter pulse widths achieve greater differential thresholds between the different nerve fibres and hence a more selective stimulus (Grill & Mortimer 1996). This has practical implications since it is usually more desirable to stimulate large, myelinated, sensory or motor nerve fibres rather than the smaller pain fibres.

DIRECT INTRADURAL NERVE ROOT STIMULATION

This method of electrical stimulation has been used in the management of voiding dysfunction in the neuropathic bladder. Four potential sites of stimulation exist where neurostimulation can be applied to stimulate voiding: the conus medullaris, the sacral anterior roots, the pelvic nerves and directly to the bladder wall itself. Developments have resulted, over the last five decades, with SARS being the most extensively investigated and showing the most promise. The principal work was carried out in the United Kingdom using an intradural technique (Brindley et al 1986, 1990) with further development as an extradural stimulator in the United States (Tanagho & Schmidt 1988; Tanagho et al 1989).

Most spinally injured patients have intact local sacral reflex arcs which can be selectively stimulated to emulate normal physiological function of the lower urinary tract. The principal aims of treatment are to restore urinary continence without the need for catheterization (Wyndaele 1992), by ensuring complete bladder emptying thereby preserving upper tract function in the long term. Improved bladder emptying reduces the risk of urinary tract infection. In addition this technique results in contraction of the gastrointestinal tract to enable better bowel evacuation and can also be used to enable sexual function. In a neurologically intact person the strong stimulus required would be extremely painful, precluding this procedure in those with intact pain pathways.

When SARS is used, simultaneous contraction of both the detrusor and urethral sphincter invariably occurs. Sphincterotomy should be approached cautiously in those considered for SARS as stress incontinence may result, especially in those whose bladder neck appears widely open on videocystometry (MacDonagh et al 1990). The Finetech-Brindley stimulator (Figs 43.5–6) makes use of the physiological finding that the urethral sphincter contracts and relaxes at a faster rate than the detrusor; the detrusor continues to contract after the stimulus has ended, whereas the sphincter relaxes, resulting in an episodic stream (Fig. 43.7).

Dorsal rhizotomy may be employed both to abolish uninhibited reflex bladder contractions, thereby improving bladder compliance and capacity, and to reduce reflex sphincter contraction during stimulation, thereby reducing detrusor-sphincter dyssynergia. Dorsal rhizotomy will reduce the risk of autonomic dysreflexia during SARS, a serious complication in tetraplegic patients, which can reduce the effectiveness of SARS. The procedure of deafferentation may however result in loss of reflex erectile, ejaculatory and defecatory function. Each individual has to be fully aware of the risks and benefits with a long-term view of their lifestyle taken, before dorsal rhizotomy is carried out.

The outcome of this procedure would appear to be good; 80–91% of patients are either satisfied and/or voiding successfully (Sauerwein 1990; Madersbacher & Fischer 1993, Koldewijn et al 1994a). The initial complication of cerebrospinal fluid leakage (Brindley et al 1986) has been largely overcome by placement of a sleeve where the cable leaves the dura and infection is a rare complication through the use of scrupulous technique and use of antibiotics both parenterally and coated on the implanted equipment. This technique does, however, require specialized neurosurgical experience.

Direct nerve stimulation continues to develop with improvements in miniaturization and the possible development of implants that may incorporate neuromodulation instead of dorsal rhizotomy. A significant improvement in quality of life can be gained by the select group of spinal injured patients through its use.

NEUROMODULATION

From their work into extradural sacral anterior root stimulation, Tanagho and Schmidt developed the first sacral neuromodulation implant which was used in

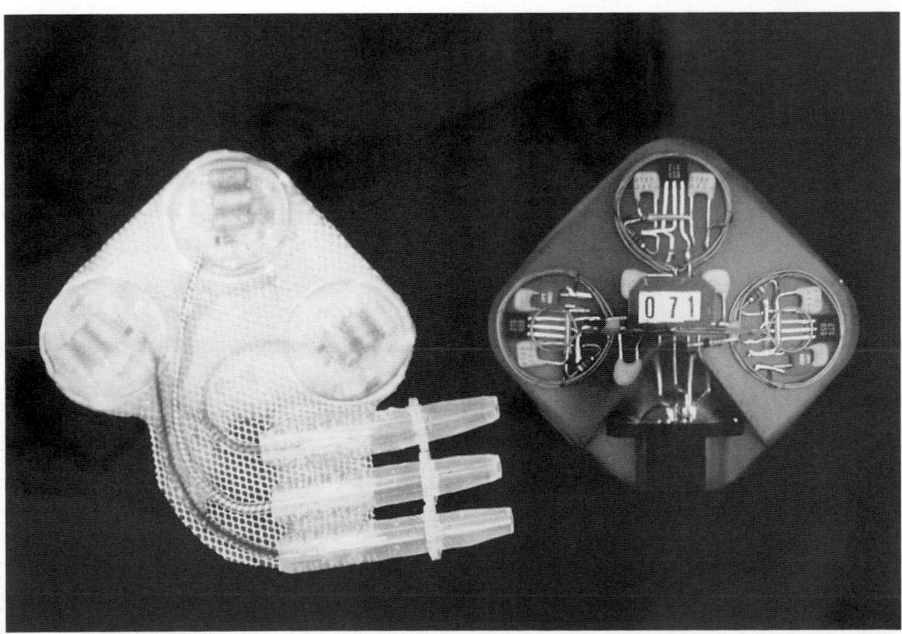

Fig. 43.5 Sacral anterior root stimulator: implanted coils that stimulate a book of electrodes (not shown) surrounding intradural sacral nerves.

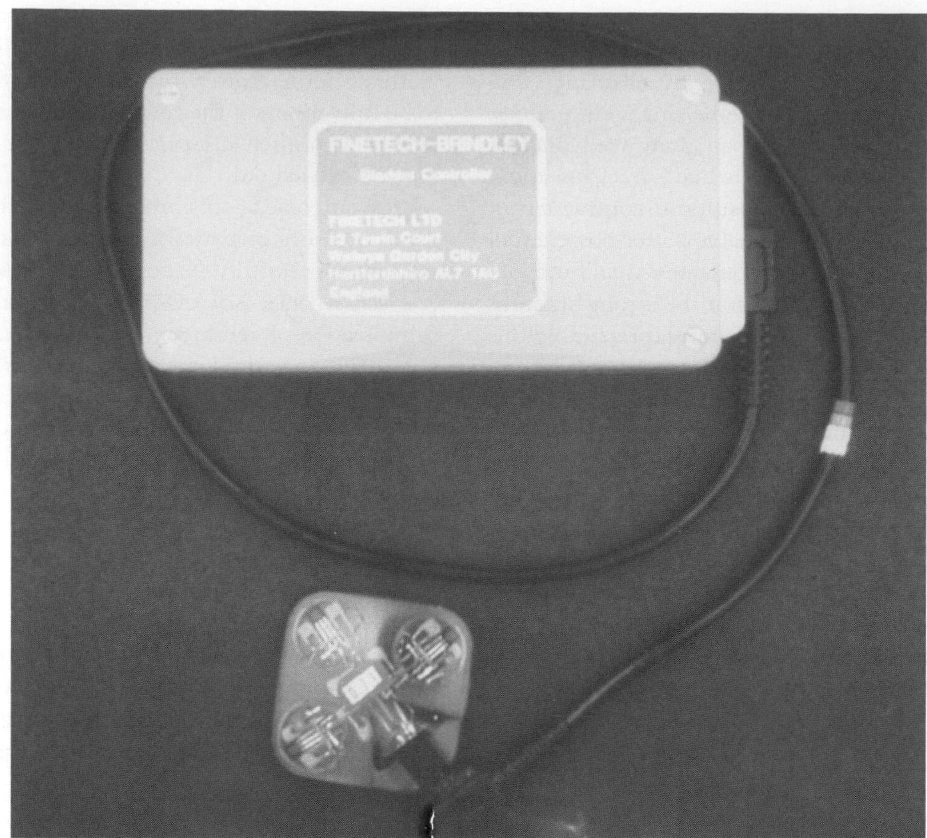

Fig. 43.6 Sacral anterior root stimulator: Finetech–Brindley device.

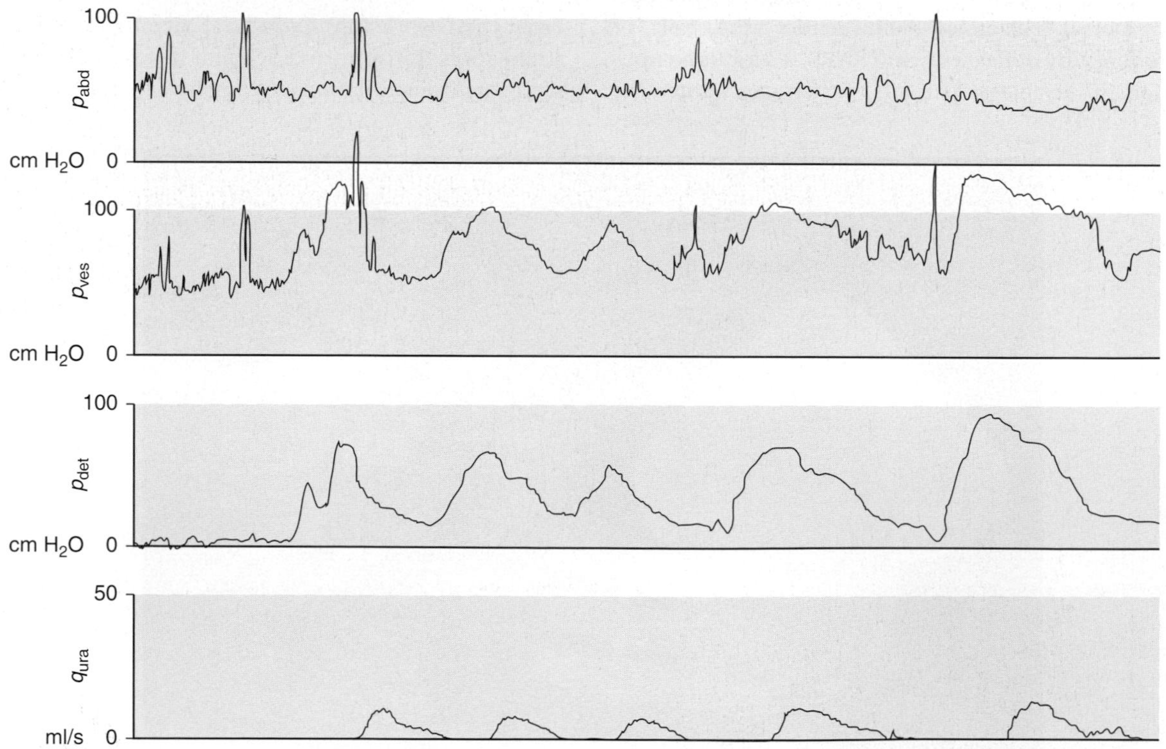

Fig. 43.7 Urodynamic print out of a patient voiding using sacral anterior root stimulation (SARS). Note 'saw-tooth' of the flow rate (Qura) each time the urethral sphincter relaxes.

1981 (Schmidt 1986). Further refinements have permitted the use of this implant in a number of urological conditions. Stimulation of sacral nerves as they emerge from the anterior surface of the sacrum, the final common pathway that contains all the afferent and efferent nerves of pelvic target organs, will potentially modulate lower urinary tract physiology. A test procedure performed as an outpatient under local anaesthetic, peripheral nerve evaluation (PNE), assesses neural integrity and the temporary response to neuromodulation using a temporary electrode. A significant improvement in urinary symptoms indicates that permanent stimulation may achieve the same result. Furthermore, an unsuccessful test is not deleterious to the underlying condition. A constant stimulus is required as the lower urinary tract condition being treated will usually return once the electrical stimulus is removed. An implanted unit provides a constant stimulus to modulate continuously the lower urinary tract, without hindrance to daily activity.

Peripheral nerve evaluation (PNE) (Fig. 43.8)

Using the landmarks of the sacrum and pelvis, an insulated needle electrode is inserted into the 3rd sacral foramen (S3) under local anaesthetic, aiming to place its conducting tip adjacent to the anterior 3rd sacral root. The sacral root is able to move within the foramen and by correct angulation of the inserted needle there is minimal risk of damage to the nerve. To date there are no reports of nerve damage or complications arising from the perforation of pelvic organs. The needle is stimulated at a set frequency (10 Hz) and pulse width (200 ms) while the voltage is gradually increased until the somatic response of a 'bellows contraction' of the levator ani and sometimes ipsilateral hallux plantar-flexion are observed and the patient feels a tightening sensation in the anal region. Stimulation of the 2nd sacral root (S2) leads to lateral hip rotation and ankle dorsiflexion and may cause inconvenient leg movement.

Having established the optimum S3 stimulus, the outer needle is used to place the temporary electrode and the needle withdrawn. The external stimulator used for acute stimulation is attached to the temporary electrode and a period of stimulation of at least 72 hours commenced. The patient adjusts the voltage to maintain the maximum tolerable sensation at all times. PNE is considered successful when symptoms improve by 50% and return to pre-test levels once the electrode is removed (to ensure there is not a

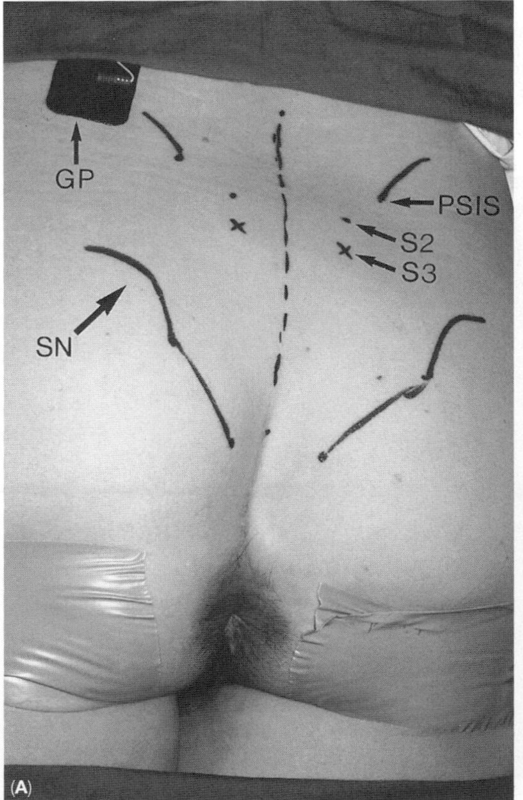

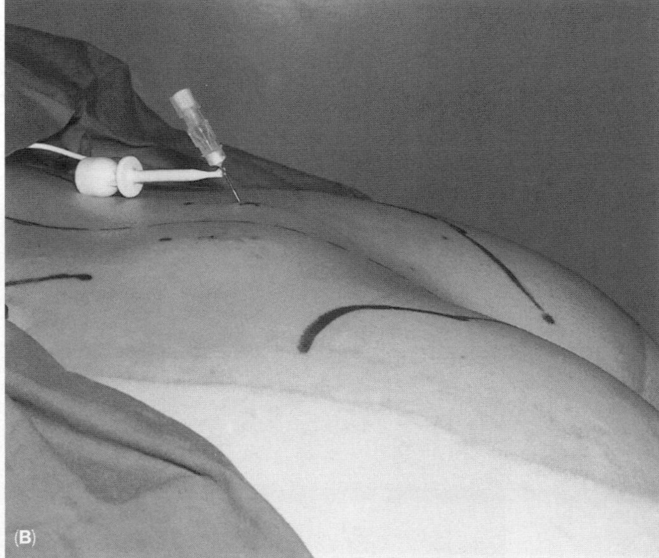

Fig. 43.8 (**A**) Peripheral nerve evaluation. GP, grounding pad; PSIS, posterior superior iliac spine; S2, 2nd sacral foramen; S3, 3rd sacral foramen. (**B**) Lateral view. Stimulating electrode at 70° to the sacral plane and entering the 3rd sacral foramen.

spontaneous, coincidental resolution of the underlying condition).

Permanent neuromodulation implant (Fig. 43.9)

A permanent electrode is placed in the foramen via a small vertical incision over the sacrum and fixed to the periosteum. The lead is tunnelled subcutaneously to the stimulator which is placed in a subcutaneous pocket over the left abdomen. The stimulator is programmed the next day and switched on. Adjustment is required over the next 2–3 months as tissues heal and electrical impedance changes. The patient can alter the voltage or switch the stimulator on/off with a hand-held device. The pulse generator lasts between 3 and 5 years and can be replaced by a simple operation. The main complication has been loss of stimulus due to lead fracture, electrode migration and loss of nerve electrode coupling.

Clinical studies

Since the initial work by Tanagho and Schmidt, a number of conditions refractory to conservative therapy have been treated with neuromodulation, with varying degrees of success. These include motor and sensory detrusor dysfunction, chronic retention in women and chronic pelvic pain, but treatment of detrusor instability has the greatest application. A greater than 90% improvement in symptoms is considered to indicate a cure while greater than 50% indicates significant improvement. The exact method of subjective assessment is sometimes unclear, making comparisons of published data difficult. Our own practice when treating detrusor dysfunction is to consider the average voided volume from the voiding diary (functional voiding capacity) first, in conjunction with urgency and leakage. The initial work by Schmidt studied patients with urge incontinence and 'dysfunctional voiding syndromes' over a 5-year period comparing his initial experience with sacral root stimulation and pudendal nerve stimulation. The best results for sacral foramen stimulation occurred with urge incontinence, where 75% of patients were treated successfully while those with voiding dysfunction had a successful outcome in 65% of men and 67% of women (Schmidt 1988a). Further studies of patients with urge incontinence have shown similar results (Thon et al 1991; Dijkema et al 1993) while a multinational study of 140 patients had 45% of patients with urge incontinence who were dry after implantation and a further 30% who had greater than 50% improvement (Janknegt et al 1997). However our experience has found that the success achieved, using the functional voiding capacity and not just frequency, is only 40% (Bryan et al 1998).

Urodynamic assessment of patients undergoing neuromodulation has found some patients to be stable but generally the improvement in symptoms and urodynamic changes have proved inconsistent. Urodynamic data demonstrates increased cystometric capacity, bladder volumes at which subjective desires to void occur and a higher volume at which the first unstable contraction occurred. The maximum pres-

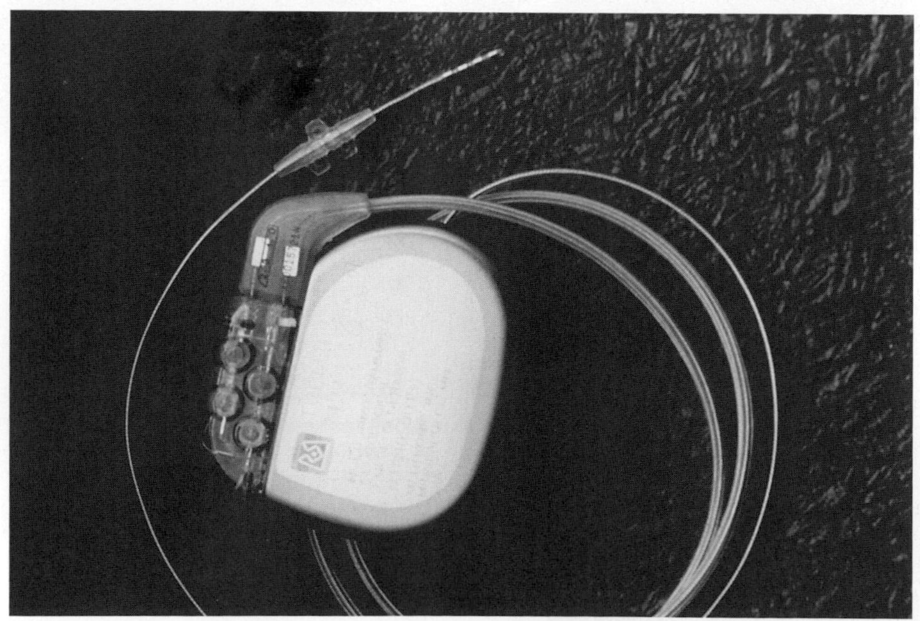

Fig. 43.9 Permanent implant for neuromodulation.

sure of unstable contractions was lowered by neuromodulation (Bosch & Groen 1995; Bosch et al 1996; Hasan et al 1996). Subjective outcomes correlate with conventional urodynamics and the more physiological ambulatory urodynamics in our own (Bryan et al 1998) and parallel studies (Bosch & Groen 1998).

Other lower urinary tract conditions have also been treated by neuromodulation but with less success. Detrusor hyperreflexia secondary to neurogenic bladder dysfunction has proved amenable to neuromodulation in both adults and children (Tanagho 1992; Hohenfellner et al 1994; Koldewijn et al 1994a; Bosch & Groen 1996). This may prove to be of more benefit when used in conjunction with sacral anterior root stimulation. Sensory disorders of the lower urinary tract (urge/frequency and pelvic pain) are less amenable to neuromodulation with 40–50% showing subjective improvement (Schmidt 1988b; Schmidt & Kaula 1996). Those who respond to PNE are likely to improve with permanent implantation (Schmidt et al 1997). Patients with interstitial cystitis show a generally poor response with under 30% subjectively improving on neuromodulation (Koldewijn et al 1994).

Long-term data on implanted devices are limited but nevertheless encouraging. Complications are rare and mainly limited to lead fracture, displacement or failure of the implant itself. Infection is rare, as long as standard precautions for insertion of a foreign body are used, and it is only occasionally necessary to move the electrode because of chronic pain (Grünewald et al 1996; Weil et al 1996; Shaker & Hassouna 1997).

CONCLUSION

Currently nerve stimulation via implants is an expensive therapy which suits only a proportion of patients. Once implanted, patients require careful long-term follow-up. Where appropriate, the Finetech-Brindley device has been developed to effect normal voiding in spinal injured patients. Neuromodulation had initial success but clearly requires further investigation in order to:

- Develop the technology and understand its mode of action further
- Improve the technique of PNE so that the minimum number of tests are required
- Develop a non-invasive technique (such as functional magnetic stimulation) to acutely suppress unstable detrusor contractions and thereby identify patients suitable for neuromodulation.

REFERENCES

Abel J, Ottesen B, Fischer-Rasmussen W, Lose G 1996 Maximal electrical stimulation of the pelvic floor in the treatment of urge incontinence: a placebo controlled study. Neurourology and Urodynamics 15: 283–284

Alexander S, Rowan O 1968 An electric pessary for stress incontinence. Lancet i: 728

Association for the Advancement of Medical Instrumentation 1980 Standard for transcutaneous electrical nerve stimulators. 1901 N Et Myer Or, Suite 602, Arlington, VA 22209

Blaivas J 1982 The neurophysiology of micturition: a clinical study of 550 patients. Journal of Urology 127: 958–963

Blaivas J 1985 Pathophysiology of lower urinary tract dysfunction. Clinics in Obstetrics and Gynaecology 12: 285–309

Bo K, Talseth T, 'Holme I 1999 Single blind, randomised controlled trial of pelvic floor exercises, electrical stimulation, vaginal cones, and no treatment in management of genuine stress incontinence in women. British Medical Journal 318: 487–493

Boone T B, Roehrborn C, Hurt G 1992 Transurethral intravesical electrotherapy for neurogenic bladder dysfunction in children with myelodysplasia: a prospective randomized clinical trial. Journal of Urology 148: 550–554

Bosch J L H R, Groen J 1995a Effects of sacral segmental nerve stimulation on urethral resistance and bladder contractility: how does neuromodulation work in urge incontinence patients? Neurourology and Urodynamics 14(5): 502

Bosch J L H R, Groen J 1995b Sacral(S3) segmental nerve stimulation as a treatment for urge incontinence in patients with detrusor instability: results of chronic electrical stimulation using a plantable neural prosthesis. Journal of Urology 154: 504–507

Bosch R, Groen J 1998 Unilateral sacral (S3) segmental nerve stimulation (neuromodulation) in patients with urge incontinence due to detrusor instability or hyperreflexia: correlation between symptomatic and urodynamic results. European Urology 33(suppl. 1): 61

Bosch J, Groen J 1996 Treatment of refractory urge urinary incontinence with sacral spinal nerve stimulation in multiple sclerosis patients. Lancet 348: 717–719

Bosch R, Groen J, Essink-Bot M 1996 Sacral segmental (S3) nerve stimulation as a treatment for urge incontinence due to detrusor instability: quality of life analysis and cost-effectiveness. Journal of Urology 155: 594a

Bradley W 1978 Innervation of the male urinary bladder. Urological Clinics of North America 5: 279–293

Brindley G S, Polkey C E, Rushton D N 1990 Sacral anterior root stimulation for bladder control in paraplegia. Paraplegia 20: 365–381

Brindley G S, Polkey C E, Rushton D N, Cardozo L 1986 Sacral anterior root stimulators for bladder control in paraplegia: the first 50 cases. Journal of Neurology, Neurosurgery and Psychiatry 49: 1104–1114

Brubaker L, Benson J T, Bent A, Clark A 1996 Transvaginal electrical stimulation is effective for treatment of detrusor overactivity. Neurourology and Urodynamics 15: 282–283

Bryan N, Byrne L, Tophill P, Chapple C 1998 Objective evidence of the effect of sacral neuromodulation. European Urology 33(supplement 1): 61

Caldwell K P 1963 The electrical control of sphincter incompetence. Lancet i: 174–175

Caldwell K P, Cook P J, Flack F C, James E D 1968 Stress incontinence in females:report on 31 cases treated by electrical implant. Journal of Obstetrics and Gynaecology of the British Commonwealth 75: 777–780

Chai T, Steers W 1996 Neurophysiology of micturition and continence. Urologic Clinics of North America 23(2): 221–236

De Araujo C, Schmidt R, Tanagho E 1982 Neural pathways to the lower urinary tract identified by retrograde axonal transport of horseradish peroxidase. Urology 19: 290–295

De Groat W C, Ryall R W 1969 Reflexes to sacral parasympathetic neurones concerned with micturition in the cat. Journal of Physiology (London) 200: 87–109

De Groat W, Saum W 1976 Synaptic transmission in parasympathetic ganglia in the urinary bladder of the cat. Journal of Physiology 256: 137–158

Del Popolo G, Lombardi G, Doggweiler R, De Scisciolo G, Tosto A 1996 Early experience with intravesical electrical stimulation in the rehabilitation of neurological bladder and non-neurological detrusor impairment. Urodinamica 6(3): 203–205

De Soldenhoff R, McDonnel H 1969 New devices for control of female urinary incontinence. British Medical Journal 4: 230

Dijkema H E, Weil E H J, Mijs P T, Janknegt R A 1993 Neuromodulation of sacral nerves for incontinence and voiding dysfunction. European Urology 24: 72–76

Doyle T P, Edwards L E, Harrison N W, Malvern J, Stanton S L 1974 Treatment of urinary incontinence by external stimulating devices. Urologia Internationalis 29: 450–457

Dray A, Metsch R 1984 Opioid receptors and inhibition of urinary bladder motility in vivo. Neuroscience Letters 47: 81–84

Ebner A, Jiang C, Lindström S 1992 Intravesical electrical stimulation – an experimental analysis of the mechanism of action. Journal of Urology 148: 920–924

Edwards L E, Malvern J 1972 Electronic control of incontinence: a critical review of the present situation. British Journal of Urology 44: 467–472

Elbadawi A 1982 Neuromorphological basis of vesicourethral function: I. Histochemistry, ultrastructure, and function of intrinsic nerves of the bladder and urethra. Neurourology and Urodynamics 1: 3–50

Elbadawi A, Schenk E 1968 A new theory in the innervation of bladder musculature. Part I. Morphology of the intrinsic vsical innervation apparatus. Journal of Urology 99: 585–587

Elbadawi A, Schenk E 1971 A new theory in the innervation of bladder musculature. Part 3. Postganglionic synapses in ureterovesico-urethral autonomic pathways. Journal of Urology 105: 372–74

Eriksen B C, Bergmann S, Mjølnerrød 1987 Effect of anal electrostimulation with the 'incontak' device in women with urinary incontinence. British Journal of Obstetrics and Gynecology 94: 147–156

Eriksen B C, Bergmann S, Eik-Nes S H 1989 Maximal electrostimulation of the pelvic floor in female idiopathic detrusor instability and urge incontinence. Neurourology and Urodynamics 8: 219–230

Erlandson B-E, Fall M, Carlsson C-A 1978 The effect of intravaginal electrical stimulation on the feline urethra and urinary bladder. Electrical parameters. Scandinavian Journal of Urology and Nephrology 44 (suppl I): 5–18

Fall M, Madersbacher H 1994 Peripheral electrical stimulation. In: Mundy AR, Stephenson T P, Wein A J (Eds) Urodynamics. Principles, practice and application, 2nd edn. Churchill Livingstone, Edinburgh, pp 495–520

Fall M, Erlandson B-E, Carlsson C-A, Lindstrom S A 1977a The effect of intravaginal electrical stimulation on the feline urethra and urinary bladder. Neuronal mechanisms. Scandinavian Journal of Urology and Nephrology, suppl. 44: 19–30

Fall M, Erlandson B-E, Sundin T, Waagstein F 1977b The effect of intravaginal electrical stimulation. Clinical experiments on bladder inhibition. Scandinavian Journal of Urology and Nephrology, suppl. 44: 41–48

Fall M, Erlandson B-E, Nilson A E, Sundin T 1977c Long-term intravaginal electrical stimulation in urge and stress incontinence. Scandinavian Journal of Urology and Nephrology, suppl. 44: 55–63

Gleason C A 1991 Electrophysiological fundamentals of neurostimulation. World Journal of Urology 9: 110–113

Godec C, Cass A 1978 Acute electrical stimulation for urinary incontinence. Urology 12: 340–342

Godec C, Cass A S, Ayala G F 1975 Bladder inhibition with functional electrical stimulation. Urology 6: 663–666

Godec C, Cass A S, Ayala G F 1976 Electrical stimulation for incontinence: technique, selection and results. Urology 7: 388–397

Grill W M, Mortimer J T 1996 The effect of stimulus pulse duration on selectivity of neural stimulation. IHEE Transactions on Biomedical Engineering 43(2): 161–166

Grünewald V, Höfner K, Becker A, Krah K, Gonnermann O, Jonas U 1996 Clinical results and complications of chronic sacral neuromodulation after four years of application. International Continence Society. Athens, 116

Habler H, Janig W, Kolzenburg M 1990 Activation of unmyelinated afferent fibres by mechanical stimuli and inflammation of the urinary bladder in the cat. Journal of Physiology (London) 425: 545–562

Harrison N W, Paterson P J 1970 Urinary incontinence in women treated by an electronic pessary. British Journal of Urology 42: 481–485

Hasan S T, Robson W A, Pridie A K, Neal D E 1996 Transcutaneous electrical nerve stimulation and temporary S3 neuromodulation in idiopathic detrusor instability. Journal of Urology 155: 2005–2011

Hohenfellner M, Schultz-Lampel D, Spranger C, Fleig P, Weinhold D, Thüroff J W 1994 Sacral neuromodulation for treatment of neurogenic bladder dysfunction. Journal of Urology 152: 511A

Hopkinson B R, Lightwood R 1967 Electrical treatment of incontinence. British Journal of Surgery 54: 802–805

Janež J, Plevnik S, Šuhel P 1979 Urethral and bladder responses to anal electrical stimulation. Journal of Urology 122: 192–194

Janež J, Plevnik S, Korošec L, Stanovnik L, Vrtačnik P 1981 Changes in detrusor receptor activity after electric pelvic floor stimulation. Proceedings of the International Continence Society, Lund, pp 22–23

Janknegt R, van Kerrebroeck P, Nijeholt A et al 1997 Sacral nerve modulation for urge incontinence: a multinational, multicenter randomized study. Journal of Urology 157(4 (supplement)): 317

Jiang C-H, Lindström S 1996 Effect of intravesical electrical stimulation on bladder mechanoreceptor sensitivity. 26th Annual Meeting of the International Continence Society, 27–30 August, Athens, Abstracts: 55

Jiang C-H, Lindström S, Mazières L 1991 Segmental inhibitory control of ascending sensory information from bladder mechanoreceptors in cat. Proceedings of the International Continence Society, Hanover. Neurourology and Urodynamics 10(4): 286–288

Jünemann Ch-P, Lue T F, Schmidt R A, Tanagho E 1988 Clinical significance of sacral and pudendal nerve anatomy. Journal of Urology 139: 74–80

Katona F, Eckstein H B 1974 Treatment of neuropathic bladder by transurethral electrical stimulation. Lancet 27: 780

Koldewijn E L, Rosier P F W M, Meuleman E J H, Koster A M, Debruyne F M J, van Kerrebroeck P 1994a Predictors of success with neuromodulation in lower urinary tract dysfunction: results of trial stimulation in 100 patients. Journal of Urology 151: 2071–2075

Koldewijn E L, van Kerrebroeck P, Rosier P F W M, Wijkstra H, Debruyne F M J 1994b Bladder compliance after posterior sacral root rhizotomies and anterior sacral root stimulation. Journal of Urology 151: 955–960

Kralj B, Plevnik S, Janko M, Vrtačnik P 1977 Urge incontinence and maximal electrical stimulation. Proceedings of the 7th Annual Meeting of the International Continence Society, Portorož, pp 16–17

Laycock J, Green R J 1988 Interferential therapy in the treatment of incontinence. Physiotherapy 74: 161–168

Laycock J, Plevnik S, Senn E 1994 Electrical stimulation. In: Schüssler B, Laycock J, Norton P, Stanton S (eds) Pelvic Floor Re-education: principles and practice. Springer-Verlag, London, pp 143–153

Lindström S, Sudsuang R 1989 Functionally specific bladder reflexes from pelvic and pudendal nerve branches: an experimental study in the cat. Neurourology and Urodynamics 8: 392–393

Lindström S, Fall M, Carlsson C-A, Erlandson B-E 1983 The neurophysiological basis of bladder inhibition in response to intravaginal electrical stimulation. Journal of Urology 129: 405–410

Luber M K, Wolde-Tsadik G 1997 Efficacy of functional electrical stimulation in treating genuine stress incontinence: a randomized clinical trial. Neurourology and Urodynamics 16: 543–551

MacDonagh R P, Forster D, Thomas D G 1990 Urinary continence in spinal injury patients following complete sacral posterior rhizotomy. British Journal of Urology 66: 618–622

Madersbacher H 1992 Intravesical electrical stimulation for the rehabilitation of the neuropathic bladder. Paraplegia 28: 349–352

Madersbacher H, Fischer J 1993 Anterior sacral root stimulation and posterior sacral root rhizotomy. Aktuelle Urologie 24: 32–35

Madersbacher H, Hetzel H, Gottinger F, Ebner A 1987 Rehabilitation of micturition in adults with incomplete spinal cord lesions by intravesical electrotherapy. Neurourology and Urodynamics 8: 366

Madersbacher H, Kiss G, Kölle D, Mair D 1995 Intravesikale Elektrostimulation zur Rehabilitation von Blasenfunktionsstörungen nach gynäkologischen Operationen. Urologe A 34 (suppl. 1): S46

Matzel K, Schmidt R, Tanagho E 1990 Neuroanatomy of the striated muscular anal continence mechanism; implications for the use of neurostimulation. Diseases of the Colon and Rectum 33: 666–673

McGuire E, Shi-Chun Z, Horwinski R, Lytton B 1983 Treatment of motor and sensory detrusor instability by electrical stimulation. Journal of Urology 129: 78–79

McKenna K, Nadelhaft I 1985 The organisation of the pudendal nerve in the male and female cat. Journal of Comparative Neurology 248: 532–549

Mitchell G 1953 Anatomy of the autonomic nervous system. Livingstone, Edinburgh

Moore T, Schofield P F 1967 Treatment of stress incontinence by maximal perineal electrical stimulation. British Medical Journal 3: 150–151

Morgan C, Nadelhaft I, deGroat W 1981 The distribution of visceral primary afferents from the pelvic nerve within Lissauer's tract and the spinal gray matter and its relationship to the sacralparasympathetic nucleus. Journal of Comparative Neurology 201: 415–440

Mortimer J T 1981 Motor prosthesis. In: Brooks V B (ed) Handbook of Physiology. Williams and Wilkins, Baltimore, pp 155–187

Olah K S, Bridges N, Denning J, Farrar D J 1990 The conservative management of patients with symptoms of stress incontinence: a randomized, prospective study comparing weighted vaginal cones and interferential therapy. American Journal of Obstetrics and Gynecology 162: 87–92

Onufrowicz B 1899 Notes on the arrangement and function of the cell groups in the sacral region of the spinal cord. Journal of Nervous and Mental Disease 26: 498–504

Peattie A B, Plevnik S, Stanton S L 1988 Vaginal cones: a conservative method of treating genuine stress incontinence. British Journal of Obstetrics and Gynaecology 95: 1049–1053

Plevnik S 1985 New method for testing and strengthening of pelvic floor muscles. In: Proceedings of the 15th Annual Meeting of the International Continence Society, London, pp 267–268

Plevnik S, Janež J 1979 Maximal electrical stimulation for urinary incontinence. Urology 14: 638–645

Plevnik S, Šuhel P, Rakovec S, Kralj B 1977 Effects of functional electrical stimulation on the urethral closing muscles. Medical and Biological Engineering and Computing 15: 155–167

Plevnik S, Homan G, Vrtačnik P 1984 Short-term maximal electrical stimulation for urinary retention. Urology 24: 521–523

Plevnik S, Janež J, Vrtačnik P, Tršinar B, Vodušek D B 1986a Short-term electric stimulation: home treatment for urinary incontinence. World Journal of Urology 4: 24–26

Plevnik S, Vodušek D B, Vrtačnik P, Janež J 1986b Optimization of the pulse duration for vaginal or anal electric stimulation for urinary incontinence. World Journal of Urology 4: 22–23

Plevnik S, Janež J, Vodušek D B 1991 Electrical stimulation. In: Krane R J, Siroky MB (eds) Clinical Neuro-urology. Little, Brown, Boston, pp 559–571

Primus G, Kramer G, Pummer K 1996 Restoration of micturition in patients with acontractile and hypocontractile detrusor by transurethral electrical bladder stimulation. Neurourology and Urodynamics 15: 489–497

Risi O, Blefari F, Milesi R, Rocchi B, Pino P 1996 Home intravesical electrostimulation in the treatment of non-neurological voiding dysfunctions. A preliminary report. Urodinamica 6(3): 201–203

Roppolo J, Nadelhaft I, de Groat W 1985 The organisation of pudendal motor neurons and primary afferent projections in the spinal cord of the rhesus monkey revealed by horseradish peroxidase. Journal of Comparative Neurology 234(475–487)

Rotembourg J L, Ghoneim M A, Fretin J, Susset J G 1976 Study on the efficiency of electric stimulation of the pelvic floor. Investigative Urology 13: 354–358

Salmons S, Vrbova G 1969 The influence of activity on some contractile characteristics of mammalian fast and slow muscle. Journal of Physiology 201: 535–549

Sand P K, Richardson D A, Staskin D R, Swift S E, Appel R A, Whitmore K E, Ostergard D R 1995 Pelvic floor electrical stimulation in the treatment of genuine stress incontinence: a multicenter, placebo-controlled trial. American Journal of Obstetrics and Gynecology 173/1: 72–79

Sauerwein D 1990 Surgical treatment of spastic bladder paralysis in paraplegic patients. Sacral deafferentation with implantation of a sacral anterior root stimulator [German]. Urologe 29: 196–203

Schiøtz H A 1994 One month maximal electrostimulation for genuine stress incontinence in women. Neurourology and Urodynamics 13: 43–50

Schmidt R A 1986 Advances in genitourinary neurostimulation. Neurosurgery 18: 1041–1044

Schmidt R A 1988a Applications of neurostimulation in urology. Neurourology and Urodynamics 7: 585–592

Schmidt R A 1988b Treatment of pelvic pain with neuroprosthesis. Journal of Urology 139(part 2): 277A

Schmidt R A, Kaula N 1996 Sacral nerve root stimulation screening efficacy in management of pelvic pain. Journal of Urology 155: 594A

Schmidt R A, Tanagho E A 1991 Clinical applications of neurostimulation. In: Krane R J, Siroky M B (eds) Clinical Neuro-urology, 2nd edn. Little Brown, Boston, pp 643–648

Schmidt R A, Gajewski J, Hassouna M, Chancellor M 1997 Management of refractory urge frequency syndromes using an implantable neuroprosthesis: a North American study. Journal of Urology 157(4 (supplement)): 317

Shaker H, Hassouna M 1997 Long term effects of neuromodulation on voiding behaviour in patients with chronic voiding dysfunction. Journal of Urology 157(4 (supplement)): 188

Sheehan D 1941 Spinal autonomic outflows in man and monkey. Journal of Comparative Neurology 45: 341–370

Sundin T, Carlsson C-A 1972 Reconstruction of several dorsal roots innervating the urinary bladder. An experimental study in cats. I. Studies on the normal afferent pathways in the pelvic and pudendal nerves. Scandinavian Journal of Urology and Nephrology 6: 176–184

Sundin T, Carlsson C-A, Kock N G 1974 Detrusor inhibition induced from mechanical stimulation of the anal region and from electrical stimulation of pudendal nerve afferents. Investigative Urology 11: 374–378

Šuhel P 1976 Adjustable nonimplantable electrical stimulators for correction of urinary incontinence. Urologia Internationalis 34: 115–123

Tanagho E 1992 Neuromodulation in the management of voiding dysfunction in children. Journal of Urology 148: 655–657

Tanagho E 1993 Concepts of neuromodulation. Neurourology and Urodynamics 12: 487–488

Tanagho E A, Schmidt R A 1988 Electrical stimulation in the clinical management of the neurogenic bladder. Journal of Urology 140: 1331–1339

Tanagho E, Meyers F, Smith D 1969 Urethral resistance: its components and implications II. Striated muscle component. Investigative Urology 7: 195–205

Tanagho E, Schmidt R A, de Araujo G C 1982 Urinary striated sphincter: what is the nerve supply? Urology 20(4): 415–417

Tanagho E A, Schmidt R A, Orvis B R 1989 Neural stimulation for the control of voiding dysfunction: a preliminary report in 22 patients with serious neuropathic voiding disorders. Journal of Urology 142: 340–345

Thon W F, Baskin L, Jonas U, Tanagho E, Schmidt R A 1991 Neuromodulation of voiding dysfunction and pelvic pain. World Journal of Urology 9: 138–141

Tršinar B, Kralj B 1996 Maximal electrical stimulation in children with unstable bladder and nocturnal enuresis and/or daytime incontinence: a controlled study. Neurourology and Urodynamics 15: 133–142

U S Department of Health and Human Services, Public Health Service, Agency for Health Care Policy and Research. Managing acute and chronic urinary incontinence. Quick reference guide for clinicians No. 2, 1996 update. Rockville, MD: AHCPR 96–0686

Vereecken R, Das J, Grisar P 1984 Electrical sphincter stimulation in the treatment of detrusor hyperreflexia of paraplegics. Neurourology and Urodynamics 3: 145–154

Vodušek D B 1990 Pudendal SEP and bulbocavernosus reflex in women. Electroencephalography and Clinical Neurophysiology 77: 134–136

Vodušek D B 1996 Evoked potential testing. Urological Clinics of North America 23: 427–446

Vodušek D B, Kralj B 1979 Change in sphincter EMG activity after strong electrical stimulation. In: Proceedings of the 9th Annual Meeting of the International Continence Society, Rome, pp 235–238

Vodušek D B, Janko M, Lokar J 1983 Direct reflex responses in perineal muscles on electrical stimulation. Journal of Neurology, Neurosurgery and Psychiatry 46: 67–71

Vodušek D B, Light J K, Libby J 1986 Detrusor inhibition induced by stimulation of pudendal nerve afferents. Neurourology and Urodynamics 5: 381–389

Vodušek D B, Plevnik S, Vrtačnik P, Janež J 1988 Detrusor inhibition on selective pudendal nerve stimulation in the perineum. Neurourology and Urodynamics 6: 389–393

Vrtačnik P, Plevnik S, Janež J 1985 Electric stimulator for short-term home treatment of urinary incontinence: assessment of fundamental requirements for output-stage design. In: Proceedings of the 15th Annual Meeting of the International Continence Society, London, pp 228–229

Weil E, Eerdmans P, Janknegt R 1996 5 year treatment of patients with severe voiding disorders, so called urological cripples, by neuromodulation. The facts. European Urology 31(supplement 1): 236

Williams P, Warwick R, Dyson M, Bannister L (eds) 1989 Gray's Anatomy, 37th edn. Churchill-Livingstone, London

Wise B G, Cardozo L D, Plevnik S, Kelleher C J, Abbott D 1993 A comparative study of oxybutynin and maximal electrical stimulation in the treatment of detrusor instability. In: Proceedings of the 23rd Annual Meeting of the International Continence Society, Rome, (Abstract) p. 236

Yamanishi T, Yasuda K, Hattori T, Suda S, Hosaka H 1996 Pelvic floor electrical stimulation in the treatment of stress incontinence: a placebo-controlled double-blind trial. Neurourology and Urodynamics 15: 397–398

Wyndaele J J 1992 Neurourology in spinal cord injured patients. Paraplegia 30: 50–53

Zoll P M, Linenthal A J 1964 External electrical stimulation of the heart. Annals of the New York Academy of Sciences 3: 932–937

Zvara P, Carrier S, Kour N-W, Tanagho E 1994 The detailed neuroanatomy of the human striated urethral sphincter. British Journal of Urology 74: 182–187

Bladder drainage

PAUL HILTON

INTRODUCTION

Catheterization of the bladder is employed in up to 20% of all patients in hospital (Stevens et al 1981) and approximately 1 in 2000 in the community (Kohler-Ockmore & Feneley 1996). It is the commonest cause of nosocomially acquired infection, accounting for at least 35% of such events in the USA (National Nosocomial Infections Study 1973), the United Kingdom (Report on the National Survey of Infection in Hospitals 1980, 1981) and elsewhere (Liedberg 1989). Catheter-associated infection is estimated to occur in approximately 1 in 40 hospital admissions (Thompson et al 1984), and it has considerable financial implications for health (Liedberg 1989; Givens & Wenzel 1980). It is perhaps the very familiarity which both medical and nursing staff feel they have with catheterization, which leads them all too often to neglect the basic principles underlying bladder drainage, and which may lead to unnecessary catheterizations, inappropriate timing of the procedure, and inadequate techniques (Jain et al 1995).

INDICATIONS

Within gynaecology

- Acute urinary retention
- Chronic urinary retention
- Pre- and peroperative use
- Postoperative use
- Bladder or urethral trauma
- Acute vulvovaginitis
- Intractable urinary incontinence
- Neurogenic bladder dysfunction
- For diagnostic purposes
- In the terminally ill

Within obstetrics

- At operative delivery
- To measure urine output

METHODS

The bladder may be drained either continuously via the urethra or a cystostomy incision, or intermittently via the urethra; the method used, and the type of catheter employed in any individual case, depends on the particular indication present. The following methods will be described:

1 Urethral
  (a) Single event
  (b) Continuous indwelling
  (c) Intermittent catheterization
2 Cystostomy
  (a) Open suprapubic cystostomy
  (b) Closed suprapubic stab
  (c) Vaginal cystostomy

URETHRAL CATHETERIZATION

Single event or 'in-out' urethral catheterization

This is most frequently performed prior to pelvic surgery or operative delivery, where catheterization is used diagnostically to measure the residual volume or during radiological or urodynamic investigation, or where the bladder is to be filled prior to the insertion of a suprapubic catheter.

Choice of catheter

It is a reasonable working rule in all aspects of bladder drainage always to use the narrowest, softest catheter that will serve the purpose (Blandy 1981); to this one might add that it should also be the shortest and the cheapest. The Nelaton or Jaques catheter with a tapered tip and one or more side-holes is most often used. The material is of little consequence in this situation in view of the short time of contact between catheter and urethra; however, a plastic or PVC construction is most usual, and a female length (20–25 cm) catheter of 8, 10 or at most 12 FG is perfectly adequate.

Continuous indwelling catheterization

A continuous indwelling urethral catheter may be indicated in any of the situations detailed above, although other modes of bladder drainage may be advantageous in specific situations; these are detailed where appropriate (see 'intermittent catheterization' and 'closed suprapubic stab cystostomy' in particular).

Choice of catheter

Once the decision to insert an indwelling catheter has been taken, the selection of the most appropriate instrument is crucial to its optimal functioning, as well as to the patient's comfort and wellbeing. The calibre, material and length of the catheter, as well as the balloon size, should be considered, and the temptation to accept the first catheter that comes to hand should be denied. The indication for catheterization itself, the quality of urine anticipated, and the proposed duration of drainage should all be borne in mind.

Catheter calibre As noted above, one should always select the narrowest catheter that will serve the desired function. If this is to drain heavily bloodstained urine a catheter of 16–18 FG may be necessary; if, however, it is purely for bladder emptying, then a calibre 12 or at most 14 FG will suffice in the short term. For longer-term bladder drainage, the problem of encrustation becomes significant, but even here catheters of greater than 16 FG can rarely be justified. Many of the problems associated with continuous urethral catheterization are a result of catheters of excessive diameter.

Catheter material In the past, catheters have been made from plastic (PVC or polyurethane) or latex. Both have been prone to encrustation with prolonged use (see Fig. 44.1), and the cytotoxicity of latex in particular causes concern (Ruutu et al 1985). Attempts have been made to reduce these problems, and hence improve the duration of satisfactory drainage, by coating latex catheters with a variety of materials, including PTFE ('Teflon') and silicone. The coating reduces the available internal diameter (see Fig. 44.2), and flow characteristics are compromised, even though encrustation may be inhibited. One hundred per cent silicone catheters have the maximum available internal diameter for a given external diameter (see Fig. 44.2). *In vitro* studies have shown that they have better flow characteristics than coated latex catheters (Griffiths & Gallanaugh, personal communication, 1984), and the incidence of associated urethritis appears to be significantly less (Nacey et al 1985). Some patients will

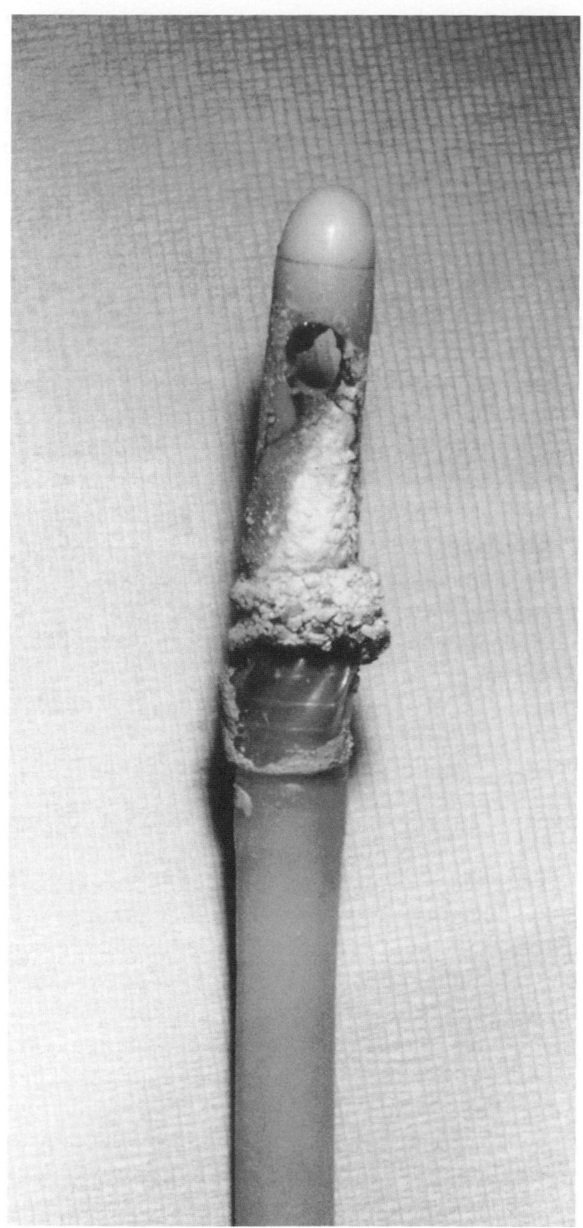

Fig. 44.1 Encrustation around eyes and balloon of Foley catheter. From Hilton (1987), with permission.

require frequent changes of catheter whatever type is used; this may be due to an increased tendency to encrustation as a result of metabolic abnormality or poor fluid intake, or repeated bypassing; for these there is certainly no advantage in silicone, and coated latex or pure latex may be perfectly satisfactory if well managed (Blannin & Hobden 1980).

Catheter length Many hospital supplies departments stock only 'male' length catheters (40–45 cm), yet the use of 'male' length catheter in a woman patient is more difficult to disguise under clothing, and easier to pull accidentally; the additional length

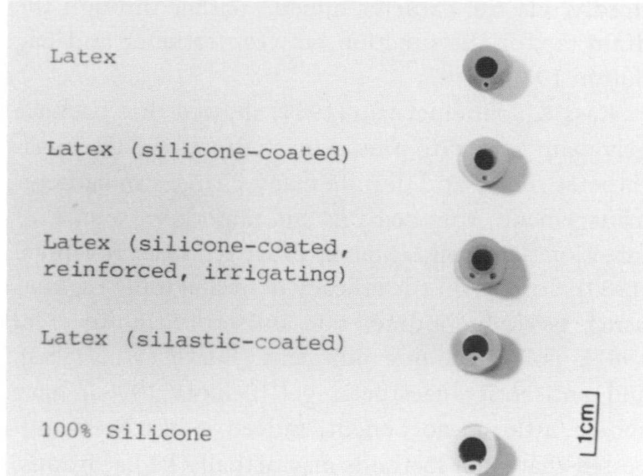

Fig. 44.2 Sections of a selection of indwelling urethral catheters (all of the same external diameter) to demonstrate variation in internal dimensions. From Hilton (1987), with permission.

gives increased potential for kinking and blockage. Female length catheters should therefore be employed in all situations where an indwelling urethral catheter is used in a woman patient.

Balloon size Foley-type catheters are available with a number of different balloon sizes: 3–5 ml (intended for paediatric use); 5–10 ml and 30–50 ml (for routine bladder drainage); 75–100 ml (for haemostatic purposes, especially following prostatectomy). The purpose of the balloon is not to achieve continence by occluding the internal meatus, but simply to retain the catheter at the bladder neck; rarely is anything other than a 5–10 ml balloon required for this purpose.

Problems of catheter management

The following problems may arise with any form of catheterization; they are included here since they are much more common with continuous indwelling urethral catheters than other types.

Catheter associated infection

Over one third of urinary tract infections seen in hospital are associated with catheterization (Tanaka et al 1997). Urinary infection is undoubtedly the most significant problem of catheter management, and even with short-term postoperative drainage over 50% may have bacteriuria and over 15% may have symptomatic urinary infection (Schiotz 1996b). There are several potential points of entry for bacteria into the urinary tract of the catheterized patient; firstly, on the outside of the catheter, at the time of insertion, secondly, by ascent in the mucus film between the catheter and urethral wall whilst indwelling, and thirdly, via the catheter lumen – either through the drain tap, or the junction between catheter and bag (Kunin 1979).

Kass & Schneiderman (1957) showed that bacteria may gain entry to the urinary tract via the pericatheter route, and despite many changes in catheter management, this remains an important source of infection (Daifuku & Stamm 1984; Schaeffer & Chmiel (1983). Studies on the efficacy of meatal toilet regimes using povidone-iodine, non-antiseptic (Burke et al 1981), poly-antibiotic ointment (Burke et al 1983), and antiseptic/anaesthetic gel (Schiotz 1996a) have shown little or no benefit, indeed it has been suggested that such methods may actually be hazardous, and encourage infection in high-risk groups.

The use of regular bladder irrigations or washouts has been advocated as a means of reducing clinical infection rates. Neomycin, chlorhexidine and noxythiolin have been suggested, although they have had little influence on infection (Brocklehurst & Brocklehurst 1978) and antibacterial solutions at least may run the risk of inducing resistance (Warren et al 1978).

The place of prophylactic chemotherapeutic agents remains controversial. In the case of long-term catheterization there is general agreement that prophylaxis is inadvisable because of the risks of persistent colonization and emergence of resistance (Turck & Stamm 1981; Kunin 1979). The same also applies to the therapeutic use of antimicrobials in patients documented to have bacteriuria, but who remain asymptomatic. In the case of short-term catheterization, particularly in the postoperative situation, prophylactic antibiotics may be used for two distinct purposes: to prevent postoperative bacteriuria in patients with sterile urine preoperatively, and to prevent septicaemia in those who come to operation with infected urine. In the first situation, there have been several studies which have documented a reduction in postoperative bacteriuria with several antimicrobial agents, e.g. nitrofurantoin, amoxycillin, co-trimaxozole and cephalosporins. These were reviewed by Slade & Gillespie (1985) who concluded that since postoperative bacteriuria is easy to treat, and rarely causes serious harm, the routine use of antibiotics is likely to do more harm than good. Where patients come to surgery with already infected urine, the literature is again discrepant, and in their review Hirschman & Inui (1980) had to conclude that the value of administering antibiotics to patients in this situation remains uncertain. It would seem, therefore, that antibiotic therapy should perhaps be reserved for those patients who develop signs and symptoms referrable to urinary tract infection, or whose catheter is likely to be removed within a few days of the recognition of bacteriuria.

The prevention of nosocomial urinary tract infection was considered by Turck & Stamm (1981) and their recommendations, with slight modification, are tabulated below:

- Avoid catheterization wherever possible
- Use a suprapubic catheter in preference to urethral
- Intermittent catheterization is preferable to indwelling
- Use aseptic techniques for insertion
- Always employ a closed sterile drainage system
- Ensure 'downhill' urine flow and anti-reflux valve in bag
- Replace catheter only if malfunctioning or obstructed
- Separate infected from non-infected cases
- Regular bacteriological monitoring
- High-volume urine flow (only when catheter free draining)

Leakage around the catheter

Bypassing, or leakage of urine around a urethral catheter, is a very common problem in long-term catheterized patients (Ferrie et al 1979; Brocklehurst & Brocklehurst 1978), of whom it may occur in over one third (Kohler-Ockmore & Feneley 1996). The simplest reason for the problem is kinking or twisting of the catheter or draining tubing, and this should be checked for immediately. If no site of occlusion is evident externally, the catheter should be gently flushed to relieve possible blockage by clot or mucosal slough. If this does not ease the problem, the catheter should be removed and examined for signs of encrustation. If encrustation is present, then in the long-term catheterized patient at least, it may be worth changing to a 100% silicone catheter.

In the absence of encrustation the most likely cause of bypassing is the occurrence of uninhibited detrusor contractions, and a course of anticholinergic drugs, e.g. oxybutynin or probanthine is often beneficial. The problem is certainly exacerbated by large balloon catheters, and the temptation to increase the volume in the balloon or to use catheters of progressively increasing calibre in an effort to occlude the bladder neck must be avoided.

Intermittent catheterization

The concept of intermittent catheterization was introduced by Guttmann & Frankel in 1966 as the most suitable method of bladder drainage in the spinal cord injured patient with a hypotonic detrusor and spastic sphincter. Clean intermittent self-catheterization or CISC was introduced by Lapides et al in 1972, in patients with outflow obstruction, but it has now found a definite place in the management of children with spinal dysraphism (Scott & Deegan 1982; Lyon et al 1975), adults with neuropathic bladders (Joiner & Lindon 1982; Hunt et al 1984), and in women with chronic voiding dysfunctions (Murray et al 1984). Early objections to the technique were based on misplaced fears of an increased risk of infection, although CISC has been shown to be associated with a reduced rate of infection as compared either to the acceptance of a large residual urine volume or to indwelling catheterization.

The optimal frequency of catheterization is a very individual factor, determined by the particular neurological or urological pathology present, the symptoms of which the patient complains, whether they pass any urine normally or are incontinent, and on their general state of health, mobility, and level of social functioning. Rates vary from weekly to 2-hourly, but most will catheterize 2–6 times per day.

Choice of catheter

Many different catheter types may be employed for CISC. In the author's experience patients are most easily taught self-catheterization using a soft plastic catheter of 12 FG (see Fig. 44.3). Low-friction catheters ('Lofric' – Astra-Meditec Ltd.) may also be used to advantage in some patients who otherwise may find the procedure uncomfortable (see Fig. 44.3). This catheter has been shown *in vitro* to lead to a 95% decrease in friction when compared to an uncoated catheter; when used for CISC 76% of patients found it preferable (Hellsten & Hjalmas 1984). For patients who have difficulties catheterizing without access to a mirror the Bruijnen Boer catheter can sometimes be used to good effect (see Fig. 44.3) (Bruijnen & Boer 1981).

CYSTOSTOMY

Cystostomy, the creation of an artificial opening into the bladder, is most often performed suprapubically, either by open operation or by a closed stab procedure. Vaginal cystostomy is included for the sake of completeness, but finds little place in current practice.

Closed suprapubic stab cystostomy

Closed suprapubic catheterization may be employed in any of the indications outlined above, but has particular advantages over the urethral route in several situations (Hilton 1988b). Following pelvic surgery, particularly for the treatment of urinary incontinence, suprapubic catheterization has the advantage

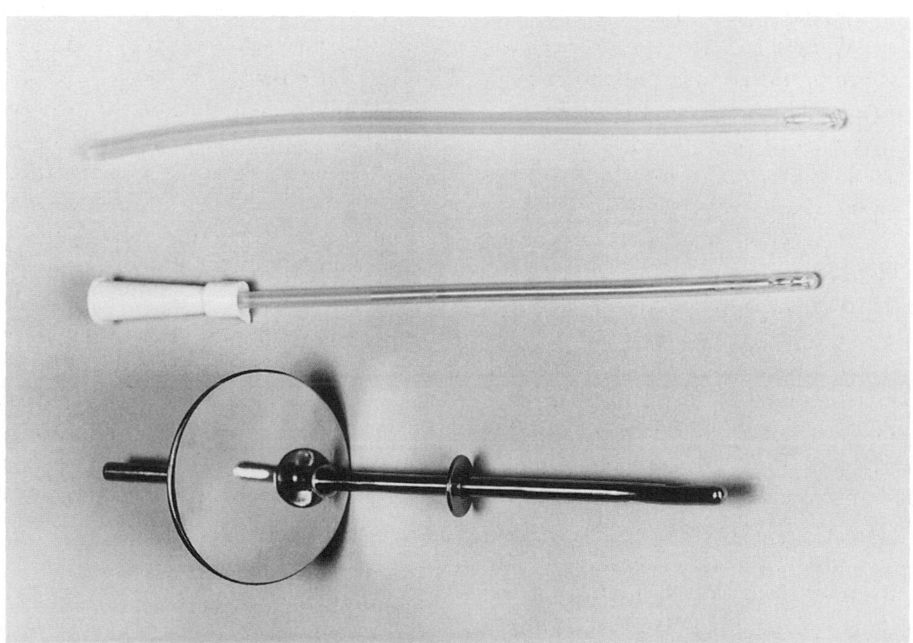

Fig. 44.3 Selection of instruments for female self-catheterization; all 12 FG. Top – PVC catheter; centre – 'low-friction' catheter; bottom – Bruijnen-Boer catheter. From Hilton (1987), with permission.

that the patient's ability to void can be tested without removing the catheter. This appreciably reduces patient discomfort, nursing time, and urinary infection, since repeated catheterizations are unnecessary (Mattingly et al 1972; Bonanno et al 1970). It has also been shown to speed the return of spontaneous voiding following incontinence surgery, presumably by allowing the more rapid resolution of periurethral oedema (Anderson et al 1982). Similarly, the pain and local swelling produced by acute vulvovaginitis may make suprapubic drainage highly desirable. Following urethral trauma, urethral or bladder neck surgery, or the repair of vesical or urethral fistulae, the presence of a catheter in the urethra, or of a catheter balloon in close proximity to the bladder neck is undesirable since it may encourage local oedema and delay healing.

Contraindications

- Inability to distend the bladder
- Gross haematuria or clot retention
- Recent cystostomy incision.

Technique

For postoperative bladder drainage the catheter will be inserted under general or regional anaesthesia; otherwise local infiltration is perfectly satisfactory. Insertion techniques vary considerably with different catheter designs (see Fig. 44.4), and the manufacturer's instructions should be studied beforehand by the operator and nursing staff.

When the catheter is to be used for postoperative drainage the bladder must be filled; using standard aseptic techniques a urethral catheter is passed and 4–500 ml saline or irrigation fluid instilled. The suprapubic area is cleansed, the point of insertion being in the midline approximately 3 cm above the symphysis. When local anaesthesia is used, the point of insertion should be infiltrated down to the bladder with 1–2% lignocaine; urine may be aspirated into the syringe to confirm correct angulation of puncture. A small stab incision made through the skin with a no. 11 scalpel blade facilitates catheter introduction; in catheters requiring a relatively high insertion force (e.g. Stamey, Argyle and Simplastic) it is advisable to incise the rectus sheath also. The catheter/trocar, assembled according to the manufacturer's instructions, is introduced through the incision with a firm thrust in a slightly caudal direction. Resistance should be minimal once the bladder is entered, and correct siting is confirmed by the free flow of urine when the catheter is aspirated, or the trocar disengaged. The catheter is advanced over the trocar until its flange is flat against the skin, and then the trocar is removed. In catheters without a fixed flange or balloon (e.g. Cystocath and Cystofix), or those with drainage holes proximal to their fixation (e.g. Stamey), it is important to ensure that all drainage holes, and not simply the trocar tip, are advanced well into the bladder. Otherwise, as the

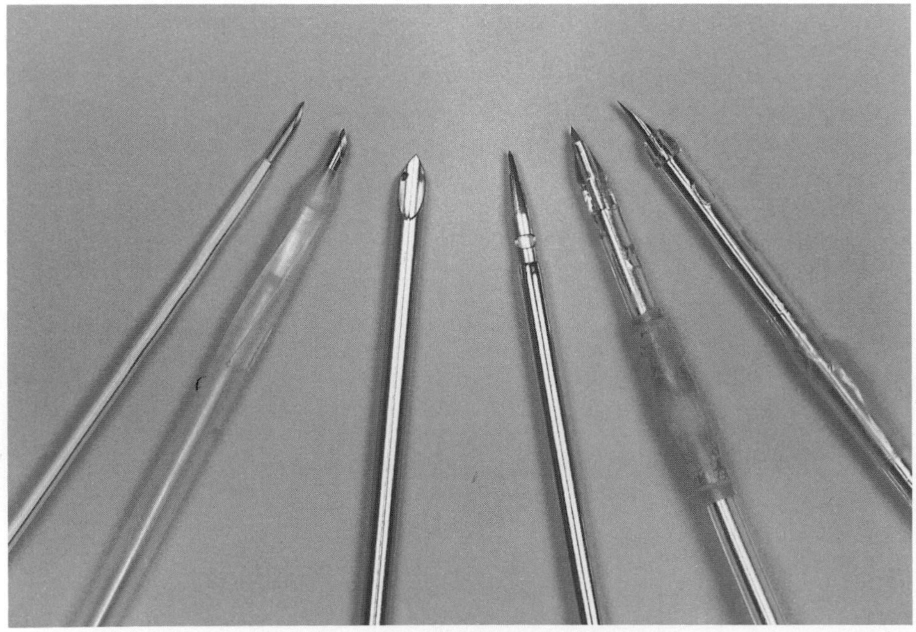

Fig. 44.4 Suprapubic catheter (or trocar) tips. Left to right, Bonanno (Becton Dickinson Ltd.), Stamey (Cook Inc.), Cystofix (B Braun Ltd.), Cystocath (Dow Corning Corp), Simplastic (Franklin Medical), Argyle Ingram (Sherwood Medical Industries). From Hilton (1987), with permission.

bladder empties, the catheter may come to lie in the retropubic space and, although initial drainage may appear satisfactory, failure may be recognized on return to the ward (see Fig. 44.5). The catheter is secured by suture, adhesive, balloon inflation or tape as appropriate and is connected to the drainage bag which should also be secured to the skin to prevent dragging. The bladder is drained, and the urethral catheter removed.

Subsequent management

The catheter should be left on continuous drainage into a closed collection system until the patient is to attempt to void. Timing will depend on the indication for catheterization, but in the situation of postoperative drainage following incontinence surgery the author's preference is for 3 days' free drainage. The adapter or drainage connection should be clamped, or the connecting three-way tap closed first thing in the morning; on no account should the catheter itself be clamped as this will encourage fracture. If the patient is unable to void, or becomes distressed, the clamp should be released to avoid overdistention of the bladder. If she achieves normal voiding the residual volume should be checked after 8 hours. The habit of checking a residual after each void is not recommended as this may give a false impression of the efficiency of micturition by masking an accumulating residual. The residual is checked by emptying the drainage bag, allowing the patient to void at her next desire, and then unclamping the catheter for 5–15 minutes (depending on catheter calibre). Although a high fluid intake may be encouraged whilst the catheter is on free drainage, this is to be avoided once the patient begins to attempt voiding. It will complicate the measurement of residual volumes (since the drainage will consist of the residual plus newly excreted urine), but more importantly will compromise detrusor contraction if muscle fibres are persistently overstretched by the high output. An intake of 1.5–2 l per 24 h is perfectly adequate. Practices vary considerably as to what constitutes an acceptable residual volume, but it is the author's practice to leave the catheter on free drainage overnight until the patient achieves an evening residual of less than 100 ml and is voiding volumes of over 200 ml. At this stage, the catheter is clamped overnight and the residual checked after voiding in the morning. If this, too, is less than 100 ml, the catheter is then left clamped for a full 24 h, and a further residual checked the following morning; if this is less than 100 ml the catheter is removed. If prophylactic chemotherapy is not employed, and it is not the author's practice to do so, urine samples should be obtained every 48 h for culture and sensitivity testing.

In the context of postoperative bladder drainage, where voiding difficulties are persistent, many regimens for encouraging voiding have been advocated. These include α-adrenoreceptor blocking drugs

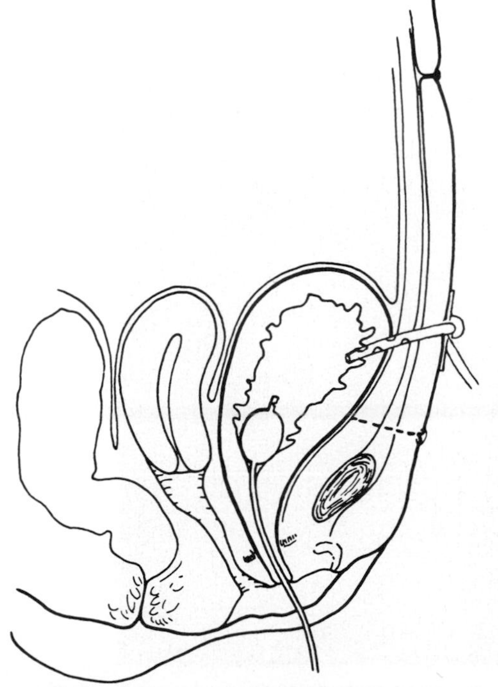

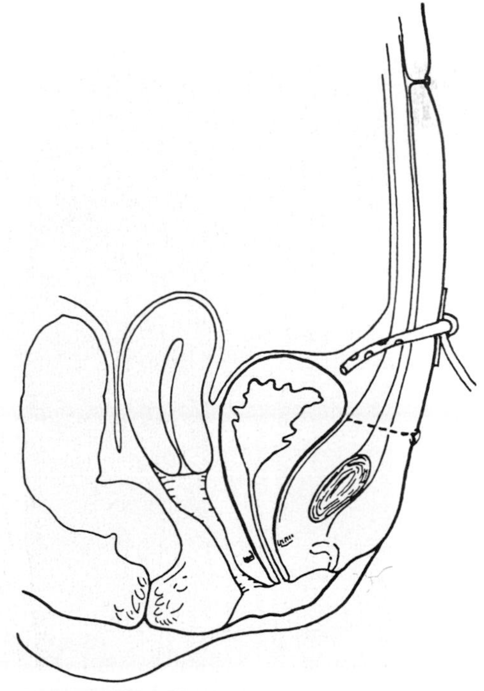

Fig. 44.5 A,B To illustrate the effects of inadequate advancement of catheter. From Hilton (1987), with permission.

(e.g. prazosin or phenoxybenzamine) which theoretically may reduce urethral tone, and cholinergic agents (e.g. carbachol and bethanechol), anticholinesterase preparations (e.g. distigmine bromide), and intravesical prostaglandin which may increase detrusor contractility. The results with all of these regimens have been inconsistent, however, and in one study the use of a benzodiazepine as night sedation was found to be the most effective pharmacotherapy in speeding the return of normal voiding following incontinence surgery (Stanton et al 1979). Undoubtedly, anxiety is a significant factor in postoperative retention, and the author's preference is to recommend discharge with a suprapubic catheter *in situ* for patients in whom voiding is delayed for more than 5 days. Whilst some patients are reluctant to take the responsibility for catheter management, the majority feel that the relief of tension which results from using their own familiar toilet facilities rather than shared hospital amenities, and the removal of the sense that they have a test to pass each time a residual volume is checked, and a deadline to meet for discharge, allows a much more rapid return to normal voiding.

Complications

Failure to enter the bladder This is rarely a problem provided the bladder is adequately distended beforehand. If free flow of urine is not observed when the catheter and stylet are disengaged, the catheter should be aspirated with a syringe; if urine is not obtained the whole assembly should be removed and re-sited after further filling. On no account must an inner trocar be advanced back into its catheter, nor should an external trocar catheter be withdrawn through its trocar; in either case perforation or fracture of the catheter may result (see Fig. 44.6).

Bowel perforation This is also most usually an indication of inadequate bladder filling. The catheter should be removed and re-sited, and antibiotic therapy instituted with metronidazole and a cephalosporin. With small calibre catheters (6–8 FG) this is usually all that is necessary, although close observation of vital signs should be kept, and evidence of peritonism sought; with larger instruments laparotomy and bowel repair should be considered mandatory (Herbert & Mitchell 1983).

Haematuria Haematuria may occur on the first day after insertion, as a result of trauma caused by catheterization, or at a later stage, due to cystitis or mucosal irritation. A catheter specimen should be cultured, but in the absence of infection haematuria usually settles spontaneously.

Detachment from the skin This is rarely a problem within the usual timescale of postoperative bladder drainage; it can usually be managed by re-suturing or taping.

Failure of drainage This may occur at any stage, and usually reflects obstruction or kinking of the catheter or drainage system; dressings and taping

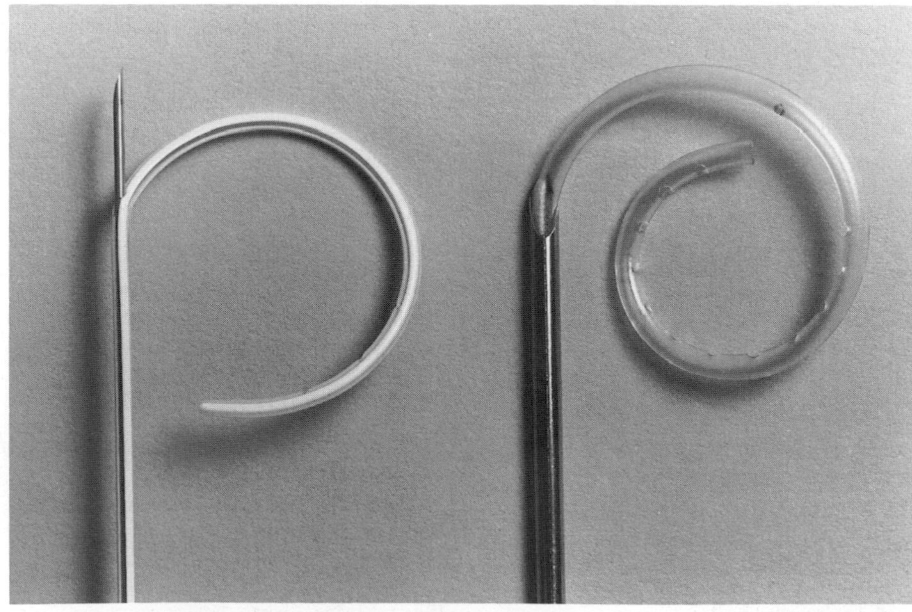

Fig. 44.6 The effects of advancing an internal trocar back through its catheter (left); the same may result with other catheter designs from withdrawal of a catheter through its external trocar (right). From Hiton (1987), with permission.

should be checked and adjusted as necessary, and the catheter should be gently flushed with sterile saline, to exclude encrustation or obstruction by clot. If no drainage results it is possible that the catheter has been extruded into the retropubic space (see insertion technique and Fig. 44.5); in the latter situation replacement is required.

Leakage around the catheter This may arise from similar reasons to failure of drainage, although it should be borne in mind that this is much less likely than with a urethral catheter, and the possibility of fracture of the catheter should be considered. This has been reported particularly with the original version of the Bonanno catheter (Drutz & Khosid 1984); if this problem is suspected the catheter should be removed and a replacement introduced. All catheters should be checked on removal; if doubt over completeness exists radiological confirmation, and if necessary cystoscopic retrieval, should be performed.

Open suprapubic cystostomy

Open suprapubic cystostomy is now seldom required in gynaecological practice. When there is difficulty in distending the bladder, where there is extensive scarring in the suprapubic area, or where permanent suprapubic drainage is to be instituted, as in the management of intractable urinary incontinence (Feneley 1983), open suprapubic cystostomy may be undertaken. As an alternative, a Foley or Malecot catheter may be inserted suprapubically either by cutting down onto a sound (Turner-Warwick 1968) or forceps, or by means of the Robertson cystotrocar (Robertson 1973). Both methods are simple and straightforward, although they are used by only 1% of gynaecologists in the British Isles (Hilton 1988a).

Vaginal cystostomy

Vaginal cystostomy has been used in the past for the drainage of the bladder following repair of a low vesicovaginal or urethrovaginal fistula; it is, however, rarely used today even in these situations, and has largely been superseded by the suprapubic approach.

REFERENCES

Anderson J, Fischer-Raumussen W, Molsted-Pedersen L, Nielsen N 1982 Suprapubic bladder drainage reduces rates of urinary infection and of impaired voiding after colposuspension/vaginal repair. Proceedings of the XIIth annual meeting of the International Continence Society. Leiden, Netherlands, pp. 96–98

Blandy J 1981 How to catheterise the bladder. British Journal of Hospital Medicine 26: 58–60

Blannin J P, Hobden J 1980 The choice of catheter. Nursing Times 76: 2092–2093

Bonanno P J, Landers D E, Rock D E 1970 Bladder drainage with the suprapubic catheter needle. Obstetrics and Gynaecology 35: 807–813

Brocklehurst J C, Brocklehurst S 1978 The management of indwelling catheters. British Journal of Urology 50: 102–105

Bruijnen C L A H, Boer P W 1981 Intermittent self-catheterisation: a new instrument. British Journal of Urology 53: 198

Burke J P, Garibaldi R A, Britt M R, Jacobson J A, Conti M, Alling D W 1981 Prevention of catheter-associated urinary tract infections. Efficacy of daily meatal care regimens. American Journal of Medicine 70: 655–658

Burke J P, Jacobson J A, Garibaldi R A, Conti M, Alling D W 1983 Evaluation of daily meatal care with poly-antibiotic ointment in prevention of urinary catheter-associated bacteriuria. Journal of Urology 129: 331–334

Daifuku R, Stamm W E 1984 Association of rectal and urethral colonisation with urinary tract infection in patients with indwelling catheters. Journal of the American Medical Association 252: 2028–2030

Drutz H P, Khosid H I 1984 Complications with Bonanno suprapubic catheters. American Journal of Obstetrics and Gynaecology 149: 685–686

Feneley R L C 1983 The management of female incontinence by suprapubic catheterisation, with or without urethral closure. British Journal of Urology 55: 203–207

Ferrie B G, Glen E S, Hunter B 1979 Long-term urethral catheter drainage. British Medical Journal 2: 1046–1047

Givens C D, Wenzel R P 1980 Catheter-associated urinary tract infections in surgical patients: a controlled study on the excess morbidity and costs. Journal of Urology, 124: 646–648

Guttmann L, Frankel H 1966 The value of intermittent catheterisation in the early management of traumatic paraplegia and tetraplegia. Paraplegia 4: 63–83

Hellsten S, Hjalmas K 1984 The low-friction catheter: a new device for urethral catheterisation. Proceedings of the XIVth annual meeting of the International Continence Society. Innsbruck, Austria, pp. 375–376

Herbert D B, Mitchell G W 1983 Perforation of the ileum as a complication of suprapubic catheterisation. Obstetrics and Gynaecology 62: 662–664

Hilton P 1987 Catheters and drains. In: Stanton S L (ed) Principles of Gynaecological Surgery. Springer-Verlag, Berlin

Hilton P 1988a Bladder drainage: a survey of practices among gynaecologists in the British Isles. British Journal of Obstetrics and Gynaecology 95: 1178–1189

Hilton P 1988b Suprapubic catheterisation. In: Procedures in Practice. British Medical Journal Publications, London, pp. 140–150

Hirschman J V, Inui T S 1980 Anti-microbial prophylaxis: a critique of recent trials. Review of Infectious Diseases 2: 1–23

Hunt G, Whitaker R H, Doyle P D 1984 Intermittent self catheterisation in adults. British Medical Journal 289: 467–468

Jain P, Parada J P, David A, Smith L G 1995 Overuse of the indwelling urinary tract catheter in hospitalized medical patients. Archives of Internal Medicine 155: 1425–1429

Joiner E, Lindon R 1982 Experience with self intermittent catheterisation for women with neurological dysfunctions of the bladder. Paraplegia 20: 147–154

Kass E H, Schneiderman L J 1957 Entry of bacteria into the urinary tracts of patients with inlying catheters. New England Journal of Medicine 256: 556–557

Kohler-Ockmore J, Feneley R C 1996 Long-term catheterization of the bladder: prevalence and morbidity. British Journal of Urology 77: 347–351

Kunin C M 1979 Detection, prevention and management of urinary tract infection. Lea & Febiger, Philadelphia

Lapides J, Diokno A C, Silber S, Lowe B S 1972 Clean intermittent self-catheterisation in the treatment of urinary tract disease. Journal of Urology 107: 458–461

Liedberg H 1989 Catheter induced urethral inflammatory reaction and urinary tract infection. An experimental and clinical study. Scandinavian Journal of Urology and Nephrology supplement 124: 1–43

Lyon R P, Scott M P, Marshall S 1975 Intermittent catheterisation rather than urinary diversion in children with meningomyelocoele. Journal of Urology 113: 409–417

Mattingly R F, Moore D, Clark D 1972 Bacteriologic study of suprapubic bladder drainage. American Journal of Obstetrics and Gynaecology 114: 732–738

Murray K, Lewis P, Blannin J, Shepherd A 1984 Clean intermittent self-catheterisation in the management of adult lower urinary tract dysfunction. British Journal of Urology 56: 379–380

Nacey J N, Tulloch A G S, Fergusson A T 1985 Catheter-induced urethritis: a comparison between latex and silicone catheters in a prospective clinical trial. British Journal of Urology 57: 325–328

National Nosocomial Infections Study 1973 National Nosocomial Infections Study, Quarterly Report – third quarter of 1971. United States Department of Health Education and Welfare, Public Health Services, Centers for Disease Control, Atlanta

Report on the National Survey of Infection in Hospitals (1980) 1981 Journal of Hospital Infection, suppl. 2

Robertson J R 1973 Suprapubic cystostomy with endoscopy. Obstetrics and Gynaecology 41: 624–627

Ruutu M, Aflathan O, Talja M et al 1985 Cytotoxicity of latex urinary catheters. British Journal of Urology 57: 82–87

Schaeffer A J, Chmiel J 1983 Urethral meatal colonisation in the pathogenesis of catheter-associated bacteriuria. Journal of Urology 130: 1096–1099

Schiotz H A 1996a Antiseptic catheter gel and urinary tract infection after short-term postoperative catheterization in women. Archives of Gynecology and Obstetrics 258: 97–100

Schiotz H A 1996b Postoperative bacteriuria and urinary tract infections in gynecological patients. Tidsskrift for Den Norske Laegeforening 116: 246–248

Scott J E, Deegan S 1982 Management of neuropathic urinary incontinence in children by intermittent catheterisation. Archives of Diseases of Childhood 57: 253–258

Slade N, Gillespie W A 1985 The urinary tract and the catheter – infection and other problems, Wiley, Chichester

Stanton S L, Cardozo L D, Kerr-Wilson R 1979 Treatment of delayed onset of spontaneous voiding after surgery for incontinence. Urology 8: 494–496

Stevens G P, Jacobson J A, Burke J P 1981 Changing patterns of hospital infections and antibiotic use. Prevalence surveys in a community hospital. Archives of Internal Medicine 141: 587

Tanaka G, Shigeta M, Usui T 1997 Statistical studies on bacteria isolated from in-patients with urinary tract infections. Nishinihon Journal of Urology 59: 1–5

Thompson R L, Haley C E, Searcy M A et al 1984 Catheter-associated bacteriuria. Journal of the American Medical Association 251: 747–752

Turck M, Stamm W 1981 Nosocomial infection of the urinary tract. American Journal of Medicine 70: 651–654

Turner-Warwick R 1968 The repair of urethral strictures in the region of the membranous urethra. Journal of Urology 100: 303–314

Warren J W, Platt R, Thomas K J 1978 Antibiotic irrigation and catheter-associated urinary tract infections. New England Journal of Medicine 299: 570–573

Diversion and undiversion

SUZIE VENN AND TONY MUNDY

INTRODUCTION

Urinary diversion can be divided for descriptive purposes into temporary diversion and permanent diversion. Temporary diversion, usually involving placement of a catheter, either percutaneously into the kidney or the bladder, or transurethrally into the bladder, or more rarely, by open operation into the ureter, will not be considered further. However, all of these techniques do have an important role to play in the management of the specific urological problems in which they are indicated; percutaneous nephrostomy and urethral and suprapubic catheterization in particular. Urinary diversion (which we will take from here on to mean permanent diversion) has a long history in the management of lower urinary tract problems. Initially, ureterosigmoidostomy was the favoured technique, implanting the ureters low into the sigmoid colon, and once this could be achieved without a significant risk of intestinal leakage, it gained in popularity. Unfortunately, it was found to be complicated in some patients by a hyperchloraemic acidosis, and in fewer patients with the development of adenocarcinoma of the colon at the ureterosigmoidostomy site. In many more patients complications involved stricturing of the ureterocolic anastomosis, leading to obstruction or to reflux of faecal matter up the ureterocolic anastomosis, causing severe recurrent urinary tract infections (Ferris & Odel 1950; Spence et al 1975).

As disillusionment with this technique set in, Bricker (1950) published his technique of ileal conduit diversion and this rapidly caught on and became the favourite means of urinary diversion for a wide range of problems for well over 20 years. Unfortunately, this too was found to have its problems, particularly with stomal stenosis or stenosis of the ureteroileal anastomosis (Schwarz & Jefs 1975). More worrying was the finding of long-term deterioration of upper urinary tract function, although in many instances this was no more than a mild degree of hydronephrosis (Shapiro et al 1975). Nonetheless, at this time Hendren (1973, 1974 and 1976) was beginning to publish his results with urinary undiversion and in any case many of the problems hitherto treated by urinary diversion, particularly in children, began to be treated by other means. Hendren (1975) also popularized Mogg's (1965) technique of colon conduit urinary diversion which seemed to be more satisfactory than the ileal conduit because a non-refluxing ureterocolic anastomosis could be performed, whereas this was difficult with an ileal conduit.

Controversies about the preferred technique of urinary diversion subsequently died down, largely because of the huge wave of enthusiasm for undiversion and for the techniques of urinary tract reconstruction that rendered diversion unnecessary in the first place. In only one area did diversion retain an unchallenged role and this was for patients having cystectomy for bladder cancer.

More recently, there has been a further wave of interest in urinary diversion and more specifically in continent urinary diversion. Having said that, paediatric urologists have continued to use the ureterosigmoidostomy technique throughout the period alluded to above in children with conditions such as bladder exstrophy who could not be reconstructed. It also continued to be used in patients having exenterations for pelvic malignant disease as this is a form of continent diversion in the sense that it is not dependent on an external appliance.

In recent years, continent diversion has come into vogue for patients where a urinary diversion is necessary because reconstruction is not feasible, to avoid the need for constant wearing of an external appliance. The patient has an external stoma, but a small, easily concealed one through which a catheter is passed to achieve intermittent bladder emptying.

Thus we have two types of urinary diversion to consider: conduit diversion, best exemplified by the ileal conduit, and continent diversion, of which there are now many types, but basically those relying on the Kock principle (Kock et al 1986) and those relying on the Mitrofanoff principle (Mitrofanoff 1980). We must not forget, of course, the ureterosigmoidostomy – the original 'continent diversion'.

CONDUIT URINARY DIVERSION

The great advantage of the conduit urinary diversion, when compared with continent urinary diversion, is that it is much simpler to perform in most instances, the exception being a straightforward Mitrofanoff procedure as described below. The problem is the external stoma and the appliance required to collect urine. This undoubtedly causes emotional problems of body image in some patients, particularly the young. Some surgeons feel that the straight ureteroileal anastomosis, which allows free reflux, is a disadvantage and would favour a colon conduit because it is non-refluxing. Although this is of great practical interest to the surgeon, is of only theoretical interest to the patient, because for her the end result is the same – a bag. In any case, the value of preventing conduit to ureter reflux is not proven, although theoretically it is obviously an advantage.

The complications recognized as relating particularly to the conduit diversion are ureteroenteric strictures in 4–8% of patients (Engel 1969). Stomal stenosis is reported as 5–10% (Emott et al 1985) and revision for other reasons (prolapse, retraction). The other complications are those of any enterocystoplasty (see below).

Because of its simplicity, the conduit diversion is likely to remain the standard diversionary procedure, particularly for patients with malignant disease.

CONTINENT DIVERSIONS

The Kock principle

The Kock principle is to form a reservoir out of 'detubularized' gut with an intussuscepted gut nipple at one end, to which the ureters are anastomosed, and a similar intussuscepted gut nipple at the other end, which is anastomosed to the skin (Fig. 45.1). The nipple intussusceptions are designed to prevent reflux up the ureters and efflux onto the abdominal wall respectively. The bladder is emptied by catheterization (Kock et al 1986).

The main problem is that the nipples are unstable and tend to unravel with time, leading to incontinence onto the abdominal wall, and revisions are therefore often necessary, even in the most experienced hands, to maintain continence. Another problem is that the technique requires around 70 cm of ileum to construct the reservoir and the two nipples. This is rather a lot of small intestine to use, particularly in children, in whom there may be potential severe nutritional and metabolic consequences.

Others have tried to overcome this by using colon instead of ileum (or a combination of the two), by using a simple tunnelled reimplantation of the ureters into the pouch to obviate the need of at least one nipple. There are also variants for providing continence at the abdominal wall end of the pouch to get rid of the other nipple. Nonetheless, the basic problems are that this requires a long section of ileum, perhaps too

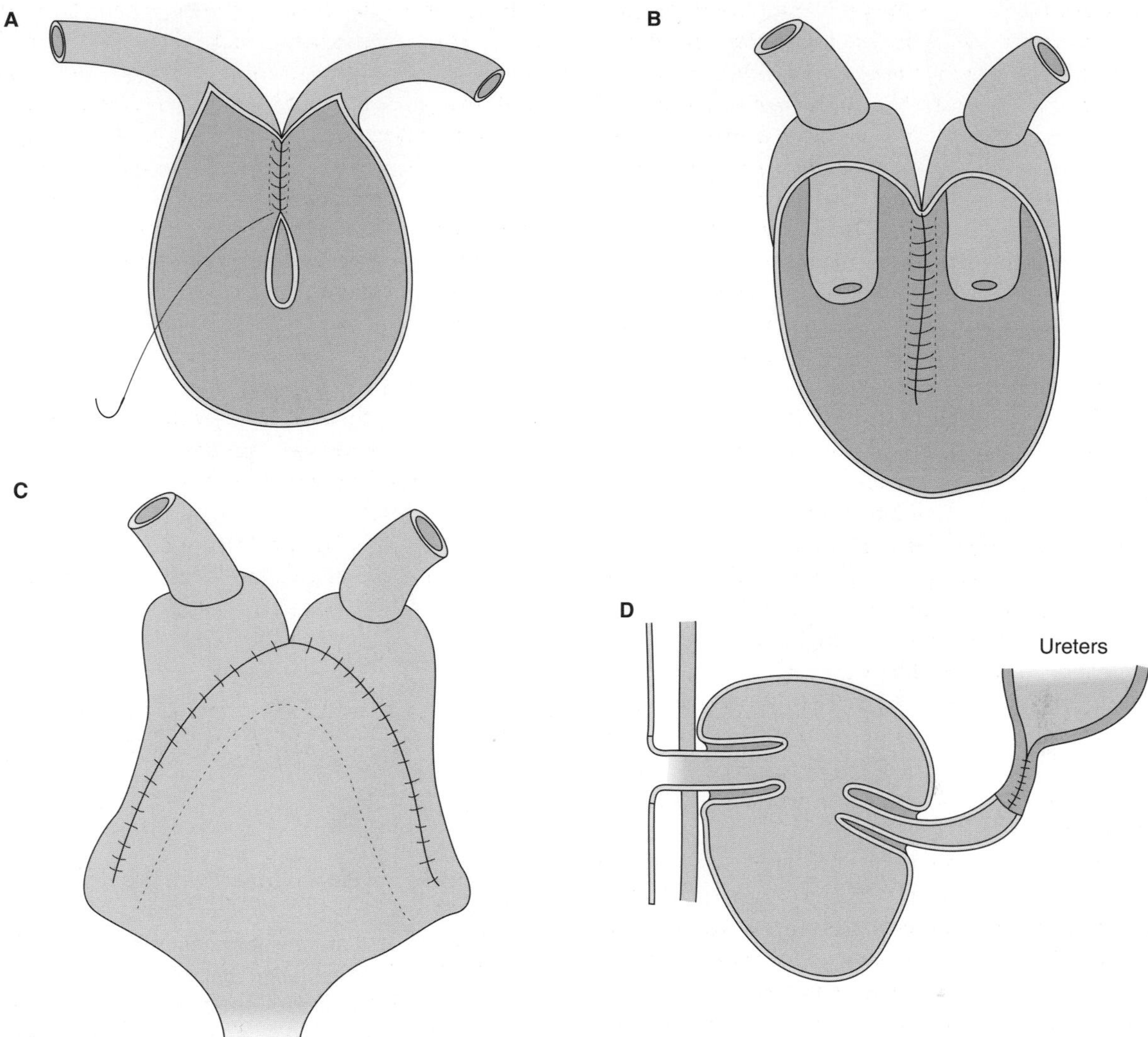

Fig. 45.1 Kock pouch. (A) The middle two quarters of a 70 cm segment of ileum are opened and sewn together. (B) The proximal and distal quarters are intussuscepted and fixed by stapling. (C) The pouch is closed. (D) The ureters are sutured to one end and the other end sewn flush to the skin.

much, and that frequent revisions are necessary to maintain a satisfactory result. Even then, problems of catheterization are common.

The Mitrofanoff principle

Mitrofanoff (1980) designed his procedure for use in children in whom he mobilized the appendix, brought the caecal end out onto the skin and then implanted the tip using a tunnel technique into the anterolateral bladder wall (Fig. 45.2). The tunnelled implantation into the bladder wall provided a flutter valve continence mechanism through which the patient could catheterize, maintaining continence by means of the valve. Apart from other considerations, one feature of the Mitrofanoff principle is that it was specifically designed to work with a natural bladder (normal, that is, in appearance, although not in the way it behaves). It is therefore useful in categories of patients other than just those having a cystectomy or in whom the bladder cannot be used, as is the case of the pouch reservoirs procedures described above. Indeed, the ideal case is a woman with chronic retention who cannot, for whatever reason, self-catheterize her urethra.

In essence, the difference between the Mitrofanoff principle and the Kock principle is that the Kock principle relies on a nipple valve to maintain continence, whereas the Mitrofanoff principle relies on a flutter valve. Another difference worth remembering is that the Kock procedure is intended to replace the bladder and urethra whereas the Mitrofanoff

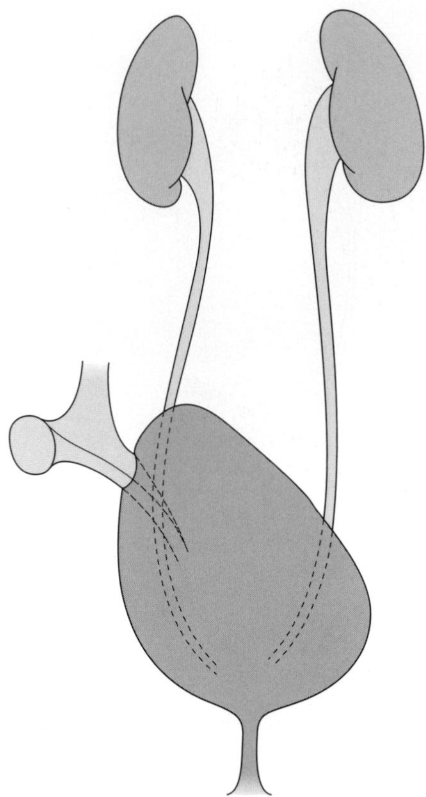

Fig. 45.2 Mitrofanoff procedure using the appendix.

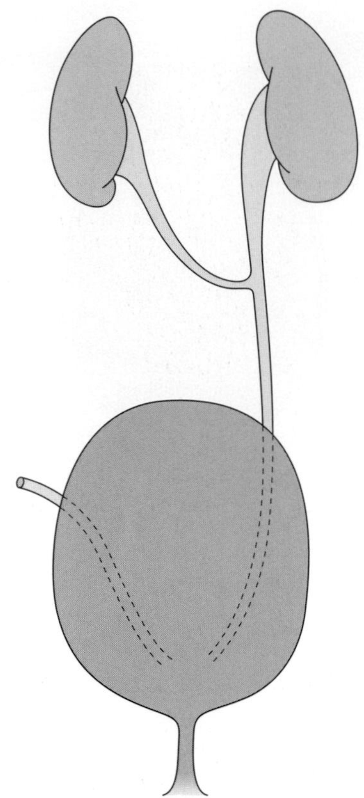

Fig. 45.3 Mitrofanoff procedure using a TUU.

procedure, as originally conceived, is intended to replace only the urethra.

If the appendix cannot be used, the ureter can be divided above the iliac vessels on one side and the proximal end swung over to the other as a transureteroureterostomy (TUU) to provide drainage into the bladder. The other end is then brought out onto the skin surface, using the natural ureterovesical junction as the continence mechanism, again emptying by intermittent self-catheterization through the stoma (Fig. 45.3). Otherwise a tapered length of small bowel can be used as in the Monti procedure (Sugarman et al 1998) (see also Fig. 45.4).

The Mitrofanoff principle has been extended from using a normal bladder drained as described above, to using a bladder augmented or even substituted by an intestinal pouch and with drainage along the lines described above, that is, using the appendix or ureter as the occasion provides (Duckett & Synder 1986).

The recto-sigmoid pouch (Mainz II)

The ureterosigmoidostomy represented the first form of continent urinary diversion. It fell out of favour due to the occurrence of hyperchloraemic acidosis and relapsing pyelonephritis with loss of kidney function.

With awareness of long-term complications of ileal conduits and the knowledge that by detubularization and reconfiguration of the intestines, a low pressure reservoir could be formed, re-interest in the use of ureterosigmoid pouches occurred. The use of efficient antireflux reimplantation of the ureters and low-pressure, adequate capacity reservoirs reduces the risk of pyelonephritis and deterioration of upper tract function. Patients have to take alkaline medication to prevent hyperchloraemic acidosis, but with continence rates of near 100% (Pajor & Kelemen 1995) this seems a small price to pay. The Mainz II (Fisch et al 1993) (see also Fig. 45.5) pouch is particularly useful when there is no distal continence mechanism available for reconstruction. The risk of malignant change in ureterosigmoidostomy is recognized (Filmer & Spencer 1990) and necessitates close long-term follow-up with yearly sigmoidoscopy from 10 years.

Complications of enterocystoplasty

These have been discussed in Chapter 20 but include:

1 Fluid and electrolyte disturbance
2 Stones

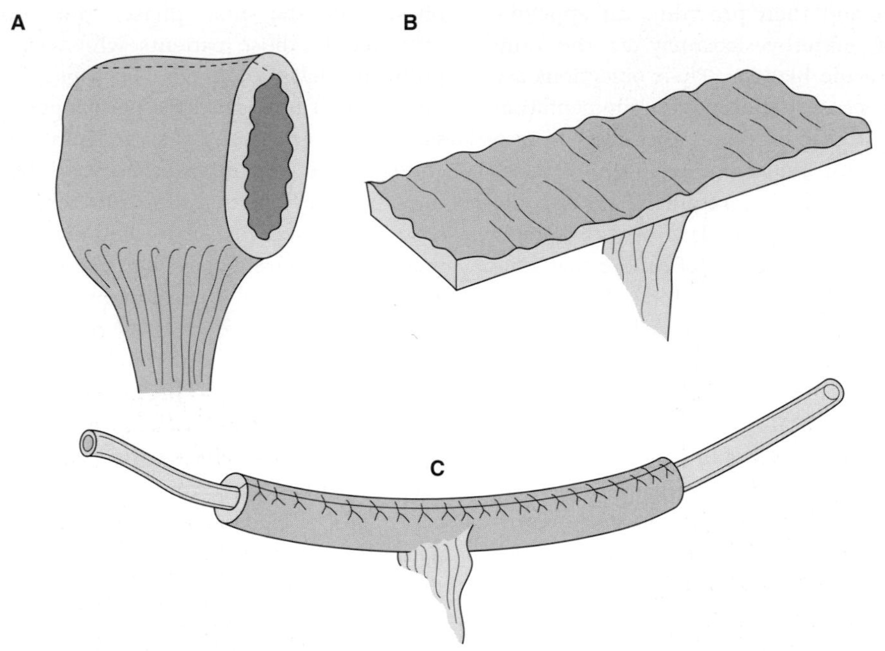

Fig. 45.4 The Monti procedure. (**A**) A 2 cm section of ileum is isolated, (**B**) opened transversely and (**C**) closed longitudinally over a catheter.

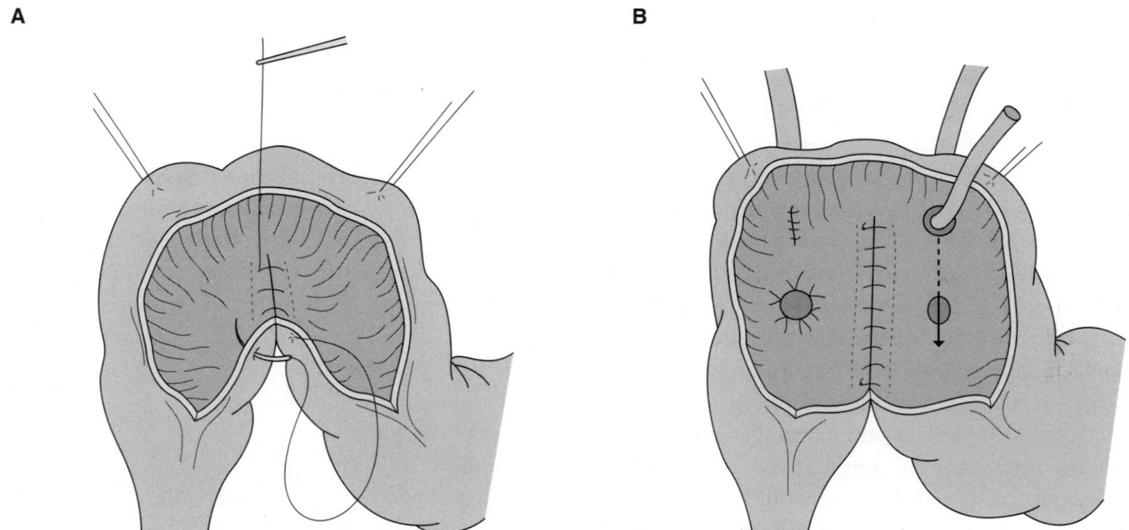

Fig. 45.5 The Mainz II rectosigmoid pouch. (**A**) The sigmoid colon and rectum are opened and anastomosed on the back wall. (**B**) The ureters are brought through into the pouch, tunnelled under the mucosa, and anastomosed.

3 Infections
4 Malignant change
5 Mucus production.

Conclusion

In the authors' view, for many patients the ileal conduit diversion will provide the most satisfactory answer to their problem because it is the simplest, it is the least prone to complications and revision procedures and because for many people managing a surface appliance is easier than managing self-catheterization. Again, it is the authors' opinion that the Kock principle is far too prone to complications and should be abandoned. On the other hand the Mitrofanoff principle, particularly when applied to a natural bladder, is a useful addition to our surgical armamentarium, particularly as indicated above for women in chronic retention who have an uncatheterizable urethra for whatever reason. The authors do, however, have reservations about going as far as some enthusiasts do in tying off the bladder neck, augmenting the bladder with gut and then providing an appendicovesicostomy or ureterovesicostomy as the only means of access to the bladder. Their objections are twofold: firstly, because patients with augmentation or substitution cystoplasties do occasionally run into problems with mucus retention, recurrent urinary infection or stone formation requiring endoscopic management. This is not possible down an appendiceal or ureteric tract of the sort of calibre that usually results from one of these procedures. The second objection is that many patients treated in this way may be candidates for reconstruction and the deliberate sacrifice of a potentially useful bladder outflow might wreck this possibility forever. Nonetheless, there are specific circumstances in which a continent diversion using the Mitrofanoff principle are positively indicated, particularly in patients with neuropathic bladders and restricted mobility, confined by long leg callipers or a wheelchair, in whom self-catheterization through an abdominal stoma would be much easier than through the urethra. Severe post-irradiation problems and following total cystourethrectomy are the two other main areas where continent diversion is positively indicated. The Mainz II pouch has a role as an alternative in patients whose outflow is not of use, to provide continence without the need for an external appliance. Long-term follow-up of the low-pressure reservoir is required before its place in diversion is established.

In summary, if a urinary tract reconstruction is not possible, a patient should be offered a choice of either an ileal conduit diversion (or perhaps a colon conduit diversion in youngsters), or alternatively a continent diversion based on the Mitrofanoff procedure leaving the patient to choose which she would prefer. In most instances it would seem that an elderly patient would prefer a conduit diversion and a younger patient the Mitrofanoff procedure, although this is a very vague generalization. Better than either would be a urinary tract reconstruction if this is at all possible, assuming one has the basic philosophy that any form of diversion is a means of last resort.

UNDIVERSION

Undiversion was popularized by Hendren who not only introduced the concept of undiversion but described several of the techniques which are now fundamental and standard techniques used routinely in almost all undiversion procedures (Hendren 1973, 1974, 1976).

Undiversion has essentially gone through three phases: in the first phase, the procedure was restricted to those patients who were diverted for problems that would now no longer be treated by diversion, at least not by a permanent type of diversion. The largest group of patients in this category are children who were diverted because of hugely dilated upper urinary tracts due to problems that were not then recognized for what they are. Such problems include vesicoureteric reflux, prune belly syndrome and vesicoureteric junction obstruction. The latter would now be treated by a relatively simple and straightforward procedure such as ureteric reimplantation. In the case of prune belly syndrome, this would not be treated surgically at all in most instances. In such patients their urinary undiversion simply involves the restoration of urinary tract continuity, where necessary correcting the underlying pathology, usually reimplanting the ureters to prevent reflux or obstruction.

The second phase was the more ambitious undiversion of patients with problems that could still now be quite reasonably treated by urinary diversion. The largest number of patients in this group are those with spina bifida and neuropathic bladder dysfunction, in whom simple restoration of urinary tract continuity would give them back the same problems they had to start off with. Thus, undiversion in this type of patient has to be combined with the establishment of normal bladder function. Sometimes, it also involves ancillary surgery either to the upper urinary tract, perhaps to remove stones or to excise a non-functioning kidney, or sometimes to other pelvic viscera if they were involved in the underlying disease process. Examples in this latter category include the major congenital malformations such as urogenital sinus and cloacal abnormalities.

The third phase is the one we are currently in, where most of the available pool of undivertible diversions have been undiverted and all that is left is those for whom diversion is the only realistic treatment option. The primary efforts of reconstructively-orientated surgeons are more directed to the primary correction of the various problems mentioned above, avoiding the need for diversion in the first place. Indeed, it is probably true to say that many of today's reconstructive surgeons cut their teeth on urinary undiversion and expanded their range of procedures from that starting point.

Undiversion therefore involves three factors: firstly, restoration of upper urinary tract continuity; secondly, restoration or creation of normal bladder function and thirdly, associated procedures.

Associated procedures to the upper urinary tract, other than simple nephrectomy or nephroureterectomy, are usually performed separately from the undiversion procedure itself. This is because the access through an anterior abdominal incision for upper urinary tract surgery other than nephrectomy or nephroureterectomy is usually inadequate, and most stone problems – the commonest reason for upper tract intervention – are better treated by percutaneous means.

Of the remaining two factors, restoration of urinary tract continuity is usually the easiest problem to deal with; establishing normal bladder function is usually more difficult, involving as it does the establishment of a good capacity low-pressure bladder with a competent bladder outflow and effective bladder emptying. This is all the more difficult because no matter how detailed the preoperative evaluation, it is never entirely satisfactory because it is based on how the bladder works at the time or at best after a few days of bladder cycling (see below), whereas the end result will only become apparent after weeks or months of use after the undiversion procedure.

Selection of patients for undiversion

Patients usually select themselves. Undiversion is still a fairly uncertain procedure as far as outcome is concerned (in that many of the postoperative problems cannot be anticipated or predicted for any specific patient) and motivation is all important. Thus, the patient should persuade the doctor to perform an undiversion, not the other way round. Unfortunately, some patients are just not suitable, however keen they are to be undiverted. This particularly applies to patients who are wheelchair bound, usually as a result of neurological disability, in whom continence is not necessarily an advantage. The main reason is the limited facilities for voiding that physically disabled people have and the surgeon's inability to guarantee a totally satisfactory result. Thus, a patient who is continent but voiding every hour to hour and a half may be delighted with the result of her operation if she is fully mobile and can get to an ordinary toilet with reasonable ease. A similar result in a wheelchair bound patient, however, may be far less than satisfactory as she will have to spend a substantial part of that hour to hour and a half finding a disabled person's toilet and then transferring from her wheelchair onto the toilet and then back off again afterwards. Thus, although we would not go as far as to say that undiversion is contraindicated in the wheelchair bound patient, we are nonetheless very hesitant about performing the procedure in such patients. For the majority of such patients, a continent diversion would be much more appropriate. With currently available surgical techniques almost anybody can be undiverted, perhaps the only exceptions being some female patients with bladder exstrophy who have had the bladder remnant totally excised and simply have no tissue available for urethral substitution. For them a continent diversion may be more suitable. That aside, almost all patients are undivertible if their general health permits (Mundy et al 1986), so technical considerations are less important than the patient's general health and mental attitude.

Most patients who are candidates for diversion will have an ileal conduit. The best screening investigations are an IVU to show the general anatomy and a loopogram to show the length and calibre of the ureters and the length of the ileal conduit. Most surgeons, ideally, would give a patient a short conduit, but most conduits are longer than intended and in any case seem to elongate with time. A long conduit is, however, an advantage to the undiverting surgeon because this is a useful source of tissue for cystoplasty.

If there is any suggestion of poor function or nonfunction on the IVU, a DMSA renal scan is indicated and if there is any suggestion of upper tract obstruction above the ureteroileal anastomosis, a DTPA or MAG III renal scan is indicated to confirm or exclude this possibility.

It is not always easy to know what the original reason for the diversion was, because many patients present for undiversion at hospitals a long way from the hospital where the original diversion procedure was performed and the notes for that earlier admission may have been lost. Even if the notes are preserved, a specific diagnosis may not be forthcoming. Obviously, clinical examination will suggest a neuropathic reason if a neuropathy exists. Otherwise, lower urinary tract assessment by videourodynamics and by endoscopy will usually give the reason when taken in conjunction with the patient's history.

A good quality videourodynamic study is extremely important. If bladder capacity is reasonably well preserved, as it often is in non-neuropathic patients, then a urodynamic assessment without previous bladder cycling may be adequate. However, a period of bladder cycling using a suprapubic catheter to fill the bladder by means of a drip over a period of a few days, may end up giving far better urodynamic assessment and much more urodynamic information. In patients with neuropathic problems, bladder cycling is less helpful, particularly when the bladder capacity is extremely restricted. However, in neuropathic bladder dysfunction the usual (but not always) underlying abnormality is an intermediate type bladder (Mundy 1986) which is best treated by a combination of an augmentation cystoplasty and placement of an artificial sphincter cuff. An artificial sphincter is by no means always necessary but a cystoplasty almost invariably is and, given that the most major part of implanting an artificial sphincter in a woman is the implantation of the cuff, particularly in the face of previous surgery and particularly when there has been a cystoplasty, it makes sense to implant the artificial sphincter cuff at the time of undiversion, even if it is subsequently not used. The only question that remains in neuropathic patients is whether they require augmentation or substitution cystoplasty and that is determined by the bladder wall thickness and the bladder capacity.

Endoscopy is necessary to be sure that the urethra is normal, to get some idea of bladder capacity to exclude intravesical pathology and for the placement of a suprapubic catheter for bladder cycling if this is indicated.

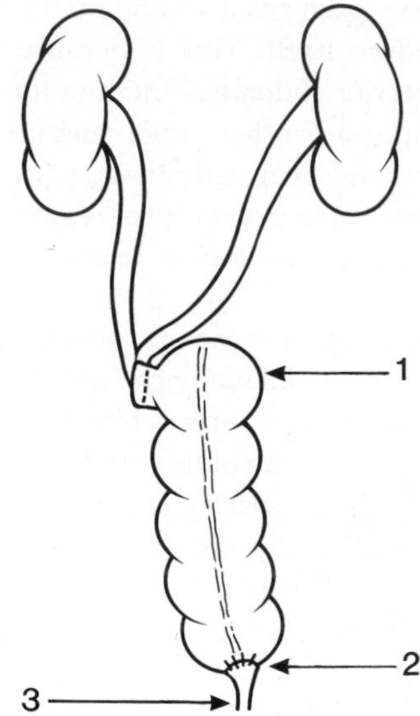

The undiversion procedure

Obviously, the ideal undiversion procedure would involve simply rejoining each ureter to the lower end to restore continuity, followed by simple correction of whatever the underlying problem was that led to the diversion in the first place. Unfortunately, this is rarely possible. Occasionally one finds a patient who was treated for reflux or vesicoureteric junction obstruction as a child by ileal conduit diversion, in whom there was such a length of tortuous, superfluous ureter that a straight end-to-end ureteroureterostomy is possible, but this is extremely rare. In most instances something has to be done to bridge the ureteric gap.

If one has a ureteric gap to bridge it is obviously easier to bridge it on one side rather than on both. For this reason the first step (conceptually at least) in most undiversion procedures is an end-to-side transureteroureterostomy, usually the end of the left into the side of the right ureter, leaving only the right ureter to connect to the lower urinary tract.

If the bladder is a write-off and a substitution cystoplasty is necessary, then obviously bridging the ureteric gap is easy because the substitution cystoplasty does all the work for you (Fig. 45.6). If, as is usually the case, there is some usable bladder left, then it should be preserved and augmented. The role of the bladder remnant is then to provide a means whereby upper to lower urinary tract continuity can be restored. There is absolutely no doubt whatsoever (in the authors' opinion at least) that if direct urothelial continuity can be restored in this way then the results are much better than if some other technique, usually some form of bowel interposition, is used.

The two main techniques for gaining upper to lower urinary tract continuity to allow implantation of the ureter into the bladder remnant are the psoas hitch and the Boari flap (Hendren 1973, 1974, 1975). The psoas hitch is the most important of the two methods because it provides not only restoration of continuity but also a stable bladder base into which the ureter can be re-implanted. This will not be subject to movement and therefore deformity as the bladder fills and empties subsequently (Fig. 45.7). The Boari flap is used to supplement the psoas hitch technique when the bladder cannot otherwise be made to reach as far as the psoas tendon so that it can be 'hitched' there and thus allow a tension-free tunnelled ureteric re-implantation into the bladder (Fig. 45.8).

Thus the basic techniques for restoration of urinary tract continuity are a TUU, usually from left to right, with re-implantation of the resulting single ureter into a psoas hitched bladder, supplemented with a Boari flap where necessary to make up for more severe deficiencies of ureteric length.

Where possible, the ureteric re-implantation should prevent vesicoureteric reflux, if only because reflux after undiversion commonly causes loin pain. It also seems desirable on pathophysiological grounds to prevent reflux as a possible source of ascending infection and back pressure on the kidney with renal deterioration as a result, but these are unproven contentions. Very occasionally, one finds a patient with such a severe deficiency of ureteric length that a psoas hitch and Boari flap will be insufficient to overcome it, but with a bladder sufficiently large to be worth preserving. One then has to consider ileal interposition to bridge the gap. This is most simply

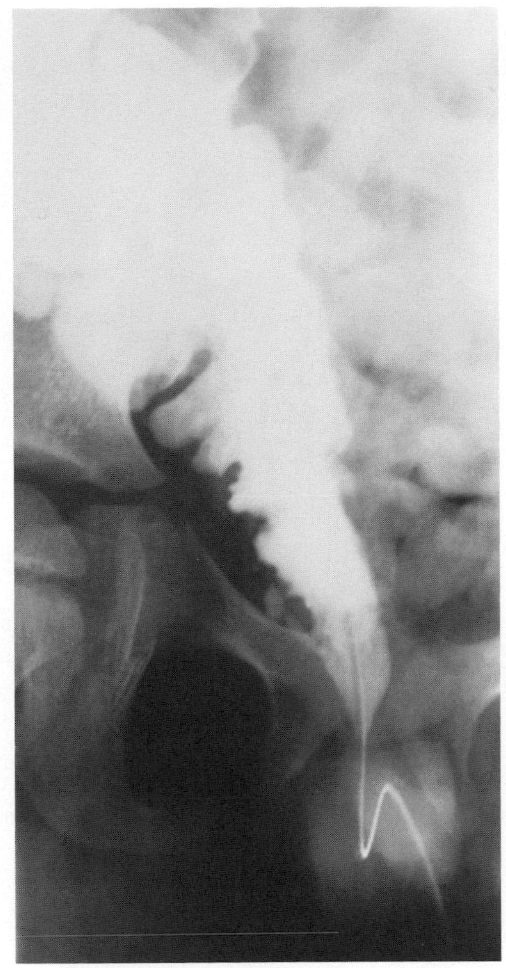

(B)

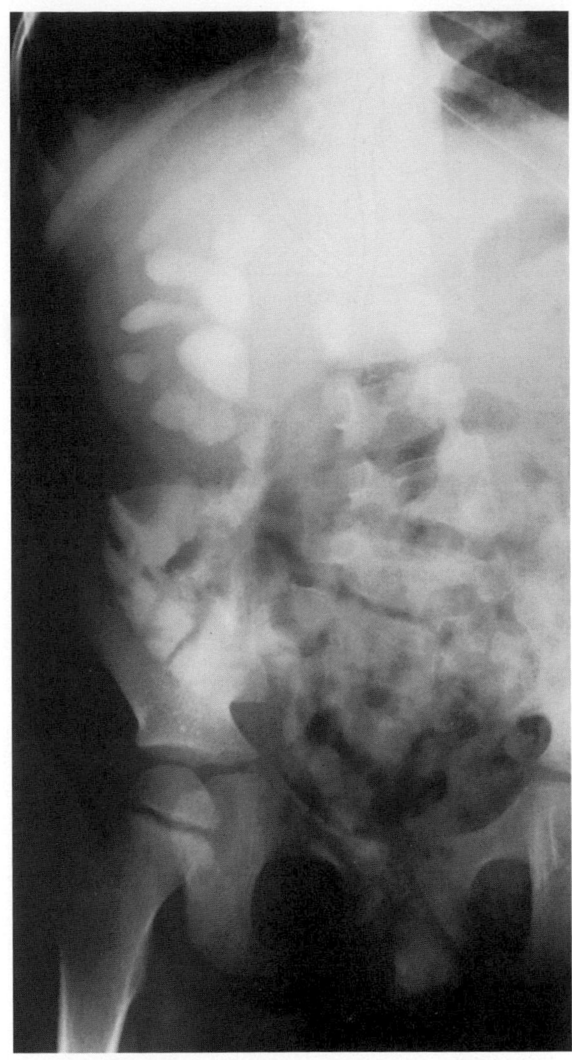

(C)

Fig. 45.6 (**A**) The appearance after substitution cystoplasty (1) emphasizing the need for a subtotal cystectomy sparing only the trigone (2) and for either sphincter balancing or substitution (with an AUS) (3). (**B**) Typical postoperative cystogram showing anastomosis of a large colonic segment to a (bilaterally incised) wide open bladder neck. Only the trigone remains to provide sensation. (**C**) A postoperative IVU film to show the appearances after such a procedure.

achieved with the ileal conduit, if that was the form of diversion the patient had had. If ileal interposition is required, it is best to shorten the loop and straighten it out as far as possible, and then to narrow it or 'tailor' it around a 14–16 F catheter and then do a tunnelled re-implantation into the psoas hitch as above (Fig. 45.9). In this case, rather than to try creating a suburothelial tunnel in the bladder, it might be easier to incise the bladder mucosa along the length of the proposed tunnel, reflect the mucosa on each side and suture the tailored ileal segment into the trench thereby created. One would then suture the urothelial flap on each side onto the surface of the tailored ileal segment, so that during the healing period re-epithelialization over the ileal segment would create a suburothelial tunnel.

Having restored continuity, all that remains from the bladder point of view is to make sure it has sufficient capacity. Augmentation cystoplasty is often necessary, even if the bladder was originally of normal capacity, because it has generally 'shrunk' during the period of diversion. If, in addition, the bladder is also hyperreflexic/unstable or poorly compliant, or both, then an augmentation cystoplasty will be required for those reasons as well. The best tissue to use for augmentation is the ileal conduit itself, opened up along its antimesenteric border and sewn onto the bladder as a patch (Figs 45.10 and 45.8D). When the bladder capacity is severely restricted then, unless the ileal conduit is unusually long, a second ileal segment may need to be mobilized, patched and laid alongside to ensure an adequate capacity. If

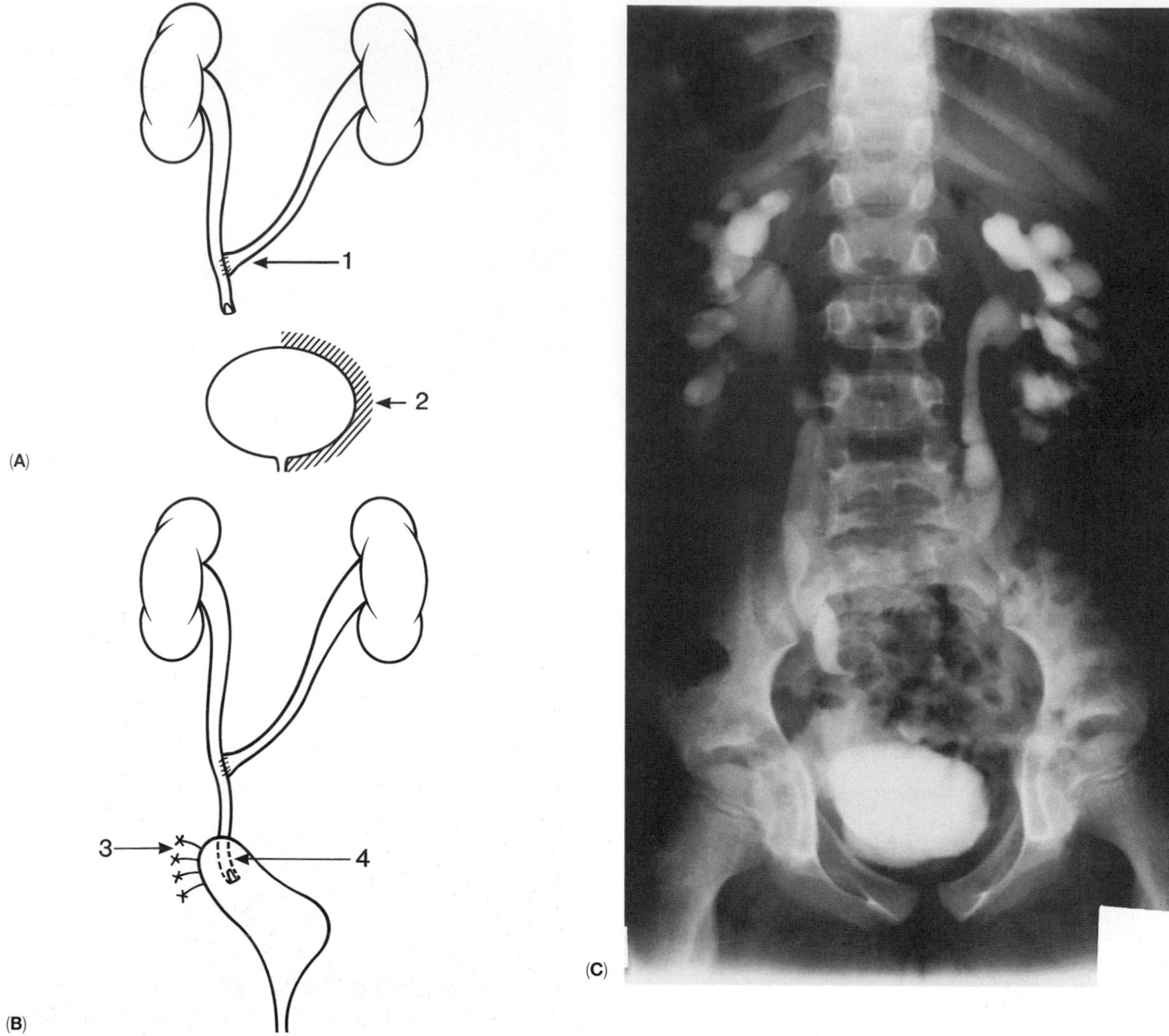

Fig. 45.7 A typical undiversion when ureteric length is adequate with TUU, psoas hitch and an antirefluxing ureteroneocystostomy (UNC). (A) TUU (1) and full mobilization of the contralateral aspect of the bladder (2) to allow: (B) A firm hitch of the bladder to the psoas (3) to allow the antirefluxing UNC (4). (C) A typical postoperative IVU film to show the TUU and psoas hitch.

the patient does not have an ileal conduit but had, for example, ureterosigmoidostomies or cutaneous ureterostomies, then rather than use a double loop of ileum it might be more satisfactory to use the caecum and ascending colon mobilized on its vascular pedicle and opened along a taenia coli. This single loop will provide enough capacity without being potentially detrimental to metabolic and nutritional function thereafter, as loss of a substantial length of terminal ileum might.

Restoration of urethral function is sometimes a problem. If the patient has relatively normal urethral function – if she was diverted, for example, because of childhood reflux or ureteric obstruction or for urge incontinence in adult life – then urethral surgery may be unnecessary. If she had simple stress incontinence with or without detrusor instability then a colposuspension-type procedure may be helpful, but unless it is certain that the urethra was normal, it seems safest to implant an artificial sphincter cuff, if not the whole device, for reasons alluded to above.

More of a problem are those patients with epispadias, exstrophy, urogenital sinus or other problems leading to a highly deficient or even absent urethra, where a urethra has to be created artificially using some other available tissue, either urothelial remnant or, where this is absent, anterior vaginal wall or a pedicled skin flap. Such techniques are beyond the scope of this chapter and the interested reader is referred elsewhere (Mundy 1988).

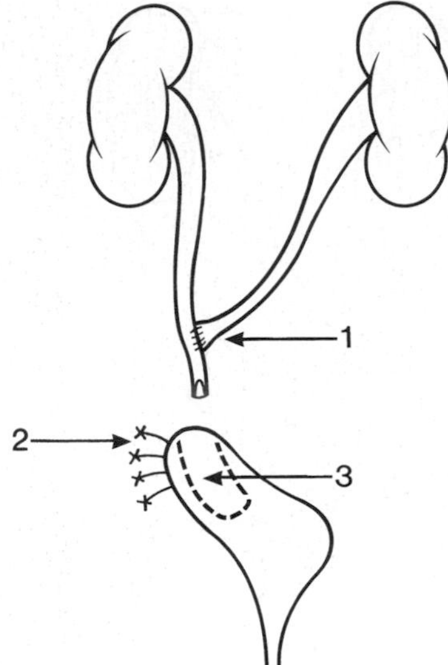

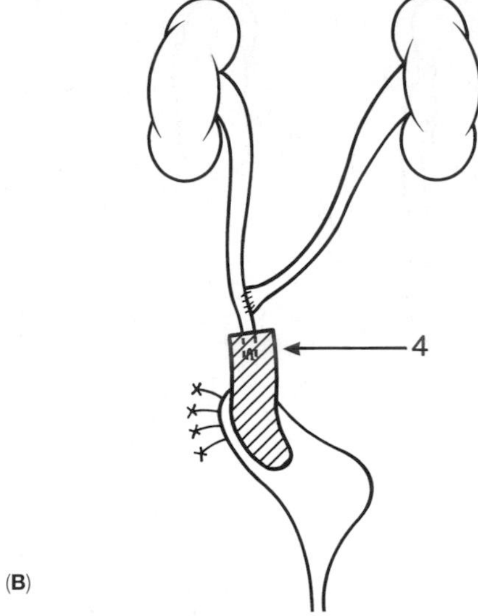

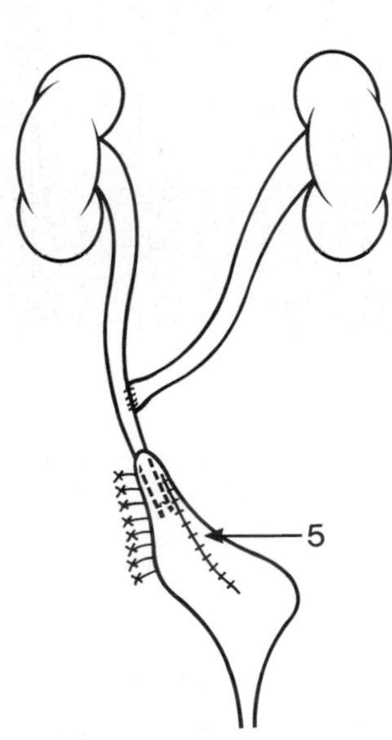

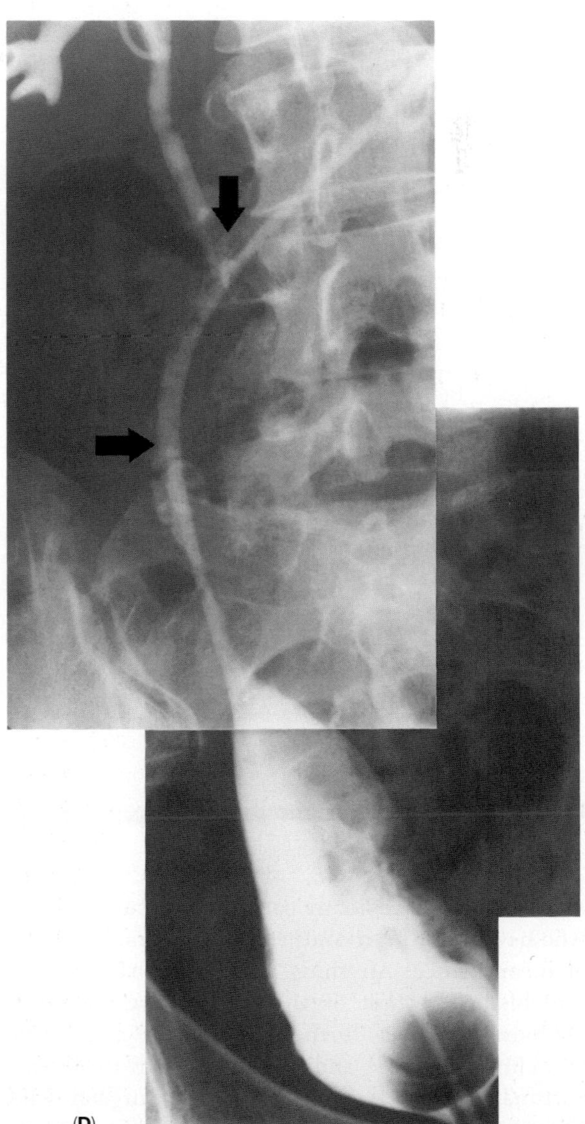

Fig. 45.8 Undiversion when the psoas hitch is insufficient to bridge the ureteric gap. (**A**) TUU (1) and psoas hitch (2) as in Figure 45.7, the Boari flap is outlined (3). (**B**) The flap is raised to allow the antirefluxing UNC (4). (**C**) The flap is closed as a tube (5) and fixed in position on the posterior abdominal wall. (**D**) Early postoperative X-ray films with nephrostomies and a trans-TUU stent still in place. The upper arrow is at the site of the TUU, the lower arrow is at the upper end of the Boari flap. In this case the bladder has been closed with an ileal patch made from the ileal conduit – hence the irregular medial border.

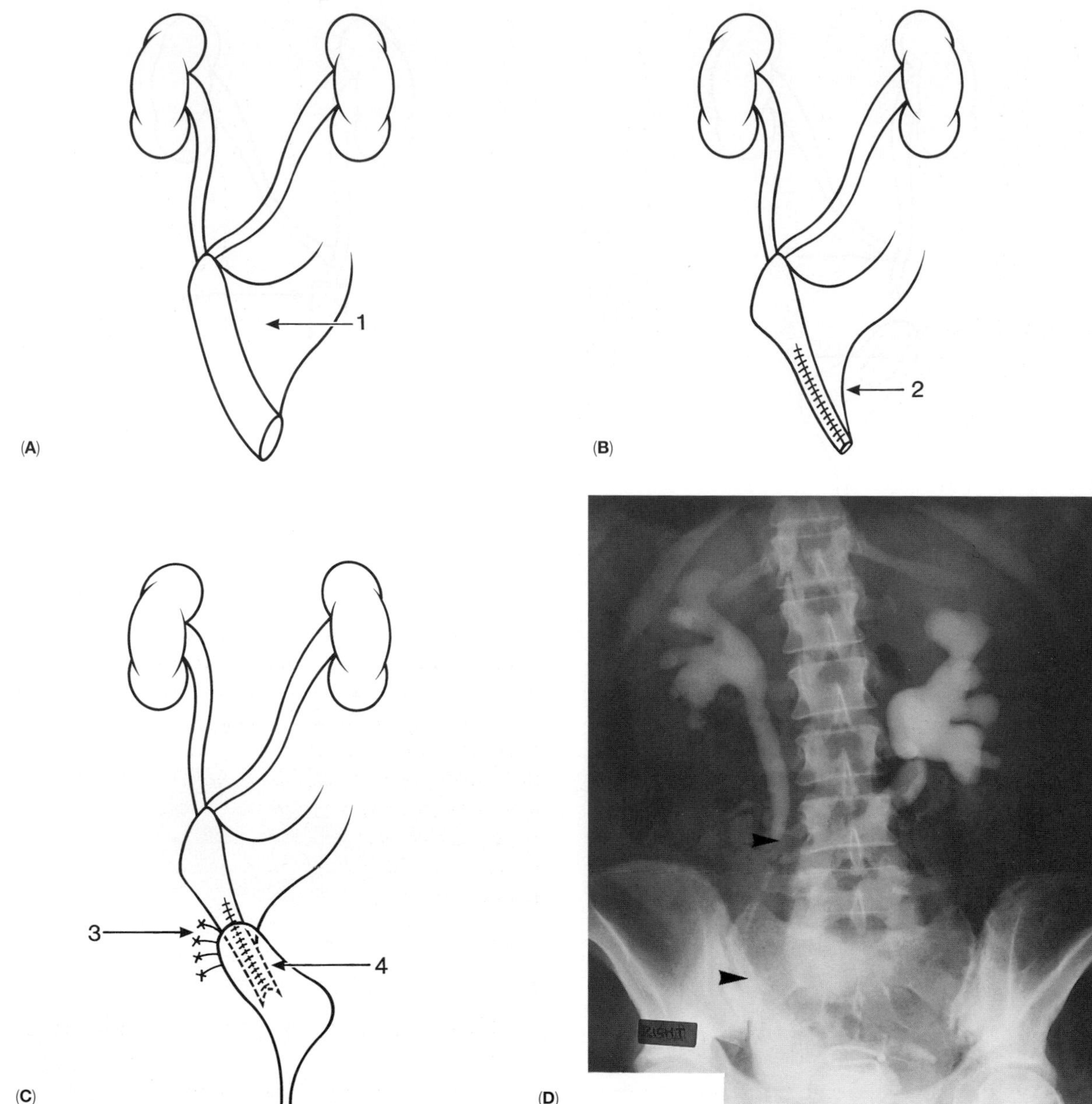

Fig. 45.9 Undiversion using a tailored segment of ileum to bridge the ureteric gap. (**A**) The ileal conduit on its vascular pedicle (1) is trimmed to an appropriate length and (**B**) tapered to a calibre of about 14 F (2). (**C**) A psoas hitch (3) then provides a stable area for an antirefluxing UNC (4). (**D**) Typical postoperative IVU film. The section between the two arrows is the ileal ureter. (The preoperative IVU showed gross obstruction with bilateral negative pyelograms only.)

Results and complications

The main complication, obviously, is failure to achieve continence. Many patients, particularly those who have never been continent, will tolerate a degree of incontinence. Anything more than that is unacceptable. Correction of the persistent abnormality obviously involves further urodynamic assessment to define the cause and the appropriate treatment. Fortunately, this is uncommon. The surgeon who encounters frequent problems with persistent incontinence after undiversion should give up doing undiversion.

More common is recurrent urinary infection due to poor bladder emptying. Here, regular or occasional intermittent self-catheterization may provide sufficient bladder emptying to reduce or eliminate recurrent urinary infections, but occasionally long-term antibiotic prophylaxis is necessary. The biggest headache of all is recurrent or persistent *Pseudomonas* infection. However, the recent introduction of ciprofloxacin has been of enormous benefit in reduc-

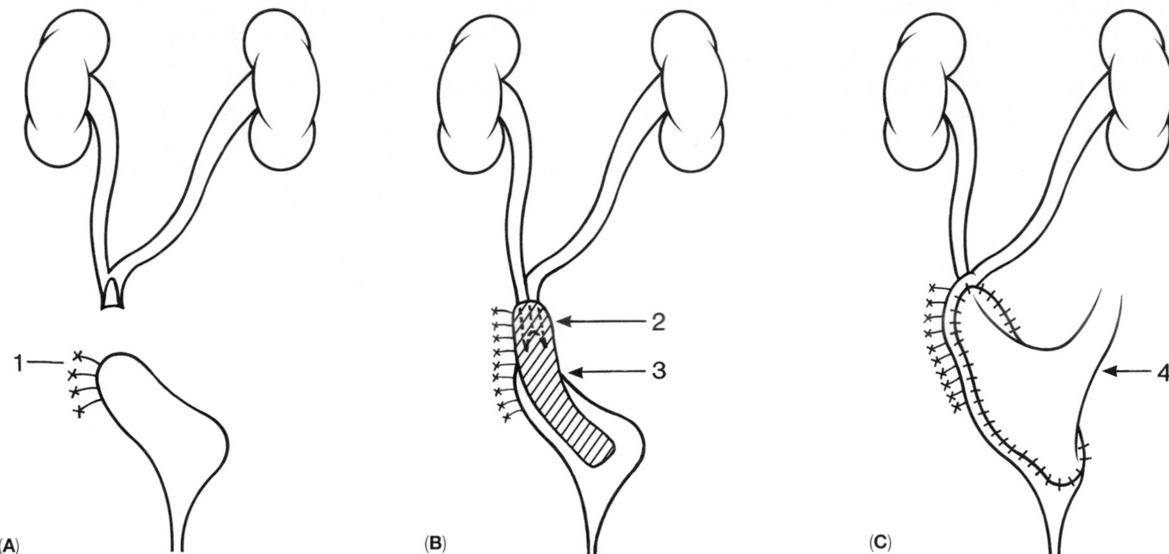

Fig. 45.10 Undiversion when the manoeuvres shown in Figure 45.8 leave a bladder with inadequate capacity. (**A**) TUU and psoas hitch (1). (**B**) Antireflux UNC (2) after a Boari flap (3). (**C**) The bladder is closed with an ileal patch formed from the ileal conduit giving in effect an augmentation cystoplasty.

ing the incidence of all forms of difficult urinary infection, particularly *Pseudomonas*.

Undiversion is major abdominal surgery and for this reason, one in every seven patients or so can be expected to develop some complication related to the surgery. Hopefully, in most instances, it will settle spontaneously without further laparotomy. Such problems include intestinal obstruction and incisional herniae. Other complications are, fortunately, rare.

Undiversion, it must be stressed, is not a procedure for amateurs. The best chance of a satisfactory undiversion is the first chance and a satisfactory result after a first time failure is difficult to achieve. In experienced hands, however, the results are satisfactory but as indicated earlier, primary reconstruction is now the rule as the pool of potentially undiverted patients has been reduced. This is assuming, of course, that the patients have reasonably easy access to a reconstructive unit.

REFERENCES

Bricker E M 1950 Bladder substitution after pelvic evisceration. Urologic Clinics of North America 30: 1511–1521

Duckett J W, Snyder H M 1986 Continent urinary diversion: variations on the Mitrofanoff principle. Journal of Urology 135: 58–62

Emott D, Noble M J, Mebust W K 1985 A comparison of end versus loop stomas for ileal conduit urinary diversion. Journal of Urology 133: 588–590

Engel R M 1969 Complications of bilateral uretero-ileal cutaneous urinary diversion. Review of 208 cases. Journal of Urology 101: 508–512

Ferris D, Odel H 1950 Electrolyte pattern of the blood after belated utero-sigmoidoscopy. Journal of the American Medical Association 142: 634–640

Filmer B, Spencer J R 1990 Malignancies in bladder augmentations and intestinal conduits. Journal of Urology 143: 671–678

Fisch M, Wammack R, Muller S C, Hohenfellner R 1993 The Mainz Pouch II (Sigma rectum pouch). Journal of Urology 149: 258–263

Hendren W H 1973 Reconstruction of previously diverted urinary tracts in children. Journal of Paediatric Surgery 8: 135–150

Hendren W H 1974 Urinary tract refunctionalisation after prior diversion in children. Annals of Surgery 180: 494–510

Hendren W H 1975 Non refluxing colon conduit for temporary or permanent urinary diversion in children. Journal of Paediatric Surgery 10: 381–398

Hendren W H 1976 Urinary diversion and undiversion in children. Surgical Clinics of North America 56: 425–449

Kock N G, Norlen L J, Philipson B M 1986 The continent ileal reservoir (Kock pouch) for urinary diversion. World Journal of Urology 3: 146–151

Mitrofanoff P 1980 Cystomie continente trans-appendiculaire dans le traitement des vessies neurologiques. Chirurgia Pediatrique 21: 297–305

Mogg R A 1965 Treatment of neurogenic urinary incontinence using colon conduit. British Journal of Urology 37: 681–686

Mundy A R 1986 The neuropathic bladder. In: Postlethwaite R J (ed) Clinical Paediatric Nephrology. John Wright and Sons, Bristol: pp. 312–328

Mundy A R 1988 Urethral substitution in females. British Journal of Urology 63(1): 80–83

Mundy A R, Nurse D E, Dick J A, Murray K H A 1986 Complex urinary undiversion. British Journal of Urology 58: 640–643

Pajor L, Kelemen Z 1995 Our experience with the Mainz Pouch II: 40 patients; follow up and complications. Annals of Urology, Paris 29: 246–249

Schwarz G R, Jeffs R D 1975 Ileal conduit urinary diversion in children: computer analysis of follow up from 2–16 years. Journal of Urology. 114: 285–288

Shapiro S R, Lebowitz R, Colodnt A H 1975 Fate of 90 children with ileal conduit urinary diversion a decade later: analysis of complications, pyelography, renal function and bacteriology. Journal of Urology 114: 289–295

Spence H M, Hoffman W W, Pate V A 1975 Exstrophy of the bladder: long term results in 37 patients treated by ureterosigmoidostomy. Journal of Urology 114: 133–137

Sugarman I D, Malone P S, Terry T R et al 1998 Transversely tubularized ileal segments for the Mitrofanoff or Malone antegrade colonic enema procedures: the Monti principle. British Journal of Urology 81: 253–256

SECTION 5
CHAPTER

46

The role of laparoscopy in urogynaecology

ANTHONY R B SMITH

INTRODUCTION

Debate about whether the abdominal or vaginal approach to pelvic reconstructive surgery is more effective has been published in the gynaecological literature since 1909 when George White first described the paravaginal repair. Fothergill (1921) suggested that gynaecologists should learn to perfect their skills in vaginal surgery before resorting to abdominal procedures. The results Fothergill published appeared to justify his view but in 1949 Marshall et al and in 1961 Burch demonstrated that better results with less risk of recurrence could be obtained by employing suprapubic procedures for the treatment of stress incontinence of urine. This has led the majority of gynaecologists to adopt the suprapubic approach to bladder neck surgery though a reluctance to move from the vaginal route has derived at least in part from concern with the increased morbidity produced by an abdominal incision.

Similarly, surgical treatment of vaginal vault prolapse can be achieved by an abdominal or vaginal approach. One randomized trial comparing sacrocolpopexy with sacrospinous fixation has been published. This demonstrated a reduced risk of recurrence with the sacrocolpopexy but sacrospinous fixation has the advantage that a laparotomy is not required (Benson et al 1996). Pereyra (1959) and Stamey (1973) described techniques for the treatment of stress incontinence which gain many of the advantages of the suprapubic approach without laparotomy. Use of a long needle to place sutures across the retropubic space from endopelvic fascia to rectus sheath fascia carries some risk of bladder perforation and cystoscopy is advised at the end of the procedure to check this has not occurred. There is no doubt that postoperative recovery is quicker and hospital stay shorter following these less invasive procedures. The short-term results are similar to the conventional Burch colposuspension but longer term follow-up has shown that the risk of recurrence is greater following the Stamey procedure (O'Sullivan et al 1995) and many surgeons now reserve these less invasive procedures for the elderly or unfit patient. It is not known why such less invasive procedures have a higher recurrence rate although probably the most common reason is that the sutures tear through either the endopelvic fascia or the rectus sheath fascia. It is possible that the reduced tissue trauma and accompanying haemorrhage and the early return to normal activity predispose to early recurrence.

Over the last decade, imaging technology has improved dramatically so that views through endoscopes can be seen with high resolution on a TV monitor. In addition, instruments have been developed which enable the surgeon to operate safely and effectively, albeit whilst working on a two-dimensional TV image. The technological developments are ongoing, as is research on three-dimensional imaging and virtual reality training equipment. These developments have led surgeons of many specialties to explore the use of endoscopic surgery in different areas of the body. In the pelvis, procedures such as colposuspension and sacrocolpopexy can be performed without resort to laparotomy. This chapter will cover the literature of laparoscopic reconstructive pelvic surgery, some of the author's own experience and the lessons and needs for the future.

COLPOSUSPENSION

The first report on laparoscopic colposuspension by Vancaillie & Schuessler (1991) demonstrated that the procedure was possible but not without technical difficulty, illustrated by two bladder injuries in this report of 9 cases. Bladder injury is the most frequently reported intraoperative problem, indicating that the technique has some inherent difficulties, but my own experience suggests that there are ways for the chance of bladder injury to be minimized. The reports published following the Vancaillie paper have no uniformity of surgical technique and many different surgical materials are used (e.g. sutures, bone anchors and meshes). Apart from bladder injury, intraoperative difficulties are little mentioned in the reports. Few details of immediate postoperative morbidity in terms of pyrexia, the need for transfusion or infective morbidity are reported. Liu (1993) reported results from a series of 58 women and found no cases of postoperative fever; all the women were able to return to work a week after surgery. Postoperative pain is not critically analysed in the published reports. In a retrospective record review in Manchester of 50 open and 116 laparoscopic colposuspensions, opiate analgesia was administered twice as frequently following open surgery, indicating that immediate postoperative pain is greater with a laparotomy incision than laparoscopic port wounds. Length of stay in hospital after surgery is difficult to compare between Europe and North America where financial imperatives dictate early hospital discharge. Postoperative voiding difficulties are often responsible for longer hospitalization after bladder neck surgery. Different catheter regimens, including routine use of intermittent self-catheterization, will influence time of discharge. In Manchester, our results show that short-term voiding difficulty is less frequent following laparoscopic surgery but, in the longer term, voiding problems are equally distributed between laparoscopic and open surgery. Table 46.1 illustrates a meta-analysis of published complications of laparoscopic colposuspension.

Objective postoperative evaluation including urodynamics is not always used, and follow-up generally ranges from 3 to 12 months. Nezhat et al (1994) described a series of 62 women who reported '100% satisfactory relief 3 months after surgery', without clarification of this terminology. Apart from Burton (1996), all the published studies are retrospective reviews. Burton performed a randomized, prospective study comparing laparoscopic with open colposuspension and demonstrated that operating time was longer, recovery time from surgery shorter and successful cure of stress incontinence was only 74% at 12 months, compared to 93% with the open approach. There was one bladder injury in each group. At 3-year follow-up the difference in success is more marked, with 60% for the laparoscopic approach compared to 94% for the open approach. The main criticism of this study, apart from the number of patients recruited, is that Burton had not gained sufficient experience in laparoscopic surgery before starting the study. It does, however, give information about what success rate a novice laparoscopic surgeon might expect to achieve if attempting laparoscopic colposuspension. More recent retrospective reports on laparoscopic colposuspension have included 2-year follow-up with different results. Lobel & Sand (1996) reported a cure rate of 89% at 3 months, 86% at 1 year and 69% at 2 years. The series included a number of different techniques and an average operating time of 190 minutes was recorded. Ross (1996) conducted a retrospective review of 40 cases over 2

Table 46.1 Meta-analysis of complications of laparoscopic colposuspension.

Haemorrhage	0.5%
Transfusion <1%	
Bladder injury	3.7%
Ureteral injury/kinking	<0.1%
Voiding dysfunction	5%
Detrusor instability	5%
Prolapse	3%
Incisional hernia	<0.1%

years and reported success rates of 98% at 6 weeks and 90% at 2 years. Thus, one series suggests a marked decline in efficacy and the other a sustained effect on longer term follow-up. It is interesting to note that Lobel and Sand frequently used a Stamey needle to assist in their technique and appear to be producing results similar to the Stamey programme with a higher risk of recurrence.

The main advantage of laparoscopic surgery is said to be the rapid postoperative recovery. This is supported by the report by Liu (1993) that all patients had returned to normal activity within a week of surgery. There is no comparative data available for open surgery in these series. It is also unknown whether it is good for the longevity of the bladder neck support for patients to return to normal activity sooner. Postoperative return to normal activity appears to vary between countries, with North American studies indicating that when there is sufficient financial pressure, early return home and to normal activity is commonplace. MacKenzie (1996) illustrated, in patients recovering from hysterectomy, that preoperative information given to patients has a major influence on time for recovery. The apparent rapid recovery following laparoscopic surgery may, at least in part, be produced by the patient's and physician's expectations. The Sheffield cholecystectomy study (1996) illustrated that when patients were blinded to the method of gall bladder removal their recovery rates were the same for open and laparoscopic techniques. A similar study is required to assess whether there is any difference in immediate postoperative recovery from colposuspension when the patients and attendant nursing staff do not know by which technique the operation was performed.

In the author's experience of over 200 cases, the main differences from open surgery are the new operative skills required and the immediate postoperative recovery. Laparoscopy is a surgical technique which all gynaecologists learn in training. Similarly, minor surgical procedures such as sterilization and minor adhesiolysis are learnt in training. The main and most difficult demand of laparoscopic colposuspension is the laparoscopic suturing. This explains why there has been a growth in the use of mesh and stapling techniques and the employment of the Stamey needle to try to overcome the suturing difficulties. Suturing skills can be learnt with training. In a review of the first 50 cases I performed the operating time halved, largely due to improved suturing skills but also due to improved familiarity of all members of the theatre team with the procedure. The laparoscopic approach now takes on average 15 minutes longer than the open approach.

Surgical technique

Position on operating table

The most convenient position, which allows the surgeon to insert fingers in the vagina to aid mobilization of the paraurethral fascia, is the reverse Trendelenberg with an assistant sitting in between the patient's legs.

Access to retropubic space

All laparoscopic surgeons need to be aware of the vessels of the anterior abdominal wall. The inferior epigastric artery is most at risk when using the transperitoneal approach.

Transperitoneal Optimal port positions for the transperitoneal approach are illustrated in Fig. 46.1. Advantages of the transperitoneal approach are as follows:

1 Intraperitoneal procedures may be performed, including treatment of enterocele
2 Larger operating field
3 There is easier access to the upper lateral vaginal wall, which is important for paravaginal repair.

Disadvantages of transperitoneal approach are as follows:

1 Risk of injury to inferior epigastric artery
2 Risk of bowel or other vascular injury with port insertion
3 Risk of bladder injury when opening peritoneum
4 Risk of hernia from port wounds
5 Intraperitoneal adhesions from previous surgery may limit access to anterior abdominal wall.

Extraperitoneal approach Under normal conditions the loose areolar connective tissue of the retropubic space can be divided easily with blunt dissection. Balloon devices are available and may prove helpful.

The main difficulty with this approach is avoiding bladder injury. Adhesions from previous pelvic surgery can lead to the bladder being adherent to the anterior abdominal wall. This can be best overcome by dissection into the retropubic space lateral to the midline at first, since most adhesions from previous surgery occur centrally and are easier to identify when the space has been opened laterally.

Mobilization of periurethral fascia

The surgeon's index finger is placed in the vagina lateral to the bladder neck whilst the bladder is

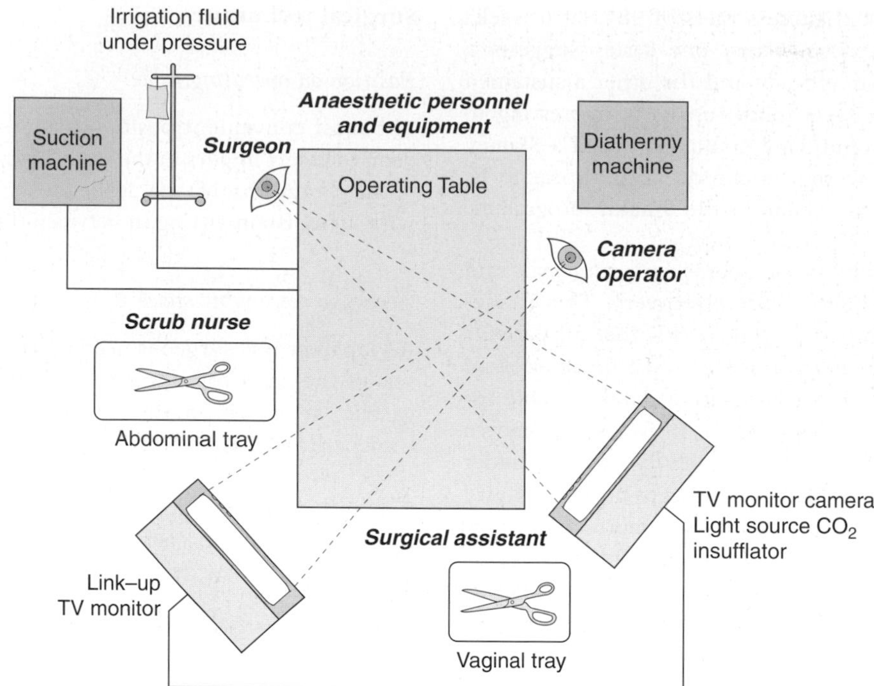

Fig. 46.1 Laparoscopy: positioning of theatre personnel and equipment.

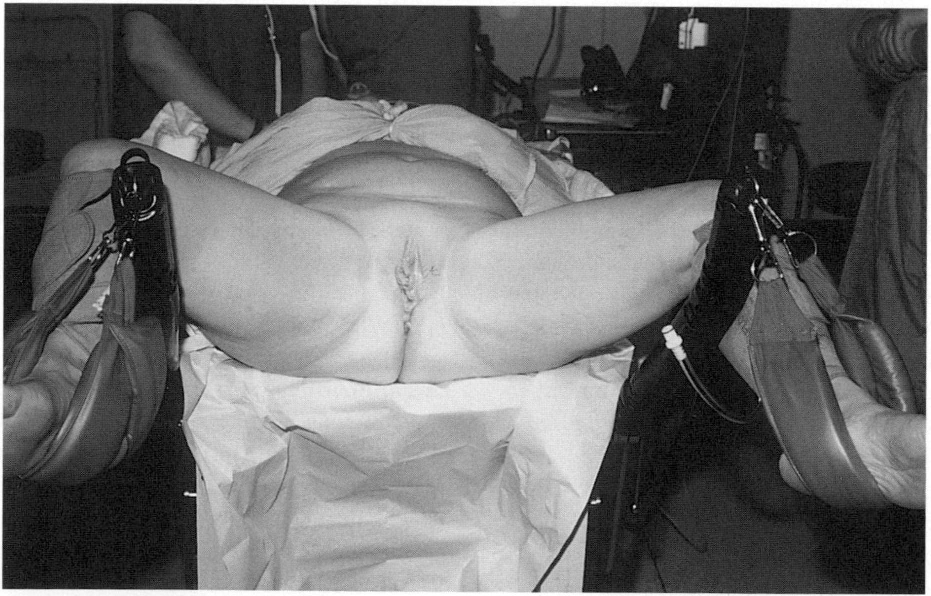

Fig. 46.2 Colposuspension: patient position.

mobilized medially with the aid of a pledget. It is advisable to tie a long suture to the pledget to avoid losing it. Disposable pledgets fixed to a holder are available.

Fixation of periurethral fascia to Cooper's ligament

Using a straight needle attached to a suture of choice, two bites of the periurethral fascia are taken and a single bite of Cooper's ligament taken and the needle withdrawn. When the tissues are poor, a full thickness bite of the fascia is advisable to reduce the risk of tearing. A Roeder knot is tied and pushed down with an assistant's finger elevating the fascia. It is not always possible to attain direct approximation of fascia to ligament, particularly when an anterior vaginal repair has been performed previously. The author places two sutures on each side to ensure a strong

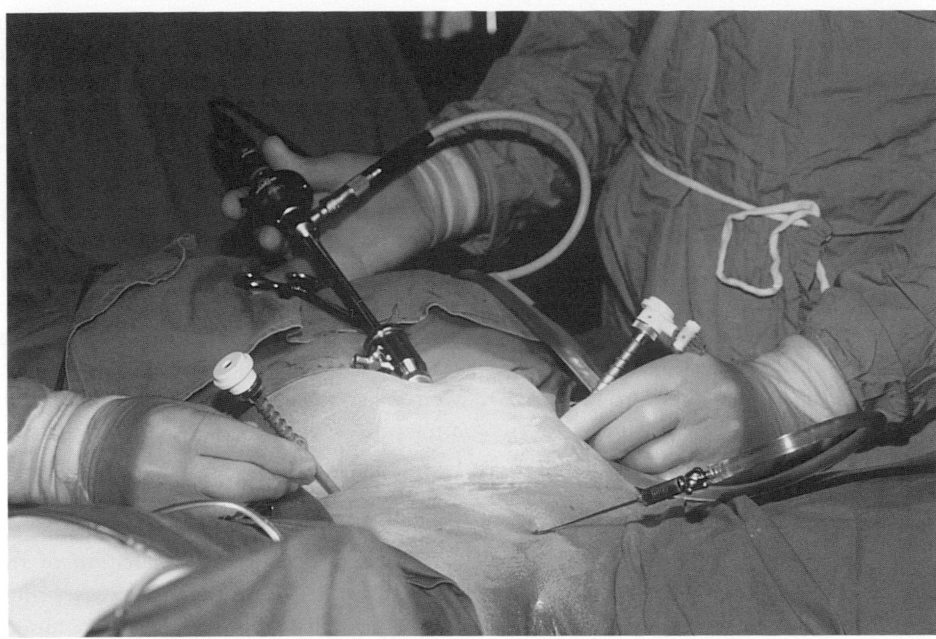

Fig. 46.3 Colposuspension: port positions.

fixation and two bites of the fascia are taken with the first suture. The main difference from open colposuspension is that a narrower area of fascia is elevated with the laparoscopic route, although the difference is not obvious on vaginal examination after the procedure.

If a paravaginal repair is performed, less bladder mobilization is required, but a curved needle is necessary to enable access for fixation of the endopelvic fascia to the fascia on the pelvic side wall.

Suprapubic catheterization

The author uses suprapubic catheterization on account of the ease of management of patients with postoperative voiding difficulties. The bladder is filled via the urethral catheter which is present throughout surgery on free drainage. The suprapubic catheter is inserted under direct vision into the bladder. A Bonnano catheter is suitable, but other types serve the purpose equally well.

Peritoneal closure

The anterior abdominal peritoneum may be closed, but this is not necessary if the peritoneal incision is large. A narrow gap in the peritoneum could lead to bowel entrapment. In 3 out of 4 cases in which the author has re-entered the peritoneal cavity some months after laparoscopic colposuspension, the peritoneum has healed normally. In one case the retropubic space remained open, but had become peritonealized.

Wound closure

There is a significant risk of hernia formation in port wounds of more than 5 mm diameter. A full thickness closure is therefore required in lateral wounds of more than 5 mm. Disposable and re-usable devices are available for this.

Postoperative care

The author clamps the suprapubic catheter 36 hours after surgery and removes the suprapubic catheter when the residual urine is less than 150 ml. In the author's experience most catheters can be removed by the fourth day, but voiding problems after this are not uncommon. Rarely, long-term intermittent self-catheterization is required.

Results

In Manchester we have found that the incidence of postoperative pyrexia is reduced from 31% to 11% and wound infection from 8% to 1%. The doses of narcotic analgesia required halved after laparoscopic colposuspension, when compared, retrospectively, to 50 women who underwent open colposuspension in the unit during a similar time period. The average time for postoperative catheterization was also reduced but voiding problems were not uncommon in both groups and so length of hospital stay (since women in the UK are reluctant to return home with a catheter in place) was only reduced by 3 days on average. At 6 months review with urodynamics the objective cure rate was similar but women said that return to normal took 9 weeks after laparoscopic colposuspension, compared to 19 weeks after open colposuspension. There was no statistical difference in the incidence of new detrusor instability on urodynamics at 6 months between the two groups. A 2-year questionnaire review has been performed which has revealed that 58% of the laparoscopic group never leak urine and 50% of the open group never leak, although 94% of the laparoscopic group said they were satisfied with the result of their surgery compared with 80% of the open group. This retrospective review is flawed in many ways, with the potential for bias (in both directions) in a number of areas but it indicates that, at 2-year follow-up of two demographically and clinically similar groups of women, there is no major difference in cure rate between the open and laparoscopic techniques and highlights the need for a randomized prospective study involving a large number of patients.

LAPAROSCOPIC SACROCOLPOPEXY

A number of abdominal procedures have been described for the treatment of vaginal vault prolapse, including anchorage of the vaginal vault to the anterior abdominal wall with fascial strips or non-absorbable sutures (Brady 1936) or elevation of the vault towards the sacrum. Several techniques for anchoring the vaginal vault to the sacrum have been described and one of the earliest was that by Lane (1962) in which a synthetic graft is sutured from the vaginal vault to the sacral promontory. Nichols et al (1970), using radiological studies, concluded that the correct axis of the vaginal vault is directed towards the hollow of the sacrum. Birnbaum (1973) described attachment of the vault to the hollow of the sacrum with Teflon mesh to achieve the correct axis. Different materials have been used to anchor the vaginal vault: Marlex mesh (Grundsell & Larsson 1984), Mersilene (Yates 1975; Addison et al 1985; Creighton & Stanton 1991) or fascia lata (Ridley et al 1976). These procedures have resulted in success rates ranging from 91%–100%.

Laparoscopic sacrocolpopexy was first reported by Nezhat et al (1994). Fifteen cases were included in which a 2.5 cm by 10 cm piece of Mersilene or Gore-Tex mesh (W L Gore & Associates, Inc, Phoenix, AZ) was sutured to the vaginal apex and sutured or stapled to the sacrum. Follow-up from 3 to 40 months is reported with 'complete relief of their symptoms' in all cases. One woman required a laparotomy for bleeding from the presacral area. In 1995, a series of 29 cases was reviewed retrospectively by Mahendran et al from Manchester (1996). In this series one recurrence of vault prolapse was reported, in follow-up ranging from 6 months to 2 years. Of interest was the finding of low rectoceles in 10 of the women when examined 6 months postoperatively, although the women were not always aware of the prolapse. In an attempt to reduce the incidence of recurrence of posterior vaginal wall prolapse I performed a number of procedures in which prolene mesh was introduced vaginally during a conventional posterior repair, thereby reinforcing the full length of the posterior vaginal wall. A series of over 35 cases illustrated that this is generally followed by an uncomplicated recovery but trimming of the mesh in the out-patient clinic was required in 1 in 4 cases. In one case a mesh was removed after a perineal abscess developed but this was thought to be related to an anal sphincter repair rather than the mesh. Subsequently a more extensive dissection between the vagina and rectum has been employed laparoscopically, enabling the mesh to be placed down to the level of the perineum without opening the vagina. This dissection can be difficult, particularly since most women have undergone previous surgery in the region. In one case, a hole was made in the rectum, but after laparoscopic repair the procedure was uneventful, as was the recovery. Since patients who have vaginal vault prolapse are often frail, elderly and obese, the benefits of laparoscopic surgery are more obvious than for colposuspension. Ross (1997) published a 12-month review of 19 women following laparoscopic surgery for post-hysterectomy 'vault eversion'. All 19 women underwent sacrocolpopexy, modified culdoplasty and Burch urethropexy. Six paravaginal and 13 posterior vaginal repairs were performed. Prolene mesh was sutured to the circumference of the vaginal apex and passed through a peritoneal tunnel to be sutured to the anterior sacral ligaments. Bladder injury occurred in three cases but all women were discharged within 24 hours of surgery and no patient had a catheter in place for more than 4 days. At one year after surgery one woman had 'mild' stress incontinence (compared to 17 preoperatively), 2 women had cystoceles and 3 rectoceles. This represents quite a high recurrence rate of lower vaginal prolapse at short-term follow-up, despite extensive repair surgery.

Technique

Once anaesthetized, the patient is placed in the reverse Trendelenberg position with the legs in Lloyd Davies stirrups. The bladder is then catheterized with a size 18 Foley catheter. A pneumoperitoneum is created by inserting a Veress needle suprapubically. A subumbilical 10 mm port is used for the laparoscope and two further ports introduced; a left lateral 5 mm port and a right lateral 12 mm port. Particular care is taken not to damage the inferior epigastric artery. These two lateral ports are used to introduce the instruments used to perform the procedure. The peritoneum over the vaginal vault is opened using the diathermy scissors and the bladder dissected anteriorly and the rectum posteriorly to expose the vaginal vault and posterior vaginal wall. This dissection is made easier by the introduction of two fingers, or a vaginal dilator, into the vagina by an assistant to elevate the vault. A prolene mesh graft is inserted into the pelvis through one of the ports. The graft is sutured to the vaginal vault using No. '0' PDS Endoknot (Ethicon, Scotland). Initially four sutures were used to secure the graft over an area 3 cm by 3 cm. With increasing experience, this area has been extended to include the whole of the posterior vaginal wall, including beyond the rectal reflection. Anchorage of the graft along the full length of the vaginal to the perineum will reduce the risk of posterior vaginal wall prolapse postoperatively. In cases where there is an obvious deficit in the upper anterior vaginal wall, this area is also covered with mesh.

The sacral promontory is identified and the peritoneum over the promontory is incised over an 8 cm vertical area using diathermy scissors, and the retroperitoneal tissue is dissected away from the periosteum of the promontory. This length incision is required to mobilize sufficient peritoneum to cover the mesh after fixation to the vagina and sacrum. Careful identification of the rectum to the left of the incision and the right internal iliac artery and right ureter is carried out during this dissection. Care is also taken with vessels running over the sacral promontory.

The graft is then secured to the sacrum using a hernia stapling device (either Autosuture–Autosuture Ltd, England – or Ethicon). The open weave type of graft has been found to be easier to suture and staple through than materials of a closer weave (e.g. Gore-Tex). The graft can be sutured to the sacral promontory, but this can be difficult. The stapler is much quicker and easier and would appear to provide a secure attachment. The authors have found that it is easier to achieve the appropriate tension in the graft by fixation to the vagina first. The vagina is then supported by a dilator while the mesh is aligned over the sacrum and the staples inserted. Any excess mesh can then be trimmed away. Having anchored the graft, the peritoneum over the graft is closed using the staples in order to close off any potential gap that could lead to an internal hernia. The patients are given an intraoperative bolus dose of Augmentin 1.2 g intravenously.

Results

A series of 29 patients who underwent laparoscopic sacrocolpopexy has been reported (Mahendran et al 1996). This paper demonstrates that the technique is safe and effective. Few intraoperative problems occurred although bladder injury occurred on two occasions, one of which occurred during colposuspension where there were adhesions from previous surgery. The mean theatre time was 123 minutes (including anaesthesia time), which is longer than

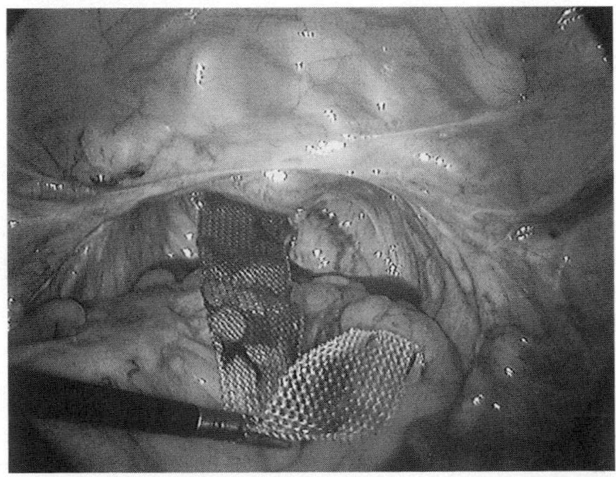

Fig. 46.4 Sacrocolpopexy: mesh secured to the vagina before fixation to sacrum.

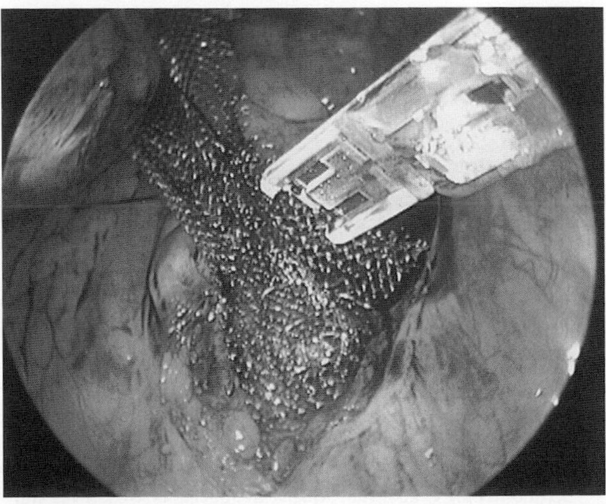

Fig. 46.5 Sacrocolpopexy: fixation of mesh to sacrum with stapler.

open surgery, although this time includes the 'learning curve' times. Postoperative recovery was markedly different from the author's experience of open surgery where ileus is not uncommon. Seventeen of the 29 cases returned home within 72 hours of surgery with a range of 1–8 days (mean 3 days). At follow-up the main problem has been of recurrence of lower posterior vaginal wall prolapse (10 cases) and it is felt that attachment of the mesh was not as low as had been thought. All women have been questioned about dyspareunia and this has not been a problem at 6 months or beyond in those women who were sexually active. Stress incontinence has been reported postoperatively and the author now performs a colposuspension when there has not been any previous retropubic surgery.

REPAIR OF ENTEROCELE AND RECTOCELE

The first published report of laparoscopic repair of enterocele in 1993 (Vancaille & Butler 1993) included 18 women in whom the enterocele repair was performed in combination with a posterior repair, a laparoscopic Burch colposuspension and in some cases a hysterectomy. In one case the enterocele repair was not possible due to intraperitoneal adhesions from previous surgery. Medial displacement of the ureter was noted in 6 of the 17 cases but no detriment to function occurred. In one case a suture was placed through the ureter but recognized and removed immediately. Most patients were discharged within 48 hours but voiding difficulties kept a few cases hospitalized for up to 5 days. Follow-up was 12 months in one case but less in the remainder. No evidence of enterocele was seen on examination but 2 of the women were troubled by dyspareunia.

A descriptive report of a new laparoscopic approach to enterocele repair (Lam & Rosen 1997) detailed a technique based upon the principles of the Zacharin abdomino-perineal repair. Forty women underwent surgery which included major concomitant surgery in 37 cases. Bladder perforation occurred in one case but the intraoperative blood loss was only 40 ml on average. Twenty-five out of the 40 women experienced low back pain postoperatively and 20 out of the 40 women complained of constipation. The average length of hospitalization was 2.2 days (range 1–7 days) and all were reported as being able to return to normal activity within 1–2 weeks. For reasons that are not made clear there are no details of further follow-up.

The only published series of laparoscopic rectocele repair included a series of 20 women in whom a polyglactin mesh was sutured into the plane between vagina and rectum (Lyons & Winer 1997). All 20 women underwent a laparoscopic colposuspension and McCall colpopexy, 16 underwent a paravaginal repair, 12 a supracervical hysterectomy, 4 a sacrocolpopexy, 3 a rectopexy and 3 a perineorrhaphy. No intraoperative problems were reported, with the average estimated blood loss being 5 ml. In no cases was there fever, anaemia or re-hospitalization and all women were discharged within 24 hours. At 12-month review no women reported dyspareunia and a '95% rate of symptom relief' is given without any details of findings on examination.

CONCLUSIONS

Laparoscopic pelvic reconstructive surgery is still in its infancy, particularly with regard to evaluation. It is clear that reproduction of the open techniques is possible but this does not equate to reproduction of results. Prospective randomized comparative studies are required for a true evaluation.

REFERENCES

Addison W A et al 1985 Abdominal sacral colpopexy with mersilene mesh in the retroperitoneal position in the management of post-hysterectomy vaginal vault prolapse and enterocoele. American Journal of Obstetrics and Gynecology 153: 140–146

Benson J T, Lucente V, McClellan E 1996 Vaginal versus abdominal reconstructive surgery for the treatment of pelvic support defects: a prospective randomized study with long-term outcome evaulation. American Journal of Obstetrics and Gynecology 175: 1418–1422

Birnbaum S J 1973 Rational therapy for the prolapsed vagina. American Journal of Obstetrics and Gynecology 115: 411–419

Brady L 1936 An operation to correct genital prolapse following panhysterectomy. American Journal of Obstetrics and Gynecology 32: 295–297

Burch J C 1961 Urethrovaginal fixation to Cooper's ligament for correction of stress incontinence, cystocoele and prolapse. American Journal of Obstetrics and Gynecology 81–281

Burton G 1996 A three year prospective randomised urodynamic study comparing open and laparoscopic colposuspension.

Continence Foundation Australia. Annual Scientific Meeting, August, Melbourne
Creighton S M, Stanton S L 1991 The surgical management of vaginal vault prolapse. British Journal of Obstetrics and Gynaecology 98: 1150–1154
Fothergill W E 1921 The end results of vaginal operations for genital prolapse. Journal of Obstetrics and Gynaecology of the British Empire 28: 251–255
Grundsell H, Larsson G 1984 Operative management of vaginal vault prolapse following hysterectomy. British Journal of Obstetrics and Gynaecology 91: 808–811
Lam A, Rosen D 1997 A new laparoscopic approach for enterocoele repair. Gynaecological Endoscopy 6: 211–217
Lane F E 1962 Repair of post-hysterectomy vaginal vault prolapse. Obstetrics and Gynecology 20: 72–77
Liu C Y 1993 Laparoscopic retropubic colposuspension (Burch procedure). Journal of Reproductive Medicine 38: 526–530
Lobel R W, Sand P K 1996 Long term results of laparoscopic Burch colposuspension. Neurourology and Urodynamics 15: 398–399
Lyons T L, Winer W K 1997 Laparoscopic rectocoele repair using polyglactin mesh. Journal of the American Association of Gynecologic Laparoscopists 4(3): 381–384
MacKenzie I Z 1996 Reducing hospital stay after abdominal hysterectomy. British Journal of Obstetrics and Gynaecology 103: 175–178
Mahendran D, Prashar S, Smith A R B, Murphy D 1996 Laparoscopic sacrocolpopexy in the management of vaginal vault prolapse. Gynaecological Endoscopy 5: 217–222
Majeed A W, Troy G, Nicholl J P et al 1996 Randomised, prospective, single-blind comparison of laparoscopic versus small-incision cholecystectomy. The Lancet 347: 989–994
Marshall V F, Marchetti A A, Krantz K E 1949 The correction of stress incontinence by simple vesicoureteral suspension. Surgery, Gynecology and Obstetrics 88: 509–518
Nezhat C H, Nezhat F, Nezhat C R 1994 Laparoscopic sacral colpopexy for vaginal vault prolapse. Obstetrics and Gynecology 84(5): 885–888
Nichols D H, Miley P S, Randall C L 1970 Significance of restoration of normal vaginal depth and axis. Obstetrics and Gynecology 36: 251–256
O'Sullivan D C, Chilton C P, Munson K W 1995 Should Stamey colposuspension be our primary surgery for stress incontinence? British Journal of Urology 4: 457–460
Pereyra A J 1959 A simplified surgical procedure for the correction of stress urinary incontinence in women. Western Journal of Surgery, Obstetrics and Gynaecology 67: 223–226
Ridley J H, Botte J M, Howlett R J 1976 A composite vaginal vault suspensions using fascia lata. American Journal of Obstetrics and Gynecology 126: 590–595
Ross J W 1996 Two year objective follow up of laparoscopic Burch colposuspension. Proceedings of the International Continence Society, Athens, pp 364–365
Ross J W 1997 Techniques of laparoscopic repair of total vault eversion after hysterectomy. Journal of the American Association of Gynecologic Laparoscopists 4(2): 173–183
Stamey T A 1973 Endoscopic suspension of the vesical neck for urinary incontinence. Surgery, Gynecology and Obstetrics 136: 547–554
Vancaillie T G, Butler D J 1993 Laparoscopic enterocoele repair – description of a new technique. Gynaecological Endoscopy 2: 211–216
Vancaillie T G, Schuessler W 1991 Laparoscopic bladder neck suspension. Journal of Laparoendoscopic Surgery 3: 169–173
White G R 1909 Cystocoele. Journal of the American Medical Association 53: 1707
Yates M J 1975 An abdominal approach to the repair of post-hysterectomy vaginal invasion. British Journal of Obstetrics and Gynaecology 82: 817–819

Bladder retraining

KATE ANDERS

INTRODUCTION

A child learns voluntary control of the bladder at an early age. A toddler is taught to recognize the symptoms of a full bladder before the reflex mechanism causes an involuntary contraction and empties the bladder inappropriately. This learning process towards continence relies on normal physiological, anatomical and neurological function, as well as a conscious requirement to become socially aware of the need to be dry.

Both parent and child will begin to identify the signs of an impending bladder contraction, thus permitting involuntary micturition to be inhibited. This gives rise to continence and allows a gradual increase in the child's bladder capacity. The process is often referred to as potty training, toilet training or bladder training.

DEFINITIONS AND PRINCIPLES

A malfunction in the voluntary control of the bladder can give rise to urinary incontinence in adult life, causing the trained process of bladder function learnt in childhood to be lost. To regain this control it is possible to instigate a regimen of bladder re-education. This is also described in the literature as bladder re-training, bladder drill or habit re-training. Other programmes of bladder re-education are often termed 'prompted' and 'timed voiding', but these do not necessarily re-train the bladder to previous or 'normal' function.

The methods of bladder re-training are most commonly used in the treatment of frequency, urgency and urge incontinence (with or without urodynamically proven detrusor instability). Techniques differ in detail, depending on the patient, her symptoms and diagnosis, and the clinician's preferences. However, the principles are similar and are based on the desire to suppress urinary urge and to extend intervals between voiding. A bladder re-training regimen is generally initiated at set voiding intervals and the patient is not allowed to void between these predetermined times, even if she is incontinent. When she remains dry, then the time interval is lengthened. This will continue until a suitable time span is achieved, usually around 3–4 hours.

Non-specific incontinence of institutionalized patients, such as the confused, mentally handicapped or elderly infirm, is frequently approached in a manner of prompted voiding. The patient is asked at regular intervals if she needs to void, and is assisted if the response is positive. In some patients continence improves, but these will need continual monitoring, prompting and praise (Schnelle 1990). Timed voiding is a fixed voiding schedule, whether the desire to void is present or not. In institutions, this is perhaps the most common approach to avoiding incontinent episodes (Ouslander & Fowler 1985).

The principle in habit re-training is to primarily adopt a timed voiding schedule, perhaps 2-hourly. This is an individualized regimen which encourages the patient not to use the toilet in between times, although she is allowed, should she be unable to delay micturition. With use of observation and charts, her voiding patterns and incontinent episodes are noted over 2 to 3 days. The regimen is then adjusted to the individual. Incontinent episodes can then be anticipated and hopefully prevented. Once she is dry, the voiding intervals can be lengthened, although they can also be shortened again, should the desired effect not be achieved.

Hadley (1986) categorized these definitions in an attempt to distinguish between the differences in voiding adjustments (see Table 47.1).

Bladder re-education has also been used in the management of stress urinary incontinence with the assistance of pelvic floor physiotherapy (see Ch. 49), with or without biofeedback. However, this will not actually improve underlying urethral sphincter incompetence, although there is some evidence that it may help reduce episodes of leakage, because the patient will keep the volume of her bladder reduced, (US Department of Health and Human Services 1992). Many professionals instigating a regimen of bladder re-training frequently advise the instruction of pelvic floor exercises, in conjunction with the proposed programme, as this can help suppress urinary urgency (Norton 1996; Wilson & Herbison 1995).

Other uses of bladder re-education are in the potential restoration of bladder tone during intermittent catheter clamping, usually within an acute setting, before removal of the catheter (bladder drainage techniques are covered in Ch. 44). Women who suffer from chronic urinary retention, with overflow incontinence, are unlikely to benefit from bladder re-training due to the nature and the aetiology of their condition. In patients with neurological deficits, bladder re-training is indicated, but this is often executed in the form of intermittent catheterization to aid bladder emptying and thus continence, rather than active re-training of the bladder to enable former function. This type of treatment is frequently supplemented with anticholinergic therapy in patients suffering from sphincter dyssynergia and detrusor hyperreflexia (Perkash 1993).

Table 47.1 Differences in scheduling adjustments of bladder re-training and related protocols.

Regimen	Change in intervoiding over course of regimen
Bladder re-training	Increased
Habit re-training	Increased or decreased
Timed voiding	Unchanged
Prompted voiding	Schedule unchanged/interval variable

REVIEW OF PROGRAMMES

Reports on bladder re-training have shown effective treatment in curing urinary frequency, urgency and urge incontinence, predominantly in patients with detrusor instability, with cure rates of 44%–90% in trials without any pharmacological assistance (Pengally & Booth 1980; Jarvis & Millar 1980). However, these successes tend to be instigated as in-patient regimens, although some deem this unnecessary (Oldenburg & Millard 1986).

A planned programme of bladder re-education was first described by Jeffcoate & Francis in 1966. They hypothesized that urinary symptoms were often psychologically influenced. In a study of 300 women with symptoms of urge incontinence, 50% of them related an emotional event surrounding the onset of their symptoms. A course of management was created for 247 of these women (women who had an organic lesion for their urinary incontinence were not used in this study), with the emphasis on discipline to eliminate the long-standing habit of atypical voiding. All patients were hospitalized in an attempt to remove outside influences which could affect their emotional status. The authors believed that the reassurance and discipline that the nursing staff could provide was invaluable to gain the continued motivation and compliance for the patients to adhere to the set programme. The bladder re-training programme which they prescribed was based on an incremental regimen of voiding so as to increase the functional capacity of the bladder. Voiding was initiated by the clock, rather than by desire, generally at 1-hour intervals to start, and the patients were unable to go to the toilet between these set times. When continence was achieved within these times, then the time span was increased by half-hourly intervals.

Success was measured by the achievement of increasing these time spans to 3.5 hours, without incontinent episodes or discomfort, in the hope that this in turn would restore lost confidence. Their cure rate was 67% after one year.

Unfortunately, voiding regimens can break down due to lack of staffing and a wish not to disturb patients at night. Patients are often motivated to set alarms at night when they are at home, but sadly many carers or relatives are not prepared to have their sleeping patterns disturbed in order to prompt patients to waken and supervise them to the toilet. This can consequently lead a patient dry by 2-hourly voids to become wet on discharge home (Castleden & Duffin 1981).

There is some controversy about whether psychological imbalance causes urinary complaints which have no pathological, anatomical or neurological origins, or whether the urinary symptoms are psychosomatic. Frewent (1978), as well as many other researchers (Willington 1975; Elder & Stephenson 1980; Macaulay et al 1987), discussed the close link between bladder and mind. They all believed a strong psychosomatic influence was to blame for urinary frequency and urgency.

In contrast, Oldenburg & Millard (1986) looked at the psychological status of 53 women before a bladder re-training programme and at the 18-month follow-up. They found that the psychological status was improved and consequently concluded that the urinary complaints were a predisposing factor in the cause of psychological distress, rather than Frewen's idea that it was the psychological distress that manifested in urinary symptoms.

Macaulay et al (1987) found that bladder training was effective in treating urinary frequency and women became less anxious and depressed. Their results showed that psychotherapy can have an impact on urinary symptoms.

Frewen in 1972 described a bladder re-training programme similar to that of Jeffcoate & Francis. He named a mode of therapy called psychomedical treatment. It involved hospitalization, a written instruction sheet which included an explanation of the complaint and treatment, drug therapy – usually anticholinergic—and a urinary frequency chart. He also recognized the continuous need for reassurance and for staff to maintain the motivation necessary in achieving the ultimate goal of restoring confidence.

His subsequent work in 1978, of 40 women with detrusor instability, showed an objective cure rate of 82.5% after 3 months. Objective outcomes were measured by the restoration of a stable bladder during cystometry. The 7 cases that failed all had predisposing emotional disturbances that were unresolved.

In 1980, Frewen suggested that women with urinary frequency and urgency, but with urodynamically stable bladders, could possibly go on to develop idiopathic detrusor instability. The idea he promoted was that if bladder re-training were instigated at this stage then the progression to detrusor instability could be prevented. Although this gives interesting thought to clinical practice, there is no evidence to substantiate it. He advocates that if a woman is aware that it is the small bladder capacity that creates her urinary symptoms, then she should be able to increase it by a re-training scheme and subsequently cure herself of these symptoms.

There has been some evidence to show the benefits of bladder re-training in women complaining of mixed urinary symptoms. Fantl et al (1991) found a 50% reduction in the incidence of incontinent episodes in 75% of the women they studied.

Interestingly, Ramsay et al (1994) randomized 60 women to either undergo urodynamics and then treatment appropriate to their diagnosis, or to have in-patient bladder re-training and pelvic floor therapy. They found little difference between the two groups after 3 months. Although this allows an attractive concept for practitioners in attempting to treat women with uncomplicated urinary complaints without prior urodynamics, there still remains a continued need to perform further long-term studies to substantiate this. Presently, urodynamic investigations still play an important role in diagnosis, treatment and objective outcomes.

PRACTICAL CONSIDERATIONS

Bladder re-training is an attractive form of treatment for urinary incontinence as this type of treatment is generally simple, reversible and low-risk, with minimal, if any, side-effects (Wilson & Herbison 1995).

The National Institute of Health consensus conference in 1989 concluded that the 'least invasive of dangerous procedure should be tried first' when attempting to treat incontinence and that 'for many forms of incontinence, behavioural therapy meets this criterion'. Bladder re-training can be a time-consuming exercise with the need for additional resources, such as nursing time, to be most effective. However, this is outweighed by the cost savings created by the reduction in laundry needs and incontinence aids, such as pads, which are used in an attempt to control urinary incontinence (Ouslander & Kane 1983; Hu 1986).

All re-education programmes for the bladder basically attempt to achieve the same goals. Described by Hadley in 1986 they:

1 Re-train the bladder to a 'normal' or improved voiding pattern so as to restore confidence
2 Avoid episodes of incontinence by timed and prompted voiding.

The first type of regimen requires active and motivated participation by the patient, who needs to be self-ambulant and mentally aware, whilst the second may need active assistance, both physically and mentally, from either the health care professional or carer.

Assessment

Common principles are found in many of the regimens or programmes used in bladder re-training. Any programme of treatment should include a careful assessment with detailed medical and surgical history. Concomitant medical disease and medications can have a high impact on the bladder and its function: e.g. cardiac disease and the use of diuretics influence urinary frequency and nocturia, especially in the elderly population. Fluid, caffeine and alcohol intake should also be noted. A physical examination and urodynamic investigations should ideally be performed to elucidate a diagnosis, and secondly to determine bladder capacity.

Possible contributing factors need to be eliminated, such as a urinary tract infection or constipation, as these will certainly impede the road to success. Suitable training programmes need to be tailored for the patient as no set programme will suit all. A detailed assessment of the patient's mental awareness, mobility, dexterity, social skills and ability to cooperate must therefore be taken into account.

Explanations

Before the onset of any programme a full explanation and instructions to all those involved must be given. Understanding that it is quite often sheer will power from the patient that makes bladder re-education work needs to be emphasized and maintained. Continuous encouragement and reassurance to restore confidence will ultimately achieve the best results. If the patient is unable to meet the criteria or falters in motivation or compliance, there is little point in continuing this type of treatment. Even in the use of prompted or timed voiding with the mentally handicapped or elderly infirm, this rule will apply, but in these cases the emphasis may point towards those supervising the programme.

Observation and monitoring

Monitoring voiding patterns at baseline and subsequently during a bladder re-education programme is fundamental in the management of urinary incontinence. The use of continence charts is widely accepted and they are of help to both patient and supervisor.

Ouslander et al (1986) advocate their use for:

- Assessment and documentation of continence status
- Identification of associated factors
- Planning and monitoring of a suitable regimen
- Assessing objective outcomes.

Continence charts are simple and easy to use, making useful modes of assessment at baseline for urinary frequency, timing and incontinence episodes (see Fig. 47.1). However, there is little room for additional information which may help in diagnosis and treatment. More complicated charts can often be impractical in an out-patient setting, but may prove more useful as a means of continued management while a regimen is instigated in an in-patient context.

Detailed charts have been developed in an attempt to create one that gives:

1 Clear differentiation between incontinent episodes, successful voiding and a dry check
2 Assessment of amount of leakage and need to change clothing etc.
3 Actual voided volume
4 Awareness of bladder sensation or incontinent episode
5 Circumstance surrounding an incontinent episode
6 Occurrence of any additional faecal incontinence.

The use of colour-coded stickers to identify episodes of incontinence and voiding has been reported to be useful in the execution of bladder re-training programmes (Autry et al 1984; Ouslander et al 1986).

The full potential of any type of continence chart can only really be achieved by adapting preferred charts to suit the needs of the clinician and the indi-

Time	Monday		Tuesday		Wednesday		Thursday		Friday		Saturday		Sunday	
6.00 am														
7.00 am														
8.00 am														
9.00 am														
10.00 am														
11.00 am														
12.00														
1.00 pm														
2.00 pm														
3.00 pm														
4.00 pm														
5.00 pm														
6.00 pm														
7.00 pm														
8.00 pm														
9.00 pm														
10.00 pm														
11.00 pm														
12.00														
Total														

☐ *Tick when using toilet* ☐ *Tick when wet*

Fig. 47.1 Continence chart.

vidual patient. Proper instruction in the use of continence charts is fundamental if they are to be a useful tool.

Fluids

Women with urinary incontinence often adjust their fluid intake in an attempt to control their symptoms. Restrictions in fluid intake can, however, have adverse effects. Frequent voiding in combination with a low urine output can result in a reduction of the bladder's functional capacity, resulting in habitual voiding at smaller volumes. Very low fluid intakes are dangerous, especially in the elderly, and should be discouraged. Dehydration can lead to electrolyte imbalance and confusion. The incidence of constipation can be increased and recurrent urinary tract infections may become common.

Women should be encouraged to consume around 1.5 litres of fluid over a 24-hour period. It is possible, though, to alter the times when fluid is taken to suit the needs of the individual woman. She may reduce her fluid intake before going to bed, if her main problem is nocturia, or drink less before going out. It is important to emphasize that this should be a reduction rather than a complete abstinence of fluid over that time.

Other considerations need to be made in the reduction of caffeine-based drinks and alcohol. Creighton & Stanton (1990) found that caffeine had an irritant effect on the bladder.

COMPLEMENTARY THERAPIES

Drug therapy

For women who experience urinary frequency, urgency and urge incontinence, pharmacological agents which increase the bladder's capacity may provide a beneficial addition to a regimen of bladder re-training.

Drug therapy commonly used in the treatment of irritative bladder symptoms include:

- Anticholinergics
- Smooth muscle relaxants
- Calcium channel blockers
- Tricyclic antidepressants
- Oestrogens
- *α*-adrenergic agonists
- Antidiuretics.

Some agents which have been recommended include oxybutynin (Tapp et al 1989; Moore et al 1990), propantheline (Holmes et al 1989) and imipramine (Castheden et al 1981). Oxybutynin is, perhaps, the most widely used in conjunction with bladder re-training.

Trials comparing bladder re-training with drug therapy are limited. Szonyi et al (1995) carried out a randomized, double-blind, parallel-group study. Sixty patients were included in the study. All were instructed in bladder re-training and randomized either to oxybutynin or to placebo. The results showed that the group taking the oxybutynin had a higher reduction in urinary urgency. The authors concluded that this may have been successful in promoting continence by delaying micturition while the bladder re-training regimen was in progress. However, these results did not allow conclusions to be drawn on the efficacy of bladder re-training.

Jarvis (1981) compared out-patient drug therapy with in-patient bladder drill in 50 women over a 4-week period. He found a significant difference in success between the two groups. In the 25 women who had bladder drill, there was an 84% cure rate, compared to only 54% in the women who were on drug therapy. He concluded that, with the advantage of fewer side-effects and an obvious better cure rate in the women studied, bladder drill was perhaps the treatment of choice.

Biofeedback

Other forms of alternative supplementary treatment include the use of biofeedback (Cardozo et al 1978). Biofeedback in the treatment of urinary urgency (detrusor instability) is a technique whereby the patient monitors her own cystometric recording, or other measurement, and observes the response of these indicators in order to control them. The only drawbacks with this type of treatment are that it is time-consuming and invasive. Studies have proved, however, that during cystometry it is possible to inhibit a detrusor contraction. Results by Cardozo et al showed a 40% cure rate in the 30 women studied, and a further 40% improvement rate in symptoms. Unfortunately, at a 5-year review (Cardozo & Stanton 1984) on 20 women, there was a high incidence of relapse.

The results are initially promising but ongoing motivation is paramount for long-term success. Biofeedback needs to be reinforced by continual training and exercise at home for it to be most effective.

Hypnotherapy and acupuncture

Other supplementary therapies include the application of hypnotherapy, which has been reported to have an 86% subjective and a 50% objective cure rate (Freeman & Baxby 1982), but this also sees a high relapse.

Acupuncture has similarly shown some positive results. It is thought that the opioid release may block or reduce the autonomic innervation of the detrusor and urethral sphincter mechanisms (Murray & Feneley 1982). Some studies have demonstrated a 76% subjective improvement (Philip et al 1988), although there is a lack of controlled trials due to the difficulty in creating a placebo. One trial comparing acupuncture to drug therapy, i.e. oxybutynin 5 mg b.d., showed no significant differences in efficacy between the two treatments. However, the women who recieved acupuncture reported fewer side-effects from their treatment (Kelleher et al 1994).

SUMMARY

There is good evidence that bladder re-training is effective in the short term. With few side-effects, if any, it would seem the treatment of choice in women with urinary frequency, urgency and urge incontinence, whether proven detrusor instability is present or not.

Long-term results, however, are very poorly reported on and many of the studies in the literature base their findings on subjective outcomes. This creates a continued need to perform long-term studies with comparable objective outcomes.

Like any form of behavioural therapy, bladder retraining requires constant encouragement, reassurance and discipline for results to be successful. Women need to be compliant and cooperative, and without tireless motivation this type of treatment will falter in its goals.

REFERENCES

Autry D, Luazon F, Holliday P 1984 The voiding record: an aid in decreasing incontinence. Geriatric Nursing: 22

Cardozo L D, Stanton S L 1984 A five year review. British Journal of Urology 50: 521–523

Cardozo L D, Abrams P D, Stanton S L et al 1978 Biofeedback in the treatment of detrusor instability. British Journal of Urology 50: 250–254

Castleden C M, Duffin H M 1981 Guidelines for controlling urinary incontinence without drugs or catheters. Age and Ageing 10: 246–249

Castleden C M, George C F, Renwick A G, Asher M J 1981 Imipramine, a possible alternative to current therapy for urinary incontinence in the elderly. Journal of Urology 125: 318–320

Creighton S, Stanton S 1990 Caffeine: does it effect your bladder? British Journal of Urology 66: 613–614

Elder D D, Stephenson T P 1980 An assessment of the Frewen regime in the treatment of detrusor dysfunction in females. British Journal of Urology 52: 467–471

Fantl J A, Wyman J F, McClish D K et al 1991 Efficacy of bladder training in older women with urinary incontinence. Journal of the American Medical Association 265: 609–613

Freeman R M, Baxby K 1982 Hypnotherapy for incontinence caused by detrusor instability. British Medical Journal 284: 1831–1832

Frewen W K 1972 Urgency incontinence. British Journal of Obstetrics and Gynaecology 79: 77–79

Frewen W K 1978 An objective assessment of the unstable bladder of psychosomatic origin. British Journal of Urology 50: 246–249

Frewen W K 1980 The management of urgency and frequency of micturition. British Journal of Urology 52: 367–369

Hadley G C 1986 Bladder training and related therapies for urinary incontinence in older people. Journal of the American Medical Association 256: 3

Holmes D M, Montz F J, Stanton S L 1989 Oxybutinin versus propantheline in the management of detrusor instability: a patient variable dose trial. British Journal of Obstetrics and Gynaecology 96: 607–612

Hu T W 1986 The economic impact of urinary incontinence. Clinics in Geriatric Medicine 2: 673–687

Jarvis G J 1981 A controlled trial of bladder drill and drug therapy in the management of detrusor instability. British Journal of Urology 53: 252–256

Jarvis G J, Millar D R 1980 Controlled trial of bladder drill for detrusor instability. British Medical Journal 281: 1322–1323

Jeffcoate T N A, Francis W J A 1966 Urgency incontinence in the female. American Journal of Obstetrics and Gynecology 94: 604–618

Kelleher C J, Rilsie J, Burton G, Cardozo L D 1994 Acupuncture and the treatment of irritative bladder symptoms in women. Journal of the British Medical Acupuncture Society V51 12: 9–12

Macaulay A J, Stern R S, Holmes D M, Stanton S L 1987 Micturition and the mind: psychological factors in the aetiology and the treatment of urinary symptoms in women. British Medical Journal 281: 540–543

Moore K H, Hay D M, Imrie A E, Watson A, Goldstein M 1990 Oxybutinin hydrocholoride (3 mg) in the treatment of women with detrusor instability. British Journal of Urology: 66: 479–485

Murray K H A, Feneley R C L 1982 Endorphins – a role in lower urinary tract function? The effect of opioid blockade on the detrusor and urethral mechanisms. British Journal of Urology 54: 638–640

National Institute of Health Conference 1989 Urinary incontinence in adults. Journal of the American Medical Association 261: 2685–2696

Norton C 1996 Nursing for continence. Beaconsfield Publishers Ltd, Beaconsfield

Oldenburg B F, Millard B F 1986 Predictions of long term outcome following a bladder retraining programme. Journal of Psychosomatic Research 30(6): 691–698

Ouslander J G, Kane R L 1983 The cost of urinary incontinence in nursing homes. Medical Care 22: 69–79

Ouslander J G, Fowler E 1985 The management of incontinence in Veterans Administration nursing homes. Journal of the American Geriatrics Society 33: 33–40

Ouslander J G, Urman H N, Uman G C 1986 Development and testing of an incontinence monitoring record. Journal of the American Geriatrics Society 34(2): 83–90

Pengally A W, Booth C M 1980 A prospective trial of bladder training as treatment for detrusor instability. British Journal of Urology 52: 463–466

Perkash I 1993 Long term urological management of the patient with spinal cord injury. Urologic Clinics of North America 20(3): 423–434

Philp T, Shah P J R, Worth P H L 1988 Acupuncture in the treatment of detrusor instability. British Journal of Urology 61: 409–493

Ramsay I, Hassan A, Hunter M, Donaldson K 1994 A randomised controlled trial of urodynamic investigations prior to conservative treatment of urinary incontinence in the female. Neurourology and Urodynamics 13: 455–456

Schnelle J F 1990 Treatment of urinary incontinence in nursing home patients by prompted voiding. Journal of the American Geriatrics Society 38(3): 373–376

Szonyi G, Collas D M, Yew Y, Ding Malone-Lee J G 1995 Oxybutinin with bladder retraining for detrusor instability in elderly people: a randomised controlled trial. Age and Ageing 24: 287–291

Tapp A J, Cardozo L D, Versi E, Cooper D 1989 The treatment of detrusor instability in post menopausal women with oxybutinin chloride: a double blind placebo controlled study. British Journal of Obestetrics and Gynaecology 97: 607–612

US Department of Health and Human Services 1992 Urinary incontinence in adults. Clinical practice guidelines. Agency for Health Care Policy and Research, US Dept. of Health and Human Services, Rockville

Willington F L 1975 Training and retraining for continence. Nursing Times 71: 500–503

Wilson D, Herbison P 1995 Conservative management of incontinence. Current Opinion in Obstetrics and Gynaecology 7: 386–392

SECTION 5
CHAPTER

48

Pads, pants and mechanical devices

KATE WANG

INTRODUCTION

As the awareness of incontinence increases, the number of companies marketing absorbent products grows. The Association of Continence Advisors directory of continence aids and appliances lists over 3000 products marketed in the UK by more than 100 companies, and the cost of pads accounts for more than half the annual Health Service expenditure on incontinence products in the UK (Cottenden 1988). While much incontinence can be cured or alleviated, treatment may take time to become effective and therefore the appropriate use of pads is an important tool in the management of the incontinent patient. The aim of the chapter is to provide an overview of three types of aids – pads, pants and mechanical devices.

PADS

Indications

The use of pads (and pants) would be indicated for patients in the following situations:

1. Those awaiting investigation
2. Those awaiting surgery
3. Those waiting for treatment to become effective
4. Those for whom investigation or active treatment is inappropriate
5. Those who have made an informed decision not to undertaken more active treatment.

Selection of pad

When selecting an absorbent product it is essential that it meets the requirements of both the patient and her incontinence, and therefore carers need a thorough knowledge about available products and should impart this to the patient. Blannin (1985) suggested three main factors to consider when choosing an incontinence aid:

1 Patient preference – the pad must be acceptable, comfortable and effective.
2 Degree of incontinence – is urine loss a dribble or a gush? How little or how much urine is lost? Is the problem greater at night or during the day? How frequently is the patient able to change the pad?
3 Mental and physical dexterity – pants that need a pad to be placed in a pouch are sometimes too difficult for some patients to cope with, either through lack of understanding or loss of dexterity.

Other points to consider are laundry facilities and disposal of pads – are there any special requirements laid down by the refuse collection department?

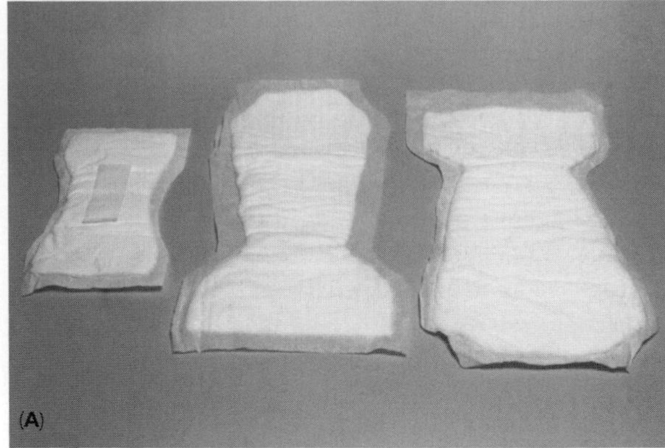

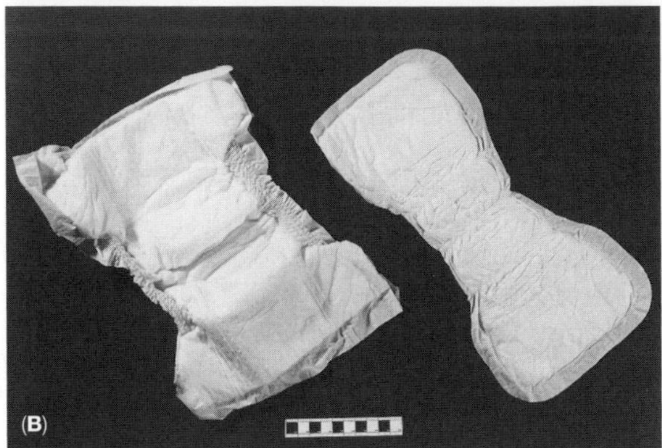

Fig. 48.1A,B A selection of disposable body-worn incontinence pads.

DISPOSABLE BODY-WORN PADS

Body-worn absorbent pads are used in conjunction with close-fitting pants or fixed into waterproof garments. They come in a range of sizes to accommodate different volumes of urine (Fig. 48.1). The simplest designs consist of a rectangle of fluff pulp encased in an envelope of liquid-permeable material known as the coverstock. This type of pad is used with pants with a waterproof layer behind the pad, e.g. the marsupial pant, which has an integral pouch to secure the pad.

A waterproof layer may be present on the aspect of the pad which is placed nearest the patient's clothing; some are rectangular shaped, but most are used with stretch net pants (Fig. 48.2). Others are shaped like all-in-one baby nappies, having such features as adhesive fastenings and elasticated legs.

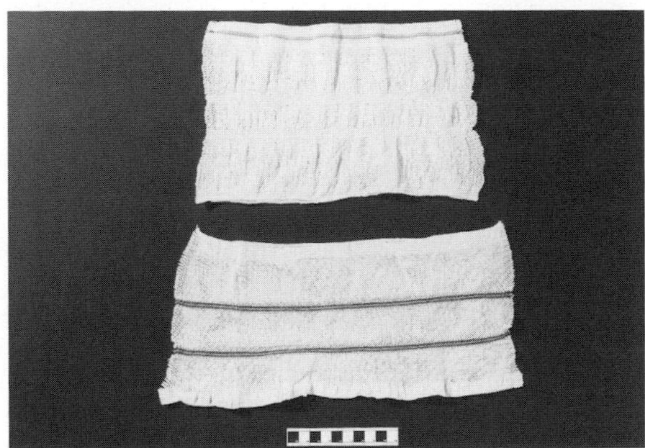

Fig. 48.2 Lightweight open-knitted stretch pants.

Pad design

Absorbents

Fluff pulp This is derived from fibres which have been pulped to remove the lignin and release the cellulosic fibres. Chemical and mechanical pulps are used in varying proportions to form fluff pulp. The advantages of fluff pulp are: (a) it is inexpensive and (b) it absorbs urine rapidly. The disadvantages are: (a) it increases pad bulk and (b) urine is squeezed out easily.

Superabsorbents The use of superabsorbent hydrogels has been the most significant development in recent years. These polymeric materials are much more absorbent than fluff pulp. Cottenden (1988), under standard laboratory conditions, found that 1 g of fluff pulp absorbed 10 g of urine, while 1 g of superabsorbent absorbed 50 g. The difference was even greater under pressure, as urine is squeezed out of fluff pulp much more easily.

The use of superabsorbents reduces pad bulk and therefore enables the production of a much more acceptable design. Hydrogels, however, have three disadvantages:

1 They are expensive,
2 Absorption is much slower, therefore 'strike-through time' (the process whereby urine passes through the coverstock and into the pad core) is lengthened, necessitating the design of some kind of reservoir to hold the urine until the hydrogel catches up.
3 Once absorption of urine and solidification takes place, its wet comfort may be seriously reduced by the slimy nature of the wet gel.

Coverstock The skin is separated from the absorbent core by a non-woven material which should be resistant to liquid penetration while allowing rapid urine passage through into the absorbent layer beneath. A coverstock should also be resistant to retrograde urine flow from the absorbent layer to the skin. Malone-Lee (1984) states that it should feel soft and dry to the wearer and it must not contribute to skin irritation or to bed sores either in the dry or wet state. Coverstocks can be made of Rayon, polyester, polypropylene or polyethylene.

Further design features

Shaping Patients view this as a key issue for comfort, prevention of leakage and maintenance of the pad in a secure position (Philp et al 1989). More companies are introducing the use of Lycra threads in the crotch area to ensure a comfortable and snug fit, thereby increasing patient security during incontinence episodes.

Wetness indicators Wetness indicators work on the same principle as those on some nappies when the pad becomes moist the wetness indicator will show the need to change the pad. This feature is meant to be used as a guide to carers.

Storage and disposal

Absorbent incontinence pads are bulky and an individual patient may need several per day. This can present storage problems in the community, particularly with infrequent deliveries of supplies, which can also lead to unnecessary hoarding of stock. In hospital, absorbent pads are classified as clinical waste and are for the most part disposed of on site by incineration. Disposal of pads for the community-based patient may present problems.

PANTS

Pants may be specifically designed to accommodate particular pads or the patient may use her own underwear, provided it will hold the pad in position to allow it to function properly. Although numerous design features are used to meet individual needs and requirements, there are four main types of pants:

1 Waterproof
2 Lightweight open-knitted stretch pants
3 Front/side-fastening or drop-front pants
4 Marsupial type pants.

Waterproof pants

These pants range from the simple traditional all-plastic to the more sophisticated waterproof variety with an inner and outer layer of nylon polyester, and are worn with a non-waterproof backed pad. The disadvantages of such pants are skin irritation, perspiration and odour. These pants create noise on movement, so that their owners become conscious of wearing them. Continued laundering may also cause the material to harden and become brittle, resulting in the garment being easily torn. Waterproof pants may fulfil the needs of some patients, particularly if extra security is needed. However, long-term continued use is inappropriate.

Lightweight open-knitted stretch pants

These pants are made of washable stretch fabric so that they conform to the shape and size of the lower torso and, to a lesser extent, cater for differences in upper thigh dimensions. They are designed to be used with a plastic-backed pad, are light to wear, easy to launder and inexpensive (Fig. 48.2).

Some of the pants in this category contain strengthening bands which run horizontally around the whole garment. There may also be colour-coded size indicators for easy identification and selection.

Front/side-fastening or drop-front pants

These pants are made of cotton and/or polyester and are suitable for users with limited manual dexterity. They open at the front or side and have velcro or press stud fastenings.

Marsupial pants

These pants are made of a hydrophobic fabric and have an internal or external pouch in the crotch area into which an absorbent pad is inserted. The pouch compartmentalizes the pad and to some extent the urine. The fabric, in theory, does not absorb or hold the urine but instead passes it through into the absorbent pad.

The innermost layer of the pants is often referred to as 'one-way' or 'stay-dry' so making the claim that the patient's skin remains dry. The Kings Fund (1987), however, found in practice that urine traversed the pad in both directions if the maximal functional capacity of the pad was reached or if excessive pressure was applied to the partially saturated pad.

The outermost layer of the pouch nearest the patient's clothing is of a waterproof material. Marsupial pants are aimed at the ambulant or semi-ambulant patient with mild to moderate urine leakage.

DISPOSABLE UNDERPADS

These range from a 5-ply to a 20-ply pad with additional fluff pulp. Most pads consist of a coverstock, an absorbent layer and a waterproof backing. The quality and technical design will influence the performance of the pad; the capacity of underpads can range from as little as 120 ml to in excess of 2 l. The variety of dimensions available should allow selection of a single pad suitable for the patient's needs.

REUSABLE BODY-WORN PRODUCTS

Developments in the reusable body-worn product market are taking place at a great rate. In 1990, only approximately 40 of these products were being marketed in the UK, however by 1993 this had increased to 70 (Philp & Cottenden 1993). Any comparison between reusable and disposable incontinence products must take into account the context in which the products will be used, the systems of supply and disposal or washing and drying, as well as relative costs and environmental issues. Philp et al (1993) found in a study that the main objection to the reusable pants and integral pad design was the inconvenience of changing, especially when users were outside the home.

Design

The object of any absorbent product is to contain urine loss. Much of the performance of a product is determined by the physical, chemical, mechanical and bacteriological properties of the material used. There are two factors governing the choice of materials: good wet comfort and good dry comfort.

Good wet comfort

A hydrophobic fabric, usually polyester, is used as it allows urine through readily to the absorbent core, while maintaining a dry surface next to the skin.

Good dry comfort

The fabric used is either cotton or a cotton/polyester mix. Cotton is good for dry comfort before voiding because it efficiently absorbs body moisture; however cotton retains urine and so remains wet against the skin after urine loss.

The choice of product will depend on the user's circumstances. If a product can be changed immediately after an incontinence episode or if urine loss is light or infrequent, a high priority may be dry comfort. However, someone who must wait for a carer to assist in changing may have different needs.

Reusables must be able to withstand frequent washing. Ideally, a normal laundering cycle should remove all urine, as well as faecal staining and bacteria. The product should also dry rapidly and retain its performance for an acceptable number of washes. The waterproof backing is particularly sensitive to damage by high temperature. In general, the more compliant the plastic the less able it is to withstand high-temperature washing and hot-air drying.

The products available are designed to cater for light, moderate and heavy urinary incontinence and can be divided into three main types of design:

1 Insert pads
2 Pad-pants (pants with integral absorbent padding (Fig. 48.3)
3 Nappy style (side-opening absorbent garments).

REUSABLE BED PADS

The development of the reusable bed pad has been concurrent with that of reusable body-worn products. They are, however, not always suitable for patients with faecal incontinence.

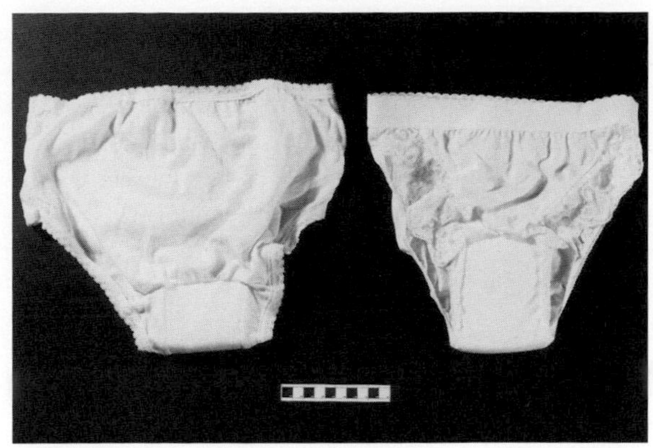

Fig. 48.3 Reusable pad-pants.

Design

Reusable bed pads consist of the following components:

1 A hydrophobic sheet used in conjunction with a disposable underpad. The aim of this product is to provide a 'stay-dry' layer between the patient's skin and the urine that has been absorbed into the underpad.
2 A hydrophobic sheet quilted to an absorbent layer of material. This design may also have an integral waterproof backing and side flaps to tuck in under the mattress.
3 A cotton upper layer with an absorbent layer beneath. This design may also have its own waterproof backing and tuck-in flaps.

Products with a 'hydrophobic' layer are intended to keep the skin dry, but this can only be achieved if no other pads, pants or clothing are between the sheet and the skin.

Norris et al (1993) showed that reusable underpads received a mixed reaction. The main criticism was leakage, and many patients did not like lying in bed naked below the waist. It was also a common complaint that products were too small.

MECHANICAL DEVICES

There are two types of mechanical device in this context: occlusive and collective.

Occlusive devices

An occlusive device inserted into the vagina or urethra, as with pads and collective methods, will merely contain the problem of incontinence rather than treating the cause.

The choice of occlusive devices is limited. Past devices include Edward's pubo-vaginal spring, first designed in 1965 and available for clinical use in 1969, and Bonnar's device. The latter was made of a soft inflatable silicone rubber, with the arms being fitted into the lateral vaginal fornices and a balloon being inflated via a small pump.

Indications for use of an occlusive device include:

1 Those waiting for other forms of treatment to become effective
2 Those waiting for surgery
3 Those who do not desire any other treatment
4 Those who are unable to receive other forms of therapy.

Designs available include the following:

1 Rocket pessary
2 Femcare sponge
3 Conveen continence guard
4 Femassist
5 Reliance urinary control insert.

Rocket pessary

This is a foam rubber vaginal tampon with a string attached for extraction. It is reusable after washing. Insertion may be difficult as it is non-rigid and has no applicator.

Femcare sponge (Fig. 48.4)

This is made from biocompatible polyvinyl alcohol (PVA), and is supplied in a dry form and must be soaked in warm water until completely softened before insertion. It, too, has a string attached for ease of extraction. The mode of action of the tampon is to apply pressure in the sagittal plane on the vesicourethral junction. The sponge may be left in position all day, however it should be removed at night.

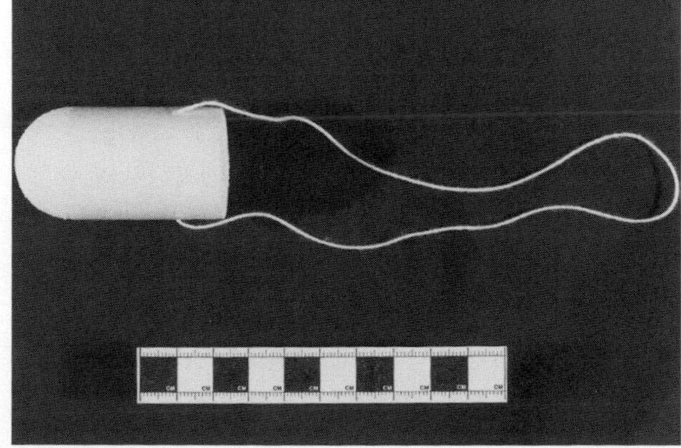

Fig. 48.4 The Femcare sponge.

Unlike the Rocket pessary the Femcare sponge is not reusable and therefore the cost implication must be considered.

Conveen continence guard (Fig. 48.5)

The guard is made of soft moulded foam plastic and is so shaped that the outer surfaces fit against the bladder neck and rectum and therefore lift the bladder slightly. It is inserted with the use of an applicator and can be worn for up to 16 hours per day. During menstruation this time period is reduced to 4–6 hours, and external sanitary protection must be used. As with the Femcare sponge, it is not reusable.

FemAssist (Fig. 48.6)

This shaped device is made of medical grade silicon and is placed over the external urethra, and is held in place by an adhesive gel. The mild vacuum action is thought to support surrounding tissue as it gently squeezes the urethra to oppose the mucosa. The device must be removed to allow urination to occur and then be reapplied. A single device can be used for up to 7 days before being discarded. Early trial results are encouraging.

Reliance urinary control insert (Fig. 48.7)

The device is manufactured from a thermoplastic elastomer and consists of an insert and applicator. Prior to using the device it must be ascertained which of the five sizes available would be appropriate. The sizing device is a sterile, single-use calibrating catheter with applicator.

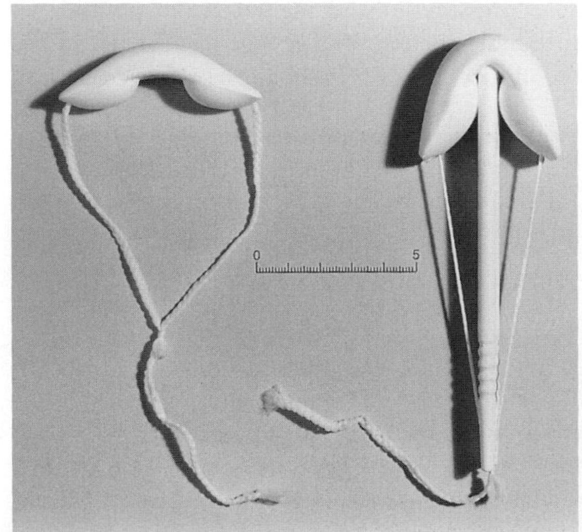

Fig. 48.5 The Conveen continence guard.

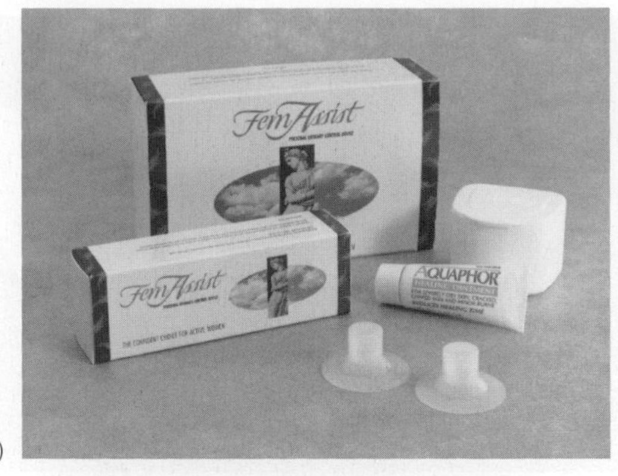

(A)

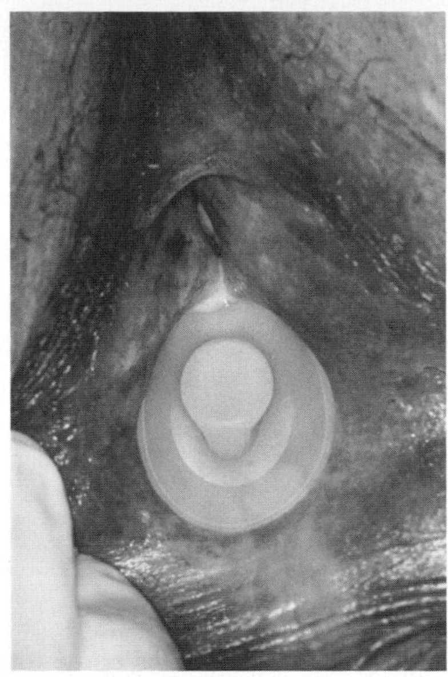

(B)

Fig. 48.6 A,B The FemAssist device.

The urinary control insert is placed into the urethra using an applicator and is kept in place by inflating a small balloon. To remove the insert a release string is pulled, the balloon deflates and the device can be removed. Staskin et al (1995) demonstrated that this device was a safe and effective alternative for the control of genuine stress incontinence in patients unsatisfied with their current management methods or for those not wishing to undergo surgery.

The urinary control insert must be removed to allow urination to take place and cannot be reused. As with other once-only use devices, the cost implication must be considered.

Collection devices

There are several collection devices (excluding urinary catheters) to choose from; most are female urinals and bedpans. Collection devices may be useful in helping the immobile patient, particularly if there is

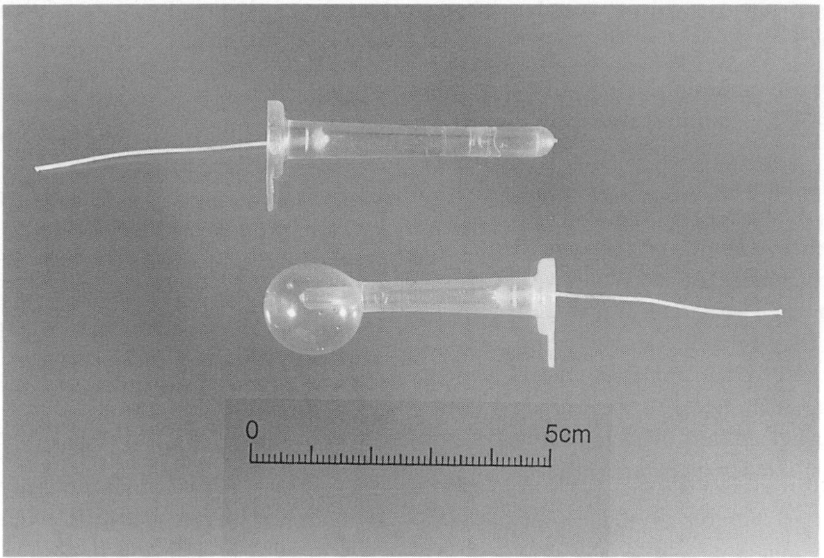

Fig. 48.7 The Reliance urinary control insert.

a problem with urinary urgency and there is no time to transfer to toilet or commode before voiding commences.

Body-worn urinals

The difficulty in attaching a collection device to the female anatomy is reflected in the paucity of devices there are on the market.

The cup-shaped devices are held in position with waist and leg straps. The devices are bulky to wear and not comfortable; there is also a great risk of leakage. Obese women would not normally be suitable for these urinals, as the limited space between the groins will cause pressure on the device against the skin, therefore risking sore and broken skin.

The disadvantages of the body-worn urinal generally render them unacceptable as a method of managing urinary incontinence in the majority of women.

Hand-held urinals

The hand-held urinal may be used where toilet facilities are not readily available or easily accessible. Choice of urinal will depend on the user's orientation, dexterity, hip abduction and quantity of urine voided. They may be used in bed, when seated or standing, depending upon the individual's abilities and needs, and the design of the urinal.

The female urinal bottle is similar in shape at the base to that of its male counterpart, but the top is shaped to fit the female vulva.

The feminal has an anatomically moulded plastic frame to which disposable plastic bags are attached. It may be used standing, sitting or lying. It is not suitable where perineal sensation is impaired or thigh abduction limited.

The femicep is made of moulded plastic and can be easily placed in position. A urinary catheter bag may be attached; the patient is therefore relieved of the necessity of disposing of the urine immediately.

The slipper bedpan has a curved rim to prevent spillage; the rubber cap is removed to allow emptying. It is suitable for bed, chair or standing.

The 'Car Loo' has a moulded plastic frame with disposable polythene bag kept in position with a plastic clip.

The 'Bridge Urinal' is shaped to the body contour and can be positioned easily. It is linked to any urinary drainage bag.

Commodes

If there is loss of manual dexterity combined with poor mobility, commodes can provide an immediate solution to the problem of an inaccessible toilet.

It is advisable to establish who is responsible for emptying the pan before it is issued; some pans can be difficult for the frail user or carer. Instructions on use and maintenance should be understood by either user or carer.

There are four main factors to consider when selecting a commode:

1 Personal preference on design
2 Size, weight, mobility and posture position of the user
3 Dependence/independence of the user, especially with regard to transfer of the user to the commode and that of emptying the commode
4 The environment where the commode will be used. In the domestic situation, it may be important that the commode strongly resembles an ordinary piece of furniture. In an institutional setting, stacking commodes may save much-needed space. Alternatively, folding commodes can be more easily taken away on visits.

The following design features should be considered when selecting a commode:

Frame Armchair or stacking, with or without upholstered backrest, armrests and detachable seats. Models resembling domestic furniture when not in use may be more acceptable in the home, but can be more difficult to clean.

Stability A heavier person may need splayed legs fixed to the floor with flanges.

Height Fixed or adjustable. The correct height for easy rising should be selected.

Armrests Fixed, swinging or detachable. Movable arms may facilitate transfer from a bed or wheelchair.

Footrests Care needs to be taken if the user has to stand on the footrests as this will cause some models to tilt forward.

Toilet seat Round or oval, with various sizes of aperture.

Commode pan Standard bedpan or rectangular pan, with or without a lid or carrying handle.

Wheels may allow flexibility of positioning, but there must be an efficient brake.

CONCLUSION

When choosing an incontinence aid, the most important issues include suitability for the individual patient, cost-effectiveness and improvement in quality of life.

REFERENCES

Blannin B 1985 A guide to selecting incontinence aids. Geriatric Medicine Feb: 20–24

Cottenden A M 1988 Incontinence pads and appliances. International Disability Studies 10: 44–47

Kings Fund Project Paper No. 65 1987. Aids for the management of incontinence

Malone-Lee J G 1984 The technology of incontinence garment manufacture. Care Science & Practice 4(2): 22–28

Norris C, Cottenden A M, Ledger D 1993 Underpad overview. Nursing Times (89): 21

Philp J, Cottenden A 1993 Picking and choosing. Nursing Times 89(30): 81–94

Philp J, Cottenden A M, Butcher, D 1989 Pads for people. Journal of District Nursing Sept: 4–6

Philp J, Cottenden A M, Ledger D 1993 A testing time. Nursing Times 89(14): 59–62

Staskin D Sant G Sand P et al 1995 Use of an expandable urethral insert for GSI – long-term results of a multicenter trial. Neurourology and Urodynamics 14(5): 420–422

SECTION 5
CHAPTER
49

Physiotherapy

JO LAYCOCK

INTRODUCTION

Physiotherapy is becoming more widely available in many countries for the conservative management of incontinence caused by pelvic muscle weakness. The main modalities in general use include pelvic floor exercises, biofeedback, vaginal cones and neuromuscular electrical stimulation. The choice of the most appropriate technique depends on thorough pelvic floor muscle assessment, available equipment and expected patient compliance to this self-help treatment.

THE PELVIC FLOOR

Providing a supportive, sexual and sphincteric function (Kegel 1956), the pelvic floor remains a mystery to many health professionals and patients. However, recent investigations (see Ch. 1) have provided insight into the anatomy and function of the pelvic floor musculature, clarifying its role in the maintenance of continence. In essence, contraction (which produces muscle shortening) of the levator ani approximates the vagina and the rectum towards the pubis, compressing and elevating the urethra and increasing the anorectal angle. Muscles exhibiting good tone will maintain these positions more effectively – even at rest; muscles which have been stretched and/or have become weak, will have to be actively contracted to support the proximal urethra and prevent descent during increased intra-abdominal pressure, until their resting tone can be improved. The tone and contractility of the external urethral sphincter also plays a crucial part in the continence mechanism, and weakness (partial denervation/re-innervation following childbirth) needs to be addressed.

It follows that if the pelvic floor muscles and external urethral sphincter are weak or fatigue easily, they will not respond adequately to the demands made on them, and strategies to implement a muscle training programme may ameliorate this dysfunction, and reduce symptoms of incontinence. The reason why the results of pelvic floor re-education are not always favourable may be due to the multifactorial aetiology of stress incontinence and, in addition, patient compliance to an exercise programme.

MUSCLE TRAINING

A muscle training programme has to satisfy the principles of overload, specificity and function, and reversibility. However, it is important not to confuse pelvic floor re-education for incontinence with the training methods described for athletes to increase their fitness, speed and performance. A well trained athlete may use maximum effort three or four times per week, with reduced training demands on other days – to allow for recovery. Pelvic floor training compares more with the rehabilitation of convalescent patients, where "a little and often" is the general rule, as patients are not generally capable of exerting great power and endurance in the early stages of their treatment. However, as the pelvic floor muscles strengthen, and using biofeedback to enhance patient effort, intensive daily pelvic floor exercises should be sufficient to have a training effect.

Overload

The response to exercise depends on muscle adaptation and this only occurs if the muscle is worked to the point of fatigue – i.e. the muscle is overloaded. It is therefore important to ascertain the amount of activity needed to produce this, by careful pelvic floor muscle assessment. It is not enough to identify the correct muscle action by vaginal palpation; the examiner must also determine the strength and endurance of the muscle.

Specificity and function

The striated pelvic floor muscles are a heterogeneous mixture of approximately 70% slow-twitch fibres and 30% fast-twitch fibres (Gilpin et al 1989), and it is proposed that specific techniques be used to activate these different fibre types. It has been shown that the slow-twitch fibres provide a postural function, and the fast-twitch fibres are recruited only when speed and power are required, such as during coughing, to quickly counteract the increased rise in intra-abdominal pressure (Gosling 1979). Long, sustained repetitive pelvic floor contractions involve slow-twitch activity, whereas fast, powerful contractions and neuromuscular electrical stimulation have been shown to recruit fast-twitch fibres.

All techniques (exercises, biofeedback, vaginal cones and neuromuscular electrical stimulation) should aim to enhance pelvic floor awareness, contractility and coordination. This in turn will increase the power and endurance of active and reflex pelvic floor contractions, leading to improved function. Consequently, teaching a patient to contract the pelvic floor muscles before and during a stress-provoking act such as coughing will assist in both urethral occlusion and in maintaining the proximal urethra within the area of transmitted abdominal pressure, thus preventing downward movement of the proximal urethra (DeLancey 1992; Mostwin et al 1993). In addition, a strong pelvic floor contraction is said to inhibit unwanted detrusor contractions (Mahoney et al 1977) and so this strategy can be used to suppress urgency and control urge incontinence.

Depending on the effort and regularity of training, it can take 3 to 6 months to detect a physiological change in muscles. However, many patients report a decrease in incontinence symptoms after only a few weeks of pelvic floor training. This may be attributed to increased muscle awareness in patients with initially good muscle contractility, but poor awareness/coordination, or it may refer to those patients whose muscular continence mechanisms (pelvic floor and urethral sphincter) are just below the threshold of continence. In these cases, a small gain in muscle contractility may be enough to restore continence.

Reversibility

If muscles are not used at their newly acquired level of fitness, the strengthening effect of training is reversed, and so it is important that patients are instructed to continue pelvic floor exercises as a lifelong habit.

PELVIC FLOOR ASSESSMENT

Digital pelvic floor muscle assessment, per vaginam, is the key to any re-education programme. The examiner should palpate the left and the right levator ani to ascertain muscle bulk and symmetry, as many women demonstrate asymmetrical pelvic floor muscles, which can result in an imbalance of muscle power. In simple terms, pelvic floor muscles need to be assessed for strength and endurance. Muscle strength is assessed by digital vaginal palpation and recorded on a modified Oxford scale (0 to 5). Endurance is recorded as the duration of a maximum contraction and the number of times the patient can repeat this before the muscle is fatigued. For example, a patient may demonstrate a grade 3 (moderate) contraction, maintained for 7 seconds and repeated 5 times; subsequent contractions would be weaker and of shorter duration. In addition, the number of fast, strong, one-second contractions is recorded; this could be any number, e.g. 8. This regimen (5 maximum contractions lasting 7 seconds followed by 8 fast contractions) becomes her daily home exercise programme. Clearly, every patient will have a different exercise programme (Laycock 1994). As treatment progresses, the exercise regimen should be altered to reflect improved muscle contractility, so that the pelvic floor muscles are always being overloaded during an exercise programme. Ideally, patients should be assessed lying and standing, as many choose to exercise standing, and it is wrong to assume that a similar voluntary contraction can be achieved in all positions.

Pelvic floor muscle assessment and the appropriate exercise regimen can also be determined using a perineometer (see Fig. 49.1), where an increase in contractile strength is registered by a higher monitor reading.

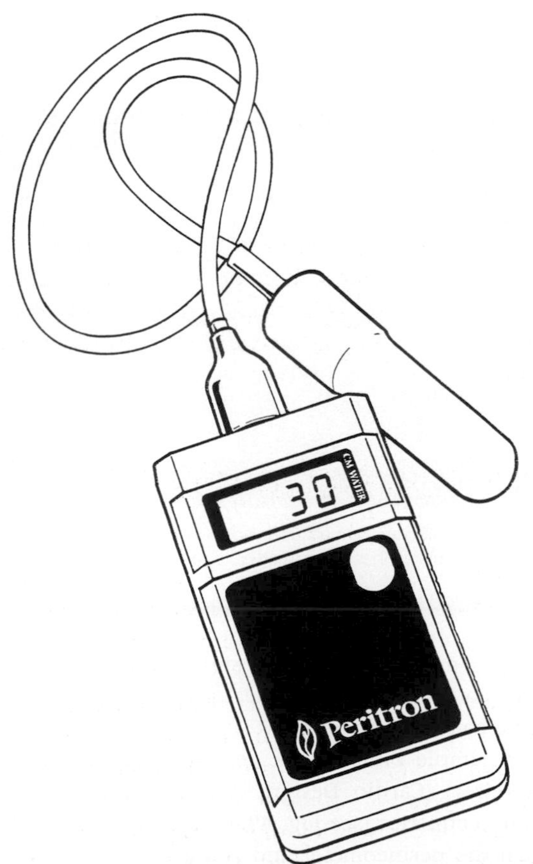

Fig. 49.1 Peritron perineometer (Cardio Design, Australia). Electronic device measuring pressure in cm H_2O.

A perineometer can only be used successfully after a digital assessment has confirmed that the correct muscle action is being carried out. Approximately 30% of patients are unable to perform a voluntary pelvic floor contraction (Bump et al 1991), and many women 'bear down' by mistake. The problem with this is the perceived increase in the perineometer reading due to the pressure of the pelvic organs on the vagina and not due to a pelvic floor contraction.

PELVIC FLOOR RE-EDUCATION

A decision has to be made on the most appropriate technique for individual patients. This will depend not only on the results of the muscle evaluation and the patient's attitude to the various devices, but also on the equipment available to the therapist. However, it has been shown that combination therapy, using modern equipment, appears to improve patient motivation and compliance to a home exercise programme, which is acknowledged as the mainstay of any pelvic floor muscle training regimen.

It is important to provide physiotherapy at least once per week for the first month for any patient on a pelvic floor re-education programme. Thereafter, less frequent treatment sessions, but still with regular monitoring of progress, should continue for 3 to 6 months.

Pelvic floor exercises

There are many ways to train skeletal muscles which can be applied to the pelvic floor muscles. After an initial warm-up of two or three submaximal contractions with instructions to 'lift and squeeze as if preventing the flow of urine', the patient is directed to perform the complete home regimen. This will consist of her previously assessed number of maximum contractions of specific length (with 4 seconds rest in between) followed by the appropriate number (enough to fatigue) of fast contractions. This regimen should be practised three to six times each day. In addition, during the day, long (up to 3 minutes) submaximal contractions can be incorporated into activities of daily living, when timing a maximum contraction would be inappropriate. Furthermore, rhythmical submaximal contractions, in time to music, can be practised to add variety to any exercise programme and can be practised sitting or standing, for several minutes. Functionally, the patient should be instructed to brace (contract) the pelvic floor muscles before and during any stress-provoking activity

– such as coughing, sneezing, standing up from sitting, or any action which may cause urine loss.

The frequency of daily pelvic floor exercises should be agreed with each patient and will depend on other commitments. All patients should have short- and long-term goals to motivate them and ensure compliance to the home exercise programme. Such aims will include increasing the strength of a contraction and the hold time, and the number of fast contractions. Monthly completion of a bladder diary will monitor the decrease in incontinence episodes and so the patient will be motivated to comply with the exercise regimen.

Klarskov et al (1986) randomized 50 consecutive women with genuine stress incontinence to either pelvic floor exercises or surgery. Subjectively, following pelvic floor training, 3 patients were cured, 14 improved and 7 were unchanged. After 12 months, 42% no longer wanted surgery, and a follow-up 4 to 8 years later showed that all patients remained satisfied with their improvement. Although results of surgery were significantly better ($p<0.01$), 1 patient was worse, 1 developed retropubic pain, 1 pelvic pain and another persistent dyspareunia and loss of libido.

Cammu & Van Nylen (1995) reported on a 5-year follow-up of 48 women previously treated with 10 weeks pelvic floor exercises for troublesome stress incontinence. They identified an overall cure or much improved rate at the end of therapy of 54%, which rose to 58% after 5 years; 13 women (27%) underwent surgery. These results suggest that some patients need a longer treatment period. Pelvic floor exercises were recommended by the patients to friends or relatives in 77% of cases.

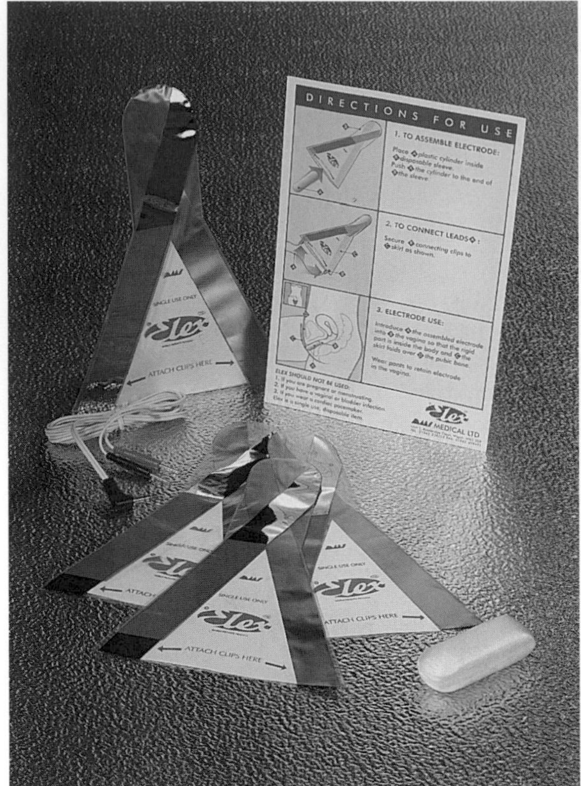

Fig. 49.2 Disposable vaginal electrode (DMI, UK) for EMG biofeedback and electrical stimulation.

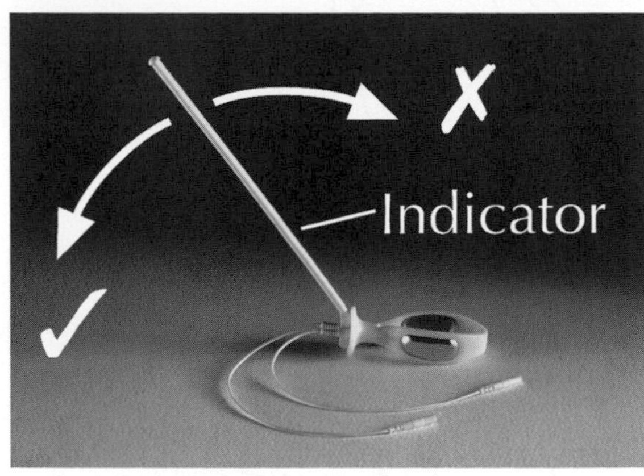

Fig. 49.3 Single-patient (multi-use) vaginal electrode (Neen HealthCare, UK) for EMG biofeedback and electrical stimulation.

Biofeedback

Converting the effect of a pelvic floor contraction to the patient, in visual or auditory format, has been shown to produce extra effort, not only in the power of contraction, but also in endurance. Biofeedback, performed lying or standing, can be provided by a simple perineometer (Fig. 49.1) or with sophisticated electronic equipment utilizing pressure and/or EMG vaginal and anal sensors. Figure 49.2 shows a lightweight, disposable vaginal electrode (DMI, UK), and Figure 49.3 shows the Periform, a lightweight, single-patient (multi-use) vaginal electrode (Neen HealthCare, UK). Both these electrodes are suitable for EMG biofeedback and electrical stimulation. The Periform, with the indicator attached, also acts as a simple biofeedback device without connection to EMG monitoring equipment. This device works on the same principle as the Q-tip test; downward (posterior) movement of the indicator signifies a correct pelvic floor contraction. The indicator moves upwards during a cough or straining.

A simple biofeedback device – PFX (pelvic floor exerciser) (Cardio Design, Australia) is available in many countries (see Fig. 49.4). This is less expensive than the perineometer and is a useful home exercise unit. Patients will respond to the challenge of increasing their previous record of muscle strength and hold time, and can exercise in the privacy of their own homes.

Shepherd et al (1983) (n=22), using a simple perineometer for biofeedback, showed that after 6 weeks, 90% of women using a home perineometer were dry or improved, compared with 55% of the control group, who practised conventional pelvic floor exercises. In addition, there were no drop-outs in the perineometer group, compared with 27% drop-outs in the control group.

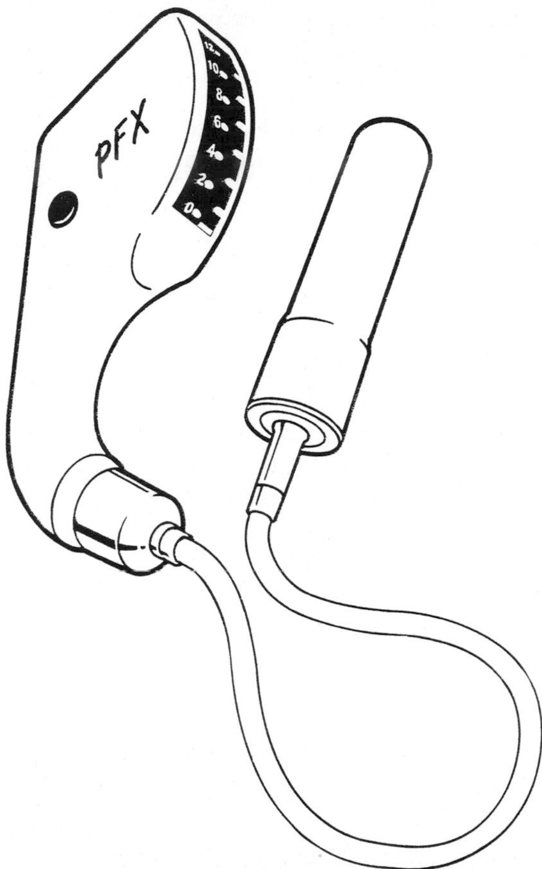

Fig. 49.4 PFX (pelvic floor exerciser). Home biofeedback unit (Cardio Design, Australia).

Vaginal cones

Introduced by Plevnik (1985), vaginal cones are available in two sizes (Seton-Scholl, UK); the cone shell opens to allow insertion of different weights (Fig. 49.5). The large, empty cone is introduced into the vagina (above the pelvic floor) and the feeling of losing the cone alerts the woman to contract her pelvic floor muscles to retain the cone. As an empty cone may be retained without any muscular effort in some patients, weights are added inside the cone, so that the patient is always required to contract the pelvic floor to prevent the cone from slipping out. When the initial individual cone size and weight has been determined for each patient, she is encouraged to walk around, up and down stairs and to cough, all the time retaining the cone by contracting her pelvic floor muscles. In addition, pelvic floor exercises with the cone in position will provide resistance to a pelvic floor muscle contraction. Extra weights are added as the muscles strengthen, and so muscle power can be increased, as with any weight-resisted body exercise. Cone therapy is practised once or twice each day for 10 minutes, and discontinued during menstruation and for 2 hours following intercourse.

Peattie et al (1988), using cone therapy, treated 39 premenopausal women with genuine stress

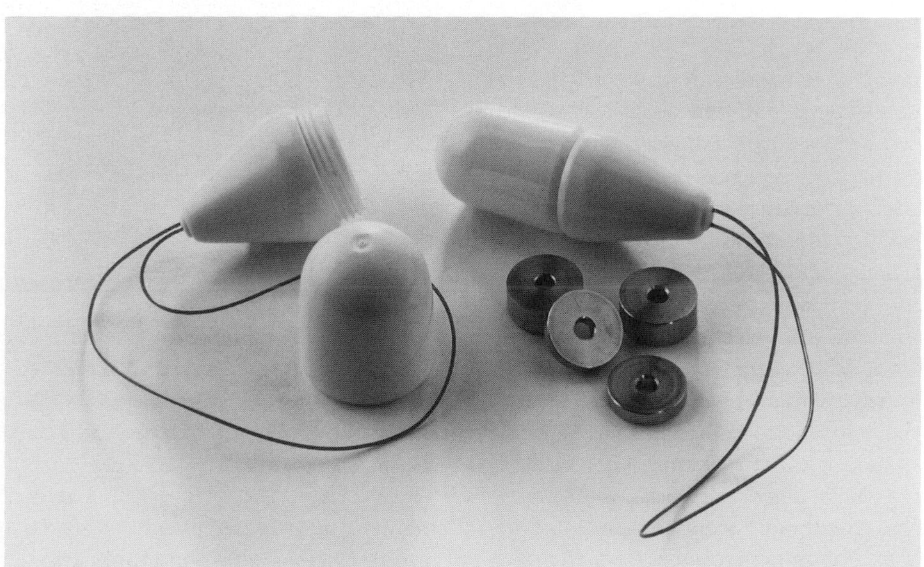

Fig. 49.5 Aquaflex cones (DePuy HealthCare, UK). Weighted vaginal cones.

incontinence who were awaiting corrective surgery, using a pad-test to measure clinical outcomes. Thirty women (77%) completed 1 month's treatment and 21/30 women (70%) reported cure or improvement.

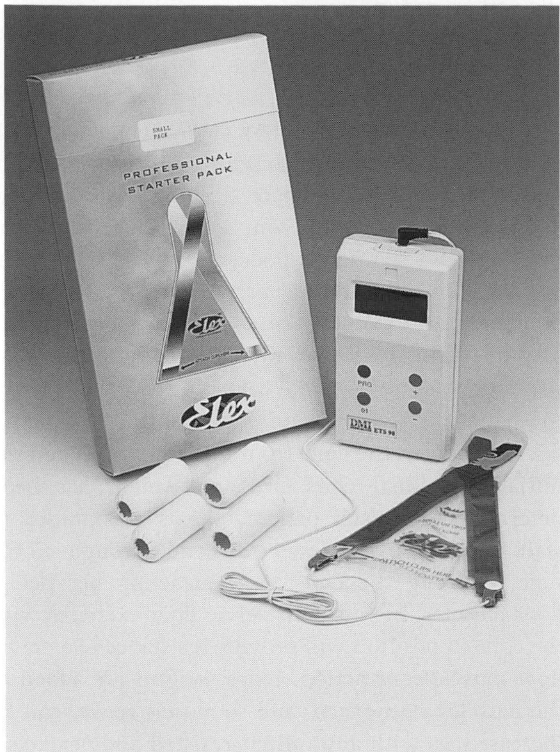

Fig. 49.6 Battery-operated, home electrical stimulation unit (DMI, UK).

When analysed with intention to treat, a total of 19 women (49%) were satisfied with treatment, 11 (28%) opted for surgery and 9 (23%) did not complete therapy. The authors did not report any adverse effects of cone therapy and recommended the treatment as a cost effective means of treating genuine stress incontinence.

Neuromuscular electrical stimulation

This treatment involves the use of a vaginally located electrode and an output of low-frequency, biphasic current of sufficient intensity to activate the pelvic floor motor units. The feeling of 'pins and needles' is quite tolerable, and patients are encouraged to increase the intensity of stimulation within their tolerance; generally, a stronger current is more effective.

With the increase in development of electrical stimulation equipment, it is now possible to provide patients with home stimulation units, and so regular (daily) treatment can be prescribed (Figs 49.6, 49.7).

Vaginal/anal stimulation at a suitable frequency (35–50 Hz) and maximum tolerated intensity (up to 80 mA), produces a contraction of the pelvic floor muscles; a frequency of 5–10 Hz and maximum intensity produces inhibition of the detrusor (Fall & Lindstrom 1991). Consequently, electrical stimulation has been successfully used in the treatment of genuine stress incontinence (Plevnik et al 1986; Sand et al 1995), and detrusor instability (Eriksen et al 1989; Fossberg

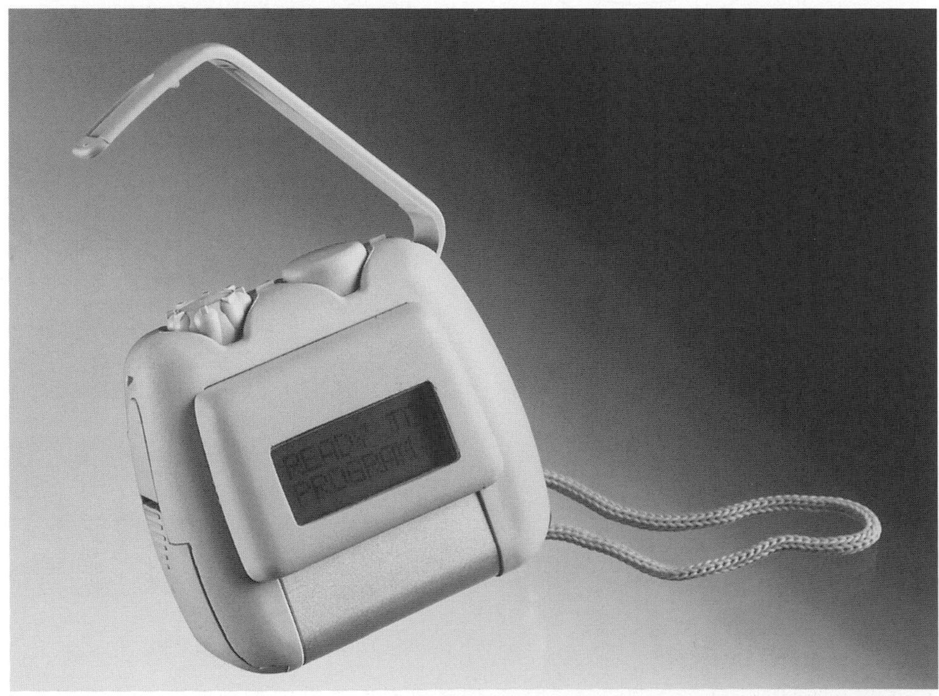

Fig. 49.7 Battery-operated, home electrical stimulation unit (Neen HealthCare, UK).

et al 1990). However, the literature can be confusing and misleading, citing different types of current, e.g. interferential therapy, faradism and functional electrical stimulation (FES). The difference between these various types of current is generally their frequency, pulse-width and pulse-shape. To date, none has outshone the other in the treatment of incontinence, but reports generally agree on a biphasic current and the choice of vaginal or anal electrodes. One-sided vaginal electrodes enable the therapist to target a weak side if asymmetry exists. When used for muscle re-education, the treatment is described as 'active assisted'. This term implies that the patient 'joins in' with the electrically stimulated muscle contraction. This technique is best achieved using the Periform vaginal electrode (see Fig. 49.3) where downward deflection of the indicator signifies adequate current intensity and a muscle contraction; further deflection indicates an 'active assisted' contraction. Electrical stimulation is not a passive treatment. Electrical stimulation is especially important for those patients who are unable to perform a voluntary contraction of the pelvic floor muscles. As up to 30% of women fall into this category, electrical stimulation is a useful addition to the physiotherapist's armamentarium.

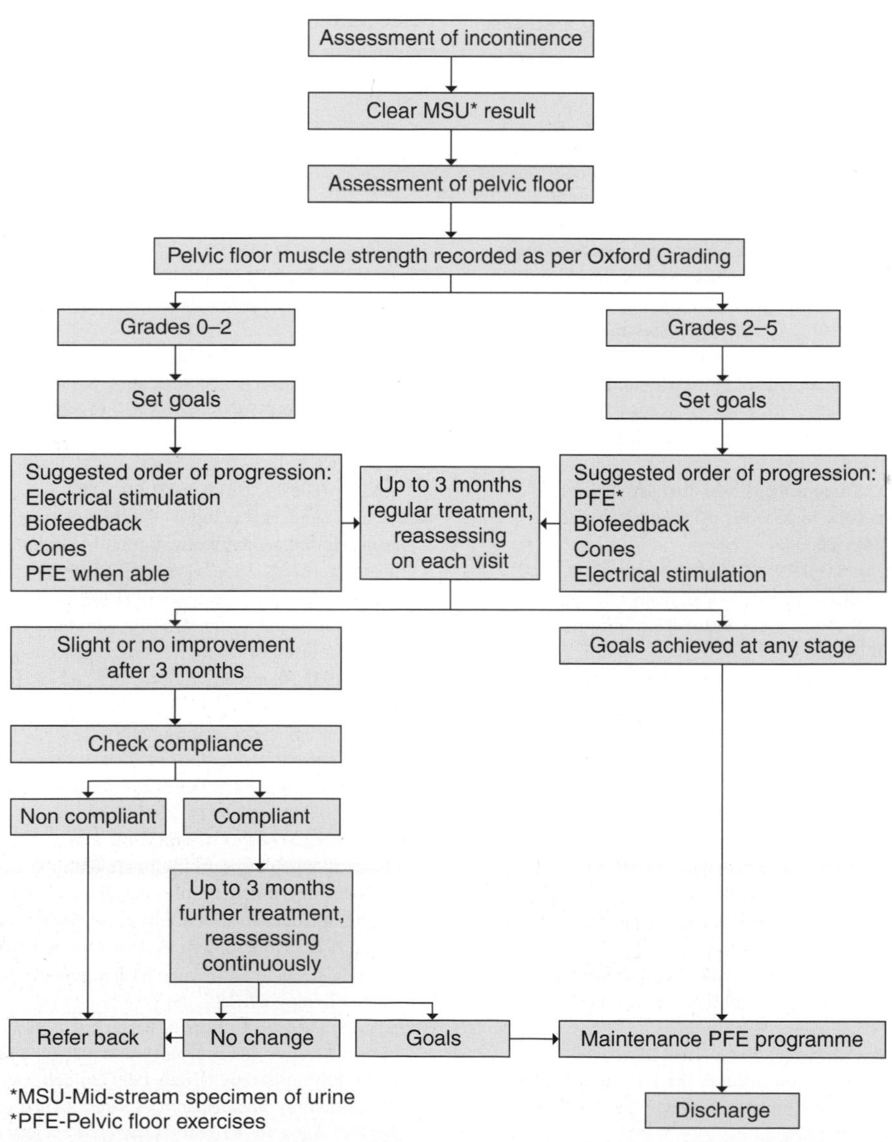

Fig. 49.8 Flowchart showing treatment options for patients with stress urinary incontinence (SUI). From Yorkshire Physiotherapy Group (in press), with permission.

SELECTION OF PATIENTS

Patients of all ages attuned to self-help should benefit from conservative management of their incontinence. Many elderly patients respond better than expected, probably because they have more time to spend on their home treatment programme. There is debate on the good prognostic features of women undergoing physiotherapy for genuine stress incontinence. Tapp et al (1988) reported that women who were most likely to succeed were premenopausal, have duration of symptoms of less than 4 years, present with a low visual analogue score on severity of symptoms and have good urethral function during stress. Hesse et al (1990) agreed with these findings and noted that severe stress incontinence (more than 10 g pad-test gain) or a history of greater than 1 year, were adverse factors. However, Bo et al (1990) reported that older women with a longer history of symptoms and lower resting urethral pressure showed greater improvement. They considered that this group of patients were better motivated to practise daily pelvic floor exercises and consequently benefitted from the treatment. Most physiotherapists believe that the greatest prognostic factor is the patient's motivation, and this is partly determined by the enthusiasm of the therapist.

Figure 49.8 suggests a method of both patient and modality selection for stress incontinence. Generally, patients with mild to moderate symptoms of short duration, with minimal genital prolapse, may succeed with pelvic floor re-education, and this should encourage clinicians to offer this treatment (where appropriate). Patients should be informed that, with perseverance and determination, they can expect a favourable outcome.

REFERENCES

Bo K, Larsen S, Kvarstein B, Hagen R H 1990 Classification and characterization of responders to pelvic floor muscle exercise for female stress urinary incontinence. Neurourology and Urodynamics 9(4): 395–397

Bump R C, Hurt W G, Fantl J A et al 1991 Assessment of Kegel pelvic muscle exercise performance after brief verbal instruction. American Journal of Obstetrics and Gynecology 165: 322–329

Cammu H, Van Nylen M 1995 Pelvic floor exercises: 5 years later. Urology 45: 113–118

DeLancey J O L 1992 Three dimensional analysis of urethral support: the hammock hypothesis. Neurourology and Urodynamics 11(4): 306–308

Eriksen B C, Bergmann S, Eik-Nes S H 1989 Maximal electrostimulation of the pelvic floor in female idiopathic detrusor instability and urge incontinence. Neurourology and Urodynamics 8: 219–230

Fall M, Lindstrom S 1991 Electrical stimulation. A physiologic approach to the treatment of urinary incontinence. Urologic Clinics of North America 18: 393–407

Fossberg E, Sorensen S, Ruuta M et al 1990 Maximal electrical stimulation in the treatment of unstable detrusor and urge incontinence. European Urology 18: 120–123

Gilpin S A, Gosling J A, Smith A R B, Warrell D W 1989 The pathogenesis of genitourinary prolapse and stress incontinence of urine. A histological and histochemical study. British Journal of Obstetrics and Gynaecology 96: 15–23

Gosling J 1979 The structure of the bladder and urethra in relation to function. Urologic Clinics of North America 6: 31–38

Hesse U, Schussler B, Frimberger J et al 1990 Effectiveness of a three step pelvic floor reeducation in the treatment of stress urinary incontinence: a clinical assessment. Neurourology and Urodynamics 9(4): 397–398

Kegel A H 1956 Early genital relaxation. New technique of diagnosis and non-surgical treatment. Obstetrics and Gynecology 8: 545–550

Klarskov P, Belving D, Bischoff N et al 1986 Pelvic floor exercises versus surgery for female stress incontinence. Urology International 41: 129–132

Laycock J 1994 Clinical evaluation of the pelvic floor. In: Schussler B, Laycock J, Stanton S, Norton P (eds) Pelvic Floor Re-education: Principles and Practice. Springer Verlag, London, pp 42–48

Mahoney D T, Laferte R O, Blais D J 1977 Integral storage and voiding reflexes. Urology IX: 95–105

Mostwin J, Sanders R, Yang A, Genadry R 1993 New insights into anatomic linkage between vaginal hypermobility and stress incontinence. Neurourology and Urodynamics 12(4): 303–304

Peattie A B, Plevnik S, Stanton S L 1988 Vaginal cones: a conservative method of treating genuine stress incontinence. British Journal of Obstetrics and Gynaecology 95: 1049–1053

Plevnik S 1985 New method of testing and strengthening of pelvic floor muscles. Proceedings of the International Continence Society, London 267

Plevnik S, Janez J, Vrtacnik P et al 1986 Short-term electrical stimulation: home treatment for urinary incontinence. World Journal of Urology 4: 24–26

Sand P K, Richardson D A, Staskin D R et al 1995 Pelvic floor electrical stimulation in the treatment of genuine stress incontinence: a multicenter, placebo controlled trial. American Journal of Obstetrics and Gynecology 173: 72–79

Shepherd A M, Montgomery E, Anderson R S 1983 Treatment of genuine stress incontinence with a new perineometer. Physiotherapy 69: 13

Tapp A J S, Cardozo L, Hills B, Barnick C 1988 Who benefits from physiotherapy? Neurourology and Urodynamics 7(3): 259–261

Yorkshire Physiotherapy Group 1999 Guidelines for the Physiotherapy Management of Stress Urinary Incontinence in Females Aged 16–65 Years. Chartered Society of Physiotherapy, London

Into practice

SECTION

6

Organisation of community continence services

CHRISTINE NORTON

INTRODUCTION

As will have become obvious from the preceding chapters in this volume, the past two decades have seen tremendous advances in our understanding of the causes of female urinary incontinence, and in our ability to diagnose and treat those patients who present to us for help. However, this is of limited usefulness if the majority of incontinent people remain too embarrassed to seek professional help or do not know how to access the help available, or if those who provide primary care services are unaware of recent advances and so fail to refer patients, or if those responsible for funding health care will not pay for continence services.

Incontinence is such a common problem (Ch. 5) that in most healthcare systems it is unrealistic, and probably undesirable, to expect that every incontinent person will have access to a specialist centre and investigations as a first option. Indeed, for countries with less developed health services, treatment of incontinence will not be a priority compared to more basic services. It is only as countries become more affluent that the relative luxury of continence services can be afforded. In countries with existing services, these have largely grown up on an *ad hoc* basis with little central planning. Much has of course depended on the prevailing health service, its organization and how it is funded, making direct comparisons difficult (Fonda et al 1994). As other countries develop services, they will have the opportunity to consider the most efficient and effective use of scarce resources, and hopefully learn from what has happened previously elsewhere.

WHY SHOULD THERE BE COMMUNITY CONTINENCE SERVICES?

There are many arguments that can be used to persuade health care planners of the importance of adequate investment in community continence services. This is a prevalent problem and the number of incontinent people is likely to increase with an ageing and increasingly dependent population. Many frail elderly people are incontinent for reasons extraneous to the urinary system (such as poor mobility, an inappropriate physical environment or lack of an individualized care regimen). It is often best to provide a first assessment for such individuals in their usual surroundings and reserve hospital or clinic referral for those who do not respond to simple measures such as treatment of constipation, modifying a diuretic medication or provision of accessible toilet facilities. A number of nationally produced guidelines have suggested an algorithmic, step-wise approach to assessment and treatment of incontinent people (Royal College of Physicians 1995; AHCPR 1997).

Incontinence is an expensive problem, not only in product usage, but, more difficult to measure, in terms of staff and carer time and morale where incontinence levels are high in nursing homes, laundry, work days lost or women who never return to the workforce because of leakage after childbirth and a whole host of other, hidden, costs. It is likely that more investment in prevention and early detection could prevent progression of symptoms for some people and prevent them from eventually becoming major users of resources (such as needing a nursing home place because incontinence can no longer be coped with at home).

Demand for services is also likely to increase in the future because of deliberate efforts, by continence organisations in particular, to stimulate public awareness and education (see below).

WHAT DO INCONTINENT PEOPLE WANT/NEED?

Too often service providers make assumptions about those that they are supposed to serve. It is only recently that we have seriously asked what people want or need, and with an embarrassing problem like incontinence, the majority of suffers have been reluctant to tell us, or to complain when things were not good. Most do not seek help anyway, and expect little when they do. In the UK the Citizen's Charter Unit chose continence as one of a series of qualitative studies into users' views on health services. Responses were mixed (NHS Executive 1994). Some people were appreciative of the compassionate treatment they had received, but others seemed bemused by the intricacies of getting help. Some typical quotes from incontinent people included:

- 'I did not tell the doctor because I am too embarrassed and he is a man'.
- 'My doctor is English and provides no interpreting service. I am too shy to use my children to interpret'.
- 'I've always been incontinent. I'm having a lot of trouble trying to find out if there's anyone I could contact. My local chemist (pharmacist) said all I have to do is see my General Practitioner (family doctor). My GP said 'No, the district nurse is for that'. She said 'No, try the social services'. The social worker told me I should see my GP.'

These experiences are by no means isolated or even uncommon. It is easy to see why some people give up and simply buy sanitary protection rather than get professional help.

The report concluded with 14 challenges for health purchasers, including catering for the needs of different client groups (e.g. disabled people and those from ethnic minorities), and involving clients in the planning of services and feedback on its quality.

A MULTIDISCIPLINARY APPROACH

For many years incontinence in the community has often been seen as a solely nursing problem, with little interest or input from other members of the multidisciplinary team. Except for a few isolated areas, the main intervention has been trying to help the individual and any carers involved cope with symptoms rather than a more therapeutic approach to try to cure the incontinence. It is still not uncommon for an elderly person presenting with incontinence to a GP to be referred directly to the district nurse 'for assessment for pads and pants', with no physical examination or further investigation considered.

In fact, incontinence is often a complex and multifaceted problem, particularly in frail or dependent individuals (Norton 1996), and it may require input from a wide variety of disciplines to tackle it effectively (Table 50.1). While it is obviously not practical for all of these specialties to physically work together, there needs to be careful consideration of who does what, preferably with protocols to guide appropriate referral and ensure good liaison. It is important to ensure that there are neither gaps nor too many overlaps in the service. In countries such as Australia, New Zealand and the UK where there is a national network of specialist continence nurses, part of that job is often to organize this liaison and integration of the service and to guide individual patients through the referral route most appropriate to their individual needs.

Some areas are starting to tackle problems of coor-

Table 50.1 Multidisciplinary teamwork – professionals potentially involved in a continence service.

Medical	Non-medical
Urologist	Continence adviser
Gynaecologist/urogynaecologist	Nurses & midwives
Physician	Health visitors
Geriatrician	Physiotherapist
Neurologist	Occupational therapist
General practitioner	Dietician
Consultant in rehabilitation	Clinical psychologist
Psychiatrist	Social worker & team
Child & adolescent psychiatrist	Learning disability team
Paediatrician	Supplies staff
Coloproctologist	Managers
Gastroenterologist	Voluntary bodies
	Users/carers

From Norton (1995).

dinating continence services by consulting on and agreeing referral criteria and pathways. Others have set up multidisciplinary clinics, such as a 'pelvic floor clinic' where gynaecologist, urologist, colorectal surgeon, physiotherapist and continence nurse work together.

AN IDEAL SERVICE?

In the UK the Royal College of Physicians (1995) set up a multidisciplinary working party which has made a number of recommendations on continence services (Table 50.2) and the Department of Health (1991) has identified the key elements of a continence service (Table 50.3) and then strongly advised Health Authorities to implement this (NHS Executive 1993). It is often difficult to define what is currently being provided in an area, as elements may be very disparate and fragmented, and provided via a wide variety of different professionals and agencies. It may be a very complex job to try to integrate all elements into a coherent service.

Unfortunately, we simply do not know the optimum way of delivering a continence service. The Department of Health in the UK has commissioned an evaluation of different models of a nursing service, with and without specialist continence advisers (Roe et al 1996). It was found that where there is a continence nurse, incontinent people are more likely to receive targeted referral to specialists such as a urologist, and are more likely to have had investigations and to receive more appropriate treatment and care for their incontinence. Patients were also more likely to report satisfaction with the service where there was a specialist nurse.

Table 50.2 Royal College of Physicians' recommendations for a continence service.

A continence service should include:

- A defined method of entry for patients referred by general practitioners, nurses, hospital staff and patients themselves
- Access to appropriate diagnostic facilities, including urodynamics and anorectal investigations
- Access to medical and surgical consultants with a special interest in incontinence
- Integration of incontinence services for children with other paediatric services
- Attention to the wishes of patients and carers
- Access to nurses and physiotherapists with special training in treatment modalities for incontinence
- A role for one or more specialist continence advisors in the education of the public and professionals in continence maintenance
- A policy concerning the purchasing and supply of containment materials and equipment in the community, in residential and nursing homes and in hospitals
- Well defined audit and quality assurance systems.

The structure required to achieve these aims might include: a designated manager, an expert advisory panel and a budget to provide staff, their training and support services, and containment materials and equipment.

From Royal College of Physicians (1995), paragraph 4.7 and 4.8.

Table 50.3 Key features of a continence service.

- Active enthusiastic medical consultant and general manager involvement
- Continence advisers (usually, but not necessarily, nurses) with management and teaching skills and a small caseload to keep their clinical skills up to scratch
- A computer to store patient information
- Active publicity work and sympathetic, knowledgeable telephone advice
- A separate budget.

From Department of Health (1991).

However, there has never been a more comprehensive examination of a total service, and at present we simply do not know if a hospital-based consultant-led clinic will achieve better and more cost-effective results than community clinics or any other model. In future, there should be local consultation and debate, with deliberate planning.

In an attempt to overcome reluctance to seek help, some continence advisors have set up 'drop-in' clinics run by nurses in user-friendly locations, such as the local health clinic (where 60% of patients presented after seeing a poster, Macaulay & Henry 1990). Other unconventional sites for continence clinics include an occupational health department in a large factory employing women (Steele & Pomfret 1992).

An open-access clinic with a computerized self-assessment proforma has been reported (Morrison et al 1992). In the first 30 months telephone advice was given to 7025 people; 1045 patients attended; 3290 professionals attended; and 1446 requests for teaching or information were dealt with. Originally a pilot project, the Resource Centre was judged a success and has received permanent funding from the Health Authority.

A comprehensive service will only work well if health care gatekeepers are educated about incontinence and know how to refer appropriately. Jolleys and Wilson (1993) found in the UK that only two-thirds of newly qualified general practitioners (GPs) had received between 1 and 4 hours total training on incontinence; one-third had no training at all. Of GPs in practice for over 5 years, 92% had received no training on incontinence, and 80% of all GPs felt that their training on the subject was totally inadequate; 92% would like specific postgraduate education on incontinence. Knowledge about incontinence was found to be poor, with 76% of GPs having 'no idea of its prevalence'. Only 30% of GPs felt very confident to diagnose and manage incontinence.

THE ROLE OF THE SPECIALIST CONTINENCE NURSE

Continence advisers were appointed in the UK throughout the 1980s with no central planning or direction. From a situation in which there were only 17 continence advisers in 1983 (Kings Fund), there are over 420 in 1998 (Continence Foundation), with nearly every purchasing authority having at least one in their area. The cynical might say that many of these posts were created in the last two decades in an attempt to limit spending on the budget for incontinence pads, which have traditionally been provided free of charge in the community, rather than because of a vision of potential clinical benefit to patients. Some new continence advisers found themselves set a task of at least saving their own salary on the pads budget. Many have been given a substantial budget with little or no financial training or clerical help. The result in a few instances has been a service almost totally focused on product supply and the mechanics of pad delivery.

The Royal College of Nursing Continence Care Forum conducted a consensus exercise amongst continence advisers (1992). This recommended that the principal functions of the continence adviser should be education, management, clinical practice and research, and that each of these elements should be recognized as equally important. At present there is no research on the most appropriate mix of these functions, or on the optimum number of continence advisers per head of population. Most areas seem to be moving towards a small team as recommended by the Department of Health (1991), rather than a lone individual. Rhodes & Parker (1993) have found that there is tremendous variation in time allocated to the different elements of the job and that non-clinical managers do not really understand what the service is about.

Hall et al (1988) have described how one continence advisor was used as a peripatetic teacher to train 10 nurses in six centres, who were subsequently able to set up their own community based continence clinics. A subjective cure rate of 30% was obtained for patients seen only by these nurses, with a further 36% 'improved'. Hospital referrals were felt to have decreased, but no statistics were given for this subjective opinion. McGhee et al (1997) found that dedicated continence staff can improve continence levels in both community and residential home settings.

Some continence advisors work via a 'link nurse' network (Gibson 1989). One nurse from each clinical unit is identified and receives additional education to enable her/him to function as a local resource consultant to colleagues. Other continence advisors work with medical specialists in educating the primary health care team. Snape et al (1992) describe a urologist, gynaecologist, geriatrician and continence advisor putting on a 'roadshow' to take education out to community professionals.

O'Brien et al (1991) found that a nurse with no previous specialist training was competent to assess and manage community patients after 3 weeks training with a continence advisor and a physiotherapist. Sixty eight per cent of women were subjectively cured or improved after nursing intervention, compared to 20% of controls. Only 20% of men were cured or improved (100% of controls were unchanged). They concluded that many incontinent people could be effectively managed by a nurse with limited additional training, reserving specialist medical help for resistant cases. These results seem to be sustained in the long term (O'Brien & Long 1995).

Other countries, such as Australia, have adopted this model of a continence nurse specialist. But there are other health care systems that make it very difficult to fund nurses working as independent practitioners across hospital and community boundaries. The education of such nurses and development of recognized training for them, has lagged behind the development of posts.

PRODUCT SUPPLY

Support for people whose incontinence does not respond to appropriate treatment will always remain important for a continence service, but should not be allowed to become its sole focus. There is a wide variety of approaches to product supply in different countries, with some putting all responsibility upon the patient, while others will provide almost any product free of charge to patients in their own home. Even where the state does agree to take responsibility for provision of incontinence products, the expenditure per head varies greatly (Norton 1992). Even where patients must purchase their own products, they will often benefit from professional guidance on choosing between the bewildering variety of products on the market (see Ch. 48).

PUBLIC AWARENESS

There is no doubt that taboos on mentioning bladders generally and incontinence in particular are gradually lifting in some cultures. Two decades ago it was almost impossible to have incontinence discussed in the media. Now women's magazines, local and national papers, radio and even television cover the subject in some countries. Many countries have run national or local public awareness campaigns, usually spearheaded by a national continence organization. Many also have confidential helplines, which can be accessed anonymously. A list of continence organizations is given in Appendix 50.1, and many are willing to share their experiences with others.

Rooker (1992) found that only one third of continence services in the UK publicize their existence directly to the public. For a taboo subject like incontinence, this must encourage the tendency not to seek professional help. Some services are, however, proactive in encouraging presentation, taking a 'roadshow' out to public venues.

There is a need to evaluate the impact of public awareness campaigns. There is some evidence that people who respond by phoning a helpline do not necessarily act on the advice that they are given (Norton et al 1995). It cannot be assumed that everyone who has a continence problem would want or welcome information. O'Brien et al (1991) found that of people who had identified themselves as incontinent of urine in a postal survey, 45% refused any help or advice. Whether this was because of genuinely not perceiving it as enough of a problem to bother about, or because of embarrassment in facing a personal consultation, is unknown.

CONCLUSIONS

A comprehensive continence service to serve an entire population will not be a solely hospital-based, doctor-led service. There is a small but growing body of evidence that clinical and cost effectiveness can be gained by having a complimentary, probably nurse-led, service based in the community. Such a specialist nurse can provide a filter for more expensive hospital services, educate community care teams, and create awareness and ease of access to enable incontinent women to obtain the most appropriate help.

INTERNATIONAL CONTINENCE ORGANIZATIONS

AUSTRALIA
Continence Foundation of Australia Ltd
AMA House, 293 Royal Parade, Parkville, Victoria 3052
Tel: (61) 3 9347 2522 Fax: (61) 3 9347 2533

AUSTRIA
Medizinische Gesellschaft für Inkontinenzhilfe Österreich
Speckbacherstrasse 1, A-6020 Innsbruck
Tel: (43) 512 58 37 03 Fax: (43) 512 58 94 76

CANADA
The Canadian Continence Foundation
PO Box 66524, Cavendish Mall, Cote St Luc, Quebec H4W 3J6
Tel: (1) 514 488 8379 Fax: (1) 514 932 3533

DENMARK
Dansk Inkontinensforening (The Danish Association of Incontinent People)
Rathsacksvej 8, 1862 Frederiksberg C
Tel: (45) 3325 5121 Fax: (45) 3325 8695

GERMANY
Gesellschaft für Inkontinenzhilfe e.V. (GIH)
Geschäftsstelle, Friedrich-Ebert-Strasse 124, 34119 Kassel
Tel: (49) 561 78 06 04 Fax: (49) 561 77 67 70

HONG KONG
Hong Kong Continence Foundation
Room 214, 2/F
Tung Ying Building, 100 Nathan Road, Hong Kong
Tel: 852 2311 2218 Fax: 852 2311 2633

INDIA
Indian Continence Foundation
C/O Bangalore Kidney Foundation, CA6, 11th Cross, 15th Main, Padmanabhanagar, Bangalore
560070, India
Fax: 91 80 6692466

ISRAEL
The National Centre for Continence in the Elderly
Rambam Medical Centre, POB-9602, Haifa 31096
Tel: (972) 485 43197 Fax: (972) 4854 2883 or 4854 2098

JAPAN
Japan Continence Action Society
Continence Centre, 103 Jurihaimu, 4–2 Zenpukuzi
1 -Chome, Suginami-Ku, Tokyo, 167
Tel: (81) 3 3301 3860 Fax: (81) 3 3301 3587

KOREA
Korea Continence Foundation
Department of Urology, Dong-A University Hospital,
3 Ga-1 Dongdaeshin-dong, Seo-Gu 602–103
Pusan City, Korea
Tel: 82 51 240 5927 Fax: 82 51 253 0591

MALAYSIA
Continence Foundation (Malaysia)
c/o University Hospital, Lembah Pantai, Kuala Lumpar 59100,
Malaysia
Fax: 603 758 6063

NETHERLANDS
Vereniging Nederlandse Incontinentie, Verpleekundigen (V N I V)
p/a Achterloseweg 33, 6044 KC Wychen
Tel/Fax: (31) 24 645 1257

NEW ZEALAND
New Zealand Continence Association Inc
41 Pembroke Street, Hamilton
Tel: (64) 7 834 3528 Fax: (64) 7 834 3532

NORWAY
NOFUS (Norwegian Society for Patients with Urologic Diseases)
Fornebuveien 10 A, N-1324 Lysaker, Norway
Tel: 47 67 59 05 35. Fax: 47 67 59 05 35

SINGAPORE
Society for Continence (Singapore)
c/o Division of Urology, Dept of Surgery, Changi General
Hospital, 2 Simei Street 3, Singapore 529889
Tel/Fax: (65) 787 0337

SWEDEN
Swedish Urotherapists
Nordenskioldsgatan 10
S-413 09, Goteborg
Tel: (46) 31 50 26 39 Fax: (46) 31 53 68 32

TAIWAN
Taiwan Continence Society
Department of Urology, Taipei Medical College
252 Wu-Hsin Street, Taipei, Taiwan

UNITED KINGDOM
Association for Continence Advice (ACA)
Winchester House, Kennington Park
Cranmer Road, London SW9 6EJ
Tel: *(44) 20 7820 8113 Fax: (44) 20 7820 0442*

The Continence Foundation
307 Hatton Square, 16 Baldwin Gardens, London EC1N 7RJ
Tel: (44) 20 7404 6875 Fax: (44) 20 7404 6876

Enuresis Resource and Information Centre (ERIC)
34 Old School House, Britannia Road, Kingswood, Bristol BS15 2DB
Tel: (44) 117 960 3060 Fax: (44) 117 960 0401

InconTact
11 Marshalsea Road, London SE1 1EP

Royal College of Nursing Continence Care Forum
c/o Royal College of Nursing, 20 Cavendish Square, London WIM OAB
Tel: (44) 20 7409 3333

UNITED STATES OF AMERICA
The Simon Foundation for Continence
PO Box 815, Wilmette, Illinois 60091
Tel: (1) 847 864 3913 Fax: (1) 847 864 9758

National Association for Continence
PO Box 8310, Spartanburg, SC 29305–8310.
Tel: (1) 864 579 7900 Fax: (1) 803 579 7902

International Foundation for Functional Gastrointestinal Disorders *(formerly International Foundation for Bowel Dysfunction)*
PO Box 17864, Milwaukee WI 53217
Tel: (1) 414 964 1799 Fax: (1) 414 964 7176.

Society of Urologic Nurses and Associates
East Holly Avenue – Box 56, Pitman NJ 08071 0056
Tel: (1) 609 256 2335 Fax: (1) 609 589 7463

REFERENCES

AHCPR 1997 Urinary incontinence in adults: clinical practice guideline, 2nd edn. Agency for Health care Policy and Research, US Department of Health and Human Services, Rockville USA

Continence Foundation 1998 Index of Continence Services. Continence Foundation, London

Department of Health 1991 An agenda for action on continence services. ML (91)1. Department of Health, London.

Fonda D, Ouslander J G, Norton C 1994 Continence across the continents. Journal of the American Geriatrics Society 42: 109–112

Gibson E 1989 Co-ordinating continence care. Nursing Times 85: 73–75

Hall C, Castleden C M, Grove G J 1988 Fifty-six continence advisors, one peripatetic teacher. British Medical Journal 297: 1181–1182

Jolleys J V, Wilson J V 1993 GPs lack confidence (letter). British Medical Journal 306: 1344

Kings Fund 1983 Action on incontinence: report of a working group. Project paper 43. Kings Fund Centre, London

Macaulay M, Henry G, 1990 Drop in and do well. Nursing Times 86(46): 65–66

McGhee M, O'Neill K, Major K 1997 Evaluation of a nurse led continence service in the south west of Glasgow. Journal of Advanced Nursing 26: 723–728

Morrison L M, Glen E S, Cherry L, Dawes H A, 1992. An open access continence resource centre for Greater Glasgow Health Board. British Journal of Urology 70: 395–398

NHS Executive 1993 Priorities and planning guidance 1994–5. Leeds, National Health Service Management Executive

NHS Executive 1994 Incontinence. London, Citizens Charter & National Health Service Executive, F50/042 1715 1P 15K

Norton C 1992 Continent's provision. Nursing Times 88(44): 76–78

Norton C 1995 Commissioning comprehensive continence services; guidance for purchasers. London, The Continence Foundation

Norton C (ed) 1996 Nursing for continence (second edition). Beaconsfield, Beaconsfield Publishers.

Norton C, Brown J, Thomas E 1995 A phone call away. Nursing Standard. 9(25): 22–23

O'Brien J, Long H 1995. Long term effectiveness of nursing interventions in primary care. British Medical Journal 311: 1208

O'Brien J, Austin M, Sethi P, O'Boyle P, 1991. Urinary incontinence: prevalence, need for treatment and effectiveness of intervention by a nurse. British Medical Journal 303: 1308–1312

Rhodes P, Parker G 1993 The role of continence advisers in England and Wales. York, Social Policy Research Unit, University of York

Roe B, Wilson K, Doll H, Brooks P 1996. An evaluation of health interventions by primary health care teams and continence advisory services on patient outcomes related to incontinence. Health Care Research Unit, University of Oxford

Royal College of Nursing 1992 The role of the continence adviser. London, Royal College of Nursing

Royal College of Physicians 1995 Incontinence: causes, management and provision of services. Royal College of Physicians, London

Rooker J 1992 Community continence services: a survey of the policies and practices of DHAs in England with respect to the provision of continence services. Labour Party, London

Snape J, Allardice A J, Lemberger R J, Pickles C J 1992 The continence roadshow a method of educating primary health care workers about services available and management of urinary incontinence. Proceedings of the 22nd Annual Meeting of the International Continence Society, Halifax, Nova Scotia

Steele W, Pomfret I, 1992. Promoting continence at work. Community Outlook January: 15–16

Training

EMMA GORTON

INTRODUCTION

Until recently, medical education has been based on a system that was driven by performance in examinations which rewarded rote learning and recall of factual information. Such a system does not encourage the development of the skills needed to acquire and appraise information in order to solve clinical problems (Towles 1998). A key element to good teaching whether at undergraduate or at postgraduate level is the ability to stimulate self-learning. The high prevalence of urinary incontinence implies that it should be included in the general training of most health care workers, and should be a major component of training of obstetricians and gynaecologists (Royal College of Physicians 1995).

Although the terms training and education are often used interchangeably in medicine, they refer to different concepts. Education is a broad concept, involving teaching and learning strategies that encourage critical thinking and the ability to solve unfamiliar problems by the application of prior knowledge (Lister 1993). This forms the main focus of the undergraduate curriculum. Training, however, refers to the acquisition of specific skills aimed at achieving technical competence and prepares the individual to respond to familiar problems and situations, often with little critical thinking. Postgraduate teaching builds on undergraduate education to train the doctor to become clinically competent (Lister 1993). Although this chapter focuses mainly on training, it is important to consider also the principles of education.

UNDERGRADUATE EDUCATION

Undergraduate medical education is undergoing major change throughout the United Kingdom with the aim of reducing information overload and making learning more problem orientated. To achieve this the curriculum is divided into a core curriculum with elective modules. The idea is that students should not be overwhelmed by a huge volume of course work, but should have time for discussion and reflection and be allowed to develop their individual interests. The emphasis is on guided self-learning with the students encouraged to take increasing responsibility for their own learning (Coles 1993). The components of the core curriculum will vary in different medical schools, and there is concern that if incontinence is not included in the core curriculum undergraduate education may diminish as it is not likely to be chosen as a special study module (Royal College of Physicians 1995).

POSTGRADUATE TRAINING

Urogynaecology is one of the five subspecialist branches of obstetrics and gynaecology, the others being fetomaternal medicine, oncology, reproductive medicine, and community gynaecology (Royal College of Obstetricians and Gynaecologists 1997b). Some basic training in each of these areas is essential for all postgraduates intending a career in obstetrics and gynaecology to ensure appropriate referral when required (Blunt & Studd 1993). Until recently such exposure has tended to be haphazard, but it was hoped that the introduction of Calman would ensure a more structured approach to training. In the latest survey of training approximately 50% of trainees said they had received basic training in urogynaecology, with slightly over 80% of those at senior registrar grade having received some training (Royal College of Obstetricians and Gynaecologists 1997a). As part of structured training, trainees are expected to complete a series of modules which are included in the basic and main log books. The log books are now used to document competencies rather than experience, and the trainee is expected to be signed off when the trainer feels that they are able to perform the skill independently. The module in urogynaecology focuses on the assessment and non-surgical management of urinary incontinence and prolapse. It is envisaged that formal teaching in this would occur in urogynaecology assessment clinics and the trainee is assessed by observation of clinical practice and formal testing. After completion of the surgical module the trainee should be able to perform vaginal prolapse surgery under indirect supervision, and suprapubic operations under direct supervision. Beyond this basic training, there is increasing pressure for generalists to have a 'special interest', and increasingly peripheral hospitals have generalists with special interest in each of the subspecialty fields (Blunt & Studd 1993).

Urodynamic training

Urodynamics remain the key to diagnosis for women with bladder symptoms. Despite their importance there is no formal training programme for the people who undertake these tests. In a recent survey of units in the United Kingdom, approximately half the respondents felt that their training had been inadequate (Hosker et al 1997). At the present time, there is no registration of urodynamic units and no requirement for certification of personnel performing urodynamics. However, training is important as the diagnosis of stress incontinence or detrusor instability depends on an interpretable cystometrogram, with good subtraction and correctly positioned transducers. In addition, good counselling skills are important as embarrassment and anxiety are more of a problem during the procedure than pain (Gorton & Stanton 1998).

Subspecialty training

Subspecialists should have specialist knowledge and expertise in dealing with the less common problems. Referral from a large population base is needed to maintain this ability, thus pure subspecialist posts should remain limited in number (Blunt & Studd 1993).

To be eligible to be considered as a centre for subspecialty training in urogynaecology a centre must have an adequate clinical workload of women with a wide range of urogynaecological problems with facilities for their investigation. In addition, there should be close links with other related specialties, such as urology, neurology, care of the elderly, colorectal surgery and an appropriately trained physiotherapist. There are currently three suspecialist training centres in urogynaecology in the United Kingdom: Kings College Hospital and St. George's Hospital, both in London, and The Liverpool Women's Hospital.

In the USA, unofficial 1–2 year training fellowships in both urogynaecology and pelvic surgery have been available for at least 20 years. Since 1997 fellowships in Urogynaecology and Reconstructive Pelvic Surgery of over 3 years duration have been eligible to apply for formal accreditation. So far 10 such programmes have been accredited. However, the American Board of Medical Specialties will not accept a discipline for certification as a subspecialty unless there are at least 25 accredited fellowships.

In Australia, urogynaecology has been recognized as a subspecialty since 1988 and there are currently three accredited centres. As with all subspecialties there are concerns about the potential risk of training too many subspecialties who would then have insufficient work to maintain their own excellence, and may take work from general gynaecologists.

The syllabus for urogynaecology training is similar in the UK, Australia and the USA. In each country the trainee is expected to gain advanced knowledge in the anatomy, physiology, pharmacology and pathophysiology of the urinary tract, lower gastrointestinal tract, pelvic floor and genital viscera. The trainee should acquire a high degree of clinical competence to be able to make a clinical diagnosis, plan and interpret investigations and treat women with a wide variety of pelvic floor and urological problems (see Appendix for details of the UK syllabus). There is a strong association between urinary and faecal incontinence (Jackson et al 1997), so there is a need for urogynaecologists to work closely with colorectal surgeons. A model that has been used at St George's Hospital is the combined clinic where patients can be reviewed by a colorectal surgeon and urogynaecologist simultaneously (Nager et al 1997). By allowing problems of all compartments of the pelvic floor to be dealt with at one visit, patient care is improved, educational opportunities are enhanced and collaborative research encouraged.

In the UK, the trainee is assessed by a midterm interview to ensure that the training is proceeding smoothly and a further interview at the end of the programme to ensure that the training objectives have been met. In Australia the trainee must produce a thesis of original research in urogynaecology and pass an examination in urogynaecology. American trainees also have to produce a thesis, but there is no formal examination.

TEACHING METHODS

Traditional didactic lectures remain one of the commonest teaching methods used throughout medical education. Lectures are useful in teaching large number of students, particularly when new material is introduced. Although often criticized in educational literature, lectures are probably superior to small group techniques for the learning of facts (Crosby 1996). To make lectures as effective as possible they should be well planned, with a clear logical order to the material so that the student can understand the basic principles of the subject. One of the main problems with lectures is the fall in student concentration with time. To help redress this problem it is useful to introduce a change in teaching style after about 20 minutes (Newble & Cannon 1994). Possibilities include questioning or testing the students or the use of a videotape segment. When a deeper approach to learning is required, however, as in the development of analytical problem solving skills or in learning to interpret urodynamic traces, then small group techniques are preferable (Crosby 1996). A small group facilitator needs to have the skills to ensure that there is active participation from all members of the group. Thus, some understanding of group dynamics is helpful (Crosby 1996). A number of small group activities have been described to encourage participation such as brainstorming, snowballing and role play.

Computers are being increasingly used in medicine, and recently have become a valuable learning resource. The Royal College of Obstetricians and Gynaecologists has developed a computer assisted learning package which enables the user to work through a number of case studies in the comfort of their own home (Pannikar 1998). The package is known as RCOG-DIALOG (Distance and Interactive Learning in Obstetrics and Gynaecology). Each of the cases is produced by an expert in the field and includes annotated figures and tables and multiple choice questions. They have been mainly developed for continuing medical education, but they are also a valuable resource for trainees.

The above techniques are useful in teaching trainees the skills needed for clinical problem solving and the interpretation of investigations; however, for surgical skill training there is no substitute for hands-on experience. Both consultants and trainees have expressed concerns that current trends to reduce junior doctors' hours and shorten training will result in a lack of surgical experience. This is further compounded by financial cuts which increase pressures on health service staff to deliver more for less, thus restricting the amount of time available in theatre for training. For example, it has been estimated that, in general surgery alone, the increased theatre time required to allow all trainees to gain adequate surgical experience during a 5-year structured programme would cost one Health Authority an extra £1.3 m (Crofts et al 1997). Theatre time can be used more efficiently if basic surgical skills such as suturing and knot tying are learnt on either fresh tissue specimens or with synthetic tissue simulation models (Thomas et al 1996).

NON-CLINICAL TRAINING

Management and teaching

Clinicians are increasingly expected to play a role in management. Although most junior doctors attend departmental meetings and are involved in administration few have any experience with contracting or organization of clinical services. Attendance at a management course is thus helpful prior to appointment as a consultant when management skills will become more important.

Until recently, few hospital doctors have had any training in effective teaching techniques. This is in contrast to general practice where training courses are mandatory for trainers and their performance is assessed. In 1994 the Standing Committee on Postgraduate Medical and Dental Education recommended improved training for all involved in medical education in the skills required for learner centred education (Standing committee on Postgraduate Medical and Dental Training 1994).

Research and audit

The ability to interpret research findings and use evidence-based medicine is essential for all doctors. Spending a period of time undertaking clinical or basic science research has been seen as the way to achieve this (Thomas 1993). In a recent survey of consultant urologists, Feneley and Feneley (1998) found that most felt that their experience had been beneficial; however, other surveys have been more critical of the role of research (Harvey et al 1992). Success in research is commonly measured by the completion of an MD or publications in peer reviewed journals. Although there is undoubtedly a need for all doctors to be able to understand research methodology, the pressure to publish has been identified as one of the factors in the poor quality of much that is published and the rise in research fraud (Altman 1994). Improved training and support have been suggested as one means of ensuring that research skills are acquired cost effectively (Gale 1995).

CONCLUSIONS

Urogynaecology training should commence in medical school, but most of the practical teaching in clinical skills, interpretation and performing urodynamics will occur after graduation. Although all obstetricians and gynaecologists must have an understanding of the causes and treatment of female urinary incontinence and prolapse there is also a need for some individuals to develop this further to offer subspecialty expertise for more complex cases. Recently this has been extended to include an interest in the posterior compartment of the pelvic floor with the establishment of combined pelvic floor clinics. Supplementary to traditional teaching methods such as lectures and small group teaching, innovative techniques, such as the use of simulation models and computer programmes can be helpful if applied appropriately.

As the non-clinical responsibilities of doctors in management, teaching, research and audit increases, training must be extended to include the skills required for these tasks.

ACKNOWLEDGEMENTS

The author would like to thank Dr P. Dwyer and Dr R. Bump for information about subspecialization in Australia and the USA respectively.

REFERENCES

Altman D G 1994 The scandal of poor medical research. British Medical Journal 308: 283–284

Blunt S, Studd J (eds) 1993 Training in Obstetrics and Gynaecology: The time for change. RCOG Press, London

Coles C 1993 Developing medical education. Postgraduate Medical Journal 69: 57–63

Crofts T J, Griffiths J M T, Sharma S, Wygrala J, Aitken R J 1997 Surgical training: an objective assessment of recent changes for a single heath board. British Medical Journal 314: 891–895

Crosby J 1996 Learning in small groups. Medical Teacher 18: 189–202

Feneley M R, Feneley R C I 1998 The contribution of research to urological training in the United Kingdom. British Journal of Urology 81: 193–198

Gale R 1995 The place of research in medical training. Joint Centre for Education in Medicine, London

Gorton E Stanton S L 1998 How unpleasant are urodynamic investigations. British Journal of Obstetrics and Gynaecology 105 (supplement) 17: 89

Harvey R F, Burns-Cox C J, Heaton K W 1992 The MD thesis in the training of a consultant physician. Journal of the Royal College of Physicians of London 26: 380–382

Hosker G L, Kilcyne P M, Lord J C, Smith A R 1997 Urodynamic services, personnel and training in the United Kingdom. British Journal of Urology 79: 159–162

Jackson S L, Weber A M, Hull T L, Mitchinson A R, Walters M D 1997 Fecal incontinence in women with urinary incontinence and pelvic organ prolapse. Obstetrics and Gynecology 89: 423–427

Lister J 1993 Postgraduate Medical Education. Nuffeild Provincial Hospital Trust London

Nager C W, Kumar D, Kahn M A, Stanton S L 1997 Management of pelvic floor dysfunction. Lancet 350: 1751

Newble D, Cannon R 1994 A Handbook for Medical Teachers, 3rd edn. Kluwer Academic Publishers, Lancaster

Pannikar J 1998 The new RCOG-DIALOG – an interactive learning experience. British Journal of Obstetrics and Gynaecology 105 (supplement) 17: 62

Royal College of Obstetricians and Gynaecologists 1997a Survey of Training. RCOG National Trainees Committee

Royal College of Obstetricians and Gynaecologists 1997b Syllabus: Subspecialisation in Urogynaecology

Royal College of Physicians 1995 Incontinence: Causes, management and provision of services. London

Standing Committee on Postgraduate Medical and Dental Education 1994 Teaching hospital doctors and dentists to teach. London

Thomas E. 1993 The role of research in the training of an obstetrician and gynaecologist. British Journal of Obstetrics and Gynaecology 100: 35–36

Thomas W E, Lee P W, Sunderland G T, Day R P 1996 A preliminary evaluation of an innovative synthetic soft tissue simulation module ('Skilltray') for use in basic surgical skills workshops. Annals Royal College of Surgeons of England 78 (supplement): 268–271

Towle A 1998 Changes in health care and continuing medical education for the 21st century. British Medical Journal 316: 301–304

Urogynaecology audit

GERALD J JARVIS

INTRODUCTION

Medical audit has been defined as the systematic critical analysis of the quality of medical care, including the procedures used for diagnosis and treatment, the use of resources, and the resulting outcome and the quality of life for the patient. The object of medical audit is to improve the quality of care provided for patients.

If audit is to be successful it should focus on the clinical processes and outcomes of care and the results should feed back into the system by which care is delivered. Audit is hence a dynamic process and follows a circular pattern called the audit cycle (Fig. 52.1). This chapter cannot complete the audit cycle but is designed to assess the current status of management of women with urinary incontinence and from this standards will be suggested; but the audit cycle loop cannot be closed until such standards have been assessed prospectively by future scientific studies.

Medical audit may take many different forms encompassing both the clinical process and the administrative process. The clinical process itself may be subdivided into the component parts of investigation and treatment and these may then be subdivided to select specific topics. Those topics chosen may be purely of local importance to the clinicians and the patients within a given area or may be of national or even international importance in assessing and laying down standards for clinical care.

The purpose of this chapter is not to select topics

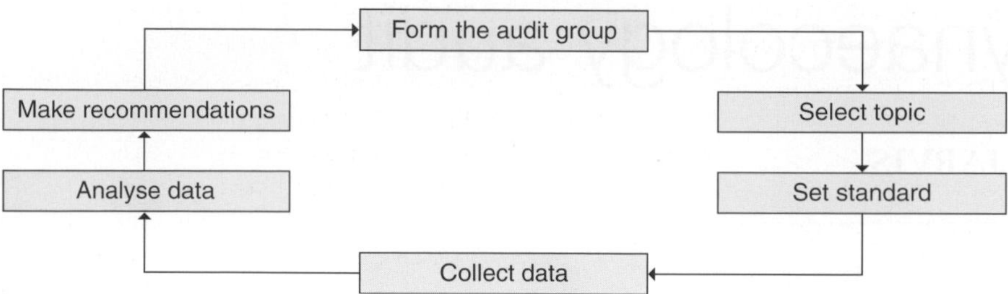

Fig. 52.1 The audit cycle.

which are too narrow but rather to assess the quality of the information upon which current practice is assessed and to make recommendations both to streamline clinical practice and to improve the quality of future information upon which practice may be modified.

HOW COMMON IS FEMALE URINARY INCONTINENCE?

That urinary incontinence in adult women leading independent lives is common is now beyond dispute. There have been numerous surveys which would suggest that the prevalence of urinary incontinence in such women varies between 14 and 45% of the population surveyed (Jolleys 1988; Lagro-Janssen et al 1991a; Brocklehurst 1993). Whichever estimate is closest to the true prevalence, urinary incontinence is undoubtedly common in apparently healthy people. The evidence is that women are more commonly incontinent than men and although the prevalence rises with increasing age, increasing parity and deteriorating general health, even young nulliparous, and otherwise totally healthy women experience urinary incontinence (Thomas et al 1980; Vetter et al 1981; Yarnell et al 1981; Brocklehurst 1993).

These and other studies have audited not only the prevalence of urinary incontinence within the apparently healthy adult female population but have also demonstrated that this collection of clinical conditions which constitute urinary incontinence has an effect on the lifestyle of at least some of these patients, and that many would welcome treatment yet are reluctant to seek it.

The effect on lifestyle will probably depend upon a woman's perception of the incontinence rather than upon the volume of urine leaked. It will vary from being a mere nuisance in some women to far more troublesome in others. Some two thirds of women for whom incontinence occurs at least weekly (and this is at least 5.7% of the adult female population) regularly wear some form of protection. They may restrict normal day-to-day activities such as shopping, travel, physical recreation, and the choice of clothing. More seriously, some of these women believe that the incontinence has affected their physical or mental health, and they may develop difficulties in relationships with family and friends. In one recent survey, one in five incontinent women were afraid that they smelt and one in nine believed that sexual activity was compromised. Only 13% of incontinent women had ever confided their problem to their spouse.

At least some of these incontinent women would welcome treatment. In one survey, 47% of incontinent women consulted a doctor (Brocklehurst 1993) and although the advice given appeared to range between the relatively useless and the particularly effective, 93% of such women considered that the advise was at least sympathetic.

Why, therefore, are these potential patients reluctant to seek advice? In one recent study only 41% of incontinent women attending a specialist unit had consulted a doctor within 1 year of their symptoms commencing, and 26% had delayed for at least 5 years (Norton et al 1988). The reasons for the delay are complex, but appear to include factors over and above the severity of the incontinence as perceived by the woman. Some women will hope that their symptoms will go spontaneously, others are either too embarrassed or ashamed to admit to the problem and discuss it with another person, whilst others are afraid of the advice that they may receive, especially should it involve surgery. Perhaps most surprisingly, a significant proportion of these women (19%) considered that it was normal to leak urine (Norton et al 1988).

How can the audit cycle be closed in this area? It is clear that at least some women who are incontinent would welcome treatment yet do not actively seek it. All nurses and doctors are aware that patients do not readily complain of the symptoms of incontinence, but may do so if some encouragement is given during discussion of other problems. Doctors in general, and gynaecologists in particular, should take a full urinary history, since some of these patients will welcome advice concerning their previously undisclosed urinary incontinence. The female population needs to be encouraged to lose the negative considerations of embarrassment, shyness, and fear of treatment, whilst being encouraged to confess their symptoms in a sympathetic environment, knowing that there is a significant chance for improvement or cure. Education of the population must be the major recommendation to close the audit loop.

WHICH PATIENTS REQUIRE INVESTIGATION PRIOR TO TREATMENT?

The vast majority of women with urinary incontinence will either have genuine stress incontinence, detrusor instability, or a combination of both. Exact figures quoted from urogynaecological units will vary depending largely upon whether or not they include patients with spinal cord trauma. If patients with such trauma are excluded, then approximately 90% of incontinent women will have one or other or both of the two major diagnoses (Jarvis 1990). In clinical practice, therefore, as in all areas of medicine, the logical step before debating treatment is to make an accurate diagnosis.

There is now a wealth of evidence that demonstrates that clinical diagnosis, when assessed objectively by a urodynamic assessment, is accurate in only about 70% of patients. Numerous studies have audited the accuracy of clinical judgement against objective urodynamic assessment. Most have taken the form of an experienced observer who knew that he or she was to be tested making a clinical diagnosis and this diagnosis was not necessarily communicated to the person who performed the urodynamic assessment. The assumption is made that the urodynamic assessment is the correct diagnosis and this is probably true so long as it is appropriately performed and fluid leakage is demonstrated during that investigation. It is possible that these studies might have underestimated the prevalence of detrusor instability and this is discussed when ambulatory monitoring is considered in the next section. However, most units do not have access to ambulatory monitoring and it has yet to be proven that the increased pickup in detrusor instability will be of clinical significance.

The best clinical practice currently available is a urodynamic assessment of some type upon which the diagnosis is made. This author has compared the relative accuracy of clinical diagnosis and objective diagnosis for both genuine stress incontinence and detrusor instability. These studies are shown in Tables 52.1 and 52.2. The range of clinical accuracy for genuine stress incontinence is 40–87%, with a meta-analysis figure of 69.2%. It might have been supposed that clinical accuracy would be significantly greater for detrusor instability than genuine stress incontinence but this is not the case. It may be seen from Table 52.2 that the range of clinical accuracy for the diagnosis of detrusor instability varied from 46 to 81% with a meta-analysis figure of 70.4%.

It is therefore clear that a history will give guidance as to the severity of the urinary incontinence but will not necessarily make the diagnosis.

This audit of clinical accuracy would lend support to the view that all patients with urinary incontinence should undergo a urodynamic assessment in order to make an objective diagnosis before treatment is offered. Is this a logical position, since urodynamic assessment is time-consuming, expensive, perhaps unpleasant or undignified, invasive, and is associated

Table 52.1 Genuine stress incontinence – clinical accuracy.

Authors	Year	Number in study	Clinical accuracy numbers	Percentage
Bent et al	1983	43	29	67
Diokno et al	1987	132	92	70
Eastwood & Warrell	1984	5	2	40
Glenning	1984	100	56	56
Haylen et al	1989	168	114	68
Jarvis & Millar	1980	41	28	68
Korda et al	1987	272	176	64
Lagro-Janssen	1991b	54	47	87
Ouslander et al	1987	39	30	77
Ouslander et al	1989	22	14	62
Sand et al	1987a	43	25	58
Summitt et al	1992	38	31	80
Versi et al	1991	113	92	81
Total		**1093**	**756**	**69.2**

Table 52.2 Detrusor instability – clinical accuracy.

Authors	Year	Numbers in study	Clinical accuracy	
			Numbers	Percentage
Bent et al	1983	40	16	46
Cantor & Bates	1980	31	25	81
Diokno et al	1987	8	4	50
Eastwood & Warell	1984	52	42	81
Jarvis et al	1980	59	46	78
Ouslander et al	1987	95	70	74
Ouslander et al	1989	22	16	74
Sand et al	1988	13	10	77
Summitt et al	1992	52	33	63
Total		**372**	**262**	**70.4**

with a small but significant incidence of postinvestigative urinary tract infection? It has been reported that some 5% of women find the investigation distasteful and dysuria may occur in 48% of patients, frequency in 39%, haematuria in 37% and bacteriologically proven urinary tract infection in up to 19% (Coptcoat et al 1988; Baker et al 1991).

Three clinical situations usually present. The first is the patient who complains of urgency and urge incontinence but denies the symptoms of stress incontinence. It is most unlikely that such a patient will have genuine stress incontinence and since she will almost certainly be treated medically rather than surgically in the first instance, it is reasonable in such patients to omit a urodynamic assessment, offer treatment, and reserve urodynamic assessment should medical therapy fail. The second concerns the patient whose only urinary symptom is stress incontinence and who vigorously denies other urinary symptoms, especially urgency or urge incontinence. It is, however, probably inappropriate to omit a urodynamic assessment in this group of patients, for three reasons:

- Having the symptom of stress incontinence as the only lower urinary tract symptom is surprisingly unusual; in one series only 12 out of 494 women with the symptom of stress incontinence had this as the sole symptom (Haylen et al 1989).
- If genuine stress incontinence is to be treated surgically and since all surgery carries a demonstrable morbidity (and sadly even mortality) it is inappropriate to offer surgery unless the incontinence can be demonstrated since approximately 4% of all patients who claim to be incontinent of urine cannot have this incontinence demonstrated (Jarvis 1990).
- Detrusor instability may coexist with genuine stress incontinence and, unless this is diagnosed, the clinician may lose the opportunity of initiating postoperative treatment for the detrusor instability in the form of either drugs or bladder retraining and the patient may blame the clinician for the occurrence of previously undiagnosed but present detrusor instability.

The logical conclusion from these audits must be that all patients should undergo a urodynamic assessment prior to surgery for genuine stress incontinence and all patients who are considered to have detrusor instability but who are not responding to treatment should also undergo a urodynamic assessment in order to confirm or refute the clinical diagnosis. It is only by following such a policy that we avoid making the mistakes of our predecessors. The classic study by Bates et al (1973) investigated 75 women who were incontinent despite surgery for their supposed genuine stress incontinence. It was found, on formal urodynamic testing, that 45% of these patients had detrusor instability without any genuine stress incontinence, whereas 30% had continuing genuine stress incontinence, and 25% had no demonstrable urinary leakage. A preoperative urodynamic assessment on women with anterior vaginal wall prolapse and who deny incontinence prior to prolapse surgery may also identify those women who are at risk of incontinence from genuine stress incontinence once their cystocoele has been replaced (Colombo et al 1996).

WHICH INVESTIGATIONS ARE THE MOST APPROPRIATE?

The wide range of urodynamic studies available are listed in Table 52.3. Clearly no patient requires all of these studies and hence some degree of selection must take place.

The choice of investigation or investigations offered to the patient will depend partly upon the clinical situation, partly upon the expectation from any given test and partly upon which tests are avail-

Table 52.3 Urodynamic investigations.

Pad weighing
Q-tip test
Filling cytometry
Ambulatory urodynamics
Videocystourethrography
Ultrasound
Urethral pressure profilometry
Fluid bridge test
Urethral electrical conductance
Pressure-flow studies
Electromyography
Sacral nerve studies
Bladder cooling test

able to the clinician. Any investigation must satisfy at least one of the following criteria:

1 To confirm that the woman is incontinent of urine
2 To give a diagnosis which is more accurate than a clinical assessment
3 To uncover any coexisting problems
4 To influence the choice of treatment.

Pad weighing is designed to quantify urine loss under standard and reproducible conditions. It will confirm that the patient is, in fact, incontinent if there is any doubt and may indicate the severity of that incontinence (Sutherst et al 1981). Most investigators believe that there is good correlation between the weight of fluid on the pad and the severity of the incontinence as described by the patient (Sutherst et al 1986; Victor et al 1987) although a minority of authors would disagree with this view (Kinn & Larsson 1987).

The major indications for a pad weighing test, therefore, in clinical practice are to quantify urine loss either before or after treatment, or to confirm incontinence on the patient prior to formal urodynamic investigation.

The **Q-tip test** has never achieved any degree of popularity in the UK but has some popularity in North America where it is considered to be an 'office procedure'. The principle of the test is that a cotton tipped swab is placed in the urethra such that its tip is at the urethrovesical junction. The patient is asked to strain and the angle of the arc made by the distal end of the Q-tip is measured. The larger the arc, the greater is the mobility of the bladder neck and the assumption is made that the more mobile is the bladder neck, the more likely it is that the cause of the patient's incontinence is genuine stress incontinence (Crystle et al 1972). More serious investigation has, however, failed to demonstrate any correlation between the degree of mobility and the differential diagnosis between genuine stress incontinence and detrusor instability (Fantl et al 1986; Karram & Bhatia 1988). This test would seem to contribute little to that already available from clinical examination.

Filling cystometry is probably the single most useful investigation in deciding whether the patient has genuine stress incontinence, detrusor instability, or both. It is a method by which the pressure–volume relationship of the bladder is measured, assessing detrusor activity, sensation, capacity, and compliance. Although the test is objective, some correlation must be sought between the findings of the test and the symptoms complained of by the patient whilst the potential underdiagnosis of detrusor instability can be reduced by ensuring that the patient assumes a standing position at some stage during the test and provocations designed to elicit positive changes (e.g. coughing, heel-rolling) should occur (Bates et al 1970; Sand et al 1987a). Any investigative regimen used to assess a patient with urinary incontinence must include a filling cystometrogram as a minimum level of investigation.

There will be some patients in whom, as it has already been stated, urinary incontinence will not be confirmed objectively. There will be other patients in whom there is a high clinical suspicion of detrusor instability yet the bladder remains stable during the filling cystometrogram. These would be the indications for **ambulatory urodynamics** in which a filling cystometrogram is performed but the patient is allowed to walk freely around the hospital area or even return home with the catheters *in situ* and the electronic recording equipment attached for a 24-hour period.

There is good evidence to show that abnormalities will be demonstrated in the majority of the subgroup of patients in whom no abnormality was demonstrated on formal filling cytometry. In up to 90% of such patients a diagnosis will be made following ambulatory cystometry. Recent studies have suggested that that diagnosis may be detrusor instability alone in 57% of patients, genuine stress incontinence alone in 30%, and both conditions coexisting in 13% (McInerney et al 1991; van Waalwijk et al 1991; Webb et al 1991). The disadvantage of this approach is that the patient leaves the urodynamic environment with approximately £1500 of electronic equipment which may become lost or damaged.

A videocystourethrogram is probably no better than a filling cystometrogram alone in distinguishing between genuine stress incontinence and detrusor instability but has the advantages of easier visualization of leakage, the assessment of the position and mobility of the bladder neck (especially after previous surgery), the estimation of residual urine, the benefit for teaching purposes, and an opportunity to diagnose morphological abnormalities such as bladder or urethral diverticulae or vesicoureteric reflux (Benness et al 1989; Shepherd 1990).

Perhaps the single most important caveat when performing videocystourethrography is that incompetence of the bladder neck on radiological screening should not be assumed to equate with incontinence. The radio-opaque medium should flow throughout the urethra if incontinence is to be diagnosed. Asymptomatic bladder neck incompetence may be demonstrated in approximately 50% of perimenopausal women and in at least 21% of young nulliparous women (Versi et al 1986; Chapple et al 1989).

The use of **ultrasound** to visualize bladder neck opening rather than X-rays has the theoretical advantage of avoiding even the low dose of irradiation; and the debate as to whether or not use of a vaginal probe will distort the information (Quinn et al 1988; Wise et al 1992) can be overcome by the use of a transrectal probe (Yamada et al 1991). However, the same caveat relating to bladder neck opening must apply and both cystourethrography and either cystourethrography or ultrasound assessment must be combined with a filling cystometrogram if an accurate assessment as to the stability of the detrusor is to be made.

The techniques of **urethral pressure profilometry**, the **fluid bridge test** and **urethral electrical conductance** are no better individually at discriminating between genuine stress incontinence and detrusor instability than is clinical judgement (Sutherst & Brown 1980; Creighton et al 1991; Versi 1990).

Pressure-flow studies are the best techniques available to study the voiding phase of micturition. The major value for uroflowmetry lies in the prediction of postoperative voiding difficulties in patients with genuine stress incontinence but no symptoms of a voiding disorder. Up to 22% of women with genuine stress incontinence have an asymptomatic coexisting voiding disorder and this may be associated with difficulty in voiding following surgery together with a longer duration of catheterization (Bergman & Bhatia 1985; Stanton et al 1983; Haylen et al 1990). The benefit of making this diagnosis should be apparent. At a minimum level, the clinician who has identified such a voiding disorder prior to surgery for genuine stress incontinence may forewarn the patient of some delay in achieving postoperative voiding and at a more serious level may wish to avoid a surgical procedure associated with a high incidence of outlet obstruction. This point is developed further below.

The techniques of **electromyography, sacral nerve studies**, and **bladder cooling** are inappropriate to routine clinical practice and should be reserved for patients in whom muscle or nerve damage is either present or suspected (Massey & Abrams 1985; Bhatia 1991; Hellstrom et al 1991).

The audit loop has been closed in the use of urodynamic assessment to assess incontinent women. Shepherd (1990) reported that when the referring consultant acted upon the recommendation of the urodynamic assessment, 72% of the patients were cured or significantly improved whereas when the treatment was at variance with that recommended by the urodynamic assessment, only 38% were cured or improved. If urodynamic studies are to influence clinical decision making, as indeed they should, the information from those studies must be robust and this requires an adequate level of training and supervision in those who carry out urodynamic studies (Hosker et al 1997).

HOW SHOULD DETRUSOR INSTABILITY BE TREATED?

The options for treatment in detrusor instability and the expectations from that treatment have already been discussed in this book. Essentially, the treatment of detrusor instability may be divided into four clear sections: patient explanation and reassurance; drug therapy; behavioural therapy; and surgery.

The two most striking conclusions from an assessment of the available literature on drug therapy are: (1) it is a relatively poor treatment modality, and (2) in those studies which have been associated with randomized and non-randomized comparative trials, the placebo effect is outstanding. So important is the placebo effect that in one study placebo was a more effective form of treatment than either flavoxate or emepronium (Meyhoff et al 1983). The placebo improvement or cure rates which can be anticipated from such trials have been listed in Table 52.4. It should be noted that drug trials tend to report the percentage of patients who have been improved rather than the percentage of patients who have been made continent and perhaps this is a reflection of the efficacy of the treatment. For instance, in five trials which assess the efficacy of oxybutynin, only one of the five quote a continent rate whereas all five quote an improvement rate. The continence rate quoted (23%) was less than half of the improvement rate (58%) and hence the limited efficacy of active treatment over placebo is real (Moore et al 1990).

What must be apparent from this survey of the literature is that any drug prescribed should be 'given

Table 52.4 Placebo effect in detrusor instability.

Authors	Year	Improvement (%)
Moore et al	1990	4
Moisey et al	1980	8
Cardozo & Stanton	1980	11
Andersen et al	1988	25
Tapp et al	1990	42
Castleden et al	1985	43
Chapple et al	1990	44
Thuroff et al	1991	45
Meyhoff et al	1983	47

the hard sell' if the maximum from the placebo effect in addition to any active effect is to be obtained.

Of all the drugs which are currently available to treat idiopathic detrusor instability in women, the single most effective agent is considered to be oxybutynin, yet there is little general agreement within the literature as to the best starting dose, the optimal dose in which to balance efficacy against side-effects, and the anticipated benefits. This author has assessed five drug trials from the literature and attempted to correlate dosage with side-effects, improvements, and continence. The data are summarized in Table 52.5. As has already been stated, only one of the five trials takes continence as an end point, the rest using improvement. Side-effects sufficient to cause the patient to stop therapy is a not uncommon finding and there is some evidence to suggest that a lower dose of oxybutynin may reduce the incidence of side-effects without prejudicing efficacy. It is clear that before the audit loop can be closed in drug therapy, more information is required on the dose–efficacy–side-effect compromise.

There are two other types of drug trial within the literature which may be important in feeding back into clinical practice. The first is the variable dosage trial where the patient titrates drug dosage against efficacy and side-effects and perhaps such a trial mimics clinical practice whilst being more difficult to perform (Massey & Abrams 1986; Milani et al 1988; Tapp et al 1989a). There is a need for greater numbers of such trials in order that research may have a more direct effect upon clinical practice. The second style of trial consists of a drug combination in the belief that lower dosages of two separate but active agents may improve efficacy without increasing side-effects (Jarvis 1981). There is, however, no such trial available in the literature which involves oxybutynin.

From the above assessment of drug studies, the importance of the placebo effect in current practice must be emphasized together with the cynicism that drug trials tend to quote improvement rates whereas, in reality, the patients and their clinicians need to know continence rates. Moreover, isolated drug trials rather than trials which compare a drug with either a placebo or an alternative treatment modality are of limited value.

Once outlet obstruction, relatively unusual in women unless they have had bladder neck surgery, has been excluded the vast majority of women with detrusor instability have to be considered as having an idiopathic aetiology. It may well be that a significant number of these patients have either psychological factors or even a psychological origin for their symptoms and it is not therefore surprising that the most effective non-surgical treatment available for idiopathic detrusor instability is behavioural.

Numerous types of behavioural therapy exist, including biofeedback, acupuncture, and hypnosis. However, the widest studied and perhaps the easiest to apply in clinical practice is the technique of bladder drill or bladder retraining. The regimens used are all variants on the same basic theme in which the essential factors are the exclusion of pathology, an explanation and reassurance for the patient, the institution of a voiding regimen based on time rather than desire, the involvement of the patient in some form of frequency-voiding chart documentation, and the institution of rewards aimed at reinforcing success.

With such regimens, the results for improvement, and more importantly for continence (together with the restoration of an unstable bladder to a stable one on urodynamic testing) are very encouraging in the short and intermediate term. The results which have been reported in the literature for women with idiopathic detrusor instability and an apparently intact

Table 52.5 Oxybutynin and detrusor instability.

Authors	Year	Dosage (mg/day)	Side-effects (%)	Improvement (%)	Continence (%)
Holmes et al	1989	15	–	61	–
Moisey et al	1980	15	17	69	–
Tapp et al	1990	15	–	62	–
Thuroff et al	1991	15	–	58	–
Moore et al	1990	9	7.5	58	23

Table 52.6 Bladder drill.

Authors	Year	Improvement (%)	Continence (%)
Elder et al	1980	86	52
Fantl et al	1981	–	79
Frewen	1982	–	86
Holmes et al	1983	85	–
Jarvis & Millar	1980	–	90
Jarvis	1981	–	84
McClish et al	1991	–	55
Mahady & Begg	1981	–	90
Millard & Oldenburg	1983	74	47
Pengelly & Booth	1980	44	32

nervous system are summarized in Table 52.6. Using such a regimen up to 90% of patients may be made continent on initial reporting. There may be a significant deterioration in these results with a recurrence of symptoms in time, but since the treatment is virtually free of any morbidity, it may be repeated with success.

Those clinicians who are involved with bladder retraining programmes will stress the importance of obtaining the patients' confidence and reinforcing success with praise and rewards if the treatment is to be effective in routine clinical practice (Jarvis & Millar 1980). What is perhaps surprising is that bladder retraining programmes may also be effective for incontinence due to genuine stress incontinence (Fantl et al 1991) although this is perhaps because the patients reinforce the bladder retraining programme with their own pelvic floor exercises.

What is even more disappointing in the audit of long-term results available for any medical treatment modality in idiopathic detrusor instability is the poor success rate in the long term. Holmes et al (1983) recorded that whilst 82.5% of patients on a bladder retraining programme were initially improved, only 40% were improved at a mean of 3 years. Cardozo & Stanton (1980) reported that whilst 80% of patients who underwent a biofeedback programme were initially cured or improved, only 27% were free of symptoms after 5 years. Aitchinson et al (1989) reported that, regardless of the initial treatment modality, at 5 years only 24% of patients were continent, a further 20% had an improvement on their presenting symptoms but 56% were unchanged.

When treating idiopathic detrusor instability medically, it would seem from the literature that the simplest form of treatment, namely drug therapy, is relatively poor but the placebo effect should be exploited. Behavioural forms of therapy are much more effective in the short and intermediate terms and perhaps should be instituted whenever drug therapy has failed but enthusiasm in the long term has to be tempered.

If medical therapy for idiopathic detrusor instability fails then there is an option for surgical intervention. There are, however, two difficulties in feeding back the results from surgical intervention into clinical practice. The first difficulty is that the patients are not comparable since they represent only a small percentage of those patients who present with detrusor instability and, what is more, they represent a percentage which conservative management has failed. The second problem is that several of the surgical modalities which have been described in the past have failed to stand the test of time. For instance, the use of subtrigonal phenol, popular in the 1980s (Ewing et al 1982), has been discredited in the 1990s (Chapple et al 1991), whilst bladder transection, promising in the 1970s and early 1980s (Essenhigh & Yeates 1973; Mundy 1980), achieved unreliable results in the intermediate term (Lucas & Thomas 1987), and now has fewer indications following the introduction of terodiline and oxybutynin.

In current practice, when surgery is indicated, clam augmentation ileocystoplasty appears to be the operation of choice. Morbidity is appreciable, however, with a significant incidence of voiding disorders, sometimes requiring clean intermittent self-catheterization. There is also a theoretical risk of the induction of a malignancy from the chronic apposition of urine with the small bowel mucosa which augments the bladder (Bramble 1982; Mundy & Stephenson 1985).

Prolonged cystodistension under regional blockade may temporarily alleviate symptoms and avoid major surgery but the success rates quoted for this procedure vary between improvement or continence in between 9 and 70% (Dunn et al 1974; Pengelly et al 1980). It is likely that the true position of this procedure is somewhere between the two; an anticipated figure which could be quoted to patients is lacking.

HOW SHOULD GENUINE STRESS INCONTINENCE BE TREATED?

Much effort has been expended in trying to find effective conservative methods of treatment for genuine stress incontinence, to avoid surgery and its subsequent complications. A review of the available literature shows that this has achieved limited success. Furthermore, there is an additional problem in assessing the results quoted within the scientific literature. As a generalization, the results for surgical treatment in genuine stress incontinence quote cure rates (objective or subjective) whilst the results for the conservative management of genuine stress incontinence, rather like drug therapy in detrusor instability, tend to quote improvement rates. This makes a comparison between conservative and surgical modalities of treatment superficially difficult. Once the clinician is aware of this situation, he or she is then able to make a more appropriate assessment of how these treatment modalities will fit into clinical practice.

Conservative therapy may be subdivided into three major groups: physiotherapy, oestrogen, and the use of adrenergic agents. Each of these will be assessed in turn, followed by a discussion of surgical treatment.

Physiotherapy

It is perhaps as useful to talk about pelvic floor physiotherapy in general as to consider surgery in general instead of breaking surgery down into its component operative procedures. There is a need, when considering different types of pelvic floor physiotherapy, as with different types of surgery, to separate the results based on subjective outcome with those based on objective outcome. It is clear that subjective improvement is always superior to objective improvement whichever of these modalities is being considered. For instance, Olah et al (1990) reported subjective improvement in 70% of patients treated with interferential therapy but only 33% continence based on pad weighing techniques.

When a course of pelvic floor exercises have been taught, the subjective improvement rates are relatively good with a range of 35–85% (Table 52.7). There are, however, very few series which look subjectively at continence rather than improvement and even less which look at continence objectively.

When continence rather than improvement is considered, the results are reduced with a subjective incidence of continence in the region of 60% being regularly quoted (Wilson et al 1987; Lagro-Janssen et al 1991b). When the stricter, but nevertheless more appropriate assessments are made using objective evidence of continence, the results become disappointing. For instance, Tapp et al (1989b) reported that only 20% of patients undergoing a course of pelvic floor exercises were objectively continent.

There is relatively little information in the literature to make the clinician favour any one of the different types of pelvic floor physiotherapy over another. Tapp et al (1989b) found no statistically significant difference in the objective continence rates between pelvic floor exercises and pelvic floor exercises augmented with faradism. Olah et al (1990) were unable to demonstrate a statistically significant difference in the subjective results when comparing interferential therapy with pelvic floor exercises augmented by the use of variably weighted cones. Wilson et al (1987) were unable to find a statistically significant difference in subjective improvement between pelvic floor exercises performed in hospital, pelvic floor exercises augmented by interferential therapy, or pelvic floor exercises augmented by faradism.

Table 52.7 Pelvic floor exercises.

Authors	Year	Improvement (%)
Burgio et al	1986	67
Burns et al	1990	54
Castledon et al	1984	64
Ferguson et al	1990	35
Henalla et al	1988	65
Lagro-Janssen et al	1991b	85
Wells et al	1991	51

The truly significant variable in pelvic floor physiotherapy appears to be the therapist rather than the modality of therapy. There can be no doubt that regular contact with an enthusiastic therapist is more likely to produce a successful outcome than is a description of treatment followed by a review several months later. Wilson et al (1987) demonstrated that 27% of patients treated by pelvic floor exercises at home were subjectively improved compared with 60% treated in hospital. Bo (1991) reported a subjective improvement following pelvic floor exercises in 17% of patients treated at home compared with 60% treated in hospital.

From this audit of pelvic floor physiotherapy, it may be concluded that in order to achieve an optimal outcome, an enthusiastic therapist should be involved in the treatment of a patient and that treatment should include regular and frequent review. Pelvic floor physiotherapy, regardless of modality, is relatively free of side-effects and whilst the overall results are not especially encouraging, those patients who are improved sufficiently to no longer require surgery must be considered as having benefited; perhaps pelvic floor physiotherapy of some type should be offered to all patients in the first instance rather than surgery. This author is only able to find one randomized trial which has compared the results of pelvic floor physiotherapy with surgery. Tapp et al (1989b) randomized patients to undergo either pelvic floor exercises, pelvic floor exercises with faradism or a Burch colposuspension. The objective continence rates 6 months after the end of therapy in each group were 20%, 13%, and 75% respectively. The other disadvantage of pelvic floor physiotherapy is that it could not be considered to be curative in that a patient who ceases pelvic floor exercises will ultimately become incontinent again.

Oestrogen

There are theoretical reasons for believing that oestrogen should improve at least some patients with genuine stress incontinence, in that a modest increase in the maximal urethral closure pressure may be demonstrated following its use (Rud 1980; Hilton & Stanton 1983; Karram et al 1989). The interpretation of the literature is made more complex by the large numbers of different oestrogens in use, many of these having different strengths and it can be difficult to judge the effect of the drug in this situation.

There has, however, been a recent meta-analysis of the use of oestrogen in the treatment of genuine stress incontinence in postmenopausal women (Fantl et al 1994). Fantl et al identified 166 articles involving the use of oestrogen in this situation but only six were controlled clinical trials and hence appropriate to study. This meta-analysis would suggest that the use of oestrogen will reduce the severity of genuine stress incontinence but will not result in the patient becoming continent. Since, at least theoretically, oestrogen may increase the blood supply to the vaginal skin and also act as a risk factor for thromboembolic disease at the time of surgery, the use of oestrogen in women with genuine stress incontinence who might undergo surgery at some stage would appear to be inappropriate in clinical practice.

Adrenergic agents

The use of α- and/or β-adrenergic agonists in the treatment of genuine stress incontinence has a limited assessment but those results which are available are poor suggesting that between 10 and 23% of patients can be made continent using either clenbutarol or phenyl propanolamine (Stewart et al 1976; Yasuda et al 1993). However, the twin disadvantages of side-effects and the need to continue these drugs for as long as continence is desired means that they are unlikely to achieve a significant place in clinical management.

Surgery

The major form of treatment for genuine stress incontinence will be surgery. Numerous different surgical procedures have been described but the majority are variants upon seven basic themes. These are the bladder buttress procedure, the Marshall–Marchetti–Krantz procedure, colposuspension, non-endoscopic bladder neck suspension (Pereyra), endoscopic bladder neck suspension (Stamey), bladder sling procedures, and periurethral injections.

Table 52.8 Objective results for surgery for genuine stress incontinence.

Procedure	Primary procedure (% continent)	Previous surgery (% continent)
Bladder buttress	67.8	–
Marshall–Marchetti–Krantz	89.5	–
Colposuspension	89.8	82.5
Non-endoscopic bladder neck suspension	75.4	75.0
Endoscopic bladder neck suspension	74.2	74.8
Bladder sling	93.9	86.1
Injectables	45.5	57.8

When assessing the results of surgery from the scientific literature, several difficulties become apparent which will limit the clinician in the modification of his or her surgical practice. In a recent review of the literature, Jarvis (1994) reported the results of over 200 studies involving over 20 000 surgical procedures. Although it is well known that objective results give generally lower success rates, but are more informative than subjective results, only 23% of the patients had been objectively assessed. From this study it was clear that the expectation of continence based on objective results was approximately 10% less than that anticipated from subjective reporting. The second problem in interpretation related to the length of follow-up before patients were reported. Some studies reported patients who had been operated upon as recently as 4 weeks prior to publication; logically surgical procedures would be reported with results at approximately 6–12 months after surgery in order to gauge the intermediate-term benefits and re-reported some 5 or 10 years later in order to gain a long-term assessment.

Of all the procedures assessed, only bladder sling procedures appear to be as effective at 5 years as they were at 6 months. The third problem related to the concept of bias within the literature. Only seven of the 213 studies identified involved a truly randomized trial which compared one surgical procedure with another. Without such studies results can not really be compared since there may be a bias of patient selection by the surgeon, a bias of surgical preference by the surgeon, a bias of surgical skill between different procedures, and possibly even a publication bias. Only 11.5% of those patients involved in objective studies or 2.7% of all patients identified were part of a randomized trial. There is a need for increased numbers of randomized trials of surgical techniques (Black & Downs 1996).

In order that the relative place of each surgical procedure can be properly identified and used to modify surgical practice, the audit loop would need to be closed by the use of a greater number of randomized trials. These should only include patients who have been objectively assessed both prior to surgery and at a set time following surgery, that set time being a minimum of 6 months. Only by such techniques will the place of each procedure and its indications be identified, and subtle alterations in surgical technique be assessed.

There is also the need to separate patients undergoing their first surgical procedure with patients who are undergoing repeat surgery, yet such a differential could be made in only 41% of patients in this study. The objective results for continence which could be anticipated for each procedure performed either as a primary procedure or following previous failed surgery is shown in Table 52.8. It should be noted that there are no satisfactory objective results for recurrent genuine stress incontinence treated by either a bladder buttress or a Marshall–Marchetti–Krantz procedure.

From Table 52.8 it may be seen that the procedures associated with the highest objective continence rates for primary surgery are the Marshall–Marchetti–Krantz procedure, colposuspension, endoscopic bladder neck suspension and the bladder sling procedure. In the presence of previous surgery, a colposuspension or a bladder sling procedure would appear to carry the most favourable results (Jarvis 1994, 1995).

When deciding which procedure to offer a patient with genuine stress incontinence, a surgeon must consider more than simply the objective continence rates assumed from the literature. Urodynamic investigation will demonstrate that not all patients have the same underlying problem. A patient whose bladder neck is very mobile, with raised intra-abdominal pressure, may be better treated by a procedure associated with some degree of elevation of the bladder neck postoperatively, such as a colposuspension or an endoscopic bladder neck suspension. A patient with limited mobility of the bladder neck preoperatively might be better treated with a bladder sling procedure. A patient with a relatively good maximal urethral closure pressure could probably be treated by any procedure, whereas a patient with a poor maximal urethral closure pressure should perhaps be treated by a bladder sling rather than any other surgical procedure (Hilton 1989b; Sand et al 1987b; Penttinen et al 1989).

Another major factor which the surgeon will need to take into account when counselling the patient is the balance between the anticipated continence rate and the complications of each procedure. The two consistent complications quoted in the literature relate to postoperative voiding disorders and to the onset of *de novo* detrusor instability. The bladder buttress procedure has an incidence of long-term voiding disorder approaching zero, but postoperative *de novo* instability may occur in up to 8% of patients (Beck et al 1991). The incidences of long-term voiding disorder and of detrusor instability are both 11% following the Marshall–Marchetti–Krantz procedure but the complication which limits the popularity of this procedure is osteitis pubis, which will occur in some 2.5% of patients (Mainprize & Drutz 1988). Following colposuspension, the mean incidence of voiding disorder is 12.5%, with a mean incidence of detrusor instability of 9.6% (Jarvis 1994). However, the complication which needs to be considered in this procedure is the incidence of genitourinary prolapse (enterocele, cystocele, or rectocele), being reported at an average of 13.6% and a range of 2.5–26.7% in patients within 5 years of this procedure (Gillon & Stanton 1984; Galloway et al 1987; Wiskind et al 1992).

There is a need for appropriate scientific evaluation of the results of surgery following a laparoscopic as opposed to an open colposuspension. Early studies suggest that the laparoscopic procedure takes longer to perform but has a lower morbidity and an equivalent cure rate (Randomski & Herschorn 1996). However, the enthusiasm for this procedure must remain guarded until longer-term results become available. There are follow-up studies for an open colposuspension which suggest a relatively modest recurrence of incontinence in excess of 10 years and these results will need to be compared with the laparoscopic procedure (Alcalay et al 1995).

There is no evidence that the objective results for an endoscopically controlled bladder neck suspension are superior to those from a non-endoscopic bladder neck suspension although cystoscopy will enable the inadvertent placing of a suture into the bladder to be noted and removed. Following endoscopic bladder neck suspension, the mean incidences of voiding disorders and of detrusor instability are both in the region of 5.8% (Jarvis 1994).

The bladder sling procedure is generally considered to be the largest of the surgical onslaughts yet is the single most effective procedure for primary genuine stress incontinence and surgeons will have to rethink their view that this procedure is primarily indicated for recurrent genuine stress incontinence.

This procedure is obstructive with a mean incidence of 12.8% (range 2–37%) and with an incidence of *de novo* detrusor instability with a mean of 16.6%.

The injection of substances into the wall of the proximal urethra is unlikely to become a first line method of treatment as judged by the results shown in Table 52.8, but it may well be that this treatment will be of particular benefit to the patient who has been improved by initial surgery yet wishes a further improvement without further formal surgery. It carries the advantage of being a relatively short procedure which could be performed as a day case on selected patients (Stanton & Monga 1997)

This audit of the place of surgery in genuine stress incontinence has demonstrated that surgery is the single most effective treatment option for these patients. Certain surgical procedures are clearly superior to others but a balance needs to be struck between efficacy and complications and these issues need to be debated with patients before a decision is made as to the operation which they will undergo. This audit also demonstrates that a patient's best chance of continence is her first operative procedure and hence careful preoperative evaluation is mandatory (Hilton 1989a).

A patient should undergo a preoperative urodynamic assessment – to demonstrate that the bladder is stable and that the procedure is appropriate – and a pressure-flow study since it would be inappropriate to perform a more obstructive procedure (colposuspension or bladder sling) on a patient with an asymptomatic voiding disorder without this being recognized and debated.

There is now an increasing and emerging industry producing devices to prevent incontinence, such as those worn either in the vagina or in the urethra. There will be a need for a critical assessment of these devices, including the major requirement for patient acceptability (Eckford et al 1996; Hahn & Milsom 1996).

HOW SHOULD TREATMENT BE PLANNED WHEN GENUINE STRESS INCONTINENCE AND DETRUSOR INSTABILITY COEXIST?

When detrusor instability and genuine stress incontinence coexist, the clinician has a choice between two lines of management which require the involvement of the patient in the decision making process. On the one hand, the clinician might choose to treat the detrusor instability medically in the first instance rather than the genuine stress incontinence surgically in the hope that the degree of improvement is so significant that the patient no longer wishes to undergo a surgical procedure. Alternatively, the surgeon may elect to treat the genuine stress incontinence surgically and offer postoperative bladder retraining or drug treatment. The choice between these options may depend upon which of the two problems is perceived (from the urodynamic assessment) as being the greater problem, and upon the patient's wishes.

What is clear from the literature, and must therefore feed back into clinical practice, are two observations. The first is that all surgery may make detrusor instability worse, if already present. Secondly, patients should be forewarned that the efficacy of surgery in the presence of detrusor instability will be less successful than if genuine stress incontinence alone is present. For instance, Eriksen et al (1990) reported that colposuspension resulted in an objectively proven continence rate of 71% if genuine stress incontinence was present with a stable bladder preoperatively, but only 33.3% if both genuine stress incontinence and detrusor instability coexisted.

HOW SHOULD VOIDING DISORDERS BE MANAGED?

As a generalization, voiding disorders in women are not well managed. This is partly because they are not always recognized and partly because there is a limited amount of scientific information which can be fed back into clinical practice.

The majority of women with a urodynamically proven voiding disorder do not have any of its classic symptoms and unless a urodynamic study is performed, either because of a clinical suspicion or for another indication, and a diagnosis is made coincidentally, the problem is often missed (Stanton et al 1983). Having been diagnosed, the management will depend in part upon the symptoms and in part upon the aetiology. It is also necessary to exclude back-pressure influences on the kidneys by measuring urea and creatinine levels and by assessing the renal anatomy using either ultrasound or intravenous urography.

The treatment options have already been described in Ch. 24. What is perhaps clear is that treatment is frequently empirical and aimed at symptomatic relief. Simpler treatment, such as drug therapy, would generally be tried before urethral dilatation, urethrotomy or even clean intermittent self-catheterization.

When a voiding disorder and genuine stress incontinence coexists, the choice of operation, as has already been described for genuine stress incontinence, needs to be such that the voiding disorder will not deteriorate. There is evidence that some surgical procedures, for example an endoscopic bladder neck suspension, will result in a lower incidence of voiding disorder postoperatively than was present preoperatively (Hilton 1989b).

WHAT IS THE PLACE FOR ARTIFICIAL SPHINCTER INSERTION?

The insertion of an artificial urinary sphincter has assumed greater importance in contemporary clinical practice, partly because of improvements in sphincter design which has made repeated surgery for the complications of sphincter insertion or mechanical breakdown less frequent. There are numerous difficulties in feeding back the conclusions from the scientific literature into clinical practice.

The first problem in such an audit relates to the observation that most studies do not distinguish in either outcome or complication between male and female patients. In 14 identified studies in which statistics are quoted, only three papers are devoted exclusively to women. Women form 15% of the patients in mixed gender studies whilst the total literature evidence from 267 women forms only 40% of the reported patients. The results from this audit become even more difficult to extrapolate into clinical practice in that not all the women have genuine stress incontinence or detrusor instability, but rather have other causes of incontinence including neural tube defects, lower urinary tract trauma, and overt neurological disease. Only one study specifically reports the results for the insertion of an artificial urinary sphincter in women with genuine stress incontinence (Duncan et al 1992).

Accepting these caveats, certain conclusions can be drawn from the literature which can guide the clinician and influence clinical practice.

1 It used to be considered that a sphincter should only be inserted in the presence of a stable bladder, but this is no longer the case since the insertion of a sphincter can be combined with a surgical procedure aimed at reducing instability, such as the clam ileocystoplasty (Whitaker 1985).
2 Most studies quote a continence rate of between 70 and 75% after sphincter insertion (Sidi et al 1984; Aliabadi & Gonzalez 1990; Montague 1992) although some authors quote higher continence rates such as 82% (Goldwasser et al 1987), and even 92% (Webster et al 1992). In as much as a specific figure for women with previous failed surgery for genuine stress incontinence is concerned, the anticipated continence rate following the insertion of an artificial urinary sphincter, based on limited numbers, may be smaller than the continence rates for sphincter insertion in general (66%; Duncan et al 1992).

A major problem which will limit the use of artificial sphincter insertion in patients is the need to explore or even replace sphincters already inserted because of cuff erosion, infection, or mechanical breakdown. Such events may be anticipated in up to 17% of women in whom a sphincter is inserted, perhaps at a rate of approximately 4% per annum (Light & Reynolds 1992; Webster et al 1992; Fulford et al 1997). These problems are particularly likely in women who have had previous pelvic radiotherapy or previous inorganic bladder sling surgery (Duncan et al 1992).

How can this data be used in clinical practice? Patients who remain incontinent despite multiple previous attempts with more conventional treatment, and perhaps patients who have a particularly low maximum urethral closure pressure are appropriate for artificial sphincter insertion. Such insertion, however, should probably take place in a small number of experienced centres in order that the experience gained from potentially difficult surgery and the management of complications can be concentrated and audited. There can be no place for the surgeon who indulges in occasional sphincter insertion.

WHAT IS AVAILABLE FOR THE LONG-TERM INCONTINENT WOMAN?

However expert the management, there will remain a subgroup of women who will be incontinent despite all that clinicians may offer. Any unit which offers treatment for incontinent women must also offer advice and support should that treatment fail. Whilst there are many places in which a continence advisor, generally with nursing experience, can play a role in earlier management protocols, perhaps this is where the expertise of such people becomes paramount.

It is not possible to quote scientific statistics in this region but clinical experience has demonstrated areas where the role of such continence advisors will feed back into clinical protocols. Such an advisor should firstly question whether or not appropriate non-surgical and surgical techniques of management have been offered and discussed with the patient. Advice on such simple matters as timed toileting, clothing, bowel habit, and a revision of intercurrent drug therapy should be offered. Such advice should reduce either the number of episodes of incontinence or the severity of those episodes. The social and hygienic effects of those episodes should also be reduced by a comprehensive knowledge of available continence and toileting aids, choosing the most appropriate for a patient's circumstances and liaising with manufacturers to suggest improvements on aids which are currently available (Mandelstam 1990). The value of such a resource cannot be overemphasized.

CONCLUSIONS

Audit, by definition, requires that the quality of information upon which clinical practice is based should be assessed critically, that the recommendations from the best practice be encompassed into routine contemporary practice and the results of such a policy should be regularly reviewed.

It behoves the clinician not only to manage his or her patients based upon both experience and upon the information available within scientific literature, but that the results from his or her own clinical practice are also known. Any clinician involved in urogynaecology (or in any other sphere of medicine) must be aware of whether the results of treatment modalities from their own practice reach the expectation in the literature. If they do not, that clinician must identify why not. Only by a knowledge of the complete scientific literature (as opposed to selected publications) can the true place of treatments be assessed and only by personal audit can the quality of the service for which we have a professional responsibility be judged.

REFERENCES

Aitchinson M, Carter R, Patterson P et al 1989 Is the treatment of urge incontinence a placebo response? British Journal of Obstetrics and Gynaecology 64: 478–480

Alcalay M, Monga A, Stanton S L 1995 Burch colposuspension: 8–10, 10–20, 20 year follow up. British Journal of Obstetrics and Gynaecology 102: 740–745

Aliabadi H, Gonzalez R 1990 Success of artificial urinary sphincter after failed surgery for incontinence. Journal of Urology 143: 987–990

Andersen J R, Lose G, Norgaard M et al 1988 Terodiline, emepronium or placebo for the treatment of detrusor over activity? British Journal of Urology 61: 310–331

Baker K R, Drutz H, Barnes M D 1991 Effectiveness of antibiotics prophylaxis in prevention of bacteruria after multichannel urodynamics. American Journal of Obstetrics and Gynecology 165: 679–681

Bates C P, Whiteside C G, Turner-Warwick R T 1970 Synchronous cine-pressure-flow-cystourethrography with special reference to stress and urge incontinence. British Journal of Urology 42: 714–723

Bates C P, Loose H, Stanton S L 1973 The objective study of incontinence after repair operations. Surgery, Gynecology and Obstetrics 136: 17–22

Beck R P, McCormick S, Nordstrom L 1991 A 25-year experience with 519 anterior colporrhaphy procedures. Obstetrics and Gynecology 78: 1011–8

Benness C J, Barnick C J, Cardozo L 1989 Is there a place for routine videocystourethrography in the assessment of lower urinary tract dysfunction? Neurourology and Urodynamics 8: 299–300

Bent A E, Richardson D A, Ostergard D R 1983 Diagnosis of lower urinary tract disorders in post menopausal patients. American Journal of Obstetrics and Gynecology 145: 218–22

Bergman A, Bhatia N N 1985 Uroflowmetry for predicting postoperative voiding difficulties in women with genuine stress incontinence. British Journal of Obstetrics and Gynaecology 92: 835–8

Bhatia N N 1991 Sphincter electromyography and electrophysiological testing. In: Ostergard D R, Bent A (eds) Urogynaecology and Urodynamics. Williams and Wilkins, Baltimore, pp 143–163

Black N A, Downs S H 1996 The effectiveness of surgery for stress incontinence in women; a systematic review. British Journal of Urology 78: 497–510

Bo K 1991 Pelvic floor muscle exercises for the treatment of women with stress urinary incontinence. Acta Obstetrica et Gynaecologica Scandinavica 70: 637–9

Bramble F J 1982 The treatment of adult enuresis and urge incontinence by enterocystoplasty. British Journal of Urology 54: 693–6

Brocklehurst J C 1993 Urinary incontinence in the community. British Medical Journal 306: 832–4

Burgio K L, Robinson J C, Engel B T 1986 The role of biofeedback in Kegel exercise training for stress urinary incontinence. American Journal of Obstetrics and Gynecology 154: 58–64

Burns P A, Pranikoff K, Nochajski T et al 1990 Treatment of stress incontinence with pelvic floor exercises and biofeedback. Journal of the American Geriatric Society 38: 341–4

Cantor T J, Bates C P 1980 A comparative study of symptoms and objective urodynamic findings in 214 incontinent women. British Journal of Obstetrics and Gynaecology 87: 889–92

Cardozo L D, Stanton S L 1980 A comparison between Bromocriptine and Indomethacin in the treatment of detrusor instability. Journal of Urology 123: 184–6

Castleden C M, Duffin H M, Mitchell E P 1984 The effect of physiotherapy on stress incontinence. Age and Ageing 13: 235–7

Castleden C M, Duffin H M, Gulati R S 1985 Double blind study of imipramine and placebo for incontinence due to detrusor instability. Age and Ageing 14: 303–6

Chapple C R, Helm C W, Blease S et al 1989 Asymptomatic bladder neck incompetence in nulliparous females. British Journal or Urology 64: 657–9

Chapple C R, Parkhouse H, Gardener C et al 1990 Double blind placebo control crossover study of Flavoxate in the treatment of detrusor instability. British Journal of Urology 66: 691–4

Chapple C R, Hampson C J, Turner-Warwick R T et al 1991 Subtrigonal Phenol injection – how safe and effective is it? British Journal of Urology 68: 483–6

Colombo M, Maggioni A, Zanett A G et al 1996 Prevention of post operative urinary stress incontinence after surgery for genitourinary prolapse. Obstetrics and Gynaecology 87: 266–71

Coptcoat M J, Reed C, Cummings J et al 1988 Is antibiotic prophylaxis necessary for routine urodynamic investigations? British Journal of Urology 61: 302–3

Creighton S M, Plevnik S, Stanton S L 1991 Distal urethral electrical conductants – a preliminary assessment of its role as a quick screening test for incontinent women. British Journal of Obstetrics and Gynaecology 98: 68–72

Crystle D, Charm L, Copeland W 1972 Q-tip test in stress urinary incontinence. Obstetrics and Gynaecology 38: 313–5

Diokno A C, Wells T J, Brink C A 1987 Urinary incontinence in elderly women. Journal of the American Geriatric Society 35: 940–6

Duncan H J, Nurse D E, Mundy A R 1992 Role of the artificial urinary sphincter in the treatment of stress incontinence in women. British Journal of Urology 69: 141–3

Dunn M, Smith J C, Ardran G M 1974 Prolonged bladder distension as a treatment of urge and urge incontinence of urine. British Journal of Urology 46: 645–52

Eastwood H D R, Warrell R 1984 Urinary incontinence in the elderly female. Age and Ageing 13: 230–4

Eckford S D, Jackson S R, Lewis P A et al 1996 The continence control pad. British Journal of Urology 77: 538–40

Elder D D, Stephenson T P, Bary P R 1980 An assessment of the Frewen regimen in the treatment of detrusor instability in females. In: Zinner N R, Sterling A M (eds) Female Incontinence. Liss, New York, pp 231–8

Eriksen B C, Hagen B, Eik-Nessh et al 1990 Long term effectiveness of the Burch colposuspension. Acta Obstetrica et Gynaecologica Scandinavica 69: 45–50

Essenhigh D M, Yeates W K 1973 Transection of the bladder with particular reference to enuresis. British Journal of Urology 45: 299–304

Ewing R, Bultitude M I, Shuttleworth K E D 1982 Subtrigonal Phenol injection for urge incontinence. British Journal of Urology 54: 689–92

Fantl J A, Hurt W G, Dunn L J 1981 Detrusor instability syndrome – the use of bladder re-training drills with or without anticholinergics. American Journal of Obstetrics and Gynecology 140: 885–90

Fantl J A, Hurt W G, Bump R C et al 1986 Urethral axis and sphincteric function. American Journal of Obstetrics and Gynecology, 140 Gynecology 155: 554–8

Fantl J A, Wyman J F, McClish D K et al 1991 Efficacy of bladder re-training in older women with urinary incontinence. Journal of the American Medical Association 265: 309–13

Fantl J A, Cardozo L, McChish D K et al 1994 Estrogen therapy in the management of urinary incontinence in post menopausal women. Obstetrics and Gynecology 83: 12–8

Ferguson K L, McKey P L, Bishop K R et al 1990 Stress urinary incontinence – effects of pelvic muscle exercises. Obstetrics and Gynecology 75: 671–5

Frewen W K 1982 A re-assessment of bladder re-training in detrusor dysfunction in the female. British Journal of Urology 54: 372–4

Fulford S C V, Sutton C, Bales G et al 1997 The fate of the modern artificial urinary sphincter with a follow up of more than ten years. British Journal of Urology 79: 713–6

Galloway N T M, Davis N, Stephenson T P 1987 The complications of colposuspension. British Journal of Urology 60: 122–4

Gillon G, Stanton S L 1984 Long term follow up of surgery for urinary incontinence in elderly women. British Journal of Urology 56: 478–81

Glenning A B 1984 Clinical symptoms and urodynamic assessment. Australian and New Zealand Journal of Obstetrics and Gynaecology 24: 95–7

Goldwasser B, Furlow W L, Barrett D M 1987 The model AS800 artificial urinary sphincter. Journal of Urology 137: 668–71

Hahn I, Milsom I 1996 Treatment of female stress urinary incontinence with a new anatomically shaped vaginal device. British Journal of Urology 77: 711–5

Haylen B T, Sutherst J R, Frazer M I 1989 Is investigation of most stress incontinence really necessary? British Journal of Urology 64: 147–9

Haylen B T, Parys B T, Anyaebunam W F 1990 Urine flow rate in male and female urodynamic patients compared with the Liverpool nomogram. British Journal of Urology 65: 683–7

Hellstrom P A, Tummela T L J, Konituri M J et al 1991 The bladder cooling test for urodynamic assessment. British Journal of Urology, 67: 275–8

Henalla S M, Kirwan P, Castleden C M et al 1988 The effects of pelvic floor exercises in the treatment of genuine urinary stress incontinence in women at two hospitals. British Journal of Obstetrics and Gynaecology 95: 602–6

Hilton P 1989a Which operation and for which patient? In: J L Drife, P Hilton, S L Stanton (eds) Micturition pp 225–246. Springer-Verlag, London

Hilton P 1989b A clinical and urodynamic study comparing the stamey bladder neck suspension and sub-urethral sling procedures. British Journal of Obstetrics and Gynaecology 96: 213–20

Hilton P, Stanton S L 1983 The use of intravaginal oestrogen cream in genuine stress incontinence. British Journal of Obstetrics and Gynaecology 90: 940–3

Holmes D M, Stone A R, Bary P R et al 1983 Bladder training – 3 years on. British Journal of Urology 55: 660–2

Holmes D M, Montz F J, Stanton S L 1989 Oxybutynin versus propantheline in the management of detrusor instability – a patient regulated variable dose trial. British Journal of Obstetrics and Gynaecology 96: 607–12

Hosker G L, Kilcoyne P M, Lord J C et al 1997 Urodynamic services, personnel and training in the United Kingdom. British Journal of Urology 79: 159–62

Jarvis G J 1981 A controlled trial of bladder drill and drug therapy in the treatment of detrusor instability. British Journal of Urology 53: 565–7

Jarvis G J 1990 The place of urodynamic investigation. In: G J Jarvis (ed) Female Urinary Incontinence. Royal College of Obstetricians and Gynaecology, London, pp 15–20

Jarvis G J 1994 Surgery for genuine stress incontinence. British Journal of Obstetrics and Gynaecology 101: 371–4

Jarvis G J 1995 Long term bladder neck suspension for genuine stress incontinence. British Journal of Urology 76: 467–9

Jarvis G J, Millar D R 1980 Controlled trial of bladder drill for detrusor instability. British Medical Journal, 281: 1322–3

Jarvis G J, Hall S, Stamp S et al 1980 An assessment of

urodynamic examination in incontinent women. British Journal of Obstetrics and Gynaecology 87: 893–6

Jolleys J V 1988 Reported incidence of urinary incontinence in women in a general practice. British Medical Journal 296: 1300–2

Karram M M, Bhatia N N 1988. The Q-tip test. Obstetrics and Gynecology 71: 807–11

Karram M M, Yeko T R, Sauer M K et al 1989 Urodynamic changes following hormone replacement therapy. Obstetrics and Gynecology 74: 208–11

Kinn A C, Larsson B 1987 Pad test with fixed bladder volume and urinary stress incontinence. Acta Obstetrica et Gynaecologica Scandinavica 66: 369–71

Korda A, Crieger M, Hunter P et al 1987 The value of clinical symptoms in the diagnosis of urinary incontinence in the female. Australian and New Zealand Journal of Obstetrics and Gynaecology 27: 149–51

Lagro-Janssen T L M, Smits A J, van Weel C 1991a Women with urinary incontinence – self-perceived worries and general practitioners knowledge of the problem. British Journal of General Practice 40: 331–4

Lagro-Janssen T L M, Debruyne F M J, Smits A J et al 1991b Controlled trial of pelvic floor exercises in the treatment of urinary stress incontinence in general practice. British Journal of Obstetrics and Gynaecology 41: 445–9

Light J K, Reynolds J C 1992 Impact of the new cuff design on reliability of the AS800 artificial urinary sphincter. Journal of Urology 147: 609–11

Lucas M G, Thomas D G 1987 Endoscopic bladder neck transection for detrusor instability. British Journal of Urology 59: 526–8

McClish D K, Fantl J A, Wyman J F et al 1991 Bladder training in older women with urinary incontinence. Obstetrics and Gynecology 77: 281–6

McInerney P D, Vanner T F, Harris S A B et al 1991 Ambulatory urodynamics. British Journal of Urology 67: 272–4

Mahady I W, Begg B M 1981 Long term symptomatic and cystometric cure of the urge incontinence syndrome using bladder re-education. British Journal of Obstetrics and Gynaecology 88: 1038–40

Mainprize T C, Drutz H P 1988 The Marshall-Marchetti-Krantz procedure – a clinical review. Obstetrics and Gynecological Survey 43: 724–9

Mandelstam D 1990 The role of the continence advisor in Female Urinary Incontinence (ed. G J Jarvis) Royal College of Obstetricians and Gynaecologists, London, pp 86–89

Massey J A, Abrams P 1985 Urodynamics of the lower urinary tract. Clinics in Obstetrics and Gynecology 12: 319–21

Massey J A, Abrams P 1986 Dose titration in clinical trials. British Journal of Urology 58: 125–8

Meyhoff H H, Gerstenberg T C, Nordling J 1983. Placebo – the drug of choice in female motor urge incontinence. British Journal of Urology 53: 129–33

Milani R, Scalanbrino S, Carrera S et al 1988 Comparison of flavoxate hydrochloride in dosages of 600 versus 1200 mg for the treatment of urgency and urge incontinence. Journal of International Medical Research 16: 244–8

Millard R J, Oldenburg B F 1983 The symptomatic urodynamic and psychodynamic results of bladder re-education programmes. Journal of Urology 130: 719–7

Moisey C, Stephenson T, Brendler C B 1980 The treatment of detrusor instability with oxybutynin. British Journal of Urology 52: 272–7

Montague D K 1992 The artificial urinary sphincter. Journal of Urology 147: 380–2

Moore K H, Hay D M, Imrie A E et al 1990 Oxybutynin hydrochloride in the treatment of women with idiopathic detrusor instability. British Journal of Urology 66: 479–85

Mundy A R 1980 Bladder transection for urge incontinence associated with detrusor instability. British Journal of Urology 52: 580–3

Mundy A R, Stephenson T P 1985 Clam ileocystoplasty for the treatment of refractory urge incontinence. British Journal of Urology 57: 641–6

Norton P A, MacDonald I D, Sedgwick P M et al 1988 Distress and delay associated with urinary incontinence-frequency, and urgency in women. British Medical Journal 397: 1187–9

Olah K S, Bridges N, Denning J et al 1990 The conservative management of patients with symptoms of stress incontinence. American Journal of Obstetrics and Gynecology 162: 87–92

Ouslander J, Staskin D, Raz S et al 1987 Clinical versus urodynamic diagnosis in an incontinence geriatric female population. Journal of Urology 137: 68–71

Ouslander J, Leach G, Staskin D et al 1989 Prospective evaluation of an assessment strategy for geriatric urinary incontinence. Journal of the American Geriatric Society 37: 715–24

Pengelly A W, Booth C M 1980 A prospective trial of bladder re-training as a treatment for detrusor instability. British Journal of Urology 52: 463–5

Pengelly A W, Stephenson T P, Milroy E J G et al 1980 Results of prolonged bladder distension as the treatment for detrusor instability. British Journal of Urology 50: 243–5

Penttinen J, Kaar K, Kauppila A 1989 Effective suprapubic operation on urethral closure. British Journal of Urology 63: 389–91

Quinn M J, Benyon J, Mortensen N J M et al 1988 Vaginal endosonography in the post-operative assessment of colposuspension. British Journal of Urology 63: 295–300

Radomski S B, Herschorn S 1996 Laparoscopic Burch bladder neck suspension – early results. The Journal of Urology 155: 515–8

Rud T 1980 The urethral pressure profile in continent women from childbearing to old age. Acta Obstetrica et Gynaecologica Scandinavica 59: 331–5

Sand P K, Hill R C, Ostergard D R 1987a Supine urethroscopic and standing cystometry. Obstetrics and Gynecology 70: 57–60

Sand P K, Bowen L W Panganiban R 1987b The low pressure urethra is a factor in failed retro-pubic urethropexy. Obstetrics and Gynecology 69: 399–402

Sand P K, Hill R C, Ostergard D R 1988 Incontinence history as a predictor of detrusor instability. Obstetrics and Gynecology 71: 257–60

Shepherd A 1990 The range of urodynamic investigations. In: Jarvis G J (ed) Female Urinary Incontinence. Royal College of Obstetricians and Gynaecologists, London, pp 21–32

Sidi A A, Sinha B, Gonzalez R 1984 Treatment of urinary incontinence with an artificial sphincter. Journal of Urology 131: 891–3

Stanton S L, Monga A K 1997 Incontinence in elderly women – is periurethral collagen an advance? British Journal of Obstetrics and Gynaecology 104: 154–7

Stanton S L, Ozsoy C, Hilton P 1983 Voiding difficulty in the female – prevalence, clinical and urodynamic review. Obstetrics and Gynecology 61: 144–7

Stewart B, Banowsky L W H, Montague D K 1976 Stress incontinence – conservative therapy with sympathomimetic drugs. Journal of Urology 116: 558–9

Summitt S L, Stovall T J, Bent A E et al 1992 Urinary incontinence – correlation of history with multichannel urodynamic testing. American Journal of Obstetrics and Gynecology 166: 1835–44

Sutherst J R, Brown M C 1980 Detection of urethral incompetence in women using the fluid bridge test. British Journal of Urology 52: 138–42

Sutherst J R, Brown M C, Shawer M 1981 Assessing the severity of urinary incontinence in women by weighing perineal pads. Lancet 1: 1128–30

Sutherst J C, Brown M C, Richmond J 1986 Analysis of the pattern of urine loss in women with incontinence as measured by weighing perineal pads. British Journal of Urology 58: 273–8

Tapp A J S, Fall M, Norgaard J et al 1989a A dose titrated multicentre study of the treatment of idiopathic detrusor instability in women. Journal of Urology 142: 1027–31

Tapp A J S, Hills B, Cardozo L D 1989b Randomized study comparing pelvic floor physiotherapy with the Burch colposuspension. Neurourology and Urodynamics 8: 356–7

Tapp A J S, Cardozo L D, Versi E et al 1990 The treatment of detrusor instability in post menopausal women with oxybutynin chloride. British Journal of Obstetrics and Gynaecology 97: 521–6

Thomas T M, Plymat K R, Blannin J et al 1980 Prevalence of urinary incontinence. British Medical Journal 281: 1243–5

Thuroff J W, Bunk E, Ebner A et al 1991 Randomized double blind multicentre trial on the treatment of frequency, urgency and incontinence related to detrusor hyperactivity. Journal of Urology 145: 183–7

van Waalwijk E S C, Remmers S, Janknegi R A 1991 Extramural ambulatory urodynamic monitoring during natural filling and normal daily activities. Journal of Urology 146: 123–4

Versi E 1990 Discriminant analysis of urethral pressure profilometry data for the diagnosis of genuine stress incontinence. British Journal of Obstetrics and Gynaecology 97: 251–9

Versi E, Cardozo L D, Studd J W W et al 1986 Internal urinary sphincter maintenance of female continence. British Medical Journal 292: 166–7

Versi E, Cardozo L D, Anand D et al 1991 Symptom analysis for the diagnosis of genuine stress incontinence. British Journal of Obstetrics and Gynaecology 98: 815–9

Vetter M J, Jones D A, Victor C R 1981 Urinary incontinence in the elderly at home. Lancet 2: 1275–7

Victor A, Larason G, Asbrink A S 1987 A simple patient-administered test of objective quantitation of the symptom of urinary incontinence. Scandinavian Journal of Urology and Nephrology 21: 277

Webb R J, Ramsden P D, Neal D E 1991 Ambulatory monitoring and electronic measurement of leakage in the diagnosis of detrusor instability. British Journal of Urology 68: 148–52

Webster G D, Perez L M, Choury J M et al 1992 Management of stress urinary incontinence using artificial urinary sphincter Urology 39: 499–503

Wells T J, Brink C A, Diokno A C et al 1991 Pelvic muscle exercises for stress urinary incontinence in elderly women. Journal of the American Geriatric Society 39: 785–91

Whitaker R H 1985 Artificial urinary sphincter. British Medical Journal 290: 1927–8

Wilson P D, Samarrai T A, Deakin M et al 1987 An objective assessment of physiotherapy for female genuine stress incontinence. British Journal of Obstetrics and Gynaecology 94: 575–82

Wise B G, Burton G, Cutner A et al 1992 Effects of vaginal ultrasound probe on lower urinary tract function. British Journal of Urology 70: 12–6

Wiskind A K, Creighton S M, Stanton S L 1992. The incidence of genital prolapse following the Burch colposuspension operation. American Journal of Obstetrics and Gynecology 167: 399–405

Yamada T, Mizuu T, Kawakami S et al 1991 Applications of transrectal ultrasound in modified Stamey procedure for stress urinary incontinence. Journal of Urology 146: 1555–8

Yarnell J W G, Voyle G J, Richards C J et al 1981 The prevalence and severity of urinary incontinence in women. Journal of Epidemiology and Community Health 35: 71–4

Yasuda K, Kawabe K, Takimoto Y et al 1993 A double blind clinical trial of a beta adrenergic agonist in stress incontinence. International Urogynecology Journal 4: 146–51

The standardisation of terminology of lower urinary tract function

Scandinavian Journal of Urology and Nephrology, Supplementum 114 (1988) Published 1988 by the Scandinavian University Press

Produced by the International Continence Society Committee on Standardisation of Terminology; Members: Paul Abrams, Jerry G Blaivas, Stuart L Stanton and Jens T Andersen (Chairman)

1. INTRODUCTION

The International Continence Society established a committee for the standardisation of terminology of lower urinary tract function in 1973. Five of the six reports[1–5] from this committee, approved by the Society, have been published. The fifth report on 'Quantification of urine loss' was an internal I.C.S. document but appears, in part, in this document.

These reports are revised, extended and collated in this monograph. The standards are recommended to facilitate comparison of results by investigators who use urodynamic methods. These standards are recommended not only for urodynamic investigations carried out on humans but also during animal studies. When using urodynamic studies in animals the type of any anaesthesia used should be stated. It is suggested that acknowledgement of these standards in written publications be indicated by a footnote to the section 'Methods and Materials' or its equivalent, to read as follows:

'Methods, definitions and units conform to the

standards recommended by the International Continence Society, except where specifically noted.'

Urodynamic studies involve the assessment of the function and dysfunction of the urinary tract by any appropriate method. Aspects of urinary tract morphology, physiology, biochemistry and hydrodynamics affect urine transport and storage. Other methods of investigation such as the radiographic visualisation of the lower urinary tract is a useful adjunct to conventional urodynamics.

This monograph concerns the urodynamics of the lower urinary tract.

2. CLINICAL ASSESSMENT

The clinical assessment of patients with lower urinary tract dysfunction should consist of a detailed history, a frequency/volume chart and a physical examination. In urinary incontinence, leakage should be demonstrated objectively.

2.1. History

The general history should include questions relevant to neurological and congenital abnormalities as well as information on previous urinary infections and relevant surgery. Information must be obtained on medication with known or possible effects on the lower urinary tract. The general history should also include assessment of menstrual, sexual and bowel function, and obstetric history.

The urinary history must consist of symptoms related to both the storage and the evacuation functions of the lower urinary tract.

2.2. Frequency/volume chart

The frequency/volume chart is a specific urodynamic investigation recording fluid intake and urine output per 24 hour period. The chart gives objective information on the number of voidings, the distribution of voidings between daytime and night-time and each voided volume. The chart can also be used to record episodes of urgency and leakage and the number of incontinence pads used. The frequency/volume chart is very useful in the assessment of voiding disorders, and in the follow-up of treatment.

2.3. Physical examination

Besides a general urological and, when appropriate, gynaecological examination, the physical examination should include the assessment of perineal sensation, the perineal reflexes supplied by the sacral segments S2–S4, and anal sphincter tone and control.

3. PROCEDURES RELATED TO THE EVALUATION OF URINE STORAGE

3.1. Cystometry

Cystometry is the method by which the pressure/volume relationship of the bladder is measured. All systems are zeroed at atmospheric pressure. For external transducers the reference point is the level of the superior edge of the symphysis pubis. For catheter mounted transducers the reference point is the transducer itself.

Cystometry is used to assess detrusor activity, sensation, capacity and compliance.

Before starting to fill the bladder the residual urine may be measured. However, the removal of a large volume of residual urine may alter detrusor function especially in neuropathic disorders. Certain cystometric parameters may be significantly altered by the speed of bladder filling (see 6.1.1.4.).

During cystometry it is taken for granted that the patient is awake, unanaesthetised and neither sedated nor taking drugs that affect bladder function. Any variations should be specified.

Specify

(a) Access (transurethral or percutaneous)
(b) Fluid medium (liquid or gas)
(c) Temperature of fluid (state in degrees Celsius)
(d) Position of patient (e.g. supine, sitting or standing)
(e) Filling may be by diuresis or catheter. Filling by catheter may be continuous or incremental; the precise filling rate should be stated.

  When the incremental method is used the volume increment should be stated. For general discussion, the following terms for the range of filling rate may be used:
  (i) up to 10 ml per minute is slow fill cystometry ('physiological' filling).
  (ii) 10–100 ml per minute is medium fill cystometry.
  (iii) over 100 ml per minute is rapid fill cystometry.

Technique

(a) Fluid-filled catheter – specify number of catheters, single or multiple lumens, type of catheter (manufacturer), size of catheter.

(b) Catheter tip transducer – list specifications.
(c) Other catheters – list specifications.
(d) Measuring equipment.

Definitions

Intravesical pressure is the pressure within the bladder.

Abdominal pressure is taken to be the pressure surrounding the bladder. In current practice it is estimated from rectal or, less commonly, extraperitoneal pressure.

Detrusor pressure is that component of intravesical pressure that is created by forces in the bladder wall (passive and active). It is estimated by subtracting abdominal pressure from intravesical pressure. The simultaneous measurement of abdominal pressure is essential for the interpretation of the intravesical pressure trace. However, artefacts on the detrusor pressure trace may be produced by intrinsic rectal contractions.

Bladder sensation. Sensation is difficult to evaluate because of its subjective nature. It is usually assessed by questioning the patient in relation to the fullness of the bladder during cystometry.

Commonly used descriptive terms include:

First desire to void

Normal desire to void (this is defined as the feeling that leads the patient to pass urine at the next convenient moment, but voiding can be delayed if necessary).

Strong desire to void (this is defined as a persistent desire to void without the fear of leakage).

Urgency (this is defined as a strong desire to void accompanied by fear of leakage or fear of pain).

Pain (the site and character of which should be specified). Pain during bladder filling or micturition is abnormal.

The use of objective or semi-objective tests for sensory function, such as electrical threshold studies (sensory testing), is discussed in detail in 5.5.

The term 'Capacity' must be qualified.

Maximum cystometric capacity, in patients with normal sensation, is the volume at which the patient feels he/she can no longer delay micturition. In the absence of sensation the maximum cystometric capacity cannot be defined in the same terms and is the volume at which the clinician decides to terminate filling. In the presence of sphincter incompetence the maximum cystometric capacity may be significantly increased by occlusion of the urethra e.g. by Foley catheter.

The *functional bladder capacity,* or voided volume is more relevant and is assessed from a frequency/volume chart (urinary diary).

The *maximum (anaesthetic) bladder capacity* is the volume measured after filling during a deep general or spinal/epidural anaesthetic, specifying fluid temperature, filling pressure and filling time.

Compliance indicates the change in volume for a change in pressure. Compliance is calculated by dividing the volume change (ΔV) by the change in detrusor pressure (ΔP_{det}) during that change in bladder volume ($C = \Delta V/\Delta P_{det}$). Compliance is expressed as ml per cm H_2O (see 6.1.1.4).

3.2. Urethral pressure measurement

It should be noted that the urethral pressure and the urethral closure pressure are idealised concepts which represent the ability of the urethra to prevent leakage (see 6.1.5). In current urodynamic practice the urethral pressure is measured by a number of different techniques which do not always yield consistent values. Not only do the values differ with the method of measurement but there is often lack of consistency for a single method. For example the effect of catheter rotation when urethral pressure is measured by a catheter mounted transducer.

Intraluminal urethral pressure may be measured:

(a) At rest, with the bladder at any given volume
(b) During coughing or straining
(c) During the process of voiding (see 4.4)

Measurements may be made at one point in the urethra over a period of time, or at several points along the urethra consecutively forming a *urethral pressure profile* (UPP).

Storage phase

Two types of UPP may be measured:

(a) Resting urethral pressure profile – with the bladder and subject at rest.
(b) Stress urethral pressure profile – with a defined applied stress (e.g. cough, strain, Valsalva).

In the storage phase the *urethral pressure profile* denotes the intraluminal pressure along the length of the urethra. All systems are zeroed at atmospheric pressure. For external transducers the reference point is the superior edge of the symphysis pubis. For catheter mounted transducers the reference point is the transducer itself. Intravesical pressure should be measured to exclude a simultaneous detrusor contraction. The subtraction of intravesical pressure from urethral pressure produces the *urethral closure pressure profile*.

The simultaneous recording of both intravesical and intra-urethral pressures are essential during stress urethral profilometry.

Specify

(a) Infusion medium (liquid or gas)
(b) Rate of infusion
(c) Stationary, continuous or intermittent withdrawal
(d) Rate of withdrawal
(e) Bladder volume
(f) Position of patient (supine, sitting or standing).

Technique

(a) Open catheter – specify type (manufacturer), size, number, position and orientation of side or end hole.
(b) Catheter mounted transducers – specify manufacturer, number of transducers, spacing of transducers along the catheter, orientation with respect to one another; transducer design e.g. transducer face depressed or flush with catheter surface; catheter diameter and material. The orientation of the transducer(s) in the urethra should be stated.
(c) Other catheters, e.g. membrane, fibreoptic – specify type (manufacturer), size and number of channels as for microtransducer catheter.
(d) Measurement technique: For stress profiles the particular stress employed should be stated e.g. cough or Valsalva.
(e) Recording apparatus: Describe type of recording apparatus. The frequency response of the total system should be stated. The frequency response of the catheter in the perfusion method can be assessed by blocking the eyeholes and recording the consequent rate of change of pressure.

Definitions (Fig. I.A: Referring to profiles measured in storage phase).

Maximum urethral pressure is the maximum pressure of the measured profile.

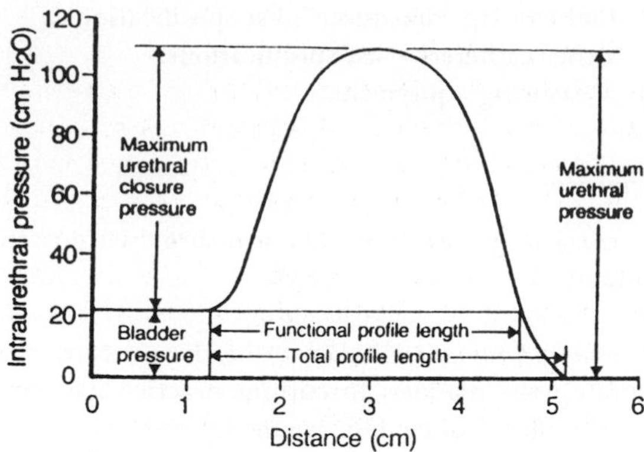

Fig. I.A Diagram of a female urethral pressure profile (static) with I.C.S. recommended nomenclature.

Maximum urethral closure pressure is the maximum difference between the urethral pressure and the intravesical pressure.

Functional profile length is the length of the urethra along which the urethral pressure exceeds intravesical pressure.

Functional profile length (on stress) is the length over which the urethral pressure exceeds the intravesical pressure on stress.

Pressure 'transmission' ratio is the increment in urethral pressure on stress as a percentage of the simultaneously recorded increment in intravesical pressure. For stress profiles obtained during coughing, pressure transmission ratios can be obtained at any point along the urethra. If single values are given the position in the urethra should be stated. If several pressure transmission ratios are defined at different points along the urethra a pressure 'transmission' profile is obtained. During 'cough profiles' the amplitude of the cough should be stated if possible.

Note: the term 'transmission' is in common usage and cannot be changed. However, transmission implies a completely passive process. Such an assumption is not yet justified by scientific evidence. A role for muscular activity cannot be excluded.

Total profile length is not generally regarded as a useful parameter.

The information gained from urethral pressure measurements in the storage phase is of limited value in the assessment of voiding disorders.

3.3. Quantification of urine loss

Subjective grading of incontinence may not indicate reliably the degree of abnormality. However it is important to relate the management of the individual patients to their complaints and personal circumstances, as well as to objective measurements.

In order to assess and compare the results of the

treatment of different types of incontinence in different centres, a simple standard test can be used to measure urine loss objectively in any subject. In order to obtain a representative result, especially in subjects with variable or intermittent urinary incontinence, the test should occupy as long a period as possible; yet it must be practical. The circumstances should approximate to those of everyday life, yet be similar for all subjects to allow meaningful comparison. On the basis of pilot studies performed in various centres, an internal report of the ICS (5th) recommended a test occupying a one-hour period during which a series of standard activities was carried out. This test *can* be extended by further one hour periods if the result of the first one hour test was not considered representative by either the patient or the investigator. Alternatively the test can be repeated having filled the bladder to a defined volume.

The total amount of urine lost during the test period is determined by weighing a collecting device such as a nappy, absorbent pad or condom appliance. A nappy or pad should be worn inside waterproof underpants or should have a waterproof backing. Care should be taken to use a collecting device of adequate capacity.

Immediately before the test begins the collecting device is weighed to the nearest gram.

Typical test schedule

(a) Test is started without the patient voiding.
(b) Preweighed collecting device is put on and first one hour test period begins.
(c) Subject drinks 500 ml sodium free liquid within a short period (max. 15 min), then sits or rests.
(d) Half hour period: subject walks, including stair climbing equivalent to one flight up and down.
(e) During the remaining period the subject performs the following activities:
    (i) standing up from sitting, 10 times
    (ii) coughing vigorously, 10 times
    (iii) running on the spot for 1 minute
    (iv) bending to pick up small object from floor, 5 times
    (v) wash hands in running water for 1 minute
(f) At the end of the one hour test the collecting device is removed and weighed.
(g) If the test is regarded as representative the subject voids and the volume is recorded.
(h) Otherwise the test is repeated preferably without voiding.

If the collecting device becomes saturated or filled during the test it should be removed and weighed, and replaced by a fresh device. The total weight of urine lost during the test period is taken to be equal to the gain in weight of the collecting device(s). In interpreting the results of the test it should be borne in mind that a weight gain of up to 1 gram may be due to weighing errors, sweating or vaginal discharge.

The activity programme may be modified according to the subject's physical ability. If substantial variations from the usual test schedule occur, this should be recorded so that the same schedule can be used on subsequent occasions.

In principle the subject should not void during the test period. If the patient experiences urgency, then he/she should be persuaded to postpone voiding and to perform as many of the activities in section (e) as possible in order to detect leakage. Before voiding the collection device is removed for weighing. If inevitable voiding cannot be postponed then the test is terminated. The voided volume and the duration of the test should be recorded. For subjects not completing the full test the results may require separate analysis, or the test may be repeated after rehydration.

The test result is given as grams urine lost in the one hour test period in which the greatest urine loss is recorded.

Additional procedures

Additional procedures intended to give information of diagnostic value are permissible provided they do not interfere with the basic test. For example, additional changes and weighing of the collecting device can give information about the timing of urine loss. The absorbent nappy may be an electronic recording nappy so that the timing is recorded directly.

Presentation of results

Specify

(a) Collecting device
(b) Physical condition of subject (ambulant, chairbound, bedridden)
(c) Relevant medical condition of subject
(d) Relevant drug treatments
(e) Test schedule.

In some situations the timing of the test (e.g. in relation to the menstrual cycle) may be relevant.

Findings

Record weight of urine lost during the test (in the case of repeated tests, greatest weight in any stated period). A loss of less than one gram is within experimental error and the patients should be regarded as essentially dry. Urine loss should be measured and recorded in grams.

Statistics

When performing statistical analysis of urine loss in a group of subjects, non-parametric statistics should be employed, since the values are not normally distributed.

4. PROCEDURES RELATED TO THE EVALUATION OF MICTURITION

4.1. Measurement of urinary flow

Urinary flow may be described in terms of *rate* and *pattern* and may be *continuous* or *intermittent*. *Flow rate* is defined as the volume of fluid expelled via the urethra per unit time. It is expressed in ml/s.

Specify

(a) Voided volume.
(b) Patient environment and position (supine, sitting or standing).
(c) Filling:
  (i) by diuresis (spontaneous or forced: specify regimen),
  (ii) by catheter (transurethral or suprapubic).
(d) type of fluid.

Technique

(a) Measuring equipment.
(b) Solitary procedure or combined with other measurements.

Definitions

(a) *Continuous flow* (Fig. I.B)

Voided volume is the total volume expelled via the urethra.

Maximum flow rate is the maximum measured value of the flow rate.

Average flow rate is voided volume divided by flow time. The calculation of average flow rate is only meaningful if flow is continuous and without terminal dribbling.

Flow time is the time over which measurable flow actually occurs.

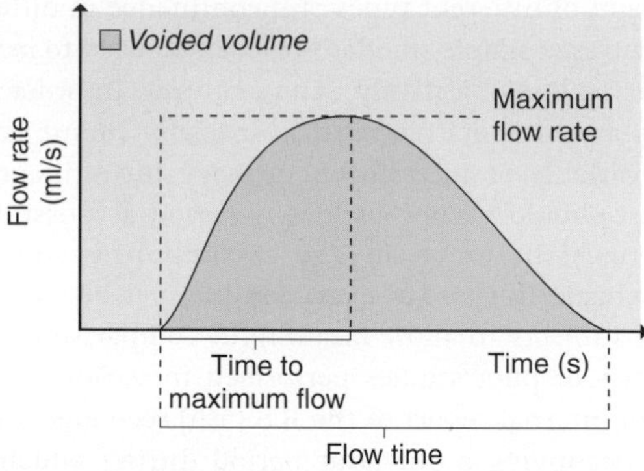

Fig. I.B Diagram of a continuous urine flow recording with ICS recommended nomenclature.

Time to maximum flow is the elapsed time from onset of flow to maximum flow.

The flow pattern must be described when flow time and average flow rate are measured.

(b) *Intermittent flow* (Fig. I.C)
The same parameters used to characterise continuous flow may be applicable if care is exercised in patients with intermittent flow. In measuring flow time the time intervals between flow episodes are disregarded.

Voiding time is total duration of micturition, i.e. includes interruptions. When voiding is completed without interruption, voiding time is equal to flow time.

4.2. Bladder pressure measurements during micturition

The specifications of patient position, access for pressure measurement, catheter type and measuring equipment are as for cystometry (see 3.1).

Definitions (Fig. I.D)

Opening Time is the elapsed time from initial rise in detrusor pressure to onset of flow. This is the initial isovolumetric contraction period of micturition. Time lags should be taken into account. In most urodynamic systems a time lag occurs equal to the time taken for the urine to pass from the point of pressure measurement to the uroflow transducer.

The following parameters are applicable to measurements of each of the pressure curves: intravesical, abdominal and detrusor pressure.

Premicturition pressure is the pressure recorded immediately before the initial isovolumetric contraction.

Opening pressure is the pressure recorded at the onset of measured flow.

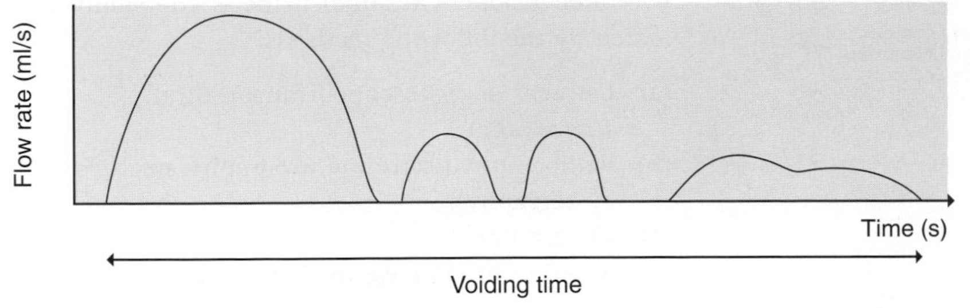

Fig. I.C Diagram of an interrupted urine flow recording with ICS recommended nomenclature.

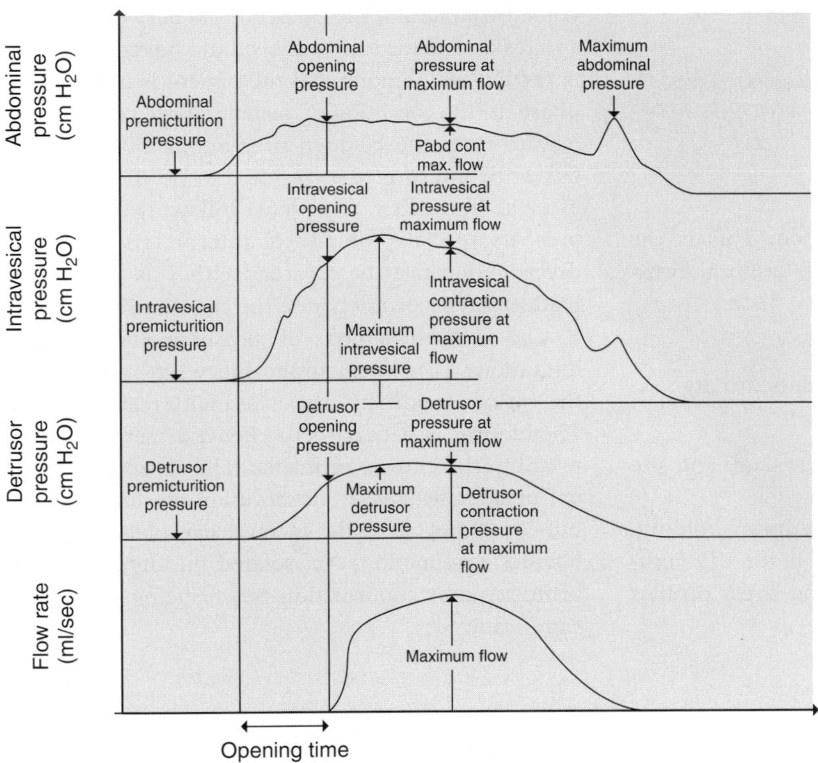

Fig. I.D Diagram of a pressure-flow recording of micturition with I.C.S. recommended nomenclature.

Maximum pressure is the maximum value of the measured pressure.

Pressure at maximum flow is the pressure recorded at maximum measured flow rate.

Contraction pressure at maximum flow is the difference between pressure at maximum flow and premicturition pressure.

Postmicturition events (e.g. after contraction) are not well understood and so cannot be defined as yet.

4.3. Pressure-flow relationships

In the early days of urodynamics the flow rate and voiding pressure were related as a 'urethral resistance factor'. The concept of a resistance factor originates from rigid tube hydrodynamics. The urethra does not generally behave as a rigid tube as it is an irregular and distensible conduit whose walls and surroundings have active and passive elements and, hence, influence the flow through it. Therefore a resistance factor cannot provide a valid comparison between patients.

There are many ways of displaying the relationships between flow and pressure during micturition; an example is suggested in the ICS 3rd Report[4] (Fig. I.E). As yet available data do not permit a standard presentation of pressure/flow parameters.

When data from a group of patients are presented, pressure-flow relationships may be shown on a graph as illustrated in Fig. I.E. This form of presentation allows lines of demarcation to be drawn on the graph to separate the results according to the problem being studied. The points shown in Fig. I.E are purely illustrative to indicate how the data might fall into groups. The group of equivocal results might include either an unrepresentative micturition in an obstructed or an unobstructed patient, or underactive detrusor

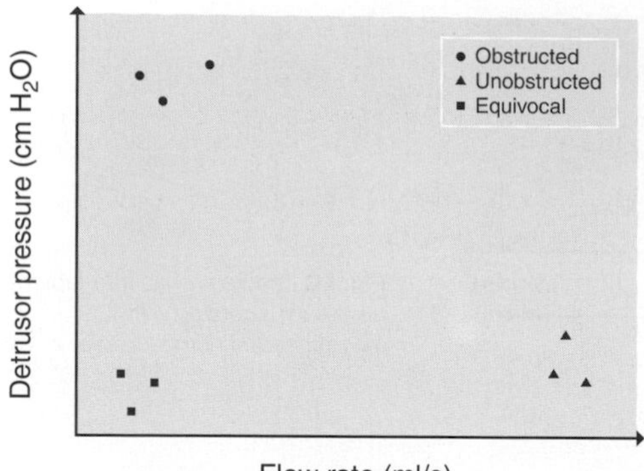

Fig. I.E Diagram illustrating the presentation of pressure flow data on individual patients in three groups of 3 patients: obstructed, equivocal and unobstructed.

function with or without obstruction. This is the group which invalidates the use of 'urethral resistance factors'.

4.4. Urethral pressure measurements during voiding (VUPP)

The VUPP is used to determine the pressure and site of urethral obstruction.

Pressure is recorded in the urethra during voiding. The technique is similar to that used in the UPP measured during storage (the resting and stress profiles 3.2).

Specify

As for UPP during storage (3.2).
Accurate interpretation of the VUPP depends on the simultaneous measurement of intravesical pressure and the measurement of pressure at a precisely localised point in the urethra. Localisation may be achieved by radio opaque marker on the catheter which allows the pressure measurements to be related to a visualised point in the urethra.

This technique is not fully developed and a number of technical as well as clinical problems need to be solved before the VUPP is widely used.

4.5. Residual urine

Residual urine is defined as the volume of fluid remaining in the bladder immediately following the completion of micturition. The measurement of residual urine forms an integral part of the study of micturition. However voiding in unfamiliar surroundings may lead to unrepresentative results, as may voiding on command with a partially filled or overfilled bladder. Residual urine is commonly estimated by the following methods:

(a) Catheter or cystoscope (transurethral, suprapubic).
(b) Radiography (excretion urography, micturition cystography).
(c) Ultrasonics.
(d) Radio-isotopes (clearance, gamma camera).

When estimating residual urine the measurement of voided volume and the time interval between voiding and residual urine estimation should be recorded: this is particularly important if the patient is in a diuretic phase. In the condition of vesicoureteric reflux, urine may re-enter the bladder after micturition and may falsely be interpreted as residual urine. The presence of urine in bladder diverticula following micturition presents special problems of interpretation, since a diverticulum may be regarded either as part of the bladder cavity or as outside the functioning bladder.

The various methods of measurement each have limitations as to their applicability and accuracy in the various conditions associated with residual urine. Therefore it is necessary to choose a method appropriate to the clinical problems. The absence of residual urine is usually an observation of clinical value, but does not exclude infravesical obstruction or bladder dysfunction. An isolated finding of residual urine requires confirmation before being considered significant.

5. PROCEDURES RELATED TO NEUROPHYSIOLOGICAL EVALUATION OF THE URINARY TRACT DURING FILLING AND VOIDING

5.1. Electromyography

Electromyography (EMG) is the study of electrical potentials generated by the depolarisation of muscle. The following refers to striated muscle EMG. The functional unit in EMG is the motor unit. This is comprised of a single motor neurone and the muscle fibres it innervates. A motor unit action potential is the recorded depolarisation of muscle fibres which results from activation of a single anterior horn cell. Muscle action potentials may be detected either by needle electrodes, or by surface electrodes.

Needle electrodes are placed directly into the muscle mass and permit visualisation of the individual motor unit action potentials.

Surface electrodes are applied to an epithelial

surface as close to the muscle under study as possible. Surface electrodes detect the action potentials from groups of adjacent motor units underlying the recording surface.

EMG potentials may be displayed on an oscilloscope screen or played through audio amplifiers. A permanent record of EMG potentials can only be made using a chart recorder with a high frequency response (in the range of 10 kHz).

EMG should be interpreted in the light of the patients' symptoms, physical findings and urological and urodynamic investigations.

General information

Specify

(a) EMG (solitary procedure, part of urodynamic or other electrophysiological investigation).
(b) Patient position (supine, standing, sitting or other).
(c) Electrode placement:
  - (i) Sampling site (intrinsic striated muscle of the urethra, periurethral striated muscle, bulbocavernosus muscle, external anal sphincter, pubococcygeus or other). State whether sites are single or multiple, unilateral or bilateral. Also state number of samples per site.
  - (ii) Recording electrode: define the precise anatomical location of the electrode. For needle electrodes, include site of needle entry, angle of entry and needle depth. For vaginal or urethral surface electrodes state method of determining position of electrode.
  - (iii) Reference electrode position.

Note: ensure that there is no electrical interference with any other machines, e.g. X-ray apparatus.

Technical information

Specify

(a) Electrodes
  - (i) Needle electrodes
    - design (concentric, bipolar, monopolar, single fibre, other)
    - dimensions (length, diameter, recording area)
    - electrode material (e.g. platinum).
  - (ii) Surface electrodes
    - type (skin, plug, catheter, other)
    - size and shape
    - electrode material
    - mode of fixation to recording surface
    - conducting medium (e.g. saline, jelly)

(b) Amplifier (make and specifications)
(c) Signal processing (data: raw, averaged, integrated or other)
(d) Display equipment (make and specifications to include method of calibration, time base, full scale deflection in microvolts and polarity)
  - (i) oscilloscope
  - (ii) chart recorder
  - (iii) loudspeaker
  - (iv) other

(e) Storage (make and specifications)
  - (i) paper
  - (ii) magnetic tape recorder
  - (iii) microprocessor
  - (iv) other

(f) Hard copy production (make and specifications)
  - (i) chart recorder
  - (ii) photographic/video reproduction of oscilloscope screen
  - (iii) other

EMG findings

(a) Individual motor unit action potentials – Normal motor unit potentials have a characteristic configuration, amplitude and duration. Abnormalities of the motor unit may include an increase in the amplitude, duration and complexity of wave-form (polyphasicity) of the potentials. A polyphasic potential is defined as one having more than 5 deflections. The EMG findings of fibrillations, positive sharp waves and bizarre high frequency potentials are thought to be abnormal.

(b) Recruitment patterns – In normal subjects there is a gradual increase in 'pelvic floor' and 'sphincter' EMG activity during bladder filling. At the onset of micturition there is complete absence of activity. Any sphincter EMG activity during voiding is abnormal unless the patient is attempting to inhibit micturition. The finding of increased sphincter EMG activity, during voiding, accompanied by characteristic simultaneous detrusor pressure and flow changes is described by the term, detrusor-sphincter-dyssynergia. In this condition a detrusor contraction occurs concurrently with an inappropriate contraction of the urethral and or periurethral striated muscle.

5.2. Nerve conduction studies

Nerve conduction studies involve stimulation of a peripheral nerve, and recording the time taken for a response to occur in muscle, innervated by the nerve under study. The time taken from stimulation of the nerve to the response in the muscle is called the 'latency'. Motor latency is the time taken by the fastest motor fibres in the nerve to conduct impulses to the muscle and depends on conduction distance and the conduction velocity of the fastest fibres.

General information

(also applicable to reflex latencies and evoked potentials – see below).

Specify

(a) Type of investigation
  (i) nerve conduction study (e.g. pudendal nerve)
  (ii) reflex latency determination (e.g. bulbocavernosus)
  (iii) spinal evoked potential
  (iv) cortical evoked potential
  (v) other
(b) Is the study a solitary procedure or part of urodynamic or neurophysiological investigations?
(c) Patient position and environmental temperature, noise level and illumination.
(d) Electrode placement: Define electrode placement in precise anatomical terms. The exact interelectrode distance is required for nerve conduction velocity calculations.
  (i) Stimulation site (penis, clitoris, urethra, bladder neck, bladder or other).
  (ii) Recording sites (external anal sphincter, periurethral striated muscle, bulbocavernosus muscle, spinal cord, cerebral cortex or other). When recording spinal evoked responses, the sites of the recording electrodes should be specified according to the bony landmarks (e.g. L4). In cortical evoked responses the sites of the recording electrodes should be specified as in the International 10–20 system.[6] The sampling techniques should be specified (single or multiple, unilateral or bilateral, ipsilateral or contralateral or other).
  (iii) Reference electrode position.
  (iv) Grounding electrode site: ideally this should be between the stimulation and recording sites to reduce stimulus artefact.

Technical information

(also applicable to reflex latencies and evoked potential – see see below)

Specify

(a) Electrodes (make and specifications). Describe *separately* stimulus and recording electrodes as below.
  (i) design (e.g. needle, plate, ring, and configuration of anode and cathode where applicable)
  (ii) dimensions
  (iii) electrode material (e.g. platinum)
  (iv) contact medium
(b) Stimulator (make and specifications)
  (i) stimulus parameters (pulse width, frequency, pattern, current density, electrode impedance in Kohms. Also define in terms of threshold e.g. in case of supramaximal stimulation)
(c) Amplifier (make and specifications)
  (i) sensitivity (mV–μV)
  (ii) filters – low pass (Hz) or high pass (kHz)
  (iii) sampling time (ms)
(d) Averager (make and specifications)
  (i) number of stimuli sampled
(e) Display equipment (make and specifications to include method of calibration, time base, full scale deflection in microvolts and polarity)
  (i) oscilloscope
(f) Storage (make and specifications)
  (i) paper
  (ii) magnetic tape recorder
  (iii) microprocessor
  (iv) other
(g) Hard copy production (make and specification)
  (i) chart recorder
  (ii) photographic/video reproduction of oscilloscope screen
  (iii) XY recorder
  (iv) other

Description of nerve conduction studies

Recordings are made from muscle and the latency of response of the muscle is measured. The latency is taken as the time to onset, of the earliest response.

(a) To ensure that response time can be precisely measured, the gain should be increased to give a clearly defined take-off point. (Gain setting at least 100 μV/div and using a short time base e.g. 1–2 ms/div).

(b) Additional information may be obtained from nerve conduction studies, if, when using surface electrodes to record a compound muscle action potential, the amplitude is measured. The gain setting must be reduced so that the whole response is displayed and a longer time base is recommended (e.g. 1 mV/div and 5 ms/div). Since the amplitude is proportional to the number of motor unit potentials within the vicinity of the recording electrodes, a reduction in amplitude indicates loss of motor units and therefore denervation. (Note: A prolongation of latency is not necessarily indicative of denervation.)

5.3. Reflex latencies

Reflex latencies require stimulation of sensory fields and recordings from the muscle which contracts reflexly in response to the stimulation. Such responses are a test of reflex arcs which are comprised of both afferent and efferent limbs and a synaptic region within the central nervous system. The reflex latency expresses the nerve conduction velocity in both limbs of the arc and the integrity of the central nervous system at the level of the synapse(s). Increased reflex latency may occur as a result of slowed afferent or efferent nerve conduction or due to central nervous system conduction delays.

General information and technical information

The same technical and general details apply as discussed above under Nerve Conduction Studies (5.2).

Description of reflex latency measurements

Recordings are made from muscle and the latency of response of the muscle is measured. The latency is taken as the time to onset, of the earliest response.

To ensure that response time can be precisely measured, the gain should be increased to give a clearly defined take-off point. (Gain setting at least 100 μV/div and using a short time base e.g. 1–2 ms/div.)

5.4 Evoked responses

Evoked responses are potential changes in central nervous system neurones resulting from distant stimulation usually electrical. They are recorded using averaging techniques. Evoked responses may be used to test the integrity of peripheral, spinal and central nervous pathways. As with nerve conduction studies, the conduction time (latency) may be measured. In addition, information may be gained from the amplitude and configuration of these responses.

General information and technical information

See above under Nerve Conduction Studies (5.2).

Description of evoked responses

Describe the presence or absence of stimulus evoked responses and their configuration.

Specify

(a) Single or multiphasic response.
(b) Onset of response: defined as the start of the first reproducible potential. Since the onset of the response may be difficult to ascertain precisely, the criteria used should be stated.
(c) Latency to onset: defined as the time (ms) from the onset of stimulus to the onset of response. The central conduction time relates to cortical evoked potentials and is defined as the difference between the latencies of the cortical and the spinal evoked potentials. This parameter may be used to test the integrity of the corticospinal neuraxis.
(d) Latencies to peaks of positive and negative deflections in multiphasic responses (Fig. I.F). P denotes positive deflections, N denotes negative deflections. In multiphasic responses, the peaks are numbered consecutively (e.g. P1, N1, P2, N2 ...) or according to the latencies to peaks in milliseconds (e.g. P44, N52, P6[[6]] ...).
(e) The amplitude of the responses is measured in μV.

5.5 Sensory testing

Limited information, of a subjective nature, may be obtained during cystometry by recording such parameters as the first desire to micturate, urgency or pain. However, sensory function in the lower urinary

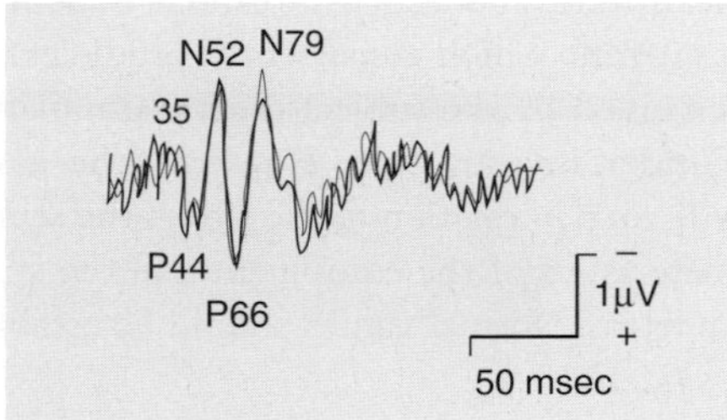

Fig. I.F Multiphasic evoked response recorded from the cerebral cortex after stimulation of the dorsal aspect of the penis. The recording shows the conventional labelling of negative (N) and positive (P) deflections with the latency of each deflection from the point of stimulation in milliseconds.

tract, can be assessed by semi-objective tests by the measurement of urethral and/or vesical sensory thresholds to a standard applied stimulus such as a known electrical current.

General information

Specify

(a) Patient's position (supine, sitting, standing, other)
(b) Bladder volume at time of testing
(c) Site of applied stimulus (intravesical, intraurethral)
(d) Number of times the stimulus was applied and the response recorded. Define the sensation recorded, e.g. the first sensation or the sensation of pulsing.
(e) Type of applied stimulus
  (i) electrical current: it is usual to use a constant current stimulator in urethral sensory measurement
    – state electrode characteristics and placement as in section on EMG
    – state electrode contact area and distance between electrodes if applicable
    – state impedance characteristics of the system
    – state type of conductive medium used for electrode/epithelial contact. *Note: topical anaesthetic agents should not be used.*
    – stimulator make and specifications
    – stimulation parameters (pulse width, frequency, pattern, duration, current density).
  (ii) other – e.g. mechanical, chemical.

Definition of sensory thresholds

The vesical/urethral sensory threshold is defined as the least current which consistently produces a sensation perceived by the subject during stimulation at the site under investigation. However, the absolute values will vary in relation to the site of the stimulus, the characteristics of the equipment and the stimulation parameters. Normal values should be established for each system.

6. A CLASSIFICATION OF URINARY TRACT DYSFUNCTION

The lower urinary tract is composed of the *bladder* and *urethra*. They form a functional unit and their interaction cannot be ignored. Each has two functions, the bladder to store and void, the urethra to control and convey. When a reference is made to the hydrodynamic function or to the whole anatomical unit as a storage organ – the vesica urinaria – the correct term is the *bladder*. When the smooth muscle structure known as the m. detrusor urinae is being discussed then the correct term is *detrusor*. For simplicity the bladder/detrusor and the urethra will be considered separately so that a classification based on a combination of functional anomalies can be reached. Sensation cannot be precisely evaluated but must be assessed. This classification depends on the results of various objective urodynamic investigations. A complete urodynamic assessment is not necessary in all patients. However, studies of the filling and voiding phases are essential for each patient. As the bladder and urethra may behave differently during the storage and micturition phases of bladder function it is most useful to examine bladder and urethral activity separately in each phase.

Terms used should be objective, definable and ideally should be applicable to the whole range of abnormality. When authors disagree with the classification presented below, or use terms which have not been defined here, their meaning should be made clear.

Assuming the absence of inflammation, infection and neoplasm, *lower urinary tract dysfunction* may be caused by:

(a) Disturbance of the pertinent nervous or psychological control system.
(b) Disorders of muscle function.
(c) Structural abnormalities.

Urodynamic diagnoses based on this classification should correlate with the patient's symptoms and signs. For example the presence of an unstable contraction in an asymptomatic continent patient does not warrant a diagnosis of detrusor overactivity during storage.

6.1. The storage phase

6.1.1. Bladder function during storage

This may be described according to:
6.1.1.1 Detrusor activity
6.1.1.2 Bladder sensation
6.1.1.3 Bladder capacity

6.1.1.4 Compliance

6.1.1.1 *Detrusor activity* In this context detrusor activity is interpreted from the measurement of detrusor pressure (P_{det}).

Detrusor activity may be:

(a) Normal
(b) Overactive

(a) *Normal detrusor function* During the filling phase the bladder volume increases without a significant rise in pressure (accommodation). No involuntary contractions occur despite provocation.

A normal detrusor so defined may be described as 'stable'.

(b) *Overactive detrusor function* Overactive detrusor function is characterised by involuntary detrusor contractions during the filling phase, which may be spontaneous or provoked and which the patient cannot completely suppress. Involuntary detrusor contractions may be provoked by rapid filling, alterations of posture, coughing, walking, jumping and other triggering procedures. Various terms have been used to describe these features and they are defined as follows:

The *unstable detrusor* is one that is shown objectively to contract, spontaneously or on provocation, during the filling phase while the patient is attempting to inhibit micturition. Unstable detrusor contractions may be asymptomatic or may be interpreted as a normal desire to void. The presence of these contractions does not necessarily imply a neurological disorder. Unstable contractions are usually phasic in type (Fig. I.G-A). A gradual increase in detrusor pressure without subsequent decrease is best regarded as a change of compliance (Fig. I.G-B).

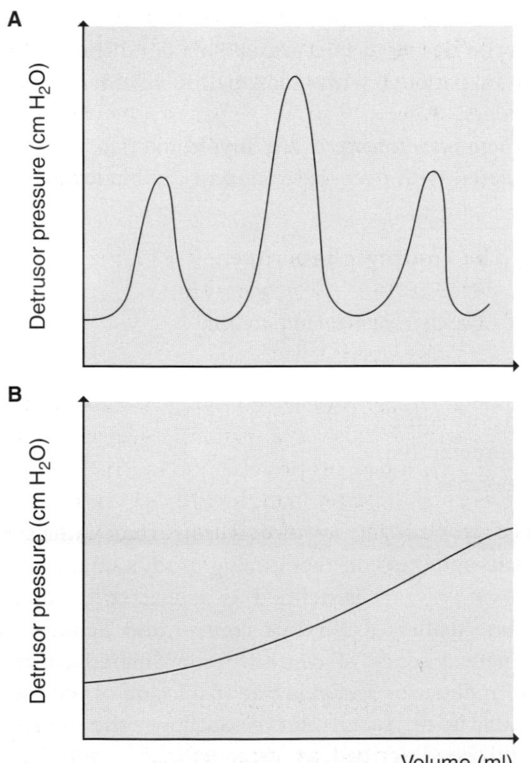

Fig. I.G Diagrams of filling cystometry to illustrate: **A**. Typical phasic unstable detrusor contraction. **B** The gradual increase of detrusor pressure with filling characterisitic of reduced bladder compliance.

Detrusor hyperreflexia is defined as overactivity due to disturbance of the nervous control mechanisms. The term detrusor hyperreflexia should only be used when there is objective evidence of a relevant neurological disorder. The use of conceptual and undefined terms such as hypertonic, systolic, uninhibited, spastic and automatic should be avoided.

6.1.1.2. *Bladder sensation* Bladder sensation during filling can be classified in qualitative terms (see 3.1) and by objective measurement (see 5.5). Sensation can be classified broadly as follows:

(a) Normal
(b) Increased (hypersensitive)
(c) Reduced (hyposensitive)
(d) Absent

6.1.1.3 *Bladder capacity* (see 3.1.)

6.1.1.4 *Compliance* is defined as: $\Delta V/\Delta p$ (see 3.1).

Compliance may change during the cystometric examination and is variably dependent upon a number of factors including:

(a) Rate of filling
(b) The part of the cystometrogram curve used for compliance calculation
(c) The volume interval over which compliance is calculated
(d) The geometry (shape) of the bladder
(e) The thickness of the bladder wall
(f) The mechanical properties of the bladder wall
(g) The contractile/relaxant properties of the detrusor

During normal bladder filling little or no pressure change occurs and this is termed 'normal compliance'. However at the present time there is insufficient data to define normal, high and low compliance.

When reporting compliance, specify:

(a) The rate of bladder filling
(b) The bladder volume at which compliance is calculated
(c) The volume increment over which compliance is calculated
(d) The part of the cystometrogram curve used for the calculation of compliance.

6.1.2. Urethral function during storage

The urethral closure mechanism during storage may be:

(a) Normal
(b) Incompetent

(a) The *normal urethral closure mechanism* maintains a positive urethral closure pressure during filling even in the presence of increased abdominal pressure. Immediately prior to micturition the normal closure pressure decreases to allow flow.
(b) *Incompetent urethral closure mechanism*. An incompetent urethral closure mechanism is defined as one which allows leakage of urine in the absence of a detrusor contraction. Leakage may occur whenever intravesical pressure exceeds intraurethral pressure (genuine stress incontinence) or when there is an involuntary fall in urethral pressure. Terms such as 'the unstable urethra' await further data and precise definition.

6.1.3. Urinary incontinence

Urinary incontinence is involuntary loss of urine which is objectively demonstrable and a social or hygienic problem. Loss of urine through channels other than the urethra is extraurethral incontinence.

Urinary incontinence denotes:

(a) A symptom
(b) A sign
(c) A condition

The symptom indicates the patient's statement of involuntary urine loss.

The sign is the objective demonstration of urine loss.

The condition is the urodynamic demonstration of urine loss.

Symptoms

Urge incontinence is the involuntary loss of urine associated with a strong desire to void (urgency).
Urgency may be associated with two types of dysfunction:

(a) Overactive detrusor function (*motor urgency*)
(b) Hypersensitivity (*sensory urgency*)

Stress incontinence: the symptom indicates the patient's statement of involuntary loss of urine during physical exertion.

'Unconscious' incontinence. Incontinence may occur in the absence of urge and without conscious recognition of the urinary loss.

Enuresis means any involuntary loss of urine. If it is used to denote incontinence during sleep, it should always be qualified with the adjective 'nocturnal'.

Post-micturition dribble and *continuous leakage* denote other symptomatic forms of incontinence.

Signs

The sign stress-incontinence denotes the observation of loss of urine from the urethra synchronous with physical exertion (e.g. coughing). Incontinence may also be observed without physical exercise. Post-micturition dribble and continuous leakage denotes other signs of incontinence. Symptoms and signs alone may not disclose the cause of urinary incontinence. Accurate diagnosis often requires urodynamic investigation in addition to careful history and physical examination.

Conditions

Genuine stress incontinence is the involuntary loss of urine occurring when, in the absence of a detrusor contraction, the intravesical pressure exceeds the maximum urethral pressure.
Reflex incontinence is loss of urine due to detrusor hyperreflexia and/or involuntary urethral relaxation in the absence of the sensation usually associated with the desire to micturate. This condition is only seen in patients with neuropathic bladder/urethral disorders.
Overflow incontinence is any involuntary loss of urine associated with over-distension of the bladder.

6.2. The Voiding phase

6.2.1. The detrusor during voiding

During micturition the detrusor may be:

(a) acontractile
(b) underactive
(c) normal

(a)*The acontractile detrusor* is one that cannot be demonstrated to contract during urodynamic studies. *Detrusor areflexia* is defined as acontractility due to an abnormality of nervous control and denotes the complete absence of centrally coordinated contraction. In detrusor areflexia due to a lesion of the conus medullaris or sacral nerve outflow, the detrusor should be described as *decentralised* – not denervated, since the peripheral neurones remain. In such bladders pressure fluctuations of low amplitude, sometimes known as 'autonomous' waves, may occasionally occur. The use of terms such as atonic, hypotonic, autonomic and flaccid should be avoided.

(b) *Detrusor underactivity*. This term should be reserved as an expression describing detrusor activity during micturition. Detrusor underactivity is defined as a detrusor contraction of inadequate magnitude and/or duration to effect bladder emptying with a normal time span. Patients may have underactivity during micturition and detrusor overactivity during filling.

(c) *Normal detrusor contractility*. Normal voiding is achieved by a voluntarily initiated detrusor contraction that is sustained and can usually be suppressed voluntarily. A normal detrusor contraction will effect complete bladder emptying in the absence of obstruction. For a given detrusor contraction, the magnitude of the recorded pressure rise will depend on the degree of outlet resistance.

6.2.2. Urethral function during micturition

During voiding urethral function may be:

(a) normal
(b) obstructive
 – overactive
 – mechanical

(a) *The normal urethra* opens to allow the bladder to be emptied.

(b) *Obstruction due to urethral overactivity*: this occurs when the urethral closure mechanism contracts against a detrusor contraction or fails to open at attempted micturition. Synchronous detrusor and urethral contraction is *detrusor/urethral dyssynergia*. This diagnosis should be qualified by stating the location and type of the urethral muscles (striated or smooth) which are involved. Despite the confusion surrounding 'sphincter' terminology the use of certain terms is so widespread that they are retained and defined here. The term *detrusor/external sphincter dyssynergia* or *detrusor-sphincter-dyssynergia* (DSD) describes a detrusor contraction concurrent with an involuntary contraction of the urethral and/or periurethral striated muscle. In the adult, detrusor sphincter dyssynergia is a feature of neurological voiding disorders. In the absence of neurological features the validity of this diagnosis should be questioned. The term *detrusor/bladder neck dyssynergia* is used to denote a detrusor contraction concurrent with an objectively demonstrated failure of bladder neck opening. No parallel term has been elaborated for possible detrusor/distal urethral (smooth muscle) dyssynergia.

Overactivity of the striated urethral sphincter may occur in the absence of detrusor contraction, and may prevent voiding. This is not detrusor/sphincter dyssynergia.

Overactivity of the urethral sphincter may occur during voiding in the absence of neurological disease and is termed *dysfunctional voiding*. The use of terms such as 'non-neurogenic' or 'occult neuropathic' should be avoided.

Mechanical obstruction: is most commonly anatomical e.g. urethral stricture.

Using the characteristics of detrusor and urethral function during storage and micturition an accurate definition of lower urinary tract behaviour in each patient becomes possible.

7. UNITS OF MEASUREMENT

In the urodynamic literature pressure is measured in cmH_2O and *not* in millimetres of mercury. When Laplace's law is used to calculate tension in the bladder wall, it is often found that pressure is then measured in dyne cm^{-2}. This lack of uniformity in the systems used leads to confusion when other parameters, which are a function of pressure, are computed, for instance, 'compliance', contraction force, velocity etc. From these few examples it is evident that standardisation is essential for meaningful communication. Many journals now require that the results be given in SI units. This section is designed to give guidance in the application of the SI system to urodynamics and defines the units involved. The principal units to be used are listed below (Table I.1).

Table I.1

Quantity	Acceptable unit	Symbol
volume	millilitre	ml
time	second	s
flow rate	millilitres/second	ml s^{-1}
pressure	centimetres of water[a]	cmH_2O
length	metres or submultiples	m, cm, mm
velocity	metres/second or submultiples	m s^{-1}, cm s^{-1}
temperature	degrees Celsius	°C

[a] The SI Unit is the pascal (Pa), but it is only practical at present to calibrate our instruments in cmH_2O. One centimetre of water pressure is approximately equal to 100 pascals (1 cmH_2O = 98.07 Pa = 0.098 kPa).

Table I.2 List of symbols

Basic symbols		Urological qualifiers		Value	
Pressure	*P*	Bladder	ves	Maximum	max
Volume	*V*	Urethra	ura	Minimum	min
Flow rate	*Q*	Ureter	ure	Average	ave
Velocity	*v*	Detrusor	det	Isovolumetric	isv
Time	*t*	Abdomen	abd	Isotonic	ist
Temperature	*T*	External		Isobaric	isb
Length	*l*	stream	ext	Isometric	ism
Area	*A*				
Diameter	*d*				
Force	*F*				
Energy	*E*				
Power	*P*				
Compliance	*P*				
Work	*W*				
Energy per unit volume	*e*				

Examples:
$P_{det,max}$ = maximum detrusor pressure
e_{ext} = kinetic energy per unit volume in the external stream

Symbols

It is often helpful to use symbols in a communication. The system in Table I.2 has been devised to standardise a code of symbols for use in urodynamics. The rationale of the system is to have a basic symbol representing the physical quantity with qualifying subscripts. The list of basic symbols largely conforms to international usage. The qualifying subscripts relate to the basic symbols to commonly used urodynamic parameters.

REFERENCES

1. Abrams P, Blaivas J G, Stanton S L et al 1986 Sixth report on the standardisation of terminology of lower urinary tract function. Procedures related to neurophysiological investigations: Electromyography, nerve conduction studies, reflex latencies, evoked potentials and sensory testing. World Journal of Urology 4: 2–5. Scandinavian Journal of Urology and Nephrology 20: 161–164
2. Bates P, Bradley W E, Glen E et al 1976 First report on the standardisation of terminology of lower urinary tract function. Urinary incontinence. Procedures related to the evaluation of urine storage: Cystometry, urethral closure pressure profile, units of measurement. British Journal of Urology 48: 39–42. European Urology 2: 274–276. Scandinavian Journal of Urology and Nephrology 11: 193–196. Urologia Internationalis 32: 81–87.
3. Bates P, Glen E, Griffiths D et al 1977 Second report on the standardisation of terminology of lower urinary tract function. Procedures related to the evaluation of micturition: Flow rate, pressure measurement, symbols. Acta Urologica Japonica 27: 1563–1566. British Journal of Urology 49: 207–210. European Urology 3: 168–170. Scandinavian Journal of Urology and Nephrology 11: 197–199.
4. Bates P, Bradley W E, Glen E et al 1980 Third report on the standardisation of terminology of lower urinary tract function. Procedures related to the evaluation of micturition: Pressure flow relationships, residual urine. British Journal of Urology 52: 348–350. European Urology 6: 170–171. Acta Urologica Japonica 27: 1566–1568. Scandinavian Journal of Urology and Nephrology 12: 191–193.
5. Bates P, Bradley W E, Glen E et al 1981 Fourth report on the standardisation of terminology of lower urinary tract function. Terminology related to neuromuscular dysfunction of lower urinary tract. British Journal of Urology 52: 333–335. Urology 17: 618–620. Scandinavian Journal of Urology and Nephrology 15: 169–171. Acta Urologica Japonica 27: 1568–1571.
6. Jasper H H 1958 Report to the committee on the methods of clinical examination in electroencephalography. Electroencephalography in Clinical Neurophysiology 10: 370–75.

Lower urinary tract rehabilitation techniques: seventh report on the standardisation of terminology of lower urinary tract function

Neurourology and Urodynamics 11: 593–603 (1992) Published 1992 by Wiley-Liss, Inc.

J T Andersen (Chairman), J G Blaivas, L Cardozo and J Thüroff

International Continence Society Committee on Standardisation of Terminology

1. INTRODUCTION

Lower urinary tract rehabilitation comprises non-surgical, non-pharmacological treatment for lower urinary tract dysfunction. The specific techniques defined in this report are listed in the contents above.

Most of the conditions for which rehabilitation techniques are employed have both a subjective and an objective component. In many instances, treatment is only capable of relieving symptoms, not curing the underlying disease. Therefore, symptoms should be quantified before and after treatment, and the means by which the physiology is altered should be clearly stated.

The applications of the individual types of treatment cited here are taken from the scientific literature and from current clinical practice. It is not within the scope of this committee to endorse specific recommendations for treatment, nor to restrict the use of these treatments to the examples given.

The standards set in this report are recommended to ensure the reproducibility of methods of treatment and to facilitate the comparison of results obtained by different investigators and therapists. It is suggested that acknowledgement of these standards, in written publications, should be indicated by a footnote to the section 'Methods and Materials' or its equivalent, to read as follows:

'Methods, definitions and units conform to the standards recommended by the International Continence Society, except where specifically noted.'

2. PELVIC FLOOR TRAINING

2.1. Definition

Pelvic floor training is defined as repetitive selective voluntary contraction and relaxation of specific pelvic floor muscles. This necessitates muscle awareness in order to be sure that the correct muscles are being utilised, and to avoid unwanted contractions of adjacent muscle groups.

2.2. Techniques

2.2.1. Standard of diagnosis and implementation

The professional status of the individual who establishes the diagnosis must be stated as well as the diagnostic techniques employed. Also the professional status of the person who institutes, supervises and assesses treatment must be specified.

2.2.2. Muscle awareness

The technique used for obtaining selective pelvic floor contractions and relaxations should be stated. Registration of electromyographic (EMG) activity in the muscles of the pelvic floor, urethral or anal sphincter, or the anterior abdominal wall, may be necessary to obtain this muscle awareness. Alternatively or additionally, registration of abdominal, vaginal, urethral or anal pressure may be used for the same purpose.

2.2.3. Muscle training

It should be specified as to whether treatment is given on an inpatient or outpatient basis. Specific details of training must be stated:

1. Patient position
2. Duration of each contraction
3. Interval between contractions
4. Number of contractions per exercise
5. Number of exercises per day
6. Length of treatment programme (weeks, months)

2.2.4. Adjunctive equipment

Adjunctive equipment may be employed to enhance muscle awareness or muscle training. The following should be specified:

1. Type of equipment
2. Mechanism of action
3. Duration of use
4. Therapeutic goals

Examples of equipment in current use are:

Perineometers and other pressure-recording devices
EMG equipment
Ultrasound equipment
Faradic stimulators
Interferential current equipment
Vaginal cones

2.2.5. Compliance

Patient compliance has three major components:

1. Appropriate comprehension of the instructions and the technique
2. Ability to perform the exercises
3. Completion of the training programme

Objective documentation of both the patient's ability to perform the exercises and the result of the training programme is mandatory. The parameters employed for objective documentation during training should be the same as those used for teaching muscle awareness.

2.3. Applications

Pelvic floor training can be used as treatment on its own, or as an adjunctive therapy, or for prophylaxis. The indications, mode of action and the therapeutic goals must be specified. Examples of indications for therapeutic pelvic floor training are incontinence and descent of the pelvic viscera (prolapse). Examples of indications for prophylactic pelvic floor training are postpartum and following pelvic surgery.

3. BIOFEEDBACK

3.1. Definition

Biofeedback is a technique by which information about a normally unconscious physiological process is presented to the patient and the therapist as a visual, auditory or tactile signal. The signal is derived from a measurable physiological parameter, which is subsequently used in an educational process to accomplish a specific therapeutic result. The signal is displayed in a quantitative way and the patient is taught how to alter it and thus control the basic physiological process.

3.2. Techniques

The physiological parameter (e.g. pressure, flow, EMG) which is being monitored, the method of measurement and the mode by which it is displayed as a signal (e.g. light, sound, electric stimulus) should all be specified. Further, the specific instructions to the patient by which he/she is to alter the signal must be stated. The following details of biofeedback treatment must also be stated:

1. Patient position
2. Duration of each session
3. Interval between sessions
4. Number of sessions per day/week/month and intervals between
5. Length of treatment programme (weeks, months)

3.3. Applications

The indications, the intended mode of action and the therapeutic goals must be specified. The aim of biofeedback is to improve a specific lower urinary tract dysfunction by increasing patient awareness, and by alteration of a measurable physiological parameter. Biofeedback can be applied in functional voiding disorders where the underlying pathophysiology can be monitored and subsequently altered by the patient. The following are examples of indications and techniques for biofeedback treatment:
Motor urgency and urge incontinence: display of detrusor pressure and control of detrusor contractions
Dysfunctional voiding: display of sphincter EMG and relaxation of the external sphincter
Pelvic floor relaxation: display of pelvic floor EMG and pelvic floor training

4. BEHAVIORAL MODIFICATION

4.1. Definition

Behavioral modification comprises analysis and alteration of the relationship between the patient's symptoms and his/her environment for the treatment of maladaptive voiding patterns. This may be achieved by modification of the behaviour and/or environment of the patient.

4.2. Techniques

When behavioral modification is considered, a thorough analysis of possible interactions between the patient's symptoms, his general condition and his environment is essential. The following should be specified:

1. Micturition complaints; assessment and quantification:
   Symptom analysis
   Visual analogue score
   Fluid intake chart
   Frequency/volume chart (voiding diary)
   Pad-weighing test
   Urodynamic studies (when applicable)
2. General patient assessment:
   General performance status (e.g. Kurtzke disability scale[1])
   Mobility (e.g. chairbound)
   Concurrent medical disorders (e.g. constipation, congestive heart failure, diabetes mellitus, chronic bronchitis, hemiplegia)
   Current medication (e.g. diuretics)
   Psychological state (e.g. psychonalysis)
   Psychiatric disorders
   Mental state (e.g. dementia, confusion)
3. Environmental assessment:
   Toilet facilities (access)
   Living conditions
   Working conditions
   Social relations
   Availability of suitable incontinence aids
   Access to health care

For behavioral modification, various therapeutic concepts and techniques may be employed. The following should be specified:

1. Conditioning techniques:
   Timed voiding (e.g. hyposensitive bladder)
   Double/triple voiding (e.g. residual urine due to bladder diverticulum)
   Increase of intervoiding intervals/bladder drill (e.g. sensory urgency)
   Biofeedback (see above)
   Enuresis alarm
2. Fluid intake regulation (e.g. restriction)
3. Measures to improve patient mobility (e.g. physiotherapy, wheelchair)
4. Change of medication (e.g. diuretics, anticholinergics)
5. Treatment of concurrent medical/psychiatric disorders
6. Psychoanalysis/hypnotherapy (e.g. idiopathic detrusor instability)

7. Environmental changes (e.g. provision of incontinence pads, condom urinals, commode, furniture protection etc.)

Treatment is often empirical, and may require a combination of the above-mentioned concepts and techniques. The results of treatment should be objectively documented using the same techniques as used for the initial assessment of micturition complaints.

4.3. Applications

Behavioral modification may be used for the treatment of maladaptive voiding patterns in patients when:

The etiology and pathophysiology of their symptoms cannot be identified (e.g. sensory urgency)
The symptoms are caused by a psychological problem
The symptoms have failed to respond to conventional therapy
They are unfit for definitive treatment of their condition

Behavioral modification may be employed alone or as an adjunct to any other form of treatment for lower urinary tract dysfunction.

5. ELECTRICAL STIMULATION

5.1. Definition

Electrical stimulation is the application of electrical current to stimulate the pelvic viscera or their nerve supply. The aim of electrical stimulation may be to directly induce a therapeutic response or to modulate lower urinary tract, bowel or sexual dysfunction.

5.2. Techniques

The following should be specified:

1. Access:
   Surface electrodes (e.g. anal plug, vaginal electrode)
   Percutaneous electrodes (e.g. needle electrodes, wire electrodes)
   Implants
2. Approach
   Temporary stimulation
   Permanent stimulation
3. Stimulation site
   Effector organ
   Peripheral nerves
   Spinal nerves (intradural or extradural)
   Spinal cord
4. Stimulation parameters
   Frequency
   Voltage
   Current
   Pulse width
   Pulse shape (e.g. rectangular, biphasic, capacitatively coupled)
   With monopolar stimulation, state whether the active electrode is anodic or cathodic
   Duration of pulse trains
   Shape of pulse trains (e.g. surging trains)
5. Mode of stimulation
   Continuous
   Phasic (regular automatic on/off)
   Intermittent (variable duration and time intervals)
   Single sessions: number and duration of, and intervals between, periods of stimulation
   Multiple sessions: number and duration of, and intervals between sessions
6. Design of electronic equipment, electrodes and related electrical stimulation characteristics:
   Electrodes (monopolar or bipolar)
   Surface area of electrodes
   Maximum charge density per pulse at active electrode surface
   Impedance of the implanted system
   Power source (implants):
      active, self-powered
      passive, inductive current
7. For transurethral intravesical stimulation
   Filling medium
   Filling volume
   Number of intravesical electrodes

5.3. Units of measurement and symbols

Parameters related to electrical stimulation, units of measurement and the corresponding symbols are listed in Table II. 1.

5.4. Applications

The aims of treatment should be clearly stated. These may include control of voiding, continence, defecation, erection, ejaculation or relief of pain. Specify whether electrical stimulation aims at:

A functional result completely dependent on the continuous use of electrical current

Modulation, reflex facilitation, reflex inhibition, re-education or conditioning with a sustained functional result even after withdrawal of stimulation

Electrical stimulation is applicable in neurogenic or non-neurogenic lower urinary tract, bowel or sexual dysfunction. Techniques and equipment vary widely with the type of dysfunction and the goal of

Table II.1 Parameters for electrical stimulation

Quantity	Unit	Symbol	Definition
Electric current	ampere	A	1 A of electric current is the transfer of 1 C of electric charge per second
Direct (DC)			Steady unidirectional electric current
Galvanic			Unidirectional electric current derived from a chemical battery
Alternating (AC)			Electric current that physically changes direction of flow in a sinusoidal manner
Faradic			Intermittent oscillatory current similar to alternating current (AC), e.g. as produced by an induction coil
Voltage (potential difference)	volt	V	1 V of potential difference between 2 points requires 1 J of energy to transfer 1 C of charge from one point to the other
Resistance	ohm	Ω	1 Ω of resistance between 2 points allows 1 V of potential difference to cause a flow of 1 A of direct current (DC) between them
Impedance (Z)	ohm	Ω	Analogue of resistance for alternating current (AC); vector sum of ohmic resistance and reactance (inductive and/or capacitative resistance)
Charge	coulomb	C	1 C of electric charge is transferred through a conductor in 1 s by 1 A of electric current
Capacity	farad	F	A condensor (capacitor) has 1 F of electric capacity (capacitance) if transfer of 1 C of electric charge causes 1 V of potential difference between its elements
Frequency	hertz	Hs(s^{-1})	Number of cycles (phases) of a periodically repeating oscillation per second
Pulse width	time	ms	Duration of 1 pulse (phase) of a phasic electric current or voltage
Electrode surface area	area	mm^2	Active area of electrode surface
Charge density per pulse	coulomb/area/time	$\mu C\ mm^{-2} ms^{-1}$	Electric charge delivered to a given electrode surface area in a given time (one pulse width)

electrical stimulation. If electrical stimulation is employed for control of a neuropathic dysfunction, and the chosen site of stimulation is the reflex arc (peripheral nerves, spinal nerves or spinal cord), this reflex arc must be intact. Consequently electrical stimulation is not applicable for complete lower motor neuron lesions except when direct stimulation of the effector organ is chosen.

When ablative surgery is performed (e.g. dorsal rhizotomy, ganglionectomy, sphincterotomy or levatorotomy) in conjunction with an implant to achieve the desired functional effect, the following should be specified.

1. Techniques used to reduce pain or mass reflexes during stimulation
   Number and spinal level of interrupted afferents
   Site of interruption of afferents
   Dorsal rhizotomy (intradural or extradural)
   Ganglionectomy
2. Techniques to reduce stimulated sphincter dyssynergia:
   Pudendal block (unilateral or bilateral)
   Pudendal neurectomy (unilateral or bilateral)
   Levatorotomy (unilateral or bilateral)
   Electrically induced sphincter fatigue
   External sphincterotomy

If electrical stimulation is combined with ablative surgery, other functions (e.g. erection or continence) may be impaired.

5.4.1. *Voiding*

When the aim of electrical stimulation is to achieve voiding, state whether this is obtained by:
Stimulation of the afferent fibres to induce bladder sensation and thus facilitate voiding (transurethral intravesical stimulation)
Stimulation of efferent fibres or detrusor muscle to induce a bladder contraction (electromicturition)

5.4.2. *Continence*

Electrical stimulation may aim to inhibit overactive detrusor function or to improve urethral closure. State whether overactive detrusor function is abolished/reduced by reflex inhibition (pudendal to pelvic nerve) or by blockade of nerve conduction. When electrical stimulation is applied to improve urethral closure, state whether this is by:
A direct effect on the urethra during stimulation
Re-education and conditioning to restore pelvic floor tone.

5.4.3. *Pelvic pain*

If electrical stimulation is applied to control pelvic pain, the nature and etiology of the pain should be stated. When pelvic pain is caused by pelvic floor spasticity, electrical stimulation may be effective by relaxing the pelvic floor muscles.

5.4.4. Erection and ejaculation

If electrical stimulation is applied for the treatment of erectile dysfunction or ejaculatory failure, the etiology should be stated. Electrically induced erection requires an intact arterial supply and cavernous tissue, and a competent venous closure mechanism of the corpora cavernosa. Electroejaculation requires an intact reproductive system.

5.4.5. Defecation

Defecation may be obtained by electrical stimulation, either intentionally or as a side-effect of electromicturition.

At present, the mechanism of action of electrically induced control of pelvic pain, erection, ejaculation and defecation are not fully understood. The clinical applications of these techniques have not yet been fully established.

6. VOIDING MANOEUVRES

Voiding manoeuvres are employed to obtain/facilitate bladder emptying. For lower urinary tract rehabilitation, voiding manoeuvres may be used alone or in combination with other techniques such as biofeedback or behavioral modification. The aim is to achieve complete bladder emptying at low intravesical pressures. The techniques employed may be invasive (e.g. catheters) or non-invasive (e.g. triggering reflex detrusor contractions, increasing intra-abdominal pressure).

When reporting on voiding manoeuvres, the professional status of the individual (s) who establishes the diagnosis must be stated as well as the diagnostic techniques employed. Also the professional status of the person(s) who institutes, supervises and assesses treatment should be specified.

6.1. Catheterisation

6.1.1. Definition

Catheterisation is a technique for bladder emptying employing a catheter to drain the bladder or a urinary reservoir. Catheter use may be intermittent or indwelling (temporary or permanent).

6.1.2. Intermittent (in/out) catheterisation

Intermittent (in/out) catheterisation is defined as drainage or aspiration of the bladder or a urinary reservoir with subsequent removal of the catheter. The following types of intermittent catheterisation are defined:

1. Intermittent self-catheterisation: performed by the patient himself/herself
2. Intermittent catheterisation by an attendant (e.g. doctor, nurse or relative)
3. Clean intermittent catheterisation: use of a clean technique. This implies ordinary washing techniques and use of disposable or cleansed reusable catheters.
4. Aseptic intermittent catheterisation: use of a sterile technique. This implies genital disinfection and the use of sterile catheters and instruments/gloves.

6.1.2.1 Techniques. The following should be specified:

1. Preparation used for genital disinfection
2. Preparation and volume of lubricant
3. Catheter specifications: type, size, material and surface coating
4. Number of catheterisations per day/week
5. Length of treatment (e.g. weeks, months, permanent)

6.1.2.2 Applications. Specify the indications and the therapeutic goals. Typical examples for the use of intermittent catheterisation are: neurogenic bladder with impaired bladder emptying, postoperative urinary retention and transstomal catheterisation of continent reservoirs.

6.1.3 Indwelling catheter

An indwelling catheter remains in the bladder, urinary reservoir or urinary conduit for a period of time longer than one emptying. The following routes of access are employed:

Transurethral
Suprapubic

6.1.3.1 Techniques. The following should be specified:

1. Catheter specifications: type, size, material
2. Preparation and volume of lubricant
3. Catheter fixation: e.g. balloon (state filling volume), skin suture
4. Mode of drainage: continuous/intermittent. For intermittent drainage specify clamping periods
5. Intervals between catheter change
6. Duration of catheterisation (days, weeks, years)

6.1.3.2 Applications. The indications and the therapeutic goals should be specified. Examples of the use of temporary indwelling catheters are:
Suprapubic catheter: after major pelvic surgery
Transurethral catheter: in order to monitor urine output in a severely ill patient

Examples of the use of permanent indwelling catheters are:
Suprapubic: candidates for urinary diversion unfit for surgery
Transurethral: severe bladder symptoms from untreatable bladder cancer

6.2. Bladder reflex triggering

6.2.1. Definition

Bladder reflex triggering comprises various manoeuvres performed by the patient or the therapist in order to elicit reflex detrusor contractions by exteroceptive stimuli. The most commonly used manoeuvres are: suprapubic tapping, thigh scratching and anal/rectal manipulation.

6.2.2. Techniques

For each manoeuvre the following should be specified:

1. Details of manoeuvre
2. Frequency, intervals and duration (weeks, months, years) of practice

6.2.3. Applications

When using bladder reflex triggering manoeuvres, the etiology of the dysfunction and the goals of treatment should be stated. Bladder reflex triggering manoeuvres are indicated only in patients with an intact sacral reflex arc (suprasacral spinal cord lesions).

6.3. Bladder expression

6.3.1. Definition

Bladder expression comprises various manoeuvres aimed at increasing intra-vesical pressure in order to facilitate bladder emptying. The most commonly used manoeuvres are abdominal straining, Valsalva's manoeuvre and Credé's manoeuvre.

6.3.2. Techniques

For each manoeuvre, the following should be specified:
Details of the manoeuvre
Frequency, intervals and duration of practice (weeks, months, years)

6.3.3. Applications

When using bladder expression, the etiology of the underlying disorder and the goals of treatment should be stated. Bladder expression may be used in patients where the urethral closure mechanism can be easily overcome.

REFERENCE

1. Kurtzke J F 1983 Rating neurological impairment in multiple sclerosis: an expanded disability status scale (EDSS). Neurology 33: 1444–1452.

APPENDIX III

The standardisation of terminology of female pelvic organ prolapse and pelvic floor dysfunction

American Journal of Obstetrics and Gynecology 175: 10–17 (1996) © 1996 Mosby-Year Book, Inc.

Richard C Bump, Anders Mattiasson, Kari Bø, Linda P Brubaker, John O L DeLancey, Peter Klarskov, Bob L Shull and Anthony R B Smith

Produced by the International Continence Society Committee on Standardisation of Terminology (Anders Mattiasson, chairman), Subcommittee on Pelvic Organ Prolapse and Pelvic Floor Dysfunction (Richard Bump, chairman) in collaboration with the American Urogynecologic Society and the Society of Gynecologic Surgeons.

CONDENSATION

A system of standard terminology for the description and evaluation of pelvic organ prolapse and pelvic floor dysfunction, adopted by several professional societies, is presented.

1. INTRODUCTION

The International Continence Society (ICS) has been at the forefront in the standardisation of terminology of lower urinary tract function since the establishment of the Committee on Standardisation of Terminology in 1973. This committee's efforts over the past two decades have resulted in the world-wide acceptance of terminology standards that allow clinicians and researchers interested in the lower urinary tract to communicate efficiently and precisely. While female pelvic organ prolapse and pelvic floor dysfunction are intimately related to lower urinary tract function, such accurate communication using standard terminology has not been possible for these conditions since there has been no universally accepted system for describing the anatomic position of the pelvic organs. Many reports use terms for the description of pelvic organ prolapse which are undefined; none of the many aspiring grading systems has been adequately validated with respect either to reproducibility or to the clinical significance of different grades. The absence of standard, validated definitions

prevents comparisons of published series from different institutions and longitudinal evaluation of an individual patient.

In 1993, an international, multidisciplinary committee composed of members of the ICS, the American Urogynecologic Society (AUGS), and Society of Gynecologic Surgeons (SGS) drafted this standardisation document following the committee's initial meeting at the ICS meeting in Rome. In late 1994 and early 1995, the final draft was circulated to members of all three societies for a one-year review and trial. During that year several minor revisions were made and reproducibility studies in six centres in the United States and Europe were completed, documenting the inter- and intrarater reliability and clinical utility of the system in 240 women.[1–5] The standardisation document was formally adopted by the ICS in October 1995, by the AUGS in January 1996, and by the SGS in March 1996. The goal of this report is to introduce the system to clinicians and researchers.

Acknowledgement of these standards in written publications and scientific presentations should be indicated in the Methods Section with the following statement: 'Methods, definitions and descriptions conform to the standards recommended by the International Continence Society except where specifically noted.'

2. DESCRIPTION OF PELVIC ORGAN PROLAPSE

The clinical description of pelvic floor anatomy is determined during the physical examination of the external genitalia and vaginal canal. The details of the examination technique are not dictated by this document but authors should precisely describe their technique. Segments of the lower reproductive tract will replace such terms as 'cystocele, rectocele, enterocele, or urethrovesical junction' because these terms may imply an unrealistic certainty as to the structures on the other side of the vaginal bulge particularly in women who have had previous prolapse surgery.

2.1. Conditions of the examination

It is critical that the examiner sees and describes the maximum protrusion noted by the individual during her daily activities. Criteria for the end point of the examination and the full development of the prolapse should be specified in any report. Suggested criteria for demonstration of maximum prolapse should include one or all of the following: (a) Any protrusion of the vaginal wall has become tight during straining by the patient. (b) Traction on the prolapse causes no further descent. (c) The subject confirms that the size of the prolapse and extent of the protrusion seen by the examiner is as extensive as the most severe protrusion which she has experienced. The means of this confirmation should be specified. For example, the subject may use a small hand-held mirror to visualise the protrusion. (d) A standing, straining examination confirms that the full extent of the prolapse was observed in other positions used.

Other variables of technique that should be specified during the quantitative description and ordinal staging of pelvic organ prolapse include the following: (a) the position of the subject; (b) the type of examination table or chair used; (c) the type of vaginal specula, retractors, or tractors used; (d) diagrams of any customised devices used; (e) the type (e.g., Valsalva manoeuvre, cough) and, if measured, intensity (e.g. vesical or rectal pressure) of straining used to develop the prolapse maximally; (f) fullness of bladder and, if the bladder was empty, whether this was by spontaneous voiding or by catheterisation; (g) content of rectum; (f) the method by which any quantitative measurements were made.

2.2. Quantitative description of pelvic organ position

This descriptive system is a tandem profile in that it contains a series of component measurements grouped together in combination, but listed separately in tandem, without being fused into a distinctive new expression or 'grade'. It allows for the precise description of an individual woman's pelvic support without assigning a 'severity value'. Second, it allows accurate site-specific observations of the stability or progression of prolapse over time by the same or different observers. Finally, it allows similar judgements as to the outcome of surgical repair of prolapse. For example, noting that a surgical procedure moved the leading edge of a prolapse from 0.5 cm beyond the hymeneal ring to 0.5 cm above the hymeneal ring denotes more meagre improvement than stating that the prolapse was reduced from Grade 3 to Grade 1 as would be the case using some current grading systems.

2.2.1. Definition of anatomic landmarks

Prolapse should be evaluated by a standard system relative to clearly defined anatomic points of reference. These are of two types, a fixed reference point and defined points which are located with respect to this reference.

(a) *Fixed Point of Reference*. Prolapse should be evaluated relative to a fixed anatomic landmark which can be consistently and precisely identified. The hymen will be the fixed point of reference used throughout this system of quantitative prolapse description. Visually, the hymen provides a precisely identifiable landmark for reference. Although it is recognised that the plane of the hymen is somewhat variable depending upon the degree of levator anti dysfunction, it remains the best landmark available. 'Hymen' is preferable to the ill-defined and imprecise term 'introitus'. The anatomic position of the six defined points for measurement should be centimetres above or proximal to the hymen (negative number) or centimetres below or distal to the hymen (positive number) with the plane of the hymen being defined as zero (0). For example, a cervix that protruded 3 cm distal to the hymen would be + 3 cm.

(b) *Defined Points*. This site-specific system has been adapted from several classifications developed and modified by Baden and Walker.[6] Six points (two on the anterior vaginal wall, two in the superior vagina, and two on the posterior vaginal wall) are located with reference to the plane of the hymen.

Anterior Vaginal Wall. Because the only structure directly visible to the examiner is the surface of the vagina, anterior prolapse should be discussed in terms of a segment of the vaginal wall rather than the organs which lie behind it. Thus, the term 'anterior vaginal wall prolapse' is preferable to 'cystocele' or 'anterior enterocele' unless the organs involved are identified by ancillary test; two anterior sites are as follows:

Point Aa. A point located in the midline of the anterior vaginal wall three (3) cm proximal to the external urethral meatus. This corresponds to the approximate location of the 'urethro-vesical crease', a visible landmark of variable prominence that is obliterated in many patients. By definition, the range of position of Point Aa relative to the hymen is –3 to +3 cm.

Point Ba. A point that represents the most distal (i.e., most dependent) position of any part of the upper anterior vaginal wall from the vaginal cuff or anterior vaginal fornix to Point Aa. By definition, Point Ba is at –8 cm in the absence of prolapse and would have a positive value equal to the position of the cuff in women with total post-hysterectomy vaginal eversion.

Superior Vagina. These points represent the most proximal locations of the normally positioned lower reproductive tract. The two superior sites are as follows:

Point C. A point that represents either the most distal (i.e., most dependent) edge of the cervix or the leading edge of the vaginal cuff (hysterectomy scar) after total hysterectomy.

Point D. A point that represents the location of the posterior fornix (or pouch of Douglas) in a woman who still has a cervix. It represents the level of uterosacral ligament attachment to the proximal posterior cervix. It is included as a point of measurement to differentiate suspensory failure of the uterosacral-cardinal ligament complex from cervical elongation. When the location of Point C is significantly more positive than the location of Point D, this is indicative of cervical elongation which may be symmetrical or eccentric. Point D is omitted in the absence of the cervix.

Posterior Vaginal Wall. Analogous to anterior prolapse, posterior prolapse should be discussed in terms of segments of the vaginal wall rather than the organs which lie behind it. Thus, the term 'posterior vaginal wall prolapse' is preferable to 'rectocele' or 'enterocele' unless the organs involved are identified by ancillary tests. If small bowel appears to be present in the rectovaginal space, the examiner should comment on this fact and should clearly describe the basis for this clinical impression (e.g., by observation of peristaltic activity in the distended posterior vagina, by palpation of loops of small bowel between an examining finger in the rectum and one in the vagina, etc.). In such cases, a 'pulsion' addendum to the point Bp position may be noted (e.g., Bp = +5 [pulsion]; see Sections 3.1(a) and 3.1(b) for further discussion). The two posterior sites are as follows:

Point Bp. A point that represents the most distal (i.e., most dependent) position of any part of the upper posterior vaginal wall from the vaginal cuff or posterior vaginal fornix to Point Ap. By definition, Point Bp is at –3 cm in the absence of prolapse and would have a positive value equal to the position of the cuff in a women with total post-hysterectomy vaginal eversion.

Point Ap. A point located in the midline of the posterior vaginal wall three (3) cm proximal to the hymen. By definition, the range of position of Point Ap relative to the hymen is –3 to +3 cm.

(c) *Other Landmarks and Measurements*. The genital hiatus (GH) is measured from the middle of the external urethral meatus to the posterior midline hymen. If the location of the hymen is distorted by a loose band of skin without underlying muscle or connective tissue, the firm palpable tissue of the perineal body should be substituted as the posterior margin for this measurement. The perineal body (PB) is measured from the posterior margin of the genital hiatus

to the midanal opening. Measurements of the genital hiatus and perineal body are expressed in centimetres. The total vaginal length (TVL) is the greatest depth of the vagina in cm when Point C or D is reduced to its full normal position. *Note:* Eccentric elongation of a prolapsed anterior or posterior vaginal wall should not be included in the measurement of total vaginal length. The points and measurements are represented in Fig. III. A.

2.2.2. Making and recording measurements

The position of Points Aa, Ba, Ap, Bp, C, and (if applicable) D with reference to the hymen should be measured and recorded. Positions are expressed as centimetres metres above or proximal to the hymen (negative number) or centimetres below or distal to the hymen (positive number) with the plane of the hymen being defined as zero (0). While an examiner may be able to make measurements to the nearest half (0.5) cm, it is doubtful that further precision is possible. All reports should clearly specify how measurements were derived. Measurements may be recorded as a simple line of numbers (e.g., –3, –3, –7, –9, –3, –3, 9, 2, 2 for Points Aa, Ba, C, D, Bp, Ap, total vaginal length, genital hiatus, and perineal body respectively). Note that the last three numbers have no + or – sign attached to them because they denote lengths and not positions relative to the hymen. Alternatively, a three-by-three 'tic-tac-toe' grid can be used to organise concisely the measurements as noted in Fig. III.B and/or a line diagram of the configuration can be drawn as noted in Figs III.C and III.D. Figure III.C is a grid and line diagram contrasting measurements indicating normal support to those of post hysterectomy vaginal eversion. Figure III.D is a grid and line diagram representing predominant anterior and posterior vaginal wall prolapse with partial vault descent.

2.3. Ordinal stages of pelvic organ prolapse

The tandem profile for quantifying prolapse provides a precise description of anatomy for individual patients. However, because of the many possible combinations, such profiles cannot be directly ranked; the many variations are too numerous to permit useful analysis and comparisons when populations are studied. Consequently they are analogous to other tandem profiles such as the TNM Index for various cancers. For the TNM description of individual patient's cancers to be useful in population studies evaluating prognosis or response to therapy; they are clustered into an ordinal set of stages. Ordinal stages represent adjacent categories that can be ranked in an ascending sequence of magnitude, but the categories are assigned arbitrarily and the intervals between them cannot be actually measured. While the committee is aware of the arbitrary nature of an ordinal staging system and the possible biases that it introduces, we conclude such a system is necessary if populations are to be described and compared, if symptoms putatively related to prolapse are to be evaluated, and if the results of various treatment options are to be assessed and compared.

Stages are assigned according to the most severe portion of the prolapse when the full extent of the protrusion has been demonstrated. In order for a stage to be assigned to an individual subject, it is essential that her quantitative description be completed first. The 2 cm buffer related to the total vaginal length in Stages 0 and IV is an effort to compensate for vaginal distensibility and the inherent imprecision of the measurement of total vaginal

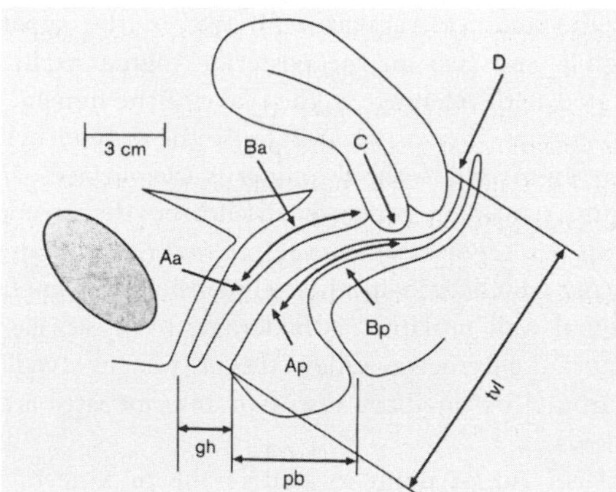

Fig. III.A The six sites (*Aa, Ba, C, D, Bp* and *Bp*), the genital hiatus (*gh*), perineal body (*pb*) and total vaginal length (*tvl*) used of pelvic organ support quantitation.

anterior wall **Aa**	anterior wall **Ba**	cervix or cuff **C**
genital hiatus **gh**	perineal body **pb**	total vaginal length **tvl**
posterior wall **Ap**	posterior wall **Bp**	posterior fornix **D**

Fig. III.B A three-by-three grid for recording the quantitative description of pelvic organ support.

length. The 2 cm buffer around the hymen in Stage II is an effort to avoid confining a stage to a single plane and to acknowledge practical limits of precision in this assessment. Stages can be subgrouped according to which portion of the lower reproductive tract is the *most distal* part of the prolapse using the following letter qualifiers: a = anterior vaginal wall, p = posterior vaginal wall, C = vaginal cuff, Cx = cervix, and Aa, Ap, Ba, Bp, and D for the points of measurement already defined. The five stages of pelvic organ support (0 through IV) are as follows:

Stage 0. No prolapse is demonstrated. Points Aa, Ap, Ba, and Bp are all at −3 cm and either Point C or D is between − TVL cm and − (TVL −2) cm (i.e., the quantitation value for point C or D is ≤ − (TVL −2) cm). Figure III.C.B represents Stage 0.

Stage I. The criteria for Stage 0 are not met but the most distal portion of the prolapse is more than 1 cm above the level of the hymen (i.e., its quantitation value is < −1 cm).

Stage II. The most distal portion of the prolapse is 1 cm or less proximal to or distal to the plane of the hymen (i.e., its quantitation value is ≥ −1 cm but ≤ +1 cm).

Stage III. The most distal portion of the prolapse is more than 1 cm below the plane of the hymen, but protrudes no further than two centimetres less than the total vaginal length in cm (i.e., its quantitation value is > +1 cm but < + (TVL −2) cm). Figure III.D.A represents Stage III-Ba and Figure III.D.B represents Stage III-Bp prolapse.

Stage IV. Essentially complete eversion of the total length of the lower genital tract is demonstrated. The distal portion of the prolapse protrudes to at least (TVL −2) cm (i.e., its quantitation value is ≥ + (TVL −2) cm). In most instances, the leading edge of stage IV prolapse will be the cervix or vaginal cuff scar. Figure III.C.A represents Stage IV-C prolapse.

3. ANCILLARY TECHNIQUES FOR DESCRIBING PELVIC ORGAN PROLAPSE

This series of procedures may help further characterise pelvic organ prolapse in an individual patient. They are considered ancillary either because they are not yet standardised or validated or because they are not universally available to all patients. Authors utilising these procedures should include the following information in their manuscripts: (a) Describe the objective information they intended to generate and how it enhanced their ability to evaluate or treat prolapse. (b) Describe precisely how the test was performed, any instruments that were used, and the specific testing conditions so that other authors can reproduce the study. (c) Document the reliability of the measurement obtained with the technique.

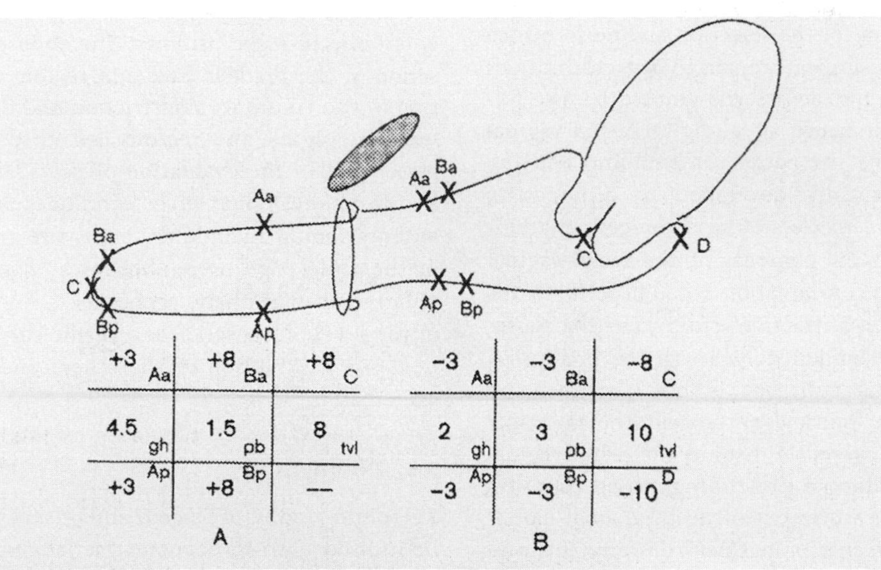

Fig. III.C **A** Example of a grid and line diagram of complete eversion of the vagina. The most distal point of the anterior wall (Point Ba), the vaginal cuff scar (Point C) and the most distal point of the posterior wall (Bp) are all at the same position (+8) and Points Aa and Ap are maximally distal (both at +3). The fact that the total vagina length equals the maximum protrusion makes this a Stage IV prolapse. **B** Example of normal support. Points Aa and Ba and Points Ap and Bp are all −3 since there is no anterior or posterior wall descent. The lowest point of the cervix is 8 cm above the hymen (−8) and the posterior fornix is 2 cm above this (−10). The vaginal length is 10 cm and the genital hiatus and perineal body measure 2 and 3 cm respectively. This represents Stage 0 support.

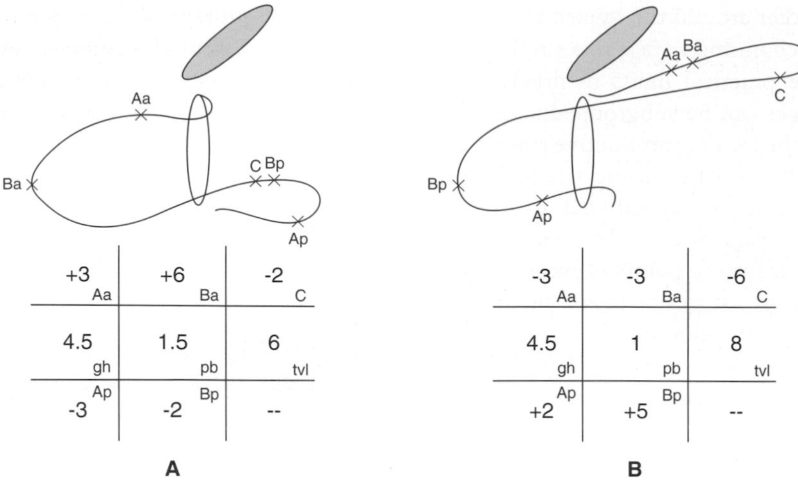

Fig. III.D A Example of a grid and line diagram of a predominant anterior support defect. The leading point of the prolapse is the upper anterior vaginal wall, Point Ba (+6). Note that there is significant elongation of the bulging anterior wall. Point Aa is maximally distal (+3) and the vaginal cuff scar is 2 cm above the hymen (C = −2). The cuff scar has undergone 4 cm of descent since it would be at −6 (the total vaginal length) if it were perfectly supported. In this example, the total vaginal length is not the maximum depth of the vagina with the elongated anterior vaginal wall maximally reduced, but rather the depth of the vagina at the cuff with Point C reduced to its normal full extent as specified in Section 2.2.1(c). This represents Stage III-Ba prolapse. **B** Example of a predominant posterior support defect. The leading point of the prolapse is the upper posterior vaginal wall, Point Bp (+5). Point Ap is 2 cm distal to the hymen (+2) and the vaginal cuff scar is 6 cm above the hymen (−6). The cuff has undergone only 2 cm of descent since it would be at −8 (the total vaginal length) if it were perfectly supported. This represents Stage III-Bp prolapse.

3.1. Supplementary physical examination techniques

Many of these techniques are essential to the adequate pre-operative evaluation of a patient with pelvic organ prolapse. While they do not directly affect either the tandem profile or the ordinal stage, they are important for the selection and performance of an effective surgical repair. These techniques include, but are not necessarily limited to, the following: (a) performance of a digital rectal-vaginal examination while the patient is straining and the prolapse is maximally developed to differentiate between a high rectocele and an enterocele; (b) digital assessment of the contents of the rectal-vaginal septum during the examination noted in 3.1(a) to differentiate between a 'traction' enterocele (the posterior cul-de-sac is pulled down with the prolapsing cervix or vaginal cuff but is not distended by intestines) and a 'pulsion' enterocele (the intestinal contents of the enterocele distend the rectal-vaginal septum and produce a protruding mass); (c) Q-tip testing for the measurement of urethral axial mobility; (d) measurements of perineal descent; (e) measurements of the transverse diameter of the genital hiatus or of the protruding prolapse; (f) measurements of vaginal volume; (g) description and measurement of rectal prolapse; (h) examination techniques for differentiating between various types of defects (e.g., central versus paravaginal defects of the anterior vaginal wall).

3.2. Endoscopy

Cystoscopic visualisation of bowel peristalsis under the bladder base or trigone may identify an anterior enterocele in some patients. The endoscopic visualisation of the bladder base and rectum and observation of the voluntary constriction and dilation of the urethra, vagina and rectum has, to date, played a minor role in the evaluation of pelvic floor anatomy and function. When such techniques are described, authors should include the type, size and lens angle of the endoscope used, the doses of any analgesic, sedative or anaesthetic agents used, and a statement of the level of consciousness of the subjects in addition to a description of the other conditions of the examination.

3.3. Photography

Still photography of Stage II and greater prolapse may be utilised both to document serial changes in individual patients and to illustrate findings for manuscripts and presentations. Photographs should contain an internal frame of reference such as a centimetre ruler or tape.

3.4. Imaging procedures

Different imaging techniques have been used to visualise pelvic floor anatomy, support defects and relationships among adjacent organs. These techniques may be more accurate than physical examination in determining which organs are involved in pelvic organ prolapse. However, they share the limitations of the other techniques in this section, i.e., a lack of standardisation, validation and/or availability. For this reason, no specific technique can be recommended but guidelines for reporting various techniques will be considered.

3.4.1. General guidelines for imaging procedures

Landmarks should be defined to allow comparisons with other imaging studies and the physical examination. The lower edge of the symphysis pubis should be given high priority. Other examples of bony landmarks include the superior edge of the pubic symphysis, the ischial spine and tuberosity, the obturator foramen, the tip of the coccyx and the promontory of the sacrum. All reports on imaging techniques should specify the following: (a) position of the patient including the position of her legs; (Images in manuscripts should be oriented to reflect the patient's position when the study was performed and should not be oriented to suggest an erect position unless the patient was erect.) (b) specific verbal instructions given to the patient; (c) bladder volume and content and bowel content, including any pre-study preparations; and (d) the performance and display of simultaneous monitoring such as pressure measurements.

3.4.2. Ultrasonography

Continuous visualisation of dynamic events is possible. All reports using ultrasound should include the following information: (a) transducer type and manufacturer (e.g., sector, linear, MHz); (b) transducer size; (c) transducer orientation; and (d) route of scanning (e.g., abdominal, perineal, vaginal, rectal, urethral).

3.4.3. Contrast radiography

Contrast radiography may be static or dynamic and may include voiding colpo-cysto-urethrography, defecography, peritoneography and pelvic fluoroscopy among others. All reports of contrast radiography should include the following information: (a) projection (e.g., lateral, frontal, horizontal, oblique); (b) type and amount of contrast media used and sequence of opacification of the bladder, vagina, rectum and colon, small bowel and peritoneal cavity; (c) any urethral or vaginal appliance used (e.g., tampon, catheter, bead-chain); (d) type of exposures (e.g., single exposure, video); and (e) magnification – an internal reference scale should be included.

3.4.4. Computed tomography and magnetic resonance imaging

These techniques do not currently allow for continuous imaging under dynamic conditions and most equipment dictates supine scanning. Specifics of the technique should be specified including: (a) the specific equipment used, including the manufacturer; (b) the plane of imaging (e.g., axial, sagittal, coronal, oblique); (c) the field of view (d) the thickness of sections and the number of slices; (e) the scan time; (f) the use and type of contrast; and (g) the type of image analysis.

3.5. Surgical assessment

Intra-operative evaluation of pelvic support defects is intuitively attractive but as yet of unproven value. The effects of anaesthesia, diminished muscle tone and loss of consciousness are of unknown magnitude and direction. Limitations due to the position of the patient must also be evaluated.

4. PELVIC FLOOR MUSCLE TESTING

Pelvic floor muscles are voluntarily controlled, but selective contraction and relaxation necessitates muscle awareness. Optimal squeezing technique involves contraction of the pelvic floor muscles without contraction of the abdominal wall muscles and without a Valsalva manoeuvre. Squeezing synergists are the intra-urethral and anal sphincteric muscles. In normal voiding, defecation and optimal abdominal-strain voiding, the pelvic floor is relaxed, while the abdominal wall and the diaphragm may contract. With coughs and sneezes and often when other stresses are applied, the pelvic floor and abdominal wall are contracted simultaneously.

Evaluation and measurement of pelvic floor muscle function includes (1) an assessment of the patient's ability to contract and relax the pelvic muscles selectively (i.e., squeezing without abdominal straining and vice versa) and (2) measurement of the force (strength) of contraction. There are pitfalls in the measurement of pelvic floor muscle function because the muscles are invisible to the investigator and because patients often simultaneously and

erroneously activate other muscles. Contraction of the abdominal, gluteal and hip adductor muscles, Valsalva manoeuvre, straining, breath holding and forced inspirations are typically seen. These factors affect the reliability of available testing modalities and have to be taken into consideration in the interpretation of these tests.

The individual types of tests cited in this report are based both on the scientific literature and on current clinical practice. It is the intent of the committee neither to endorse specific tests or techniques nor to restrict evaluations to the examples given. The standards recommended are intended to facilitate comparison of results obtained by different investigators and to allow investigators to replicate studies precisely. For all types of measuring techniques the following should be specified: (a) patient position, including the position of the legs; (b) specific instructions given to the patient; (c) the status of bladder and bowel fullness; (d) techniques of quantification or qualification (estimated, calculated, directly measured); and (e) the reliability of the technique.

4.1. Inspection

A visual assessment of muscle integrity, including a description of scarring and symmetry, should be performed. Pelvic floor contraction causes inward movement of the perineum and straining causes the opposite movement. Perineal movements can be observed directly or assessed indirectly by movement of an externally visible device placed into the vagina or urethra. The abdominal wall and other specified regions might be watched simultaneously. The type, size and placement of any device used should be specified as should the state of undress of the patient.

4.2. Palpation

Palpation may include digital examination of the pelvic floor muscles through the vagina or rectum as well as assessment of the perineum, abdominal wall and/or other specified regions. The number of fingers and their position should be specified. Scales for the description of the strength of voluntary and reflex (e.g., with coughing) contractions and of the degree of voluntary relaxation should be clearly described and intra-and inter-observer reliability documented. Standardised palpation techniques could also be developed for the semi-quantitative estimation of the bulk or thickness of pelvic floor musculature around the circumference of the genital hiatus. These techniques could allow for the localisation of any atrophic or asymmetric segments.

4.3. Electromyography

Electromyography from the pelvic floor muscles can be recorded alone or in combination with other measurements. Needle electrodes permit visualisation of individual motor unit action potentials, while surface or wire electrodes detect action potentials from groups of adjacent motor units underlying or surrounding the electrodes. Interpretation of signals from these latter electrodes must take into consideration that signals from erroneously contracted adjacent muscles may interfere with signals from the muscles of interest. Reports of electro-myographic recordings should specify the following: (a) type of electrode; (b) placement of electrodes; (c) placement of reference electrode; (d) specifications of signal processing equipment; (e) type and specifications of display equipment; (f) muscle in which needle electrode is placed; and (g) description of decision algorithms used by the analytic software.

4.4. Pressure recording

Measurements of urethral, vaginal and anal pressures may be used to assess pelvic floor muscle control and strength. However, interpretations based on these pressure measurements must be made with a knowledge of their potential for artefact and their unproven or limited reproducibility. Anal sphincter contractions, rectal peristalsis, detrusor contractions and abdominal straining can affect pressure measurements. Pressures recorded from the proximal vagina accurately mimic fluctuations in abdominal pressure. Therefore it may be important to compare vaginal pressures to simultaneously measured vesical or rectal pressures. Reports using pressure measurements should specify the following: (a) the type and size of the measuring device at the recording site (e.g., balloon, open catheter, etc.); (b) the exact placement of the measuring device; (c) the type of pressure transducer; (d) the type of display system; and (e) the display of simultaneous control pressures.

As noted in Section 4.1, observation of the perineum is an easy and reliable way to assess for abnormal straining during an attempt at a pelvic muscle contraction. Significant straining or a Valsalva manoeuvre causes downward/caudal movement of the perineum; a correctly performed pelvic muscle contraction causes inward/cephalad movement of the perineum. Observation for perineal movement should be considered as an additional validation procedure whenever pressure measurements are recorded.

5. DESCRIPTION OF FUNCTIONAL SYMPTOMS

Functional deficits caused by pelvic organ prolapse and pelvic floor dysfunction are not well characterised or absolutely established. There is an ongoing need to develop, standardise, and validate various clinimetric scales such as condition-specific quality of life questionnaires for each of the four functional symptom groups thought to be related to pelvic organ prolapse.

Researchers in this area should try to use standardised and validated symptom scales whenever possible. They must always ask precisely the same questions regarding functional symptoms before and after therapeutic intervention. The description of functional symptoms should be directed toward four primary areas: (1) lower urinary tract, (2) bowel, (3) sexual, and (4) other local symptoms.

5.1. Urinary symptoms

This report does not supplant any currently approved ICS terminology related to lower urinary tract function.[7] However, some important prolapse related symptoms are not included in the current standards (e.g., the need to manually reduce the prolapse or assume an unusual position to initiate or complete micturition). Urinary symptoms that should be considered for dichotomous, ordinal, or visual analogue scaling include, but are not limited to, the following: (a) stress incontinence, (b) frequency (diurnal and nocturnal), (c) urgency, (d) urge incontinence, (e) hesitancy, (f) weak or prolonged urinary stream, (g) feeling of incomplete emptying, (h) manual reduction of the prolapse to start or complete bladder emptying, and (f) positional changes to start or complete voiding.

5.2. Bowel symptoms

Bowel symptoms that should be considered for dichotomous, ordinal or visual analog scaling include, but are not limited to, the following: (a) difficulty with defecation, (b) incontinence of flatus, (c) incontinence of liquid stool, (d) incontinence of solid stool, (e) faecal staining of underwear, (f) urgency of defecation, (g) discomfort with defecation, (h) digital manipulation of vagina, perineum or anus to complete defecation, (i) feeling of incomplete evacuation and (j) rectal protrusion during or after defecation.

5.3. Sexual symptoms

Research is needed to attempt to differentiate the complex and multifactorial aspects of 'satisfactory sexual function' as it relates to pelvic organ prolapse and pelvic floor dysfunction. It may be difficult to distinguish between the ability to have vaginal intercourse and normal sexual function. The development of satisfactory tools will require multidisciplinary collaboration. Sexual function symptoms that should be considered for dichotomous, ordinal, or visual analog scaling include, but are not limited to, the following: (a) Is the patient sexually active? (b) If she is not sexually active, why? (c) Does sexual activity include vaginal coitus? (c) What is the frequency of vaginal intercourse? (d) Does the patient experience pain with coitus? (e) Is the patient satisfied with her sexual activity? (f) Has there been any change in orgasmic response? (g) Is any incontinence experienced during sexual activity?

5.4. Other local symptoms

We currently lack knowledge regarding the precise nature of symptoms that may be caused by the presence of a protrusion or bulge. Possible anatomically based symptoms that should be considered for dichotomous, ordinal or visual analog scaling include, but are not limited to, the following: (a) vaginal pressure or heaviness; (b) vaginal or perineal pain; (c) sensation or awareness of tissue protrusion from the vagina; (d) low back pain; (e) abdominal pressure or pain; (f) observation or palpation of a mass.

ACKNOWLEDGEMENTS

The subcommittee would like to acknowledge the contributions of the following consultants who contributed to the development and revision of this document: W. Glenn Hurt, Bernhard Schüssler, L. Lewis Wall.

REFERENCES

1. Athanasiou S, Hill S, Gleeson C, Anders K, Cardozo L 1995 Validation of the ICS proposed pelvic organ prolapse descriptive system. Neurourology and Urodynamics 14: 414–415 (abstract of ICS 1995 meeting).
2. Schüssler B, Peschers U 1995 Standardisation of terminology of female genital prolapse according to the new ICS criteria: inter-examiner reproducibility. Neurourology and Urodynamics 14: 437–438 (abstract of ICS 1995 meeting).
3. Montella J M, Cater J R 1995 Comparison of measurements obtained in supine and sitting position in the evaluation of pelvic organ prolapse (abstract of AUGS 1995 meeting).
4. Kobak W H, Rosenberg K, Walters M D 1995 Interobserver variation in the assessment of pelvic organ prolapse using the draft International Continence Society and Baden grading systems. (abstract of AUGS 1995 meeting).
5. Hall A F, Theofrastous J P, Cundiff G C et al 1996 Inter-and intra-observer reliability of the proposed International Continence Society, Society of Gynecologic Surgeons, and American Urogynecologic Society pelvic organ prolapse classification system. American Journal of Obstetrics and Gynecology (submitted through the program of the Society of Gynecologic Surgeons 1996 meeting).
6. Baden W, Walker T 1992 Surgical repair of vaginal defects. Philadelphia: Lippincott, pp 1–7, 51–62
7. See this volume, Appendix I.

The standardisation of terminology and assessment of functional characteristics of intestinal urinary reservoirs

Neurourology and Urodynamics 15:499–511 (1996) © 1996 Wiley-Liss, Inc.

Joachim W. Thüroff, Anders Mattiasson, Jens Thorup Andersen, Hans Hedlund, Frank Hinman Jr., Markus Hohenfellner, Wiking Månsson, Anthony R Mundy, Randall G Rowland, and Kenneth Steven

Produced by the International Continence Society Committee on Standardisation of Terminology (Anders Mattiasson, chairman) Subcommittee on Intestinal Urinary Reservoirs (Joachim W Thüroff, chairman)

1. INTRODUCTION

In 1993, the International Continence Society (ICS) established a committee for standardisation of terminology and assessment of functional characteristics of intestinal urinary reservoirs in order to allow reporting of results in a uniform fashion so that different series and different surgical techniques can be compared.

This report is consistent with earlier reports of the International Continence Society Committee on Standardisation of Terminology with special reference to the collated ICS report from 1988 (see Appendix I, pp 631–646).

As the present knowledge about physiological characteristics of intestinal urinary reservoirs is rather limited in regard to normal and abnormal reservoir sensation, compliance, activity, continence, and other specifications, some of the definitions are necessarily imprecise and vague. However, it was felt that this report still would be capable of stipulating the standardised assessment of intestinal urinary reservoirs and reporting of the results in order to accumulate more information about physiological characteristics of intestinal urinary reservoirs and to establish precise definitions of normal and abnormal conditions. With increased knowledge and better understanding of intestinal urinary reservoirs, this report will have to be updated to become more specific.

It is suggested that in written publications, the acknowledgement of these standards is indicated by a footnote to the section Methods and Materials or its equivalent: 'Methods, definitions and units conform

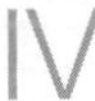

to the standards recommended by the International Continence Society, except where specifically noted.'

2. TERMINOLOGY OF SURGICAL PROCEDURES

Up to now, when different surgical procedures for constructing an intestinal urinary reservoir are described, conflicting terminology is often used. This section defines the terminology of surgical procedures used throughout the report. These definitions may not be universally applicable to the published scientific literature to date, viewed in retrospect, but represent a standardised terminology for surgical procedures for the future.

Definitions

Bladder augmentation is a surgical procedure for increasing bladder capacity. This may be accomplished without other tissues (e.g., autoaugmentation) or with incorporation of other tissues such as intestine (enterocystoplasty, intestinocystoplasty), with or without changing the shape of such intestine (i.e., detubularisation and reconfiguration), and with or without resection of a portion of the original bladder.

Bladder replacement – see 'Bladder Substitution.'

Bladder substitution (Bladder Replacement) is a surgical procedure for in situ (orthotopic) total substitution/replacement of the bladder by other tissues such as isolated intestine. After subtotal excision of the original bladder (e.g., in interstitial cystitis) the intestinal urinary reservoir may be connected to the bladder neck (bladder substitution to bladder neck) and after complete excision of the original bladder (radical cystoprostatectomy), the reservoir may be connected to the urethra as a continent outlet (bladder substitution to urethra). If indicated, the urethral closure function may be surgically supported in addition (e.g., sling procedure, prosthetic sphincter, periurethral injections). Alternatively, an orthotopically placed urethral substitute/replacement, e.g., from intestine may be used as a continent outlet for a complete substitution of the lower urinary tract.

Continent anal urinary diversion is a surgical procedure for continent urinary diversion utilising bowel in continuity or isolated bowel as a reservoir and the anus as a continent outlet.

Continent cutaneous urinary diversion is a surgical procedure for continent urinary diversion providing an urinary reservoir, e.g., from intestine and a continence mechanism, e.g., from intestine for formation of a continent heterotopically placed (e.g., cutaneous) outlet (stoma).

Enterocystoplasty (bladder augmentation with intestine) – see 'Bladder Augmentation'.

Intestinocystoplasty (bladder augmentation with intestine) – see 'Bladder Augmentation'.

3. ASSESSMENT

3.1. Experimental assessment

For reporting animal studies, the principles and standards for experimental scientific publications should be followed. Species, sex, weight, and age of the animals must be stated, as well as type of anesthesia. If chronic experiments are performed, the type of treatment between the initial experiment and the evaluation experiment should be stated. Raw data should be presented and, when applicable, the type of statistical analysis must be stated. For standardisation of urodynamic evaluation see 4 and 5.

3.2. Patient assessment

The assessment of patients with intestinal urinary reservoirs should include history, frequency/volume chart, physical examination, and evaluation of the upper urinary tract.

3.2.1. History

The history must include etiology of the underlying disease (i.e., congenital anomaly, neurogenic bladder dysfunction, lower urinary tract trauma, radiation damage, bladder cancer or other tumours of the true pelvis) and indication for constructing an intestinal urinary reservoir (e.g., radical surgery for malignancy in the true pelvis, low bladder capacity/compliance, upper tract deterioration due to vesicoureteral obstruction or reflux, urinary incontinence). Information must be available on the duration of previous history of the underlying disease, previous urinary tract infections, and relevant surgery.

The history should also provide information on dexterity and ambulatory status of the patient (i.e., wheelchair bound, paraplegia, or tetraplegia). Information on sexual and bowel function must be reported in respect to the status prior to applying an intestinal urinary reservoir.

The urinary history must report symptoms related

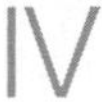

to both the storage and evacuation functions of the lower urinary tract with special reference to the technique of evacuation (i.e., spontaneous voiding with or without abdominal straining, Valsalva or Credé manoeuvres, intermittent catheterisation). Problems of evacuation due to mucus production or difficulty with catheterisation must be reported. Incidence of urinary infections must be reported in respect to the incidence prior to construction of an intestinal urinary reservoir.

3.2.2. Specification of surgical technique

The surgical technique must be specified stating the applied type of urinary reservoir and origin of gastrointestinal segments used (e.g., stomach, ileum, cecum, transverse colon, sigmoid colon, rectum), length and shape (e.g., tubular, detubularised) of bowel segments, the technique of urethral implantation (when applicable) and the type of the continent outlet (i.e., original urethra, functionally supported urethra, anal sphincter, catheterisable continent cutaneous outlet). If an intussusception nipple valve is applied, technique of fixation of the intussusception (i.e., sutures, staples) should be stated.

Additional and combined surgical procedures in the true pelvis must be reported, such as hysterectomy, colposuspension, excision of vaginal or rectal urinary fistulae, or resection of rectum. Information of adjuvant treatment, such as pharmacotherapy, physiotherapy, or electrical stimulation, must be available.

3.2.3. Frequency/volume chart

On the frequency/volume chart the time and volume of each micturition are reported along with quantities of fluid intake. It must be stated if evacuation was prompted by the clock or by sensation. In addition, episodes of urgency and incontinence have to be reported. The frequency/volume chart can be used for the primary assessment of symptoms of urgency, frequency, and incontinence and for follow-up studies.

3.2.4. Physical examination

Besides general, urological, and, when appropriate, gynecological examination, the neurological status should be assessed with special attention to sensitivity of the sacral dermatomes, sacral reflex activity (anal reflex, bulbocavernosus reflex), and anal sphincter tone and control.

3.2.5. Evaluation of the upper urinary tract

Evaluation of renal function and morphology must be related to the status prior to constructing an intestinal urinary reservoir. Studies of renal morphology can be based on renal ultrasound, intravenous pyelography, and radioisotope studies. Quantification of findings should be recorded by using accepted classifications of upper tract dilatation [Emmett and Witten, 1971], renal scarring [Smellie et al., 1975], and urethral reflux [Heikel and Parkkulainen, 1966]. Renal function should be assessed by measuring the serum concentration of creatinine and, if indicated, by creatinine clearance and radioisotope clearance studies.

3.2.6. Other relevant studies

Reported complications of urinary diversion into an intestinal reservoir include electrolyte and blood-gas imbalance, malabsorption syndromes, urolithiasis, urinary tract infection, and development of a secondary malignancy. Follow-up evaluation should include relevant tests when applicable and indicated, and reports should state the results of such studies as serum electrolyte concentrations, analysis of blood gases, serum levels of vitamins A, B12, D, E, K, and folic acid, serum levels of bile acids, urine osmolality and pH, urine excretion of calcium, phosphate, oxalate, and citrate, colonisation of urine, and findings on endoscopy and biopsy of the urinary reservoir.

4. PROCEDURES RELATED TO THE EVALUATION OF URINE STORAGE IN AN INTESTINAL URINARY RESERVOIR

4.1. Enterocystometry

Enterocystometry is the method by which the pressure/volume relationship of the intestinal urinary reservoir is measured. All systems are zeroed at atmospheric pressure. For external transducers the reference point is the superior edge of the symphysis pubis for bladder augmentation, bladder substitution or continent anal urinary diversion, and the level of the stoma for continent cutaneous urinary diversion. Enterocystometry is used to assess reservoir sensation, compliance, capacity, and activity. Before filling is started, residual urine must be evacuated and measured. Enterocystometry is performed with the patient awake and unsedated, not taking drugs that may affect reservoir characteristics. In a urodynamic follow-up study for evaluation of adjutant treatment

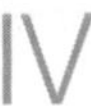

(e.g., pharmacological therapy) of an intestinal urinary reservoir, mode of action, dosage, and route of administration (enteral, parenteral, topical) of the medication have to be specified.

As an intestinal urinary reservoir starts to expand when permitted to store urine, time intervals between surgery for construction of the intestinal urinary reservoir, its first functional use for storage of urine and urodynamic testing must be stated. For reporting of functional characteristics of an intestinal urinary reservoir, the time interval between surgery and enterocystometric assessment must be stated to account for postoperative expansion of the reservoir.

As several intestinal segments used in urinary reservoirs react to gastric stimuli, time interval between food ingestion and the urodynamic evaluation should be stated. Reporting of pressure/volume relationships of an intestinal urinary reservoir should be obtained at standardised filling volumes or standardised pressures, which must be stated in absolute numbers.

Specify

a) Access (transurethral, transanal, transstomal, percutaneous);
b) Fluid medium;
c) Temperature of fluid (state in degrees Celsius);
d) Position of patient (supine, sitting or standing);
e) Filling may be by diuresis or catheter. Filling by catheter may be continuous or stepwise: the precise filling rate should be stated. When the stepwise filling is used, the volume increment should be stated. For general discussion, the following terms for the range of filling rate should be used:
   i) up to 10 ml per minute is slow fill enterocystometry ('physiological' filling);
   ii) 10–100 ml per minute is medium fill enterocystometry;
   iii) over 100 ml per minute is rapid fill enterocystometry.

Technique

a) Fluid-filled catheter – specify number of catheters, single or multiple lumens, type of catheter (manufacturer), size of catheter, type (manufacturer), and specifications of external pressure transducer;
b) Catheter mounted microtransducer – list specifications;
c) Other catheters – list specifications;
d) Measuring equipment.

Definitions

Total reservoir pressure is the pressure within the reservoir.

Abdominal pressure is taken to be the pressure surrounding the reservoir. In current practice it is estimated from rectal or, less commonly, intraperitoneal or intragastric pressures.

Subtracted reservoir pressure is estimated by subtracting abdominal pressure from total reservoir pressure. The simultaneous recording of the abdominal pressure trace is essential for the interpretation of the subtracted reservoir pressure trace as artefacts of the subtracted reservoir pressure may be produced by intrinsic rectal contractions or relaxations.

Contraction pressure (amplitude) is the difference between maximum reservoir pressure during a contraction of an intestinal urinary reservoir and baseline reservoir pressure before onset of this contraction. Contraction pressure may be determined from the pressure curves of total reservoir pressure or subtracted reservoir pressure. For assessment of functional significance of such activity of an intestinal urinary reservoir, pressure and volume must be stated for the first, atypical, and the maximum contraction. The frequency of contractions should be stated at a specified volume.

Leak point pressure is the total reservoir pressure at which leakage occurs in the absence of sphincter relaxation. Leakage occurs whenever total reservoir pressure exceeds maximum outlet pressure so that a negative outlet closure pressure results.

Reservoir sensation is difficult to assess because of the subjective nature of interpreting fullness or 'flatulence' from the bowel segments of the intestinal urinary reservoir. It is usually assessed by questioning the patient in relation to the sensation of fullness of the intestinal urinary reservoir during enterocystometry.

Commonly used descriptive terms are similar to conventional cystometry:

First desire to empty

Normal desire to empty (this is defined as the feeling that leads the patient to empty at the next convenient moment, but emptying can be delayed if necessary);

Strong desire to empty (this is defined as a persistent desire to empty without the fear of leakage);

Urgency (this is defined as a strong desire to empty accompanied by fear of leakage or fear of pain);

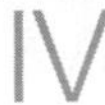

Pain (the site and character of which should be specified).

Maximum enterocystometric capacity is the volume at strong desire to empty. In the absence of sensation, maximum enterocystometric capacity is defined by the onset of leakage. If the closure mechanism of the outlet is incompetent, maximum enterocystometric capacity can be determined by occlusion of the outlet, e.g., by a Foley catheter. In the absence of both sensation and leakage, maximum enterocystometric capacity cannot be defined in the same terms and is the volume at which the clinician decides to terminate filling, e.g., because of a risk of over-distension. *Functional reservoir capacity* or evacuated volume is assessed from a frequency/volume chart (urinary diary). If a patient empties the urinary reservoir by intermittent catheterisation, functional reservoir capacity will be dependent on presence or absence of sensation and/or leakage. Thus, when reporting functional reservoir capacity the following should be stated:

a) Mode of evacuation (e.g., spontaneous voiding, intermittent catheterisation);
b) Presence/absence of sensation of fullness;
c) Presence/absence of leakage;
d) Timing of evacuation (e.g., by sensation, by the clock, by leakage).

Maximum (anaesthetic) anatomical reservoir capacity is the volume measured after filling during a deep general or spinal/epidural anaesthetic, specifying fluid temperature, filling pressure and filling rate. *Compliance* describes the change in volume over a related change in reservoir pressure. Compliance (C) is calculated by dividing the volume change (ΔV) by the change in subtracted reservoir pressure (ΔP_s) during that change in reservoir volume ($C = \Delta V/\Delta P_s$). Compliance is expressed as ml per cmH_2O.

4.2. Outlet pressure measurement

It should be noted that even under physiological conditions the evaluation of the competence of the closure mechanism of a continent outlet by measuring intraluminal pressures under various conditions is regarded as an idealized concept. Moreover, measurements of intraluminal pressures for functional evaluation of a continent outlet do not allow comparison of results between different closure mechanisms, which are in use with different types of intestinal urinary reservoirs. In addition, similar closure mechanisms may behave differently when used in different types of intestinal urinary reservoirs.

Therefore, urodynamic measurements of a continent outlet always have to be related to symptoms of the patient as assessed by history, frequency/volume chart, and, when applicable, measurement of urine loss.

The rationale of performing outlet pressure measurements is not to verify continence or degree of incontinence but to understand how different closure mechanisms work, which urodynamic parameters reflect their competence or dysfunction, and how their function is related to the characteristics of a reservoir.

In current urodynamic practice, intraluminal outlet pressure measurements are performed by a number of different techniques which do not always yield consistent values. Not only do the values differ with the method of measurement but there is often a lack of consistency for a single method – for example, the effect of catheter rotation when outlet pressure is measured by a catheter mounted microtransducer.

Measurements can be made at one point in the outlet (stationary) over a period of time, or at several points along the outlet consecutively during continuous or intermittent catheter withdrawal forming an outlet pressure profile (OPP). OPPs should be obtained at significant filling volumes of an intestinal urinary reservoir, which must be standardised and stated.

Two types of OPP can be measured:

a) Resting outlet pressure profile – with the urinary reservoir and the subject at rest;
b) Stress outlet pressure profile – with a defined applied stress (e.g., cough, strain, Valsalva manoeuvre).

The outlet pressure profile denotes the intraluminal pressure along the length of the closure mechanism. All systems are zeroed at atmospheric pressure. For external transducers the reference point is the level of the continence mechanism. For catheter mounted transducers the reference point is the transducer itself. Intrareservoir pressure should be measured to exclude a simultaneous reservoir contraction. The subtraction of total reservoir pressures from intraluminal outlet pressures produces the outlet closure pressure profile.

Specify

a) Infusion medium;
b) Rate of infusion;
c) Stationary, continuous or intermittent catheter withdrawal;

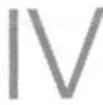

d) Rate of withdrawal;
e) Reservoir volume;
f) Position of patient (supine, sitting or standing);
g) Technique (catheters, transducers, measurement technique and recording apparatus are to be specified according to the 1988 ICS report; see Appendix I).

Definitions

Maximum outlet pressure is the maximum pressure of the measured profile.

Maximum outlet closure pressure is the difference between maximum outlet pressure and total reservoir pressure.

Functional outlet profile length is the length of the closure mechanism along which the outlet pressure exceeds total reservoir pressure.

Functional outlet profile length (on stress) is the length over which the outlet pressure exceeds total reservoir pressure on stress.

Pressure 'transmission' ratio[1] is the increment in outlet pressure on stress as a percentage of the simultaneously recorded increment in the total reservoir pressure. For stress profiles obtained during coughing, pressure 'transmission' ratios can be obtained at any point along the closure mechanism. If single values are given, the position in the closure mechanism should be stated. If several transmission ratios are defined at different points along the closure mechanism, a pressure 'transmission' profile is obtained. During 'cough profiles' the amplitude of the cough should be stated if possible.

4.3. Quantification of urine loss

On a frequency/volume chart, incontinence can be qualified (with/without urge or stress) and quantified by the number, type, and dampness (damp/wet/soaked) of pads used each day. However, subjective grading of incontinence may not completely disclose the degree of abnormality. It is important to relate the complaints of each patient to the individual urinary regimen and personal circumstances, as well as to the results of objective measurements.

In order to assess and compare results of different series and different surgical techniques, a simple standard test can be used to measure urine loss objectively in any subject. In order to obtain a representative result, especially in subjects with variable or intermittent urinary incontinence, the test should occupy as long a period as possible; yet it must be practical. The circumstances should approximate to those of everyday life, yet be similar for all subjects to allow meaningful comparison.

The total amount of urine lost during the test period is determined by weighing a collecting device such as a nappy, absorbent pad, or condom appliance. A nappy or pad should be worn inside waterproof underpants or should have a waterproof backing if worn over a continent stoma. Care should be taken to use a collecting device of adequate capacity.

Immediately before the test begins the collecting device is weighed to the nearest gram.

In the 1988 collated report on 'Standardisation of Terminology of Lower Urinary Tract Function' (see Appendix I), the ICS has offered the choices to conduct a pad test either with the patient drinking 500 ml sodium-free liquid within a short period (max. 15 min) without the patient voiding before the test or after having the bladder filled to a defined volume. Because there is a great variation in the functional capacity of different types of intestinal urinary reservoirs and since some types of closure mechanism of the outlet physiologically have a leak point and others have no leak point, it is recommended that the reservoir is emptied by catheterisation immediately before the test and refilled with a reasonable volume of saline, which must be standardised and be stated in absolute numbers. A typical test schedule and additional procedures are described in the 1988 ICS report (Appendix I). Specifications for presentation of results, findings, and statistics from the 1988 ICS report are applicable (Appendix I).

[1]The term 'transmission' is in common usage and cannot be changed. However, transmission implies that forces transmitted to the closure mechanism are generated completely by extrinsic activities. Such an assumption is not yet justified by scientific evidence. A role for intrinsic muscle activity cannot be excluded for the urethra and the anus and their intrinsic sphincter mechanisms, while it is unlikely to be of significance in any of the surgically constructed closure mechanisms of a continent outlet.

The terms 'passive transmission' and 'active transmission' have been introduced to describe different processes in respect of the source of extrinsically generated forces and the mode of transmission. 'Passive transmission' is taken to be the result of forces, which are generated by striated muscles distant from the closure mechanism (e.g., diaphragm, abdominal wall muscles) and are 'passively' transmitted through surrounding tissues to the closure mechanism in the same way they are transmitted to all other intraabdominal tissues and organs. 'Active transmission' is taken to be result of forces, which are generated by striated muscles in direct anatomical contact with the closure mechanism (e.g., pelvic floor muscles with urethra or anus, and abdominal wall muscles with a continent cutaneous outlet) and are directly 'transmitted' to the closure mechanism.

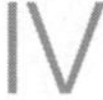

5. PROCEDURES RELATED TO THE EVALUATION OF EVACUATION OF AN INTESTINAL URINARY RESERVOIR

5.1. Mode of evacuation

The mode of evacuation of an intestinal urinary reservoir varies as some patients may have a surgically constructed closure mechanism requiring catheterisation (e.g., continent cutaneous urinary diversion) and some patients may have a reservoir with a physiological sphincter mechanism (e.g., bladder augmentation, bladder substitution to bladder neck or to urethra, continent anal urinary diversion), through which they may be able to evacuate urine spontaneously. However, as catheterisation may also be required after bladder augmentation or bladder substitution to bladder neck or to urethra, it must be stated by what means the reservoir is emptied (e.g., spontaneous evacuation with or without Valsalva or Credé manoeuvres and/or intermittent catheterisation).

If intermittent catheterisation is necessary, whether it is performed on a regular basis or only periodically, the intervals between catheterisations must be stated.

Measurements of urinary flow, reservoir pressures during micturition and residual urine apply only to patients with bladder augmentation or bladder substitution to bladder neck or to urethra who void spontaneously. However, as there is no volitional initiation of contraction of an intestinal urinary reservoir, spontaneous evacuation is different from voiding by a detrusor contraction.

In patients with an intestinal urinary reservoir, evacuation is initiated by relaxation of the urethral sphincteric mechanisms and/or passive expression of the reservoir by abdominal straining or Valsalva or Credé manoeuvres. Therefore, measurements of flow and micturition pressures must be interpreted with great caution in respect of the diagnosis of an outlet obstruction.

5.2. Measurements of urinary flow, micturition pressure, residual urine

For specifications of measurements of urinary flow, reservoir pressures during micturition and residual urine the 1988 ICS report is applicable (Appendix I) The specifications of patient position, access for pressure measurement, catheter type, and measuring equipment are as for enterocystometry (see 4.1).

6. CLASSIFICATION OF STORAGE DYSFUNCTION OF AN INTESTINAL URINARY RESERVOIR

Dysfunction of an intestinal urinary reservoir has to be defined in respect to indications and functional intentions of incorporating bowel into the urinary tract. The rationale of using an intestinal urinary reservoir is to improve or provide storage function by:

a) Reducing bladder hypersensitivity;
b) Providing/enlarging reservoir capacity;
c) Providing/improving reservoir compliance;
d) Lowering bladder pressures/providing low reservoir pressures;
e) Improving/providing the closure function of the outlet.

It is not a primary goal of surgery to maintain or provide the capability of spontaneous voiding; intermittent catheterisation is required for evacuation of the reservoir in all cases of continent cutaneous diversion and in many other situations. The need to evacuate a urinary reservoir by intermittent catheterisation is not regarded as a failure in bladder augmentation and bladder substitution to bladder neck or to urethra, even though the majority of patients may evacuate urine spontaneously.

Consequently, the classification of dysfunctions of an intestinal urinary reservoir relates to the storage phase only. Problems of storing urine in an intestinal urinary reservoir may be related to dysfunction of the reservoir or dysfunction of the outlet. The classification is based on the pathophysiology of dysfunction as assessed by various urodynamic investigations. The urodynamic findings must be related to the patient's symptoms and signs. For example, the presence of reservoir contractions in an asymptomatic patients with normal upper tract drainage does not warrant a diagnosis of reservoir overactivity unless the contractions cause urine leakage or other problems defined below.

6.1. Reservoir dysfunction

The symptoms of frequency, urgency, nocturia, and/or incontinence may relate to dysfunction of an intestinal urinary reservoir and should be assessed by enterocystometry, which is an adequate test for evaluation of the pathophysiology of a reservoir dysfunction (see 4.1). Abnormal findings may relate to sensation, compliance, capacity, and/or activity of an intestinal urinary reservoir.

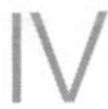

6.1.1. Sensation

Sensations from an intestinal urinary reservoir as assessed by questioning the patient during enterocystometry can be classified in qualitative terms. Often these symptoms are associated with contractions of the reservoir as shown by enterocystometry or fluoroscopy. However, up to now there is insufficient information about an isolated hypersensitive state of the bowel of an intestinal urinary reservoir. If symptoms such as frequency, urgency, and nocturia are persisting after bladder augmentation or bladder substitution to bladder neck (e.g., in interstitial cystitis), they are likely to derive from remnants of the original lower urinary tract, which have not been replaced by intestine, if enterocystometry is otherwise normal.

6.1.2. Capacity/Compliance

Capacity of an intestinal urinary reservoir is determined by sensation and/or compliance. For definitions of reservoir capacity and compliance ($\Delta V/\Delta P$), see 4.1. Compliance describing the change in volume over a related change in reservoir pressure is likely to reflect a different physiology when determined in an intestinal urinary reservoir as compared to the urinary bladder. The calculation of compliance will reflect wall characteristics of an intestinal urinary reservoir such as distensibility only after a process of 'unfolding' of an empty intestinal urinary reservoir has been completed and stretching of the walls begins to take place, which is different in the normal urinary bladder. Compliance may change during the enterocystometric examination and is variably dependent upon a number of factors including:

a) Rate of filling;
b) The part of the enterocystometrogram curve used for compliance evaluation;
c) The volume interval over which compliance is calculated;
d) The distensibility of the urinary reservoir as determined by mechanical and contractile properties of the walls of the reservoir.

During normal filling of an intestinal urinary reservoir little or no pressure changes occur and this is termed 'normal compliance.' However, at the present time there is insufficient data to define normal high, and low compliance. When reporting compliance, specify:

a) The rate of filling;
b) The volume at which compliance is calculated;
c) The volume increment over which compliance is calculated;
d) The part of the enterocystometrogram curve used for the calculation of compliance.

The selection of bowel segments, the size of bowel (diameter, length), and the geometry (shape) of a reservoir after bowel detubularisation and reconfiguration determine capacity of an intestinal urinary reservoir [Hinman, 1988]. For a given length of bowel, reconfiguration into a spherical reservoir provides the largest capacity. The distensibility of bowel wall, as assessed in experimental models, varies between bowel segments (i.e., large bowel, small bowel, stomach) and with orientation (longitudinal, circumferential) of measurement within a bowel segment [Hohenfellner et al., 1993]. However, the relative contributions of wall distensibility (influenced by selection of bowel segments) and of geometric capacity (influenced by size of selected bowel and reservoir shape after detubularisation and reconfiguration) in determining the capacity of an intestinal urinary reservoir are not yet precisely understood. Low capacity of an intestinal urinary reservoir may relate to bowel size (diameter/length) and/or configuration of bowel segments in the reservoir (e.g. tubular, inadequate detubularation, and reconfiguration).

6.1.3. Activity

In intact bowel segments, peristaltic contractions are elicited at a certain degree of wall distension. As a result of detubularisation and reconfiguration of bowel segments in an intestinal urinary reservoir, such contractions do not encompass the whole circumference of a reservoir. Net pressure changes in the reservoir are determined by the mechanical and muscular properties of both the contracting and the non-contracting segments of the reservoir. Contractions of segments of an intestinal urinary reservoir may be observed by fluoroscopy but may not increase subtracted reservoir pressure if the generated forces are counterbalanced by other segments of a urinary reservoir which relax and distend. Some contractile activity of an intestinal urinary reservoir is a normal finding on enterocystometry or fluoroscopy.

Overactivity of an intestinal urinary reservoir is defined as a degree of activity which causes lower urinary tract symptoms and/or signs of upper tract deterioration in the absence of other causes of upper tract damage such as urethral obstruction or reflux. Symptoms such as abdominal cramping, urgency, frequency, and/or leakage may be related to reservoir activity seen during enterocystometry and thus establish the diagnosis of an unacceptable degree of reservoir activity ('overactivity'). Signs of impaired upper tract drainage may be associated with elevated subtracted reservoir pressures on enterocystometry due to an early onset, high amplitudes, and/or frequency of contractions and thus establish the diagnosis of overactivity even if subjective symptoms are not experienced.

However, since a precise definition of normal and increased activity of a urinary reservoir from intestine is not yet established, the frequency of contractions should be reported at a specified volume and the pressure/volume relationships should be stated for the following defined contractions of the reservoir:

a) First contraction;
b) Contraction with maximum contraction pressure (amplitude);
c) Typical contraction.

The diagnosis of overactivity of an intestinal urinary reservoir should not be made until a reasonable interval – which must be stated – has elapsed after surgery, since an intestinal urinary reservoir expands after surgery, when permitted to store urine, and since some of the reservoir activity subsides with time with an increase of capacity.

6.2. Outlet dysfunction

The symptoms of incontinence and/or difficulties with catheterisation may relate to dysfunction of the outlet of an intestinal urinary reservoir and should be assessed in terms of pathophysiology. Leakage may occur if total reservoir pressure exceeds outlet pressure so that the result is a negative outlet closure pressure as assessed by outlet pressure profiles (see 4.2). For such an event, volume and total reservoir pressure at onset of leakage (leak point pressure) must be stated.

Leakage may occur with a functioning closure mechanism because of an excessive reservoir pressure increase due to contractions of the intestinal urinary reservoir (overactivity) or overdistension of the reservoir (overflow).

The definition of incompetence of a closure mechanism is different for a closure mechanism which physiologically has a leak point from that for a closure mechanism without a leak point.

A closure mechanism which physiologically has a leak point (e.g., the urethral sphincter, some types of closure mechanism in continent cutaneous urinary diversion) is incompetent if it allows leakage or urine in the absence of contraction of the intestinal urinary reservoir (overactivity) or overdistension of the reservoir (overflow) as assessed by enterocystometry (see 4.1). A closure mechanism which normally has no leak point (e.g. an intussusception nipple) is incompetent if it permits leakage of urine independent of results of enterocystometry.

REFERENCES

Emmett J L, Witten D M 1971 Urinary stasis: The obstructive uropathies, atony, vesicoureteral reflux, and neuromuscular dysfunction of the urinary tract. In: Emmett J L, Witten D M (eds): Clinical urography. An atlas and textbook of roentgenologic diagnosis. Vol. 1, 3rd edn. Philadephia, London, Toronto: Saunders, p 369

Heikel P E, Parkkulainen K V 1966 Vesicoureteric reflux in children. A classification and results of conservative treatment. Annals of Radiology 9: 37

Hinman F Jr 1988 Selection of intestinal segments for bladder substitution: physical and physiological characteristics. Journal of Urology 139: 519

Hohenfellner M, Büger R, Schad H et al 1993 Reservoir characteristics of Mainz-pouch studied in animal model. Osmolality of filling solution and effect of Oxybutynin. Urology 42: 741

Smellie J M, Edwards D, Hunter N, Normand ICS, Prescod N 1975 Vesico-ureteric reflux and renal scarring. Kidney International 8: 65

The standardisation of terminology of lower urinary tract function: pressure–flow studies of voiding, urethral resistance and urethral obstruction

Neurourology and Urodynamics 16: 1–18 (1997) Published 1997 by Wiley-Liss, Inc.

Derek Griffiths (subcommittee chairman), Klaus Höfner, Ron van Mastrigt, Harm Jan Rollema, Anders Spångberg, Donald Gleason and Anders Mattiasson (overall chairman)

International Continence Society Subcommittee on Standardisation of Terminology of Pressure–Flow Studies

1. INTRODUCTION

This report has been produced at the request of the International Continence Society. It was approved at the twenty-fifth annual meeting of the society in Sydney, Australia.

The 1988 version of the collated reports on standardisation of terminology, which appeared in *Neurourology and Urodynamics*, vol. 7, pp. 403–427 (see also Appendix I), contains material relevant to pressure-flow studies in many different sections. This report is a revision and expansion of Sections 4.2 and 4.3 and parts of Sections 6.2 and 7 of the 1988 report. It contains a recommendation for a provisional standard method for defining obstruction on the basis of pressure-flow data.

2. EVALUATION OF MICTURITION

2.1. Pressure-flow studies

At present, the best method of analysing voiding function quantitatively is the pressure-flow study of micturition, with simultaneous recording of abdominal, intravesical and detrusor pressures and flow rate (Fig. V.A).

Direct inspection of the raw pressure and flow data before, during and at the end of micturition is essential, because it allows artefacts and untrustworthy data to be recognised and eliminated. More detailed analyses of pressure-flow relationships, described below, are advisable to aid diagnosis and to quantify data for research studies.

The flow pattern in a pressure-flow study should be representative of free flow studies in the same

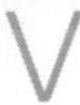

patient. It is important to eliminate artefacts and unrepresentative studies before applying more detailed analyses.

Pressure-flow studies contain information about the behaviour of the urethra and the behaviour of the detrusor. Section 2.2 deals with the urethra. Detrusor function is considered in Section 2.3.

2.1.1. Pressure and flow rate parameters

Definitions See Fig. V.A and Table V.2; see also Table I.2 (page 648).

Maximum flow rate is the maximum measured value of the flow rate. Symbol Q_{max}.

Maximum pressure is the maximum value of the pressure measured during a pressure-flow study. Note that this may be attained at a moment when the flow rate is zero. Symbols: $P_{abd, max}$, $P_{ves, max}$, $P_{det, max}$.

Pressure at maximum flow is the pressure recorded at maximum measured flow rate. If the same maximum value is attained more than once or if it is sustained for a period of time, then the point of maximum flow is taken to be where the detrusor pressure has its lowest value for this flow rate; abdominal, intravesical and detrusor pressures at maximum flow are all read at this same point. Flow delay (see Section 2.1.2) may have a significant influence and should be considered. Symbols: $P_{abd, Qmax}$, $P_{ves, Qmax}$, $P_{det, Qmax}$.

Opening pressure is the pressure recorded at the onset of measured flow. Flow delay should be considered. Symbols: $P_{abd, open}$, $P_{ves, open}$, $P_{det, open}$.

Closing pressure is the pressure recorded at the end of measured flow. Flow delay should be considered. Symbols: $P_{abd, clos}$, $P_{ves, clos}$, $P_{det, clos}$.

Minimum voiding pressure is the minimum pressure during measurable flow (see Fig. V.A). It may be, but is not necessarily, equal to the opening pressure or the closing pressure. Example: minimum voiding detrusor pressure, symbol: $P_{det, min, void}$.

2.1.2. Flow delay

When a pressure-flow study is performed, the flow rate is measured at a location downstream of the bladder pressure measurement and so the flow rate measurement is delayed. The delay is partly physiological, but it also depends on the equipment. It may depend on the flow rate.

When considering pressure-flow relationships, it may be important to take this delay into account, especially if there are rapid changes in pressure and flow rate. In current practice an average value is estimated by each investigator, from observations of the delay between corresponding pressure and flow rate changes in a number of actual studies. Values from 0.5 to 1.0 s are typical.

Definition
Flow delay is the time delay between a change in bladder pressure and the corresponding change in measured flow rate.

2.1.3. Presentation of results

Pressure-flow plots and the nomograms used for analysis should be presented with the flow rate plotted along the *x*-axis and the detrusor pressure along the *y*-axis (see Fig. V.A).

Specify
The value of the flow delay that is used.

2.2. Urethral resistance and bladder outlet obstruction

2.2.1. Urethral function during voiding

During voiding urethral function may be

(a) normal or
(b) obstructive as a result of
  (i) overactivity or
  (ii) abnormal structure.

Obstruction due to urethral overactivity occurs when the urethral closure mechanism contracts involuntarily or fails to relax during attempted micturition in spite of an ongoing detrusor contraction. Obstruction due to abnormal structure has an anatomical basis, e.g., urethral stricture or prostatic enlargement.

2.2.2. Urethral resistance

Urethral resistance is represented by a relation between pressure and flow rate, describing the pressure required to propel any given flow rate through the urethra. The relation is called the *urethral resistance relation* (URR).

An indication of the urethral resistance relation is obtained by plotting detrusor pressure against flow rate. The most accurate procedure, which requires a computer or an *x*/*y* recorder, is a quasi-continuous plot showing many pairs of corresponding pressure and flow rate values (Fig. V.B). A simpler procedure, which can be performed by hand, is to plot only two or three pressure-flow points connected by straight lines; for example, the points of minimum voiding pressure and of maximum flow may be

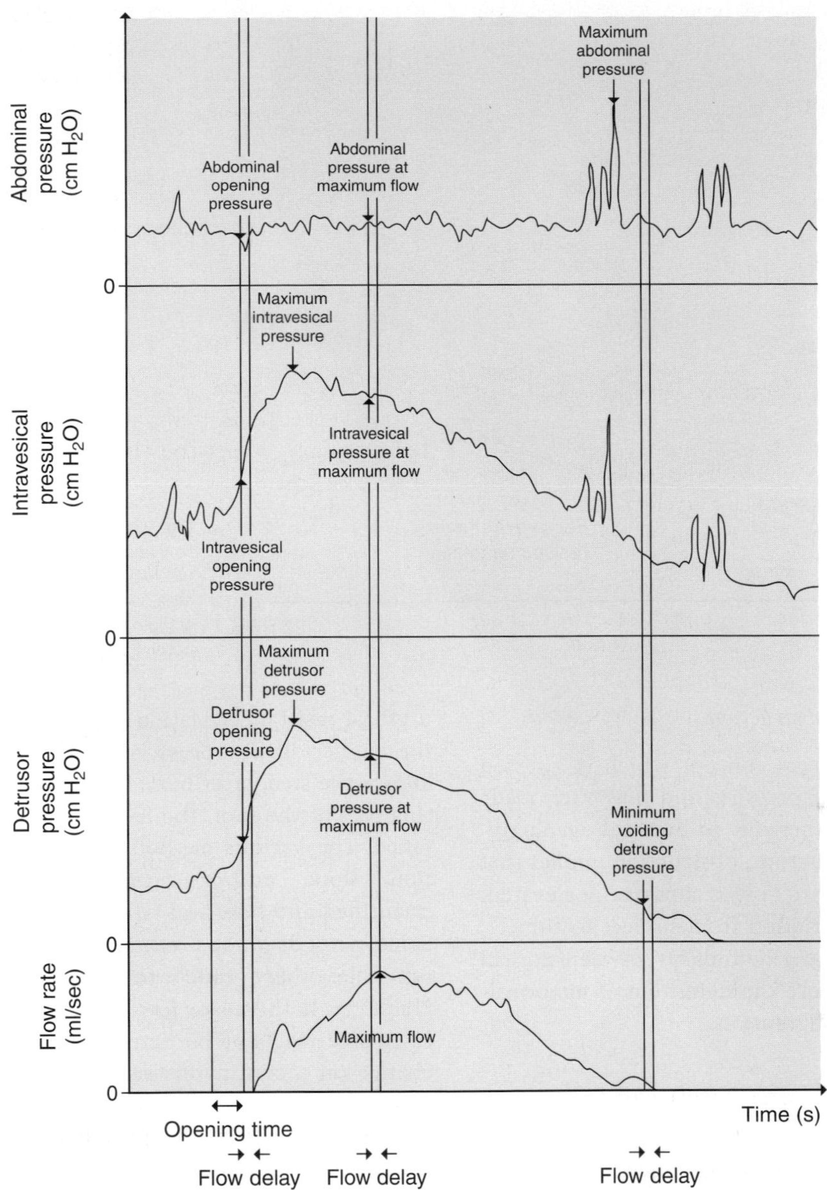

Fig. V.A Diagram of a pressure-flow study with nomenclature recommended in this report.

selected. In whatever way the plot is made, flow delay should be considered.

A further simplification is to plot just one point showing the maximum flow rate and the detrusor pressure at maximum flow. Flow delay should be considered.

Methods of analysing pressure-flow plots are further discussed below.

2.2.3. Urethral activity

Ideally, the urethra is fully relaxed during voiding. The urethral resistance is then at its lowest and the detrusor pressure has its lowest value for any given flow rate. Under these circumstances the urethral resistance relation is defined by the inherent mechanical and morphological properties of the urethra and is called the *passive urethral resistance relation* (Fig. V.B).

Urethral activity can only increase the detrusor pressure above the value defined by the passive urethral resistance relation. Therefore, any deviations of the pressure-flow plot from the passive urethral resistance relation toward higher pressures are regarded as due to activity of the urethral or periurethral muscles, striated or smooth.

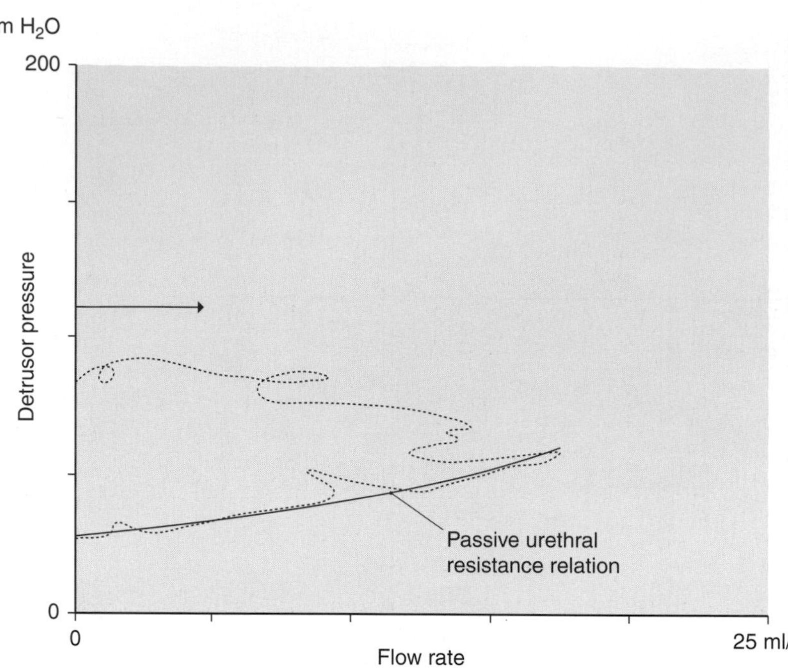

Fig. V.B Plot of detrusor pressure against flow rate during voiding (broken curve), providing an indication of the urethral resistance relation (URR). The continuous smooth curve is an estimate of the passive urethral resistance relation.

2.2.4. Bladder outlet obstruction

Obstruction is a physical concept which is assessed from measurements of pressure and flow rate, made during voiding. Whether due to urethral over-activity or to abnormal structure, obstruction implies that the urethral resistance to flow is abnormally elevated. Because of natural variation from subject to subject, there cannot be a sharp boundary between normal and abnormal. Therefore the definition of abnormality requires further elaboration.

2.2.5. Methods of analysing pressure-flow plots

The results of pressure-flow studies may be used for various purposes, for example for objective diagnosis of urethral obstruction or for statistical testing of differences in urethral resistance between groups of patients. For these purposes methods have been developed to quantify pressure-flow plots in terms of one or more numerical parameters. The parameters are based on aspects such as the position, slope or curvature of the plot. Some of these methods are primarily intended for use in adult males with possible prostatic hypertrophy.

Some methods of analysis are shown in Table V.1.

Quantification of Urethral Resistance In all current methods, urethral resistance is derived from the relationship between pressure and flow rate. A commonly used method of demonstrating this relationship is the pressure-flow plot. The lower pressure part of this plot is taken to represent the passive urethral resistance relation (see Fig. V.B). In general, the higher is the pressure for a given flow rate, and/or the steeper or more sharply curved upward is this part of the plot, the higher is the urethral resistance. The various methods differ in how the position, slope, and/or curvature of the plot are quantified and how and whether they are combined. Some methods grade urethral resistance on a continuous scale; others grade it in a small number of classes (Table 1). If there are few classes, small changes in resistance may not be detected. Conversely, a small change on a continuous scale may not be clinically relevant.

Some methods result in a single parameter; others result in two or more parameters (Table V.I). A single parameter makes it easy to compare different measurements. A larger number of parameters makes comparison more difficult but potentially gives higher accuracy and validity. If there are too many parameters, however, accuracy may be compromised by poor reproducibility.

Choice of Method Some methods in Table V.I are intended primarily to quantify urethral resistance. Others are intended only for the diagnosis of obstruction. Methods that quantify urethral resistance on a scale can also be used to aid diagnosis of obstruction by comparison with cutoff values. In every case an equivocal zone may be included.

Because of their underlying similarity, all the above methods classify clearly obstructed and clearly unobstructed pressure-flow studies consistently, but

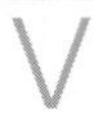

Table V.1 Methods of analysing pressure-flow plots

Method	Aim	Number of *p/Q* points	Assumed shape of URR	Number of parameters	Number of classes or continuous
Abrams-Griffiths nomogram[1]	diagnosis	1	n/a	n/a	3
Spångberg nomogram[2]	diagnosis	1	n/a	n/a	3
URA[3,4]	resistance	1	curved	1	continuous
linPURR[5]	resistance	1[a]	linear	1	7
Schäfer PURR[6]	resistance	many	curved	2	continuous
CHESS[7]	resistance	many	curved	2	16
OBI[8]	resistance	many	linear	1	continuous
Spångberg *et al.*	resistance	many	linear or curved	3	continuous + 3 categories
DAMPF[9]	resistance	2	linear	1	continuous
A/G number[10]	resistance	1	linear	1	continuous

[a]Schäfer uses 2 points to draw a linear relation but the point at maximum flow determines the resistance grade.

there is some lack of agreement in a minority of cases with intermediate urethral resistance.

Any of the methods of analysing pressure-flow studies may be useful for a particular purpose. In selecting a method, investigators should consider carefully what their aims are and which method is best suited to attain them.

Identification of Optimum Methods For a subsequent report the International Continence Society will compare the above methods with each other and may also develop new methods, with the aim of reaching a consensus on their use. The Society will continue to seek better ways of clinically validating these methods. The following procedure has been agreed on.

Making use of good-quality data stored in digital format, the following databases will be examined:

1. Pressure-flow studies in untreated men with lower urinary tract symptoms and signs suggestive of benign prostatic obstruction.
2. Pressure-flow studies repeated after a time interval with no intervention.
3. Pressure-flow studies before and after TURP.
4. Pressure-flow studies before and after alternative therapeutical intervention that causes a small change in urethral resistance.

Database 1 will be used to determine which existing or new methods adequately describe the actual pressure-flow plots of male patients with lower urinary tract symptoms. Database 2 will be used to determine the reproducibility of the various methods. Database 3 will be used to determine in which groups of patients TURP significantly reduces urethral resistance, and hence which patients are indeed obstructed. Database 4 will be used to test the sensitivity of the various methods to small changes of urethral resistance.

On the basis of these analyses, the International Continence Society will attempt to identify:

(i) A simple and reproducible method with high validity of diagnosing obstruction.
(ii) A sensitive and reproducible method with high validity of measuring urethral resistance and changes in resistance.

Provisional Recommendation Pending the results of these procedures, it is recommended that investigators reporting pressure-flow studies in adult males, particularly those with benign prostatic hyperplasia, use one simple standard method of analysis in addition to any other method that they have selected, so that results from different centres can be compared. For this provisional method it is recommended that urethral resistance is specified by the maximum flow rate and the detrusor pressure at maximum flow, i.e., by the pair of values (Q_{max}, $P_{det,\ Qmax}$). A provisional diagnostic classification may be derived from these values as follows:

- If $(P_{det,\ Qmax} - 2Q_{max}) > 40$ the pressure-flow study is obstructed.
- If $(P_{det,\ Qmax} - 2Q_{max}) < 20$ the pressure-flow study is unobstructed.
- Otherwise the study is equivocal.

In these formulae pressure and flow rate are expressed in cmH_2O and ml/s respectively. This method is illustrated graphically in Fig. V.C. It may be referred to as the *provisional ICS method for definition of obstruction.*

The equivocal zone of the provisional method (Fig. V.C) is similar but not identical to those of the

Abrams-Griffiths and Spångberg nomograms and to the region defining linPURR grade II. For micturitions with low to moderate flow rates it is consistent with cutoff values used to define obstruction in the URA and CHESS methods.

2.3 The detrusor during micturition

During micturition the detrusor may be

(a) Acontractile
(b) Underactive
(c) Normal

(a) The acontractile detrusor is one that cannot be demonstrated to contract during urodynamic studies.
(b) Detrusor underactivity is defined as a detrusor contraction of inadequate magnitude and/or duration to effect complete bladder emptying in the absence of urethral obstruction. (Concerning the elderly see (c)). Both magnitude and duration should be considered in the evaluation of detrusor contractility.
(c) Normal detrusor contractility. In the absence of obstruction, a normal detrusor contraction will effect complete bladder emptying. Detrusor contractility in the elderly may need special consideration.

For a given detrusor contraction, the magnitude of the recorded pressure rise will depend on the outlet resistance. In general, the higher the detrusor pressure and/or the higher the flow rate, the stronger is the detrusor contraction. The magnitude of the detrusor contraction may be approximately quantified by means of a nomogram applied to the pressure-flow plot or by calculation.

Table V.2 Qualifiers that can be used to indicate pressure and flow variables relevant to voiding

Qualifiers	
At maximum flow	Q_{max}
During voiding	void
Opening	open
Closing	clos
Examples	
$P_{det,\ Qmax}$	Detrusor pressure at maximum flow
$P_{det,\ min,\ void}$	Minimum voiding detrusor pressure
$P_{ves,\ open}$	Intravesical opening pressure
$P_{ves,\ clos}$	Intravesical closing pressure

When possible, qualifiers should be printed as subscripts (see above). Note that the preferred symbol for pressure is lower-case *p*, while the symbol for flow rate is capital (upper-case) *Q*.

3. ADDITIONAL SYMBOLS

Qualifiers that can be used to form symbols for variables relevant to voiding are shown in Table V.2. These are additions to those in Table 2 of the 1988 standardisation report.

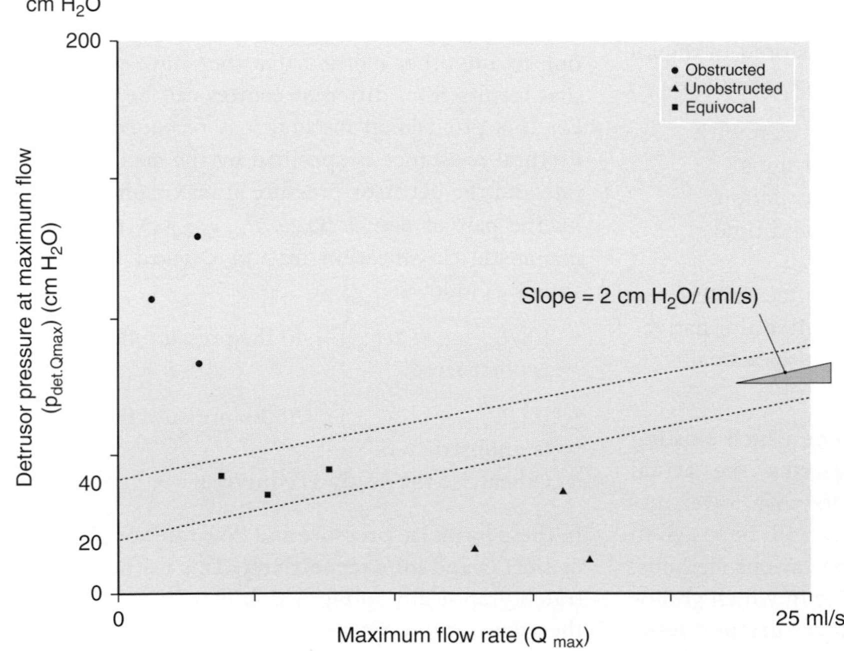

Fig. V.C Provisional ICS method for definition of obstruction. The points represent schematically the values of maximum flow rate and detrusor pressure at maximum flow for 9 different voids, 3 in each class.

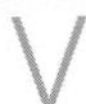

REFERENCES

1. Abrams P H, Griffiths D J 1979 The assessment of prostatic obstruction from urodynamic measurements and from residual urine. British Journal of Urology 51: 129–134
2. Spångberg A, Teriö H, Ask P, Engberg A 1991 Pressure/flow studies preoperatively and post-operatively in patients with benign prostatic hypertrophy: estimation of the urethral pressure flow relation and urethral elasticity. Neurourology and Urodynamics 10: 139–167
3. Griffiths D, Van Mastrigt R, Bosch R 1989 Quantification of urethral resistance and bladder function during voiding, with special reference to the effects of prostate size reduction on urethral obstruction due to benign prostatic hypertrophy. Neurourology and Urodynamics 8: 17–27
4. Rollema H J, van Mastrigt R 1992 Improved indication and follow-up in transurethral resection of the prostate (TUR) using the computer program CLIM. Journal of Urology 148: 111–116
5. Schäfer W 1990 Basic principles and clinical application of advance analysis of bladder voiding function. Urology Clinics of North America 17: 553–566
6. Schäfer W 1983 The contribution of the bladder outlet to the relation between pressure and flow rate during micturition. In: Hinman F Jr (ed) Bening prostatic hypertrophy. New York: Springer-Verlag, pp. 470–496
7. Höfner K, Kramer A E J L, Tan H K, Krah H, Jonas U 1995 CHESS classification of bladder outflow obstruction. A consequence in the discussion of current concepts. World Journal of Urology 13: 59–64.
8. Kranse M, Van Mastrigt R 1991 The derivation of an obstruction index from a three parameter model fitted to the lowest part of the pressure flow plot. Journal of Urology 145: 261A
9. Schäfer W 1995 Analysis of bladder-outlet function with the linearized passive urethral resistance relation, linPURR, and a disease-specific approach for grading obstruction: from complex to simple. World Journal of Urology 13: 47–58
10. Lim G S, Abrams P 1995 The Abrams-Griffiths nomogram. World Journal of Urology 13: 34–39

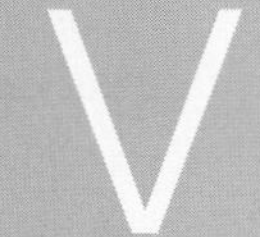

Standardisation of outcome studies in patients with lower urinary tract dysfunction: a report on general principles from the Standardisation Committee of the International Continence Society

Neurourology and Urodynamics 17:249–253 (1998) © 1998 International Continence Society

Anders Mattiasson, Jens Christian Djurhuus, David Fonda, Gunnar Lose, Jørgen Nordling, and Manfred Stöhrer

Anders Mattiason served as Coordinating Chairman. The other authors served as chairmen of the respective Outcome Subcommittees on Lower Urinary Tract Dysfunction: Children, Frail Elderly, Women, Men, and Neurogenic Dysfunction.

INTRODUCTION

Scientific evaluation of the outcome of therapeutic interventions in patients is not possible without assessment both before and after the intervention. The methods and measurements used must conform to set criteria in order that they may be applied to all interventions so that comparison between studies may be made. They must be valid, accurate, precise, reliable, and repeatable using a test-retest variation. Evaluations should be properly directed, such that the right variable is measured. Even though methods of intervention and evaluation may vary, certain domains of measurement should be represented and a multidimensional approach undertaken. The time scale for evaluations and interventions and the composition of the study group are important factors, so that some standardization exists, enabling understanding of the results by other investigators and comparison between studies.

Unfortunately, no consensus of opinion presently exists on the way in which studies should be performed, including interventions and evaluations, nor on how the results thus obtained should be represented. The scientific basis for many methods is also frequently unclear. A recent American survey of the literature on outcome in genuine stress incontinence classified almost all of the investigations as unsatisfactory and only a few as excellent. We thus have a dilemma between what we 'know' as based on reliable scientific data, and what we 'believe' based on clinical practice. This emphasises the poor investigative technique and reporting presently in use and the need for the standardisation of outcome measures.

STANDARDISATION OF OUTCOME STUDIES

In 1993, the International Continence Society set up subcommittees within the frame of the Standardisation

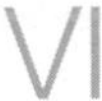

Committee in order to standardise outcome studies in patients with lower urinary tract dysfunction:

1. Children,
2. Frail Elderly,
3. Women,
4. Men, and
5. Neurogenic Dysfunction.

Each of these specific subcommittees was asked to make recommendations on how outcome studies should be performed in their respective fields. In this general report, common principles and outlines are discussed. These should be seen as recommendations rather than guidelines, representing a move towards a more rational and uniform presentation of outcome studies. In the separate reports from respective subcommittees, more specific recommendations are given.

DEFINITION OF OUTCOME MEASURES

No single measure can fully express the outcome of an intervention. It is necessary for outcome to incorporate improvement and deterioration in function, complications of the intervention, socioeconomic data, and the effect on quality of life. Both subjective and objective measurements should be included and bias eliminated where possible. It should be emphasised that frequently the perception of the patient, doctor, or therapist are at variance, and hence the choice and application of measurement tool is all the more important.

An intervention might have both primary and secondary outcome objectives. The primary objective might be an anatomical change (e.g., surgery), while the secondary objective might be functional (e.g., continence).

ENDPOINTS

In order for maximum information to be obtained, it is important that the correct endpoints are chosen and defined at the beginning of the study. This involves the stating of a null hypothesis, although other factors may be of importance and should be included where appropriate. Endpoints should be chosen so that they are relevant and may be incorporated into practice at the end of the study. The time frame of the intervention and its expected outcome should be considered when designing a study. Long-term outcome should be measured whenever possible. Statistical expertise is vital and should be applied from the beginning of the study.

OUTCOME MEASURES

Directed, accurate measures are necessary in order to reflect the degree of change or improvement with a high degree of correlation.

The groups of measures generally termed objective, subjective, compliance, quality of life, and socioeconomic can also be grouped into domains of interest. The use of domains describes another perspective, with the interests of the involved parts weighted according to their perceived importance. Certain measurements are not easy to make because of dearth of presently available instruments and a lack of agreement about which tool is most appropriate. At present, there is also a lack of correlation between the various measures mentioned.

Urinary incontinence as a symptom, a sign, and a condition is here redefined as far as the condition part is concerned. The condition 'urinary incontinence' is comprised of the passage of urine through the urethra at an inappropriate point in time, and is thus not, as previously suggested, a part of the underlying pathophysiological process itself. Urinary incontinence is thus a consequence and not a cause, and this is valid for both the symptom, the sign, and the condition parts.

Outcome in studies of lower urinary tract function and dysfunction should be described using:

- Patient's observations (symptoms)
- Quantification of symptoms (e.g., urine loss)
- Physician's observations (anatomical and functional; compliance)
- Quality-of-life measures
- Socioeconomic evaluations.

Patient- and physician-observed measures should be regarded as compulsory in all outcomes of lower urinary tract dysfunction; compliance measurements from patients and healthy volunteers should be given, and quality-of-life and socioeconomic data included when available. These data should be increasingly incorporated into study designs, so that the picture becomes complete.

EVALUATION AND GRADING OF OUTCOME

Although the ideal result of treatment should be cure and normalisation, outcome may sometimes be better described as a degree of improvement in addition to measuring cure. Even if the elimination of symptoms often is the goal for a treatment and thus comprises the expected outcome, some other aspects have to be considered. 'Cure' usually refers to a single dimension. That a patient becomes symptom-free does not mean that the underlying pathophysiological process is completely reversed. The patient might experience normalisation, but structural as well as functional changes might remain. Examples of such remaining changes could be displacement of the bladder neck, a subnormal intraurethral pressure, a hyperactive bladder, or a hyperplastic prostate. When a given treatment is directed against symptoms and not against the pathophysiological process itself, we can of course never expect to cure. An alternative measure could therefore use the terms 'responders' and 'nonresponders,' which describe less extreme degrees of improvement than those implied by cure and normalisation. However, it may be necessary to divide this into degrees of response, so that differentiation may be made between maximum responders and minimal responders who gain only small benefit from the intervention. The size of such a response should exceed the value of the test-retest variation as performed and reported by the investigators.

REPORTING OF OUTCOME STUDIES

The editors of journals considering outcome studies on patients with lower urinary tract dysfunction for publication are recommended to include a passage referring to this document in their instructions for authors.

FUTURE DIRECTIONS

Considerable effort is needed to describe the way in which various measures correlate with each other. It may be a considerable time before final decisions can be made on what outcome means for different patient groups. This requires a multidimensional and multidisciplinary approach, including the continuous and active participation of all the members of our International Continence Society.

CONCLUSIONS AND RECOMMENDATIONS

Data from five groups of measures should be represented in every scientific investigation of outcome in patients with lower urinary tract dysfunction:

- Patient's observations (symptoms)
- Quantification of symptoms (e.g., urine loss)
- Physician's observations (anatomical and functional; compliance)
- Quality of life
- Socioeconomic data.

- Measurements should be directed and accurate.
- A null hypothesis should be formulated.
- Endpoints should be defined.
- A grading of response should be measured, using the terms 'responders' and 'nonresponders.'
- A multidimensional, multidisciplinary approach should be used.

Addendum

Was the study in any part supported by commercial interest?

Acknowledgements

The authors thank Drs. Andrew Fantl, Matthew Zack, and Linda Cardozo for valuable contributions to this report.

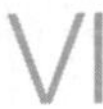

Appendix

Practical points for outcome studies in patients with lower urinary tract dysfunction*

Purpose of the study
What are the reasons for this particular study?
What do the investigators want to show?

Patient groups
Definition of patient groups
Inclusion/exclusion criteria

Disease/disorder
Causal or symptomatic treatment?
Arrest of a process?
Reversible changes?

Intervention
Description of the intervention
Intervention related complications, morbidity, and mortality

Study design and controls
Intervention studies should have a control group and should be randomised
Define endpoints
Define response criteria
Nature of trial, e.g., double-blind, placebo controlled, crossover
Adverse events, dropouts

Methods of measurement
Characterisation of methods, test-retest data in the hands of the investigators
Change in circumstances or procedures prior to and after intervention
Interindividual variation (+ differences between centers in multicenter trials)
Normal values

Statistics
Power of the study
Reason for choice of statistical method
Compliance
Statistician involved?

Time scale
Why was outcome evaluated at a particular time in relation to the intervention?
Long-term outcome?

Expected outcome
Degree of improvement
Risk-benefit analysis
Patient expectations
Quality-of-life effects
Socioeconomic factors

Interpretation of data
Comparison with outcome in other studies
Unexpected/adverse findings
Limitations
Clinical significance
Theoretical importance
Possible ways of improving the study
Conclusions for future investigations

*Whenever an outcome study on lower urinary tract dysfunction is planned, a series of questions should ideally be considered and appropriately addressed in the manuscript at the time of submission for publication. The above list serves only as a reminder. More specific information concerning the different topics is represented in the reports from the subcommittees. ICS terminology should be used wherever practicable.

Outcome measures for research in adult women with symptoms of lower urinary tract dysfunction

Neurourology and Urodynamics 17:255–262 (1998) © 1998 International Continence Society

Gunnar Lose, J Andrew Fantl, Arne Victor, Steen Walter, Thelma L Wells, Jean Wyman, and Anders Mattiasson

Produced by the Standardisation Committee of the International Continence Society, A, Mattiasson, Chairman. Subcommittee on Outcome Research in Women, G. Lose, Chairman.

INTRODUCTION

The purpose of this communication is to offer the clinical and research communities an initial attempt at incorporating outcome measurements within identifiable domains, as well as providing initial information as to the reliability of those measurements most commonly used.

Scientific evaluation of the outcome of therapeutic interventions is based on assessment before and after treatment. However, the reliability of methods and measurements used in the evaluation is often poor or unclear, which makes interpretation of outcome difficult. The reliability of a test depends on the accuracy and reproducibility of the method. The diagnostic accuracy is determined by verifying test results against a reference ('gold') standard that defines true disease status. The predictive value of a measure is considered the most important. Since it may be impossible to establish a final true diagnosis, reliability must in some cases be measured by reproducibility, which is determined by comparing results of

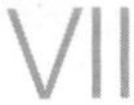

repeated examinations of the same patient.[1] Reproducibility for tests where the result is given on a continuous scale may be expressed as bias with the 95% confidence limit [Bland and Altman, 1986], while for binary tests the kappa coefficient, which adjusts the observed agreement for expected chance agreement, is used [Gjørup, 1997].

Urinary incontinence is defined as 'a condition in which involuntary urine loss is a social or hygienic problem and is objectively demonstrable.' It represents a multidimensional phenomenon with wide-reaching effects which may be quantified within various areas or domains. These areas or domains include:

1. The patient's observations (symptoms)
2. Quantification of symptoms (e.g., urine loss)
3. The clinician's observations (anatomical and functional)
4. Quality of life
5. Socioeconomic measures.

Outcome measures should be selected within the context of a specific study.

The ideal combination or measurement 'in aggregate,' particularly if belonging to different domains, will enhance the overall significance and value of the study results. A multidimensional approach is important, since the effect of intervention depends on the outcome measure chosen and may vary significantly between various domains and even within a certain domain.

DOMAIN OF SYMPTOMATOLOGY

Symptoms

General and condition-specific. Here are included a respondent's overall opinion of the condition (incontinence) and/or one or more characteristics of the condition, e.g., frequency, quantity, or magnitude. Different methods to obtain this measure include: a question with a forced choice, a graded response, a statement with a Likert scale agree-disagree response, and a statement with a visual analog graded scale response.

Recommendations/comments

There is no general symptom (opinion) measure with established methodologic reliability. Therefore, researchers should clearly describe their instrument and procedure and provide reliability data or indicate their absence.

DOMAIN OF SYMPTOM QUANTIFICATION

Diary (frequency/volume chart) [Larsson and Victor, 1988; Larsson et al., 1991; Wyman et al., 1988]

This entails a self-monitored record of selected lower urinary functions kept for specific time periods. Selected variables include episodes of incontinence/pad use frequency (diurnal and nocturnal), voiding/toileting frequency (diurnal and nocturnal), total voided volume, mean voided volume, and largest single void. Accuracy depends on the patient's ability to follow instructions but is still difficult to assess because there is no gold standard against which the test result can be compared. Reproducibility depends on the parameter used and improves with an increase in the number of days that self-recording is obtained.

The highest reproducibility has been found for mean voided volume.

The circumstances under which a diary is kept should be approximate to those of everyday life, and should be similar before and after intervention to allow for meaningful comparison.

Recommendations/comments

A diary kept for a minimum of three days is recommended as an outcome measure.

Pad-weighing tests [Lose and Versi, 1992; Victor, 1990]

Pad tests can be divided into short-term tests, generally performed under standardized conditions as office tests, and long-term tests, generally performed by the patient at home during 24–48 hr.

Accuracy is difficult to assess. Reproducibility is generally poor, but improves if the circumstances are standardized as much as possible. For long-term tests, the test period should be sufficiently long.

[1] Other terms might have been chosen to denote accuracy and reproducibility. Terms such as precision, validity, observer or interrater variability, observer error, and efficacy have been used. At the moment it does not seem possible to establish a commonly accepted terminology. Readers of papers about reliability must therefore in each case examine the author's use of the terms.

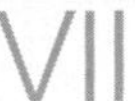

Recommendations/comments

Pad-weighing offers a potential for quantifying the degree of incontinence. For short-term tests, the experimental conditions should be described. Standardized bladder filling volumes are generally recommended. For long-term tests, the time period should be as long as practical.

DOMAIN OF CLINICIAN'S OBSERVATIONS

Pelvic muscle activity

This is the force of voluntary pelvic muscle contraction determined in direct (digital or air pressure) or indirect (surface electromyography) measures.

Accuracy is difficult to assess. Test-retest data are mainly based on correlations analysis, which is problematic to interpret.

Recommendations/comments

At this time there is no conclusive information as to the potential of muscle activity as an outcome measure.

Researchers should clearly describe their instrument and procedure and provide reliability data or indicate their absence.

Cystometry

Cystometry variables include sensation, compliance, capacity, and activity of the bladder. The investigation can be carried out in a stationary or ambulatory setting. Data obtained are method-dependent.

Accuracy is difficult to assess, since variation in various parameters is significant [Lose and Thyssen, 1996; Sørensen et al., 1988; Sørensen, 1988].

Recommendations/comments

It is recommended that authors provide reproducibility data or indicate their absence.

Uroflowmetry

Normal female voiding produces a bell-shaped curve on uroflowmetry. Voiding dysfunctions may give rise to an intermittent or multiple peaked flow, suggesting either abdominal straining, unsustained bladder contractions, intermittent sphincter contractions, or bladder outlet obstruction.

Maximum and average flow are directly dependent upon voided volume. Consequently, interpretation and comparison of flow rates require that the voided volume is taken into account. Various nomograms are available. Flow rate depends to a lesser extent on age and sex, while parity, weight, menstrual cycle phase, or menopause status seem not to influence flow rate [Fantl et al., 1982].

A certain test-retest variation exists in terms of flow rates and pattern [Sørensen et al., 1988; Sørensen, 1988].

Recommendations/comments

Uroflowmetry represents a simple initial test to assess the emptying phase of the lower urinary tract. However, researchers should describe their methodology and provide reproducibility data or indicate their absence.

Pressure-flow study

This represents the simultaneous study of urine flow and intravesical or detrusor pressure during voluntary voiding. Graphic plotting of pressure-flow data enables classification of individual patients into one of the following groups: obstructed, equivocal, or unobstructed patterns.

In patients with an irregular micturition pattern, the technique should be accomplished with simultaneous EMG recording to allow differentiation between abdominal straining, intermittent detrusor contraction, or detrusor/sphincter dyssynergia. Pressure-flow data are subject to significant test-retest variation [Lose and Thyssen, 1996].

Recommendations/comments

Researchers should describe their methodology and reproducibility data or indicate their absence.

Electromyography

Electromyographic (EMG) recordings are performed to examine the activity (behavior) of pelvic and sphincter muscles during different maneuvers, particularly during bladder filling and voiding. This type of EMG is also called kinesiologic EMG. Both surface and intramuscular electrodes may be used for recording. Surface electrodes are more nonselective and may be used for assessing the overall behavior of the muscle bulk underlying the electrodes. Intramuscular electrodes (needle or wire) provide more selective recordings of higher quality, but reflect only the activity of a small muscle volume.

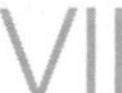

Electromyographic techniques (concentric-needle EMG, single-fiber EMG) allow acquisition of electrophysiologic parameters that define a striated muscle as normal or abnormal. With concentric-needle EMG, muscle denervation and reinnervation can be assessed by recording of spontaneous activity and motor-unit action potentials. Single-fiber EMG reveals muscle changes due to reinnervation by recording muscle-fiber density [Flink, 1997; Vodusêk, 1996].

The reliability of EMG recordings is poorly determined.

Recommendations/comments

Surface electrodes can be used to identify striated muscle activity during different maneuvers, particularly during bladder filling and voiding, and also as a biofeedback therapeutic technique.

Intramuscular electrodes can be used in the more precise studies to identify the activity patterns of individual striated muscles. Special needle electrodes are required to assess denervation and reinnervation of the pelvic floor muscles and striated sphincters.

Researchers should describe their methodology and reproducibility data or indicate their absence.

Nerve stimulation

This entails neurophysiological tests involving stimulation of nervous system structures.

Electrical and magnetic stimulators are used to depolarize nervous structures (particularly the pudendal nerve and its branches, sacral roots, and the motor cortex). Recordings are obtained both from pelvic floor muscles and striated sphincters, but also from nerve structures, particularly over the somatosensory cortex. Several tests exist and can be broadly grouped into evoked potentials and reflex responses.

The reproducibility of several tests is fairly acceptable if the tests are performed under standardized conditions, but no overall accepted standards for individual tests as yet exist.

Recommendations/comments

The clinical usefulness of these tests has not yet been clarified. They seem to be helpful in research. Researchers should describe their methodology and their laboratories' normal values. They should indicate reproducibility data or indicate their absence.

Urethral pressure measurement

Conceptually, urethral closure pressure represents the ability of the urethra to prevent urine leakage. Technically, it represents the difference between the pressure at one given point in the urethra and the simultaneously recorded pressure in the bladder.

Measurements of urethral closure pressure may be made at one point in the urethra over a period of time (continuous urethral pressure recording), or at several points along the urethra consecutively, forming a urethral pressure profile (UPP). These measurements can be made at rest or during exertion.

The results of urethral pressure measurements are highly influenced by methodological and biological factors and have been found to have significant test-retest variability. The overlap between both the static and dynamic urethral closure measurements in continent and incontinent women is significant [Lose, 1997].

Recommendations/comments

Urethral pressure profile parameters are of limited value in the assessment of urethral sphincter function. Urethral pressure measurement may be useful in evaluating local pathology (e.g., diverticulum and stricture), in assessment of changes with intervention, and in therapeutic selection (e.g., intrinsic sphincter deficiency).

Imaging

Imaging techniques in terms of radiography, ultrasound, and magnetic resonance imaging (MRI) are used to provide morphological and functional information on the lower urinary tract and the pelvic floor. Until now, as with conventional radiology, neither ultrasound nor MRI appeared to provide conclusive and discriminatory diagnostic information. Scant information is available on reproducibility of measurement, while significant inter- and intraobserver variation in the assessment of radiography pictures has been reported.

Recommendations/comments

At this time, imaging techniques are of limited value as outcome measures in female incontinence. Researchers should clearly describe their instrument and procedure and provide reliability data or indicate their absence.

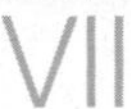

DOMAIN OF QUALITY-OF-LIFE MEASUREMENTS

Health-related quality of life (HRQOL) is a multidimensional construct that refers to an individual's perceptions of the effect of a health condition or disease and its subsequent treatment. Primary domains of HRQOL include physical, psychological, and social functioning, overall life satisfaction/well-being, and perceptions of health status. Secondary domains include somatic sensations (symptoms), sleep disturbance, intimacy and sexual functioning, and personal productivity (e.g., household, occupational, volunteer, or community activities).

Three measurement approaches are commonly used to assess HRQOL: generic, condition-specific, and dimension-specific. Generic HRQOL instruments are designed to be used across multiple disease states or conditions, and allow for comparisons across groups by having established age and gender norms. Condition-specific instruments are designed to measure the impact of a particular disease or condition. These instruments tend to be more responsive than generic instruments in detecting treatment effects. Symptom scales are considered condition-specific; generally, these scales should include measurement of the presence of a symptom as well as its 'bothersome' or 'troublesome' nature. The majority of generic and condition-specific instruments are multidimensional, i.e., they measure more than one aspect of HRQOL. Dimension-specific instruments, in contrast, are designed to assess a single component of HRQOL, such as emotional distress. The trend in assessing HRQOL outcomes has been toward the use of a multidimensional generic and/or condition-specific instrument, supplemented with dimension-specific instruments, as needed [Grimby et al., 1993; Shumaker et al., 1994; Wagner et al., 1996; Naughton and Wyman, 1997].

Recommendations/comments

The selection of an HRQOL instrument should be based upon the purpose of the study. Descriptive or epidemiological studies should consider both generic and condition-specific instruments. Intervention studies should include a condition-specific instrument. Dimension-specific instruments should be used when more detail about a specific subdomain of HRQOL is desired. Researchers should define HRQOL as it is conceptualized for their study, clearly describe their instrument(s) and data collection, and provide reliability data if available.

It is recommended that researchers select instruments with reliability and sensitivity. In adopting HRQOL instruments, we recommend comparing results obtained in the study population with published norms. If a new condition-specific instrument will be used in a study, adequate pretesting should be done to establish its clinimetric characteristics (e.g., reliability and sensitivity).

DOMAIN OF SOCIOECONOMIC COSTS

Cost-effectiveness analysis is a method to decide on the relative merits of alternative courses of action by comparing costs to achieve a given health effect. Costs can be divided into direct and indirect costs. Direct costs are all costs incurred in the routine care, diagnosis, treatment, and management of adverse consequences associated with treatment or with being incontinent, which can be assessed from the market value of goods and services. Indirect costs are those incurred as a result of being incontinent or of having to care for someone who is incontinent. These opportunity costs, e.g., time lost enjoying leisure activity or engaging in productive effort, are more difficult to quantify, and thus, are usually not measured. If morbidity and mortality are considered, they should be converted to a monetary value.

Effectiveness is characterized as a specific health outcome, e.g., disease prevented or cured, function restored, or symptoms alleviated.

Direct costs are all costs incurred in routine care, diagnosis, treatment of incontinence, and management of adverse consequences associated with treatment or with being incontinent. Indirect costs are those incurred as a result of being incontinent or having to care for someone who is incontinent. These opportunity costs, e.g., time lost enjoying leisure activity or engaging in productive effort, are more difficult to quantify, and thus, are usually not measured.

Recommendations/comments

The types of costs and how they are determined should be clearly articulated. Typical resource uses to be collected in a study include:

1. Clinician's time/service
2. Laboratory and imaging studies
3. Treatment expenses (e.g., procedural charges, medication costs)
4. Supplies (disposable and reusable products)
5. Side and adverse effects and their management

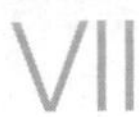

6. Travel costs to obtain health care
7. Loss of wages from receiving health care or surgery.

CONCLUSIONS

Research on lower urinary tract symptoms in adult women remains impaired by lack of standardization of outcome variables. The use of primary and secondary outcomes on different areas or domains should help overcome some of these difficulties. However, it is imperative that investigators focus attention on these issues. Studies leading to the development and standardization of outcomes should be entertained. Success in this regard will not only enhance knowledge of actual treatment strategies but stimulate the development of new ones.

REFERENCES

Bland J A, Altman D G (1986) Statistical method for assessing agreement between two methods of clinical measurement. Lancet 1: 307–310

Fantl J A, Smith P S, Schneider V, Hurt W G, Dunn L J (1982) Fluid weight uroflowmetry in women. Am J Obstet Gynecol 145: 1017–1024

Flink R (1997) Clinical neurophysiological methods for investigating the lower urinary tract in patients with micturition disorders. Acta Obstet Gynecol Scand [Suppl] 166: 50–58

Gjørup T (1997) Reliability of diagnostic tests. Acta Obstet Gynecol Scand [Suppl] 166: 9–14

Grimby A, Milson L, Molander U, Wiklund I, Ekelund P (1993) The influence of urinary incontinence on the quality of life of elderly women. Age Ageing 22: 82–89

Larsson G, Victor A (1988) Micturition patterns in a healthy female population, studied with a frequency/volume chart. Scand J Urol Nephrol [Suppl] 144: 53–57

Larsson G, Abrams P, Victor A (1991) The frequency/volume chart in detrusor instability. Neurourol Urodyn 10: 533–543

Lose G (1997) Urethral pressure testing. Acta Obset Gynecol Scand [Suppl] 166: 39–42

Lose G, Thyssen H (1996) Reproducibility of cystometry and pressure-flow parameters in female patients. Neurourol Urodyn 15: 302–303

Lose G, Versi E (1992) Pad-weighing tests in the diagnosis and quantification of incontinence. Int Urogynecol J 3: 324–328.

Naughton M J, Wyman J F (1997) Quality of life of geriatric patients with lower urinary tract dysfunctions. Am J Med Sci 314: 219–224

Shumaker S A, Wyman J F, Uebersac J, McClish D K, Fantl J A (1994) Health-related quality of life measures for women with urinary incontinence: The urogenital Distress Inventory and the Incontinence Impact Questionnaire. Quality Life Res 3: 291–306

Sørensen S (1988) Urodynamic investigations and the reproducibility in healthy postmenopausal females. Scand J Urol Nephrol [Suppl] 114: 42–47

Sørensen S, Gregersen H, Sørensen M (1988) Long term reproducibility of urodynamic investigation in healthy females. Scand J Urol Nephrol [Suppl] 114: 35–41

Victor A (1990) Pad weighing tests – A simple method to quantitate urinary incontinence. Ann Med 22: 443–447

Vodusêk D B (1996) Evoked potential testing. Urol Clin North Am 23: 427–446

Wagner T H, Patrick D L, Bueschina D P (1996) Quality of life of persons with urinary incontinence. Development of a new measure. Urology 47: 67–73

Wyman J F, Choi S C, Harkins S W, Wilson M S, Fantl J A (1988) The urinary diary in evaluation of incontinent women: A test-retest analysis. Obstet Gynecol 71: 812–817

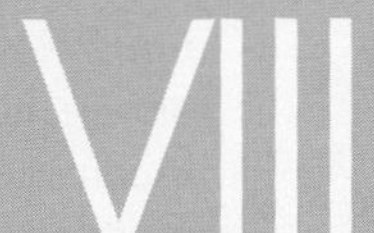
APPENDIX VIII

Outcome measures for research of lower urinary tract dysfunction in frail older people

Neurourology and Urodynamics 17:273–281 (1998) © 1998 International Continence Society

D Fonda, N M Resnick, J Colling, K Burgio, J G Ouslander, C Norton, P Ekelund, E Versi, and A Mattiasson

Produced by the Standardisation Committee of the International Continance Society, A. Mattiasson, Chairman. Subcommittee on Outcome Research in Frail Older People, D. Fonda, Chairman.

INTRODUCTION

The aim of this paper is primarily to provide a framework for investigators conducting research on incontinence in frail older people. Since it is difficult to precisely define 'frailty,' the definition used in this paper is 'any person over age 65 years with incontinence of urine who does not leave their place of residence without assistance of others, or a person with dementia, or a person who has been admitted to a long-term care facility.' These people usually suffer from multiple medical conditions and disabilities (comorbidity), which results in them becoming homebound or institutionalized. Because they require the assistance of others to perform some or all of the most basic activities of daily living (ADLs), including bathing, dressing, toileting, and ambulating, results from younger populations or from older people without disabilities cannot necessarily be extrapolated to this population. For this population there is little validated research showing long-term efficacy of treatment for urinary incontinence.

If incontinence develops in healthy older people, its management is generally similar to the approach taken in younger individuals, except that greater caution should be taken when pharmacological intervention is being considered because of the susceptibility of older people to adverse drug reactions. This paper therefore does not focus on the fit older person, and in the absence of data to the contrary, the same outcome measures should be used as for adults of the same sex [Mattiasson et al., 1998]. This paper deals with lower urinary tract dysfunction with a major emphasis on incontinence. Nocturia is a significant problem for older people, and the principles alluded to in this paper cover this area.

Because of the frailty of this population, all patients being considered for entry into a research protocol should be assessed for coexisting reversible or modifiable (comorbid) factors such as fecal impaction, confusional states, functional disabilities, or use of medication which may be contributing to incontinence or might affect the outcome of the study. No patient should receive another intervention until such transient causes have been addressed. The extent of invasive testing should balance study requirements with the benefits, risks, and inconvenience to the patient.

Research in this population is difficult because of:

The heterogeneity of this population, resulting in difficulty in designing studies that account for comorbidity, drug use, intercurrent illness, and shorter life expectancy
Lack of standardized terminology to define and measure cure and improvement
Lack of validated research tools to measure baseline and outcome variables in the frail elderly
Lack of long-term follow-up to gauge impact, durability, and applicability of the intervention
Lack of information of the natural history of incontinence in this group.

CONSIDERATIONS IN STUDY DESIGN

General principles in designing a study on lower urinary tract dysfunction have been published elsewhere and apply equally in this group [Mattiasson et al., 1998]. Below are listed some additional considerations for research in incontinence involving the frail elderly.

Baseline clinical data

The following baseline clinical data should be considered when designing a study in the frail older population. Relevant information should be included in the final report of the study's findings.

Descriptive data
- Type of setting of the study, e.g., home, nursing home
- Patient-staff ratio (where staff are involved in the management protocol)
- Usual continence care
- Direct and indirect costs of current care
- Patient, family, and/or staff expectations
- Age and gender
- Description of care givers (e.g., training, qualifications)
- System incentives or disincentives that may influence management options (e.g., government funding).

Symptoms and investigations
- Type of symptoms
- Duration of symptoms
- Response to prior treatment (e.g., pharmacological, surgical, behavioral)
- Midstream urine for culture and sensitivities
- Postvoid residual urine estimation.

Associated factors
- Environmental factors that might contribute to incontinence (e.g., distance to toilet, use of continence aids or appliances)
- Associated comorbid conditions that might be contributing to incontinence or the effectiveness of intervention
- Bowel status (e.g., constipation, incontinence)
- Functional level of the patients (by use of a standardized scale such as Barthel or Katz ADL scales [Katz et al., 1963, Mahoney et al., 1965])
- Cognitive state/function of the patients (by use of a standardized scale such as the Mini-mental Scale Examination [Folstein et al., 1979])
- Concurrent medications that could contribute to incontinence or affect outcome of treatment (e.g., sedatives, diuretics, alcohol)
- Fluid intake.

Description of study design

Details of study design should be provided, including methodology, recruitment, inclusion and exclusion criteria, interventions, outcome measures to be used, and statistical methods. Further information has been provided on guidelines for study design by the ICS [Mattiasson et al., 1998].

Outcome data

To determine the effect of an intervention, accurate, valid, and meaningful outcome variables are needed. It is most important to define the major endpoints prior to commencing studies. Baseline diagnostic data should be gathered in order to characterize the patient's condition and to document the severity of incontinence (see Outcome Measurements, below). The selection of an outcome variable depends on the nature of the intervention being studied, e.g., pharmacological, surgical, or behavioral. Successful short-term interventions should, wherever possible, have long-term follow-up provided (at least 12 months) in order to gauge more accurately their impact, durability, and relevance in this frail population.

There are age-specific influences on lower urinary tract function, and normative data are generally lacking in this frail population. In addition, test-retest

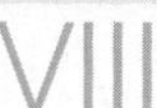

reliability and sensitivity to change of the more invasive measures of lower urinary tract function are poorly documented in the frail elderly. It is, therefore, the belief of the committee that it is not appropriate to repeat invasive measures at follow-up in this frail population unless these measures are fundamental in understanding components of the intervention being studied.

The following information, which could impact on outcome, should wherever possible be addressed and reported at time of follow-up:

Number and reason for dropouts and deaths (i.e., were they trial-related?)
Compliance issues (by patients, staff, or caregivers), such as compliance to exercise programs, toileting protocols, or drug use
Type of bladder training or toileting programs (if any)
Other intercurrent treatment not directly related to bladder function that might impact on outcome
Medication which might impact on incontinence/continence
Socioeconomic data, including impact of the intervention on the patient
Changes in caregiver or staff status or numbers
Cost of treatment
Cost-benefit data
Patient and/or caregiver satisfaction with the intervention
Risk-benefit data

Recommendations/comments

Because comorbidity and drug use contribute to the presence and severity of continence in this population, they should be addressed and/or stabilized before patients are enrolled. In any research project, it is essential to clearly determine endpoints at the outset.

OUTCOME MEASUREMENTS

In this section, the key outcome areas are identified and recommendations are made which may be of use to researchers. In keeping with the format of the ICS Outcomes Standards Reports, outcome measurements for frail elderly people are covered under the following five headings: patient observations and symptoms; documentation of the symptoms; anatomical and functional measures; quality-of-life measures; and socioeconomic measures.

Measurement of patient observations and symptoms

History alone is insufficient in diagnosing the etiology of bladder dysfunction. In the frail older person this is compounded by the age-associated decline in cognitive function and increase in depression. Caregivers may be able to provide important supplementary or supportive information. One study has recently validated a nonurodynamic-based diagnostic algorithm [Resnick et al., 1996].

Recommendations/comments

Research in this group should not be based solely on patients' subjective reporting of symptoms. Patient-derived symptoms response as an outcome measure should be supplemented where necessary by data derived from caregivers.

Documentation of urine loss

Bladder diaries

Bladder diaries are simple and noninvasive and have the potential to be reliable and sensitive to therapeutic intervention, especially when completed by competent staff. However, accuracy of self-report data is always a matter of concern, and interpretation of what constitutes clinical vs. statistical significance is difficult. Bladder diaries have not been validated when completed by the frail housebound or institutionalized elderly, although they may prove accurate for the cognitively intact and motivated frail older person. Bladder diaries completed by others such as caregivers or staff (wet checks), or pad weighing, are alternatives (see below).

Recommendations/comments

Bladder diaries should be a useful outcome measure for hospitalized or institutionalized older people. The usefulness of bladder diaries as an outcome measure when completed by the frail elderly or their 'untrained' carers has not yet been validated.

Pad-weighing tests

Difficulties with determining wetness can be overcome by weighing pads before and after specified time intervals. To standardize the pad tests, the ICS introduced the 1-hr pad-weighing test, which measures urine loss as weight gain of perineal pads under standardized conditions [Abrams et al., 1988]. Only

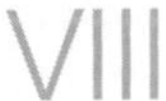

one relevant study of the 1-hr pad-weighing test in frail elderly could be identified. The 24-hr inpatient measurement of urine leakage of frail elderly patients by staff was more feasible and sensitive than the 1-hr pad test; reducibility was not directly assessed [Griffiths et al., 1991]. The 48-hr home pad test with patients weighing their own pads has been shown to be reliable for quantifying urine loss in cognitively intact and reasonably independent (but not 'frail') elderly incontinent women; reproducibility was not assessed [Ekelund et al., 1988].

The principal advantages in performing pad tests at home are simplicity, cost-effectiveness (as hospital personnel are not required), and the relaxed environment, which reproduces more accurately the conditions leading to incontinence when compared with the relatively unfamiliar hospital or clinic setting. It is important to provide the patient with careful written and oral instructions before attempting the test. Certain forms of handicap, such as dementia, reduced mobility, physical handicap, fecal incontinence, or defective vision, pose problems which could in some cases be compensated for by involving a caregiver in the test procedure. It should be noted that some pads leak, further reducing reliability and accuracy of this test.

Recommendations/comments

Pad-weighing offers the potential for quantifying the degree of incontinence in older patients and can be useful in the hospital setting. Further data are still required to establish its usefulness in the frail elderly, especially in those confined to home.

Wet checks

Wet checks consist of examining the patient at regular intervals for leakage. Such checks are a commonly used measure of incontinence in nursing home residents. At least 10 clinical studies of frail incontinent elderly have been published using wet checks as an outcome measure. The exact method of determining wet or dry status is not well-described in any of the studies, while the frequency of checks varied from 1–4 hourly. Nonetheless, despite these limitation, wet checks appear to be a reliable means of documenting incontinence [Hu et al., 1989; Colling et al., 1992, 1995]. However, it should be noted that in one study, when an electronic monitor was used to document incontinence, there was considerable disagreement noted with caregivers underreporting wet episodes [Colling et al., 1995]. The Incontinence Monitoring Record (which is a record of whether the patient is wet on regular checking), particularly the colored form, has been shown in one study to be a reliable documentation tool when completed by nurses' aides [Ouslander et al., 1986].

Although these instruments are practical, understandable, and commonly used outcome measures, the following should be considered:

- It is difficult to get ward staff to reliably check and record wetness. Hence for research purposes, dedicated research staff may be needed to record these data.
- It is sometimes difficult to correctly identify wet absorbent products now, because many of them have materials which 'wick' away the moisture, making it impossible to see and even difficult to feel moisture.
- Many institutes now require the use of universal precautions in handling of body fluids, which would include performing wet checks. If litmus paper is used to identify moisture, a false negative can result unless it is placed where it is likely to pick up the urine. Conversely, a false positive can occur when moisture from the skin shows up on litmus paper.
- Wet checks are intrusive and invasive to patients, and in some cases may actually stimulate patients to void.
- Absolute pad counts are not a reliable outcome measure, as it is most difficult to impose consistent criteria for changing of pads.
- While the electronic monitor shows promise of increasing the accuracy of identifying wet episodes, its use has not yet been well-studied in the frail elderly and it is not yet available commercially.

Recommendations/comments

The wet-check method of assessing incontinence appears to be both a practical and reliable tool to assess outcome in dependent older patients, provided attention is given to the above considerations. Compliance of staff necessitates education and close supervision. The more frequent the 'checking,' e.g., hourly, the more likely the data will be reliable for the actual number of wet episodes.

Anatomical and functional measurements

'Simple' cystometry

Simple cystometry is a relatively inexpensive form of single-channel water cystometry, which can be performed without specialized equipment in an outpatient clinic, acute hospital, nursing home, or home setting. It is not so feasible and accurate in the severely cognitively impaired. The procedure is generally well-tolerated and adds little time to that needed for a postvoid residual determination by catheterization. While studies have shown comparability of results from simple and multichannel cystometry in an outpatient setting, this has not been demonstrated in institutional settings [Ouslander et al., 1988; Fonda et al., 1993]. The major disadvantage is the lack of an abdominal pressure measurement. Adequate data on the test-retest reliability of simple cystometry do not exist. There are no data to support the usefulness of simple cystometry as an outcome measurement, nor in predicting responsiveness to various interventions or in elucidating the mechanism of action of interventions for geriatric incontinence.

Recommendations/comments

Simple cystometry has not been validated as an outcome measure for research in frail patients.

Multichannel urodynamics

The few available studies indicate that, when carefully performed, multichannel urodynamic testing of the frail elderly is feasible and safe, and reproducibly yields the same diagnosis. Fluoroscopic monitoring appears to increase its accuracy by facilitating detection of the low-pressure involuntary contractions that are more common in the frail elderly. However, compared with urodynamic evaluation of more robust individuals, testing in this population is technically more difficult to conduct, is less available, requires additional personnel, and is probably more susceptible to artifact. Furthermore, normative data are lacking for this population.

Few investigators have employed multichannel urodynamics as an outcome measure in the frail elderly. Cystometric capacity and reduced bladder sensation (both measured after therapy) have been shown to correlate with response to oxybutynin treatment [Griffiths et al., 1996]. In a small study, response to prostatectomy correlated with the severity of obstruction on initial pressure/flow testing, despite persistence of unstable contractions in all patients but one [Gormley et al., 1993].

Recommendations/comments

Complex urodynamic testing has not been evaluated sufficiently to determine its utility as an outcome measure in the frail elderly.

Pelvic muscle strength

Pelvic muscle exercises may be of value in management of incontinence, either by increasing pelvic muscle strength or as a form of biofeedback. The force of voluntary pelvic muscle contraction can be determined directly (digitally or by air pressure) or indirectly (surface electromyography). For the frail elderly there are no validated data on the measurement of pelvic muscle strength as an outcome measure following teaching of pelvic floor exercises.

Recommendations/comments

At present, measurement of pelvic muscle strength before and after treatment has not been validated as a useful outcome measure for frail older patients.

Ultrasound

Estimation of residual urine is an important adjunct to investigation of older patients, especially before addition of drugs that may impair bladder emptying. Estimation of postvoid residual by a portable ultrasound device has been shown to correlate well with that measured by catheterization [Griffiths et al., 1992]. Sensitivity may not be so good when volumes are greater than 200 ml as measured by catheter, in which case repeated measurements may be necessary to exclude a very high postvoid residual [Ouslander et al., 1994]. Improvement in the equipment's design since this study may have improved its accuracy.

Recommendations/comments

Use of ultrasound for residual urine estimation offers much potential as a convenient noninvasive research tool for frail older people, especially for drug or surgical interventions that may affect bladder emptying. Further studies are required to validate the newer portable models.

Quality-of-life measurements

Health-related quality of life (HRQL) is a multidimensional concept that refers to an individual's evaluation and satisfaction with his/her physical, social, and psychological health, as well as total well-being. This can be measured by a generic or condition-specific instrument. HRQL is important to measure, because a patient's life quality may improve even without change in degree of incontinence; conversely, improved continence status may not result in improved life quality. Unfortunately, few HRQL instruments have been tested for reliability, validity, and responsiveness in incontinent populations, let alone in a frail elderly population.

Recommendations/comments

There is a need to develop tools to measure HRQL for frail elderly incontinent people.

Socioeconomic measurements

Economic impact of continence interventions can be measured by cost, cost-benefit, and cost-effectiveness. To be of real value, all costs related to actual health expenditure should be estimated before and after the intervention. This includes those related to treatment (e.g., drugs, surgery, nursing time on bladder training) and those related to managing any incontinence (e.g., pads, skin care products, laundry, caregiver time).

Cost-benefit is even more difficult to assess, as it is unclear how to define 'benefit' in this population. For example, Schnelle et al. [1995] showed modest improvement in the degree of incontinence, but at increased cost compared to usual care. Is it better to be 'socially continent' (dry with the assistance of pads or aids) and only occasionally disturbed by staff to change pads, or to be toileted frequently and be less wet at a greater staff cost but with a need to still wear pads?

Costs also include more nebulous areas which are borne by society as a whole rather than the health care system, such as work days lost for caregivers, impact of incontinence on the caregivers, or need for institutional care. While it is often stated that incontinence is a major factor in referral for institutional care, there are few convincing data to support this assertion.

Recommendations/comments

There is a need to develop tools to help evaluate cost, cost-benefit, and cost-effectiveness for this population.

CONCLUSIONS

Research methodology for studying incontinence in the frail and housebound elderly is fraught with pitfalls. This has compromised the usefulness of past research. There is a great need for basic research to validate practical and useful outcome measures that will allow meaningful results to be obtained. In addition, an understanding is required of the importance of defining clinical rather than statistical significance.

REFERENCES

Abrams P, Blaivas J G, Stanton S L, Andersen J T (1988) The standardisation of terminology of lower urinary tract function. Scand J Urol Nephrol [Suppl] 114: 5–19.

Colling J, Ouslander J G, Hadley B J. Campbell E (1992) The effects of patterned urge response toiletting (PURT) on urinary incontinence among nursing home residents. J Am Geriatr Soc 40: 135–141

Colling J, Hadley B J, Campbell E, Eisch J, Newman D (1995) 'Continence Program for Care Dependent Elderly. Final Report.' NIH-NCNR-NR 01554. Bethesda, M D

Ekelund P, Bergstrom H, Milsom I, et al. (1988) Quantification of urinary incontinence in elderly women with the 48-hour pad test. Arch Gerontol Geriatr 7: 281–287

Folstein M F, Folstein S, McHugh P R (1975) Mini Mental State: A practical method for grading the cognitive state of patients for the clinician. J Psychiatr Res 12: 189–198

Fonda D, Brimage P J, D'Astoli M (1993) A comparison of simple cystometry and multichannel cystometry in the assessment of urinary incontinence in an elderly outpatient population. Urology 42: 536–540

Gormley E A, Griffiths D J, McCracken P N. Harrison G M, McPhee M S (1993) Effect of transurethral resection of the prostate on detrusor instability and urge incontinence in elderly males. Neurourol Urodyn 12: 445–453, 1993

Griffiths D J, McCracken P N, Harrison G M (1991) Incontinence in the elderly: Objective demonstration and quantitative assessment. Br J Urol 67: 467–471

Griffiths D J, McCracken P N, Harrison G M, Gormley E A (1992) Characteristics of urinary incontinence in elderly patients studied by 24 hour monitoring and urodynamic testing. Age Ageing 21: 195–201

Griffiths D J, McCracken P N, Harrison G M, Moore KEN (1996) Urge incontinence in elderly people: Factors predicting the severity of urine loss before and after pharmacological treatment. Neurourol Urodyn 15: 53–57

Hu T-W, Igou J F, Kaltreider D L, et al. (1989) A clinical trial of a behavioral therapy to reduce urinary incontinence in nursing homes. JAMA 261: 2656–2662

Katz S, Ford A, Moskowitz R, et al. (1963) The index of ADL: A standardized measurement of biological and psychosocial function. JAMA 185: 914–919

Mahoney F I, Barthel D W (1965) Functional evaluation: The Barthel Index. Md State Med J 14: 61–65

Mattiasson A, Djurhuus J C, Fantl A, Fonda D, Nordling J,

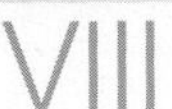

Stohrer M (1998) Standardization of outcome studies in patients with lower urinary tract dysfunction: A report on general principles from the Standardisation Committee of the International Continence Society. Neurourol Urodyn (this issue).

Ouslander J G, Uman H N, Uman G C (1986) Development and testing of an incontinence monitoring record. J Am Geriatr Soc 34: 83–90

Ouslander J G, Leach G E, Abelson S, Staskin D R, Blaustein J, Raz S (1988) Simple versus multichannel cystometry in the evaluation of bladder function in an incontinent geriatric population. J Urol 140: 1482–1486

Ouslander J G, Simmons S, Tuico E, Nigam J G, Fingold S, Bates-Jensen B, Schnelle J F (1994) Use of a portable ultrasound device to measure post-void residual volume among incontinent nursing home residents. J Am Geriatr Soc 42: 1189–1192.

Resnick N M, Brandeis G H, Baumann M M, Morris J N (1996) Evaluating a national assessment strategy for urinary incontinence in nursing home residents: Reliability of the Minimum Data Set and validity of the Resident Assessment Protocol. Neurourol Urodyn 15: 583–598

Schnelle J F, Keeler E, Hays R D, Simmons S, Ouslander J G, Siu A L (1995) A cost value analysis of two interventions with incontinent nursing home residents. J Am Geriatr Soc 43: 1112–1117

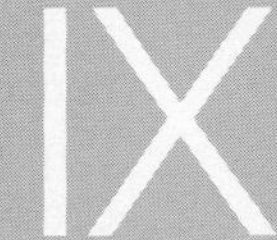

The standardisation of terminology in neurogenic lower urinary tract dysfunction

Neurourology and Urodynamics 18:139–158 (1999) © 1999 International Continence Society

Manfred Stöhrer, Mark Goepel, Atsuo Kondo, Guus Kramer, Helmut Madersbacher, Richard Millard, Alain Rossier, and Jean-Jacques Wyndaele

Produced by the Standardization Committee of the International Continence Society, A. Mattiasson, Chairman. Subcommittee on Terminology in Patients with Neurogenic Lower Urinary Tract Dysfunction. M. Stöhrer, Chairman.

1. INTRODUCTION

This report has been produced at the request of the International Continence Society. It was approved at the twenty-eighth annual meeting of the Society in Jerusalem.

The terminology used in neurogenic lower urinary tract dysfunction developed over the years, defined by neurologists, neurological, and urological surgeons. Because of the particular intents of each specialist, confusion exists on the various terminologies used and on their definitions. The International Continence Society did not define in detail the procedures and conditions in neurogenic lower urinary tract dysfunction. During our discussions the need for standardization of this terminology became obvious.

This report follows the earlier standardization report for lower urinary tract dysfunction [Abrams et al., 1988, 1990] and is adapted to the specific group of patients with neurogenic lower urinary tract dysfunction. Terms defined in the earlier report are marked (*) and their definitions not repeated here. New or adapted definitions follow *the terms in italics*.

Any pertinent texts repeated from the earlier report are marked (with shading). If they are not repeated completely, this is marked by the term (abbreviated).

Recently, the International Continence Society published a dedicated standardization report on pressure-flow studies [Griffiths et al., 1997]. This adapts and extends the earlier report with respect to pressure and flow plots and the analysis of the results and provides a provisional standard. Some new definitions are added, some existing ones changed, and some others no longer used. (Changed) definitions from this second report are marked differently ($^{+}$).

Two more reports from the International Continence Society are in preparation and bear a relationship to the present report: A general report on Good Urodynamic Practice [Schäfer et al.] and a dedicated report on Standardization of Ambulatory Urodynamic Monitoring [Van Waalwijk et al.]. This document is intended to be complementary to the mentioned reports and to be consistent in particular with the recommendations in the report of Schäfer et al.

Neurogenic lower urinary tract dysfunction is lower urinary tract dysfunction due to disturbance of the neurological control mechanisms. Neurogenic lower urinary tract dysfunction thus can be diagnosed in presence of neurological pathology only.

2. CLINICAL ASSESSMENT

Before any functional investigation is planned, a basic general and specific diagnosis should be performed. In the present context of neurogenic lower urinary tract dysfunction, part of this diagnosis is specific for neurogenic pathology and its possible sequelae. The clinical assessment of patients with neurogenic lower urinary tract dysfunction includes and extends that for other lower urinary tract dysfunction.

The latter should consist of a detailed history, a frequency/volume chart and a physical examination.

In urinary incontinence, leakage should be demonstrated objectively. These data are indispensable for reliable interpretation of the urodynamic results in neurogenic lower urinary tract dysfunction.

2.1 History

2.1.1 General history

The general history should include questions relevant to neurological and congenital abnormalities as well as information on previous urinary infections and relevant surgery. Information must be obtained on medication with known or possible effects on the lower urinary tract. The general history should also include the assessment of menstrual, sexual, and bowel function, and obstetric history.

Symptoms of any metabolic disorder or neurological disease that may induce neurogenic lower urinary tract dysfunction must be checked particularly. Presence of spasticity or autonomic dysreflexia must be noted. A list of items of particular importance is

- Neurological complaints
- Congenical anomalies with possible neurological impact
- Metabolic disorders with possible neurological impact
- Preceding therapy, including surgical interventions
- Present medication
- Continence/incontinence (see urinary history)
- Bladder sensation (see urinary history)
- Mode and type of voiding (see urinary history)
- Infections of the lower urinary tract
- Defecation, including possible faecal incontinence (see defecation history)
- Sexual function (see sexual history)

2.1.2 Specific history

2.1.2.1 Urinary history. The urinary history must consist of symptoms related to both the storage and the evacuation functions of the lower urinary tract.

Specific symptoms and data must be assessed in neurogenic lower urinary tract dysfunction and if appropriate be compared with the patients' condition before the neurogenic lower urinary tract dysfunction developed.

Specify:

a) Urinary incontinence
   - Predictability of the occurrence of incontinence
   - Type of incontinence: Urge incontinence*, stress incontinence*, other incontinence
   - Position or condition when incontinence occurs (supine/sitting/standing/moving/bedwetting only)
   - Control of the incontinence: Medication, pads, external appliances, penile clamp, urethral plug, pessary, catheterisation
   - Extent of the incontinence: Pad number or weight or estimated volume per 24 hour period, frequency/volume chart*

b) Bladder sensation*:
   - Absent*
   - Specific bladder sensation (desire to void*, urgency*, pain*)
   - General sensation related to bladder filling (abdominal fullness, vegetative symptoms, spasticity)

bb) If specific bladder sensation exists:
   - Normal*, hypersensitive*, or hyposensitive*
   - Can urgency be suppressed?
   - If yes, as effective as before the neurogenic condition?

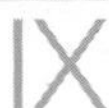

bbb) If the patient has normal bladder sensation:
- Timing and duration of the sensation
- Ability to initiate voiding voluntarily
- Need for abdominal straining or other triggering to initiate or sustain voiding

c) Mode and type of voiding:
- Voiding position (standing, sitting, supine)
- Continuous* or intermittent flow*
- Residual urine*
- Initiation of voiding:
  - Voluntary voiding
  - Reflex voiding*: spontaneous or triggered (state type and area of triggering). Remark: Some patients with uncontrollable reflex voiding may use a condom urinal and a urine bag
  - Voiding by increased intravesical pressure (state mode of pressure increase: abdominal strain or Credé). Remark: Credé is contraindicated in children; also in adults when pressure exceeds 100 cm H_2O
  - Passive voiding by decreased outlet resistance (state mode: removal of urethral and/or vaginal appliances, sphincterotomy, TUR bladder neck, artificial sphincter)
  - Sacral root electrostimulation

c1) If the patient has an artificial sphincter:
- Implant date and date(s) of revision surgery
- Micturition frequency
- Cuff pressure
- Number of pump strokes
- Cuff closure time
- Continence or stress incontinence with closed sphincter

c2) If the voiding is induced by sacral root electrical stimulation:
- Implant date and date(s) of revision surgery
- Location of electrodes (roots used)
- Stimulation parameters
- Micturition frequency
- Duration of voiding stimulation
- 'Double voiding' stimulation

c3) If the patients empties the bladder by catheterisation, residual urine is assessed to check also the effectiveness of the catheterisation

c31) Intermittent catheterisation: Emptying of the bladder by catheter, mostly at regular intervals. The catheter is removed after the bladder is empty. The procedure may be *sterile intermittent catheterisation*: Use of sterile components or *clean intermittent catheterisation*: At least one component is not sterile. *Intermittent self-catheterisation* is performed by the patient.
- Type, size, and material of catheter (conventional, hydrophylic)
- Use of lubricating jelly (intra-urethral or on catheter only) or soaking (sterile saline, tap water)
- Disinfection of meatus

c32) An *indwelling catheter* is permanently introduced into the bladder. An external urine collecting device is used.
- Transurethral or suprapubic approach
- Type, size, and material of catheter
- Type of collecting device and associated materials (anti-reflux valves)
- Interval between changes of collecting device

d) *Urinary diary* (Frequency/volume chart*) The frequency/volume chart is a specific urodynamic investigation recording fluid intake and urine output per 24 hour period. The chart gives objective information on the number of voidings, the distribution of voidings between daytime and night-time and each voided volume. The chart can also be used to record episodes of urgency and leakage and the number of incontinence pads used.

The urinary diary is also useful in patients who perform intermittent catheterisation. A reliable urinary diary cannot be taken in less than 2–3 days. The urinary diary permits the assessment of voiding data under normal physiological conditions.

- Time and volume for each voiding or catheterisation
- Total volume over the period of the recording or 24 hour volume
- Diurnal variation of volumes
- *Functional bladder capacity*: average voided volume
- *Voiding interval*: average time between daytime voidings
- *Continence interval*: average time between incontinence episodes or between last voiding and incontinence (assessed only during daytime)
- The fluid intake may also be recorded

Only for patients who use catheterisation it is also feasible to assess:

- Residual urine
- *Total bladder capacity*: Sum of functional bladder capacity and residual urine

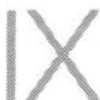

2.1.2.2 Defecation history. Patients with neurogenic lower urinary tract dysfunction may suffer from a related neurogenic condition of the lower gastro-intestinal tract. The defecation history also must address symptoms related to the storage and the evacuation functions and specific symptoms and data must be compared with the patient's condition before the neurogenic dysfunction developed.
Specify:

a) Faecal incontinence:
  - Extent (complete, spotting, diarrhoea, flatulence)
  - Pads use (type and number)
  - Anal tampons (number)

b) Rectal sensation:
  - Filling sensation
  - Differentiation between stool, liquid stool and flatus
  - Sensation of passage

c) Mode and type of defecation:
  - Toilet use or in bed
  - Frequency of defecation
  - Duration of defecation
  - Use of oral or rectal laxatives
  - Interval between laxatives and defecation
  - Use of enema (frequency, amount used)
  - Antegrade continence enema (date of surgery, date(s) of revision, frequency of stomal dilation, frequency of washout)
  - Initiation of defecation:
    - Voluntary or spontaneous
    - After digital stimulation
    - Mechanical emptying (patient or caregiver)
    - Sacral root electrical stimulation

c1) If the defecation is induced by sacral root electrical stimulation:
  - Implant date and date(s) of revision surgery
  - Location of electrodes (roots used)
  - Stimulation parameters
  - Continuous or interrupted stimulation (interval)
  - Combination with other treatment (laxatives or rectal mucosal stimulation)

2.1.2.3 Sexual history. The sexual function may also be impaired because of the neurogenic condition.
Specify:
Males:

a) Sensation in genital area and for sexual functions (increased/normal/reduced/ absent)
b) Erection:
  - Spontaneous or inducible by psychogenic stimuli
  - Mechanical or medical initiation (state method or drug)
  - Sacral root electrical stimulation

b1) If the erection is induced by sacral root electrical stimulation:
  - Implant date and date(s) of revision surgery
  - Location of electrodes (roots used)
  - Stimulation parameters
  - Leg clonus (absent/present)
  - If erection is insufficient: Use of supportive treatment

c) Intercourse (erection sufficient or extra mechanical stimulation)
c1) If the erection is insufficient state tumescence, rigidity, duration
d) If the patient has a penile implant:
  - Implant date and date(s) of revision surgery
  - Type of prosthesis
  - Result of implantation
  - Frequency of use

e) Ejaculation:
  - Natural (normal, dribbling, semen quality and appearance)
  - Artificial:
    - Vibrostimulation, electro-ejaculation, intrathecal drugs (frequency. results)
    - Semen analysis (most recent, result)

Females:

a) Sensation in genital area and for sexual functions (increased/normal/reduced/absent)
b) Arousal or orgasm inducible (psychogenic or mechanical stimuli)

2.2 Physical examination

2.2.1 General physical examination

Attention should be paid to the patient's physical and possible mental handicaps with respect to the planned investigation. Impaired mobility, particularly in the hips, or extreme spasticity may lead to problems in patient positioning in the urodynamics laboratory. Patients with very high neurological lesions may suffer from a significant drop in blood pressure when moved in a sitting or standing position. Subjective indications of bladder filling sensations may be impossible in retarded patients.

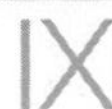

2.2.2 Neurourological status

Specify:

- Sensation S_2-S_5 (both sides): Presence (increased/normal/reduced/absent), type (sharp/blunt), afflicted segments
- Reflexes: Bulbocavernous reflex, perianal reflex, knee and ankle reflexes, plantar responses {Babinski} (increased/normal/reduced/absent)
- Anal sphincter tone (increased/normal/reduced/absent)
- Anal sphincter and pelvic floor voluntary contractions (increased/normal/reduced/absent)
- Prostate palpation
- Descensus of pelvic organs

2.2.3 Laboratory tests

- Urinalysis (infection treatment, if indicated and possible, before further intervention)
- Blood laboratory, if necessary
- Free flowmetry and assessment of residual urine (mostly sonographic; by catheter in patients catheterising or immediately preceding a urodynamic investigation). Because of natural variations, multiple estimations are necessary (at least 2–3)
- Quantification of urine loss* by pad testing, if appropriate
- Imaging:

Sonography: Kidneys (size, diameter of parenchyma, pelvis, calyces)
Ureter (dilation)
Bladder wall (diameter, outline, trabeculation, diverticulae or pseudodiverticulae)

X-ray: Cystography, excretion urography, urethrography, clearance studies, if necessary.
Apart from the data in sonography, attention must be paid to urinary stones, spinal anomalies, reflux, bladder neck condition, and urethral anomalies.

MRI: Accordingly

3. INVESTIGATIONS

In patients with neurogenic lower urinary tract dysfunction, and particularly when detrusor hyperreflexia* might be present, the urodynamic investigation is even more provocative than in other patients. Any technical source of artifacts must be critically considered. The quality of the urodynamic recording and its interpretation must be ensured [Schäfer et al.].

In patients at risk for autonomic dysreflexia, blood pressure assessment during the urodynamic study is advisable.

In many patients with neurogenic lower urinary tract dysfunction, assessment of maximum (unaesthetic) bladder capacity* may be useful. The rectal ampulla should be empty of stool before the start of the investigation. Medication by drugs that influence the lower urinary tract function should be abandoned at least 48 hours before the investigation (if feasible) or otherwise be taken into account for the interpretation of the data.

3.1 Methods

In neurogenic lower urinary tract dysfunction a combination of urodynamic investigations is mostly warranted. Some comments on the use of a single investigation are listed (see also Section 4). Urodynamic investigation should be performed only when the patient's free flowmetry and residual data are available (see Section 2.2.3) if the patient's condition permits these tests.

*3.1.1 Measurement of urinary flow**

Care must be taken in judging the results in patients who are not able to void in a normal position. Both the flow pattern* and the flow rate* may be modified by this inappropriate position and by any constructions to divert the flow.

*3.1.2 Cystometry**

Cystometry is used to assess detrusor activity, sensation, capacity, and compliance. As an isolated investigation this is probably only useful for follow-up studies of treatment.

3.1.3 Leak point pressure measurement [McGuire et al., 1996]

There are two kinds of leak point pressure measurement. The detrusor leak point pressure is a static test and the abdominal leak point pressure is a dynamic test. The pressure values at leakage should be read exactly at the moment of leakage.

The *detrusor leak point pressure* is the lowest value of the detrusor pressure* at which leakage is observed in the absence of abdominal strain or detrusor contraction.

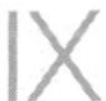

Detrusor leak point pressure measurement assesses the storage function and detrusor compliance, in particular in patients with neurogenic lower urinary tract dysfunction, with low compliance bladder (see below) or with reflex voiding. High detrusor leak point pressure puts these patients at risk for upper urinary tract detorioration or might cause secondary damage to the bladder. A detrusor leak point pressure above 40 cm H_2O appears hazardous [McGuire et al., 1996].

The *abdominal leak point pressure* is the lowest value of the intentionally increased intravesical pressure* that provokes urinary leakage in the absence of a detrusor contraction. The abdominal pressure increase can be induced by coughing (*cough leak point pressure*) or by Valsalva (*Valsalva leak point pressure*) with increasing amplitude. Multiple estimations at a fixed bladder volume (200–300 ml in adults) are necessary.

For patients with stress incontinence, the abdominal leak point pressure measurement gives an impression of the severity (slight or severe) or the nature (anatomical or intrinsic sphincter deficiency) of incontinence.

With the assumption that the intravesical pressure in abdominal leak point pressure is caused only by the abdominal pressure, vaginal pressure or rectal pressure may also be used to record the intravesical pressure. This will obviate the need for intravesical catheterisation.

3.1.4 Bladder pressure measurements during micturition and pressure-flow relationships**

Most types of obstructions caused by neurogenic lower urinary tract dysfunction are due to urethral overactivity* (detrusor/urethral dyssynergia*, detrusor-{external}-sphincter dyssynergia*, and detrusor/bladder neck dyssynergia*). This urethral over-activity will increase the detrusor voiding pressure above the level that is needed to overcome the urethral resistance+ given by the urethra's inherent mechanical and anatomical properties. Pressure-flow analysis mostly assesses the amount of mechanical obstruction* caused by the latter properties and has limited value in patients with neurogenic lower urinary tract dysfunction.

3.1.5 Electromyography (often combined with cystometry/uroflowmetry)*

Depending on the location of the electrodes, the electromyogram records the function of

- External urethral and/or anal sphincter
- Striated pelvic floor muscles

Owing to possible artefacts caused by other equipment used in a urodynamic investigation, its interpretation may be difficult.

*3.1.6 Urethral pressure measurement**

Urethral pressure measurement has a limited place in the diagnosis of neurogenic lower urinary tract dysfunction. The following techniques are available:

- Resting urethral pressure profile*
- Stress urethral pressure profile*
- Intermittent catheter withdrawal (to cope with massive reflex contractions)
- *Continuous urethral pressure measurement*: the catheter sensor or opening is placed at about the point of maximum urethral closure pressure* and left there over time. This records time variations of urethral pressure and responses to various conditions of the lower urinary tract

3.1.7 Video urodynamics

Definition: Combination of lower urinary tract imaging during filling and voiding with urodynamic measurements.

3.1.8 Ambulatory urodynamics

An ambulatory urodynamic investigation is defined as any functional investigation of the urinary tract utilizing predominantly natural filling of the urinary tract and reproducing normal subject activity [Van Waalwijk et al.]. The recording of an ambulatory urodynamic investigation is comparable to Holter EKG and the patient is more or less in a situation of daily life. More detailed information on standardization of ambulatory urodynamics is found in the specific report [Van Waalwijk et al., submitted].

3.1.9 Provocative tests during urodynamics

- Coughing, triggering, anal stretch
- Ice water test
- Carbachol test
- Acute drug tests

3.1.10 Maximum (anaesthetic) bladder capacity measurement

The volume measured after filling during a deep general or spinal/epidural anaesthetic.

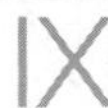

3.1.11 Specific uro-neurophysiological tests

- Electromyography (in a neurophysiological setting)
- Nerve conduction studies*
- Reflex latency measurements*
- Evoked responses*
- Sensory testing*

3.2 Measurement technique

3.2.1 Measurement of urinary flow

Specify:
0) Type of voiding:
  - Spontaneous voiding: Voluntary or reflex voiding
  - Triggered voiding or sacral root electrostimulation:
    Type of triggering

a) Voided volume
b) Patient environment and position (supine, sitting or standing)
c) Filling:
  i) By diuresis (spontaneous or forced; specify regimen)
  ii) By catheter (transurethral or suprapubic)
d) Type of fluid

Technique:
a) Measuring equipment
b) Solitary procedure or combined with other measurements

3.2.2 Cystometry

All systems are zeroed at atmospheric pressure. For external transducers the reference point is the level of the superior edge of the symphysis pubis. For catheter mounted transducers the reference point is the transducer itself.

If a different type of catheter is used in follow-up cystometries the findings in Rossier and Fam [1986] may be of interest.

Specify:
a) Access (transurethral or percutaneous)
b) Fluid medium (liquid or gas)

Gas filling should not be used in patients with neurogenic lower urinary tract dysfunction. State type and concentration of liquid used (for example, contrast medium, isotonic saline).

c) Temperature of fluid (state in degree Celsius)

In neurogenic lower urinary tract dysfunction a body-warm filling medium is advised.

d) Position of patient (e.g., supine, sitting, or standing)

Offer the patient the individually most comfortable position, particularly when voiding.

e) Filling may be by diuresis or catheter. Filling by catheter may be continuous or incremental; the precise filling rate should be stated

When the incremental method is used the volume increment should be stated.
For general discussion, the following terms for the range of filling may be used:

i) Up to 10 ml per minute is slow fill cystometry ('physiological' filling)
ii) 10–100 ml per minute is medium fill cystometry
iii) Over 100 ml per minute is rapid fill cystometry

A physiological filling rate or alternatively a maximum filling rate of 20 ml per minute is advised in neurogenic lower urinary tract dysfunction to prevent provocation of detrusor hyperreflexia or other sequelae of faster filling. From ambulatory urodynamics data the impression arises that the mentioned filling rates should be reconsidered [Klevmark, 1997].

Technique:
a) Fluid-filled catheter – specify number of catheters, single or multiple lumens, type of catheter (manufacturer), size of catheter
b) Catheter tip transducer – list specifications
c) Other catheters – list specifications
d) Measuring equipment

3.2.3 Leak point pressure measurement

Specify:
a) Location and access of pressure sensor (intravesical – transurethral or percutaneous, vaginal, or rectal)
b) Position of patient (for instance supine, sitting, or standing)
c) Bladder filling by diuresis or catheter (state type of liquid)
d) Bladder volume during test, also in relation to maximum cystometric capacity*

Technique:
a) Mode of leak detection (observation, alarm nappy, meatal or urethral conductance measurement, or other)
b) Catheters – list specifications, type (manufacturer) and size
c) Measuring equipment for pressure and, if applicable, for leak detection

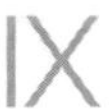

3.2.4 Bladder pressure measurements during micturition and pressure-flow relationships

The specifications of patient position, access for pressure measurement, catheter type, and measuring equipment are as for cystometry (see Section 3.2.2)

If urethral pressure measurements during voiding* are performed, the specifications are according to those in urethral pressure measurement (see Section 3.2.6).

If other assessments of the relation between pressure and flow are used (for example stop test, urethral occlusion, condom urinal occlusion) the specifications should be equivalent, according to the technique used.

3.2.5 Electromyography

The extensive specifications in the earlier report are appropriate in a neurophysiological setting. They are condensed here for practical use during urodynamics.

Specify:

a) EMG (solitary procedure, part of urodynamic or other electrophysiological investigation)
b) Patient position (supine, standing, sitting or other)
c) Electrode placement (surface electrodes or intramuscular electrodes)
   i) sampling site (abbreviated)
   ii) recording electrode: location (abbreviated)
   iii) reference electrode position

Note: Ensure that there is no electrical interference with any other machines, for example, X-ray apparatus.

Technique:

a) Electrodes:
   i) Needle electrodes: type, size, material (abbreviated) The same holds for other types of intramuscular electrodes (for example enamel wire)
   ii) Surface electrodes: type, size, material, fixation, conducting medium (abbreviated)
b) Amplifier (make and specifications)
c) Signal processing (data: raw, averaged, integrated or other)
d) Display equipment (abbreviated)
e) Storage (abbreviated)
f) Hard copy production (abbreviated)

3.2.6 Urethral pressure measurement

Because of its limited place in neurogenic lower urinary tract dysfunction, the reader is referred to the earlier standardization report [Abrams et al., 1988, 1990] for the specifications.

3.2.7 Video urodynamics

Specify imaging system (fluoroscopy, ultrasound). Further specifications according to the type of urodynamic study.

3.2.8 Ambulatory urodynamics

Specifications according to the type of urodynamic study.

3.2.9 Provocative tests during urodynamics

Specify type of test, type of trigger, or drug used. Further specifications according to type of urodynamic study.

3.2.10 Maximum (anaesthetic) bladder capacity measurement

Specify fluid temperature, filling pressure, filling time, type of anaesthesia, anaesthetic agent, and dosage.

3.2.11 Specific uro-neurophysiological tests

Electromyography (see Section 3.2.5)
Nerve conduction studies, reflex latency measurements, evoked responses
Specify:

a) Type of investigation (abbreviated)
b) Is the study a solitary procedure or part of a urodynamic or neurophysiological investigation?
c) Patient position and environmental temperature, noise level and illumination
d) Electrode placement (abbreviated)

Technique:
a) Electrodes (abbreviated)
b) Stimulator (abbreviated)
c) Amplifier (abbreviated)
d) Averager (abbreviated)
e) Display equipment (abbreviated)
f) Storage (abbreviated)
g) Hard copy production (abbreviated)

Sensory testing
Specify:
a) Patient position (supine, sitting, standing, and other)
b) Bladder volume at time of testing

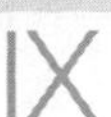

c) Site of applied stimulus (intravesical and intraurethral)
d) Number of times the stimulus was applied and the response recorded. Define the sensation recorded, for example the first sensation or the sensation of pulsing
e) Type of applied stimulus (abbreviated)

3.3 Data

3.3.1 Measurement of urinary flow

- Voided volume*
- Maximum flow rate*
- Flow time*
- Average flow rate*
- Time to maximum flow*
- Flow pattern, includes the statement of continuous or intermittent voiding
- Voiding time*, when the voiding is intermittent
- *Hesitancy*: The occurrence of significant delay between the patient's voluntary initiation of micturition as signalled for example by pushing the marker button on the flow meter and the actual start of flow (note the flow delay⁺)

3.3.2 Cystometry

- Intravesical pressure
- Abdominal pressure
- Detrusor pressure
- Infused volumes at:
  - First desire to void* or other sensation of filling
  - Normal desire to void* or other sensation that indicates the need for a toilet visit
  - *Reflex volume*: Starting of first hyperreflexive detrusor contraction
  - Urgency
  - Pain (specify)
  - Maximum cystometric capacity (in patients with abolition of sensations, this is defined as the volume at which the investigator decides to stop filling)
  - Autonomic dysreflexia (specify)
- Compliance* $\{\Delta V/\Delta p_{det}\}$ (ml/cm H_2O) is mostly measured between (specify):
  - Reference value: Detrusor pressure at empty bladder (start of filling)
  - Measurement value: The (passive) detrusor pressure:
    - At maximum cystometric capacity in patients with existing sensation and without urine loss
    - At the start of the detrusor contraction leading to the first significant incontinence in patients with failing sensation or significant incontinence

➡ When a different volume range is used this should be specified in particular

A problem in the calculation of the compliance occurs when Δp_{det} is negative or zero: the defined calculation then gives a negative or infinite compliance. The first is physically impossible, the last gives little information. *In the compliance calculation a minimum value of 1 cm H_2O is used for Δp_{det}.* This means that the maximal possible value of the compliance will be equal to the volume range over which the compliance is calculated.

- *Break volume*: the bladder volume after which a sudden significant decrease of compliance is observed during the remainder of the filling phase (mind the distinction between passive detrusor pressure and detrusor contraction). It is yet unclear whether this observation is consistent in patients with neurogenic lower urinary tract dysfunction with or without detrusor hyperreflexia. When true, this might indicate that the detrusor is in a different state after the break volume

3.3.3 Leak point pressure measurement

- Minimum of measured pressure for first observation of leakage

3.3.4 Bladder pressure measurements during micturition and pressure-flow relationships

- Opening time* (note the flow delay)
- Opening pressure* (note the flow delay)
- Maximum pressure*
- Pressure at maximum flow⁺ (note the flow delay)
- Closing pressure⁺ (note the flow delay)
- Minimum voiding pressure⁺ (note the flow delay)

All pressure values will be estimated for intravesical, abdominal and detrusor pressure separately. They will not only differ in amplitude, but often also in timing. The detrusor pressure is generally the most important one. The maximum pressure values may be attained at a moment where the flow rate is zero [Griffiths et al., 1997].

3.3.5 Electromyography

- Recruitment patterns, * particularly in relation to specific stimuli (bladder filling, hyperreflexive

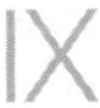

contractions, onset of voiding, coughing, Valsalva, etc.)
- If individual motor unit action potentials are recorded: duration (msec) and amplitude (mV) of spontaneous activity, fibrillations, positive sharp waves, and complex repetitive discharges. Complexity and polyphasicity (descriptive or number)

3.3.6 Urethral pressure measurement

One parameter describing the contribution of the urethra to continence is the functional profile length*, the length of the urethra over which the urethral pressure exceeds intravesical pressure.

The functional profile length should reflect the length of the urethra that contributes to the prevention of leakage. In the female, this concept is straightforward, but in the male, the length of the bulbous and penile urethra will often add significantly to the functional profile length. The infra-sphincteric part of the urethra however contributes little, if any, to continence. The functional profile length in men thus is much greater than in women, without the associated implication that this greater length indeed is functional in maintaining continence. This functional part of the urethra probably extends down from the bladder to the junction from sphincteric to bulbous urethra, but this junction is often difficult to detect on the curve.

The contribution of the bulbous and penile urethra also show a large variance between patients and between several assessments in the same man. Therefore a third urethral length parameter is used, the *urethral continence zone*: the length of the urethra between the bladder neck and the point of maximum urethral pressure [Gleason et al., 1974] (Fig. IX.A).

- Resting urethral pressure profile:
  - Maximum urethral pressure*
  - Maximum urethral closure pressure
  - Functional profile length (not mandatory in men)
  - Urethral continence zone (not mandatory in women)
- Stress urethral pressure profile: above parameters and
  - Pressure 'transmission' ratio*
- Intermittent withdrawal: above parameters and
  - Relaxing time before measurement is read
- Continuous urethral pressure measurement. This study is probably best represented by the measured curve. Urethral pressure variations in relation to specific stimuli (bladder filling, hyperreflexive contractions, onset of voiding, coughing, Valsalva, etc.) may be described separately

3.3.7 Video urodynamics

- According to type of urodynamic study
- Morphology:
  - Configuration and contour of the bladder during filling and voiding
  - Reflux, occurrence, and timing:
    - Into the upper urinary tract
    - Into the adnexa (for instance the prostate, the ejaculatory duct)
  - Bladder neck during filling and voiding phases

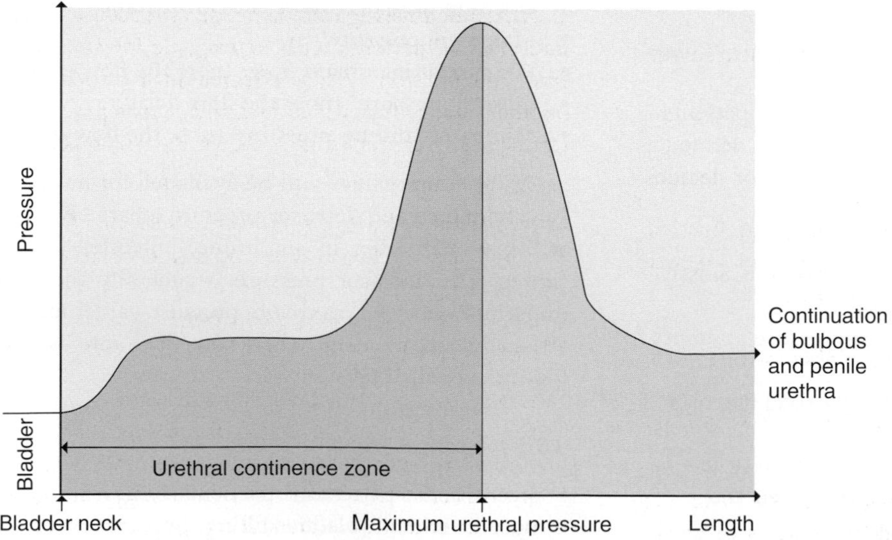

Fig. IX.A Schematic measurement of urethral continence zone in men.

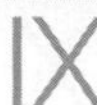

- Configuration of proximal urethra during filling and voiding, urethral kinking
- Bladder or urethral descensus

3.3.8 Ambulatory urodynamics

According to type of urodynamic study

3.3.9 Provocative tests during urodynamics

Response of the lower urinary tract function to the provocation. Compare with situation without provocation

3.3.10 Maximum (anaesthetic) bladder capacity measurement

Anatomical maximum volume that bladder will accommodate

3.3.11 Specific uro-neurophysiological tests

- Electromyography (see Section 3.3.5)
- Nerve conduction studies:
  - Latency time* (abbreviated)
  - Response amplitude* (abbreviated)
- Reflex latency measurement:
  - Response time* (abbreviated)
- Evoked responses:
  - Single or multiphasic response*
  - Onset of response* (abbreviated)
  - Latency to onset* (abbreviated)
  - Latency to peaks* (abbreviated)
  - The amplitude of the responses is measured
- Sensory testing:
  - Sensory threshold* (abbreviated)

3.4 Typical manifestations of neurogenic lower urinary tract dysfunction

3.4.1 Filling phase

- Hyposensitivity or hypersensitivity
- Vegetative sensations for example goose flesh, sweating, headache, and blood pressure increase (particularly in patients with autonomic dysreflexia)
- *Low compliance*: Compliance value lower than 20 ml/cm H_2O
  - Cause: Neural or muscular (described before as hypertonic bladder)
- *High volume bladder*: A bladder that can be filled to far over functional bladder capacity in non-anaesthetised condition without significant increase in pressure (described before as hypotonic bladder). The use of the terms excessive or very high compliance to describe this situation is discouraged, as a high value of compliance will also be measured at lower volumes when only a slight increase in pressure occurs during filling
  - Cause: Neural or muscular
- Detrusor hyperreflexia, spontaneous or provoked; classified according to maximal detrusor pressure as *low-pressure hyperreflexia* or *high-pressure hyperreflexia*. Because of its clinical implications, as a practical guideline a value of 40 cm H_2O is proposed as cut-off value between low-pressure and high-pressure hyperreflexia [McGuire et al., 1996]
- *Sphincter areflexia*: No evidence of reflex sphincter contraction during filling, particularly at higher volumes, or during physical stress

3.4.2 Voiding phase

- Detrusor areflexia*
- *External sphincter hyperreflexia*: involuntary activity (for example, intermittently) of external sphincter during voiding other than detrusor sphincter dyssynergia
- Detrusor sphincter dyssynergia
- Detrusor bladder neck dyssynergia

4. CLINICAL VALUE AND CLASSIFICATION OF URODYNAMIC INVESTIGATION

Urodynamic investigation is needed for accurate evaluation of all patients with neurogenic lower urinary tract dysfunction. When effected in a standardised manner, it produces standardised and reproducible results (cf. [Schäfer et al.]). After the evaluation, its results must be summarised and evaluated:

1. Neurological background (type/duration of neurological disease or lesion) and characteristics of uro-neurophysiological tests
2. Characteristics of filling function
3. Characteristics of voiding function

In the conclusive evaluation the condition of the upper urinary tract and the incontinence care in incontinent patients must also be taken into account. Core investigation of patients with neurogenic lower urinary tract dysfunction will include:

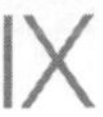

1. History
2. Urine culture
3. Flow rate and post-void residual (multiple estimations)
4. Filling and voiding cystometry

Not all urodynamic procedures are equally important in the diagnosis of patients with neurogenic lower urinary tract dysfunction. The following list is an indication of the place of each procedure in these patients.

0: Urinary diary: Semi-objective quantification of the physiological lower urinary tract function. Advisable.
1: Free uroflowmetry and assessment of residual urine: First impression of voiding function. Mandatory before any invasive urodynamics is planned.
2: Cystometry. The only method to quantify filling function. Limited significance as a solitary procedure. Powerful when combined with bladder pressure measurement during micturition and even more in video urodynamics. Necessary to document the status of the lower urinary tract function during the filling phase.
3: Leak point pressure measurement. Detrusor leak point pressure: Specific investigation if high pressures during the filling phase might endanger the upper urinary tract or lead to secondary bladder damage. Abdominal leak point pressure: Less important in neurogenic lower urinary tract dysfunction. Useful for patients with stress incontinence.
4: Bladder pressure measurements during voiding and pressure-flow relationships. Pressure measurements reflect the co-ordination between detrusor and urethra or pelvic floor during the voiding phase. Even more powerful in combination with cystometry and with video urodynamics. Necessary to document the status of the lower urinary tract function during the voiding phase. Pressure-flow analysis is aimed at assessing the passive urethral resistance relation[+] and as such of less importance in neurogenic lower urinary tract dysfunction.
5: Urethral pressure measurement. Limited applicability in neurogenic lower urinary tract dysfunction.
6: Electromyography: Vulnerable to artefacts when performed during a urodynamic investigation. Useful as a gross indication of the patient's ability to control the pelvic floor. When more detailed analysis is needed, it should be performed as part of a uro-neurophysiological investigation.
7: Video urodynamics: When combined with cystometry and pressure measurement during micturition probably the most comprehensive investigation to document the lower urinary tract function and morphology. In this combination the first choice of invasive investigations.
8: Ambulatory urodynamics: Should be considered when office urodynamics do not reproduce the patient's symptoms and complaints. May replace office (not video) urodynamics in future when all parameters from office urodynamics are available in ambulatory urodynamics too.
9: Specific uro-neurophysiological tests. Advised as part of the neurological work-up of the patient. Elective tests may be asked for specific conditions that became obvious during patient work-up and urodynamic investigations.

5. SUPPLEMENTAL INVESTIGATIONS

5.1 Endoscopic procedures

Endoscopic investigation of the lower urinary tract may be necessary in a limited number of patients. The indication must be very restrictive.

5.2 Other investigations to define the neurological status

Specific investigations to assess the neurological status of the patient may also be necessary in individual cases.

ACKNOWLEDGEMENTS

The authors used the 'Manual Neuro-Urology and Spinal Cord Lesion: Guidelines for Urological Care of Spinal Cord Injury Patients' prepared by the Arbeitskreis Urologische Rehabilitation Querschnittgelähmter for the German Urological Society as a starting point for their discussions. The authors thank Dr. Clare Fowler and Dr. Derek Griffiths for valuable discussions during the production of this report.

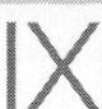

REFERENCES

Abrams P, Blaivas J G, Stanton S L, Andersen J T 1988 Standardization of terminology of lower urinary tract function. The International Continence Society Committee on Standardization of Terminology. Neurourol Urodynam 7: 403–427. Scand J Urol Nephrol 114(suppl): 5–19

Abrams P, Blaivas J G, Stanton S L, Andersen J T 1990 Standardization of terminology of lower urinary tract function. The International Continence Society Committee on Standardization of Terminology. Int Urogynecol J 1: 45–58

Gleason D M, Reilly R J, Bottacini M R, Pierce M J 1974 The urethral continence zone and its relation to stress incontinence. J Urol 112: 81–88

Griffiths D J, Höfner K, van Mastrigt R, Rollema H J, Spångberg A, Gleason D 1997 Standardization of terminology of lower urinary tract function: pressure-flow studies of voiding, urethral resistance, and urethral obstruction. Neurourol Urodynam 16: 1–18

Klevmark B 1997 Ambulatory urodynamics. Letter to the editor. Br J Urol 79: 490

McGuire E J, Cespedes R D, O'Connell H E 1996 Leak-point pressures. Urol Clin North Am 23: 253–262

Rossier A B, Fam B A 1986 5-microtransducer catheter in evaluation of neurogenic bladder function. Urology 27: 371–378

Schäfer et al. Good urodynamic practice. In preparation

Van Waalwijk van Doorn E, Anders K, Khullar V, Kulseng-Hanssen S, Pesce F, Robertson A, Rosario D, Schäfer W Standardization of ambulatory urodynamic monitoring. First draft report of the standardization sub-committee of the ICS for ambulatory urodynamic studies. Neurourol Urodynam (submitted).

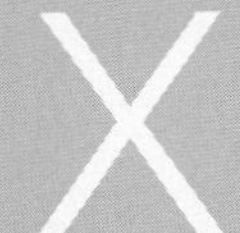

Standards of efficacy for evaluation of treatment outcomes in urinary incontinence: recommendations of the Urodynamic Society

Neurourology and Urodynamics 16:145–147 (1997) © 1997 Wiley-Liss, Inc.

Jerry G Blaivas, Rodney A Appell, J Andrew Fantl, Gary Leach, Edward J McGuire, Neil M Resnick, Shlomo Raz, and Alan J Wein

1. **Purpose** – The purpose of this document is to provide minimal standards by which the efficacy of therapy for urinary incontinence may be assessed. The standards were developed by a committee of the Urodynamic Society. They have been approved by both the American Urologic Association and the Urodynamic Society and are the official recommendations of those organizations. It is intended that these standards will be adopted by clinical and basic science researchers, the FDA, the peer review process, specialty and sub-specialty organizations, the health care industry, the regulatory agencies and ultimately by clinicians.

The accompanying document 'Definition and Classification of Urinary Incontinence: Recommendations of the Urodynamic Society' was drafted to encourage that a uniform lexicon be used when reporting the results.

2. **General considerations**: All clinical trials should consist of a pre and post treatment evaluation which adheres to these standards.

Post treatment evaluation of surgical, prosthetic and implantation therapies should be conducted no less often than 1, 6, and 12 months after treatment. Evaluation should be done at yearly intervals thereafter and continued as long as possible, preferably for at least five years.

At each post-treatment interval, the following data should be recorded:

- the total number of patients treated during that time interval
- the total number of patients actually evaluated during that time interval
- the total number of patients lost to follow up during that time interval
- the reasons why patients were lost to follow up

2.1 Some therapies (such as most pharmacologic agents) exert their effect only during active treatment. These should be evaluated at intervals dictated by the expected outcome, but no less often than monthly.

2.2 After a successful pilot study, all drug therapies should be double blind and placebo controlled.

2.3 Whenever repeated therapies are contemplated (such as periurethral injections) the indications for retreatment and the time interval since the last treatment should be specified. Efficacy

assessment should be done at a specific time interval after the last treatment. The protocol should further specify the criteria by which treatment success or failure is determined.

3. **Pretreatment evaluation** should consist of:

3.1 Structured micturition history and/or questionnaire including at least:
- number of micturitions/day
- number of micturitions/night
- number of incontinent episodes/day
- number of incontinent episodes/night
- type of incontinence (stress, urge, unconscious, continuous leakage)
- Description of voiding (emptying) symptoms

3.2 Structured physical examination with full bladder including at least:

3.2.1. Neurourologic exam:
- perianal sensation
- anal sphincter tone and control
- bulbocavernosus reflex
- brief screening neurologic exam to discriminate normal, paraplegic, quadriplegic, hemiplegic, dementia, etc.

3.2.2 (Women) vaginal exam:

Demonstration of urinary leakage
- spontaneous/continuous
- synchronous with stress
- after stress

Presence and degree of:
- cystocele
- urethrocele
- uterine prolapse
- enterocele
- rectocele

3.2.3. (Men) prostate exam:
- Size and consistency of prostate

Demonstration of urinary leakage
- spontaneous/continuous
- synchronous with stress
- after stress

3.3. Micturition diary – self reported by patient.
- time of micturition
- time and type of incontinence
- voided volume

3.4. Pad test – a quantitative or semi-quantitative pad test should be done to estimate the amount of urinary loss.

3.5. Urodynamics – Videourodynamics is the most comprehensive method of evaluation. The minimum evaluation should consist of:
- Cystometry (liquid) with simultaneous measurement of vesical and abdominal pressure for determination of detrusor pressure.
- Synchronous detrusor pressure/uroflow study
- Simple uroflow
- Assessment of the relative contribution of urethral hypermobility and intrinsic sphincter deficiency such as the Q-tip test and leak point pressure.
- Estimation of post-void residual urine e.g., by ultrasound or catheterization.

4. **Post-treatment evaluation**. The method by which data collection was accrued should be specified, e.g., prospective or retrospective chart review, independent researcher, etc. The interval between the time of evaluation and the last treatment should be specified (e.g. for injection therapy). The evaluation should consist of:

4.1 The patient's opinion of treatment outcome and its impact on quality of life.

4.2 Structured micturition history and/or questionnaire at each follow up.

4.3 Structured physical examination with full bladder at least once during follow up.

4.4 Micturition diary at each follow up.

4.5 Pad test at each follow up.

4.6 Uroflow at least once during follow up.

4.7 Estimation of post void residual urine at least once during follow up.

4.8 Other urodynamic techniques are optimal.

APPENDIX XI

Definition and classification of urinary incontinence: recommendations of the Urodynamic Society

Neurourology and Urodynamics 16:149–151 (1997) © 1997 Wiley-Liss Inc.

Jerry G Blaivas, Rodney A Appell, J Andrew Fantl, Gary Leach, Edward J McGuire, Neil M Resnick, Shlomo Raz, and Alan J Wein

1. **Purpose** – The purpose of this document is to provide a uniform lexicon for describing urinary incontinence. This lexicon was developed by a committee of the Urodynamic Society and conforms to the terminology established by the ICS standardization committee [Abrams et al., 1988]. It has been approved by both the American Urologic Association and the Urodynamic Society and is the official recommendation of these organizations.

1.2 Urinary incontinence is the involuntary loss of urine – It denotes:

1.2.1. A symptom – The symptom indicates the patient's (or caregiver's) statement of involuntary urine loss.

1.2.2. A sign – The sign is the objective demonstration of urine loss.

1.2.3. A condition – The condition is the pathophysiology underlying incontinence as demonstrated by clinical or urodynamic techniques.

2. **Conditions causing urinary incontinence:** Conditions may be presumed or definite. Definite conditions are documented by urodynamic techniques. Presumed conditions are documented clinically. For example, a neurologically normal woman who complains of urge incontinence despite a normal cystometrogram will be considered to have presumed detrusor instability provided that sphincter abnormalities and overflow incontinence have been excluded. If the cystometrogram documents involuntary detrusor contractions, the diagnosis is definite detrusor instability. When reporting results it should be clearly stated whether the conditions causing urinary incontinence were definite or presumed. The technique by which the condition is documented should always be specified.

2.1. Bladder abnormalities causing urinary incontinence:

2.1.1. Detrusor overactivity – Detrusor overactivity is a generic term for involuntary detrusor contractions. This term should be used when the etiology of the involuntary detrusor contractions is unclear.

2.1.1.1. Detrusor instability – This denotes involuntary detrusor contractions which are not due to neurologic disorders.

2.1.1.2. Detrusor hyperreflexia – This denotes involuntary detrusor contractions which are due to neurologic conditions.

2.1.2. Low bladder compliance – Low bladder compliance denotes an abnormal (decreased) volume/pressure relationship during bladder filling. At the present time there are no clear cut, well defined normal values for compliance.

2.2. Sphincter abnormalities causing urinary incontinence – There are two generic types of sphincter abnormalities – urethral hypermobility and intrinsic sphincter deficiency. The two conditions may coexist. At the present time there are no well defined objective methods to distinguish the two.

2.2.1. Urethral hypermobility – In urethral hypermobility, the basic abnormality is a weakness of the pelvic floor. During increases in abdominal pressure there is abnormal descent of the vesical neck and proximal urethra. If the urethra opens concomitantly, stress urinary incontinence ensues. Urethral hypermobility is often present in women who are not incontinent. Thus, the mere presence of urethral hypermobility is not sufficient to make a diagnosis of a sphincter abnormality unless incontinence is also demonstrated.

2.2.2. Intrinsic sphincteric deficiency – This denotes an intrinsic malfunction of urethral sphincter itself.

2.3. Overflow incontinence – Overflow incontinence is leakage of urine at greater than normal bladder capacity. It is associated with incomplete bladder emptying due to either impaired detrusor contractility or bladder outlet obstruction.

2.4. Extraurethral incontinence – This denotes leakage of urine from a source other than the urethra. It may be due to urinary fistula or ectopic ureter.

3. **Signs and symptoms of incontinence:**

3.1. Urge incontinence:

3.1.1. Symptom – The symptom urge incontinence is the complaint of the involuntary loss of urine associated with a sudden, strong desire to void (urgency).

3.1.2. Sign – The sign urge incontinence is the observation of involuntary urinary loss from the urethra synchronous with an uncontrollable urge to void.

3.1.3. Condition – The condition urge incontinence is due to detrusor overactivity.

3.2. Stress incontinence

3.2.1. Symptom – The symptom stress incontinence is the complaint of involuntary loss of urine during coughing, sneezing, or physical exertion such as sport activities, sudden changes of position, etc.

3.2.2. Sign – The sign stress incontinence is the observation of loss of urine from the urethra synchronous with coughing, sneezing, or physical exertion.

3.2.3. Condition – The condition stress incontinence is due to sphincter abnormalities.

3.3. Unconscious (Unaware) incontinence

3.3.1. Symptom – The symptom unconscious incontinence is the involuntary loss of urine which is unaccompanied by either urge or stress. The patient may be aware of the incontinent episode by feeling wetness.

3.3.2. Sign – The sign unconscious incontinence is the observation of loss of urine without patient awareness of urge or stress.

3.3.3. Condition – The condition unconscious incontinence may be caused by detrusor overactivity, sphincter abnormalities, overflow or extraurethral incontinence.

3.4. Continuous leakage

3.4.1. Symptom – The symptom continuous leakage is the complaint of a continuous involuntary loss of urine.

3.4.2. Sign – The sign is the observation of a continuous urinary loss.

3.4.3. Condition – The condition may be caused by sphincter abnormalities or extraurethral incontinence.

3.5. Nocturnal enuresis

3.5.1. Symptom – The symptom nocturnal enuresis is the complaint of urinary loss which occurs only during sleep.

3.5.2. Sign – The observation of urinary loss during sleep.

3.5.3. Condition – The condition may be caused by a sphincter abnormality, overflow incontinence, detrusor overactivity, or extraurethral incontinence.

3.6. Post-void dribble:

3.6.1. Symptom – The symptom post-void dribble is the complaint of a dribbling loss of urine which occurs after voiding.

3.6.2. Sign – The sign post-void dribble is the complaint of a dribbling loss of urine which occurs after voiding.

3.6.3. Condition – The condition underlying post-void dribble has not been adequately defined, but is thought to be due to retained urine in the urethra distal to the sphincter in men. In women it may be caused by retained urine in the vagina or in a urethral diverticula.

REFERENCES

Abram P A, Blaivas J G, Stanton S L, Andersen J T 1988 Standardization of lower urinary tract function. Neurourol Urodynam 7: 403.

Index

10 0318003 X
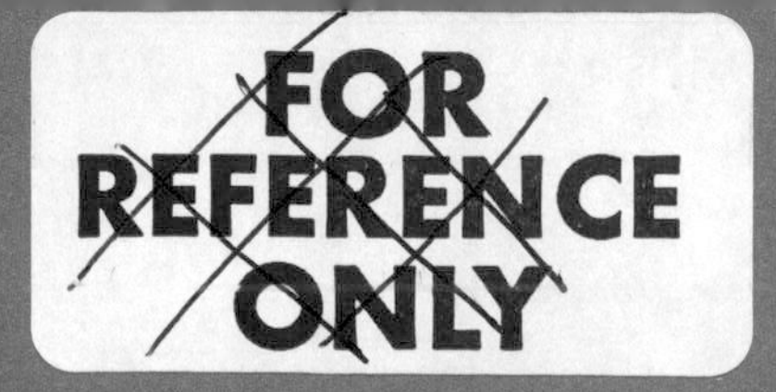
FOR
REFERENCE
ONLY